Principles and Practice of

Burn Care

Principles and Practice of
Burn Care

Second Edition

Editor-in-Chief

Sujata Sarabahi
MBBS MS MCh DNB MNAMS
Professor
Consultant and Head
Department of Burns and Plastic Surgery
VMMC and Safdarjung Hospital
New Delhi, India

Editors

VK Tiwari
MBBS MS MCh
Professor
Consultant Plastic Surgeon and
Dean, NDMC Medical College
Ex-Medical Superintendent and
Ex-Head
Department of Plastic Surgery
ABVMC and RML Hospital
New Delhi, India

Arun Goel
MBBS MS MCh FICS
Consultant Plastic Surgeon
Formerly, Consultant and
Head of Unit (Superannuated)
Department of Burns, Plastic,
Maxillofacial and Microvascular Surgery
Lok Nayak Hospital and Associated
Maulana Azad Medical College
New Delhi, India
(Professor of Plastic Surgery,
University of Delhi)

Suvashis Dash
MBBS MS MCh
Assistant Professor
Department of Plastic Surgery
AIIMS
New Delhi, India

Foreword

SP Bajaj

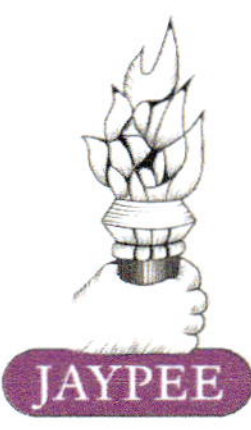

JAYPEE

JAYPEE BROTHERS MEDICAL PUBLISHERS
The Health Sciences Publisher
New Delhi | London

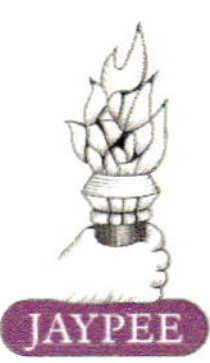

Jaypee Brothers Medical Publishers (P) Ltd

Headquarters
EMCA House
23/23-B, Ansari Road, Daryaganj
New Delhi 110 002, India
Landline: +91-11-23272143, +91-11-23272703
+91-11-23282021, +91-11-23245672
E-mail: jaypee@jaypeebrothers.com

Overseas Office
JP Medical Ltd.
83, Victoria Street, London
SW1H 0HW (UK)
Phone: +44-20 3170 8910
E-mail: info@jpmedpub.com

Corporate Office
Jaypee Brothers Medical Publishers (P) Ltd.
4838/24, Ansari Road, Daryaganj
New Delhi 110 002, India
Phone: +91-11-43574357
Fax: +91-11-43574314
E-mail: jaypee@jaypeebrothers.com

EU GPSR Authorised Representative
Logos Europe, 9 rue Nicolas Poussin
17000, La Rochelle, France
Phone: +33 (0) 6 67 93 73 78
E-mail: Contact@logoseurope.eu

Website: www.jaypeebrothers.com
Website: www.jaypeedigital.com

Inquiries for bulk sales may be solicited at: jaypee@jaypeebrothers.com

Principles and Practice of Burn Care* / *Sujata Sarabahi

First Edition: 2010

Second Edition: 2025, Reprint: **2026**

ISBN: 978-93-5696-770-0

Printed in India

DEDICATION

To
My parents,
who made me what I am today

To
My husband,
whose constant moral support gave me the base on which I worked

To
My children, Rohan and Arushi,
whose patience and love helped me to continue

To
My father-in-law,
who inspired me to write this book initially

Last but not the least,

To
My readers and students,
who appreciated the efforts put in and benefited from the book. They actually motivated me and helped me to revise it and bring out this second edition

Contributors

Aakanksha Goel MBBS MS DrNB(Plastic Surgery) MNAMS
Consultant Plastic Surgeon
Divine Aesthetic Surgery
Formerly Specialist
Department of Burns, Plastic, Maxillofacial and Microvascular Surgery
Lok Nayak Hospital
New Delhi, India

Suhas V Abhyankar MBBS MS MCh DNB
Professor and Head
Department of Plastic Surgery
Dr DY Patil School of Medicine
Nerul, Navi Mumbai
Honorary Consultant
Masina Hospital and BJ Wadia Hospital
Mumbai, Maharashtra, India

Akanksha Mohanty MBBS MD DNB
Senior Resident
Department of Obstetrics and Gynaecology
VMMC and Safdarjung Hospital
New Delhi, India

Amrita More MBBS MS DNB MRCS MCh
Associate Professor
Department of Burns and Plastic Surgery
VMMC and Safadrjung Hospital
New Delhi, India

Anoop S MBBS MS(General Surgery) MRCS(Edinburgh) MCh DrNB(Plastic Surgery)
Consultant Plastic Surgeon
MOSC Medical College
Kochi, Kerala, India

Archana Sinha MBBS MS MCh
Associate Professor
Department of Burns and Plastic Surgery
VMMC and Safdarjung Hospital
New Delhi, India

Arun Goel MBBS MS MCh FICS
Consultant Plastic Surgeon
Formerly, Consultant and Head of Unit (Superannuated)
Department of Burns, Plastic, Maxillofacial and Microvascular Surgery
Lok Nayak Hospital and Associated Maulana Azad Medical College
New Delhi, India
(Professor of Plastic Surgery, University of Delhi)

Arvind Vartak MBBS MS MCh
Honorary Plastic Surgeon and Ex-Head
Department of Plastic Surgery
Ben Jerbai Wadia Hospital
Mumbai, Maharashtra, India

Atul Kumar Shah MBBS MS MCh MPhil LLB PGDip(Medical Law and Ethics)
Consultant—Burns, Plastic Cosmetic and Medicolegal Expert
Vadodara, Gujarat, India

BC Shankar MS
Consultant Plastic Surgeon
Ex-Associate Director of Biomedical Group Bhabha Atomic Research Centre (BARC)
Mumbai, Maharashtra, India

Bhavya Krishna MBBS MD
Assistant Professor
Department of Anesthesia and Intensive Care
VMMC and Sadarjung Hospital
New Delhi, India

Chandrakant MBBS MD
Formerly, Head
Department of Forensic Medicine
Safdarjung Hospital
New Delhi, India

Deepak Nanda MBBS MS MCh
Professor and Consultant
Department of Burns and Plastic Surgery
VMMC and Safdarjung Hospital
New Delhi, India

Deepthi Nair MBBS MD
Professor and Head
Department of Microbiology
VMMC and Safdarjung Hospital
New Delhi, India

Deepti Gupta MBBS MS MCh
Associate Professor
Department of Burns and Plastic Surgery
VMMC and Safdarjung Hospital
New Delhi, India

Harish Chellani MBBS MD
Distinguished Scientist
Society for Applied Studies
Former Head
Department of Pediatrics
VMMC and Safdarjung Hospital
New Delhi, India

JC Suri MBBS MD DTCD DNB FNCCP
Consultant Pulmonologist and
Sleep Care Specialist
Fortis Hospital, Vasant Kunj
Ex-Head
Department of Pulmonary Medicine
Safdarjung Hospital
New Delhi, India

Karoon Agrawal MBBS MS MCh
Consultant Plastic Surgeon
National Heart Institute
Ex-Head
Department of Burns and
Plastic Surgery
VMMC and Safdarjung Hospital
New Delhi, India

Komal Tripathi MBBS MS MCh
Assistant Professor
Department of Burns and
Plastic Surgery
VMMC and Safdarjung Hospital
New Delhi, India

Lukesh Patil MBBS MS MCh
Consultant Plastic and Cosmetic
Surgeon
Kokilaben Dhirubhai Ambani Hospital
Navi Mumbai, Maharashtra, India

Madhuri Gore MBBS MS
Consultant Surgeon
Ex-Head
Department of Surgery
LTMC and General Hospital
Mumbai, Maharashtra, India

Mamta Sikroria MBBS MS MCh
Consultant
Joint Director and Ex-Head
Department of Burns and Plastic
Surgery
JLN Hospital and Research Institute
Bhilai, Chhattisgarh, India

Maneesh Singhal MBBS MS MCh FACS
FRCS(Glasgow)
Professor and Head
Department of Plastic Reconstructive
and Burn Surgery
AIIMS
New Delhi, India

Manish Kumath MBBS MD
Director Professor
Department of Forensic Medicine
VMMC and Safdarjang Hospital
New Delhi, India

Mary Babu MSc PhD
Ex-Head Biomaterials Division
Central Leather Research Institute
(CLRI)
Chennai, Tamil Nadu, India

MK Sen MBBS DTCD FNCCP MD
Consultant Pulmonologist
ESIC Medical College and Hospital
Faridabad, Haryana, India

Mula Rohit Babu MBBS MS MCh
Assistant Professor
AIIMS Hyderabad
Hyderabad, Telangana India

N Shanmuganathan M Pharma PhD
Assistant Professor
Department of Pharmaceutics
Sri Ramachandra College of Pharmacy
Sri Ramachandra University
Chennai, Tamil Nadu, India

PK Bilwani MBBS MS MCh
Director
Gujarat Burns Hospital and
Research Centre
Ex-Head
Department of Burns and Plastic
Surgery
NHL Municipal Medical College
Ahmedabad, Gujarat, India

PK Verma MBBS MD
Professor and Head
Department of Critical Care
ESIC Medical College and Hospital
Faridabad, Haryana, India

Poonam Gupta MBBS MD
Professor and Consultant
Anaesthetist
Specialist in Critical Care
VMMC and Safdarjung Hospital
New Delhi, India

Pramod Kumar MBBS MS MCh DNB MBA
Ex-Consultant and Head
Department of Plastic Surgery
King Fahad Central Hospital
Jizan, Kingdom of Saudi Arabia
Ex-Head
Department of Plastic Surgery
Kasturba Medical College
Manipal, Karnataka, India

PS Bhandari MBBS MS MCh
Senior Consultant Plastic Surgeon
and Head
Kailash Deepak Hospital, Karkardooma
Formerly Head (Superannuated)
Department of Burns, Plastic,
Maxillofacial and Microvascular
Surgery
Lok Nayak Hospital and Associated
Maulana Azad Medical College
New Delhi, India

Ramyaa Lakshmi TS MSc
Assistant Professor
Department of Zoology
Thiagarajar College
Madurai, Tamil Nadu, India

Raghav Rajesh Mago MBBS MS MCh
Associate Professor
Department of Plastic Surgery
KEM Hospital
Mumbai, Maharashtra, India

Rahul M MS MCh DrNB(Plastic Surgery)
Assistant Professor
MOSC Medical College
Kochi, Kerala, India

R Raja ShanmugaKrishnan MBBS
MS DNB MRCS
Consultant Plastic Surgeon
Ganga Hospital
Coimbatore, Tamil Nadu, India

Rajiv Kohli MD FICP
Senior Consultant Physician
Formerly Head, Dialysis Unit
(Superannuated)
Department of Medicine
Lok Nayak Hospital and Associated
Maulana Azad Medical College
New Delhi, India

Rakesh Kain MBBS MS MCh
Professor
Department of Burns and Plastic Surgery
VMMC and Safdarjung Hospital
New Delhi, India

Ravi Chittoria MBBS MS MCh MBA MNAMS DSc PhD
Professor
Department of Burns and Plastic Surgery, JIPMER
Puducherry, India

Ravindra Tah MBBS MS MCh
Consultant Plastic Surgeon
Mediways Hospital
Mohan Dai Oswal Cancer and General Hospital
Professor and Head
Department of Surgery and Plastic Surgery
BJS Dental College
Ludhiana, Punjab, India

Reisha Rijal MBBS MD
Senior Resident
Department of Forensic Medicine
VMMC and Safdarjung Hospital
New Delhi, India

Rekha Bharti MBBS MD FICOG
Professor
Department of Obstetrics and Gynaecology
VMMC and Safdarjung Hospital
New Delhi, India

Rojaleen Das MBBS MD
Assistant Professor
Department of Laboratory Medicine
AIIMS
New Delhi, India

RP Narayan MBBS MS MCh FICS
Consultant Plastic Surgeon
ESIC Medical College and Hospital
Faridabad, Haryana
Ex-Head
Department of Plastic Surgery
VMMC and Safdarjung Hospital
New Delhi, India

Sameek Bhattacharya MBBS MS DNB
Professor and Head
Department of Burns and Plastic Surgery
ABVMC and RML Hospital
New Delhi, India

Savita Arora MBBS MS MCh
Professor
Consultant
Department of Burns and Plastic Surgery
VMMC and Safdarjung Hospital
New Delhi, India

Shailesh Ranade MBBS MS MCh
Consultant Plastic Surgeon
Bhatia Hospital
Mumbai, Maharashtra, India

Shankar Sriniwasan MS MCh
Head of Burns and Plastic Surgery
Wadia Hospital for Children
Hiranandani Hospital
Mumbai, Maharashtra, India

Shivangi Saha MBBS MS MCh
Assistant Professor
Department of Plastic Reconstructive and Burn Surgery
AIIMS
New Delhi, India

SP Bajaj MBBS MS MCh FRCS MNASc
Consultant Plastic Surgeon
Jaipur Golden Hospital
Former Head
Department of Burns and Plastic Surgery
Safdarjung Hospital (Superannuated)
New Delhi, India

S Raja Sabapathy MBBS MS MCh DNB FRCS MNAMS
Director, Ganga Hospital and Chairman
Division of Plastic Surgery, Hand and Microsurgery
Ganga Hospital
Coimbatore, Tamil Nadu, India

Sugandha Arya MBBS MD
Consultant Pediatrician and Neonatologist
VMMC and Safdarjung Hospital
New Delhi, India

Sujata Sarabahi MBBS MS MCh DNB MNAMS
Professor
Consultant and Head
Department of Burns and Plastic Surgery
VMMC and Safdarjung Hospital
New Delhi, India

Suvashis Dash MBBS MS MCh
Assistant Professor
Department of Plastic Surgery
AIIMS
New Delhi, India

Thakur Thussu MBBS MS MCh
Consultant Plastic Surgeon
Fortis Hospital
Palampur, Himachal Pradesh, India

VK Tiwari MBBS MS MCh
Professor
Consultant Plastic Surgeon and Dean, NDMC Medical College
Ex-Medical Superintendent and Ex-Head
Department of Plastic Surgery
ABVMC and RML Hospital
New Delhi, India

V Suman Babu MBBS MS MCh
Associate Professor
Burns and Plastic Surgery
ABVIMS and RML Hospital
New Delhi, India

Foreword

Nearly a decade and half back, in 2010, Dr Sujata Sarabahi edited a multiauthored book *"Principles and Practice of Burn Care"*, published by Jaypee Brothers Medical Publishers (P) Ltd., New Delhi, India. Within a short period, this book became a Bible for all the students and surgeons involved in burn care in India, rather in whole of Indian Subcontinent. This book covers everything from history, epidemiology, pathophysiology, and clinical management of burns to the management of mass casualties and how India has planned for their management. Last but not least management of postburn sequelae is covered in detail for the burn victim to return to society. All the authors are authorities in their own subjects.

In 2023, it was felt to review the book again and put down all the advancements which have taken place since last publication. All the aspects that have become obsolete have been taken off and all the relevant advancements have been added to avoid an unnecessary increase in the volume of the book.

In the last 15 years, there has been great improvements in the dressing materials which help both by comforting the patient and at the same time prevent infection. A detailed analysis of these dressing materials and their application has been beautifully put in the new edition.

An attempt has been made to talk about skin banking which has grown quite considerably in India in the last two decades. This will certainly help many burn centers to start a skin bank and thus reduce the cost of burns management till the wound is ready to accept the skin graft.

Dermal substitutes are now available in great numbers and this has been discussed in quite detail including use and advantages vis-à-vis cost involved. Chapter on burns of hand and their reconstruction is nicely updated.

Burns of special types like electrical burns have been updated. Giving importance to the venous thrombosis vis-à-vis arterial damage and early immediate flap cover to provide alternative venous channels to save the limb is also discussed and controversy on this subject is beautifully explained. Similarly, in chemical burns, an explanation of phenol burns and hydrofluoric acid burns is given in quite detail, which is normally not available in burns literature and this would help to save many lives.

Chapters on disaster management and radiation injury are unique and will help readers in managing these cases in very critical situations.

Overall, this new edition has got all the good of the last edition which have been updated to the present thinking. I am sure that this edition will be equally liked by the readers—both students and established burn surgeons.

My good wishes and compliments to Dr Sujata Sarabahi for bringing out such an excellent book.

SP Bajaj
MBBS MS MCh FRCS MNASc
Consultant Plastic Surgeon
Jaipur Golden Hospital
Former Head
Department of Burns and Plastic Surgery
Safdarjung Hospital (Superannuated)
New Delhi, India

Preface to the Second Edition

Since the publication of the first edition, the landscape of burn care has undergone significant evolution. Technological advancements, coupled with interdisciplinary collaboration, have propelled the field forward, offering new insights and approaches to managing burn injuries. This second edition serves as a testament to the ongoing progress in the field, incorporating updated chapters, expanded knowledge, and a diverse array of contributions from both seasoned experts and emerging talents.

For practicing surgeons, this book offers a comprehensive resource that reflects the latest evidence-based practices and guidelines in burn care. From wound healing techniques to pain management strategies, each chapter has been meticulously curated to provide practical insights and actionable recommendations for optimizing patient outcomes. Additionally, the integration of visual enhancements, such as illustrations, line diagrams, flowcharts and tables, enhances comprehension and serves as valuable educational tools for surgeons at all stages of their careers. Majority of the chapters have been updated and revised with the latest developments and innovations in the last 14 years after the publication of the first edition and few chapters have been completely rewritten by new authors.

For students entering the field of burn care, this book serves as an invaluable learning companion. In fact, the inspiration to bring out a new edition came after many students, who had not only learned about burn care, managed their patients during their residency and cleared their examinations after reading this book as their primary textbook, expressed deep appreciation for the contents of the first edition. This second edition is therefore dedicated to all plastic surgery residents of our country.

One of the hallmarks of this edition is the inclusion of contributions from both seasoned experts and budding talents in the field of burn care. By synthesizing the expertise of experienced practitioners with the fresh perspectives of young authors, it offers a holistic view of burn management that spans from fundamental principles to cutting-edge advancements. By embracing diversity in perspectives and experiences, we enrich our collective understanding and foster innovation in patient care. The visual enhancements not only elucidate complex concepts but also serve as valuable educational tools for readers at all levels of expertise.

I express my gratitude to all my authors and especially Dr Suvashis Dash without whom this mammoth task could not have been completed. My sincere thanks to Dr Arun Goel who has contributed very significantly in consistently editing and proofreading all the chapters once again and giving necessary timely suggestions in an effort to make it free of errors.

I thank my family and friends who have enthusiastically supported me and helped me to finish this work.

I extend my heartfelt gratitude to all the contributors—both old and new—who have generously shared their expertise and experiences in shaping this edition. Special thanks to the publisher, M/s Jaypee Brothers Medical Publishers (P) Ltd, New Delhi, India, for their unwavering support and commitment to excellence.

As we embark on this journey of exploration and discovery, let us reaffirm our dedication to advancing the field of burn care and improving the lives of those affected by these devastating injuries. May this second edition serve as a beacon of knowledge and inspiration for burn surgeons, physicians, and healthcare professionals worldwide. Jai Hind and Good Luck to all our readers, wherever they may be.

Sujata Sarabahi

Preface to the First Edition

Burns is the most serious injury ever inflicted on mankind. This appears to be the price of civilization which man is paying today. India is amongst the few countries of the world where the incidence of burns is showing a rising trend even though it is on the decline in the Western world. Management of burns is difficult and time consuming. Apart from being a costly treatment, it is also a heart-breaking experience for any specialist treating a burn victim and rehabilitating him back to the society is equally difficult.

Over the centuries, we have discovered how to use new technological innovations and scientific advances to the greater advantage of victims of burns, fire, bomb blast and other terrorist crimes. However, in view of the continuously changing circumstances, it becomes imperative for burn surgeons, physicians and other para-medicals to constantly learn to change and accept changes and keep themselves updated at all the times with the new skills and techniques in the management of burn patients. We cannot afford to remain silent, inactive or resilient even in the treatment of minor accidental burn cases which otherwise receive scant attention by the hospital staff possibly because they are not dangerous to life or due to lack of interest on their part.

In the 21st century we are learning to evaluate new products and technologies more realistically. In short we are re-discovering the wisdom of our ancestors and learning to value the efforts made by others so far in modifying and improving our methods and skills in burn care. Regular studies and continuous research in various fields have proven to be the right investment in improving every aspect of human life—so why not for burn injury?

Though a burn specialist treats burn patients, but the modern treatment of major burns depends upon multidisciplinary team approach which includes anesthetist, medical specialist, pulmonologist, nutritionist, physiotherapist and occupational therapist. Each of them helps in providing a holistic approach towards treating and rehabilitating a burn patient.

This book brings together the knowledge and clinical experience of many of the specialists from all over the country, who have made outstanding contributions in the field of burn care. An attempt has been made to deliver comprehensive information about the treatment of a burn victim in all its aspects from the experiences and expertise of these surgeons and physicians serving in the battlefield of burns, i.e., The Burn Units; thus gaining and giving opportunities to learn from the best. This book emphasizes not only on the treatment and rehabilitation of burns but also the pathophysiology of burns and its prevention. It was not an easy task and required constant follow up to get others associated in producing this book.

I am thankful to all the contributors who are experts in their own fields for sharing their knowledge and experiences which have been reflected in their contributions, which I am sure will be beneficial to all the postgraduate and practicing burn surgeons who will be reading this book.

I have personally inserted photographs of many interesting cases in various chapters in addition to the photographs provided by the contributors in order to make the topic more interesting and easy to comprehend.

A book of this magnitude cannot be brought out single handedly. Dr Arun Goel, Dr VK Tiwari and Dr LC Gupta have been associated in editing this book and their help and support cannot be acknowledged in words. Without them, it would not have been possible to bring out this book which is complete in every sense, whether it is in the text content, pictorial depiction or practical case management protocol.

I am grateful to Dr SP Bajaj, who has been my guide and a father figure in burn management in India, for his valuable suggestions and encouragement at every step.

I am also thankful to my residents specially Dr Jeethendran Iyer for providing help in procuring the case photographs and Dr Geetika Khanna for providing the histological slides.

I must especially thank my publisher M/s Jaypee Brothers Medical Publishers (P) Ltd. especially Shri Jitendar P Vij (Chairman and Managing Director), Mr Tarun Duneja (Director, Publishing) for having recognized the merits of the presented material and to have come forward enthusiastically for publishing the book.

Lastly, I am thankful to my family for their moral support in helping me complete this book.

JAI HIND and Good Luck to my readers whoever and wherever they are.

Sujata Sarabahi

Acknowledgments

I am deeply indebted and grateful to the following individuals for their invaluable assistance in writing this book, now in its second edition—a significant achievement in itself.

I would like to extend my heartfelt thanks to Dr VK Tiwari and Dr Arun Goel for their help in revising and editing, as well as for their timely advice for the book. Their insightful suggestions and unwavering support have greatly enriched the quality of this work. I also wish to thank Dr Suvashis Dash and Dr Mula Rohit Babu, who were my students and are now faculty members themselves, who helped me at every step, in updating chapters, finding references, and creating tables and figures and were instrumental in accomplishing this enormous task of bringing out a new edition that will benefit many more students and colleagues.

I am extremely thankful to Shri Jitendar P Vij (Group Chairman), Mr Ankit Vij (Managing Director), Mr MS Mani (Group President), Ms Chetna Malhotra (Senior Director—Professional Publishing, Marketing, and Business Development), Ms Pooja Bhandari [Director—Production (Books and Journals)], and Mr Akhilesh Saxena (Publishing Coordinator) of Jaypee Brothers Medical Publishers (P) Ltd., New Delhi, India, for their constant encouragement. My sincere thanks also go to Shri Ramesh Krishnamachari of M/s Jaypee Brothers Medical Publishers.

Finally, I express my profound gratitude to my patients, whose management and treatment outcomes have been my greatest teachers. Their contributions have been invaluable, transforming my thoughts into words on paper.

Sujata Sarabahi

Contents

SECTION 3: LOCAL CARE OF BURN WOUND

SECTION 4: BURNS OF SPECIAL TYPES

SECTION 5: BURNS OF SPECIAL SITES

SECTION

1

General Considerations

CHAPTER 1

History, Epidemiology, and Prevention of Burns

Ravi Chittoria

OVERVIEW

Burn injuries represent one of the most important public health problems faced by both developing as well as industrialized nations today. Burn injuries may be intentional or nonintentional but intent is sometimes difficult to determine. Burns or thermal injuries occur when hot liquids (scalds), hot solids (contact burns), or flames (flame burns) destroy some or all of the different layers of cells which form the human skin and even deeper tissues. For traditional reasons, skin injuries due to ultraviolet radiations or radioactivity, electricity and chemicals, as well as respiratory insults resulting from smoke inhalation, are considered as fire/burn injuries. Burns represent an extremely stressful experience for both the burn victims as well as their families. An extensive burn profoundly affects the patient's physique, psyche, financial situation, and family. Patients suffering from extensive burn injuries frequently die while others suffer from painful and prolonged physical recovery. In different communities and countries, the etiological factors responsible for burn injuries vary considerably, hence, a careful analysis of the epidemiological factors in different places is needed before the planning and implementation of a sound prevention program. This chapter highlights the history, epidemiology, and prevention strategies for burns in both the developed and developing countries especially pertaining to Indian scenario.[1,2]

HISTORY OF BURNS

"Those who fail to read history are destined to suffer the repetition of its mistakes". "You have to learn what others have done because you will not live long enough to make all the mistakes yourself".

INTRODUCTION

Burn trauma is as old as the discovery of fire in the history of mankind. Medicine is built on the best of the past. Thus, a study of "History of Burns" contributes to a review of accomplishments and errors, false theories and misinformation, and mistaken interpretations. The history of burns, especially in India, is very fascinating. It teaches us where we started from, where we stand today, in what direction we are marching, and guides us for the future.[1,2]

HISTORY OF BURNS IN THE ANCIENT AGES

World History

The philosopher Santayana said, "Those who cannot remember the past are condemned to repeat it". In an address to the Royal College of Surgeons, Churchill remarked, "The longer you look back, the further you can look forward". In considering the history of the treatment of burn injuries, one might quote Adam MacDougall, who in 1819 stated that "It would equally exceed the bounds of convenience and utility to particularize all the remedies that have been recommended in the treatment of accidents of this kind". Hippocrates (430 BC) used swine's semen, resin, bitumen and Oak bark solutions in the treatment of burns. Chinese (600–500 BC) used extracts of tea leaves. Smith papyrus mentions (1500 BC) that Egyptians use of gum and goat's milk mixed with mother's milk and strips soaked in oil. Celsius (ancient Rome) advocated honey and bran. Glen (ancient Rome) described vinegar or wine in the treatment of burns **(Table 1)**.[1-3]

TABLE 1: Burn treatment history.

Neanderthal man	Extracts of plants
Smith papyrus (1500 BC, Egyptians)	Gum and goat's milk mixed with mother's milk
Chinese (600–500 BC)	Extracts of tea leaves
Hippocrates (430 BC)	Swine's semen, resin and bitumen
	Oak bark solutions
Celsius (ancient Rome)	Honey and bran
Rhases (9th century)	Cold water
Pare (1517–1596)	Excision and ointments
David Cleghorn (1792)	Vinegar and chalk poultice
Edward Kentish (1797)	Pressure dressings
Syme (1827)	Wool dressings
Lisfranc (1835)	Calcium-chloride dressings
Passavant (1858)	Saline baths
Joseph Lister (1875)	Boric acid and carbolic acid
Tomasalis (1897)	Salt water injections
Wallace (1949)	Exposure treatment
Keswani MH (1984, India)	Boiled potato peel (BPP) bandage

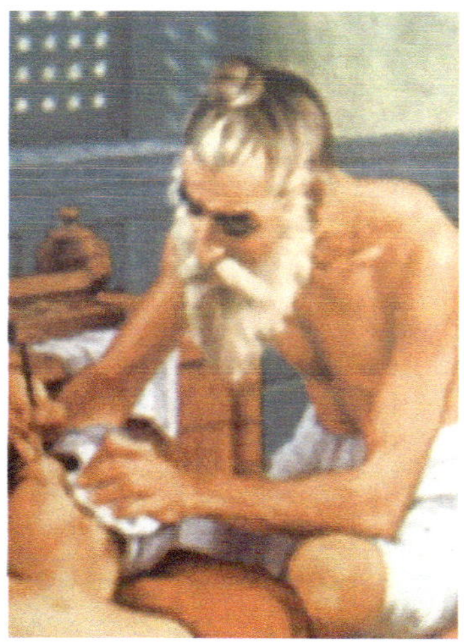

FIG. 1: Sushruta at work.

Indian History

Fire injuries in India have been common right from the ancient times. Suicide by fire out of insult was one of the common reasons. In Shiva Purana, it is mentioned that Lord Shiva's consort Sati had jumped into the sacred fire after being insulted by her father Daksha. Another reason for suicide by fire was "Sati Pratha" a common tradition of committing suicide by widows. It is well known that "Plastic Surgery" originated in India in the Vedic Period about 3500 BC. Among the many distinguished names in Hindu medicine, that of Sushruta, the "Father of Ancient Plastic Surgery" stands out in prominence **(Fig. 1)**. Sushruta was the son of the sage Vishwamitra, contemporary of Rama of Ramayana. He compiled the surgical knowledge of his time in his classic "Sushruta Samhita". It is believed that this classic was compiled between 800 BC and 400 AD. Sushruta was the first to classify burns into four degrees: (1) Singeing, (2) Blister, (3) Superficial, and (4) Deep burns.[1-3]

HISTORY OF BURNS IN THE MIDDLE AGES

World History

The British at the Battle of Crecy in 1346 were the first to use gunpowder and this development gave rise to many medical problems including those associated with the treatment of burns. The stimulus of the war experience initiated new and experimental types of treatment. In 1596, Clowes wrote a treatise on gunpowder burns. He did not differentiate the depth of burns but rather described multiple types of treatment on different parts of the body. He suggested oily dressings containing many drugs, did not open the blisters, and was an advocate of bleeding. Ambroise Pare (1517–1596) described about excision and ointments. Fabricus Hildanus (1610), who wrote De Combustionibus, classified burns into three categories and also showed pictorially the early successful surgical release of hand contractures. Pare clearly described the differences between second- and third-degree burns that frequently developed contractures. Richard Wiseman, in 1676, wrote several "chirurgical treatise" and discussed splinting to avoid contractures. He advised refrigerants or calefactive medicaments. Kentish (1797) described pressure dressings as a relief for pain and in his essay on burns promised to "rescue the healing art from empiricism and to reduce it to established laws". David Cleghorn (1792) used vinegar and chalk poultice for burns treatment. The use of ice and ice water for analgesia and the prevention of edema was explained by H Earle (1799) in his essay "the means of lessening the effects of fire on the human body". Syme (1827) used wool dressings. Lisfranc (1835) described calcium chloride dressings. In 1823, the Edinburgh Medical Journal published two papers on postmortem finding in two burn deaths. One patient had a gastric ulcer and another gastric congestion. Multiple lectures at this time were describing perforation of the stomach following burn deaths and there was increased interest in studying both the pathology and treatment of thermal injuries. Cotton dressing over burns was first discussed in a Glasgow Medical Journal in 1928. Readers were told how to apply dressing and were cautioned against changing them more than once daily. Dupuytren (1832), the brilliant French surgeon, made multiple contributions to burn research, including the documentation of the degree of injury to depth and the description of the phases of the post-burns course—irritation, inflammation, suppuration, and exhaustion. Sir George Ballingall, in 1833, gave one of the best descriptions of death from burn sepsis; "sinking in a hectic state, exhausted by a profuse discharge of matter from an extensive separating surface". In a landmark decision in 1848, the managers of the Royal Infirmary in Edinburgh designated one building for all burn cases and this became known as the "burns hospital". Passavant (1858) gave concept of saline baths. In 1875, Joseph Lister recommended boric acid and carbolic acid for burn wounds in order to kill bacteria. In 1881, Tappeiner of Munich studied autopsies of burn deaths and recognized the concentration of blood, increased hemoglobin concentration and decreased blood and water volume. The appreciation by Tappeiner of burn pathology was a significant event. Thomasalis (1897) described use of saltwater injection **(Fig. 1)**.[1-3]

Indian History

The history of burns in India in medieval period is that of decline in India and lull in European countries. The natural feeling of fear for operations grew and love for medicines increased. The governments prohibited and neglected the practice of surgery. The famous Buddhist scripture Mahāagga Jatak enjoined strict prohibition of surgery and extended the terror of hell both for the surgeon and the patient. "Manusmriti" prescribed special rituals by way of purifications of surgeons, who were looked down upon as unclean. Later during the Rajput, Muslim and Maratha periods, Ayurvedic (Hindu), and Unani (Arabic) systems of medicine were practiced by Vaids and Hakims, respectively. The Vaids were purely physicians and the practice of surgery was restricted only to incision of abscess, dressing of wounds, and treatment of bone and joint injuries by barbers and bone-setters. Not much information is available in literature related to burn injuries.[1-3]

HISTORY OF BURNS IN THE MODERN AGE

World History

Major advances were made in burn care in the 19th century. Physicians described excision of burnt tissue and skin grafting, which led to an important publication in JAMA (1905) advocating for early skin grafting.[4] In 1905, Steve noted the importance of intravenous saline for resuscitation and wrote an article in the Journal of the American Medical Association advocating early skin grafting. The understanding of burn pathology took a great leap forward when Underhill (1930) studied a group of patients burned in a theater fire in 1921. He analyzed the content of blister fluid and determined that burn shock was due to fluid loss and not toxins (a popular theory of that time). The Coconut Grove Fire in Boston in 1942 resulted in extensive studies by Cope and Moore on the diagnosis and treatment of burn shock. Controversies over the best method to treat the burn wound persist to the present day. Dressings remained popular until Wallace in 1949 advocated exposure treatment for burns of the face, buttock, and perineum. Formulas gradually evolved to calculate fluid losses. Evans (1952) used burn skin surface area and weight as the principal variable. The Brooke formula was a modification of the Evans formula and utilized salt, colloid, and water. Moyer and Associates (1965) recommended only Ringer's lactate solution, yielding alert, oriented patients even when the body surface area burn was large. The pattern of triage of burn patients changed dramatically in the 1960's. The US Army Research Unit was initially guided by Pulaski and Artz, who stressed patient care as well as clinical and laboratory burn related research. Critically injured patients, civilian and military, were referred to the center and the concept of the multidisciplinary burn team evolved. The major milestone in topical burn therapy was the application of solutions of silver compounds or salts, which played an important role in reducing the rate of burn wound sepsis and mortality. Silver sulfadiazine was developed by Charles Fox in the 1960s and has become the mainstay of topical antimicrobial therapy due to its success in controlling infection and minimal side effect profile. Mafenide acetate (sulfamylon) briefly was a viable alternative to the use of silver compound solutions in the treatment of infections but due to its carbonic anhydrase inhibitory effects which can lead to systemic acidosis, its use was all but discontinued except in cases of treatment of invasive wound infections. The other common silver-based therapy was silver nitrate, described by Moyer et al. in 1965. Silver-based topical treatments were successful in controlling infections especially *Pseudomonas aeruginosa* infections.[5] In 1962, the Shriners fraternal organization in the United States began development of three burn centers affiliated with universities and dedicated specifically to the care of burned children. These centers served as role models that have completely altered burn care around the world. Their superb survival statistics made others realize that patients with large burns were not automatically doomed but had a chance of survival if cared for in a specialized center. Laboratory and clinical research in burn injury improved other areas of trauma care as well. It became obvious that the burn patient with multisystem involvement was the perfect trauma model. The universality of the burn problems provided a reason for better international cooperation and exchange of ideas. In 1960, the first international congress on research in burns was held in Washington, DC. At the second meeting in 1963, The International Society for Burn Injuries (ISBI) was founded, and it has been conducting meetings every 4 years. The American Burn Association (ABA) was founded in 1968. The society's membership was unique in that it consisted of all the members of the burn team, including nonphysicians (dieticians, physical and occupational therapists, nurses, and psychologists).[3]

Indian History

Burns became alarmingly frequent in India in the modern age of industrialization. To pour kerosene over the clothes and then set them on fire is the most common form of committing suicide or murder. There are also innumerable instances of accidental burning caused by clothes catching fire on low stoves or open gas rings; the loose flowing end of "*sarees*" and "*dupatta*" of Indian women increases this danger enormously. Open fires in winter are an added hazard. Acid burns of the face are frequently the result of blind jealousy. Suicidal burns among Hindu women are usually fatal because of its extent. Practice of tradition of "Sati Pratha" declined in this period. Most of the burn cases in India are treated by general surgeons and general practitioners in small cities and rural areas because plastic surgeons are few and settled mostly in metro cities. These general surgeons and general practitioners have negligible facilities and have no forum to exchange, enhance or update their knowledge. The initial local treatment on admission to hospitals varies according to the area involved in the burns—face, front of chest, and abdomen are routinely treated by the exposure method. Burns of extremities and fingers alone are dressed. The majority of hospitals do not have the "Stryker Frame" and hence only circumferential body burns are dressed. Resistant strains of organisms have increased in recent years due to excessive use of antibiotics. Surgeons are not in favor of keeping grafts exposed from the start. Skin grafts are dressed with pressure pads for a week and then kept exposed. To keep the donor area exposed was attempted by many but were not satisfied by this method. In fact, dressing of the donor area is retained for a fortnight during which the part heals. Severe cases of contractures of the flexor creases like the neck, axilla, and elbow are released and skin grafted. Free grafts are preferred to tube pedicles as the relief is quick as well as complete.[6]

In India, many plastic surgeons have contributed in the development of Burns Unit and management in modern era. Dr Noshir H Antia, the 3rd generation trained Plastic Surgeon under Sir Harold Gillies, was the first surgeon to start a unit at Grant Medical College and associated JJ Hospital, Mumbai, in 1959. In 1964, Tata Trusts provided a substantial grant to carry out two projects—one on leprosy and other on burns. In 1963, Safdarjung Hospital, New Delhi started a department of burns, plastic, and maxillofacial surgery with Dr JL Gupta as its head. Professor Antia felt that they should have a forum and thus, a Burn Association of India (BAI) was formed at JJ Group of hospitals, Bombay in 1972. Dr MH Keswani was the Secretary. Later under leadership of Dr Keswani the BAI flourished with contributions like Boiled Potato Peel (BPP) dressings, prevention campaigns by way of radio and TV talks, small documentary ads, "School Education Program" in burns, etc. "Pour water on Burns" has received worldwide popularity. "AGNIVARTA" is a quarterly publication of "BAI" devoted to the problems concerning "burns". Burn injury is a disease of the poor at least in our country. Dr Keswani gave various modifications to reduce the cost of burns treatment like common homemade curd (called yogurt in the US) as a de-sloughing agent, butter milk diet (BMD) as cheap high calorie high protein diet, X-plasty of Vartak as a simple operation of release of contracture, Vartak's wheel as mesh graft dermatome, cellophane dressing for donor area, simple operation cum bath trolley, etc. Dr Keswani has to his credit the setting up of the first children's burn unit in India and India's first skin bank at Bai Jerbai Wadia Hospital in Parel, Mumbai, in 1975 and 1978, respectively.[7-9]

In 1990, Prof JL Gupta convened a meeting at Pragati Maidan, New Delhi. A very active and detailed discussions and consultations were held among Prof JL Gupta, Prof Mathangi Ramakrishnan, Prof JK Sinha, Prof SP Bajaj, Prof SK Bhatnagar, Prof RK Keswani, Prof Siti Roy Choudhary, Prof PK Bilwani, Prof Madhuri Gore, Prof DLN Prasad, Prof Swarna Arora, and Prof Anil Chadha and many others. This historic and significant meeting led to the birth of National Academy of Burns India (NABI).[10] The NABI mainly aims at preparing and making available a suitable appropriate and latest information relevant to all those concerned with burn care. Recognizing the services of Prof JL Gupta in the field of burns in the country, he was unanimously named as the Patron of NABI. Prof SN Sharma was the choice for the founder Presidentship. Dr SP Bajaj became the founder Secretary. The academy brought out an annual journal named "Indian Journal of Burns" with Dr Rajeev B Ahuja and Dr Arun Goel as an editor and an assistant editor, respectively. They worked for 5 years (1993–1997) before passing on the task to others. The first volume was brought out in 1993 and the journal is being regularly published. While NABI is an association of burn care professionals (doctors, nurses, therapists, etc.), BAI even included persons like businessmen, old recovered burn victims, etc., who were ready to serve the cause of burns in their own way.

Dr JL Gupta gave guidelines for planning a Burns Unit.[11] Subsequently, many Burn Units have been developed successfully in various Institutions and Medical Colleges like Burn Unit in the Department of Plastic Surgery at Kasturba Medical College, Manipal, Karnataka, IPGME&R, Kolkata, etc. Of all the existing Burns Units in India, special mention is made of Burns Unit of Safdarjung Hospital, New Delhi which is the largest burn unit in the country and which has been modernized and equipped with all modern "burn care infrastructure facilities". "Early Tangential Excision and skin grafting", "Rescuer Burns", "Policy of antibiotics in burns", etc., have been popularized extensively by the Burns Unit of Manipal, Karnataka.[12,13]

In India, Burn injuries due to fireworks on the occasion of "Diwali" are very common. Safety tips related to fireworks have been explained by Anjali Burma.[14] The Government Health System is not able to keep pace with population growth in recent years. Although major burn accidents are decreasing in relation to the population growth, the actual number of burn cases is on the increase. Gradually, more and more teaching hospitals started separate burn wards. Possibly, about 60% of them are managed by the "General Surgery" services and the rest by a Burn and Plastic Surgeon. The requirement for more burn beds encouraged many nongovernment groups into establishing burn management centers. Many of these centers have well-equipped wards, trained support staff, and enthusiastic burn specialists. These specialists have been instrumental in maintaining the prevention and rehabilitation programs concerning burns.

RECENT ADVANCES

What have been the outstanding features of burn injuries in the last 25 years? It is the best understanding of burn pathophysiology that is the most remarkable feature of last quarter of a century. The second important feature is the realization that the care of Burns is a team effort, the leader of the team being the one, who can lead the team most inspiringly, a person with vision, with dedication and with tenacity. It would not be fair to single out any one individual for all the advances. Half a century ago, the most common cause of death following a burn >20% was surgical shock, at least in India. With a better understanding of postburn surgical shock, it is possible to treat this rationally and efficiently. The mortality from this cause has reduced considerably. Generalized infection of the tissues (septicemia) is the single most common cause of death following burns, at present. Better drugs and their widespread availability have helped us to control infection to some extent. However, while these drugs are useful, they have many undesirable side effects, some of them are lethal. Moreover, the cost of these drugs is prohibitive. They have encouraged resistant strains to develop and they have put the clock back in many instances. Postburn sequelae need correction. These have been satisfactorily corrected by reconstructive surgeons and in many instances by interested general surgeons. Early postburn rehabilitation has been encouraged, but much progress needs to be made in this direction in this country. When the hands are burned, it is a severe blow to the person's economic viability. Better methods of rehabilitation need to be developed. Unfortunately, over the last 25 years, not much progress has been made in this area. It costs approximately US $1,000 per patient per day to provide satisfactory care in the Western world. This is clearly not possible in India and in many of the developing countries. Prevention of burns is the only logical solution. This is not easy and is time-consuming. Easy or not, we have no option(s). We must prevent burns. Fortunately, the BAI, which was formed in 1972, has been doing precisely that. Burns prevention has to be propagated zealously by everyone who is able to do so, especially doctors, nurses, paramedical workers, social workers, teachers, surviving burns patients, and the media—in fact, it should be a national responsibility. India is a country with tremendous problems—those of population explosion, education, malnutrition, unemployment, and many more. Our hopes lie in a unified approach to work together and solve some if not all of these problems.[15]

EPIDEMIOLOGY OF BURNS

"I keep six honest serving men; they taught me all I know. Their names are 'WHAT', 'WHY', 'WHEN', 'HOW', 'WHERE', and 'WHO'."

INTRODUCTION

Epidemiology has been defined by John M Last in 1988 as: "The study of the distribution and determinants of health-related states or events in specified populations and the application of this study to the control of health problems". Epidemiology began with Adam and Eve, both trying to investigate the qualities of the "forbidden fruit". Epidemiology is derived from the word epidemic (epi = among; demos = people; logos = study), which is a very old word dating back to the third Century BC. Burn injuries and their related morbidity, disability, and mortality represent a public health problem of increasing importance in developing countries. Developing countries have a high incidence of burn injuries, creating a formidable public health problem. Epidemiological studies of burn injuries are a prerequisite for effective burn prevention programs because each population seems to have its own epidemiological characteristics and knowledge of the epidemiology of burns is needed to select target groups for preventive actions.[16] The precise global occurrence rate of burn injury is unknown but according to the World Health Organization at least 265,000 deaths are attributed to burns and fires per year. Severe burn injuries are not only physically debilitating but affect different organ systems leading to high morbidity and mortality rates and thus benefit from interdisciplinary treatment The risk of burn death and/or burn injury are greatest among the developing countries due to older buildings, lower safety standards, absence of smoke detectors, and faulty electrical gadgets among others.[17,18] For the last 10 years, interest has risen in the advancements of global burn care. Due to the invention of multiple new dressings, treatment has proved to be very effective in a way that healing is promoted as well. On a global scale, overall morbidity and mortality of burn wound infections, secondary sepsis, or tissue invasion have decreased in recent years as the growth of bacteria on a wound surface can be controlled and eradicated more effectively. Significant differences regarding number of dressing changes till healing for superficial burns could be detected in Africa, where more dressing changes were needed until healing. Asia also noted a higher number of dressing changes. This could again be due to different treatment standards in different regions.[19]

BURN REGISTRY

The ABA commissioned Jeffrey T Suffle and Byron of the University of Utah Health Center, Salt Lake City, Utah, USA, to develop a computer program to assist burn units to collect data useful for patient care and prevention. The ABA graciously permitted the ISBI to distribute a version of this program, adapted for use internationally, to ISBI members free of charge.[20]

USES OF BURN DATA

Burn data are useful to:

- Define the burn problem.
- Determine the most common ways that people are burned.
- Evaluate the effectiveness of medical care for burn patients.
- Identify which burn hazards should be targeted by burn prevention programs.
- Examine the economic impact of burn injuries and burn treatment.[20]

SOURCES OF BURN DATA

The sources of burn data vary, depending upon the severity of the burn injury:[20]

- *For burn deaths:* Collect information from hospitals and local, regional, or national vital statistics registries. Many people die immediately of fire and burn injuries and do not receive medical care.
- *For serious burns:* Collect information from hospitals; decide whether to collect data only on burn patients admitted to the hospital, or on all patients seen at the hospital. If there are several hospitals treating burn patients from the defined population, Collect data from all these hospitals. Referral patterns may distort the true profile of burns in that population.
- *For less severe burns:* Collect information from health clinics, doctors' offices, visiting nurses or any other medical treatment service. A good sampling plan will make this task easier.
- *For burns of all levels of severity occurring in a community:* Collect information through a community survey, asking residents in face-to-face or telephonic interviews to recall circumstances of burn injuries suffered by family members. Questions about burn injuries could be added to a larger multipurpose community survey.
- *For burns associated with building fires:* Contact the local fire service for information about fires in which people were killed or injured. Remember, this is not a good source for clothing ignition burns, scalds, contact, electrical, or chemical burns.

STANDARD CODING OF BURN INJURY DATA

Most countries use the World Health Organization's International Classification of Disease (ICD) codes for coding data on hospital discharge records, although there are other coding schemes. For example, the Nordic countries use a coding scheme called NOMESCO. The ICD system contains two sets of codes for burn data. The first set classifies what type of fire or burn injury was sustained:[20]

Code	Type of burn
940–949	Burn injuries
986–987	Smoke inhalations
692.71	Sunburn
910–919	Superficial injuries (friction burns are among these codes)

The second set of codes is the ICD E-codes (External Cause of Injury) which classify the causes of burn. These are four-digit codes, with the fourth digit often capturing important burn information:[20]

Code	Cause of burn
E890–899	Burns caused by fire and flames
E923	Accident caused by explosive material (includes fireworks and explosive gases; not all injuries coded here are burns)
E924	Accident caused by hot substance or object, caustic material and steam
E925	Accident caused by electric current (burns or electrocution)
E926	Exposure to radiation E958.1, .2 suicide (by burns or scalds)
E965–968	Homicide and assault (965.6, 967, 968.0, 968.3 related to burns)
E988.1, .2	Undetermined if accidentally or purposely inflicted
E990, 996	War

NATURE OF DATA NEEDED TO STUDY BURN EPIDEMIOLOGY[20]

How Big is Our Burn Problem?

Determine the number of people who have been burned. Do not ignore burn deaths, especially those who die before coming to the hospital. Counts of nonfatal burns are made easier in areas where computerized hospital discharge records are coded using the ICD codes or another standard coding scheme. Count the number of patients with a burn injury diagnosis, coded using "type of burn" codes.

How are Our People Getting Burned?

Determine the number of people burned by specific causes of burns, such as clothing ignition or scalds. Collect information which will permit patients to be classified using "cause of burn" codes. Perfect workable coding depends upon accurate, useful information in the medical record. This includes details about the circumstances of the burning, ignition sources, and other product involvement, where the event happened, and the activities of the people involved and demographic information about the patient. This often requires an interview with the patient, a family member or someone present at the burn episode. Make sure that this information is written in the medical record, coded and, whenever possible, entered into computerized hospital discharge records.

How can We Prevent Burns?

Analyze data describing the common causes of burn injuries in the population to identify high-risk groups such as young children and high-risk activities, such as meal preparation.

How can We Evaluate the Success of Our Prevention Programs?

The precise nature of the data required depends upon the prevention program and the research design of the evaluation.

Information about Larger Populations

It is important to know certain characteristics of the defined population, whether this be a village, a region, or a country. Important characteristics are the number of people in the population and the age distribution of these people. If your country collects and publishes census data, these provide an excellent source of information to use to describe risk factors for burns in your population.

Burn Rates

Burn epidemiology uses rates of burn injury or deaths. A rate is calculated by dividing the number of burn injuries sustained during a specified time period by the number of people in a population during that same period. It is expressed, for example, as "burns per 100,000 populations per year". One must use burn rates to compare the burn problem in communities or countries with different-sized populations. A densely populated community may have many more burns but a relatively lower burn rate than a sparsely populated region. A lower burn rate signifies a lesser burn problem. It is important to know the age distribution of the defined population because burn risk is age-related. A population with a lower median age will have higher rates even if its adults have an equal or slightly lower risk than a population with a higher median age.

Usefulness of Burn Data from a Single Hospital

If only one hospital treats patients with serious burns in a defined population and if one is interested only in serious burns, the vital statistics registry and this hospital are the two appropriate data sources for fatal and serious burn injuries, respectively, for that population. If the hospital is one among many serving a single population, one cannot draw any conclusions about the population's burn problem by studying only one hospital. However, even without collaboration with other local hospitals, it can be valuable to analyze burn data from a single hospital. Individual hospitals can provide useful information about a specific circumstance which causes burns and can provide "cases" for a "case-control" study. One cannot, however, draw conclusions about the population's burn problem.

EPIDEMIOLOGY OF BURNS IN INDIA

National Burns Registry

One of the major activities of the NABI is to maintain a National Burns Registry. Various data are collected from centers engaged in management of "burns". This is, however, a voluntary effort and has so far not reached to all places. In a few years with continued efforts and support from all areas, National Burns Registry of NABI will be able to truly reflect the scene of burns problem in India.[21]

Extent of Problem (Mortality and Morbidity)

Over 100,000 people are affected by burns in India annually and 20,000 of them die according to rough estimates.[22] In 1991, the reported deaths were 22,306. A survey of almost 3,500 hospital admission over the past few years supplemented by intermittent published reports over the past 30 years indicated a mortality rate of between 25 and 49% for adults and between 6 and 20% for children (0–10 years old).[23] 10% of all accidental deaths and 7% of all suicides in India are caused by fire. Although incidence of burn trauma is on the decline in the developed nations, it is still rising in India and is second largest killer after road traffic accidents. Thousands of victims of burns are being mutilated, disfigured, and handicapped every year.[24] The cost of burns is both visible and invisible. In India, the cost of burns ranges from $25 to $300 a day. To this may be added the loss of wages of the patient and of those who have to be away from work to care for him or her during hospitalization. The other visible cost is in the scarring and deformity, of loss of hair and body-pigment and alterations in skin texture. There is also a loss of physical skill which leads to demotion at the place of work and makes one less fit or unfit in domestic life. The invisible cost is in the pain the patient undergoes, both physical and emotional, the emotional trauma of itching, of scarring and intolerance to heat. Neither the trauma of patient's psyche nor the imperceptible alterations of the patient's personality can be measured. And then, there is loss of time—of time lost from studies, of vanished opportunities in social life, like marriage or career promotion. And finally, one has to remember the cost to the patient's family—to the husband who loses a beloved wife, to the child who becomes motherless, to a young wife who becomes widowed, and to the aged parents who lose their support. In India, society is structured differently and the cost borne by the patient's family is truly immense and immeasurable.[25]

Age and Sex Distribution

The age distribution revealed by various studies in India shows that more than half the cases are aged between 21 and 40 years. In children, the lack of coordination and unawareness of dangerous substances play an important role in the occurrence of burns. High incidence among young adults may be explained by the fact that they are generally active and exposed to hazardous situations both at home and at work.[26-28] Male predominance in the younger age group (5–10 years) might be explained by the inquisitive and exploring nature of boys of this age. As regard sex distribution, the female preponderance in the age group 20–40 years concurs with reports from other developing countries and might be explained by the involvement of females in domestic activities and dowry deaths too. However, figures from industrialized countries are clearly lower than those reported from developing countries. This may be due to the relatively lower percentage of occupational and recreational burns or due to better home safety with safer cooking and heating devices in industrialized countries.[29-31]

Sociocultural Factors

Sociocultural factors are among the major causes of different age and sex predisposition of developing countries like India compared to other developed nations. The majority of the patients belong to low socioeconomic status (69.6%), while 21.8% are from middle and only 8.6% are of high socioeconomic status. 42.6% belong to an urban area while the rest are from rural areas. Arrival time to hospital after the incidence is variable, only few patients (9.7%) arrive within 6 hours of the incidence. The majority (61.8%) reached the hospital between 6 and 24 hours; those reaching the hospital after 24 hours contribute about 28.5%. In general, being unemployed, a low socioeconomic status, alcohol and tobacco use, and drug consumption or being a victim of crime or assaults are independent risk factors for burns throughout all regions.[32-34]

Etiology

An extensive study was done by the Department of Burns, Plastic, and Maxillofacial Surgery, Safdarjung Hospital, New Delhi.[35] Analysis of the causes of 9,927 burn cases is given in **Table 2**.

It is seen that the vast majority in these are dry burns, by direct contact with either flash or flame. The second most common are scalds. This is because of conditions which are peculiar to the villages in our country. Most of the cooking is done at the floor level with open fire. Stoves, coal, and wood are commonly used. Often large families live and cook in the same room. If there is a kitchen, it is small, crowded, and ill-designed. The storage shelves lie above the *chulha/angithi* (a kind of open oven used in India) or stove, so that while getting up to pick up an article from the shelf, any loose garment can easily catch fire. The lamps used for illumination are made of an ordinary glass bottle or tin can, with cotton wick and kerosene oil. They are either kept on the floor or on any shelf. They can be easily upset and result in an oil fire. The majority of the population lives in villages in thatched houses which easily catch fire. Accidents at home form the major bulk and the common causes are:

- Loose clothing like "*saree*" and "*dupatta*", mostly made of synthetic, inflammable material.
- Spilling and spraying of kerosene oil from pressure stove is more common than actual bursting of it. The jet of oil under pressure catches fire immediately.
- Hot food stuff and liquids carry a constant danger to children and infants, particularly in overcrowded rooms. They often fall in the steaming food, cooking utensils, and hot water buckets and tubs.
- It is common to heat water in a tin with its lid in position. As the lid is handled, the steam under pressure inflicts severe scalds of face, neck, and upper chest wall.

After flame and scalds, electrical burn is the third most common cause of burns in India. The electric appliances used are substandard and are used without any regard to safety measures. Electrical burns while flying kite is very common in India especially in young children.

TABLE 2: Showing incidence of different types of burns.

Causes of burns	%
Dry burns	51.64
Scalds	33.35
Electric burns	3.59
Chemical burns	2.97
Petrol burns	2.36
Coal tar burns	0.79
Industrial burns	0.75
Miscellaneous	4.55

Circumstances of the Injury

There has been a change in the pattern of burn injuries as far as circumstances of the burn injury are concerned. Recent study shows that majority of burn injuries, i.e., >85% occurs in homes. Kitchen-related activities are most often responsible for burns in domestic setup. Flames represent the most common agent of burn injuries (75.1%). Among the flame burns, kerosene pressure stove is the most common source. Chimney and liquid petroleum gas (LPG) burns rank the second most common source of flame injuries. Most of the burn injuries are accidental (67.7%), followed by homicidal (13.4%) and suicidal (18.9%). Adult males are most at risk for burns at the workplace (faulty electrical wiring, flames, and scalds), whereas women are at higher risk of burns at home, particularly in the kitchen given that these gender-related stereotypes are still "alive" in many regions.[36]

Epidemiology of Pediatric Burns

Pediatric burns differ from adult burn injuries in many aspects and need separate consideration. Only few pediatric burn units exist in India. Most of the children with burns are treated in a common Burns Unit. Epidemiological studies on childhood burn injuries in India are very scant. Information on the exact magnitude of burn injuries has not been well documented. It is known, however, that burn hazards are present in the daily life of children. Household activities, including cooking, are expected of girls early in their lives. According to one of the epidemiological studies of pediatric burns, various risk factors attributed to burn injuries in children are low socioeconomic conditions, poor living conditions, illiteracy, overcrowding, and floor level cooking, on either kerosene pressure stove or an open fire. These pressure stoves are sometimes of shoddy construction and commonly malfunction leading to explosive disintegration. The overcrowded conditions cause young children to play in the vicinity of the cooking area leading to scalds from spilled hot fluids or foods. Preexisting diseases and malnutrition afflict a considerable number of patients, particularly children injured in slum areas, thereby ensuring that patients have a reduced ability to compensate for the physiological stress inherent in a severe burn. The ridiculous first aid measures like application of ink, cowdung, hen's blood, *haldi* (turmeric), honey, and other homemade remedies, surprisingly, are still frequently used. Delay in transportation and initiation of treatment due to lack of education, lack of transportation facilities, and lack of economic support are still prevalent.[37] According to the recent study of 500 pediatric burns, majority (24%) of burns occur in children between 1 and 2 years age group. Male to female sex ratio was 1.38:1. Burn injury occurred predominantly during winter. Most common type of burn was scalds which occurred mainly in domestic circumstances. Mortality rate was 10.4%. Mortality rate was high in patients having >40% total body surface area (TBSA) involvement. Parental occupation, family size, and the first aid did not affect the mortality rate.[38] Babies and children under the age of 1 year are at most risk from burns from bed-netting and sleepwear, but also due to faulty electrical wiring or simple devices such as mosquito coils.[39-41]

PREVENTION OF BURNS IN INDIA

"The only thing more expensive than education is ignorance. Prevention is better than cure."

INTRODUCTION

Burn injuries are universal and incidence is on the increase with the complexities of modern living and industrialization. As most of the burns occur either at home or at the place of work, it becomes important to know about "burn prevention". In order to bring down the incidence of burn, education programs are oriented to bring the changes of culture pattern, change in the way of life, change of rules and regulations at workplace, change in dangerous substandard gadgets, and change of habits. Prevention does not mean only to reduce the incidence but also to reduce the depth and severity of the burn. The majority of data are from high-income countries and are directly related to access to healthcare resources, differences in environments, and the resources of the various healthcare systems. In lower-income countries, fewer resources, geographical constraints and cost limit data collection, and access to healthcare. Additionally, cultural factors such as open-air cooking areas and loose clothing (e.g., *sarees*), domestic violence, and dowry deaths contribute to regional variation.[42]

RISK FACTORS

Before preventive measures are discussed, it is important to know about the risk factors especially in Indian scenario. Various risk factors are as follows:[43]

At Home

In India, most of the burn injuries occur at home, especially in the kitchen. Various risk factors are floor-level cooking, substandard kerosene pressure stove, loosely worn garments (*sarees* and *dupatta*), low level of electric plug points, long over hanging flex of kettle, overhanging tablecloth over which hot food or beverages are kept, carelessly kept match boxes within reach of children, substandard pressure cookers, etc.

At Work

Inadequate safety measures, overwork, and fatigue are common risk factors at workplace.

At Play

During Diwali, Indians play with fire crackers and celebrate the festival with lights. Inferior quality of crackers and carelessness during their bursting are important risk factors.

RESEARCH DESIGNS FOR BURN PREVENTION

Given below are the broad outlines of four research designs which may be helpful in planning and implementing burn prevention programs and their evaluation.[44,45]

Nonexperimental Descriptive Study

Purpose

To determine dimensions of a serious burn problem in a defined population.

Tasks

- Define the population of interest, determine numbers and age distribution, if possible.
- Decide on a time period. Include at least 1 year, since in most locations, burn injuries have seasonal variations.
- Decide on the level of burn severity. Include all deaths and people hospitalized for a burn injury and may be those treated and released from hospital or clinic.
- Identify all hospitals treating burn patients in the defined population. Request permission to review medical records or request hospital staff's help to provide data.
- Use a standardized burn form to collect all available information. Record as much information as is available on the circumstances surrounding the burn episode. The ISBI Burn Registry computer software is a useful tool for collecting and recording burn data.
- Prepare report to include rates:
  - Death rates [(number of deaths/number in population) × 1,000,000], expressed as deaths per million persons.
  - Injury rates [(number of injuries/number in population) × 1,000,000], expressed as injuries per million persons.

Calculate rates for the following categories:
  - Age groups
  - Gender
  - Type of burn (flame, scald, and other)
  - Severity (depth and extent of burn)
- Identify the most common circumstances and/or products causing injury (e.g., pressure stoves, clothing, and ignition).
- Plan a prevention program to address these problems. A review of literature may reveal which strategies have been effective.

Pre-experimental Design: One Group Pretest–Posttest Design

Purpose

To document change associated with a prevention program.

Cautions

There is no control for natural time trends, societal forces and factors other than the intervention which influence burn rates.

Tasks

1. Conduct the descriptive study to determine the burn problem in a defined population. Determine rates for those types of burn injuries and those age groups expected to be affected by the program.
2. Design or adapt a burn prevention program which addresses a significant burn problem.
3. Repeat the descriptive study and compare burn-type and age-specific rates before and after the intervention.

Note: If the prevention intervention has already been instituted, as it often is with safety standards or regulations, the descriptive studies of burns before and after implementation are retrospective and may be conducted simultaneously. Burns are relatively rare occurrence and are known to have yearly fluctuations. For this reason, it is well to collect data for several years before and after intervention.

Quasi-experimental Design: Nonequivalent Control Group Design

Purpose

To measure the effectiveness of a burn prevention program.

Tasks

- Conduct the descriptive study to determine the burn problem in two communities. These communities should be comparable in size, age distribution, and socioeconomic variables.
- Select a burn prevention program, proven to be effective in other locations, which addresses a burn problem shared by both defined communities.
- Randomly select one community as experimental and one as control. Conduct the prevention program in the experimental community.
- Repeat the descriptive study in both populations and compare burn-type and age-specific rates. A successful program would be indicated by significantly lower burn rates in the experimental community with rates essentially unchanged in the control community.

Experimental Design: A Case-control Study

Purpose

To measure the effectiveness of a burn prevention program, for example, whether a new inexpensive kerosene stove, recently introduced into a community, has reduced the likelihood that someone will be burned.

Tasks

- Identify "cases", that is, patients treated for burn injuries caused by stoves.
- Interview the patient or family member to determine the type of stove used by the patient. Determine fuel source, whether or not stove is the "new design".
- Select appropriate "control" for each case. This is the most difficult task of a case-control study to find persons comparable to the case in all things except the type of stove used in the home. It is well to find multiple controls for each case, drawn from different categories. For instance, a hospital "control" could be a person admitted to the hospital the same day for an illness rather than an injury, who is the same gender, same socioeconomic status and in the same age group as the burn patient. A neighborhood "control" could be a person living on the same road, within a certain number of houses, who is the same gender, same socioeconomic status and in the same age group as the burn patient.
- Interview each "control" to determine the type of stove used. Determine fuel source, whether or not stove is the "new design".

- Analyze data using simple 2 × 2 table, categorizing subjects along two axes: positive or negative for burn injuries associated with stoves and positive or negative for exposure to "new stove". Success would be achieved if those using the new stove were significantly less likely to be in the burn category.

EVIDENCE THAT BURN PREVENTION CAN SUCCEED

- Throughout history, whole cities have burned down, cities like Rome, London, and Chicago, to name but a few. Today, such massive fires are rare; when they do occur, they are associated with war and natural disasters. There are many reasons why whole cities do not burn down: More fire-safe construction methods and materials, fire-safety-related building codes and standards, professional fire services, and water delivery systems.
- Fewer children are being burned when their clothes catch fire. There are many reasons: Sleepwear flammability standards, the introduction of new, less flammable fibers and fabrics and more close-fitting designs for girls' clothing. This pattern has not been seen in all countries, particularly not in those countries like India where girls and women commonly wear flowing dresses (*sarees*) made of cotton and rayon.
- Fewer people in the USA are dying in residential fires, due in part to the widespread adoption of smoke detectors which warn residents of deadly smoke.
- Electrical burns of the mouth were all but eliminated in Denmark when a defective electrical cord for a popular vacuum cleaner was recalled and replaced.[46]

COMMON ELEMENT IN SUCCESSFUL BURN PREVENTION PROGRAMS

A consumer product or the environment is made safer for everyone by using prevention programs. Although it might seem easier to teach people to act safely in an unsafe environment, it does not usually work that way. Put your energy into making a safer environment. Burns can happen to anyone, but some groups are at greater risk: the very young or very old, the poor and people with disabilities or who are impaired by drugs or alcohol. These groups are the hardest to reach with educational messages or are less able to adopt safe practices, even if they hear the educational messages.[46]

BASIC PRINCIPLE UNDERLYING BURN PREVENTION STRATEGIES

Keep people separated from excessive heat. This may appear simplistic, but it is fundamental. A person cannot be burned unless a person and a heat source come into contact.[46]

- *Separate with a barrier:* For example, insulate the outer surfaces of stoves and heaters to prevent contact burns; install fences to keep trespassers away from electrical power stations; use sun block creams, umbrellas and roofs to protect people from sunburn.
- *Separate by location:* For example, keep children out of the kitchen or away from the cooking area.
- *Separate by time:* For example, permit trucks carrying volatile fuel to be driven through tunnels only during hours of low-traffic volume.

SEQUENCE OF TASKS FOR BURN PREVENTION PROGRAMS

The Haddon Matrix (assessing pre-event, event-related, and post-event factors) should be considered when constructing prevention programs as the matrix helps to organize interventions for appropriate upstream, midstream, and downstream targets. This approach can be applied at a regional level or even at a case level. There are six major tasks within a burn prevention program:[46]

1. Document the problem
2. Set goals
3. Consider possible strategies
4. Design the intervention
5. Implement program
6. Evaluate program

Above tasks can be exemplified by study program conducted in India by Injury Prevention Workers to protect the people of India from burns caused by fireworks; a secondary success was increasing the use of cool water as first aid for burns.

Document the Problem

Determine the size and nature of the burn problem in your community. Make sure you get good information about what causes these burns and what products and circumstances are involved, e.g., in India, researchers found out that the "cone fountain" fireworks were involved in most of the injuries sustained during Diwali, the festival of lights.[44]

Set Goals

Decide what you want to accomplish in your prevention program. Have single and specific goals, not multiple and broad ones, e.g., in India, researchers decided to prevent injuries caused by "cone fountain" fireworks.

Consider Possible Strategies

Use the "public health model", following the example of public health specialists who consider three factors (agent, host, and environment) when trying to eradicate diseases. Energy (be it thermal, electrical, chemical, or ultraviolet radiant energy) is the "agent" for the burn injury. Host is person at risk. Environment includes both social and physical environment. Here is an example how planners in India have addressed host, agent, and environmental factors when designing their programs:

Host (person at risk)	Teach proper use of fireworks
Agent (energy source)	Redesign "cone fountain" fireworks or ban them
Environment (social and physical)	Restrict sale of these fireworks to professionals and/or restrict locations where they can be used

Design the Intervention

Decide how your goal will be accomplished. Be specific about what is to be done, who is to do it, in what time-frame, with what resources, e.g., in India, researchers decided to mount a media campaign during Diwali, to teach people to handle "cone fountain" fireworks safely and to pour water on burn.

Implement Program

Gather the necessary resources to implement your program and get to work. This means finding financial support if necessary and hiring people or finding volunteers to perform appointed tasks and to monitor progress. It means regular review of progress and brainstorming on how to correct elements of the program that is not working. It means hard work. In India, researchers got financial support and technical expertise from a local insurance company and advertising firm which made television spots about safe handling of "cone fountain" fireworks and about cool water as first aid for burns. Television spots, print advertisements, and brochures were prepared. The television ran the spots just before and during Diwali.

Evaluate Program

Evaluation is the key to progress. This is true of surgical procedures, infection control, skin replacements, and prevention practices. It indicates what is effective and what is not, what should be duplicated, what should be redesigned and what should be dropped. Evaluation is complex, but easier when the goals of the program are very clear. The bottom line is fewer burn injuries. Evaluators try to determine if there are fewer burns after the program, linked to measurable changes in behaviors, products or the environment. In India, researchers found no significant difference in the number of people injured by "cone fountain" fireworks during Diwali after the media program. However, they found significant increases in the number of patients who used cool water for first aid for burns. Thus, this program had mixed results.[47]

GENERAL GUIDELINES FOR POTENTIALLY EFFECTIVE BURN PREVENTION ACTIVITIES

Burn prevention efforts must be tailored to the characteristics of specific burn risks. It is not possible to prevent all burns simultaneously. Burn prevention specialists must be patient and systematic, addressing one type of burn at a time. The best strategy to prevent scald burns will not reduce the number of flame or chemical burns.

Kerosene Lamps and Stoves

In homes throughout the lower income nations, the most common flame burn risk is associated with kerosene lamps and stoves. These two appliances are in constant use for cooking and lighting. Burns occur when these appliances malfunction and kerosene sprays out while people attempt to clean and fix them. One study from India reported that a kerosene stove was involved in 80% of the flame burn injuries treated at a burn unit. Customary cooking at floor level was cited as an additional risk factor. Flame burns would be reduced dramatically worldwide if people used efficient, safe, and inexpensive kerosene lamps and stoves placed above floor level. Keep children out of kitchen. Avoid storing cooking material across the stove. Avoid bending over the flame to put out fire. Avoid keeping stove near gas cylinder.[48]

Flammable Fabrics

In many higher income countries, clothing ignition burns have become quite rare and those which do occur are often linked with flammable liquids. Reasons for this reduction include: flammability standards for children's nightwear, a trend toward closer-fitting garments for women and girls and the redesign of ignition sources, such as space heaters. However, clothing ignition is a major problem in countries where women's traditional dress is loosely draped (*sarees*) and made of cotton or rayon. The beauty of these garments and pride in the traditional dress has made it unlikely that reductions seen elsewhere will occur. These garments combined with floor-level cooking, place women at very high risk. Research is needed in the development of inexpensive flame-resistant materials that can be used in the manufacture of *sarees* and other traditional women's clothing. While cooking, the women should be encouraged to wear only those designs of traditional dress which fit closer to the body and are thus, less likely to catch fire at the stove. Avoid using "*saree*" or "*dupatta*" to handle hot vessels.[48]

Cigarette

Lighted tobacco products, primarily cigarettes, are the major cause of fire deaths in higher income countries, e.g., approximately 50% in Sweden,[49] 33% in Canada, and 25% in the USA.[50] In Japan, smoking materials cause 14% of fire-deaths, second only to incendiary suicide (23%).[51] In the USA, the Center for Fire Research at the National Institute for Standards and Technology has developed a test method to measure compliance with a performance standard to reduce cigarette ignition propensity. Once this standard is adopted, death and injury from cigarette-ignited fires should drop dramatically around the world. It is necessary that all cigarettes manufactured, imported or exported, and/or sold within a country meet the performance standard for reduced cigarette ignition propensity. Home-owners must install smoke detectors in all owner-occupied and rented homes. Educate people not to smoke in bed or under influence of alcohol and drugs. Extinguish all cigarettes before throwing. Redesign cigarette to make them fire safe. Ban use of cigarette at places like petrol pump.

Hot Liquids

Do not keep hot liquids/foods near the edge of table. Keep them out of the reach of children. The temperature of the hot water heater should be set at 124°F. Check temperature of water before bathing children. Never leave a child unattended in the bathroom. Avoid leaving unattended hot liquids. Do not use loose pressure cooker rubber (casket). Do not carry hot water on a slippery floor. Avoid carrying hot liquids when children are around. Do not pour water in an empty hot car radiator, wait to cool or keep the face away from the radiator while pouring water.[51]

Liquid Petroleum Gas Leak

Windows and door should be kept open. Do not light a match or switch on the electric light. Call Gas Company or Fire Department.[51]

Fire Works/Fire Crackers

Fire crackers should be ignited from a distance and those which fail to burst should not be inspected from close distance because it can burst at any time. Do not wear easily flammable fabrics while playing with fire crackers. Do not leave children to play with firecrackers unsupervised. Redesign fire crackers with safety measures. Ban dangerous fire crackers. Use fireworks in the open ground only.[51]

Crowded Places (Theater)

Heat and smoke detectors should be installed. A well-designed fire escape plan should be available. Fire brigade and police telephone numbers should be kept near phone. Fire extinguishers, water, and sand should be available readily.[51]

Electric Burn

Educate children not to touch wires and electrical appliances. Do not handle electric appliances with wet hands and bare feet. Unplug electric appliances when not in use. Use standard company electric appliances. Plug point should be placed at higher level out of the reach of children and it should be covered with a cap. There should be no dangling cords. All flawed cords should be replaced with redesigned cords. Keep electric appliances away from the water. Hot iron should not be left unattended within reach of children. Avoid open plug point. Avoid open bathrooms if immersion rod is used to heat water. The rescuer must be careful so that he does not become a part of the electrical circuit in attempting to free a person still in contact with a live wire. Use dry wood and push the patient away from current source.

When flying a kite, it is important to remember the 3 Cs of kite safety: Caution, Courtesy, and Common sense. By keeping these three items in mind at all times, you will make your recreational time more enjoyable, and safer.[52]

Here are some extra tips for making your kite outing a safe one:

- Choose a flying site at least 3 miles (5 km) away from airfields; also stay away from roads and railway lines.
- Never fly your kite near electrical pylons, overhead power cables, or overhead lines of any kind.
- If your kite becomes entangled, do not attempt to free it yourself. Seek help from your local authorities.
- Do not fly your kite in electrical storms. The kite will act as a lightning conductor, causing injury and even death.
- Be aware of casual observers. They could be unaware of the potential dangers involved in kite flying.
- Flying kites on larger lines can cause line burns on your hands, so be sure to wear gloves.

- Always be aware of who or what is behind you as well as in front of you.
- Know your skill level, limitations, and strengths. Do not fly anything too large for the conditions or try any complicated moves in crowded areas.[53,54]

SUMMARY

Burn injuries in a developing nation like India are still a major problem. Poverty, illiteracy, lack of funds and lack of burn education, etc., are the major hurdles in solving the problem of burns in India. The only answer is "burn prevention". It is not quick, cheap, or easy. If it were, the burn problem would have been eliminated long ago. Be prepared to make long-term plans to gather public support for safer product designs and for codes and regulations which are often necessary for effective burn prevention. Be prepared to rethink strategies halfway through a project. Be prepared for a struggle. But know that burns are preventable.

A final word: "Prevention takes time, energy, and money but ultimately, it is the solution to the world's burn problem". "Vision is nothing but a dream that is backed by the drive to achieve it".

REFERENCES

1. Bhatia S.L. Ind J Med Hist. 1957;2:70.
2. Bhishagratna KKL. An English translation of the Sushruta Samhita. Based on Original Sanskrit text in three volumes. Calcutta: KL Bhishagratna; 1907.
3. Salisbury RE. Chapter 23: Thermal Burns. In: McCarthy JG, May JW, Littler JW (Eds). Plastic Surgery, Vol. 1. Philadelphia: WB Saunders Company; 1990. pp. 787-8.
4. Lee RC. Chapter 18: Acute management of burn and electrical trauma. In: Song DH, Neligan PC (Eds). Plastic Surgery—Lower Extremity, Trunk and Burns, (Vol 4), 4th edition. Netherland: Elsevier Publication; 2018. p. 392.
5. Lee KC, Joory K, Moiemen NS. History of burns: The past, present and the future. Burn Trauma. 2014;2:169-80.
6. Maneksha RJ. Chapter 4: Plastic Surgery in the Tropics. Hyderabad, Andhra Pradesh: Orient Longman Limited; 1976.
7. McDowell F. The source book of Plastic Surgery. Baltimore: Williams and Wilkins Company; 1977. pp. 65-85.
8. Gupta JL. Past, present and future of Plastic Surgery in India. Indian J Plast Surg. 1991;24:1-9.
9. Rana RE, Arora BS. History of plastic surgery in India. J Postgrad Med. 2002;48:76-8.
10. Sarabahi S. Chapter 1: History, Epidemiology and Prevention of Burns. In: Sarabahi S (Ed). Principles and Practice of Burn Care, 1st edition. New Delhi: Jaypee Brothers Medical Publishers (P) Ltd.; 2010.
11. Gupta JL. Planning a Burns Unit. Agnivarta. 1997;14:8-14.
12. Chatterjee SS. Department of plastic surgery, IPGME&R, Kolkata. Indian J Plast Surg. 2004;37:77-9.
13. Prasanna M, Singh K, Kumar P. Early tangential excision and skin grafting as a routine method of burn wound management: an experience from a developing country. Burns. 1994;20: 446.
14. Burma A. Fireworks: Fun or Folly. Agnivarta. 1997;14:3-7.
15. Park K. Chapter 3: Principles of epidemiology and epidemiologic methods. In: Park K (Ed). Park's textbook of Preventive and Social Medicine, 19th edition. Jabalpur, India: M/s Banarsidas Bhanot Publishers; 2007.
16. WHO. ACCIDENTS in childhood; facts as a basis for prevention. World Health Organ Tech Rep Ser. 1957;118:1-40.
17. Wang Y, Beekman J, Hew H, Jackson S, Issler-Fisher A, Parungao R, et al. Burn injury: challenges and advances in burn wound healing, infection, pain and scarring. Adv Drug Deliv Rev. 2018;123:3-17.
18. Smolle Ch, Cambiaso-Daniel J, Forbes A, Wurzer P, Hundeshagen G, Branski LK, et al. Recent trends in burn epidemiology worldwide: a systematic review. Burns. 2017;43:249-57.
19. Jenkins ATA. Young Smart dressings for the prevention of infection in pediatric burns patients. Expert Rev Anti Infect Ther. 2010;8:1063-65.
20. McLoughlin E. A simple guide to burn epidemiology. International Society for Burn Injuries in collaboration with the World Health Organization. Burns. 1995;21:217-20.
21. Kumar P, Chirayil PT, Chittoria R. Then and now: burns in India. Burns. 2000;26:63-81.
22. Amor AJ. World Health. 1979.
23. Govt of India, Health Information of India 1993, DGHS, New Delhi.
24. Kharbanda S. Social Welfare. 1933;30:22.
25. Keswani MH. Evertte Idris Evans Memorial Lecture delivered in the US on March 16, 1996 by Manohar H. Keswani, Honorary Secretary, Burns Association of India.
26. Subrahmanyam M. Topical application of honey in treatment of burns. Br J Surg. 1991;78:497-8.
27. Ytterstad B, Sogaard AJ. The Harstad Injury Prevention Study: prevention of burns in small children by a community-based intervention. Burns. 1995;21:259-66.
28. Sen R, Banerjec C. Survey of 1000 admissions to a burns unit, SSKM Hospital, Calcutta. Burns. 1981;7:357-60.
29. Adesunkanmi K, Oyelami OA. The pattern and outcome of burn injuries at Wesley Guild Hospital, Ilesha, Nigeria: A review of 156 cases. J Trop Med Hyg. 1994;97:108-12.
30. El-Muhtaseb H, Qaryoute S, Ragheb SA. Burn injuries in Jordan: a study of 338 Cases. Burns Incl Therm Inj. 1983;10:116-20.
31. Jay KM, Bartlett RH, Danet R, Allyn PA. Burn epidemiology: A basis for burn prevention. J Trauma. 1977;17:943-7.
32. Kamel FA. Some epidemiological features of burn patients admitted to the emergency department of the Main University Hospital and to Ras El-Teen Hospital in Alexandria [MPH thesis]. Burns. 1995;21:24-8.
33. Eadie PA, Williams R, Dickson WA. Thirty-five years of pediatric scalds: Are lessons being learned? Br J Plast Surg. 1995;48:103-5.
34. Green AR, Fairclough J, Sykes PJ. Epidemiology of burns in childhood. Burns. 1984;10:368-71.
35. Gupta JL, Tiwari IN. Burns-Thermal and Chemical. Chapter 16. Plastic Surgery in the Tropics. Hyderabad, Andhra Pradesh: Orient Longman Limited; 1976. pp. 163-6.

36. Jaiswal AK, Aggarwal H, Solanki P, Lubana PS, Mathur RK, Odiya S. Epidemiological and socio-cultural study of burn patients in M.Y. Hospital, Indore, India. Indian J Plast Surg. 2007;40:158-63.
37. Kumar P, Chirayil PT, Chittoria R. Ten years epidemiological study of pediatric Burns in Manipal, India. Burns. 1999;25:1-4.
38. Verma SS, Srinivasan S, Vartak AM. An epidemiological study of 500 pediatric burn patients in Mumbai, India. Indian J Plast Surg. 2007;40:153-7.
39. Rybarczyk MM, Schafer JM, Elm CM, Sarvepalli S. A systematic review of burn injuries in low- and middle-income countries: epidemiology in the WHO-defined. African Region Afr J Emerg Med. 2017;7:32-6.
40. Stokes MAR, Johnson WD. Burns in the third World: an unmet need. Ann Burns Fire Disasters. 2017;30:243-6.
41. Nischwitz SP, Luze H, Kotzbeck P, Kamolz LP. Electrical burns and their consequences. Burns. 2020;46:982-4.
42. Dhanraj P. Thermal Injury (Chapter 13). In: Dhanraj P (Ed). Plastic Surgery Made Easy. New Delhi: Jaypee Brothers Medical Publishers (P) Ltd.; 2006. pp. 355-61.
43. Kumar P. Causes and Prevention of Burns (Chapter 1). In: Kumar P (Ed). Fundamentals of Burns Management. Hyderabad, India: Paras Medical Publisher; 1998. pp. 2-5.
44. Campbell DT, Stanley JC. Experimental and Quasi-experimental Designs for Research. Chicago: Rand McNally College Publishing Company; 1996.
45. Hulley SB, Cummings SR. Designing Clinical Research: An Epidemiological Approach. Baltimore: Williams & Wilkins; 1998.
46. McLoughlin E. A simple guide to burn prevention. International Society for Burn Injuries in collaboration with the World Health Organization. Burns. 1995;21:226-9.
47. Mohan D, Varghese M. Fireworks cast a shadow on India's festival of lights. World Health Forum. 1990;11:323-6.
48. Sawhney CP. Flame burns involving kerosene pressure stoves in India. Burns. 1989;15:362-4.
49. Hall JR. Fire in the USA and Sweden: International Fire Comparison Report No. 7. Quincy, MA: National Fire Protection Association; 1997.
50. Hall JR. Fire in the USA and Canada: International Fire Comparison. 1992.
51. Keswani MH. The prevention of burning injury. Burns. 1986;12:533-9.
52. Tiwari VK, Sharma D. Kite flying: a unique but dangerous mode of electrical injury in children. Burns. 1999;25:537-9.
53. Kumar P. Clinical Forensic evidence in burns: Rescuer Burns. Burns. 2007;33:1071.
54. Haddon W. The changing approach to the epidemiology, prevention, and amelioration of trauma: the transition to approaches etiologically rather than descriptively based. Inj Prev. 1999;5:231-5.

CHAPTER

2

Anatomy of the Skin

Sujata Sarabahi

INTRODUCTION

Skin is the largest organ, covering a surface area of 1.5–2.0 m^2 in an adult. In burns, although there is direct damage by the causative agent to this outer protective layer of the body, almost all the other organ systems are indirectly involved, in addition. Before considering the pathophysiology of burn wound, it is imperative to understand the anatomy and physiology of normal skin as both are disrupted following burns.

The skin consists of a thin outer layer which is cellular and derived from the ectoderm—the epidermis—and an inner thicker fibrous layer which originates from the mesoderm—the dermis **(Figs. 1 and 2)**. The two layers are separated by a basement membrane or basal lamina. Nerve endings are present throughout both the layers. The connective tissue of the dermis provides a firm structural base for the skin. Underneath the skin lie the subcutaneous tissues, muscle, and bone. The thickness of skin is variable in different anatomical areas of the body, in different sexes, and at different ages in the same individual. This produces differing depths of burn injury in different parts of the body and at different ages from a given temperature and time of exposure. In general, the skin of infants, children, and elderly is thinner as compared to that of adults. Thus, the burns may be deeper in children and elderly with the same agent causing a comparatively superficial injury in adults. Males have thicker skin as compared to females.

The skin of the scalp, palm, and soles is thickest (2 mm thick) compared to the rest of the body, whereas it is thinnest on the eyelids (0.5 mm thick) and external genitalia. This is because of the difference in the degree of keratinization of the epidermis. The degree of keratinization of skin is largely under genetic control. However, intermittent mechanical pressure or abrasion stimulates the adventitious production of keratinized cells

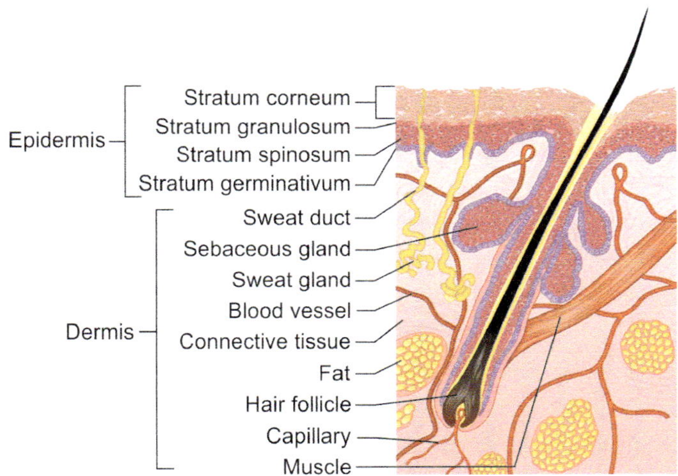

FIG. 1: Diagrammatic representation of anatomy of skin.

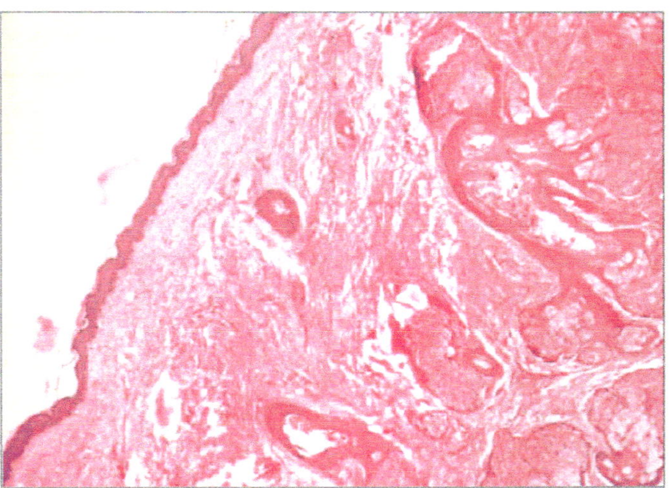

FIG. 2: Normal skin on histopathological examination.

Courtesy: Dr Geetika Khanna. Director Professor of Pathology and Principal, VMMC and Safdarjung Hospital, New Delhi.

which enhances stress-resisting properties of the skin. The interface between the epidermis and dermis is marked by peg and socket or ridge and groove interdigitations which along with specialized anchoring structures linking the epidermis to the dermis prevent the epithelium from being stripped off the surface of the dermis by shearing forces.

ANATOMY OF EPIDERMIS

Normal epidermis is a terminally differentiated, stratified squamous epithelium divided into five distinct layers, each of which represents different stages in the development of the fully mature cells of the outermost layer—the *stratum corneum* (as we go from the innermost layer to the outermost layer). The thickness of stratum corneum varies in different parts of the body and it is subjected to constant shedding. It consists of several rows of cornified, non-nucleated dead cells containing keratin. This layer forms a barrier on the surface of the skin, protecting the underlying living cells from damage by trauma and desiccation.[1]

The *stratum lucidum* lies immediately deep to the stratum corneum and is found only in the skin of the soles of feet and palm of hand as a thin eosinophilic band. The *stratum granulosum* is the next layer of flattened nucleated cells containing a precursor of keratin called keratohyalin granules. The fourth layer is the *stratum spinosum* which is a prickle cell layer containing several layers of polyhedric and cylindrical cells.

The deepest layer is the *stratum basale* or the germinal layer of the epidermis. This consists of a single layer of pigment granules containing cuboidal- or columnar-shaped cells called keratinocytes which are in a state of high mitotic activity. These epidermal stem cells in the basal layer divide to form transient amplifying cells which then migrate suprabasally, stop dividing, and undergo terminal differentiation. This process of maturation and migration from the basal layer to the outermost layer takes about 26–42 days. The keratinocytes are attached to each other by desmosomes which can be broken and reformed allowing the mature keratinocytes to migrate upward. The desmosomes of the stratum corneum are also degraded before desquamation so that there is shedding of outer layers of epidermis as deeper layers move outward. The time taken for the deepest layer of stratum corneum to reach the outermost layer and desquamate is approximately 14 days. Thus, the normal epidermis completely replaces itself in 45–75 days.

Within the germinative layer of the epidermis, there are three other cell types, namely the melanocytes, Langerhans cells, and Merkel's cells.

Melanocytes are dendritic cells which produce pigment granules called melanosomes which contain melanin pigment. Majority of these melanocytes are located at the dermoepidermal junction beneath the basal cells and some lie in the dermis. Embryonically, melanocytes are derived from the neural crest and they migrate to the epidermis. The dendritic processes of the melanocytes contain the melanosomes and once their tips are sheared off, they are phagocytosed by the keratinocytes. Thus, the pigment is transferred from the melanocytes to the keratinocytes.

The rate of melanin production, transfer to keratinocytes, and degradation of melanosomes determine the degree of skin pigmentation. The ratio of melanocytes to epidermal cells is 1 in 5 on the face and 1 in 20 in the buttocks. The average ratio of melanocyte to keratinocyte in the body varies from 1:4 to 1:10. The relative number of melanocytes is approximately equal for men and women and for all races. The difference in color between races is not due to difference in the number of melanocytes but due to the activity, rate, and production of melanin. For example, individuals with darker skin have very large melanosomes which are fully melanized as compared to individuals with fairer skin who have smaller and less melanized melanosomes. This is to be kept in mind when choosing a donor area for procuring the skin graft. There will be a definite difference in color when skin from an area of higher melanosomes content is grafted onto areas that have a smaller number of melanosomes.

Melanin protects the epidermis from the harmful effects of the ultraviolet rays of sun by forming a protective layer around the nucleus of the keratinocyte so that these rays do not damage the DNA in the nucleus. A higher amount of melanin, thus, protects the skin from sun burn which is a first-degree epidermal burn of skin on increased exposure to sunlight.

Langerhans cells are also dendritic cells found in the epidermis but devoid of melanin. They contain rod-like Langerhans granules, some of which are in continuity with the external membrane of the cell. Their function is still unclear. Recent research has shown that these cells are a type of phagocytic cells and they provide a "trap" for various contact antigens and present them to T cells for destruction. Thus, they protect the internal structures from the potentially infectious agents in the external environment.

Merkel cells are found in the basal part of the epidermis of hairy skin. They are in close contact with the tactile sensory nerve endings terminating in the basal part of the epidermis. Thus, they play an important role in the sensory processes.

The basement membrane at the dermoepidermal junction is a highly organized structure of protein that anchors the epidermis to the dermis. It consists of grooves on the epidermal side which fit into projections from the dermis called dermal papillae. A number of microfilaments insert into this basement membrane and get aggregated in the adjacent papillary dermis resulting in structures called "rete pegs" or "rete ridges" which are seen as invaginations into the papillary dermis to increase the surface area. These resist the shearing forces between the epidermis and dermis. Any gap due to shearing between epidermis and dermis can produce a blister as is seen following superficial dermal burns.

ANATOMY OF EPIDERMAL APPENDAGES

The functions of human skin are further affected by certain cutaneous appendages which are of ectodermal origin. These are the hair follicles, sebaceous glands, apocrine glands, and sweat glands.

Hair Follicle

Hairs are found on nearly all parts of the human body except the palm of hands and sole of feet, glans penis, the inner surface of prepuce and clitoris, and labia majora and minora. The hair has a root which is the part inside the skin and a shaft which is projecting outside the skin. The root of the hair has a proximal enlargement, the hair bulb, which is set in an invagination of the epidermis and superficial portion of the dermis called the hair follicle. The hair follicle commences on the skin surface with a funnel-shaped opening and then passes obliquely downward to become dilated at its end which corresponds to the hair bulb. The ducts of one or more sebaceous glands open into the follicle near the skin surface. In the hair bulb, there is a small conical vascular prominence or papilla which is continuous with the dermal layer of the follicle and is supplied with myelinated and nonmyelinated nerve endings. The nutrition to the hair is derived from the capillaries in this papilla.

The hair follicle has two coats—an outer coat which is mainly fibrous tissue and is continuous with the dermis and an inner coat or root sheath which is closely adherent to the root of the hair and is basically a continuation of the epidermal cell layer. Since the hair follicle is primarily composed of epidermal tissue, it has a significant role in re-epithelialization of burn wounds.

The hair bulb is molded over the papilla and consists of polyhedral cells which are undifferentiated and rapidly dividing. The products of these rapidly dividing cells are the inner root sheath and hair which move outward toward the surface of the skin.

The hair shaft is a dead cornified structure which extends from the follicle above the skin surface. The shaft consists from within outward, the medulla, the cortex, and the cuticle. The color of the hair depends on the amount of melanin and its distribution in the cortex. Blond hair has few melanosomes, while gray hair does not have melanosomes due to a relative absence of melanocytes.

The terminal hair follicle has three phases in its growth cycle, the active phase or anagen, the involuting phase or catagen, and the resting phase or telogen. The hair follicles produce hair independent of each other.

In burns, unless the wound is very deep or full thickness, the epidermal tissue lining the hair follicles is still available in the depths of the dermis in the wound site to generate new epithelium. The hair also traps air and provides insulation, though this is true only for the scalp.

Sebaceous Glands

Sebaceous glands are small sacculated glands arising from an epithelial bud from the outer hair root sheath. They are found in most parts of the skin, more abundant in the scalp and face while being absent in the palms of hands and soles of feet. Each gland has a single duct which emerges from a cluster of oval or piriform alveoli. Each alveolus has a basement membrane enclosing a number of epithelial cells. The marginal cells are small and polyhedral and in continuation with the cells lining the ducts. The remainder of the alveolus is filled with larger cells containing fat. In the center, the cells are broken up leaving a cavity filled with a mass of fatty matter called sebum cutaneum. Since the sebaceous glands produce their secretions by complete fatty degeneration of their central cells, they are classified as holocrine glands. Commonly, their ducts open into the hair follicles. Occasionally, they open onto the general surface. Sebum acts as a natural lubricant for the hair and skin and thus protects them from desiccation. It has bactericidal action as well. Their secretory activity is under hormonal control, especially androgens. Following a burn injury, if the sebaceous glands are damaged or the raw area is split skin grafted, the new skin may not be able to secrete enough sebum to lubricate the skin. Hence, a frequent application of moisturizing creams/bland oil is required to prevent the dried skin from cracking and subsequent infection.

Sweat Glands

Sweat glands are present in the skin of almost every part of the body and are classified into two types: Eccrine and apocrine.

The eccrine glands are more numerous. They consist of a single tube which is coiled into a spherical or oval ball called a body in its deep part which is situated in the deeper layers of the dermis or in subcutaneous tissues. The duct traverses the dermis and epidermis and opens onto the surface of the skin by an aperture. The size and number of glands vary in different parts of the body. They are large in the axilla and groin where the amount of perspiration is more. They are also numerous in palm and sole. The tube consists of two layers—an outer layer of fine areolar tissue which is continuous with the superficial layer of dermis and an inner epithelial layer consisting of cubical or polyhedral cells. Between the basal aspects of these cells and the basement membrane, there is an incomplete layer of myoepithelial cells, which help in the expression of secretions from the gland by virtue of their contractile property. The ducts are composed of a basement membrane lined by two to three layers of polyhedral cells. These eccrine sweat glands are merocrine in nature, that is, they produce their thin watery secretions without epithelial cell disintegration.

Apocrine sweat glands are present in the axilla, eyelids, nipple, areola, periareolar region of the breast, and external genitalia. They are in close association with hair follicles and produce thick secretions. They contain a coiled secretory gland in the lower dermis and a straight excretory duct. Their secretions are sterile and odorless within the duct but once excreted onto the surface of the skin, bacteria degrade them resulting in body odor.

The primary stimulus for the production of sweat is heat. The thermoregulatory center in the hypothalamus is responsible for sweat production in an effort to maintain body temperature, as sweating helps in dissipating heat. A patient who has sustained deep dermal or full-thickness burns loses majority or all of his eccrine sweat glands and if significant body surface area is involved in these burns, the patient's rate of sweating becomes inefficient. Thus, these patients may not be able to regulate their body temperature by sweating in hot and humid surroundings leading to a rise in their core body temperature.

ANATOMY OF DERMIS

The dermis is also called corium. It is a tough, flexible, and highly elastic structure. It is very thick in the palm of hands (1.6 mm) and soles of feet and very thin in the eyelids (0.4 mm), scrotum, and penis. It consists of mainly connective tissue with varying numbers of elastic and collagen fibers, numerous blood vessels, lymphatic vessels, and nerves. The fibroblasts are the "master cells" of the dermis which produce the collagen fibers, elastic fibers, and ground substance. Collagen forms approximately 77% of the dry weight of dermis and provides tensile strength to it. 85% of the collagen is type I and 15% is type II collagen. Elastic fibers are interwoven within the network of collagen fibers. The connective tissue in the dermis is arranged in two layers: Superficial papillary dermis and deeper reticular dermis.

Papillary dermis consists of numerous papillae which are highly sensitive vascular conical projections, which project perpendicularly into corresponding pits on the undersurface of the epidermis. Each papilla consists of small closely interlacing bundles of fine fibrillar tissue with a few elastic fibers and within this, there is a capillary loop. In some papillae, especially on the palms and fingers, there are tactile corpuscles. The papillary dermis primarily consists of small loosely distributed elastic and collagen fibrils with a greater proportion of interfibrillar gel and connective tissue that encloses the microcirculation and lymphatic network below the papillary projections.

Reticular dermis is the thicker part of dermis and is more acellular and avascular compared to papillary dermis. It consists of strong interlacing bands of white fibrous tissue and some yellow elastic fibers. The collagen bundles are arranged mainly parallel to the skin surface, and some are perpendicularly arranged forming a lattice work. This arrangement of collagen fibers in the reticular dermis provides skin with extensibility in different directions. The directions taken by the parallel bundles of collagen fibers form the cleavage lines of the skin. Surgical incisions given along the direction of cleavage lines heal with minimal scar tissue, whereas incisions perpendicular to these lines cause retraction of the severed fibers, leading to a broad scar. With increasing age, the yellow elastic fibers atrophy and skin loses its elasticity and becomes wrinkled.[2,3]

Following burns, if only the epidermis is involved, they heal without any scarring of the skin. However, as the deeper layers of skin are involved, depending on the depth of the dermis involved, the skin always heals with scarring. Again, depending on the amount of collagen production and the arrangement of collagen fibers, there can be either hypertrophic scarring or keloid formation **(Figs. 3A to C)**. Details of the pathophysiology of postburn scar formation have been described in Chapter 6 on "Wound Healing in Burns".

Deep to the reticular layer is the subcutaneous areolar tissue which contains fat. In many regions, the skin is separated from the deep fascia or other structures by loose areolar tissue, and in these sites, the skin is freely movable over the deeper structures. Elsewhere, however, the skin may be firmly anchored to structures like the periosteum over subcutaneous parts of bones or to deep fascia in regions related to movements of underlying joints where it leads to permanent creases in the skin known as flexure lines, for example, palm of hand and flexure surface of digits.

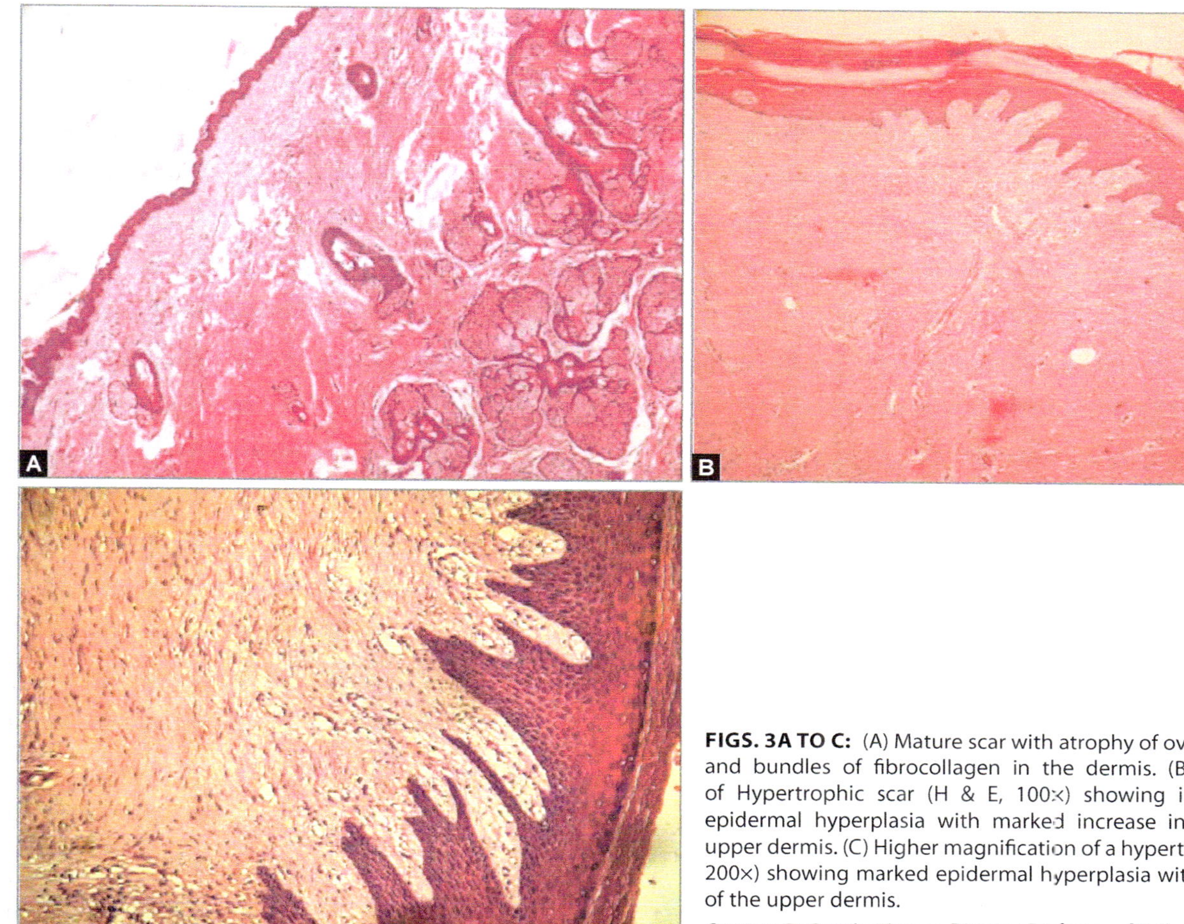

FIGS. 3A TO C: (A) Mature scar with atrophy of overlying epidermis and bundles of fibrocollagen in the dermis. (B) Histopathology of Hypertrophic scar (H & E, 100×) showing increased keratin, epidermal hyperplasia with marked increase in collagen in the upper dermis. (C) Higher magnification of a hypertrophic scar (H & E, 200×) showing marked epidermal hyperplasia with collagenization of the upper dermis.

Courtesy: Dr Geetika Khanna. Director Professor of Pathology and Principal, VMMC and Safdarjung Hospital, New Delhi.

BLOOD SUPPLY OF SKIN

The blood supply and drainage of skin lie along well-determined pathways which depend upon the metabolic requirement of various cellular components. The most active areas of the skin are the epidermis and its appendages and the dermal papillae which contain active fibroblasts and sensory endings of cutaneous nerves. The reticular layer is highly fibrous and contains few active cells; therefore, its metabolic requirement is low. There are two vascular plexuses—one at the dermal-subcutaneous junction called rete cutaneum and one in the papillary dermis called rete subpapillare or superficial plexus. These are connected by vertical vascular channels. In the papillary plexus, there is a network of arterioles, capillaries, and venules which provide a large amount of blood supply to this layer. Capillaries extend from this layer toward the base of epidermis within the dermal papillae and loop back to the flat venous plexus which lies immediately beneath the rete subpapillare which drains into venous plexus at dermis-subcutaneous junction via another intermediate plexus in the middle of reticular dermis. Various capillaries in the dermis around glands and hair follicles also drain into these three venous plexuses at different levels in the skin.[4]

Apart from providing nutrition to the skin, the cutaneous vasculature has an important function of thermoregulation. Another important role of micro-circulation is in the inflammatory process seen in the skin following any kind of trauma which helps in the healing process. Following burns involving only superficial layers of skin, the microvascular circulation in the deeper layer is intact. Therefore, the deeper vascular bed of the skin has the potential to heal rapidly as it promotes the re-epithelialization process.

LYMPHATIC DRAINAGE OF SKIN

The lymphatic drainage of skin is via numerous blindly ending lymphatic vessels which terminate in the dermis near the base of epidermis and drain first into a dermal network in the papillary layer and then into another network in the middle of the reticular layer and finally into a network at the junction of dermis and subcutaneous tissues. Deeper to this, there are wide channels with valves which drain into the main lymphatics of the area.

INNERVATION OF SKIN

Skin is richly supplied by myelinated and nonmyelinated sensory fibers of craniospinal nerves and via nonmyelinated autonomic fibers which supply blood vessels, sweat glands, and hair follicles. The nerves penetrate the superficial fascia and ramify through the reticular and papillary layers of the dermis forming nerve plexuses around hair follicles in both the reticular dermis and the papillary dermis. Most of the nerve fibers end in the dermis and some penetrate into the basement membrane.

The skin contains sensory organs for all the principal sensations, such as touch, pain, temperature, pressure, itch, and tickle. There are mainly six types of sensory receptors in the skin:

1. Free terminals or free nerve endings form majority of the sensory receptors found in the epidermis and dermis. They are related to sensations of itch and pain and fine discrimination for sensory stimuli in digits. As the name suggests, they contain one or more axons enclosed in an extension of Schwann cell which is then covered with a basal lamina.
2. Merkel cells are special cells found in the epidermal ridges having attachments next to keratinocytes. They act as mechanoreceptors for the sensation of touch.
3. Meissner's corpuscles are found mainly in the papillary dermis of palm and sole, responsible for the sensation of touch and relative pressure associated with touch.
4. Pacinian corpuscles are present in the deep layers of dermis in palm and palmar subcutaneous tissue and near periosteum of proximal phalanges. They are responsible for the sensation of vibration and signal for local changes of blood flow.
5. Pilo-Ruffini corpuscles are sensory receptors which encircle the hair follicles, and therefore, they respond to changes in pressure on skin sensed by movements of hair follicles. They are also responsible for the sensation of warmth.
6. Krause's end bulbs are widely distributed in superficial layers of the dermis and are end organs for cold sensation. Patient sustaining burns may lose some or all of these sensory receptors depending on the depth of burns. As a result, they may lose some of the sensations in the affected areas.

FUNCTIONS OF SKIN[5]

- The most important function of the skin is its ability to act as a physical barrier preventing bacteria and other organisms from entering it. It also serves as a water barrier and thus maintains fluid balance in the body. Following burns, the integrity of skin is disrupted allowing loss of fluids from the body and entry of organisms into the body. Thus, hypovolemia and infection are the two major complications to be tackled by a burn surgeon.
- Skin also regulates heat exchange and helps body temperature homeostasis. When the cutaneous vessels dilate the blood flow to skin is increased, the amount of heat transmitted to the body surface is also increased. When cutaneous vessels constrict, blood flow to the skin is decreased with a consequential decrease in heat loss from the body. In this way, the body temperature is maintained.
- Similarly, perspiration from the skin surface also controls the body temperature. The rate of evaporative water loss from the burned skin surface is directly proportional to the extent and depth of burns. This evaporative water loss enhances the heat loss from the body as well. Approximately 580 kcal is required for the evaporation of 1 L of water from the body surface. The excessive heat loss from the body surface of a burn victim causes a severe metabolic drain as well because this is accompanied by hypermetabolism. This evaporative water loss can be estimated by the following formula:
- Evaporative water loss (mL/h) = (25 + %TBSA burn) × BSA m^2

  (BSA; body surface area; TBSA: total body surface area)
- The stratum corneum of the skin has the ability for selective permeability allowing absorption of some substances and acting as a barrier to others, while hair follicles and eccrine glands only allow percutaneous absorption. A concentration gradient is required to allow the percutaneous absorption of substances across stratum corneum. This is also affected by the relative hydration of stratum corneum. Lipid and lipid-soluble substances pass through the skin easily compared to hydrophilic organic compounds. A gaseous compound such as carbon monoxide can also get absorbed by the skin when present in high concentrations.
- Through its various sensory receptors, the skin transmits sensory feedback from the environment.
- Last but not the least, the skin has a sophisticated immune system which plays an important role in host

defenses. Whenever skin is exposed to a new antigen, activated antigen expressing Langerhans cells migrate from the skin to lymph nodes, where they activate naïve T cells which then become memory T cells and express new surface markers that allow them to accumulate preferentially in the skin in response to cutaneous injury.

SUMMARY

Knowledge of the detailed anatomy and physiology of skin is a must for a better understanding of the mechanisms of alterations produced in burns, the management of burn patient as a whole, and the causation and minimization of scars.

REFERENCES

1. McGrath JA, Eady RAJ, Pope FM. Anatomy and organization of human skin. In: Burns T, Breathnach S, Cox N, Griffiths C (Eds). Rook's Textbook of Dermatology, Vol. 1, 7th edition. Oxford: Blackwell; 2004. pp. 3.1-3.84 (Chapter 3).
2. Archer CB. Functions of the skin. In: Burns T, Breathnach S, Cox N, Griffiths C (Eds). Rook's Textbook of Dermatology, Vol. 1, 7th edition. Blackwell; 2004. pp. 4.1-4.12 (Chapter 4).
3. Murphy GF. Histology of the skin. In: Elder DE, Elenitsas R, Johnson BL Jr, Murphy GF (Eds). Lever's Histopathology of the Skin, 9th edition. Philadelphia: Lippincott William and Wilkins; 2005. pp. 9-58 (Chapter 3).
4. James WD, Berger TG, Elston DM Skin. Basic structure and function. Andrew's Diseases of the Skin Clinical Dermatology, 10th edition. Canada: Saunders Elsevier's; 2006. pp. 1-14.
5. Chu DH, Haake AR, Holbrook K, Loomis CA. The structure and development of skin. In: Freedberg IM, Eisen AZ, Wolff K, Austen KF, Goldsmith LA, Katz SI (Eds). Fitzpatrick's Dermatology in General Medicine, 6th edition. New York: McGraw Hill; 2003. pp. 58-88 (Chapter 6).

CHAPTER

3

Burns: Etiology and Classification

Sameek Bhattacharya, V Suman Babu

INTRODUCTION

Since the discovery of fire, man has been on a relentless quest for energy. This pursuit is driven by the expansion and progress of human civilization. The benefits of fire reaped by man have paralleled the fatalities and disabilities caused by it. The magnitude of this devastating injury has increased with the ability to harness higher energy source, use of fire in most activities of life and its application as a destructive modality. Hence, the epidemiological profile of burn injury has changed with time and advancement of the society. The incidence of burn injury directly reflects the imbalance between the use of fire and the level of fire safety consciousness of a society. Therefore, any preventive strategy must be preceded by adequate and reliable data collection about the cause and circumstances of injury. Burns are classified on the basis of cause, degree of burn, and total body surface area (TBSA) involved.

CLASSIFICATION ACCORDING TO ETIOLOGY

Burn injury leads to local and systemic clinical features following exposure to very high temperature, electrical energy, chemical, and radiation.

Thermal Burns

The most common cause of burns is thermal, caused by flame, blast, contact with hot objects, and hot liquids. Thermal damage to skin is primarily a function of energy transfer from heat source to the body. The heat transmission depends on the temperature of the source, conductivity of the tissues, insulation such as hair and keratin layer and the clothing. The thermal threshold of human skin is about 70°C.

Flame Burns

Flame burns account for over 80% of the total burn cases in India and other developing countries **(Fig. 1)**.[1] This is at variance with the western data where scalds are the predominant cause. More than 85% of the flame burns in our country are attributed to accidents of which mishaps in the kitchen account for over 60%.[1] In contrast, space heating and house fires are the predominant causes in the west.[2] The high incidence of cooking accidents is ascribed to unsafe heating appliances, floor level cooking, and wearing of loose-fitting clothes. The major killer among these is the kerosene pressure stoves, which work on aerosolized kerosene oil **(Fig. 2A)**. In the event of carbon-choked burner holes, vigorous pumping of the stove suddenly opens up the holes expressing out a large volume of kerosene aerosol which ignites into fireball **(Fig. 2B)**.

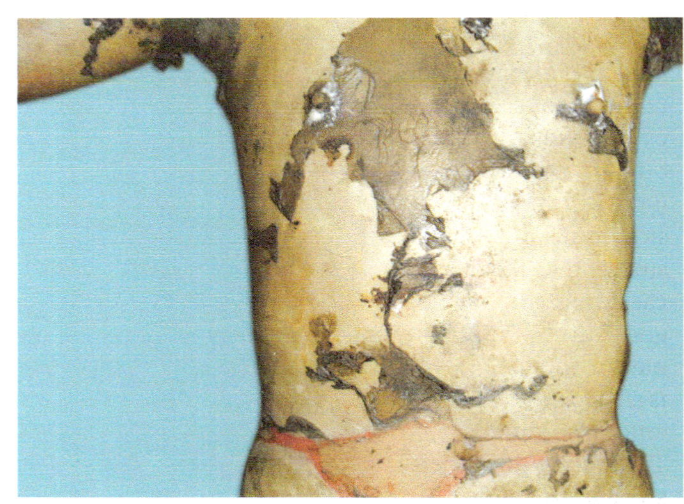

FIG. 1: Flame burns leading to extensive injury.

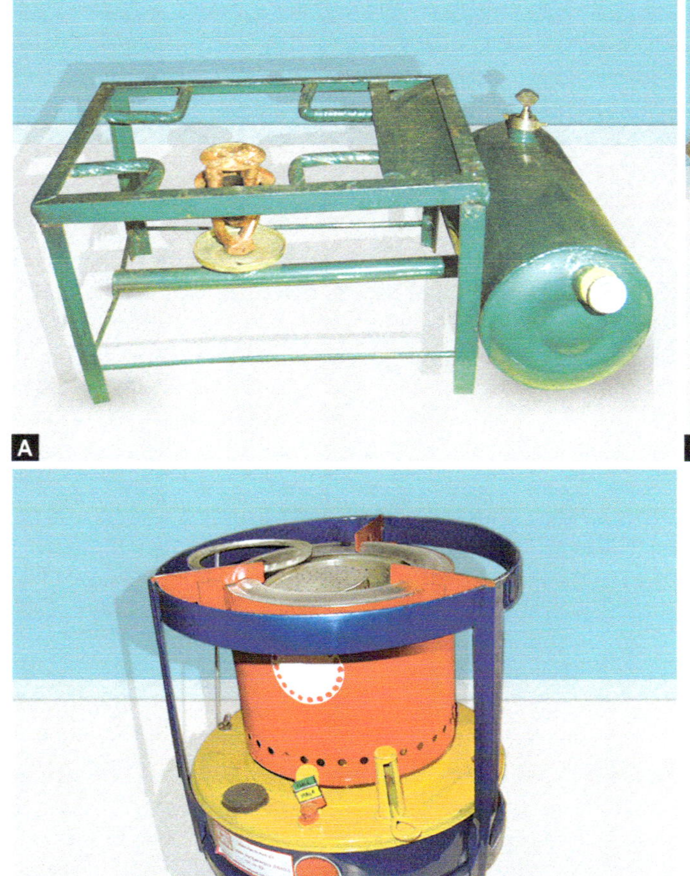

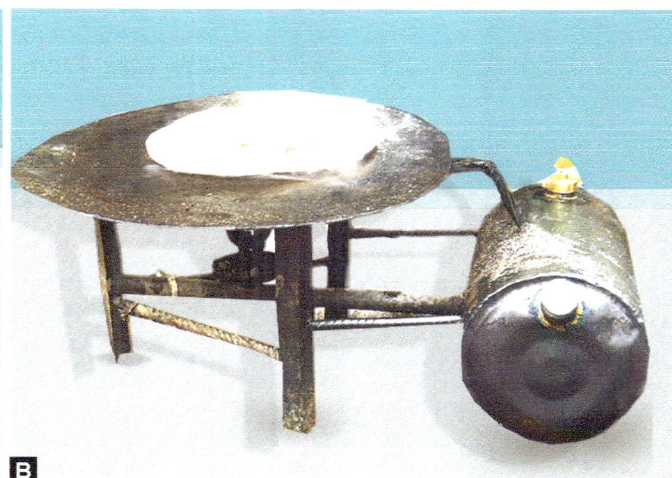

FIGS. 2A TO C: (A) Kerosene pump stove. (B) Kerosene pump stove in action—it is a pressure stove in which continuous pumping aerosolizes the kerosene. If the burner holes are choked and suddenly open up by vigorous pumping of the stove, there is a release of large volume of kerosene aerosol which ignites into a fireball when the stove burner is lit. This is wrongly labeled as "stove burst". (C) Kerosene "wick" stove—safer than pump stove.

This event is frequently labeled as "stove burst". A safer version of the kerosene stove is "wick" stove which works by capillary action **(Fig. 2C)**. Another frequent mishap in kitchen is liquid petroleum gas (LPG) leak. The leak can be from a cracked tubing, faulty regulator, or from an unignited burner. The LPG gas, being heavier than air, does not diffuse out of the ventilators and instead gets settled over the floor. In the event of an ignition, be it lighting of the burner or even switching on of the electric light or exhaust fan, the expressed gas bursts into flames. Although LPG stoves are labeled as safer appliances than kerosene pump stoves, LPG mishaps generally involve a larger number of casualties compared to the latter where only the operator gets burnt **(Fig. 3)**. In addition to the inherent unsafe nature of these devices, lack of basic safety consciousness is also to be blamed in these accidents. A frequent practice among the underprivileged class is floor level cooking. The loose-fitting clothes of the housewife catch fire when she stands up near the stove to pick up something from the overhead kitchen shelves. Another frequent cause of domestic fire accidents is home-made kerosene oil lamps to lighten the house in absence of electricity. These are kept on overhead locations, get tripped by domestic pets, igniting the spilled kerosene oil on unsuspecting victims below.

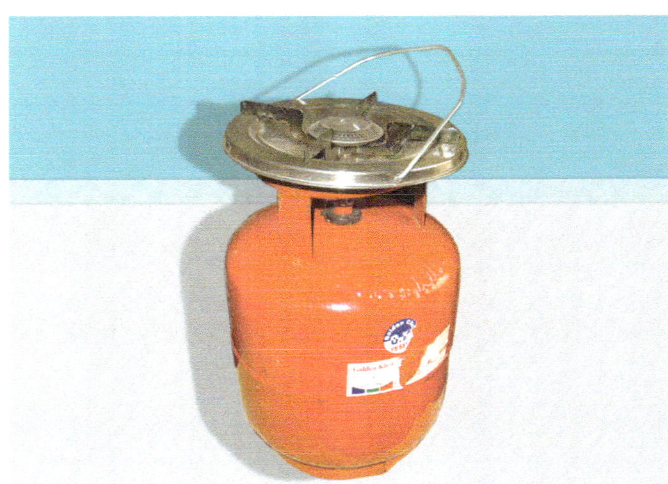

FIG. 3: Liquid petroleum gas (LPG) stove.

Homicidal burns account for about 10% of all flame burns.[1] The common mode of this aggression is to douse the victim with kerosene and then set on fire. This frequently results in extensive and deep burns as the victim is generally restrained. Suicidal burns, around 5% of all flame burns, frequently involve kerosene/petrol doused over the body by the individual herself/himself in a fit of anger and then set on fire.[1]

Flame burns on the whole are more frequent in the age group of 16–55 years. Also, there is a definite female predominance among flame burns which is more so in the productive age group of 16–35 years. This is obvious as traditionally females are engaged in the unsafe kitchens. Homicidal and suicidal burns are also more frequent among females.

Scald Burns

Scalds or burns due to hot liquids account for >50% of all burn admission in the developed world **(Fig. 4)**.[2] In contrast scalds constitute only 15% of all burn admissions in India.[1] In both scenario, scalds are more frequent in children. In the developed world, the incidence of flame burns is far less compared to the developing countries because of better safety features in the kitchens.

In contrast, incidence of scalds remains high in the west as children are less protected with working parents in nuclear families. In developing countries, on the other hand, children are relatively better off with nonworking mothers and in joint families. The incidence of scalds peaks around the age group of 3–5 years. This is the time when the child is highly mobile, inquisitive, lacks awareness regarding hazards and devoid of experiences to cope up with them. Most of the accidents take place when the child is unattended, or parents are momentarily distracted or engaged with hot liquid with the child in their arms. The extent of scald burns depends on the temperature, volume and density of the liquid, age of the child, and the absorbing ability of the garment. A small amount of boiling water causes a higher percentage of age TBSA burn in a small child compared to an adult. Also, hot water absorbed by the clothes worn spreads and involves a larger area and causes deeper burns as the exposure time is longer. The sticky sugar syrup, oil or "*ghee*" and thick gravy cause deeper burns as they can be extremely hot and stick to the skin. Due to their thin skin, children suffer from full thickness scald burns more frequently than adults. The most common circumstances of scalds in developed world are during bath followed by kettle. On the contrary, Indian children get scalded while the mother is handling hot food or water with child in her lap or around her. Children also get burnt when they "reach and pull" containers of hot liquid kept on tables. They either pull tablecloth or the container itself. If the container falls over the child, face and upper trunk get burnt. If the liquid splashes on the floor, the legs get burnt. The sitting child gets perineal and thigh burns if it falls on his/her lap. A toddler sometimes tumbles into a large hot liquid container suffering from 100% burn injuries. Overall, the boys get scald injuries more frequently as compared to female children. Although most scalds are accidental, a small definite percentage has been attributed to child abuse in the west. Such cases are a rarity in India. Thermal burns in adults are also mostly accidental. The accidents occur, while preparing tea or gravy or boiling milk and from spillage from hot water bottle. Steam burns are caused by faulty pressure cookers and on forcibly opening car radiators. Scalds and steam burns are also seen in boiler rooms of factories, ships, and steam locomotives. Steam having a high latent heat causes severe burns and can cause upper airway edema on inhalation.

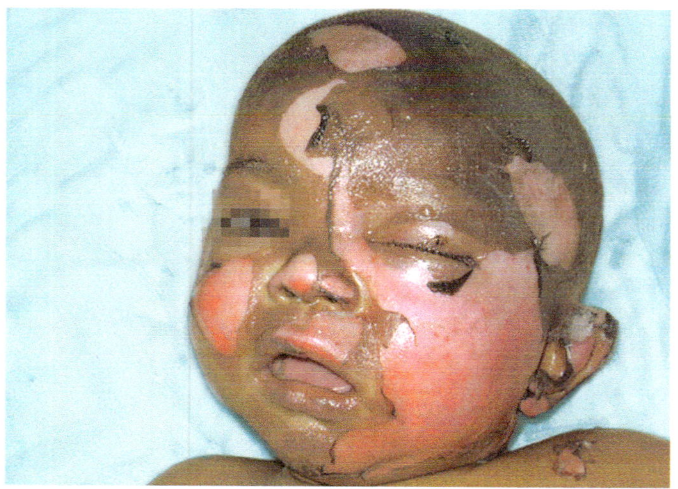

FIG. 4: Scalds over face of an infant due to accidental spilling of hot tea.

Thermal Contact Burn

Thermal contact burns are caused by touching hot objects. Unlike flame and scald burns the injury is always localized to the area of contact. Depending on the temperature and duration of contact the burns can be very deep. In domestic settings, contact thermal burn is caused by touching hot utensils, room heating coils, light bulbs, bike silencers, etc. Contact burns are frequently seen in epileptics who fall on stoves or hot objects during an attack. Due to postictal unconsciousness, the prolonged contact may lead to very deep burns up to bone. Contact burn injuries are also seen in insensate hands and feet. Contact thermal burns in factories are caused by hot machine parts, molten metals, and coal tar. These burns are also seen in case of torture and commonly used modalities are hot metals, cigarette butts, etc.

Blast Injury

Other than warfare, blast burns happen in abundance during Diwali and other festive occasions. The ill-defined legalities regarding sale and use of firecrackers and lack of safety consciousness among people, explain the high incidence of such injuries. Most of the victims are males and are in the age group of 10–25 years. The victims are mostly foolhardy "bravehearts" or unsupervised children. Although the firework operator is more frequently injured, about 15% of the victims are bystanders. Most incriminating firecrackers are *"bomb", "anar",* and igniting of collected firework powder accounting for > 60% of cases.[3] The injuries are sustained whenever the explosion is either delayed or earlier than expected. Hands and the face are mostly affected. A "bomb" or an *"anar"* exploding in the hand causes extensive damage and disruption and even loss of digits. An explosion on the face of an inquisitive child stooping over a lighted cracker not only involves the face but also damages the eyes. The ocular injury can range from reactive conjunctivitis, corneal abrasion, and perforations. Misdirected rockets accounting over 10% of cases always affect unsuspecting bystanders who get burnt when their clothes catch fire. Firecrackers like *"phooljhari"* and *"zameen chakri"* account for minority of injuries which are purely thermal burns **(Fig. 5)**.[3]

In addition to the scattered cases, mass burn casualties due to fire in firecracker factories, storage depots, and markets are also reported during Diwali. Adjoining residential buildings and parked motor vehicles may also come in range of these fires.

Electrical Burn

Electrical burns account for only 5% of the burn cases but are generally extremely devastating.[4] Majority of the cases are males and are in the age group of 10–30 years. Electrical injury is broadly divided into low- and high-tension injury, the demarcating voltage being 1,000 volts.[4] The injury is also classified as flash or contact burn depending on the mode of injury **(Figs. 6A and B)**. Flash burn mimics thermal burn and contact burn is manifested by deeper tissue destruction. The low-tension injury is

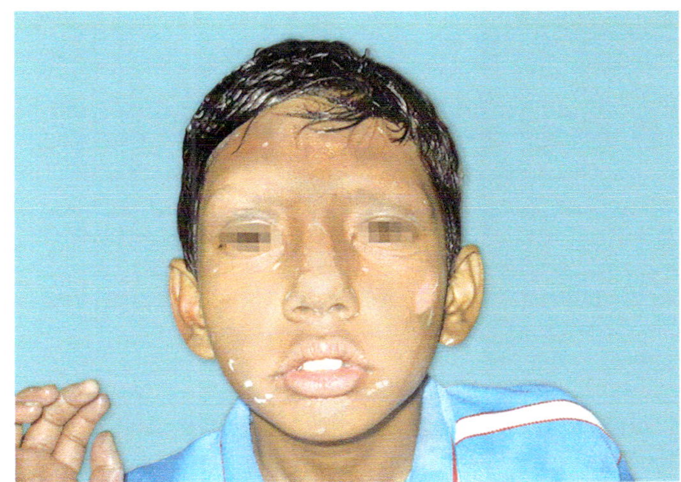

FIG. 5: Firecracker injury causing thermal burns of face.

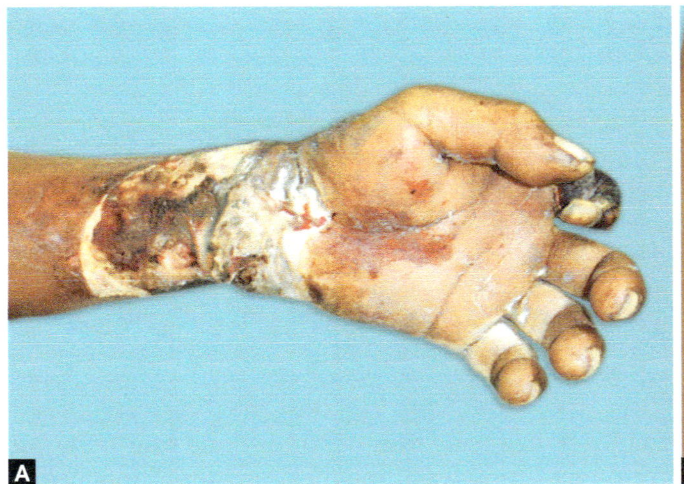

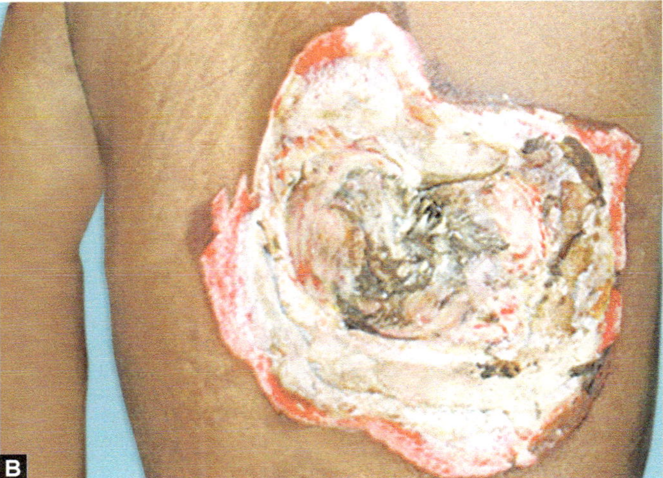

FIGS. 6A AND B: (A) Electrical contact burn to hand and wrist. (B) Electrical contact burn due to contact with high-tension wire on back of trunk.

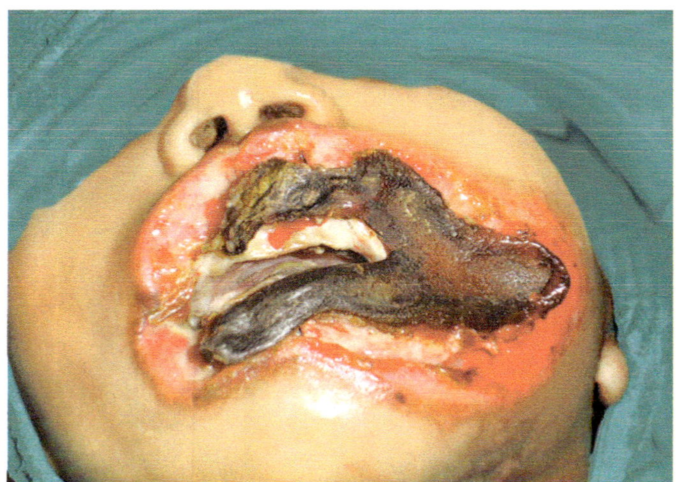

FIG. 7: A child with loss of tissues of face due to electrical contact burn by chewing of electrical wire in mouth.

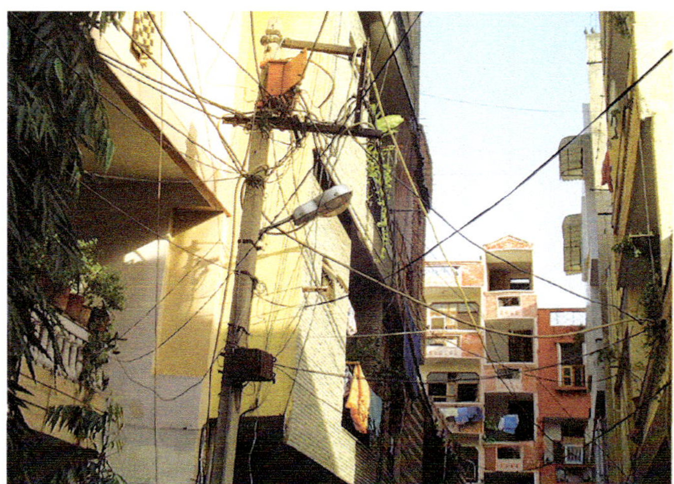

FIG. 8: Unauthorized residential areas near electrical pole with wires running close to the balcony of the houses.

generally seen in domestic settings and is characterized by flash burn on the surface with varying degrees of deeper tissue destruction depending on the site and duration of contact. Such mishaps happen with unprofessional handling and repairing of meter boxes, switchboards and domestic electrical appliances. Although most victims are young males, children get electric burn when they try to mouth or handle a livewire or poke finger in a plug socket **(Fig. 7)**.

High-tension burns are commonly seen in linemen working on high-tension wires and in factory settings. Such injuries are also seen in cases of attempted illegal tapping of electricity from high-tension wires. These cases are on the rise due to mushrooming of unauthorized dwellings near high-tension cables **(Fig. 8)**. Construction workers in these areas are also frequent victims. High-tension injury has also been reported from fallen live cables lying in agricultural fields and from passengers traveling on roof top of electrified trains. Young children are known to get injured while flying kites, when the thread comes in contact with high-voltage electric lines. This is more common in rainy season **(Fig. 9)**.[5]

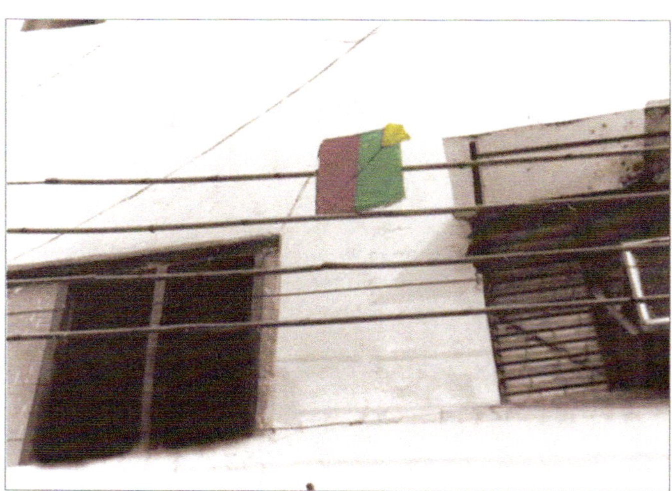

FIG. 9: Kite entangled in electric wires—common cause of electrical injury in children during kite flying.

Chemical Burn

Chemical burn is nonimmunological destruction of the skin due to acute exposure to hazardous chemicals. Unlike other forms of burn, there is extensive and deeper damage owing to prolonged exposure and continuous reaction of the chemical with tissues. More than 25,000 chemicals are known to cause chemical burns and they are broadly classified according to their chemical nature **(Table 1)**.[6] Chemical burns are reported in industrial accidents, civilian mishaps, and chemical warfare. The chemicals involved in civilian injuries are acids (40%), inorganic products (30%), alkalis (20%), and organic products (10%).[1] During warfare, the most common chemical implicated is phosphorus followed poisonous gases like phosgene and dimethyl sulfoxide (DMSO). Hence, the incidence and pattern of chemical burn varies with countries, societies, and situation. Overall incidence of chemical burn is about 2–4% of all burn admissions during peace time. In the industrialized western world, majority are reported as accidents from factories handling hazardous chemicals and the victims being male adults of working age. On the contrary, in developing countries like India most of the chemical burns are of nonindustrial nature. Most of the

TABLE 1: Different types of chemical which can cause burns.

Chemical nature	Agent
Acids	• Hydrochloric acid • Nitric acid • Hydrofluoric acid • Chromic acid • Sulfuric acid
Alkalis	• Sodium hydroxide • Potassium hydroxide • Calcium oxide • Metallic sodium • Metallic potassium • Sodium hypochlorite
Inorganic	• Phosphorus • Cyanide
Organic	• Phenol • Lysol • Cresol

domestic accidents are due to mishandling of household acid cleaners which are frequently stored in discarded mineral water bottles and victims are both adults and children. In addition to homes children also get chemical injury while working in school laboratories. Homicidal vitriolage accounts for a major share of chemical burns in India, while such cases are rare in the west. The majority of victims of this depraved aggression are women who reject the advances or proposals of local goons. The accidental as well as homicidal chemical injuries commonly involve face, upper trunk, and upper extremities. Loss of vision due to ocular damage is also frequently reported **(Fig. 10)**. The agents responsible for chemical injury are listed according to their mechanism of action in **Table 2**.[1,6]

Radiation Burn

Incidence of radiation injury during peace time is far lower than other types of burn. These mishaps are reported from the thermonuclear explosions, nuclear reactor accidents, radiography industries, and X-ray departments. Burn injury from nonionizing radiations like radio and microwaves are rare and minimal as they have minimal tissue penetration. Minor burns are reported with prolonged exposure to microwaves. On the contrary ionizing radiation like γ-rays, X-rays, and high-energy particles like protons penetrates deeply into tissues causing serious burn injuries. There have been around 50 radiation accidents reported till date other than "Three Mile Island" and Chernobyl nuclear reactor mishaps and Hiroshima Nagasaki bombings.[1,7]

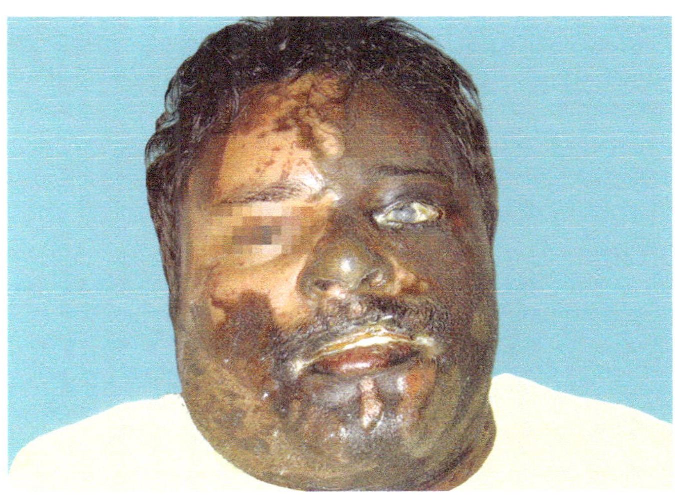

FIG. 10: Chemical burns of face involving eye.

Laser Burns

Laser burns are mostly thermal burns, where the heat created during the employment of the laser for medical purposes—such as hair removal or resurfacing of vascular or pigmented lesions—dissipates into the normal skin and results in skin burns. The amount of energy that the laser releases will determine how much skin damage occurs. Consequently, these can be deep dermal burns, which require a lot of energy to cure, or superficial burns, which are more prevalent. When combustible materials such as dry gauze, alcohol, perfume, nail polish, and oxygen used for anesthesia are present in the operating field, laser-related fires have also been documented. Hence, fire extinguishers should be always available nearby **(Fig. 11)**.

Friction Burns

Burns due to friction are one of the most common nonthermal burns. In majority of the cases, they are associated with mechanical injury, which may be more severe than the burns. Usually, friction causes partial thickness burn in a small body surface area which is ignored. Whenever there is friction between two objects, like between a body part and a machine or tire or road, the relatively delicate object, i.e.. the skin bears the brunt of the mechanical trauma in the form of abrasion, laceration, or avulsion. Hence, most often the burn takes a back seat and the mechanical injury becomes the priority **(Fig. 12)**.

CLASSIFICATION ACCORDING TO BURN DEPTH ESTIMATING BURN DEPTH

In addition to etiological categorization, a burn injury is also classified on the basis of depth. Whereas, etiological classification dwells on the epidemiology,

TABLE 2: Mechanism of action of various chemical agents.

Mechanism of action	Agents	Use	Effect
Oxidation	• Chromic acid • Sodium hypochlorite • Potassium permanganate	• Bleach, chlorinator • Disinfectant	• Corrosive type damage • Does not penetrate deep
Dehydration	• Sulfuric acid • Hydrochloric acid • Oxalic acid	• Toilet cleaner • Toilet cleaner • Rust remover	• Coagulative necrosis by cellular desiccation and exothermic reaction • Dry eschar prevents deep penetration
Denaturation	• Hydrofluoric acid • Tannic acid	• Rust remover • Metal cleaner	Denature and forms salt with vital cell proteins
Corrosion	• Sodium, potassium, and ammonium hydroxide • Phenol	• Drain, Oven cleaner • Paint remover • Disinfectant	• Liquefactive necrosis and saponification by combining with protein and lipids • Soft burn and deep penetration
Vesicant	• Gasoline • Chlorodiethyl sulfide (Mustard gas)	• Fuel • Chemical warfare	• De-fattening properties produce tissue amines and local tissue anoxia • Local irritation, blister, and corrosive damage on prolonged exposure
Self-ignition	• Methyl bromide • White phosphorus • Yellow phosphorus	• Insecticide • Military ammunition • Fire works • Flares	Thermal burn, particles get embedded in skin with blast and cause pain and prolonged damage

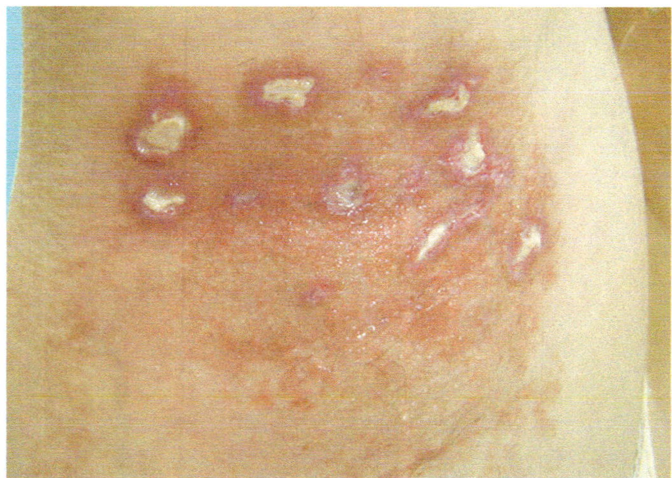

FIG. 11: Laser burns in axilla—laser used for hair removal.

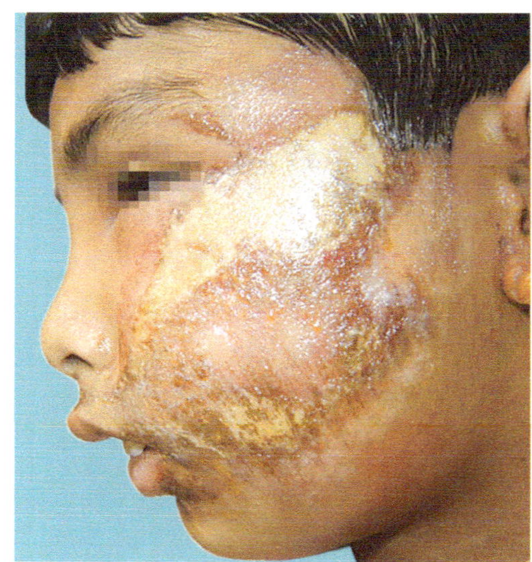

FIG. 12: Friction burns of face in a young boy.

classification based on burn depth is purely prognostic. Burn depth determination and its exact categorization are fundamental in electing a conservative or surgical modality of management. Although the prognostic importance of burn depth was postulated by Jean de Vigo in 1483, Peter Lowe, in 1597, was the first to classify burns into *"superficial, average, and great"*. Fabricus, in 1610, classified burns into three degrees and was first to recognize erythema, vesication, and eschar formation. Later Heister in 1743 and Richter in 1799 recognized four degrees of burn but were highly subjective as pain in addition to erythema eschar formation and vesication. The classical classification of burn depth was propounded by Dupuytren in 1832, which is as follows:

First degree: Erythema without vesication

Second degree: Vesication, loss of epithelium and inflammation

Third degree: Destruction of papillary dermis

Fourth degree: Destruction of whole dermis

Fifth degree: Eschar formation of all superficial parts and muscle

Sixth degree: Carbonization of whole limb

Dupuytren never described the morphology of third- and fourth-degree burns. After years of controversy, a general consensus dawned with the classification of Boyer and Ginnard, in 1855, who categorized burns in three degrees based on erythema, vesication, and eschar formation. Ironically, it was almost identical to the postulation of Fabricus of 1610. This classification is still followed with slight modifications. Snonnenburg and Tschmarke, in 1915, added fourth degree as carbonization which was added to the above classification. In 1944, Converse and Robb-Smith classified burns anatomically and described as "superficial (partial skin loss), deep (total skin loss), and mixed". This system was further refined by Jackson in 1953. He subdivided "partial skin loss" into "superficial skin loss (sup SL) and deep skin loss (deep SL)". He suggested that former heals from hair follicle remnants and latter heals from sweat gland and deep hair follicle remnants.

Burns, in this context, is basically involvement of epidermis and some amount of dermis and purely epidermal burn which is mostly seen in sun burn **(Fig. 13)** is not dealt in this context. The general consensus on classification of burn depth is on the basis of dermal thickness involvement which ranges from partial thickness to full thickness. Burns involving superficial papillary dermis are termed as "superficial partial thickness burn" and those extending into the deeper reticular dermis are called "deep partial thickness burn". To categorize a burn as partial thickness, some amount of dermis must be spared with its viable epidermal elements in hair follicle and glands, facilitating healing by epithelialization. On the contrary, a burn involving the whole of dermis is termed as "full-thickness burn" which needs skin grafting as spontaneous epithelialization is not possible due to the lack of epidermal adnexal elements. A parallel terminology also used in this context is degree of burn. Epidermal burns are termed as "first-degree burn" and as mentioned earlier are not considered in this context. Partial thickness burn is synonymous with second-degree burn and is further subclassified into second-degree superficial dermal and second-degree deep dermal based on the same criteria of involvement of dermal thickness mentioned above.

Full-thickness burns are third-degree burns. The modality of categorizing based on depth is purely clinical and subjective based on the clinical picture of the wound and symptoms. In superficial partial thickness or second-degree burns, vesication is primary feature **(Figs. 14 and 15)**. This is due to subepidermal fluid collection and post deroofing, a bright pink and moist dermis is seen. Such bullae are not seen in deep partial thickness burn as the burnt epidermis and the reticular dermis sticks to the wound and give a waxy white appearance **(Figs. 16A and B)**. In full-thickness burns, the whole devitalized skin is adherent as a parchment like eschar

FIG. 13: Epidermal burn or sunburn.

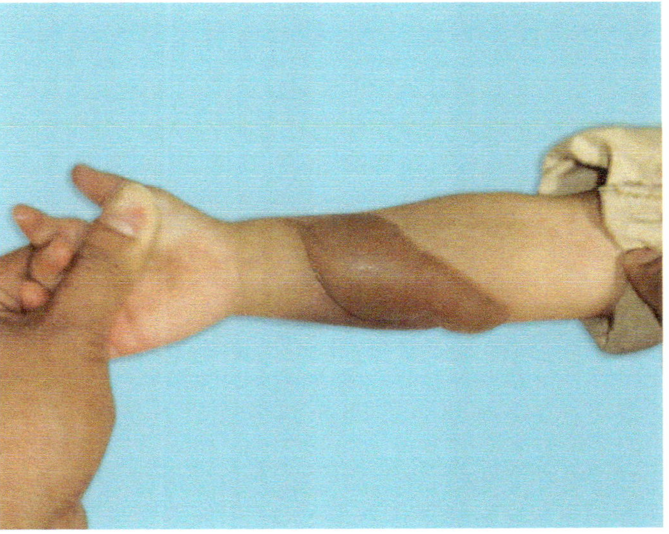

FIG. 14: Superficial partial thickness or superficial dermal burns showing blisters.

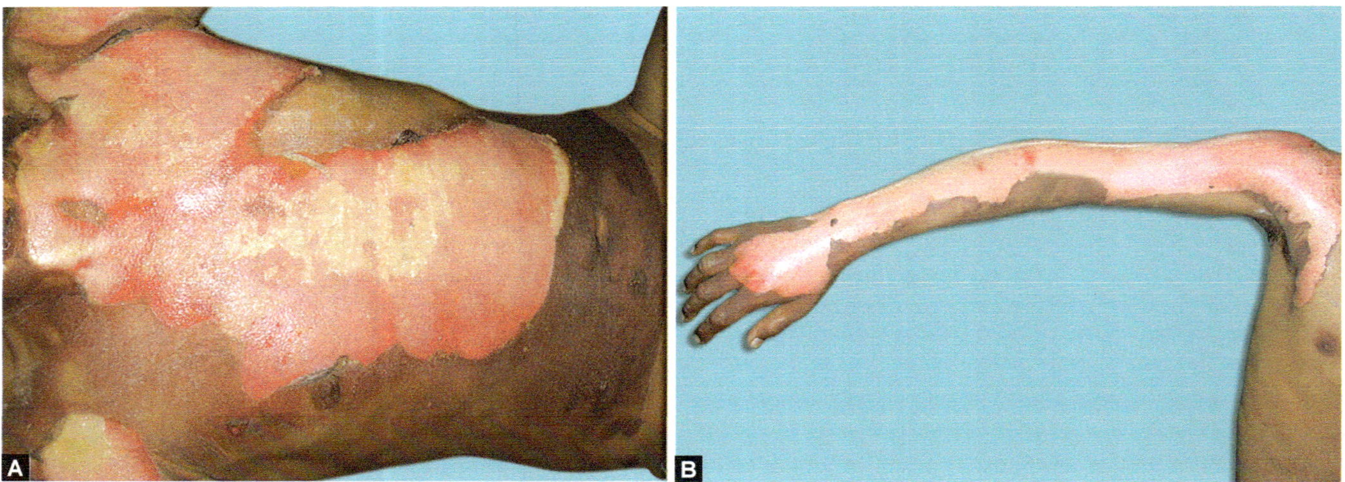

FIGS. 15A AND B: (A) Superficial dermal burns over chest and abdomen after debridement of blisters with moist red look. (B) Superficial dermal burns involving arm after removal of loose dead skin. The areas blanch on pressure with brisk capillary refill.

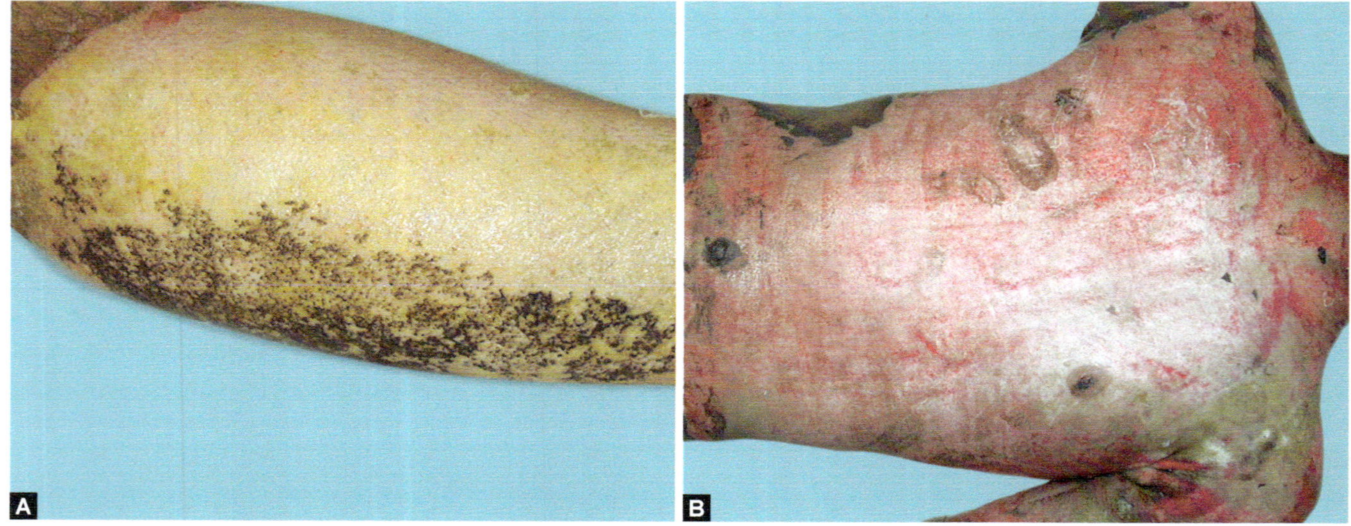

FIGS. 16A AND B: (A) Deep dermal or deep partial thickness burns involving forearm with waxy white look. (B) Deep dermal burns of chest and abdomen with mixed red and white wet look with areas that blanch on pressure but capillary refill is sluggish or absent.

on the wound **(Figs. 17 and 18)** with thrombosed vessels shining through the dead skin **(Fig. 19)**. The depth of burn can also be judged by the involvement of hair follicles. In deeper burns, there is easy pluckability of hair signifying their devitalization. Similarly, pain in the burn wound is inversely proportional to the amount of dermal involvement as nerve endings are destroyed in deeper burns. The pink appearance which blanches on pressure in a superficial burn indicates the rich capillary arborization in the superficial dermis and hence deep partial thickness burns are relatively pale or waxy white and do not blanch on pressure. The blanching test should always be done as a deeper burn can also be fallaciously erythematous due to fixation of erythrocytes leaked out of the destroyed capillaries. Such a picture is frequently seen in children who have thin skin. A subdermal burn damages muscle, bone, and interstitial tissue as is usually seen in electrical contact burns **(Fig. 20)**. They are termed "fourth-degree burns".

A workable classification with interchangeable terms is given in **Table 3**. While using this system, it is prudent to note that burn wound is in a perpetual state of change depending upon tissue perfusion and infection. A wound categorized as superficial dermal on admission, may convert into deep dermal burn because of inadequate fluid resuscitation and wound infection. Hence, repeated and

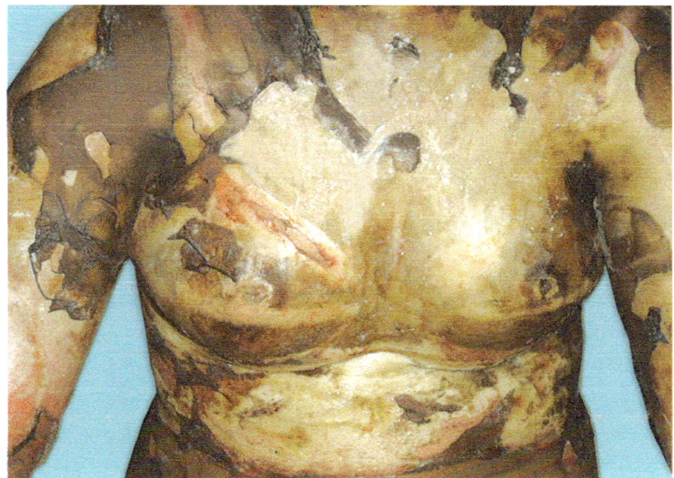

FIG. 17: Deep burns over chest and arms.

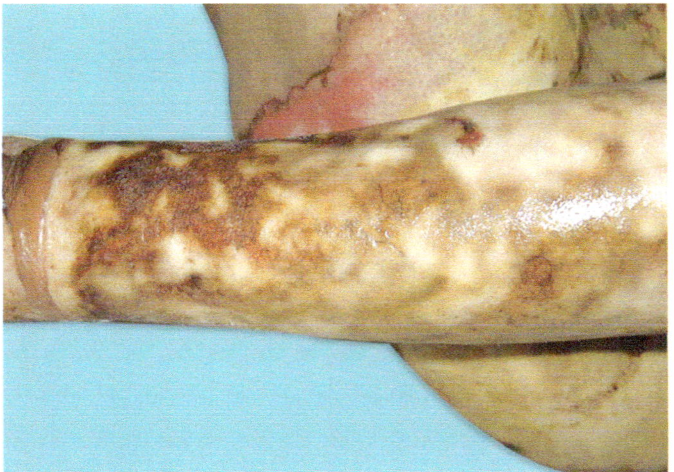

FIG. 18: Deep burns over arm and thighs.

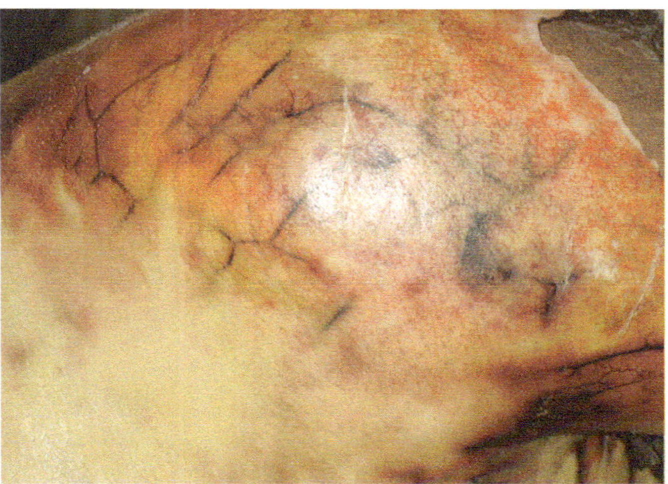

FIG. 19: Deep or full thickness burns over shoulder with dry translucent eschar with thrombosed vessels.

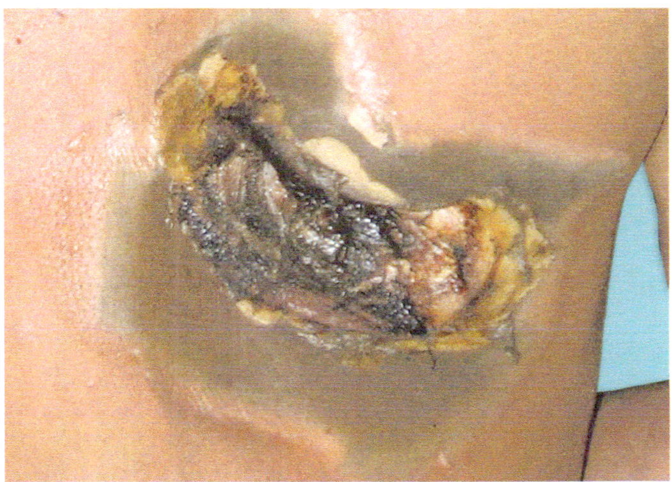

FIG. 20: Deep electrical contact burn involving skin, subcutaneous tissue, muscle, and bone.

TABLE 3: Clinical classification of burns.

Burns	Involvement	Features	Depth
First degree (sun burn)	Epidermis	• Erythema only • Heals in < 5 days	Partial thickness
• Second degree ◦ Superficial dermal or Superficial partial thickness	• Epidermis and papillary dermis	• Extremely painful • Blister formation • Wet, glistening pink • Heals in 10–15 days	• Partial thickness
◦ Deep dermal or deep partial thickness	• Epidermis, papillary dermis and part of reticular dermis	• Less painful, waxy white appearance • Heals in 3–5 weeks	• Partial thickness
Third degree	Entire thickness of skin	• Painless Inelastic, translucent, parchment like eschar with visible thrombosed veins • Require skin grafting	Full thickness
Fourth degree	Skin, subcutaneous tissue, muscle, and carbonization of limb or gangrene	Thick eschar to gangrene	Full thickness

regular assessment is always rewarding diagnostically. The term "eschar" needs to be defined, which is synonymous with third-degree burn. But, the waxy white layer seen in second degree deep dermal or deep partial thickness burn should also be regarded as "soft eschar". This layer is formed by dead papillary and reticular dermis and needs to be excised in tangential excision.

It is obvious that this clinical classification system of burns, based on visual examination, is fraught with subjectivity and high experience requirement. There is an ongoing quest.

ASSESSMENT OF BURN DEPTH

Clinical assessment is the most common technique to assess the depth of a burn wound; however, it is accurate in only 60–75% of the cases, even when carried out by an experienced burn surgeon.[8,9] Numerous attempts using thermographic, infrared and ultraviolet imaging, radioisotope scanning, Doppler laser flux measurement and visual digital imaging have been reported.[10-15] Unfortunately, none have risen out of research journals into user-friendly modality due to economic reasons.

Some people consider punch biopsy of burned tissue followed by histological evaluation to be the gold standard for depth diagnosis, using it as a benchmark to compare various diagnostic techniques.[16,17] A biopsy reveals the structural integrity of cellular and interstitial proteins as well as the patency of dermal vessels; denatured proteins and blocked vasculature are signs of devitalized tissue.[18] There has been contention that whereas collagen denaturation indicates full-thickness, microvascular damage indicates partial-thickness burns.[19] The constraints include tissue shrinking, sampling inaccuracy, and the intrusive nature of the operation.

MEASUREMENT OF TISSUE PERFUSION

Thermography

Thermography relies on measuring the temperature of burn wounds to determine their depth. Thermography can inversely correlate temperature with depth by taking use of the theory that deeper wounds are cooler than more superficial ones due to reduced vascular perfusion at the wound surface.[20] Heat loss by evaporation to the environment introduces systematic inaccuracy into this technique by making wounds appear falsely deep. Additionally, thermography performed within 3 days of the burn injury yields the best findings because accuracy is lost if wounds start to granulate.[21]

Vital dyes and UV light illumination followed by 360–400 nm UV light illumination over the burned area help to visualize depth; however, fluorescein fluorescence cannot distinguish between superficial and deep partial-thickness burns or identify live tissue that is hidden by eschar. This is because fluorescein fluorescence only partially penetrates soft tissue.[22] Renal clearance and capillary leak constrain fluorescein dosage in addition to diagnostic constraints.[23]

Indocyanine Green Video Angiography

Indocyanine green (ICG) video angiography using ICG makes it possible to record dynamic variations in tissue perfusion. Data from ICG video angiography can be used to estimate skin vitality with high sensitivity because tissue necrosis is associated with decreased microcirculation.[24] ICG-video-angiography offers the benefit of being able to correlate structure (coagulated dermal vessels) with function (limited local perfusion), in addition to its diagnostic utility.[25] The primary drawback of ICG video angiography is the way in which blood, bandages, and topical ointments affect the results it generates. Haslik et al. claim that these surface-level materials can significantly overestimate the depth of burn wounds by reducing absorption readings by 63 ± 36%.[26] To prevent this loss of accuracy, current practice standards recommend removing all topical medications from a wound completely at least 10 minutes prior to ICG-video-angiography. Comparing ICG video angiography to other cutting-edge methods for assessing burn depth, its application is restricted due to its high cost and requirement for complex infrastructure.

Laser Doppler Techniques

Based on the Doppler principle, which asserts that mono-frequency light pulses change in frequency when reflected off moving objects, laser Doppler flowmetry and laser Doppler perfusion monitoring (LDPM) are possible. When focused on moving blood cells, laser light will show a frequency shift that is proportionate to the tissue perfusion.[25] Flowmetry can diagnose burn depth with an accuracy of 90–97%, but clinical examination alone can only diagnose burn depth with an accuracy of 66%.[27,28] Doppler probes are painful, necessitate direct touch, and increase the risk of infection and healing time in cases of severe burns. Despite its excellent accuracy, flowmetry is a suboptimal approach because of these technical limitations.

Since laser Doppler imaging (LDI) and laser Doppler perfusion imaging (LDPI) rely on optics, factors such as wound infection, topical medications, heterogeneity and curvature of tissues, and ambient light can all negatively impact depth measurements.[29-31]

The development of new, human-not-yet-proven procedures, cost containment, and additional research on LDI and ICG video angiography will all be critical to the future of depth evaluation in burn wounds. Noncontact ultrasound and optical measurements hold the potential to provide quick, noninvasive diagnostic procedures with low patient morbidity. Conversely, nuclear imaging offers the potential for greater diagnostic precision at the cost of a small amount of morbidity. Clinical trials including human patient populations will be necessary for additional hypothesis confirmation as future animal models better prove the effectiveness of these approaches.

ESTIMATION OF BURN SIZE

The amount of body surface area involved in burns, expressed as a percentage of the total body surface area (%TBSA), is the key to the estimation of fluid requirement to treat shock and is also an important prognostic factor. The extent of burn is estimated by Wallace's Rule of Nine. According to this system head and neck account for 9%, each upper limb and each lower limb constitute 9% and 18%, respectively. The anterior and posterior trunk constitutes 18% each and external genitalia account for 1%. The estimation is different in children owing to the larger proportion of the head. Hence in a child, head and neck account for 18% and the lower limb constitute 13.5% each. Proportion of upper limb and trunk remains same as adult. A more accurate estimation system is the Lund and Browder Chart which can be used for all age groups and also compensates for variable body size and shape **(Table 4)**. Estimation of extent of scattered and irregular areas in all age groups is done by Rule of Palm or Hand. The palm of an individual with fingers and thumb adducted account for 1%.

Rule of Five in Burns[32]

Rule of "five": Lynch and Blocker gave a formula to estimate how badly burnt toddlers are. Anatomic regions are those that make up 5% or its multiples of the surface area of the body. As a result, it functions exceptionally well in newborns, where the head and neck, the front and posterior parts of the trunk each makes 20%, and each limb makes up 10% of the total. As a child gets older, his/her lower limb surface area grows and his/her head and trunk surface areas decrease, therefore this is significantly altered for older kids. apiece upper limb is 10%, the anterior trunk is 20%, and the head, posterior trunk, and lower limbs are 15% each.

TABLE 4: Lund and Browder's chart for estimating area of burns.

Area	Birth to 1 year	1–4 years	5–9 years	10–14 years	15 years	Adult	2nd°	3rd°	TBSA
Head	19	17	13	11	9	7			
Neck	2	2	2	2	2	2			
Anterior trunk	13	13	13	13	13	13			
Posterior trunk	13	13	13	13	13	13			
Right buttock	2.5	2.5	2.5	2.5	2.5	2.5			
Left buttock	2.5	2.5	2.5	2.5	2.5	2.5			
Genitalia	1	1	1	1	1	1			
Right upper arm	4	4	4	4	4	4			
Left upper arm	4	4	4	4	4	4			
Right lower arm	3	3	3	3	3	3			
Left lower arm	3	3	3	3	3	3			
Right hand	2.5	2.5	2.5	2.5	2.5	2.5			
Left hand	2.5	2.5	2.5	2.5	2.5	2.5			
Right thigh	5.5	6.5	8	8.5	9	9.5			
Left thigh	5.5	6.5	8	8.5	9	9.5			
Right leg	5	5	5.5	6	6.5	7			
Left leg	5	5	5.5	6	6.5	7			
Right foot	3.5	3.5	3.5	3.5	3.5	3.5			
Left foot	3.5	3.5	3.5	3.5	3.5	3.5			
Total	**100**	**100**	**100**	**100**	**100**	**100**			

(TBSA: total body surface area)

Estimation of Burns in Amputees

When measuring TBSA in amputees, the current formulae are imprecise, which results in imprecise fluid estimation in certain situations. Chauhan et al.[33] have developed a novel technique that incorporates a "correction factor (CF)" to account for the amputated parts when estimating TBSA burns in patients who have undergone significant amputations. The idea was that in an amputee, the body surface areas that were not burned should be assigned a percentage corresponding to their residual body surface area, which should be regarded as 100%. Depending on the degree of amputation, the authors created a straightforward and fast-calculating approach that may be utilized in an emergency and involves a CF. This is how the adjustment factor is computed:

Percent TBSA in an amputee = % TBSA calculated with existing system × CF

Where "CF" is the correction factor = 100/(100 – % loss of body part due to amputation).

The details of the calculation are illustrated in the following hypothetical example:

A 60 kg male with bilateral forequarter amputation presents with burns to anterior trunk.

Based on the Lund and Browder chart, the percentage of TBSA in each upper limb is 9.5%. Thus, 81% of the TBSA remains in a bilateral forequarter amputee. For this patient, the remaining body surface area should be regarded as 100% TBSA.

The CF is calculated as below:
CF = 100/(100 – % of lost body part)
CF = 100/(100 – 19)
CF = 100/81 = 1.23

According to Lund and Browder chart, anterior trunk TBSA burnt is 13%. According to our suggested calculation, his anterior trunk would make 13 × 1.23 = 16% of the TBSA. Hence, this patient should be treated as 16% TBSA burn, and the fluid, calories, and protein requirement must be calculated accordingly. The method has been named by the authors as the "Safdarjung method" of TBSA estimation in major amputees, as it was conceived by the authors while working at this hospital.

CLASSIFICATION ACCORDING TO SEVERITY OF BURNS (TABLE 5)

The severity categorization of burn is done by taking into consideration extent and depth. This classification is useful for establishing admission criteria and is indispensable in triaging in event of a fire disaster. The categorization is as follows.

TABLE 5: Classification of burns as per their severity.

Grade	Criteria
Critical burns	• Partial thickness burns > 25% total body surface area (TBSA) • Full thickness burns > 10% • Burns of special sites like hands, face, and perineum • Burns with associated injury or any preexisting illness and old age • Electrical burns • Burns complicated by respiratory tract involvement
Moderate burns	• Partial thickness burns 15–25% TBSA • Full thickness burns 1–3% TBSA
Minor burns	Partial thickness burns < 10–15% TBSA

Critical Burn

- Partial thickness burn > 25% TBSA in adult, > 15% TBSA in children, and > 5% TBSA in infants.
- Full thickness burn > 10% TBSA in adults and > 3% TBSA in children and infants.
- Burns of hand, face, and perineum
- Burns with associated head injury, thoracic or abdominal trauma, old age, and preexisting systemic illness
- Burns with associated inhalation injury
- Electrical burn

Moderate Burns

- Partial thickness burn 15–25% TBSA in adults and 10–15% TBSA in children and infants.
- Full thickness burn 3–10% TBSA in adults and 1–3% TBSA in children and infants.

Minor Burns

- Partial thickness burn < 15% TBSA burn in adults and < 10% TBSA in children and infants.
- Full thickness burn < 3% TBSA in adults and up to 1% TBSA in children and infants.

Grading of Burns

A further refinement to this system was propounded by Kumar (1993) by including the percentage of deep burn as an additional criterion **(Table 6)**.[34] He included deep partial thickness and full thickness burn as "deep" burn and estimated "burn depth index (DI)" by calculating the fraction of "deep" burn out of the total extent of burn.

TABLE 6: Prognostic grading of burns as per their severity.

Grade	Criteria
I Minor burn	• Erythema ○ <15% TBSA (<0.5 DI) ○ <15% TBSA (>0.5 DI)
II Moderate burn	• 15–30% TBSA (<0.5 DI) • 15–30% TBSA (>0.5 DI)
III Major burn	• 30–65% TBSA (<0.5 DI) • 30–65% TBSA (>0.5 DI) • >65% TBSA (<0.5 DI) • >65% TBSA (>0.5 DI) • Burns of hands, face, and perineum • Electrical burns • Associated injury • Head injury, fracture • Chest and abdominal injury • Pre-existing illness and old age • Inhalation injury

(TBSA: total body surface area; DI: depth index of burns)

$$\text{Depth index (DI) of burn} = \frac{\text{Total \% of deep burn}}{\text{Total \% total body surface area (TBSA) burn}}$$

A severity and prognostic grading taking into consideration the extent, depth and DI is given in **Table 6**. Unlike the previous grading this system helps to determine the prognosis, quantum of deformity, and the need for skin grafting.

Although the basic purpose of these classifications is to guide the treatment modality, but most often burns are still categorized simply as superficial and deep where early excisional surgery is not routinely practiced.

A knowledge of the etiology and mode of burn injury is important for devising preventive strategies whereas classification based on extent and depth guides management protocol and determines prognosis.

FACTORS AFFECTING PROGNOSTIC GRADING OF BURNS

The main factors include age, burn surface area involved, burn depth, and inhalational injury.

Baux Score[35]

System used to predict the chance of mortality due to burns.

Original Method

The score is expressed as:

Baux score = (% of body surface burned) + (patient's age)

The score is a comparative indicator of burn severity, with a score over 140 considered as being unsurvivable, depending on the available treatment resources.

Modified Method

It took into account the effect of inhalation injury. It was found that inhalation injury resulted in an increase of around 17 on the Baux score.

Modified Baux score = (% of body surface burned) + (patient's age) + 17

Recent analysis of mortality in burn units worldwide has shown that for well performing units the lethal dose 50 (LD50) for major burns has significantly improved and the best units have a modified Baux score of 130–140. This means that all burns in children (except 100% TBSA full-thickness burns) should be considered survivable injuries and actively treated. The Baux score has been shown to be effective in predicting outcomes in 87% of presenting patients aged 60 years and above.[36]

Burn Index and Prognostic Burn Index

The prognostic burn index (PBI = BI + age) and the burn index (BI, burn area of full skin thickness + 0.5 remaining burn area) are the two indices that the Japanese Society for Burn Injuries have recommended. The limited availability of original papers and clinical validation of indices resulting from small group studies published in Chinese and Japanese are linked to the assessment's lack of wider acknowledgment in international recommendations.[37,38] Both indicators were assessed in a cohort of 17,185 Japanese patients in 2015. It was discovered that there was a significant correlation between the PBI and mortality, with the link being strongest for values >85.[39]

Lethal Dose 50

Lethal dose 50, burn size with a lethality of 50% of patients. It is also called "lethal area 50 (LA50)" and reflects the quality of the resuscitation process and medical burn care.[40] It has been used as an indicator of the quality of burn care. So, it can be compared between different time periods to estimate how the quality of medical care has changed. It can be compared between various centers too. In the 1940s, LA50 in the United States has been reported as 40%,[41] and increased to approximately 60% in the 1970s.[42] Between 1991 and 1993 in 28 burn centers, the LA50 for young adults was 81% TBSA[43] and currently is about 90%.[42] LA50 for developing countries is lower than this.[44] Advanced age, female gender, inhalational injury, and burn extension determined by TBSA% were significantly associated with higher mortality. There was a significant difference in LA50 between patients with inhalation injury and those without. Inhalation injury results in severe lung-induced morbidity and mortality. The aim at present is to improve the LA50 in the developing countries also which will reflect the improvement in burn care standards in these countries.

SUMMARY

Burns are classified on the basis of etiology, depth and percentage of body surface area involved. Classification based on burn depth is purely prognostic. The amount of dermal thickness involvement and the viable epidermal elements in hair follicle and glands determine the healing process. Various methods to assess the burn depth include thermography, indocyanine green video angiography and laser doppler techniques. These techniques are based on measurement of tissue perfusion. The amount of body surface area involved in burns (% TBSA), is the key to the estimation of fluid requirement to treat shock and is also an important prognostic factor. Severity categorization of burn is done by taking into consideration extent and depth and burns and classified as critical, major and minor burns. This classification is useful for establishing admission criteria and is indispensable in triaging in event of a fire disaster. There are various methods to determine the prognosis in burns. These include Baux score, Burn index, prognostic burn index and LD50. Classification of burns is therefore the first step toward successful management of burns .

REFERENCES

1. Ahuja RB, Bhattacharya S. An analysis of 11,196 burn admissions and evaluation of conservative management techniques. Burns. 2002; 28:555-61.
2. Settle JAD. Principles and Practice of Burns Management. New York: Churchill Livingstone; 1996.
3. Mehta DR, Suri MP, Patel CK, Agrawal AB, Vora HJ, Raibagkar SC. Fireworks Injuries—Epidemiology & Prevention. Indian J Burns. 2004;12:48-50.
4. Bajaj SP, Tah R, Kohli JS. An overview of Electrical Burn. Indian J Burn. 1998;6:10-7.
5. Bajaj SP, Tiwari VK, Kohli JS, Pande S. Profile of Electrical Burn Admitted in Burn Unit of Safdarjung Hospital. Indian J Burn. 1998;6:31-4.
6. Bit UK, Sinha PK, Chowdhudary SR. Chemical Burn. Indian J Burns. 1994;2:18-23.
7. Narayan RP. Radiation Burn. Indian J Burn. 2003;11:32-3.
8. Monstrey S, Hoeksema H, Verbelen J, Pirayesh A, Blondeel P. Assessment of burn depth and burn wound healing potential. Burns. 2008;34:761-9.
9. Serrano C, Boloix-Tortosa R, Gómez-Cía T, Acha B. Features identification for automatic burn classification. Burns. 2015;41: 1883-90.
10. Cole RP, Jones SG, Shakespeare PG. Thermographic assessment of hand burns. Burns. 1990;16:60-3.
11. Wyllie FJ, Sutherland AB. Measurement of surface temperature as an aid to the diagnosis of burn depth. Burns. 1991;17:123-7.
12. Barsley RE, West MH, Jair JA. Forensic photography ultraviolet imaging of wounds on skin. Am J Forensic Med Pathol. 1990;11:300-8.
13. Bennett JE, Kingman RO. Evaluation of burn depth by use of radioactive isotopes—An experimental study. Plastic Reconstr Surg. 1957;20:261-72.
14. Niazi ZBN, Callis JB, Heimbach DM. New laser Doppler scanner, a valuable adjunct in burn depth assessment. Burns. 1993;19: 485-9.
15. Carmen S, Begona A, Gomez-Cia T, Acha JI, Roa LA. A computer assisted diagnostic tool for the classification of burns by depth of injury. Burns. 2005;31:275-81.
16. Heimbach D, Engrav L, Grube B, Marvin J. Burn depth: a review. World J Surg. 1992;16:10-5.
17. Pape SA, Skouras CA, Byrne PO. An audit of the use of laser Doppler imaging (LDI) in the assessment of burns of intermediate depth. Burns. 2001;27:233-9.
18. Watts AM, Tyler MP, Perry ME, Roberts AH, McGrouther DA. Burn depth and its histological measurement. Burns. 2001;27: 154-60.
19. Chvapil M, Speer DP, Owen JA, Chvapil TA. Identification of the depth of burn injury by collagen stainability. Plast Reconstr Surg. 1984;73:438-41.
20. Lawson RN, Gaston JP. Temperature measurements of localized pathological processes. Ann N Y Acad Sci. 1964;121:90-8.
21. Liddington MI, Shakespeare PG. Timing of the thermographic assessment of burns. Burns. 1996;22:26-8.
22. Atiyeh BS, Gunn SW, Hayek SN. State of the art in burn treatment. World J Surg. 2005;29:131-48.
23. Still JM, Law EJ, Klavuhn KG, Island TC, Holtz JZ. Diagnosis of burn depth using laser-induced indocyanine green fluorescence: a preliminary clinical trial. Burns. 2001;27:364-71.
24. Kamolz LP, Andel H, Haslik W, Donner A, Winter W, Meissl G, et al. Indocyanine green video angiographies help to identify burns requiring operation. Burns. 2003;29:785-91.
25. Essex TJH, Byrne PO. A laser Doppler scanner for imaging blood flow in skin. J Biomed Eng. 1991;13:189-94.
26. Haslik W, Kamolz LP, Andel H, Winter W, Meissl G, Frey M. The influence of dressings and ointments on the qualitative and quantitative evaluation of burn wounds by ICG video-angiography: an experimental setup. Burns. 2004;30:232-5.
27. Park DH, Hwang JW, Jang KS, Han DG, Ahn KY, Baik BS. Use of laser Doppler flowmetry for estimation of the depth of burns. Plast Reconstr Surg. 1998;101:1516-23.

28. Holland AJ, Martin HC, Cass DT. Laser Doppler imaging prediction of burn wound outcome in children. Burns. 2002;28:11-7.
29. Jeng JC, Bridgeman A, Shivnan L, Thornton PM, Alam H, Clarke TJ, et al. Laser Doppler imaging determines need for excision and grafting in advance of clinical judgment: a prospective blinded trial. Burns. 2003;29:665-70.
30. Droog EJ, Steenbergen W, Sjoberg F. Measurement of depth of burns by laser Doppler perfusion imaging. Burns. 2001;27:561-8.
31. Anselmo VJ, Zawacki BE. Multispectral photographic analysis. A new quantitative tool to assist in the early diagnosis of thermal burn depth. Ann Biomed Eng. 1977;5:179-93.
32. Lynch JB, Blocker V. The rule of five in estimation of extent of burn. In: Converse JM (Ed). Reconstructive plastic surgery, 1st edition. Philadelphia, New York: WB Saunders Co.; 1964. p. 208.
33. Chauhan N, Agrawal K, Kumar S. The "Safdarjung Method" of Estimation of Total Body Surface Area (TBSA) Burns in Major Amputees. Indian J Plast Surg. 2020;53(2):303-5.
34. Kumar P. Burn depth index and classification of burn casualties. Burns. 1993;19:252.
35. Osler T, Glance LG, Hosmer DW. Simplified estimates of the probability of death after burn injuries: Extending and updating the baux score. J Trauma. 2010;68(3):690-7.
36. Wibbenmeyer L, Amelon MJ, Morgan LJ, Robinson BK, Chang PX, Lewis r, 2nd; et al. Predicting survival in an elderly burn patient population. Burns. 2001;27(6):583-90.
37. Chien-Hua C, Hsu M, Yeh F, Jin-Teh L, Chih-Huang H, Rong-Hwuang F. The effects of burn size, age, inhalation injury and burn depth on the mortality of major burn patients. J Reconstr Plast Surg Assoc Repub China. 1998;7:111-8.
38. Yasuda K, Henmi H, Yamamoto Y, Mashiko K, Ohtomo Y, Ohtsuka T. Nutritional management and assessment on extensively burned patients. Jpn J Burn Inj. 2019;11:134-8.
39. Tagami T, Matsui H, Fushimi K, Yasunaga H. Validation of the prognostic burn index: a nationwide retrospective study. Burns. 2015;41:1169-75.
40. Jie X, Qingyan M, Zheng WY. Comparable results between standardization methods and regression analysis in predicting mortality rate among samples with burns. Burns. 2003;29(3): 247-55.
41. Saffle JR. Predicting outcomes of burns. N Engl J Med. 1998;338(6):387-8.
42. Kasten KR, Makley AT, Kagan RJ. Update on the critical care management of severe burns. J Intens Care Med. 2011;26(4): 223-36.
43. Saffle JR, Davis B, Williams P. Recent outcomes in the treatment of burn injury in the United States: a report from the American Burn Association Patient Registry. J Burn Care Rehabil. 1995;16 (3 Pt 1):219-32.
44. Khashaba HA, Al-Fadhli AN, Al-Tarrah KS, Wilson YT, Moiemen N. Epidemiology and outcome of burns at the Saud Al Babtain Burns, Plastic Surgery and Reconstructive Center, Kuwait: our experience over five years (from 2006 to 2010). Ann Burns Fire Disast. 2012;25(4):178-87.

CHAPTER

4

Pathophysiology of Burn Shock

Arvind Vartak, Suhas V Abhyankar

INTRODUCTION

Burn is the most common form of injury that afflicts human beings. An extensive burn is the severest form of trauma. Burn injury is the most painful of all injuries and the most complicated to treat, most expensive to manage. It leaves behind permanent memories, both physical and psychological. Over the last several decades, a better understanding of physiological changes which occur following a burn injury has led to great improvements in treatment. This has significantly improved the results by reducing the morbidity and mortality.

Following a severe burn, the patient passes into a state of shock.[1] The success in adequate management of shock can be achieved with anticipation, recognition, and suitable treatment of shock. Hypovolemic shock is a disparity between the circulating blood volume and the capacity of the vascular tree (the intravascular compartment). Neurogenic shock appears as a state of profound mental and physical depression consequent to severe physical injury and/or an emotional disturbance (Stedman's 1976).[2] In case of burn injury, this may be a result of intense pain associated with emotional disturbance immediately after the burn injury. It is characterized by pallor, dizziness, restlessness, and rarely unconsciousness. This state passes off spontaneously and usually is not noticed by the time the patient reaches a burn care facility. It does not need any specific treatment.

PATHOPHYSIOLOGICAL CHANGES FOLLOWING BURNS

Acute burn injury causes a cascade of events due to the release of damage-associated molecular patterns (DAMPs) and pathogen-associated molecular patterns (PAMPs) which in turn causes:

- Hypovolemic shock and vascular leak
- Immune and inflammatory responses
- Metabolic changes **(Flowchart 1)**

Hypovolemic shock and vascular leak are responsible for tissue edema, tissue injury, risk of bacterial infection, and increase in burn depth and severity.

Immune and inflammatory responses affect monocytes, T cells, macrophages, and neutrophils. Monocytes cause an increase in interleukin 6 (IL-6), IL-10, tumor necrosis factor (TNF), and prostaglandin E (PGE) levels; they decrease class II major histocompatibility complex (MHC) expression and also decrease antigen presentation. T cells are responsible for increased levels of IL-4 and IL-10 and decreased levels of IL-2 interferon-gamma (IFN-γ) and decreased proliferation. Macrophages cause decrease in phagocytosis and bacterial activity. Neutrophils also show a similar effect.

Metabolic changes occurring in the body due to burn injury will show an effect on catabolism, insulin resistance, muscle protein degradation, and lipolysis resulting in hypermetabolism. Hypermetabolism is also responsible for immunosuppression. Severe immunosuppression and bacterial multiplication result in systemic inflammatory response syndrome (SIRS) and/or sepsis leading to multiorgan dysfunction initially, and if not treated at this stage, it may lead to multiorgan failure and death.

Hypovolemic shock appears as a result of loss of liquid component of the blood (plasma) into the tissues leading to edema formation in surrounding tissues. After burn injury, there is an immediate transient decrease in the blood flow in the involved tissues. This is followed by pronounced arterial vasodilatation in the patent

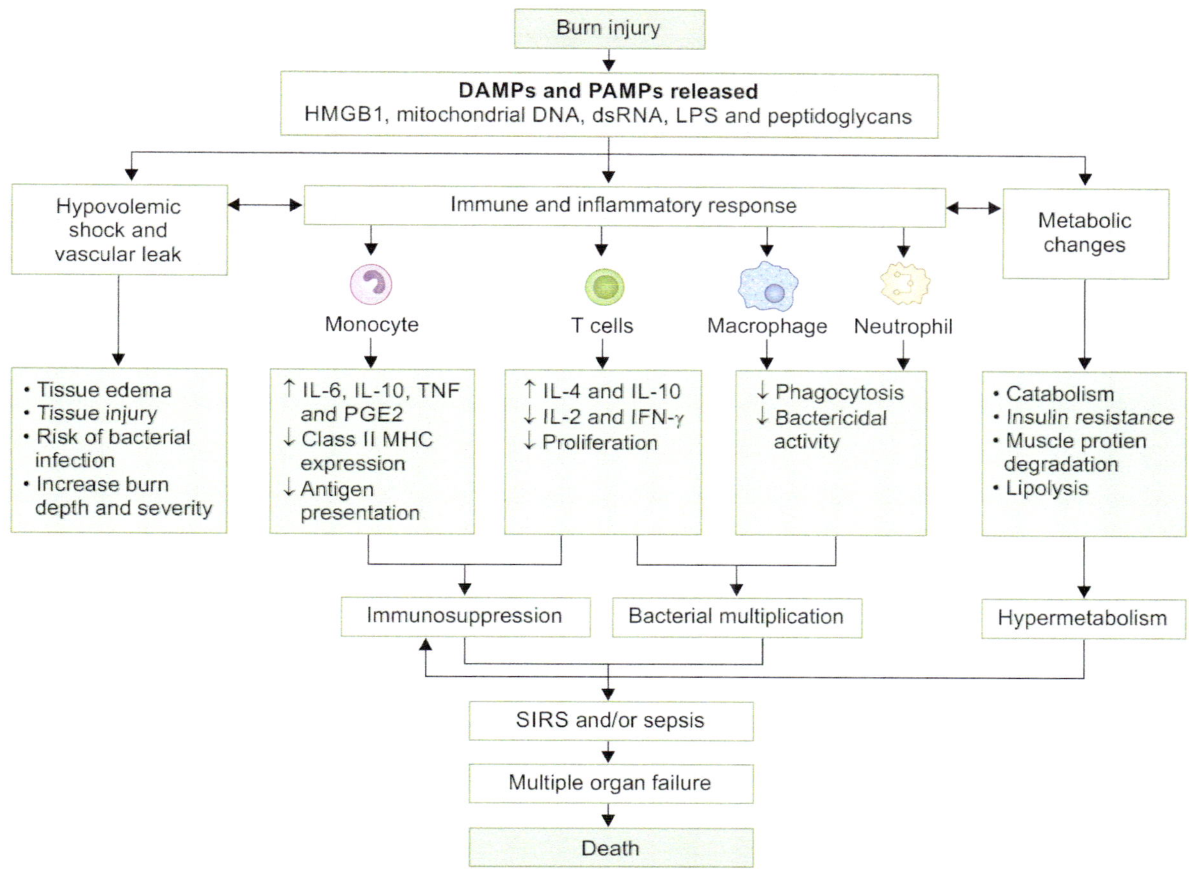

FLOWCHART 1: Hypermetabolic state in burns.[3]

(DAMPs: damage-associated molecular patterns; HMGB1: high mobility group box 1; IFN-γ: interferon-gamma; LPS: lipopolysaccharide; MHC: major histocompatibility complex; PAMPs: pathogen-associated molecular patterns; PGE: prostaglandin E; SIRS: systemic inflammatory response syndrome; TNF: tumor necrosis factor)

microcirculation. Cotran[4] demonstrated through electron micrographic studies that the burn induces an endothelial cell gap in capillary microvasculature. This leads to increased capillary permeability from the intravascular to the extravascular compartment. It has been demonstrated that fluorescein-labeled dextran with a molecular weight of around 150,000 extravasates from postcapillary venules within 10 minutes after a thermal injury.[5] This leads to burn edema. In extensive burns, due to a large volume of fluid lost from the intravascular compartment, systemic hypovolemia develops. This causes a fall in the pressure at the arterial end of the capillary network. In an untreated or inadequately treated burn injury, edema formation is retarded. After adequate resuscitation is performed, circulation is restored. With restoration of the blood flow, edema formation begins as a result of gradual, prolonged fluid flux into interstitial spaces.

The changes in a burn wound take place due to the effect of the heat and are superimposed by acute inflammatory reaction.[6] There is rapid edema formation which reaches its peak in 1–3 hours postburn. Increased permeability may prolong up to 16 hours postburns. Severe interstitial edema formation may cause significant ischemia due to the compression of subdermal vessels and can lead to progression of necrosis. This leakage from the intravascular to the extravascular compartment may continue for even 24 hours. Baxter[7,8] feels that the increased capillary permeability following a burn injury continues for about 24–36 hours and recommends that the colloids should be avoided for the first 24 hours.

Capillary permeability increases severely, following direct exposure to heat and in response to certain substances released in the tissues which include histamine and serotonin, leading to loss of fluid from the intravascular compartment to the extravascular compartment. These changes can occur even in unburnt tissues. This increased permeability in unburnt tissues like skin and muscles may remain elevated for as long as 12 hours after the burn injury for molecules of the size of albumin. The sustained increase in water content and elevated lymphatics flow in these tissues are probably caused by sustained hypoproteinemia.[6]

In superficial dermal burns, the fluid eventually exudes out of the wound in the form of blisters. There is a preponderance of albumin in this exudate due to the smaller size of albumin molecules. This permits their escape into the extravascular compartment more easily. Sometimes, clotting occurs in blister fluid indicating that large fibrinogen molecules have also leaked out of the vascular tree. This loss of protein-rich fluid from plasma after burn leads to a clinical condition of shock. The protein content of the exudate may be as high as 80% of plasma levels[9] **(Table 1)**.

After 24–36 hours, the capillary endothelial integrity returns spontaneously. The large molecules of colloids which leaked into the interstitial spaces cannot be brought back into the circulation. This additional colloid load has to be handled by the lymphatics. Under normal circumstances, the lymph returns to the circulations in a volume comparable to the intravascular pool. About 50% of circulating plasma protein is carried daily by lymphatics. Following a burn injury, quite obviously, the lymphatic system is put to a very severe increase in its workload and cannot function efficiently. This occurs due to an increase in the volume as well as the process of coagulation due to leakage of fibrinogen and its products in interstitial spaces leading to lymphatic obstruction.[6]

Extensive extracellular edema after the burn injury may occur as a result of increased capillary hydrostatic pressure.

Reduction in protein concentration of plasma causes reduction in colloidal osmotic pressure and together with lymphatic blockage and increased permeability of capillaries leads to leakage of protein-rich fluid into the extravascular compartment. Dilatation of capillaries causes a dramatic fall in peripheral resistance and an increase in blood flow. The altered endothelial permeability leads to the leakage of larger protein molecules into the interstitial compartment.[6]

In the absence of treatment, the natural defense mechanisms of the body counter the development of shock in the following ways:

- Proportionately less loss of protein than that of electrolytes. This leads to a relative increase in plasma osmotic pressure, which reduces further leakage.
- By withdrawing fluid from the extracellular space of undamaged tissues which may be the result of increased osmotic pressure
- By general visceral vasoconstriction, reducing the volume of the vascular compartment

TABLE 1: Comparison of plasma and blister fluid.

	Plasma (g%)	Blister fluid (g%)
Albumin	3.9	3.7
Globulin	2.6	1.3
Total proteins	6.5	5.0

- Development of intense thirst leads to increased ingestion of fluids and rapid absorption from the gut.

By these mechanisms, the body may be able to compensate for the rate of fluid loss in minor and moderate burns. The patient may pass safely through the shock phase.

However, in extensive burns, the rate of loss outweighs these in-built defense mechanisms and the plasma volume continues to fall. When untreated or inadequately treated, the patient may progress into a state of irreversible shock.

Edema formation is retarded in larger injury as a result of systemic hypovolemia until adequate fluid resuscitation is carried out. On many occasions, loss of plasma volume occurs in excess of replaced fluid despite massive infusion over several hours.

In minor and moderate burns, it may be possible to achieve the replacement of lost fluid by oral ingestion alone. In extensive burn injury, however, the rate of loss of fluid from the intravascular compartment is so high that it may not be possible to replace the fluid at the rate at which it is lost by the oral route alone. Replacement by the intravenous route is then necessary. Adults with 25% or more burn surface area (BSA) require intravenous replacement of lost fluids. Children and elderly patients are likely to require aggressive resuscitation even with a burn injury as little as 10% BSA.

It will be useful to understand the fluid shift in normal tissues. Under physiological conditions, the high pressure in the arterial end of capillaries causes the filtration of plasma into the tissue interstitial spaces. At the venous end of the capillaries, this fluid is partially reabsorbed and returns to circulation. The remaining fluid is handled by the lymphatic system which drains finally to the venous system **(Table 2)**.

SYSTEMIC EFFECTS

Burn injury is only to the skin; however, secondary involvement of all organs can occur as a result of reduced tissue perfusion due to a state of shock. In untreated severely burned patients, the changes become more severe and widespread and finally lead to death due to multiorgan failure.

TABLE 2: Pathophysiologic effects of major burn shock.

System	Early	Late
Cardiovascular	↓ CO due to decreased circulating blood volume, impaired cardiac contractility ↑ Systemic vascular resistance (SVR)	↑ CO due to sepsis ↑ CO may be 2–3 times > baseline hypertension, tachycardia ↑ SVR
Respiratory	Upper airway obstruction due to edema Lower airway obstruction due to edema, bronchospasm, particulate matter ↓ FRC ↓ Pulmonary compliance ↓ Pulmonary edema (as a consequence of overzealous resuscitation)	• Bronchopneumonia • Tracheal stenosis, laryngeal damage (as complication of intubation) ↓ Chest wall compliance
Renal	↓ Renal blood flow ↓ GFR: due to a. ↓ Circulating blood volume b. Myoglobinuria c. Hemoglobinuria	↑ Renal blood flow ↑ GFR 2° to ↑CO Tubular dysfunction
Hepatic	↓ Function due to ↓ circulating blood volume, hypoxia, hepatotoxins	↑ Functions due to hyper metabolism, enzyme induction, ↑ CO ↑ Functions due to sepsis-drug interaction Hepatitis
Coagulation and hematology	Hemoconcentration Hemolysis ↓ Platelets ↑ Fibrin split products, consumptive coagulopathy, anemia	Anemia
Infection and immunity	Impaired immune function (burn wound sepsis, pneumonia)	Multiple organ failure, endotoxemia
Neurologic	Encephalopathy Seizures ↑ ICP	Encephalopathy Seizures ICU psychosis
Metabolic	↓ Ionized calcium Impaired thermoregulation	↑ Metabolic rate ↑ CO_2 product and O_2 utilization
Gastrointestinal	Stress ulceration (Curling's ulcer) Impaired intestinal barrier function Endotoxemia	Stress ulceration (Curling's ulcer) Impaired intestinal barrier formula Endotoxemia
Skin	↑ Heat, fluid, electrolyte loss	Contractures, scar formation
Pharmacokinetics	Altered volume of distribution	Tolerance to narcotics, sedatives, enzyme induction, altered receptors Drug interaction

(↓: decrease in; ↑: increase in; CO: cardiac output; FRC: functional residual capacity; GFR: glomerular filtration rate; ICP: intracranial pressure; ICU: intensive care unit)

Source: Adopted and modified from: McLennan N, Heimbach DM, Cullen BF. Anesthesia for major thermal injury. Anaesthesiology. 1998;84:749-70.

In severe burns, inflammation, hypermetabolism, muscle wasting, and insulin resistance affect all organs. The phases of burn resuscitation are:

- Resuscitation (or hypodynamic) phase
- Hyperdynamic and hypermetabolic phase

There is an initial phase of resuscitation, sometimes referred to as the hypodynamic period, which lasts for around 24-72 hours.[10,11] During this phase, increased vascular permeability, fluid changes that cause intravascular volume loss, and the development of edema are all present. Both direct vascular heat injury and the release of inflammatory mediators cause an increase in vascular permeability.[10] Reduced capillary oncotic pressure is the result of increased vascular permeability, which causes intravascular fluid and plasma proteins to move into the interstitial space.[10,11] As a result, more fluid enters the interstitial space, which causes edema to develop.[10] Proteins from the damaged skin surface and the edema fluid are lost as a result of hypoproteinemia.[10] Within 2–3 hours following a 40% TBSA burn, the vascular compartment may lose up to half of its entire plasma water content.[10] Within the first 12–24 hours, hemoconcentration due to intravascular hypovolemia occurs.

After 24–72 hours, a hyperdynamic and hypermetabolic flow phase begins.[12] This phase is characterized by an increase in cardiac output, a decrease in peripheral vascular resistance, an increase in heart rate, and a decrease in vascular permeability.[10]

In severe burns, inflammation, hypermetabolism, muscle wasting, and insulin resistance affects all organs as discussed below.

CARDIOVASCULAR SYSTEM

As a result of the reduction of plasma volume, vasoconstriction, and decrease in venous return, there is a marked *fall in cardiac output* in patients with severe burn. There is severe tachycardia. With proper fluid replacement, the cardiac output promptly returns to normal. Without adequate fluid therapy, the cardiac output continues to fall at a slower rate until death occurs as a result of multiorgan failure.

As a result of vasoconstriction and increased heart rate, *blood pressure* is maintained till late and is *not a reliable guide* for the assessment of the state of shock. Moreover, in these patients, due to the formation of severe edema, blood pressure readings cannot be taken accurately.

RESPIRATORY SYSTEM

Smoke inhalation injuries are common in patients with head and face burn injuries.[13] In postburn period, increased vascular permeability, release of inflammatory mediators, and reactive oxygen species lead to the development of edema. Mucosal injury and increased secretion of the upper respiratory tract cause decreased gaseous exchange. Upper respiratory tract edema has the potential to worsen, leading to bronchospasm and airway blockage that peaks in 24–48 hours.[10] In addition, during the first 24 hours, there may be laryngospasm, ulceration, bleeding, and mucosal congestion.

Severe reduction in microcirculation in the *lungs* through rapid and continuous blood flow in larger vessels is noticed. The ventilation rate increases and is usually proportional to the severity of burn injury and declines gradually. Oxygen consumption also increases but is not affected by the ventilation rate if the respiratory exchange is not impaired. On the other hand, inhalation injuries cause severe edema of the upper respiratory tract due to the direct thermal component of hot air. The lower respiratory tract can be chemically irritated due to injuries from noxious chemicals, such as cyanide and carbon monoxide which escape.[14] On arterial blood gas analysis, these changes become apparent as the partial pressure of oxygen drops; hence, hypoxemia is an indicator of inhalational injury unless otherwise proved. It must be kept in mind that in the early phases of inhalational injury, the oxygen level may appear near normal. Excess exudates rich in protein, inflammatory cells, and necrotic debris are produced by the injured mucosal cells leading to further dysfunction of the respiratory tract.[10] This is discussed in detail in the Chapter 11 "Respiratory Tract Injury in Burns". *Interstitial edema* is present in varying degrees which later leads to a classical condition called acute respiratory distress syndrome (ARDS). Both these conditions lead to inadequate oxygen transfer resulting in marked hypoxia in various organs.[10]

RENAL SYSTEM

Kidneys are most likely to be damaged by persistent shock. Secretion of urine is a valuable guide to renal function and indirectly to the blood flow of kidneys and thus to tissue perfusion in general. The most common factor in burn-related acute kidney injury is due to either hypovolemia or hypervolemia early during resuscitation or late as a result of infection.[15] It has been reported that early AKI is linked to early multiple-organ dysfunction and an increased risk of death.[16] Although there are many contributing factors, the systemic inflammatory response that follows a septic episode, such as widespread vasodilation and a hypercoagulable condition, is largely responsible for late AKI.[15]

During the shock phase, there is a marked rise in antidiuretic hormone (ADH). This results in conservation of body fluids when oligemia is present. Antidiuresis may be the combined effect of ADH, hypovolemia, and reduction of plasma flow due to the release of vasoactive substances.[17] After a prolonged, uncontrolled shock, renal failure ensues. After about 48–72 hours, if hypovolemia is adequately corrected, reabsorption of interstitial fluids starts, the level of antidiuretic hormone (ADH) falls, and the phase of diuresis starts.

HEPATIC SYSTEM AND PANCREAS

Vasoconstriction, oligemia, and a decrease in cardiac output can all have a direct or indirect impact on the visceral organs such as liver and pancreas. Because of the liver damage brought on by oligemia, the liver enzymes [serum glutamic-oxaloacetic transaminase (SGOT), serum glutamic pyruvic transaminase (SGPT), and alkaline phosphatase] rise quickly in the postburn period, peak in 2–3 days, and continue to remain at high levels for 4–6 weeks after burns. They are highly sensitive markers of injury to liver cells. It has been demonstrated that hepatic edema development is correlated with liver injury.[17,18] After 2–7 days following burn, there is a notable increase in liver weight.[19] This is a result of edema development of the liver. The 1st week following damage sees a considerable increase in liver size and weight, which peaks 2 weeks later.

ENDOCRINE SYSTEM

In the *endocrine* system, there are variable changes in the different hormonal levels. There is a decrease in insulin production in the early postburn period lasting for 2–3 weeks. Glucagon is elevated, but fasting blood sugar is not grossly increased. Growth hormone increases in the first 2 weeks and then decreases to a lower level which is still above normal for another 6–8 weeks. This can lead to a slight increase in blood glucose levels. The adrenocorticotropic hormone (ACTH) level increases proportional to burn size, especially in children. Cortisol levels increase two- to four-fold. The gonadotrophic hormones are only slightly affected.

The effects of thermal injury on the microvasculature of the skin are discussed in the pathophysiology of the burn wound.

NEUROLOGICAL SYSTEM

For a considerable amount of time, the brain continues to get a major contribution from blood flow, and consciousness is not lost until later. Increased intracranial pressure and the development of cerebral edema are caused by cellular hypoxia in the later phase.[20,21] Agitation, disorientation, ataxia, atypical posture, brief loss of consciousness, convulsions, and even shock are additional indications of central nervous system malfunction.[22]

Following a deep burn, new nerve fibers usually migrate from the wound bed or sprout collaterally from the nearby unaffected area, resulting in cutaneous nerve regeneration.[21] However, this process has flaws leading to issues in the nerve regeneration mechanism. According to reports, 36% of sufferers of serious burns experience chronic agony and 71% experience altered sensation.[21]

GASTROINTESTINAL SYSTEM

In the *intestines,* vasoconstriction may be so intense that the blood flow may be inadequate and decreases nearly 60% of baseline to satisfy the needs of cells of capillary walls. As many as 36–70% of individuals may get intra-abdominal hypertension (IAH) or secondary abdominal compartment syndrome (ACS), which are possible after effects of systemic burn damage. Reduced abdominal wall compliance from circumferential body burns and tension brought on by pain or discomfort can both affect intra-abdominal pressure (IAP).[22,23]

Absorption of fluid from the intestine cannot occur, peristalsis ceases, and *paralytic ileus* develops. At this stage, the patient who is intensely thirsty starts vomiting after any attempt at drinking fluids and this important defense mechanism fails. Presence of peristalsis indicates that the visceral circulation is adequate. Similarly in the stomach, the intense vasoconstriction and hemoconcentration resulting in microthrombi may lead to acute ischemic damage to gastric and duodenal mucosa resulting in acute mucosal lesions called "Curling's ulcer."[24]

SKELETAL MUSCLE

The main location of peripheral glucose disposal and a key component in metabolic control is skeletal muscle.[25] After a burn, the skeletal muscle continues to operate, supplying energy for more critical processes including the production of acute phase proteins and the growth of new skin.[25,26] Protein breakdown causes muscle atrophy, which is why burn patients frequently develop cachexia.[25-27]

ANEMIA IN BURN PATIENT

The term anemia generally pertains to reduction below normal of the concentration of oxygen-transporting capacity of a designated volume of blood and is generally expressed as the amount of hemoglobin in 100 mL of blood.[2]

Following extensive burn, plasma is rapidly lost from the intravascular compartment to the extravascular compartment and causes a significant rise in hemoglobin and hematocrit levels. This slows down the blood circulation, particularly in the zone of stasis leading to local tissue anoxia.[28] Hence, blood transfusions are not advisable at this stage. Hemoconcentration can have deleterious effect on the zone of stasis where the circulation in the tissues has already slowed down.

After the initial rise of hemoglobin and hematocrit levels, a patient with extensive burn injury becomes rapidly anemic. Lowered hemoglobin can lead to tissue hypoxia, retard wound healing, and hamper the "take" of skin grafts.

In a burn patient, anemia can develop due to various causes/mechanisms:[29]

- Red cells are destruction destroyed as a result of direct heat during the process of burning.

- The red cells which are not destroyed but are exposed to heat are rendered unduly fragile. They are sooner or later removed from circulation earlier than the expected balance life span of these RBCs.
- Overzealous resuscitation leads to overhydration, and consequent hemodilution gives rise to a false anemic state.
- Bacterial toxins can cause hemolysis, particularly the invasive infection by various hemolytic organisms, sometimes leading to massive red cell destruction.
- Severe hemorrhage at the dressing changes (particularly when the dry dressing is used) during removal of adherent dressing at the stage when the granulation tissue in the wound has started developing after the necrotic tissue has come out.
- Thrombocytopenia leads to an increase in the bleeding tendency all over the body which may result in bleeding from the wound, mucous membrane, lungs, gastrointestinal tract, and in fact, anywhere in the body
- Inadequate assessment of blood loss and resultant inadequate blood transfusions during operative procedures such as escharotomy, debridement of granulation tissue, skin grafting operation, primary or secondary excision of the burn wound, etc.
- Poor nutritional status of patients with extensive burns
- Biochemical and morphological alterations in red cells and hemoglobin lead to their reduced efficiency in oxygen transport

SUMMARY

Acute burn injury triggers complex pathophysiological responses due to the release of DAMPs and PAMPs. These responses include hypovolemic shock, vascular leak, immune and inflammatory changes, and metabolic alterations. Hypovolemic shock results from significant fluid loss,increased capillary permeablity leading to tissue edema and decreased cardiac output, followed by systemic hypovolemia which affects all organs. Immune response alterations involve monocytes, T cells, macrophages, and neutrophils, causing changes in cytokine levels, reduced antigen presentation, and impaired phagocytosis, which lead to immunosuppression and higher infection risk. Metabolic changes are marked by hypermetabolism, characterized by increased catabolism, insulin resistance, muscle protein degradation, and lipolysis, further exacerbating immunosuppression, which if not managed timely contribute to SIRS and sepsis, potentially resulting in multiorgan dysfunction and failure.

REFERENCES

1. Kramer GC, Nguyen TT. Pathophysiology of burn shock and burn edema. In: Herndon DN (Ed). Total Burn Care. London: WB Saunders Company Ltd; 1996. pp. 44-52.
2. Parker W. Stedman's Medical Dictionary, 23rd edition. Baltimore: The William and Wilkins Company; 1976.
3. Jeschke MG, van Baar ME, Choudhry MA, Chung KK, Gibran NS, Logsetty S. Burn injury. Nat Rev Dis Primers. 2020;6(1):11.
4. Cotran RS. The delayed and prolonged vascular leakage in inflammation II. An electron microscope study of the vascular response after thermal injury. Am J Pathol. 1965;46:589-620.
5. Aggarwal SJ, Diller KR, Yeung HK, Baxter CR. Local macromolecular extravasation in thermal burns quantified by fluorescent video microscopy and computer vision. J Burn Care Rehabil. 1994;15(2):104-20.
6. Arturson G. Pathophysiology of the burn wound and pharmacological treatment: The Rudi Hermans Lecture. Burns 1996;22:255-74.
7. Baxter CR. Fluid therapy of burns. J Trauma. 1967;7:69-73.
8. Baxter CR. Fluid volume and electrolyte changes in early post burn period. Clin Plast Surg. 1974;1:693-709.
9. Muir IFK, Barklay TL, Settle JAD. Burns and Their Treatment, 3rd edition. London: Butterworths; 1987. p. 178.
10. Vaughn L, Beckel N. Severe burn injury, burn shock, and smoke inhalation injury in small animals. Part 1: Burn classification and pathophysiology. J Vet Emerg Crit Care (San Antonio). 2012;22:179-86.
11. Demling RH. The burn edema process: Current concepts. J Burn Care Rehabil. 2005;26:207-27.
12. Bittner EA, Shank E, Woodson L, Martyn JA. Acute and peri operative care of the burn-injured patient. Anaesthesiology. 2015;122:448-64.
13. Swanson JW, Otto AM, Gibran NS, Klein MB, Kramer CB, Heimbach DM, et al. Trajectories to death in patients with burn injury. J Trauma Acute Care Surg. 2013;74(1):282-8.
14. You K, Yang HT, Kym D, Yoon J, HaejunYim, Cho YS, et al. Inhalation injury in burn patients: Establishing the link between diagnosis and prognosis. Burns. 2014;40(8):1470-5.
15. Fagan SP, Bilodeau M-L, Goverman J. Burn intensive care. Surg Clin North Am. 2014;94:765-79.
16. Mosier MJ, Pham TN, Klein MB, Gibran NS, Arnoldo BD, Gamelli RL, et al. Early acute kidney injury predicts progressive renal dysfunction and higher mortality in severely burned adults. J Burn Care Res. 2010;31(1):83-92.
17. Jeschke MG. The hepatic response to thermal injury: Is the liver important for postburn outcomes? Mol Med. 2009;15:337-51.
18. Jeschke MG, Micak RP, Finnerty CC, Herndon DN. Changes in liver function and size after a severe thermal in jury. Shock. 2007;28:172-7.
19. Hermans G, De Jonghe B, Bruyninckx F, Van den Berghe G. Interventions for preventing critical illness polyneuropa thy and critical illness myopathy. Cochrane Database Syst Rev. 2014;1:CD006832.

20. Wilkinson. Cross reference from "Physiological responses to burn Injury." In: Davies JWL (1982). London: Academic Press; 1982. p. 262.
21. Blais M, Parenteau-Bareil R, Cadau S, Berthod F. Concise review: tissue-engineered skin and nerve regeneration in burn treatment. Stem Cells Transl Med. 2013;2:545-51.
22. Song XM, Li JG, Wang YL, Liang H, Huang Y, Yuan X, et al. Effect of vagus nerve stimulation on thermal injury in rats. Burns. 2010;36(1):75-81.
23. Vaughn L, Beckel N, Walters P. Severe burn injury, burn shock, and smoke inhalation injury in small animals. Part 2: diagnosis, therapy, complications, and prognosis. J Vet Emerg Crit Care (San Antonio). 2012;22:187-200.
24. Burke BA, Latenser BA. Defining intra-abdominal hypertension and abdominal compartment syndrome in acute thermal injury: A multicenter survey. J Burn Care Res. 2008;29:580-4.
25. Porter C, Herndon DN, Sidossis LS, Børsheim E. The impact of severe burns on skeletal musc e mitochondrial function. Burns. 2013;39:1039-47.
26. Hosokawa S, Koseki H, Nagashima M, Maeyama Y, Yomogida K, Mehr C, et al. Title efficacy of phosphodiesterase 5 inhibitor on distant burn-induced muscle autophagy, microcirculation, and survival rate. Am J Physiol Endocrinol Metab. 2013;304(9):E922-33.
27. Porter C, Herndon DN, Børsheim E, Chao T, Reidy PT, Borack MS, et al. Uncoupled skeletal muscle mitochondria contribute to hypermetabolism in severely burned adults. Am J Physiol Endocrinol Metab. 2014;307(5):E462-7.
28. Jackson DM. The diagnosis of the depth of burning. Br J Surg. 1953;40:588-96.
29. Davies JWL. Anemia and red cell disorders. In: Physiological Responses to Burning Injury, London: Academic Press; 1982. p. 650.

CHAPTER

5

Pathophysiology of Burn Wound

Arvind Vartak, Suhas V Abhyankar

INTRODUCTION

Skin is the largest organ in the body. It is made of the epidermis and the dermis. In the dermis, there is an ingrowth of epidermal elements such as sweat glands, sebaceous glands, and hair follicles **(Fig. 1)**.

The epidermis consists of stratified squamous epithelium. The deepest layer consists of tall columnar cells. As they approach the surface, they flatten. The outer layer is continuously shed off as dead cells and forms a keratin layer, which is continuously replaced from underneath.

The dermis is formed mainly by the fibrous connective tissue and ingrowths of various epidermal structures from outside, namely sweat glands, sebaceous glands, and hair follicles. Blood flow to the skin comes through capillaries arising from the subdermal plexus of blood vessels, which bring nutrients to the skin. It also contains nerve endings, which provide sensation to the skin.

The characteristics of the skin vary from place to place depending on the function of the part of the body.

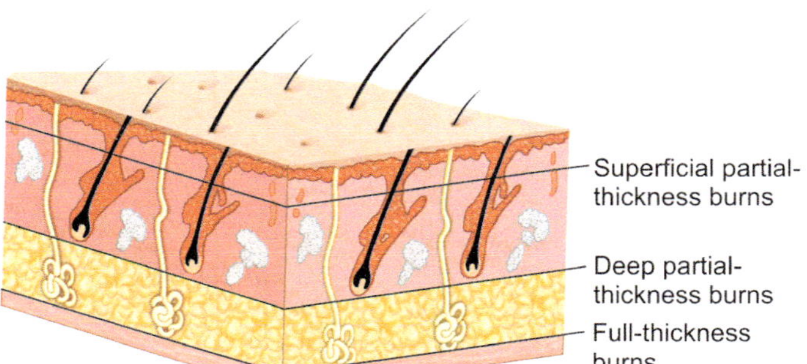

FIG. 1: Diagrammatic representation of the anatomy of the skin and classification of burn injury in relation to the depth of burn—superficial partial-thickness, deep partial-thickness, and full-thickness.

Thus, the skin of the upper eyelid is very thin, while that of the sole is very thick. It can be different even in the same part of the body; e.g., the skin of the palm is thick while that on the dorsal aspect of the hand is thin and very loose, so free movements of the fingers and the hand are possible.

Heat destroys a greater or lesser depth of the skin, depending upon the intensity and duration of exposure. When the burn injury causes partial-thickness damage, the epithelium from the epidermal appendages grows to the surface of the viable dermis underneath the devitalized layers. The dead tissue separates and is shed off after the healing underneath is complete.

The greater the depths of the burn, the lesser the epidermal structures available to grow and develop a new epidermis. Thus, the superficial burns heal rapidly, while the deeper partial-thickness burns take a longer time to heal, maybe even 3–6 weeks. Full-thickness burns, however, heal either by contraction, if very small, or with a contracture formation if large and opposite joints. They may not heal at all over rigid areas of bone, e.g., the skull, unless surgical intervention is done in the form of skin grafting.

The burn wound, although it damages only the skin cover of the body, is the cause of a variety of widespread complications in the body involving almost all organ systems, initially as a result of oligemia and later due to septic and other complications.

FUNCTIONS OF THE SKIN

The skin acts as a protective barrier and prevents invasive infections. When this barrier is broken, microorganisms from outside can invade the body. When large areas of skin are damaged, it can lead to bacteremia or even septicemia.

Skin also helps in retaining body fluids. When large areas of skin are damaged, plasma leaks out. This can result in a state of hypovolemic shock. This loss can sometimes be so large that a correction by intravenous infusion becomes necessary, and the replacement of fluids by the oral route alone is not enough. This lost fluid contains various salts, leading to an electrolyte imbalance.

Body temperature is regulated by dilatation or constriction of blood vessels in the dermis. Vasoconstriction reduces heat loss, while vasodilatation increases it. Sweating helps cool the body in a hot climate.

The sebaceous glands secrete a fatty substance that lubricates the skin, keeps it soft, and protects it from drying. The nerve endings are the defense mechanism of the body through various sensations, which perceive touch, pain, pressure, changes in temperature, etc.

Skin also helps with the immune responses of the body. Rickatts et al.[1] also postulated that the skin has self-sterilizing abilities.

The transfer of thermal energy to the skin occurs in various ways, like conduction (in a case of contact burn), convection (when there are currents of hot air or liquid), and radiation (by the transfer of heat without involving the medium through which it occurs, like in a case of sunburn or from a bonfire.[2]

Moritz and Henriquez[3] demonstrated that the transfer of heat from the surface to the deeper layers leads to cellular necrosis, depending upon the temperature and the duration of exposure.

The heat required to cause skin burns.

- *Full-thickness*:
  - At 44°C in 6 hours
  - At 52°C in 6 minutes
  - At 59°C in 1 minute
  - At 62°C in 30 seconds
  - At 67°C in 20 seconds
  - At 71°C in 10 seconds
- *Partial-thickness*:
  - At 70°C in 1 second

Ofeigsson[4] conclusively demonstrated that the use of water as a cooling agent for the burn wound is beneficial. His animal experiments showed that the general condition of the treated animals was far better than that of the controls.

There are much less secondary infections. Water cooling arrests and causes retrogation of the degenerative process of the skin and underlying tissues, thus significantly shortening the period of healing. He also showed that the superficial temperature of the scalded skin of controls takes several minutes to fall, thus causing longer exposure to heat (longer than what we believe). He also warned that extensive burns treated with ice water can cause hypothermia. This is likely to be true in cold countries and in northern India in the winter.

Cotran[5] carried out electron micrographic studies and showed that a burn induces endothelial cell gaps in the capillary microvasculature. This leads to increased capillary permeability from the intravascular compartment to the extravascular compartment, leading to burn edema.

When injured, the skin repairs itself by:

- The growth of the epidermis from the margins of unburnt skin
- Epidermal growth from intradermal epidermal adnexal elements, namely sweat glands, sebaceous glands, and hair follicles

HISTOPATHOLOGY OF BURN WOUNDS

Burn injuries have been classified into partial-thickness burns and full-thickness burns in relation to the anatomical involvement of the layer of skin involved **(Fig. 1)**.

In a partial-thickness burn, the whole of epidermis and part of dermis are burned **(Figs. 2 and 3)**. The epithelial elements from the remaining part of the dermis grow over the surface between the viable dermis and the superficial necrotic layer, which finally leads to healing. The necrotic layer separates and is finally shed off.

The partial-thickness burn is further classified as superficial partial- and deep partial-thickness burns. Superficial partial-thickness burns heal rapidly in up to 3 weeks due to the greater availability of epidermal adnexal elements in them.

In deep, partial-thickness burns, however, these epidermal elements are much less in number and obviously take a longer time to heal, maybe up to 6 weeks **(Figs. 4 and 5)**.

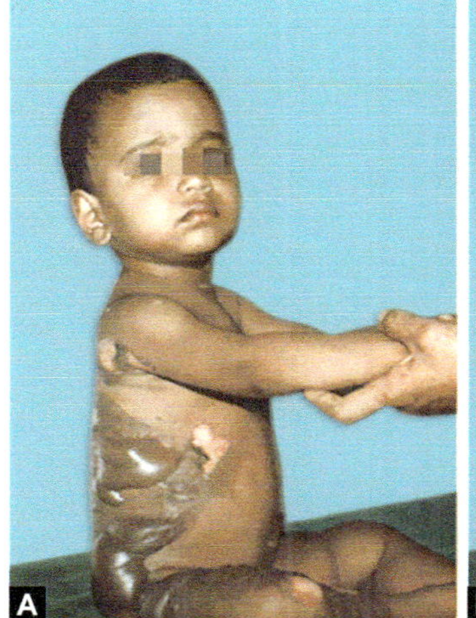

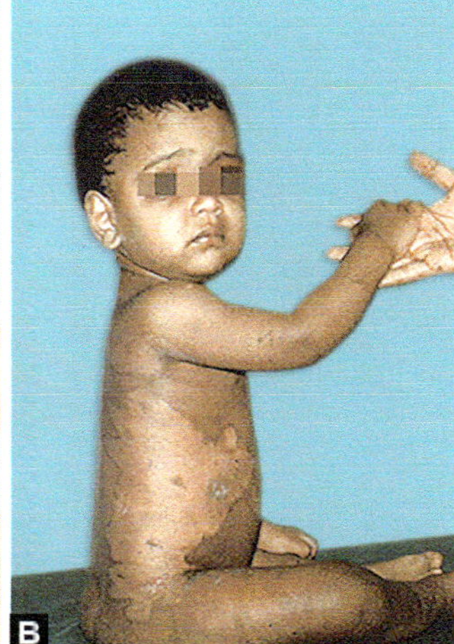

FIGS. 2A AND B: Superficial burns. (A) Note the characteristic large blisters; (B) Rapid healing in 10 days postburn.

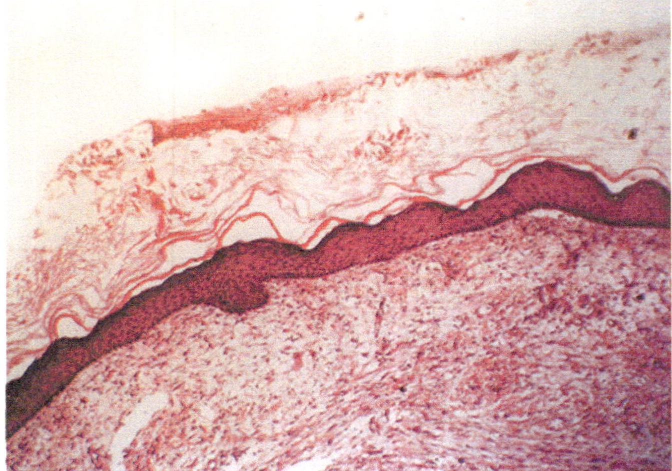

FIG. 3: Histological appearance (20×) of burn wound treated with boiled potato peel bandage. 11th postburn day. Re-epidermalization is quite evident between the slough on the surface and the viable dermis underneath.

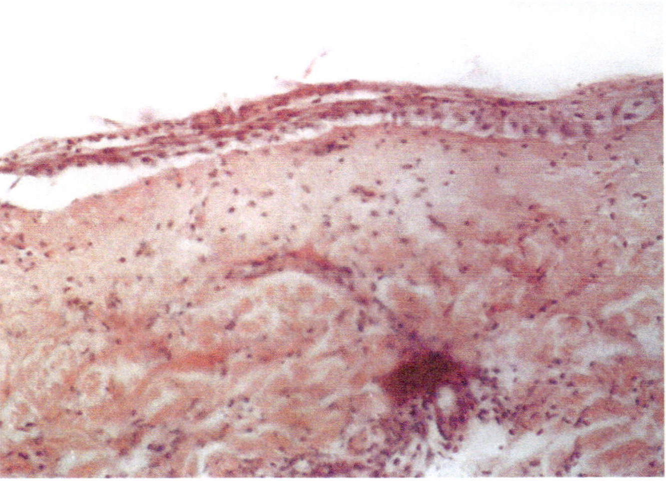

FIG. 5: Histological appearance (40×) of burnt skin on the second postburn day shows thin, sloughed-off epidermis. There is marked dermal edema with neutrophilic infiltration all over.

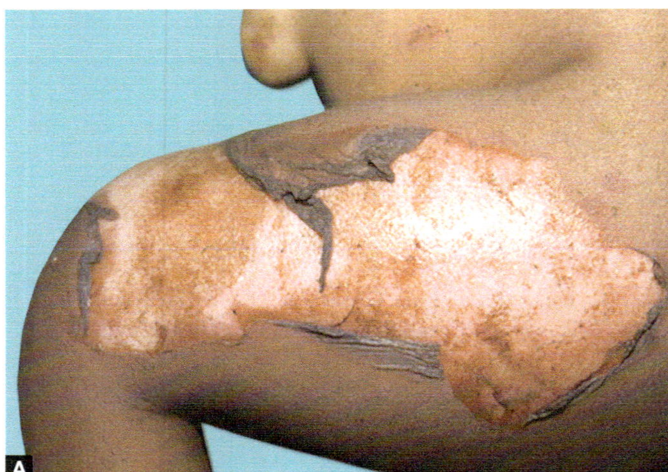

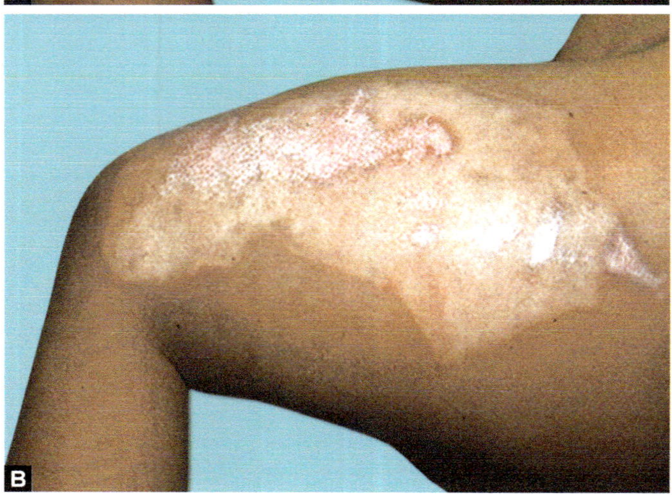

FIGS. 4A AND B: Deep burns. (A) Appearance 2 days postburn; (B) Complete healing in 3 weeks.

In a full-thickness burn, the entire thickness of the skin, involving the whole of epidermis and dermis, is damaged. The epithelial elements are destroyed. Healing cannot take place at all. However, in small full-thickness burn wounds, healing can occur from peripheral unburnt skin and wound contraction. Larger burns can heal only after skin grafting or contracture formation **(Fig. 6)**.

Following a full-thickness burn, the dead and necrotic skin gradually gets separated from the underlying viable tissues and is shed off. The resulting raw area gets covered with granulation tissue, a tissue developed from the capillary network **(Fig. 7)**, over which a skin graft can be applied for complete healing of the wound. Immediately underneath the granulation tissue, a thin fibrous layer is formed, which gradually undergoes thickening.

Figure 7 illustrates the character of granulation tissues under a microscope, with resultant micro pockets (shown with an arrow). These need to be cleared by debridement of the granulation before the application of the skin graft to ensure a better "take" of the graft **(Fig. 8)**.

Jackson[6] described three zones in the damaged burn tissue **(Fig. 9)**:

1. Zone of coagulation is the central zone with complete coagulative necrosis of the tissue cells, which become completely nonviable and obviously cannot recover with any treatment.
2. Zone of stasis is on the periphery of the zone of coagulation, where a significant reduction in microcirculation occurs following damage to the tissues and their arterioles, venules, and capillaries. The circulation is sluggish. This zone can recover after adequate resuscitation and proper wound care.

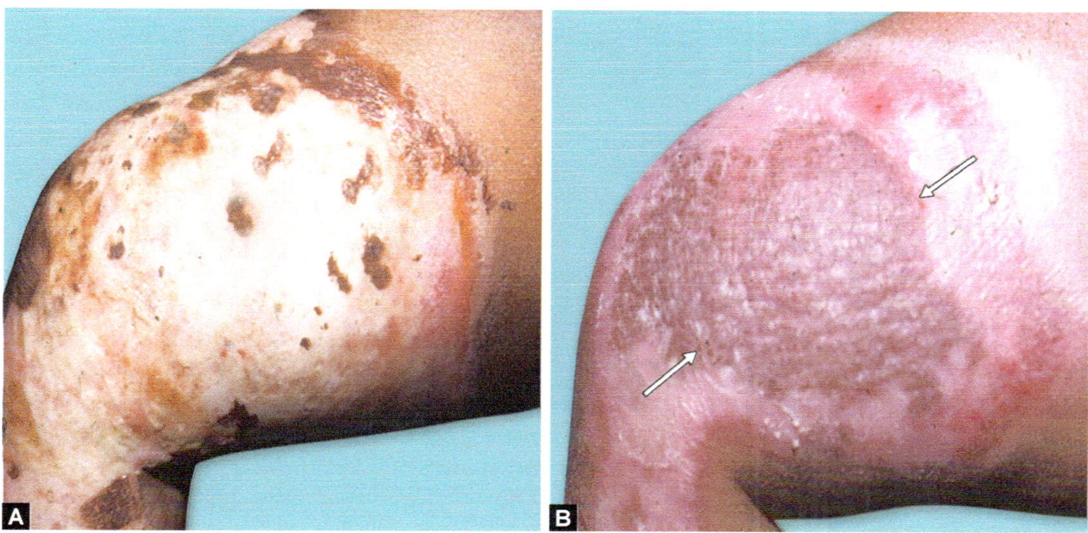

FIGS. 6A AND B: Full-thickness burns. (A) Appearance 1 week postburn; (B) Healing after skin grafting. Skin graft is marked by arrows.

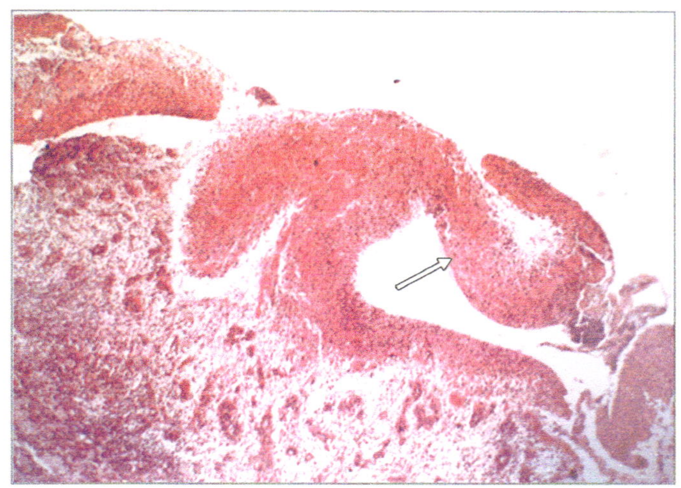

FIG. 7: Histological appearance of granulation tissue as seen under a microscope (40×). Note the pockets within the granulation tissue (shown by an arrow).

This can result in the healing of the burn wound. With inadequate resuscitation initially and due to invasive sepsis later, this zone can get converted into a zone of coagulative necrosis.

3. Zone of hyperemia is the outermost zone, peripheral to the zone of stasis, due to intense vasodilatation. This eventually recovers following adequate resuscitation with the passage of time.

Zawaki[7] demonstrated that the zone of stasis begins to recover in about 16–24 hours postburn. Oxygen consumption returns to this zone as early as the fourth postburn day and exceeds normal by 7–14 days when resuscitation is adequate and drying of the wound is prevented. When a burn wound is exposed to air, dehydration of tissues occurs, and the process of reversal of stasis is minimal or absent. Deep partial skin loss or whole skin loss occurs when the dermis is allowed to dry. The retention of blister skin or coverage with allograft or xenograft prevents dehydration of the dermis and helps the healing process favorably **(Fig. 10)**.

Zawaki[8] showed that when the drying of a burn wound is prevented, epithelium migrates toward the surface around the necrotic hair follicles **(Fig. 2)** soon after the circulation in the viable tissue returns. He also showed that the zone of stasis begins to recover in about 16–24 hours, and circulation returns in a few days postburn. When drying is prevented, oxygen consumption returns to this zone as early as the fourth postburn day.

Winter[9] showed that the scab that forms over the exposed wound decreases the possibility of migration of keratinocytes, ultimately causing impairment in the process of wound healing. On the other hand, Zawaki[10,11] demonstrated that the occlusive dressings, which do not allow the wound to dry, also allow the tissue to retain its viability.

Lawrence[12] stressed that this perinecrotic zone (zone of stasis) can be saved by applying a cover of suitable dressing. If left without proper covering, the epithelial elements in the dermis are lost due to dehydration. Zawaki[10,11] supported this hypothesis. Janzekovic[13] demonstrated that early excision of the necrotic tissue and a cover with a skin graft improved the outcome in burn patients.

Groves and Lawrence[14] demonstrated a significant improvement in the quality and quantity of dermal tissue in healed burns treated by tangential excision

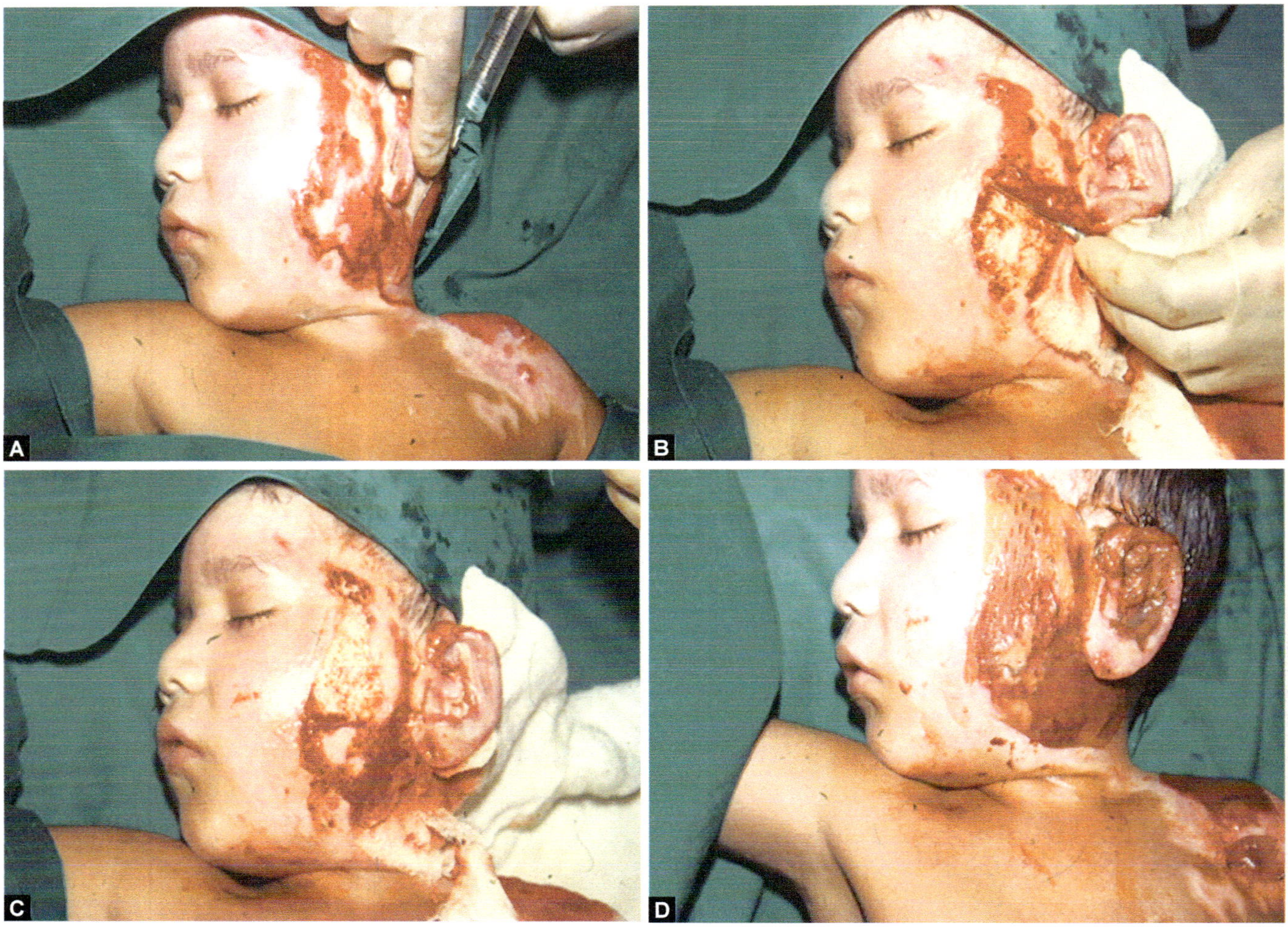

FIGS. 8A TO D: Unhealthy granulation tissue. (A) Injection of saline-adrenaline 1:100,000 to prevent blood loss; (B) Debridement of granulation tissue; (C) Wound ready for skin grafting after debridement; (D) After complete healing.

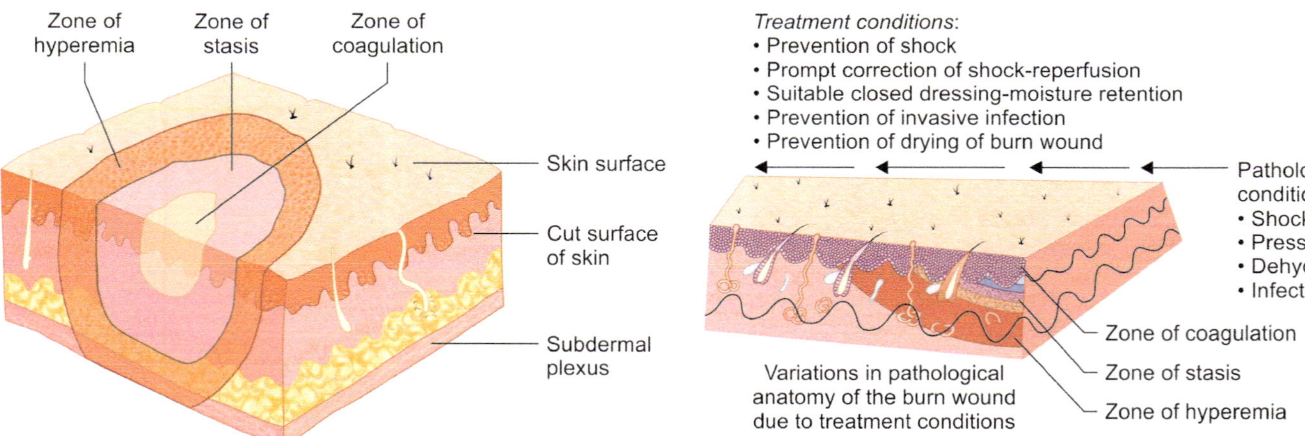

FIG. 9: Diagrammatic representation of three zones as described by Dr Douglas Jackson.

FIG. 10: Changes in the burn wound that can occur due to various pathological conditions and as a result of a response to adequate treatment.

and autografting in comparison with vapor-permeable material. The studies by Lawrence[12] have also demonstrated that a polyurethane film can prevent loss of epithelium in an experimentally tangential excised burn wound.

Hinman and Maiback[15] showed that impermeable and semipermeable materials prevent the desiccation of the wound and indirectly help the process of healing **(Fig. 10)**. Keswani et al.[16] demonstrated conclusively that the use of a moisture-retaining dressing made from boiled potato peel (BPP) did improve the quality of healing and shorten the period of healing. Compared with the treatment with plain gauze, the application of potato peel dressing reduced or eliminated desiccation, hastened epithelial regeneration, and promoted rapid healing. Pain relief after BPP bandage was significant **(Figs. 11 and 12)**.

The burn eschar is essentially dried, devitalized skin covering the burn wound. Eschar does not provide protection from infection. However, it is a good medium for the growth of bacteria in the necrotic tissues. The property of the skin to prevent loss of fluids like plasma and its components is absent in eschar due to its high degree of permeability.[17]

The necrotic tissue anywhere in the body allows bacterial colonization. The extensive burn itself is a large quantity of necrotic tissue on the body. The appreciation of this fact has led to the idea of removal of this tissue as

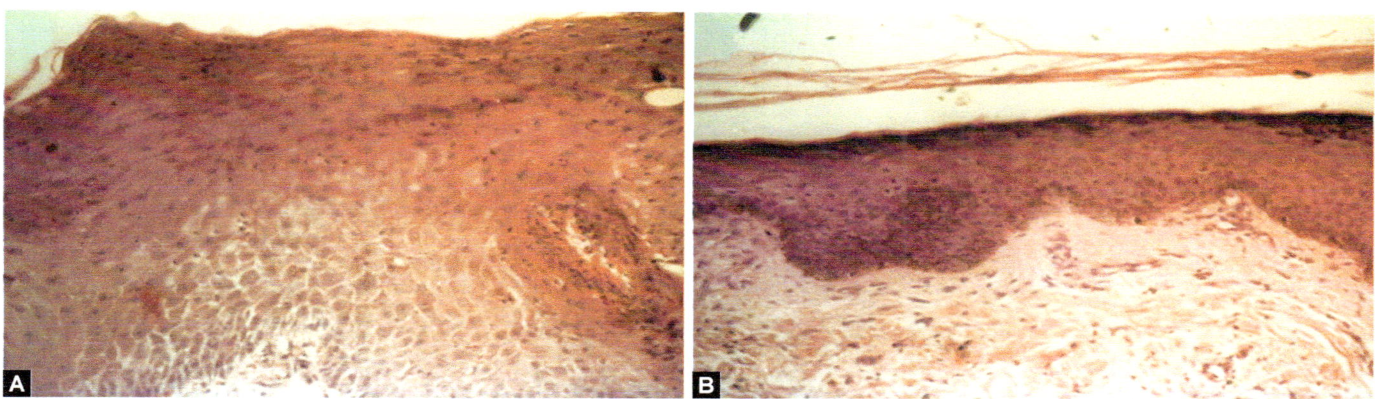

FIGS. 11A AND B: Histological appearance (40×) after complete healing on 21st postburn day. (A) Treated with boiled potato peel shows orderly stratification with a basal layer of columnar epithelium; (B) Area treated with gauze and silver sulfadiazine cream shows complete healing with dysplastic stratification and a basal layer of cuboidal cells.

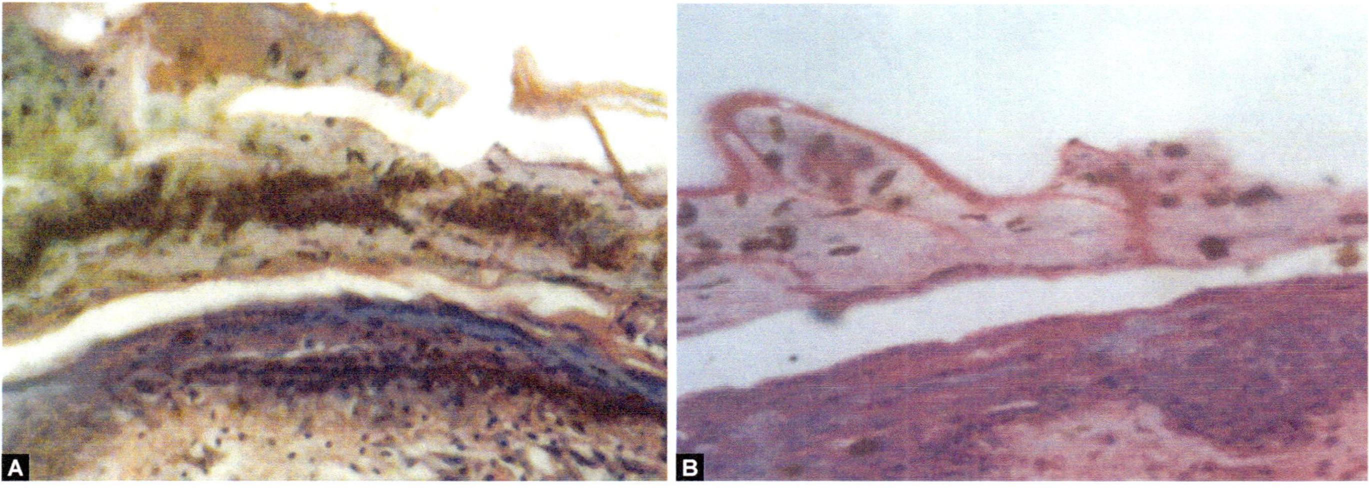

FIGS. 12A AND B: Histological appearance (40×) 7th postburn day. (A) Encrustation on the surface regeneration of the epidermis with dysplastic stratification of the epidermis; (B) The section shows the moist slough on the surface following boiled potato peel dressing. Note the more orderly stratification of the epidermis.

early as possible (primary excision) with the hope that septic complications can be avoided after the removal of burned skin. This is expected to lead to a marked improvement in the patient's condition and an improved survival rate.

Hermans[18] reported that the use of occlusive dressings using hydrocolloid material improved the quality of healing due to rapid re-epithelization, a low incidence of infection, and good cosmetic results. This led to a better quality of life for the burn patient after healing.

Hermans[19] stressed that desiccation of the burn wound leads to the formation of a scab, which decreases the migration of keratinocytes, which eventually leads to impaired wound healing. On the other hand, the occlusive dressing with retention of moisture would not allow the wound to dry out and would allow the tissues in the zone of stasis to retain their viability.

Semipermeable and impermeable dressings like synthetic films, "BPPs", skin allografts, or hydrocolloids prevent the desiccation of the wound and provide protection to the zone of stasis **(Figs. 13 and 14)**. The authors are using polyethylene drape as a dressing material in the second layer after a gauze piece dipped in topical antimicrobials since the last 25 years **(Fig. 15)**.

Some dressings (like cotton gauze) adhere to the wound bed and cause damage to the newly growing

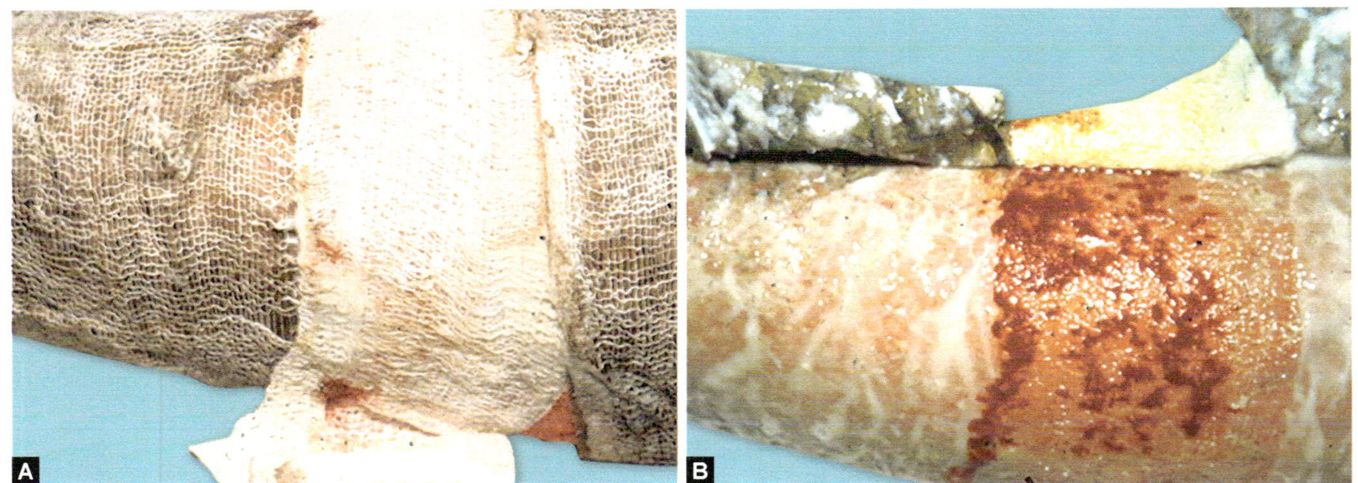

FIGS. 13A AND B: (A) Burn injury treated with boiled potato peel bandage. The middle part of the wound is treated with gauze. (B) Note areas of bleeding from the wound treated with gauze and resultant hemorrhage when the gauze dressing is removed. Other areas are undamaged due to moisture retention and nonadherence.

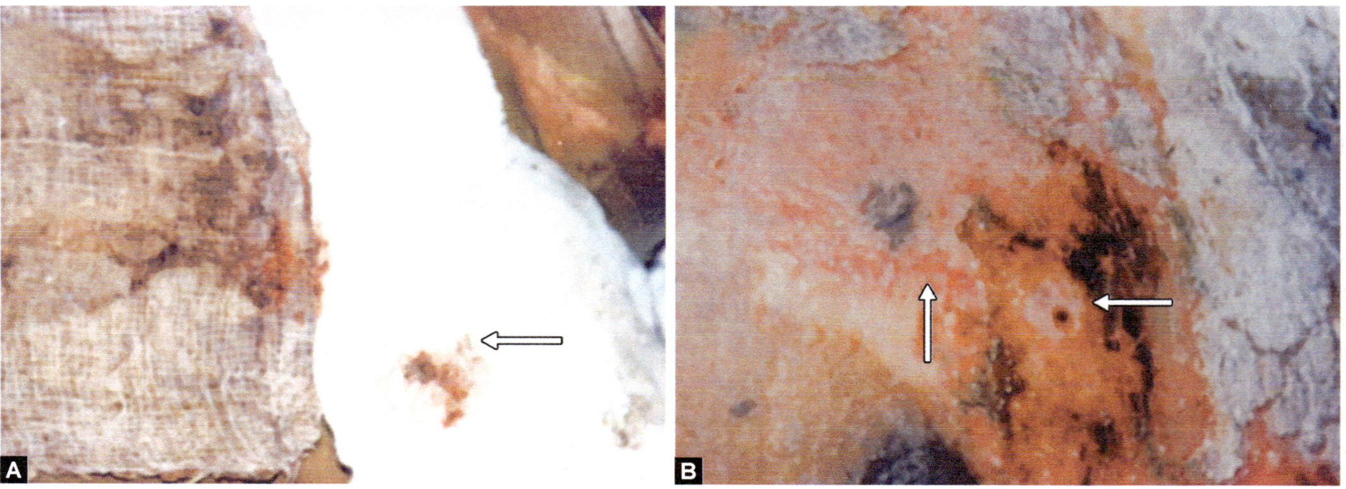

FIGS. 14A TO D: *Continued*

Continued

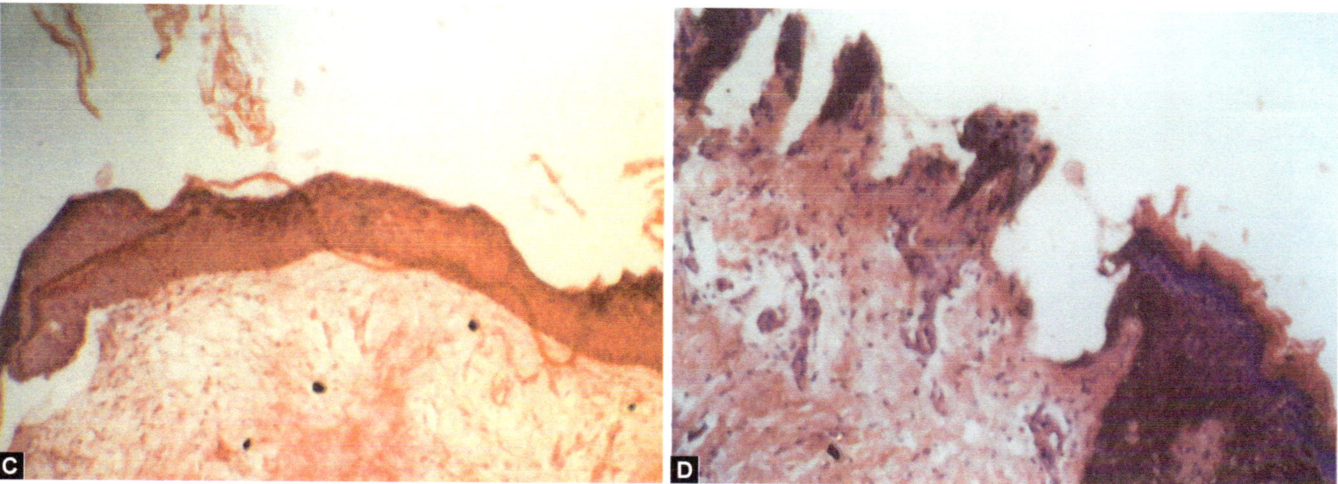

FIGS. 14A TO D: (A) Burn injury on the chest, right side treated with BPP dressing and left side treated with gauze; (B) Note the bleeding on the left side after the dressing change (horizontal arrow); (C) Complete healing of the epidermis can be seen on the side treated with a BPP bandage; (D) Note the broken epidermis in the area treated with gauze.
(BPP: boiled potato peel)

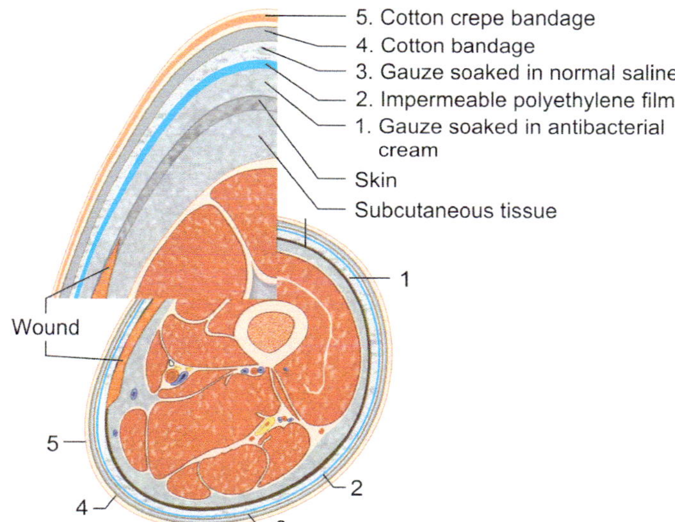

FIG. 15: Polyethylene drape closed dressing layers.[20]

epidermis and the granulation tissue. When the dressing is removed during the dressing changes, there is intense pain and bleeding from the wound bed. This clearly indicates that such dressings may cause significant damage to the healing tissues **(Figs. 13 and 14)**. Occlusive dressings, especially those that have the ability to retain moisture, do not adhere to the wound bed. There is no pain or bleeding during the dressing changes, which indirectly helps in the faster healing of the burn wound **(Figs. 16 to 18)**.

When the dressing becomes dry and firmly adheres to the burn wound, destruction of growing neoepithelium occurs during the change of dressing and delays the process of wound healing.

This epidermal damage is observed during the change of dressing using gauze or similar materials. There is bleeding from the wound and also severe pain, indicating mechanical damage.[9]

Hermans[19] has shown that the infection rate under the occlusive dressings is lower than that under the conventional dressing. *Pseudomonas aeruginosa* disappears in a moist wound environment, and the wounds do heal in spite of bacterial contamination.

Lawrence and Lilly[21] have shown that dressings provide a physical barrier for microorganisms and against bacterial contamination. This helps reduce the overall bacterial load, which the host defense mechanisms have to deal with.[3]

WOUND HEALING OF THE DONOR AREAS

Donor areas also heal in the same manner as burn wounds, i.e., by epithelial migration from the lining of epidermal appendages. Donor sites of the split skin graft are very painful, in the same way as superficial burns, because of exposed nerve endings. When these donor sites are treated with occlusive dressings, they heal satisfactorily and do not cause any problems

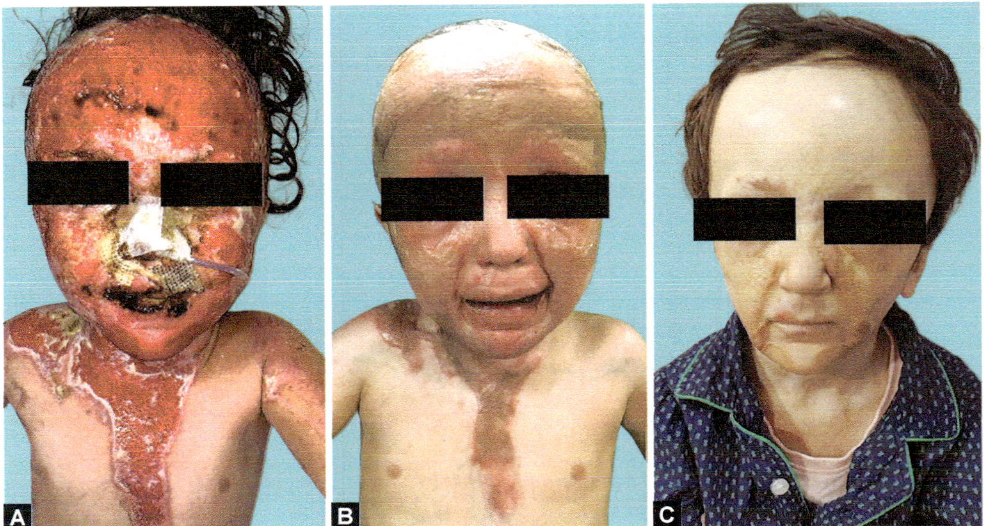

FIGS. 16A TO C: Pediatric facial burns treated with occlusive dressing: (A) 15 days postburn at the time of admission; (B) At the time of discharge; (C) 3 years after surgery.

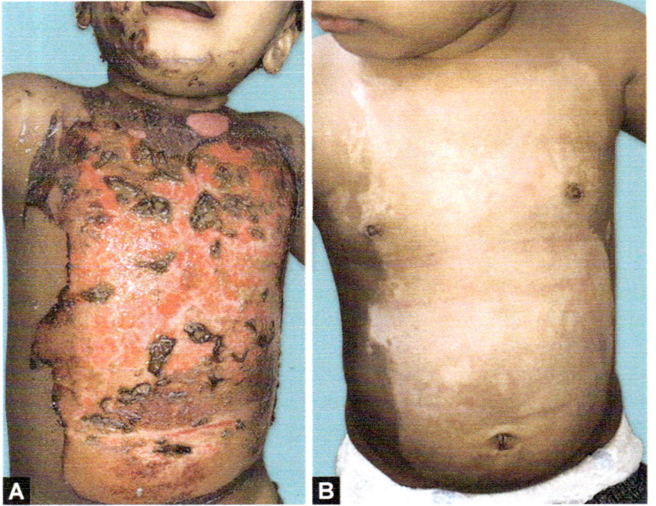

FIGS. 17A AND B: Pediatric chest burns treated with occlusive dressings. (A) 3 days postburn; (B) 2 months after discharge.

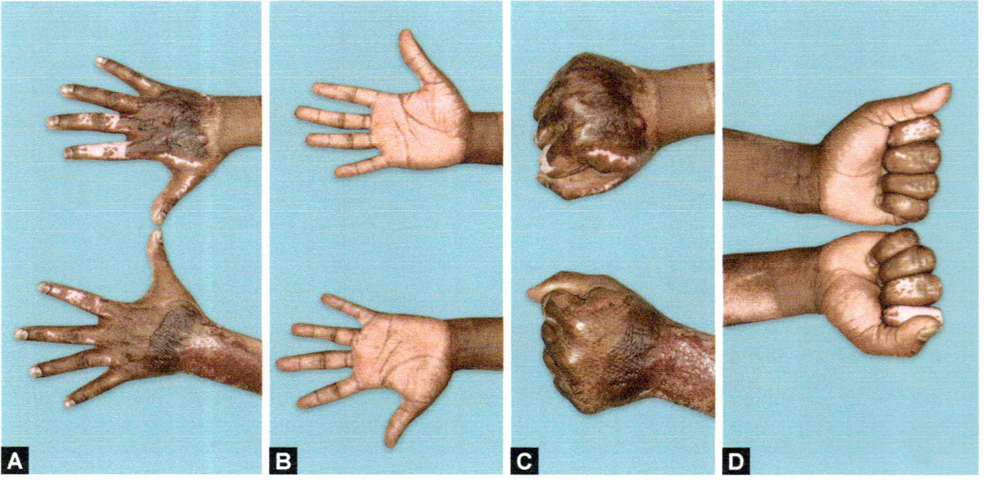

FIGS. 18A TO D: Hand burns treated with occlusive dressings—after complete healing postoperative.

(**Figs. 19A and B**). Occlusive dressing, on the other hand, helps with rapid healing and significant relief of pain.[19,22] The authors have used dry collagen, nonadhesive silver foam dressing (**Figs. 20A and B**), and cadaveric grafts (**Figs. 21A and B**). All these different dressing materials reduce the pain and promote early healing.

SUMMARY

Burn wounds can result from thermal, chemical, electrical, or radiation injuries, leading to varying degrees of tissue damage classified into first, second, and third-degree burns. The pathophysiology of burn wounds involves initial protein denaturation and cellular destruction,

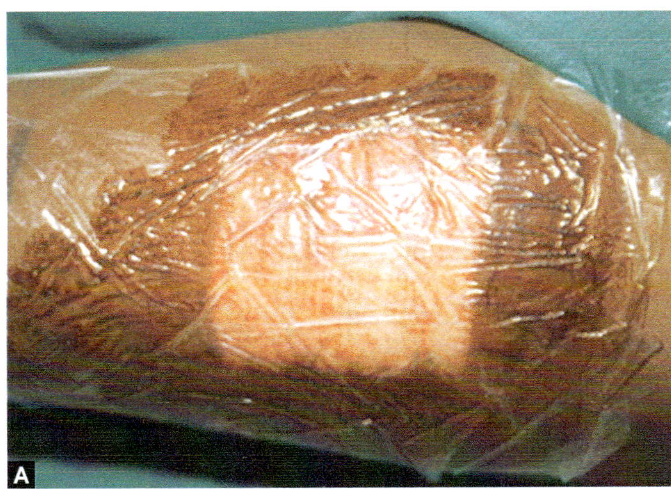

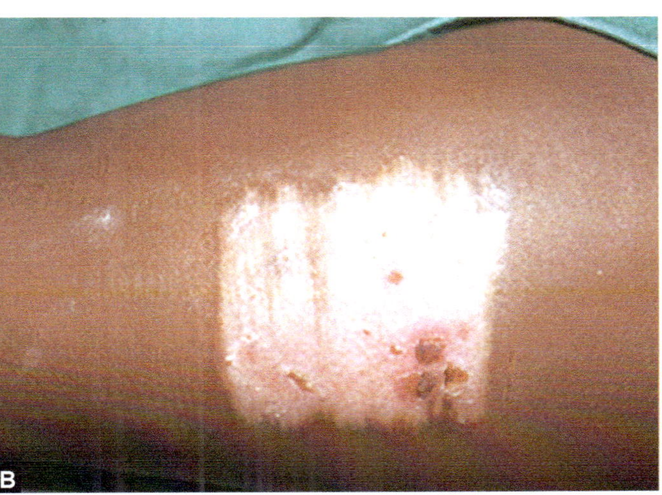

FIGS. 19A AND B: (A) Donor area of a split skin graft treated with cellophane paper; (B) After complete healing on the 10th day.

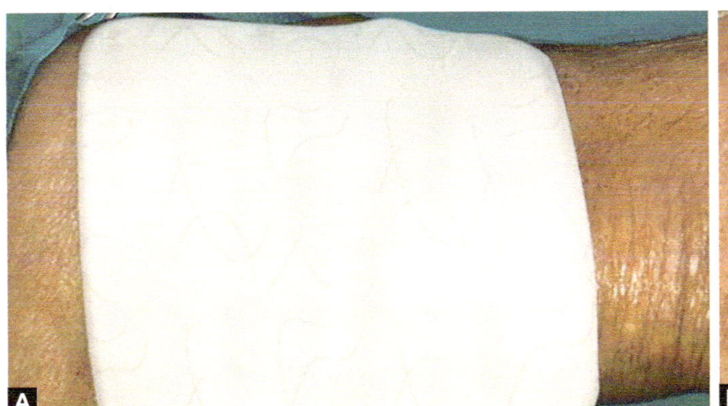

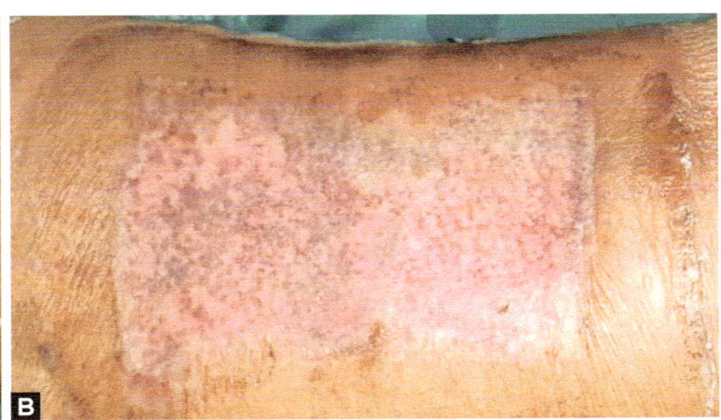

FIGS. 20A AND B: (A) Donor area of a split skin graft treated with a nonadhesive silver foam dressing; (B) After complete healing.

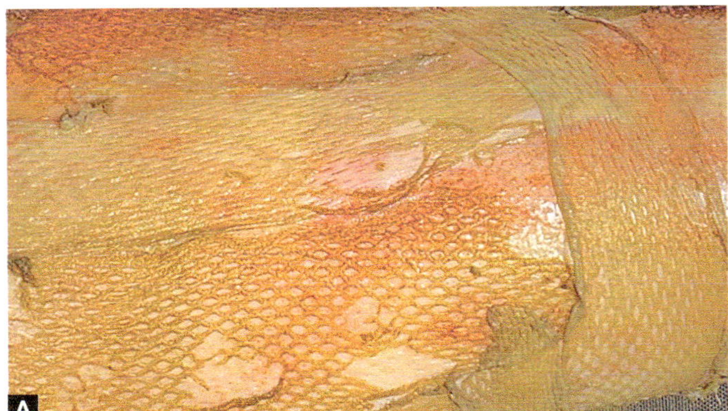

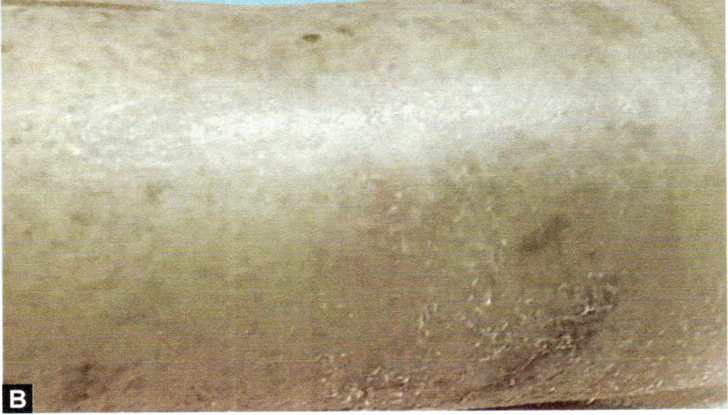

FIGS. 21A AND B: (A) Donor area of a split skin graft treated with human skin allograft (cadaver skin); (B) After complete healing.

triggering an inflammatory response characterized by the release of cytokines and growth factors, increased vascular permeability, and infiltration of immune cells such as neutrophils and macrophages. This inflammatory response results in edema, erythema, and pain.

Histopathologically, burn wounds exhibit distinct zones of injury: the central zone of coagulation with irreversible damage, the surrounding zone of stasis with reduced perfusion and salvage potential, and the outer zone of hyperemia with increased blood flow and minimal damage. Microscopically, burns show coagulation necrosis, cellular debris, and inflammatory infiltrates. Superficial burns affect the epidermis, while deeper burns extend into the dermis and subcutaneous tissue, showing extensive tissue destruction.

The healing of burn wounds progresses through three overlapping phases: Inflammation, proliferation, and remodeling. During the inflammatory phase, immune cells clear debris and pathogens. The proliferative phase involves re-epithelialization, granulation tissue formation, and angiogenesis. Keratinocytes migrate to cover the wound, while fibroblasts produce collagen and extracellular matrix to support new tissue. In the remodeling phase, collagen reorganization and scar formation occur, aiming to restore skin integrity and function. Proper wound care and treatment are crucial to support these processes and prevent complications such as infection, hypertrophic scarring, and contractures. The use of early excision and skin grafting can expedite healing and reduce the risk of complications.

This comprehensive understanding of the pathophysiology, histopathology, and healing of burn wounds is essential for effective management and optimal recovery of burn patients.

REFERENCES

1. Rickatts CR, Squire JR, Topley E. Human skin lipids with particular reference to the self-sterilizing power of the skin. Clin Sci Mol Med. 1951;10:89–111.
2. Williams WG, Philips L. Pathophysiology of the burn wound. In: Herndon DN (Ed), Total Burn Care. London: WB Saunders Company; 1996. p. 64.
3. Moritz AR, Henriquez FC. Studies of thermal injury II: The relative importance of time and surface temperature in the causation of cutaneous burns. Am J Pathol. 1947;23:695-720.
4. Ofeigsson OJ. Water cooling: First-aid treatment for scald burns. Surgery. 1965;57(3):391-00.
5. Cotran RS. The delayed and prolonged vascular leakage in inflammation II. An electron microscope study of the vascular response after thermal injury. Am J Pathol. 1965;46:589-620.
6. Jackson DM. The diagnosis of the depth of burning. Br J Surg. 1953;40:588-96.
7. Zawaki BE. Reversal of capillary stasis and prevention of necrosis in burns. Ann Surg. 1974;180:98-102.
8. Zawaki BE. The local effects of burn injury. In: Boswick JA Jr. (Ed). The Art and Science of Burn Care. Rockville, MD: Aspen Publishers; 1987. p. 27.
9. Winter GD. Effect of air drying and dressings on surface of a wound. Nature. 1993;197:91.
10. Zawaki BE. The natural history of reversible burn injury. Surg Gynecol Obstet. 1974;139:867.
11. Zawaki BE. Reversal of capillary stasis and prevention of necrosis in burns. Ann Surg. 1974;139:98.
12. Lawrence JC. The perinecrotic zone in burns and its influence on healing. Burns. 1975;1:197-206.
13. Janzekovic Z. A new concept in early excision and grafting of burns. J Trauma. 1970;10:1103-8.
14. Groves AR, Lawrence JC. The tangential excision of burns: an experimental study using an animal model. Injury, 1971;3(1):30-9.
15. Hinman CD, Maiback H. Effect of air exposure and occlusion on experimental human skin wounds. Nature. 1963;200:377.
16. Keswani MH, Vartak AM, Patil A, Davies JWL. Histological and bacteriological studies of burn wounds treated with boiled potato peel dressings. Burns. 1990;16 (2):137-43.
17. Pruitt BA, Moncrief JA. Current trends in burn research. J Surg Res. 1967;7:280-93.
18. Hermans MHE, Hermans RP. Duoderm, an alternative for the treatment of smaller burns. Burns. 1986;12:214.
19. Hermans MHE. Treatment of burns with occlusive dressings: Some pathophysiological and quality of life aspects. Burns. 1992;18(Suppl 2):S15-8.
20. Vartak AM. Care of the burn wound: As I do it. Indian J Burns. 2016;24:3-7.
21. Lawrence JC, Lilly HA. Bacterial barrier properties of hydrocolloid dressing in vitro. In: Ryan TJ (Ed). Beyond Occlusion, Wound Care Proceedings. London: Royal Society of Medical Sciences; 1988. p. 75.
22. Vartak AM, Keswani MH, Patil AR, Savitri Sr, Fernandis Sr B. Cellophane-a dressing for split-thickness skin graft donor sites. Burns. 1991;17(3):239-42.

BIBLIOGRAPHY

1. Boswick JA. The Art and Science of Burn Care. Aspen Publishers; 1987.
2. Carrougher GJ. Burn Care and Therapy. Mosby 1998
3. Davies JWL. Physiological Responses to Burning Injury. Washington, DC: Academic Press; 1982.
4. Hanumadas ML, Ramkrishnan M. Handbook on Burn Management. New Delhi: Jaypee Brothers Medical Publishers; 1991.
5. Herndon DN. Total Burn Care. Philadelphia: W B Saunders; 1996.
6. Settle JAD. Principles and Practice of Burns Management. London: Churchill Livingstone; 1996.

CHAPTER

6

Wound Healing in Burns

N Shanmuganathan, Ramyaa Lakshmi TS, Mary Babu

"You were advised his flesh was capable of wounds and scars".

—William Shakespeare, Henry IV

INTRODUCTION

A burn injury is caused by damage to skin and other deeper tissues by extreme heat, flame, and contact with heated objects or chemicals. Burn depth is generally categorized as first, second, or third degree. The treatment of burn wounds depends on the depth, extent, and location of the burn as well as some additional factors.

A first-degree burn is superficial and has characteristics similar to a typical sun burn. The skin is red in color and sensation is intact. In fact, it is usually painful and damage is limited to the epidermis characterized by erythema and hyperemia. Second-degree burns extend into the dermis to varying depths, involving papillary dermis alone or along with reticular dermis. In third-degree burns, the damage progresses to the point of death of full thickness of skin. They are painless due to damage to nerve endings, exposing subcutaneous fat layer. It should be noted that the skin is the body's first defense against infection by microorganisms. Any damage to the skin predisposes a burn victim to infections not only at the site of the wound but also systemically. In addition to depth, the extent of the burn, i.e., the total body surface area (TBSA) burnt is also significant. This is measured in terms of percentage of TBSA burnt. Burns that cover >15% of the total body surface in adults can lead to hypovolemic shock requiring hospitalization for intravenous fluid resuscitation and wound care.

Location of burn on the body is even more important than the above factors as far as wound healing is concerned. In acute stage, burns of the face or signs of burns to the nose or mouth may require urgent guarding of the patient's airway, as edema can result in life-threatening obstruction of the airway. Full thickness burns that extend circumferentially around limbs require their surgical release, escharotomy, to prevent gangrene of distal limb. Deep dermal burns heal with hypertrophic scarring (HTS) while full thickness burns, if not split skin grafted on raw areas lead to contractures.

FACTORS AFFECTING WOUND HEALING

There are several factors that affect the wound healing either beneficially or adversely. Any attempt to improve healing or prevent complications of healing should concentrate on the causes of the impairment.

Age

Age affects many aspects of wound repair. Several investigations have shown that rate of healing appears to slow down with increasing age. The fibroblast proliferation is at a slower rate in older individuals and they also have a decreased synthetic capability. The soluble collagen decreases and insoluble cross-linked collagen increases with age. The amount of elastin increases but the numbers of elastic fibers decrease to make skin less elastic. Possibly, in the earlier stages of life, wound healing is faster as compared to older individuals as it more closely resembles tissue regeneration seen in simpler animals. As a result, older patients require prolonged hospitalization compared to younger patients.

Infection

The effects of infection on tissue repair can be divided into local or systemic effects. Several bacterial strains (*Pseudomonas* and *Staphylococcus aureus)* have been found to impair wound healing and nosocomial infections are common in burn patients which include antibiotic-resistant strains like methicillin-resistant *Staphylococcus aureus* (MRSA) and *Candida* fungi. Bacterial contamination leads to an increased inflammatory response with release of more cytokines to attract more of the cells needed for wound repair. However, the wound becomes overwhelmed with virulent microorganisms and the bacterial proteases and the products of inflammatory cells lead to local tissue damage.

Nutrition

One of the major breakthroughs in the survival of burn patients has been made possible through aggressive nutritional support. Early nutritional support helps in reducing the duration of hospitalization of patients, especially adults. Extreme consumption of carbohydrates and fat may lead to systemic inflammation and immunosuppression respectively whereas an adequate consumption of proteins plays vital roles in the process of wound healing.

Vitamins and Trace Elements

Some vitamins are clearly important for normal tissue repair. Vitamin C is essential for normal collagen synthesis and deficiency leads to defects in connective tissue and impaired wound healing. Vitamin A induces fibroblasts to differentiate and to enhance collagen synthesis. Topical application of vitamin A may also improve healing. Vitamin E is a potent antioxidant and is likely to improve healing.

Deficiencies in trace elements can also lead to problems in wound healing. These trace elements are actually metals that are required for enzyme functions. Iron, zinc, copper, manganese, and selenium are the most important trace metals during the process of healing as they are involved from the initial days of healing at different stages imparting specific functions.

Oxygen

Oxygen is very essential to healing and it has been found that higher levels of oxygen may be even more beneficial. The treatment of wounds with hyperbaric oxygen is based on this hypothesis.

Steroids

The most notorious drugs associated with altered healing are steroids. Steroids are powerful inhibitors of the inflammatory response and, therefore, have the potential to inhibit wound healing. Collagen synthesis and fibrosis are inhibited with steroid use.

Chemotherapeutic Agents

They act by killing rapidly growing cells with the hope of eliminating proliferating cancer cells. However, the healing wound also requires cellular proliferation. Thus most of the chemotherapeutic agents used, locally or systematically, impair healing.

Radiation

The impairment in wound healing seen after acute radiation exposure is also due to inhibition of proliferating cells. Radiation may cause chronic vasculitis that impairs local blood supply and predisposes the patient to impaired healing.

Local factors pertain mainly to persistence of debris within the wound, for example, devitalized tissues, clots, foreign material including sutures and bacterial contamination. These can act as a physical barrier to the ordered development of granulation tissue and collagen deposition or may exaggerate the evoked inflammatory response. Ultimately, this can change the way the tissues heal, changing primary to secondary healing or resolution to organization. Local tissue hypoxia, either chronic (e.g., caused by radiation enteritis, atherosclerosis, or diabetic microvascular disease) or more acute (e.g., caused by vascular damage or tight sutures) may compromise healing. If wound is not closed primarily it will heal but more slowly than those held together by sutures.

Patients with uncontrolled diabetes suffer from a variety of problems in healing. High blood sugar levels decrease both neutrophil chemotaxis and phagocytic ability. Additionally, a sugar-rich environment favors microbial growth, further interfering with healing.

WOUND HEALING: GENERAL

A wound is a break in the epithelial integrity of the skin and may be accompanied by disruption of the structure and function of underlying normal tissues. A wound may result from precise disruption of tissue by the surgeon's knife (incision) or there may be widespread damage of tissues (e.g., after major musculoskeletal trauma and burns). A wound may also result from a contusion, laceration, or an abrasion. The continuity of the skin must be restored expeditiously as it plays a crucial role in maintaining homeostasis.

Wound healing is a highly complex physiological process. It involves the interplay of various cellular and biochemical components, which drive the repair cascade. Hemostasis is an extremely intricate physiological mechanism. The repair cascade is triggered by the interaction of multiple cellular and molecular components. Furthermore, a number of enzyme pathways activate during tissue repair and aid in tissue healing. Blood components extravasate when blood vessels are damaged due to tissue injury. Following this, blood coagulation and platelet aggregation occur, which produces a fibrin-rich clot that plugs the wound's discontinuity and restores hemostasis. After that, inflammatory cells start to migrate to the wound site and debride the wound. This initiates the inflammatory stage of the healing process of wounds. The development of new blood vessels, or angiogenesis, within the granulation tissue that has just begun to form, comes next. The granulation tissue then changes into a scar, which is the end result of the healing process.

While the creation of tissues with the same structure and functions as an intact skin would be the ideal outcome of coordinated healing, regeneration is rare (with significant exceptions such as early fetal recuperation). However, healing does produce a good structural and functional outcome—although one that is not exactly the same. It appears that several growth factors and cytokines secreted at the wound site tightly control the processes involved in wound healing. Changes that impede prompt, regulated healing processes increase tissue damage and delay healing.

WOUND HEALING: TYPES

Primary healing (healing by first intention) occurs when a wound is closed within 12–24 hours of its creation (e.g., clean surgical incision and clean laceration). The wound edges are approximated directly using sutures, tissue glue, tapes, or a mechanical device. Because of an appropriate balance between all phases of the healing process [including cellular proliferation, collagen metabolism, activity of matrix metalloproteinase (MMP), and degradation of the extracellular matrix (ECM)], the wounds heal well and proceed rapidly toward complete closure.

Secondary healing: When there is a significant loss of soft tissues in a wound, such as after a laparotomy or substantial trauma, secondary healing, also known as healing by second intention, takes place. The original tissue architecture cannot be restored by epithelial cell regeneration alone. Granulation tissue grows inward from the wound edge, and ECM accumulates as collagen is laid down **(Fig. 1)**. Hence, following wound contraction and epithelialization, these full-thickness wounds close. For instance, significant skin abnormalities might contract to 5–10% of their initial size in just 6 weeks. Myofibroblasts are believed to be essential to this kind of repair because of their structural similarities to smooth muscle cells and fibroblasts.

They start to show up in the wound within 3 days after injury, and reach their peak number in 10–21 days. Secondary intention healing is slower, more likely to result in functional restriction, and contractures, especially over joints.

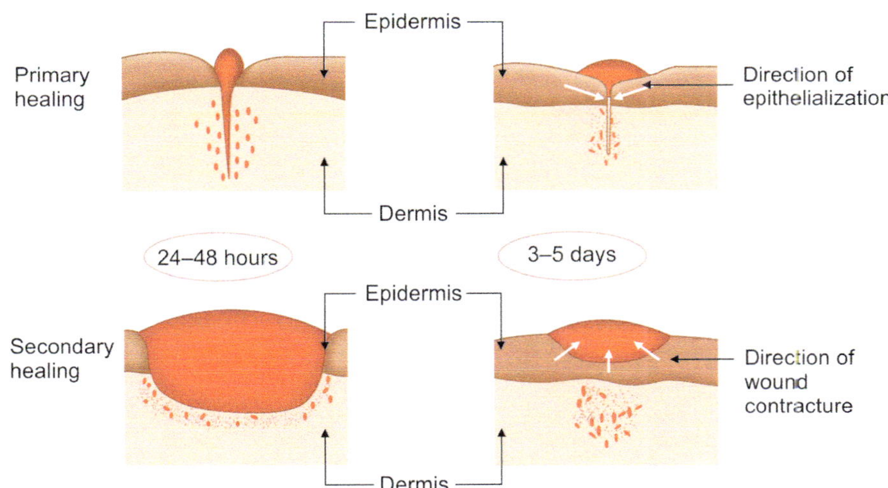

FIG. 1: Primary and secondary healing.

Source: Adapted from: Halloran CM, Slavin JP. Pathophysiology of wound healing. Surgery (Oxford). 2002;20(5):i-v.

Injuries including superficial dermal burns, donor sites for split-thickness skin grafts, and abrasions involving both the epidermis and the papillary layer of the dermis can heal of their own. Healing occurs purely by epithelialization from the epidermal appendages and anatomical and physiological restoration is virtually complete. Healing of some very deep dermal and full thickness burns require skin grafting or else a contracture forms.

PHASES IN WOUND HEALING

Inflammatory Phase

One of the body's first natural response to damage is inflammation, which works quite well. It is a crucial outcome of damage and one that typically results in tissue healing and functional restoration. Vascular and cellular responses are two subtypes of the inflammatory response. Cardinal symptoms of inflammation, such as redness, swelling, and heat, are produced early in the wounding process by local vasodilatation, blood and fluid extravasation into the extravascular space, and blockage of lymphatic outflow. This acute inflammatory response typically lasts for 24–48 hours, but in certain circumstances, it can last up to 2 weeks. Tissue injury causes blood vessel disruption and bleeding. Platelets adhere, aggregate, and release many mediators to facilitate coagulation. Although hemostasis is the major function of blood coagulation, a secondary but equally important function of platelets is to initiate the healing cascade via release of chemo-attractants and growth factors. At the same time, the clot provides a matrix scaffold for the recruitment of cells to an injured area. In response to these important mediators, leukocytes, including neutrophils and macrophages infiltrate the wounded area and assist in cleaning and removing damaged tissue debris and foreign particles. Once in the wound site, activated macrophages release several important growth factors and cytokines, initiating granulation tissue formation **(Fig. 2)**.

Cellular Response and Inflammation

Leukocyte infiltration into the damaged area characterizes the cellular response of inflammatory phase. At the site of injury, neutrophils and monocytes predominate throughout the early stages of inflammation. Monocytes and neutrophils start to migrate from capillaries into the injured tissue soon after the damage, with neutrophils arriving in large quantities first. As inflammation progresses, tissue-derived monocytes, or macrophages, become more prevalent and neutrophil counts decrease. Mast cells and chemotactic substances generated during hemostasis draw neutrophils and monocytes to the

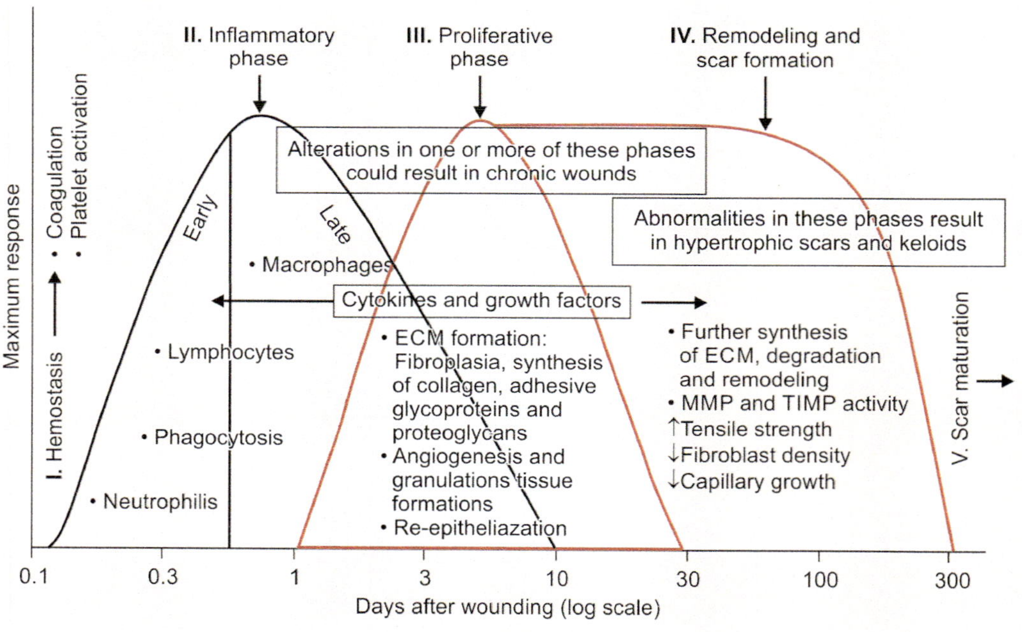

FIG. 2: Phases of wound healing.

(ECM: extracellular matrix; MMP: metalloproteinases; TIMP: tissue inhibitors of metalloproteinases)

Source: Adapted from Clark RA. In: Goldsmith LA (Ed). Physiology, biochemistry, and molecular biology of the skin, 2nd edition, Vol. I. New York: Oxford University Press; 1991. p. 577.

wound. Important intercellular adhesion molecules are also upregulated by coagulation-related chemotactic factors, including fibrinopeptides released by fibrinogen, kallikrein, and fibrin breakdown products. Other sources of chemotactic signals for the recruitment of leukocytes include substances generated by mast cells, such as tumor necrosis factor (TNF), histamine, proteases, leukotrienes (LTs), and cytokines [interleukins (ILs)]. Strong leukocyte chemotactic factors include growth factors such as platelet-derived growth factor (PDGF) and TGF-κ. Neutrophils' cell surface integrin receptors improve cell-matrix connections once they reach the wound site. As a result, bacteria and damaged matrix proteins in the wound bed that may extrude with eschar can be killed and phagocytosed by neutrophils. Neutrophil infiltration typically lasts a few days; however, wound contamination increases the amount of time neutrophils are present in the wound and can cause a delay in healing. During the later stages of the inflammatory phase, monocytes migrate into tissue gaps and develop into bigger phagocytic macrophages, which quickly take over as the main cell type. Some of the same chemoattractants that draw neutrophils also draw monocytes to the wound site. Monocyte-specific chemoattractants such macrophage inflammatory protein-1 and monocyte chemoattractant protein-1 produce signals that aid in the recruitment of monocytes. Specific chemoattractants for monocytes include collagen fragments, fibronectin fragments, and thrombin, which are byproducts of ECM disintegration. The most significant regulatory cells in the inflammatory response are thought to be macrophages. Macrophages scavenge tissue debris, phagocytose harmful organisms, digest and kill them, and eliminate any neutrophils that remain. Bacterial, cellular, and tissue phagocytoses are achieved by attaching to the extracellular membrane and then releasing physiologically active oxygen intermediates and enzymatic proteins, which cause further destruction.

Chemical Mediators of Inflammation

Numerous chemical compounds play a role in both initiating and managing inflammation. Together, these substances function as either antagonists or protagonists of inflammation. These are classified as follows: arachidonic acid metabolites of prostaglandins (PGs) and LTs; cytokines and growth factors; free radicals of nitric oxide and oxygen-derived free radicals; vasoactive amines of histamine and serotonin, plasma proteases of kinins and complements; plasma proteins of the coagulation system (**Fig. 3**). The following stage of healing is facilitated by macrophage-secreted PDGF and epidermal growth factor (EGF).

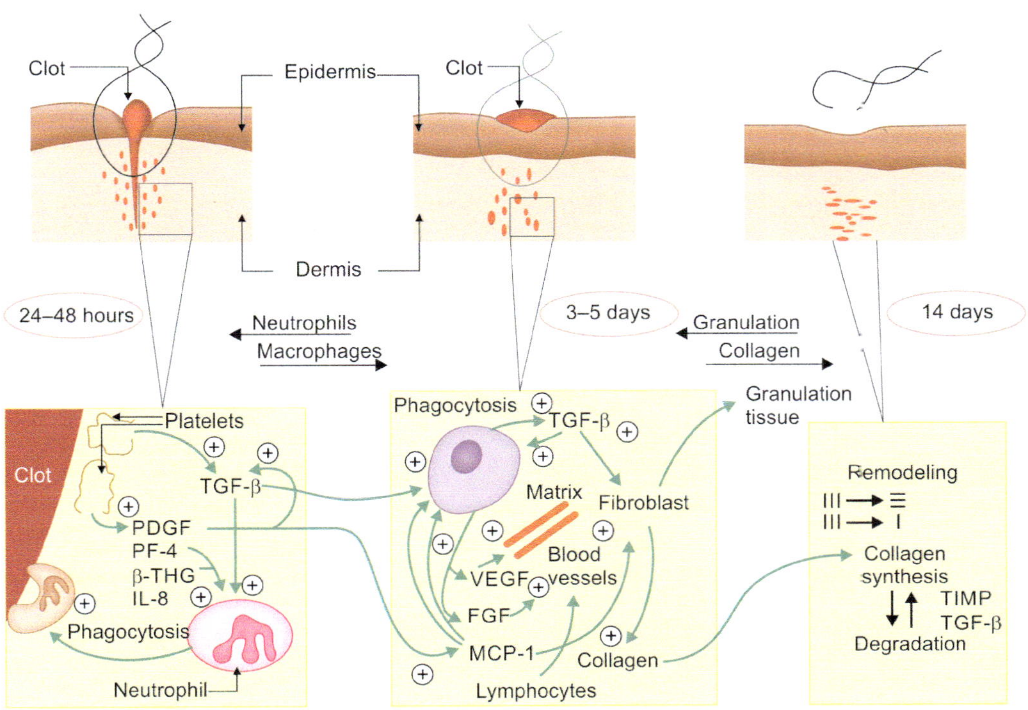

FIG. 3: Cytokines and healing.

(FGF: fibroblast growth factor; IL: interleukin; MCP-1: monocyte chemoattractant protein-1; PF-4: platelet factor-4; PDGF: platelet-derived growth factor; TGF-β: transforming growth factor-beta; THG: tetrahydrogestrinone; TIMP: tissue inhibitor of metalloproteinase; VEGF: vascular endothelial growth factor)

Source: Adapted from Halloran CM, Slavin JP. Pathophysiology of wound healing. Surgery (Oxford). 2002;20(5):i-v.

Proliferative Phase

The initial inflammatory responses to injury provide the necessary framework to the subsequent production of a new functional barrier. In this phase of healing, cellular activity predominates. The major events during this phase are the creation of a permeability barrier (i.e., re-epithelialization), the establishment of appropriate blood supply (i.e., angiogenesis), and reinforcement of the injured dermal tissue (i.e., fibroplasia).

Re-epithelialization (Fig. 4)

The process of healing in a cutaneous injury that restores the continuity in the epidermis is called re-epithelialization. There is migration of neighboring epidermal keratinocytes into wound, growth of keratinocytes utilized to supplement the advancing and migrating epithelial tongue, differentiation of the neoepithelium into a stratified epidermis, and the restoration of an intact basement membrane zone (BMZ) that joins the dermis and epidermis.

Keratinocyte Migration

An initial step in the re-epithelialization of wounds is keratinocyte migration. Within 24 hours of an epidermal defect, the keratinocytes begin to migrate from the free margins of the skin defect. In partial skin defects thickness, keratinocyte migration happens not only from the edges of the wound but also from the residual skin appendages. Hair bulb or the germinative part of the hair is the reservoir of keratinocytes and during wound healing epidermal stem cells originate from here.

A number of processes must occur within keratinocytes in preparation for migration. Approximately 12 hours after wounding, a series of events, such as flattening and elongation of keratinocytes, development of pseudopod-like projections of lamellipodia, loss of cell-cell and cell-matrix contacts, retraction of intracellular tonofilaments, and formation of actin filaments at the edge of their cytoplasm, occurs. Although keratinocytes are migrating, their proliferative potential is inhibited. Migrating basal keratinocytes may express selective cell surface markers such as CD44 and some markers usually expressed by squamous cells.

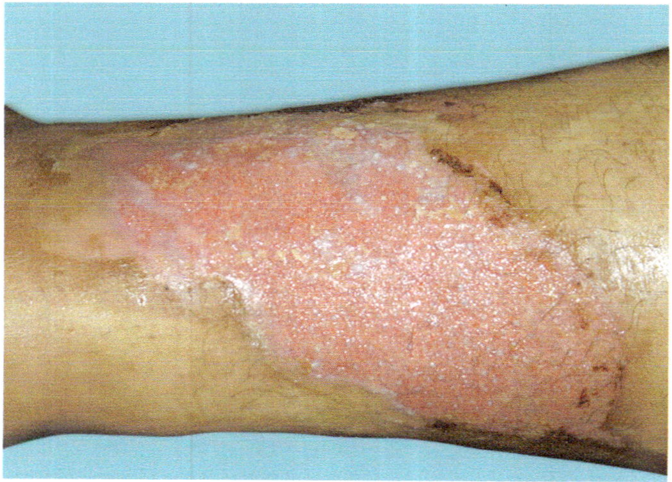

FIG. 4: Superficial dermal burns on lower leg showing re-epithelialization. The epithelial buds can be seen over the surface.

Several elements have been implicated in keratinocyte migration, including the ECM, integrin receptors, MMPs, and growth factors. An early provisional matrix formed by fibrin, fibronectin, and type V collagen enables keratinocytes to migrate and dissect under eschar and debris that may be covering the wound. Keratinocytes use their surface integrin receptors to interact with a fibronectin-rich provisional matrix. The direction of migration is also regulated by the binding of keratinocytes to integrin receptors on the newly formed collagen molecules in the wound bed. Dissociation of this binding allows the keratinocytes to migrate forward. MMPs also play an important role in keratinocyte migration by their involvement in this dissociation. MMPs, such as MMP-9, are produced by migrating keratinocytes which particularly break down type-IV collagen and laminins in the basement membrane. This enables cells to move into the wound after leaving the basement membrane. MMP-1 breaks down keratinocyte adhesion to fibrillar collagen and promotes keratinocyte migration in wounds.

Keratinocyte Proliferation

Re-epithelialization also involves increased proliferation of keratinocytes located near the cells of the tongue of the migrating front. This proliferating source of keratinocytes ensures an adequate supply of cells to migrate and cover the wound. When migration ceases, possibly as a result of contact inhibition, keratinocytes reattach themselves to the underlying substratum, reconstitute the basement membrane, and then resume the process of terminal differentiation to generate a stratified epidermis. One can observe that there are single-layered keratinocytes toward the wound center whereas there are multiple-layered or stratified keratinocytes near the wound edges. Proliferation is followed by differentiation, as evidenced by the significantly elevated proliferative index at the wound center. The wound margin is where the neoepidermal differentiation (keratins 1/10, filaggrin, and loricrin) and dermoepidermal junction regeneration (laminin 5 and collagen IV) are more advanced. It has been demonstrated that keratinocyte migration, proliferation, and re-epithelialization are significantly influenced by EGF, keratinocyte growth factor, and TGF-α.

Restoration of the BMZ: Skin integrity and function cannot be considered as restored unless there is an intact basement membrane zone (BMZ) between the epidermis and dermis. The BMZ reforms 7–9 days following re-epithelialization. The BMZ forms an adhesive structure because the inferior or lower portion anchors fibrils to stabilize the attachment to the underlying dermis, while the superior features act as an attachment site for basal keratinocytes through the creation of a hemidesmosome-anchoring filament complex. The various hereditary blistering illnesses known as epidermolysis bullosa serves as proof of the significance of BMZ. Blister development and ulcer formation are caused by mutations of one of several BMZ proteins, such as hemidesmosome collagen XVII in atrophic epidermolysis bullosa and deficiency of collagen VII anchoring fibrils in dystrophic epidermolysis bullosa.

Collagen and laminins are the two main ECM proteins that make up the BMZ of skin. The most prevalent component, collagen IV, creates a three-dimensional lattice network in the zone and is also known as the electron-dense or lamina densa. From the lamina densa to the upper papillary dermis, collagen VII proteins—also referred to as anchoring fibrils—form an anchoring plaque. Collagen XVII, also called bullous pemphigoid antigen (sometimes referred to as bullous pemphigoid antigen-2 or bullous pemphigoid antigen 180), is a 180 kDa transmembrane protein that is found on the hemidesmosome complex of basal keratinocytes. It is another significant type of collagen. The main noncollagenous ECM constituents of a variety of BMZs found in human tissues are laminins. Within the BMZ of the dermoepidermal junction, there exist several laminins. The two main laminins in skin BMZ, laminin 5 (a3b3c2) and laminin 10 (a5b1c1), are made up of a, b, and c subunits and have been discovered to be actively involved in wound repair. Following a lesion, keratinocytes in the front edge migrate and deposit laminin 5, which acts as a trail for other keratinocytes to follow. Laminin 10, a novel laminin member found in the lamina densa, has just been described. It was also shown that a significant laminin of cutaneous microvascular blood vessels is laminin 10. Hair growth abnormalities and discontinuities in the BMZ lamina densa were seen in the skin of mice lacking laminin 10.

Reconstitution of the Dermis

After an injury, dermal reconstitution starts about 3–4 days later. It is clinically characterized by the formation of granulation tissue, which involves the angiogenesis (the formation of new blood vessels) and fibroplasia (the accumulation of fibroblasts and ground matrices). By providing scaffolding and contact guidance for cells to migrate into wound spaces and for angiogenesis and fibroplasia to occur in an attempt to replace the injured dermal tissue, the fibrin clot, which is rich in fibronectin, contributes to the formation of the provisional ECM that supports the formation of granulation tissue.

Fibroplasia

The term "fibroplasia" refers to a process in which fibroblasts proliferate, migrate into wound fibrin clots, and form new collagen and other matrix proteins which are involved in the development of granulation tissue. Fibroblasts in the wound margins multiply as a first response to injury, and by day 4 or so, they start to move into the clot's provisional matrix, where they deposit a collagen-rich matrix made of collagen, proteoglycans, and elastin. After migrating inside the wound, the fibroblasts progressively adopt profibrotic phenotypes and shift their primary role to the production of proteins. Fibroblasts engage in wound contraction and are also modulated into various myofibroblast phenotypes.

Collagen and fibronectin, two structural components of the early ECM, operate as a reservoir for growth factors and cytokines as well as a scaffold for contact guiding, which helps in the production of granulation tissue. One of the main ingredients of the gel-like substance that is first produced and increases fibroblast activity is fibronectin, a glycoprotein. Fibronectin gives fibroblasts an adherent foundation for cell migration and enables them to attach to the ECM. In addition, the fibronectin matrix mediates wound contraction and acts as a scaffold for collagen fibrils. A portion of the major fibroblastic chemotactic factors come from the wound's macrophages. PDGF and TGF-κ may both increase the expression of integrin receptors and promote fibroblast migration. Among other factors, fibroblast migration and proliferation are regulated by EGF and fibroblast growth factor. Another factor that promotes fibroblast multiplication is the low oxygen and acidic environment in the center of wound. This stimulus decreases as angiogenesis advances with the creation of new vasculature and an enhanced ability to deliver oxygen.

Angiogenesis

Angiogenesis refers to new vessel growth by the sprouting of preexisting vessels adjacent to the wound. As in most normal adult tissues, dermal blood vasculatures remain quiescent. In response to the injury, microvascular endothelial cells initiate an angiogenic process consisting of activation of endothelial cells. Newly generated vessels supply growing tissues with nourishment and oxygen while also taking role in the creation of granulation tissue.

Furthermore, for inflammatory cells to penetrate the site of damage, they must interact with blood vessels. Cytokines, or physiologically active chemicals, are also produced and secreted by endothelial cells during angiogenesis.

Angiogenesis is characterized by directed migration, several mitogenic stimuli and phenotypic changes in endothelial cells.

Cytokines released by macrophages stimulate angiogenesis during wound healing, as do low-oxygen tension, lactic acid and biogenic amines produced in the wound. Several growth factors have been shown to play critical roles in wound angiogenesis, including vascular endothelial growth factor (VEGF), angiopoietins, fibroblast growth factor, and TGF-β. VEGF, also known as vascular permeability factor, which exerts its biologic activity predominantly on endothelial cells, is a key mediator of angiogenesis.

Formation of the Extracellular Matrix

Besides providing turgor to soft tissues and rigidity to bone, ECM supplies a substratum for cell adhesion and critically regulates the growth, movement, and differentiation of the cells within it. The ECM consists of fibrous structural proteins (collagens and elastin) and an interstitial matrix composed of adhesive glycoproteins embedded in a proteoglycan and glycosaminoglycan (GAG) gel. The seemingly random array of interstitial matrix in connective tissues soon becomes highly organized around epithelial cells, endothelial cells, and smooth muscle cells, forming the specialized basement membrane (which directs cell polarity and is required for the orderly renewal of the epithelial tissue).

Fibroblasts produce collagens, which are the most prevalent protein family in the body. They are essential to the healing of wounds because they give all tissues strength and integrity to all the tissues. Collagen synthesis is stimulated during the proliferative and remodeling stages by PDGF, basic fibroblast growth factor, TGF-β, IL-1, and TNF. The three protein α-chains that make up collagens are braided into a triple helix that resembles a rope. Each α-polypeptide has a glycine molecule at every third position, which allows the separate chains to interweave firmly. About 20 different forms of collagen are formed by >30 different α-chains, some of which might be exclusive to cells and tissues. Most of the connective tissue in wound healing is made up of collagen types like I, III, and V that form fibrils because of the triple helices' lateral crosslinking; other collagen types like type IV are nonfibrillar and end up as parts of the basement membrane. Adhesive glycoproteins, which include fibronectin, laminin, and thrombospondin, are structurally varied proteins that connect the elements of the ECM to one another and to cells.

- Fibronectin is a disulfide-linked heterodimer (400 kDa) and is connected to basement membranes, pericellular matrix, and cell surfaces. It may attach to cell integrins and has specialized domains that bind to a variety of ECM components, including collagen, fibrin, and proteoglycans. Cell adhesion, migration, and spread can be directly mediated by adhesive matrix proteins like fibronectin. Through the activation of intracellular signaling pathways, fibronectin also increases the sensitivity of specific cells (such as endothelium) to the proliferative action of growth factors.
- Integrins are a family of α/β heterodimeric glycoproteins that mediate cell-cell and cell-matrix adhesion. They are important in the integration of function between the ECM and the cytoskeleton.

Proteoglycans consist of GAGs (e.g., dermatan sulfate and heparan sulfate) linked to a protein backbone; they help to regulate the structure and permeability of the ECM. Proteoglycans can modulate the growth and differentiation of cells (e.g., syndecan binds ECM collagen, fibronectin, thrombospondin and basic fibroblast growth factor and associates with the intracellular actin cytoskeleton to maintain the normal morphology of epithelial sheets). GAGs without a protein core (e.g., hyaluronan) are important constituents of the ECM.

Formation of granulation tissue in 3–5 days (indicative of optimal healing) is well established. Granulation tissue has a pink, soft, and granular gross appearance (such as that seen beneath the scab of a skin wound). Histologically, it is denoted by proliferating fibroblasts and loops of capillaries in a loose ECM. This phase is characterized by angiogenesis or formation of new blood vessels from preexisting vessels at the site of injury (neovascularization).

Remodeling Phase

The process of remodeling involves the matrix deposition and subsequent alterations over time. During the proliferative phase, granulation tissue rich in type III collagen and blood vessels replaces the fibrin clot formed in the early inflammatory phase, and this process continues until the end, when a collagenous scar primarily composed of type I collagen and much less developed blood vessels replaces the original clot. The alteration in the composition of the ECM is one of the features of wound remodeling. Collagen fibers give dermal tissue its structure, strength, and stiffness. Collagen makes up about 80% of the dry weight of proteins. In healthy adults, type I collagen accounts for approximately

80% while type III collagen constitutes 10% of collagens in the dermis.

During the initial stages of wound healing, type III collagen—which is mostly produced by fibroblasts in granulation tissue—is present in large quantities, just like in the fetal dermis. After 48–72 hours, type III collagen is first seen and reaches its peak secretion in 5–7 days.

Early in the healing process, the total amount of collagen grows and reaches its peak 2–3 weeks following the injury. The dermis eventually reverts to the stable preinjury phenotype, which is primarily composed of type I collagen, over a duration of 1 year or more. Tensile strength, a functional measure of collagen, rises to 40% of its preinjury strength at 1 month and keeps rising for an year, eventually reaching 70% of its preinjury strength. As a wound heals, type-III collagen degradation and type-I collagen synthesis rise, resulting in a steady turnover of collagen. The synthesis of new collagen and the lysis of old collagen are closely regulated processes that enable this conversion in the dermis, and MMPs play a major role in this process. The biomechanical stress and strain applied to a healed wound can serve as the catalyst for this conversion. MMPs are produced during wound healing in response to cytokines, growth factors, and ECM cell interaction. Normally, MMPs are either undetectable or present at low levels in resting tissue.

The final phase of wound healing is resolution. It involves remodeling of ECM and contraction of the wound. Contraction of the wound occurs after formation of the granulation tissue and requires the fibroblasts to assume a myofibroblast phenotype. Remodeling of the ECM, which leads to the conversion of granulation tissue to scar tissue, follows this, and is dependent on the continual synthesis and degradation of collagen fibrils. All of these repair processes involve regulating mechanisms with participation of metalloproteinases which are involved in regulating cytokines and chemokines, which are mostly produced by resident cells (fibroblasts, endothelium, and epithelium), and these are what shape inflammation. By cleaving these mediators from the cell surface, processing them to boost their activity, or degrading them, MMPs can activate these mediators and block inflammatory signals. In order to encourage re-epithelialization, MMPs can also break parts of cell-matrix and cell-cell junctions inside the epithelium. Moreover, MMPs have a role in remodeling the ECM of scars through direct proteolytic destruction of proteins like collagen or indirectly through their influence on cell behavior. In addition to having an impact on the control of inflammation, ECM modification is essential to the resolution of wound healing.

As a result, MMPs are important regulators of several aspects of tissue repair. By studying more about these enzymes and how they interact with their substrates, we can improve our understanding of wound healing and identify new treatment avenues.

FETAL VERSUS ADULT

The process of wound healing is intricate and involves the migration, proliferation, and differentiation of cells as well as the production of ECM and remodeling of matrix. Several of these mechanisms are shared by both wound healing and development. Significant distinctions between the healing of wounds in adults and fetuses have been shown in various studies. In a fetus, healing happens quickly through a regenerative process without leaving scars, but in an adult, scarring results, which frequently limits tissue function and prevents further growth. The sterile aqueous fetal environment, the developmental stage of the fetus, or a combination of these elements may influence the fetal response to a lesion. The adult's regular tissue architecture is disrupted by the vast, parallel bundles of collagen that are characteristic of scar tissue. These bundles are observed running across the wound site, roughly at right angles to the basement membrane. Therefore, one of the primary distinctions between adult and fetal wound healing is the regulation and organization of collagen fibrillogenesis. The creation of collagen fibrils is a complicated process that is still not fully understood. The same fibrils contain collagen types I, III, and V, and interactions between them in vitro will change the size of the fibrils. Collagen fibrillogenesis is probably also influenced by interactions with other macromolecules. Fibronectin and proteoglycans both change the size of fibrils.

Studies have revealed that fetal wounds contain high quantities of hyaluronic acid, and that adding hyaluronic acid to an adult tympanic membrane lesion reduces scar formation and modifies the degree of collagen organization within the wound. These findings raise interesting questions about the role of GAGs. Sulfated GAGs and collagen interactions can change how fibrils develop in the fetal wound. Fetal collagen fibrils in chicks and cows had small diameters during development, but at mid-gestation, a significant increase in collagen fibril size was accompanied by a drop in hyaluronic acid and an increase in chondroitin sulfate content. Differentiations in the cellular and extracellular milieu that affect the process of fibrillar differentiation in the primary wound "scaffolding" into which fibroblasts migrate and lay down collagen fibrils may therefore be related to the different patterning of collagen fibrils in healing fetal (regeneration of normal dermal pattern) and adult (scar consisting of parallel and densely packed collagen fibrils at right angles to the epithelial surface) wounds.

Adult wounds, on the other hand, exhibit delayed fibroblast migration into a denser, more resistant wound matrix. Instead of migrating into the wound scaffold's body, fibroblasts in these wounds appear to migrate more readily up and down the wound borders. The forces of wound contracture produced by myofibroblasts and the "stiffer" matrix within the adult wound can change the orientation of collagen fibrils, causing an aberrant, scar-like orientation to form. Furthermore, compared to the adult dermis, the fetal (and neonatal) dermis's ECM is less well organized, changes more quickly, and contains fewer differentiated cells; these characteristics may contribute to the fetus's scar-free healing pattern.

The expression of cytokeratin indicates that the epithelium of the adult oral mucosa is more like that of a fetus. Adult oral mucosal fibroblasts display many embryonic traits, and the oral mucosa, like fetal skin and amniotic fluid, is constantly submerged in fluid (saliva) that is rich in growth factors and antibacterial agents.

A study is still needed to fully understand the state of epithelial differentiation and potential interactions between epithelial and mesenchymal during wound healing. An aqueous sterile environment (amniotic fluid) rich in growth factors and other factors, differences in tissue oxygenation, wound metabolism and pH, degree of tissue tension from function, presence or absence of acute inflammation, rapidity of wound closure, degree of inflammatory response, maturity and competence of the immune system, degree of organization and differentiation of the wounded tissues, composition and organization of the ECM, etc., are just a few of the many factors that contribute to the slow transition between fetal and adult wound healing.

Furthermore, the possibility of fetal wounds scarring also depends on the size and nature of the wound (deep and large excisional wounds scar), the tissue injured (internal tissues, such as the diaphragm, and scar), and the species involved. For example, rabbit fetuses do not heal their wounds appropriately, likely because of the high concentration of maternal immunoglobulin in their amniotic fluid during placentation. There are several and subtle distinctions between the healing of wounds in fetuses and adults. Studies point to many potential experimental manipulations of the healing adult wound to minimize scarring: increase cell migration by including more tenascin, create an early wound scaffold that is more open to promote fibroblast migration and the regeneration of the normal orientation of the reticular collagen fibers. This can be achieved by adding exogenous GAGs and proteoglycans, or by clonally expanding or transplanting fibroblasts with embryonic characteristics to the wound site, such as from the oral mucosa. A more fetal-like, scar-free pattern of adult wound healing might be possible by changing just one or two of the (main) factors that differentiate fetal and adult healing.

PIGMENT CHANGES IN SKIN FOLLOWING BURNS

The nature and extent of pigmentary changes in burned areas are not always predictable. The usual observation is that hyperpigmentation **(Fig. 5)** occurs after superficial burns whereas hypopigmentation/depigmentation is seen following deeper burns **(Figs. 6 and 7)**. Similarly, donor sites, where thin skin grafts are harvested, tend to hyperpigment later on. Whereas, if thick grafts are harvested, the donor area becomes hypopigmented. These changes are more noticeable in individuals with dark skin. There is enough literature on this subject as it has been extensively studied because the post-burn pigmentary changes are a cause of considerable concern to the patients.

The pathophysiology for these pigmentary changes can be explained if the anatomy of normal skin is understood. The color of normal skin is determined by the number of melanocytes, the amount of melanin synthesized and its distribution and transfer to a keratinocyte. The melanocytes contain organelles called melanosomes, in which melanin is synthesized and then transferred to keratinocyte via cell-to-cell contact between melanocyte and keratinocyte. This is called an epidermal-melanin unit.

In case of superficial burns, the superficial layer of keratinocytes and melanocytes are destroyed but the melanocytes in the deeper layers of epidermis and dermis are still intact. They become overactive in

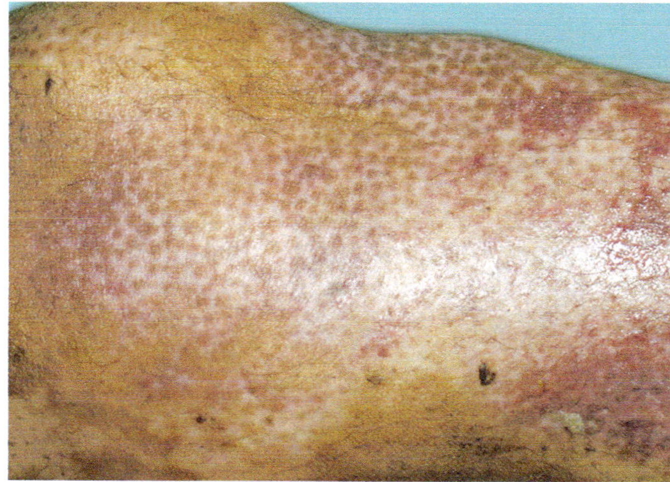

FIG. 5: Hyperpigmentation starting to appear in the scar.

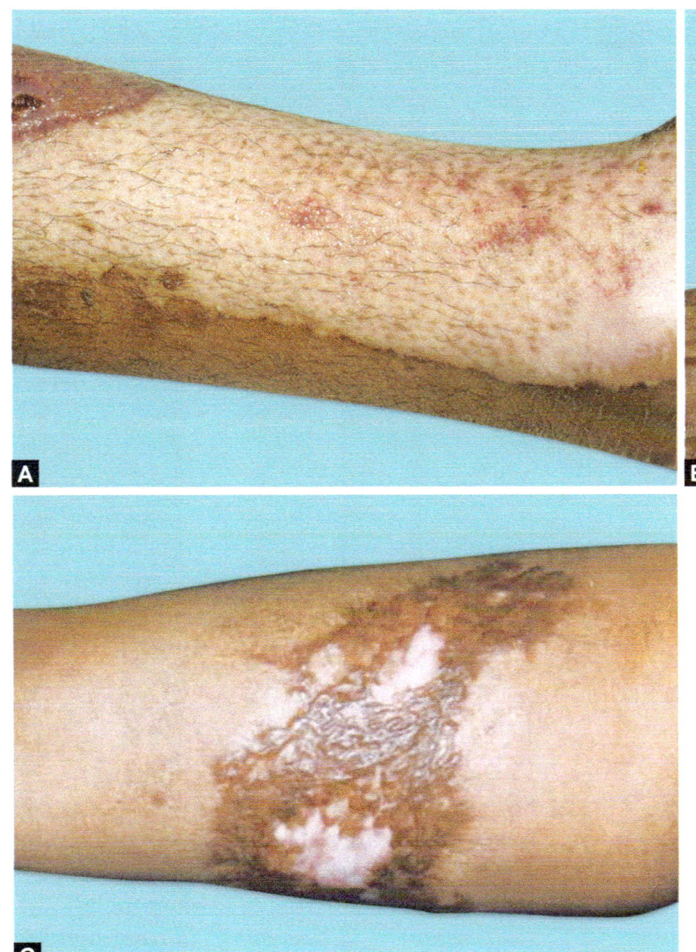

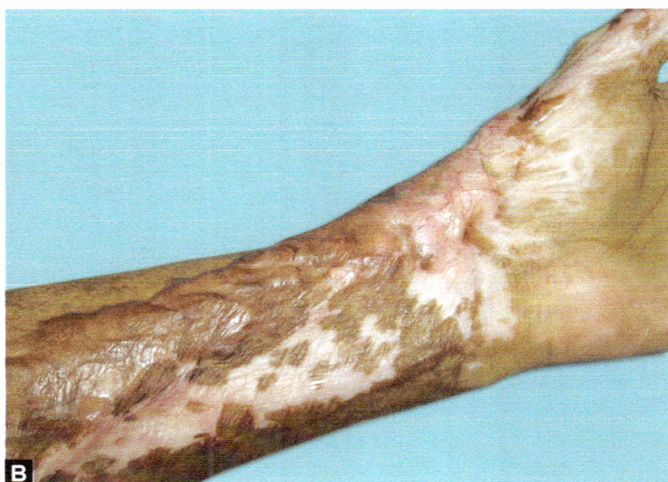

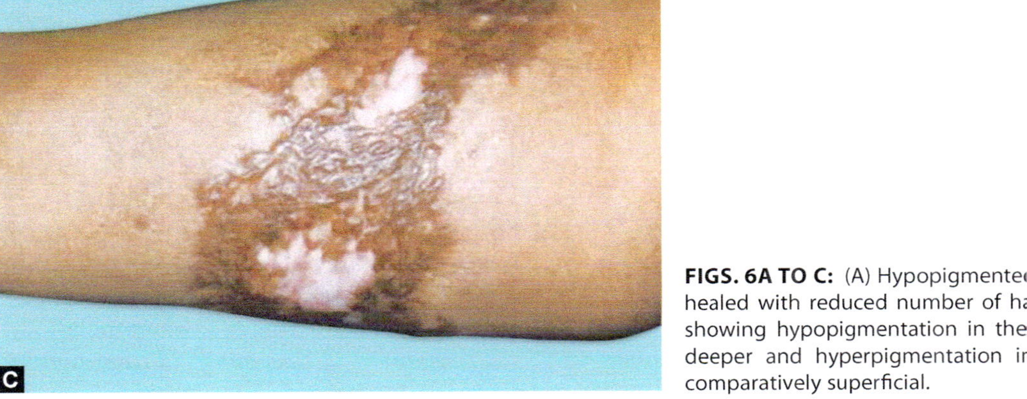

FIGS. 6A TO C: (A) Hypopigmented area immediately after wound healed with reduced number of hair. (B and C) Hypertrophic scar showing hypopigmentation in the center where the wound was deeper and hyperpigmentation in the periphery where it was comparatively superficial.

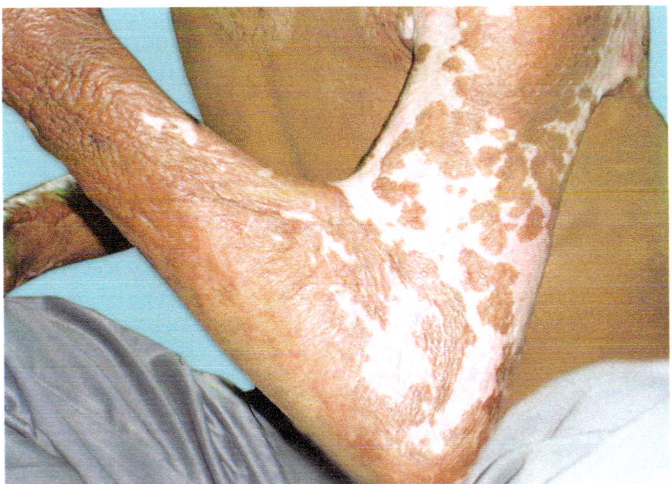

FIG. 7: Post-burn contracture of elbow with hypopigmentation in the scar.

response to the trauma of burns and stimulus of healing and probably synthesize more melanin. This leads to hyperpigmentation. This is also affected by the innate skin color, sun responsiveness of the individual's skin, and amount of ultraviolet light exposure.

In case of deeper burns there are only a few melanocytes left in the deeper layers of dermis. Therefore, there is a deficiency of melanin leading to hypopigmentation or depigmentation in these areas after they heal. Only the residual melanocytes lining the intact hair follicles in the depth of the dermis migrate upward to the basal layer of surface regenerating epidermis and give color to the healed skin which is deficient compared to surrounding healthy skin. Following skin grafting of raw areas, the re-innervation of the graft alters the melanocyte control and also increases the number of melanosomes in the epidermal-melanin unit leading to hyperpigmentation of the grafted areas.

HYPERTROPHIC SCARS AND KELOIDS

The word scar was derived from the Greek word *eschara*, meaning place of fire (fireplace). Scars are areas of fibrous tissue that replace normal skin or other tissues after injury.

A scar results from the biological process of wound repair in the skin and other tissues of the body. Thus, scarring is a natural part of the healing process. With the exception of very superficial lesions, every wound (e.g., after accident, disease, or surgery) results in some degree of scarring.

Hypertrophic scarring, also known as fibroproliferative disorder, is one of the predominant forms of complication reported in patients suffering from severe burn injury. Scar tissue is not identical to the tissue which it replaces and is usually of inferior functional quality. For example, the sweat glands and hair follicles do not grow back in the scarred skin **(Fig. 8)**.

Examples of disfiguring scars include hypertrophied scars and keloids. In both keloid as well as HTS, the wounds heal overzealously above the skin surface. The difference between a keloid and a hypertrophied scar is that whereas the former continues to enlarge beyond the original size and shape of the wound, the latter enlarges within the confines of the original wound **(Figs. 9 and 10)**. Although both can be red and raised, keloids continue to grow while HTSs tend to regress over time. Both can recur after surgical excision; however, keloids recur more commonly. HTSs are far more common than keloids and may occur in persons of any age or at any site and tend to regress spontaneously. In general, they are more responsive to treatment. Keloids occur more frequently in Black persons, being 5–15 times more common in Black as compared to Whites. They may occur in persons of any race with a proven tendency to keloid formation. This predilection for keloid formation in persons of certain races is not observed with HTS. Keloids are more prevalent in persons aged 10–30 years while HTSs occur in individuals of any age. In general, the risk for either type of abnormal scar diminishes with age. Furthermore, the propensity for keloid formation can be familial, genetically transmitted as an autosomal dominant or recessive trait. For example, ear piercing custom prevalent in many cultures of the world, including India, can give rise to keloids **(Fig. 11)**.

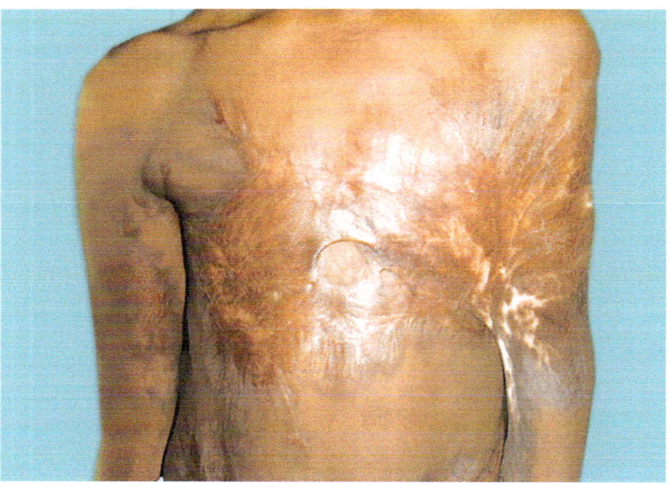

FIG. 8: Post-burn scarring of chest with contracture of axilla. The scar is showing areas of both hypo- and hyperpigmentation.

Etiology

Abnormal scar formation is unique to humans and as such, animal model research has not produced much significant information to further the understanding and treatment of keloids and HTS. Despite numerous studies, no uniformly accepted theory or explanation indicates as to what initiates keloid or hypertrophic scar formation.

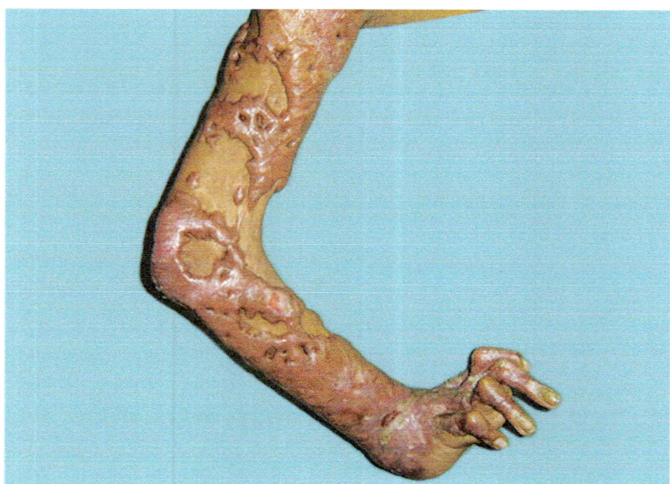

FIG. 9: Post-burn keloid in arm with severe dorsal contracture of hand.

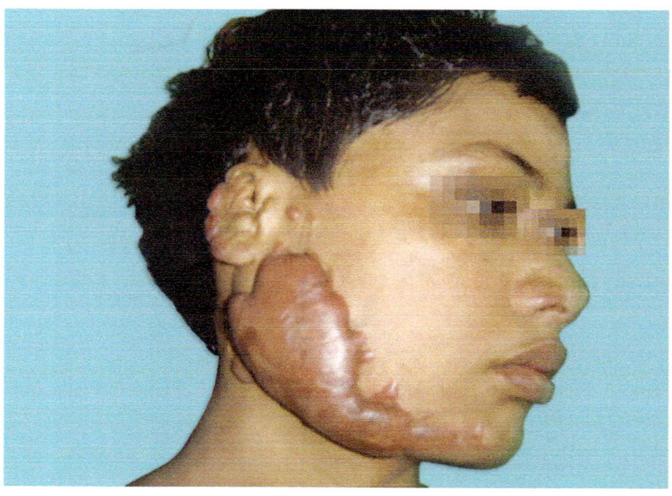

FIG. 10: Severe hypertrophic scarring over right side of face following scalds.

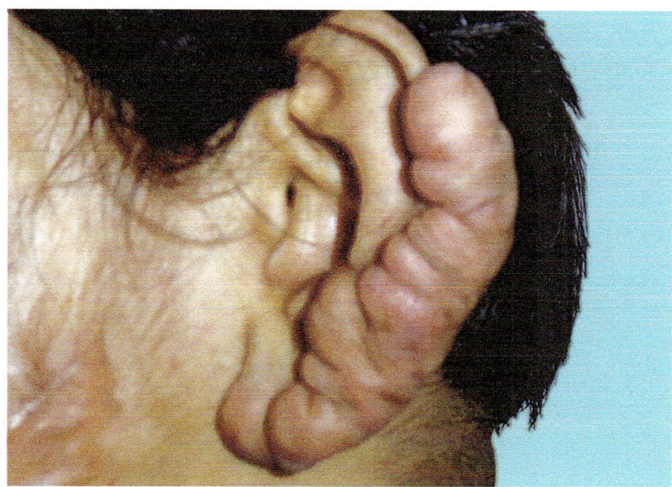

FIG. 11: Keloid over helical rim following burns.

Several genetic and environmental causes have been implicated in the etiology of keloid and HTS. In both, an excessive accumulation of collagen occurs either from increased collagen synthesis or decreased collagen degradation. Proposed causes for abnormal scar formation include foreign body reaction and bacterial infections. Almost all abnormal scars are associated with tattoos, burns, injections, bites, vaccinations, trauma, surgery, or infection. Skin tension is frequently implicated in hypertrophic scar formation. Abnormal scar healing commonly involves areas of high-skin tension, such as the anterior chest, shoulders, and upper back. Other factors implicated in the etiology of these scars include wound infection or anoxia, a prolonged inflammatory response and wound orientation different from the relaxed skin tension lines.

Immunologic alterations have been demonstrated in abnormal scars. Specifically, irregular immunoglobulin and complement levels, increased TGF-β and mast cells have been found in them. Additionally, decreased tumor necrosis factor and IL-1 levels have been found in these scars.

Pathophysiology

Although multiple factors are involved in their formation, studies indicate that keloid and hypertrophied scars result from increased collagen production and decreased collagen degradation. It was earlier demonstrated that levels of the collagen-related enzyme prolyl hydroxylase are elevated in keloid-affected skin compared to normal skin. Prolyl hydroxylase is required for the hydroxylation of proline during collagen synthesis suggesting that collagen overproduction occurs with keloids.

Collagen production is elevated in keloid biopsy samples and in cultured fibroblasts derived from keloids. Additional studies show that increased collagen production by cultured fibroblasts derived from keloids persists throughout their in vitro life span. No significant differences in DNA content or cellularity are found when keloid dermis is compared with normal dermis. This suggests that each fibroblast is producing more collagen rather than an increase occurring in the number of fibroblasts producing a normal amount of collagen. In keloid formation, excessive collagen production by fibroblasts may be due to the wound environment.

Abnormal wound healing in susceptible individuals can result in the formation of keloids that have an elevated content of ECM material compared to normal scars. Keloid-derived fibroblasts exhibit as much as a fourfold increase in the rate of fibronectin biosynthesis compared to fibroblasts from normal dermis and normal scars. Altered biosynthesis is due to an increase in the steady-state level of fibronectin messenger ribonucleic acid (mRNA). The level of fibronectin gene expression that is responsible for this increase has been identified. Thus, altered degradation of fibronectin mRNA is unlikely to contribute to overproduction of fibronectin in keloids. Keloid scars are often identified with tumor-like properties like anaerobic glycolysis, invasion, and often recurrent.

The overproduction of fibronectin and type I collagen in keloids and HTS implicates altered regulation of ECM components as an important aspect of these wound healing pathologies.

Contrary to the increased collagen production theory, keloids and HTS may also result from a decrease in collagen degradation. Levels of the collagenase inhibitor-α-2 macroglobulin have been shown to be decreased in keloids.

The HTS also has within them a large number of fibroblasts with contractile filaments in the cytoplasmic matrix and a deeply indented nucleus, indicating contraction of the cells. These fibroblasts with contractile properties are called myofibroblasts because they are structurally similar to smooth muscle cells. There is a marked increase in the number of these myofibroblasts in the granulation tissue and immature scars especially in the deep dermal portion of the HTS. As these myofibroblasts contract, the stress on the adjoining collagen fibrils is released causing them to form compact collagen nodules which are seen in the depth of the dermis. The contracting myofibroblasts in the deeper dermis also cause the "piling up" of the scar as it is forced outward. The increased number of myofibroblasts with their contractile properties also exerts sufficient force to cause severe distortion of facial structures and joint contractures as the new collagen fibers in the wound may fuse together in the position of comfort.

Clinical Examination

On clinical examination, keloids and HTS are raised above the skin level. HTSs are self-limited; they hypertrophy within the confines of the wound **(Fig. 12)**. Initially, hypertrophied scars can be raised, red, pruritic, and even painful; however, over time, they become pale and flat. Hypertrophied scars appear worst at 2 weeks to 2 months.

Medical Management of Hypertrophic Scarring and Keloids

Burn victims encounter adverse effects on the quality of life due to both HTS and keloid. No single therapeutic modality is best for all HTS and keloids. The location, size, and depth of the lesion, the age of the patient, and the past response to treatment determine the type of therapy used. Prevention is the key. The therapeutic treatment of HTS and keloids includes compression therapy, intralesional corticosteroid injections, cryosurgery, excision, radiation therapy, laser therapy, interferon therapy, 5-fluorouracil (5-FU), doxorubicin, bleomycin, verapamil, retinoic acid, imiquimod 5% cream, tamoxifen, tacrolimus, botulinum toxin, and other promising therapies such as TGF-β, and recombinant human (rh) IL-10 (rhIL-10), which are directed at decreasing collagen synthesis.

Prevention

Avoid performing nonessential cosmetic surgery in patients known to form keloids; however, the risk is lower among patients who have only earlobe lesions. Close all surgical wounds with minimal tension. Incisions should not cross joint spaces. Avoid making mid-chest incisions and ensure that incisions follow skin creases whenever possible.

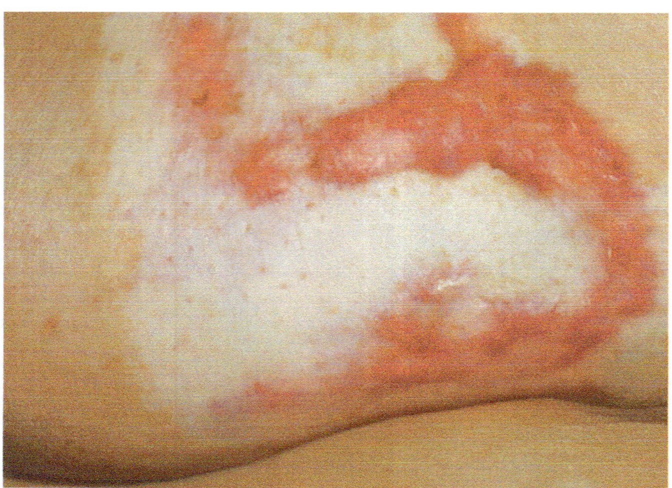

FIG. 12: Raised, red hypertrophic scar over chest following burns.

Standard Treatments

These include occlusive dressings, compression therapy and intralesional corticosteroid injections. Occlusive dressings include silicone gel sheets and dressings, nonsilicone occlusive sheets, and Cordran tape. These measures have been used with varied success. Antihypertrophic effect of silicone gel sheets appears to result from a combination of occlusion and pressure (especially when associated with pressure garments) and hydration. Studies to determine whether silicone compound itself affects the maturation of the scar have been inconclusive. Compression therapy involves pressure, which has long been known to have thinning effects on skin. Reduction in the cohesiveness of collagen fibers in pressure-treated HTS has been demonstrated by electron microscopy. Studies have shown that pressures of 15–40 mm Hg can be applied by custom-made pressure garments and this reduces the reddish discoloration in the scar and also flattens and softens them after 6–12 months of continued application.

Corticosteroids, specifically intralesional corticosteroid injections, have been the mainstay of treatment. Corticosteroids reduce excessive scarring by reducing collagen synthesis, altering glucosaminoglycan synthesis and reducing production of inflammatory mediators and fibroblast proliferation during wound healing. The most commonly used corticosteroid is triamcinolone acetonide in concentrations of 10–40 mg/mL administered intralesionally with a 25- to 27-gauge needle at 4–6 weeks intervals.

Recent Innovations

Newer treatments for keloids and HTS include intralesional interferon, 5-FU, doxorubicin, bleomycin, verapamil, retinoic acid, imiquimod 5% cream, tacrolimus, tamoxifen, botulinum toxin, TGF-b3, and rhIL-10.

Radiation Therapy

Using radiotherapy to treat keloids remains controversial. Although many studies have demonstrated efficacy and decreased recurrence rates, the safety of radiotherapy has been questioned. In one retrospective study of superficial X-ray therapy of 24 excised keloids, the author reported a recurrence rate of 53%. Use of iridium Ir^{192} interstitial irradiation after excisional surgery resulted in a 21% recurrence rate after 1 year. Excisional surgery and preoperative hyaluronidase solution (150 U/mL sodium chloride) followed by external radiation (7.2–10.8 Gy) had a 0% recurrence rate. Adjunctive high-dose rate brachytherapy (^{192}Ir) used after excision and closure resulted in a 12% recurrence rate after 26 months. When excisional surgery is followed by postoperative radiation therapy, the total fractionated dose should be a minimum of 12 Gy, according to a comparative study showing a higher recurrence rate for patients treated with total doses < 12 Gy.

Other Potential Therapies

Additional potential therapeutic options for treating hypertrophic and keloidal scarring that have been shown in vitro to affect collagen synthesis include the use of proline-cis-hydroxyproline and azetidine carboxylic acid, tranilast (anti-allergic drug shown to decrease collagen and GAG synthesis) and pentoxifylline (inhibits DNA replication).

In addition, wounds treated with anti-TGF-β compounds healed with minimal scar tissue formation without affecting wound tensile strength. A possible candidate for affecting wounds via the neutralizing effect of TGF-β is the proteoglycan termed decorin.

Surgical Management of Hypertrophic Scarring and Keloids

Cryotherapy

Cryosurgical media (e.g., liquid nitrogen) affects the microvasculature and causes cell damage via intracellular crystals, leading to tissue anoxia. Generally, 1, 2, or 3 freeze-thaw cycles lasting 10–30 seconds each are used for the desired effect. Treatment may need to be repeated every 20–30 days. Care is taken to administer liquid nitrogen in short application periods because of the possibility of reversible hypopigmentation. Cryotherapy can cause pain and permanent depigmentation in selected patients. As a single modality, cryosurgery led to total resolution with no recurrences in 51–74% of patients after 30 months of follow-up observation.

Excision

For the excision of small HTS, closure with minimal tension, paralleling the relaxed skin tension lines is carefully planned.

Use buried sutures when necessary for layered closure and to reduce tension. Whenever feasible, apply pressure dressings and garments during the immediate postoperative period to wounds of patients in whom HTS and keloid formation occur. Decreased recurrence rates have been reported with excision in combination with other postoperative modalities, such as radiotherapy, injected interferon, or corticosteroid therapy. Excisional surgery alone has been shown to yield a 45–100% recurrence rate and should very rarely be used as a solitary modality, although excision in combination with adjunct measures can be curative. Most studies in which excisional surgery was combined with injected steroids indicated <50% recurrence.

Shaving and over-grafting have been used for severe HTS which causes functional restriction also. This involves shaving the hypertrophic scar by using a manual skin grafting knife till the entire fibrous tissue is removed and healthy reticular dermis is reached, over which a thin skin graft is applied. This usually helps in releasing of minor contractures as well.

Laser Therapy

Ablation of keloids and HTS using a carbon dioxide laser (10,600 nm) can cut and cauterize the lesion, creating a dry surgical environment with minimal tissue trauma. When used as a single modality, the carbon dioxide laser was associated with recurrence rates of 39–92% and when it was combined with postoperative steroids injection, it was associated with recurrence rates of 25–74%.

The argon laser (488 nm), similar to the carbon dioxide laser, can induce collagen shrinkage via generation of excessive localized heat. The argon laser has demonstrated recurrence rates of 45–93%. The pulsed dye laser (585–595 nm) provides photothermolysis, resulting in microvascular thrombosis. Beginning in the 1980s, authors noted that scars became less erythematous, more pliable, and less hypertrophic after treatment with the 585 nm pulsed dye laser. The findings were later confirmed using objective measurements of erythema by reflectance spectrometry readings, scar height, and pliability measurements. Because of its efficacy, safety, and relatively low cost, the pulsed dye laser remains the laser treatment of choice for HTS. Hyper- or hypopigmentation may result due to the application of pulsed dye laser in the case of dark skins.

Tissue Engineering Approach

Besides the above-mentioned treatment strategies, tissue engineering platforms have shown promising alternatives in the last few decades. Repair and regeneration of damaged tissues using cells or artificially fabricated matrices and/or specific biochemical substances is the primary application of tissue engineering. Various tissue-engineered matrices have been widely investigated for the management of burn wounds as follows.

Hydrogel Dressings and Scaffolds

Due to the expeditious development in the field of tissue engineering and biomaterials in the last decades, tissue-engineered biological dressings including hydrogels have progressively shown great potential in the management of burn wounds. Four important applications of hydrogels employed in burn wound healing are: (i) delivering anti-infection agents; (ii) delivering therapeutic carriers; (iii) skin-tissue engineer scaffolds; and (iv) prehospital burn first aid. For instance, *Acticoat*™, a commercially available silver-coated antimicrobial barrier dressing, can fight and eradicate bacterial infection. Similarly, antimicrobial agents such as silver-sulfadiazine, mupirocin, colistin, ε-poly-L-lysine, and minocycline were incorporated into hydrogels and extensively investigated for their efficiency in healing burn wounds. In addition, therapies that can boost wound closure and scar reconstruction need to be applied to the wound beds. Growth factors, small signaling molecules, angiogenic factors, and antimicrobial drugs can be delivered in a sustained manner with the help of hydrogel dressings. Further, these hydrogel/scaffold dressings can also be employed as a first-aid measure in the case of burn wounds. Some of the commercially available first-aid hydrogel/scaffold dressings including Neoheal®, Simpurity™, DermaGauze™, Suprasorb® G, and Kendall® are ultimately used for burn wound management.

Various Therapeutic Delivery Vehicles

Generally, hydrogel and scaffold dressings are widely employed as therapeutic delivery vehicles. However, the advancement of nano-drug delivery systems (NDDSs) in the last few decades has brought alternative insights into the repair and regeneration of wounded skin tissue. These drug delivery platforms ensure the sustained release of drugs, protection from drug degradation, and also induce skin repair. Liposomes, lipid nanoparticles, nanofibers, nanodroplets, metal-organic frameworks, and nanogels are recently emerging NDDSs through which one can deliver growth factors, small molecules, and even oxygen. On the other hand, microspheres, microneedle patches, and microbubbles are being widely investigated microcarriers for the controlled as well as sustained release of therapies on the wounded site.

Cell-based Therapy

With the introduction of cell-laden collagen gels, cell-based therapies for wound healing started emerging as a potential strategy. Numerous stem cells have been employed for wound healing namely bone-marrow-derived mesenchymal stem cells (BMSCs), adipose-derived stem cells (ASCs), hair follicle stem cells (HFSCs), epidermal stem cells (ESCs), sweat gland-derived stem cells (SGSCs), and induced pluripotent stem cells (iPSCs). Chronic wounds with complications like senescent cells and failure in ECM production can be treated with cellular constructs. The re-establishment of cellular processes and stimulation toward regenerative pathways are the main functions of cell-based therapies. Most cell-based therapies are available in the form of tissue-engineered constructs. The following section explains various tissue-engineered cellular therapeutic constructs **(Fig. 13)**.

Tissue-engineered Skin Constructs

Recently, the applications of subcutis as a gliding layer have been extensively investigated for the resilience of scarred skin. It was Rheinwald and Green, who first reported a successful technique to culture keratinocytes from single-cell suspensions of human epidermal cells in the year of 1975. At that time, this method had the potential to save lives since it accelerated wound closure among individuals who had suffered extensive deep burns. Thereafter, the application of cultured epithelial autograft (CEA) as confluent sheets were widely employed to ensure burn wound closure permanently. However, the expansion rate of keratinocytes is a major limiting factor of this technique. On the other hand, the contribution of Yannas and Burke in developing dermal substitutes emerged a new era in wound healing. Their contribution resulted in the commercial availability of the *Integra Dermal Regeneration Template*, which is currently used as a dermal substitute composed of a silicone layer for the management of acute burns and scar reconstruction. Likewise, a single layer of dermal substitute comprising

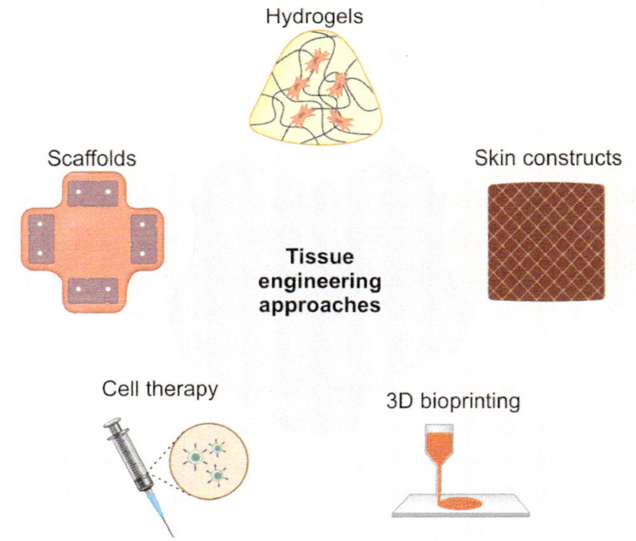

FIG. 13: Recent advancements in the field of tissue engineering for the treatment of burn wounds and scar reconstruction.

of bovine collagen and elastin known as *MatriDerm®* can be applied in a one-step procedure for burn wounds and scar reconstruction. *AlloDerm®* and *Glyaderm®* are commercialized allografts that can be permanent dermal replacements since they have natural collagen, elastin, and basement membrane structures. *Apligraf®*, *OrCel®*, and *PermaDerm®* are important commercial products of cell-based skin constructs. Later, tremendous development in the fields of three-dimensional (3D) printing and 3D bioprinting has been enrooting several research for the fabrication of 3D bioprinted skin constructs. In-situ 3D bioprinting has also been reported in this modern era that would potentially as well as effectively manage burn wounds in the near future.

Gene Therapy

The mechanism of wound healing can be effectively modified by the application of oligonucleotide nanotherapeutics. The growth in the area of DNA genotyping augments researchers and clinicians to understand more information on the genetic components of scarring from burn patients suffering from the hypertrophic scar. Tunable expression of targeted transgenes can induce rapid healing process even in the case of nonhealing chronic wounds. According to the theories of gene therapy, it would be a promising alternative strategy to manage several diseases including HTS. Because of the limited success of the direct application of growth factors due to their sensitivity and stability, delivering functional genes has been emerging as an alternative strategy. Scientists have fabricated a variety of gene-activated matrices that are also known as DNA-incorporated matrices, by incorporating vector/plasmid DNA responsible to code certain growth factors. For instance, scientists have fabricated a liposome matrix incorporated with plasmid DNA encodes. However, extensive investigations need to be performed to identify gene targets to attenuate scar formation after burn injury. Identifying the essential genes/gatekeepers which are responsible for the induction and progression of scar formation would pave a promising path toward gene therapy for this disease.

CONTRACTURES

A contracture **(Figs. 14 and 15)** is a tightening of skin that may affect the underlying muscles and tendons, limiting the joint mobility. Contractures develop when normal elastic connective tissues are replaced with inelastic fibrous tissue. This makes the tissues resistant to stretching and prevents normal movements of the affected area. Physical therapeutic measures can aid in controlling burn scar contractures. If these treatments do not control the effects of contractures, surgical intervention is required. After the release of contracture, a skin graft or a flap cover is provided. The management of this post-burn complication is discussed in Chapter 34 in detail in this volume. Conservatively, managed deep dermal burn wounds and delayed skin grafting of full-thickness burns commonly end up in various kinds of scar deformities and contractures. This significantly restricts physical and social rehabilitation of a burn victim.

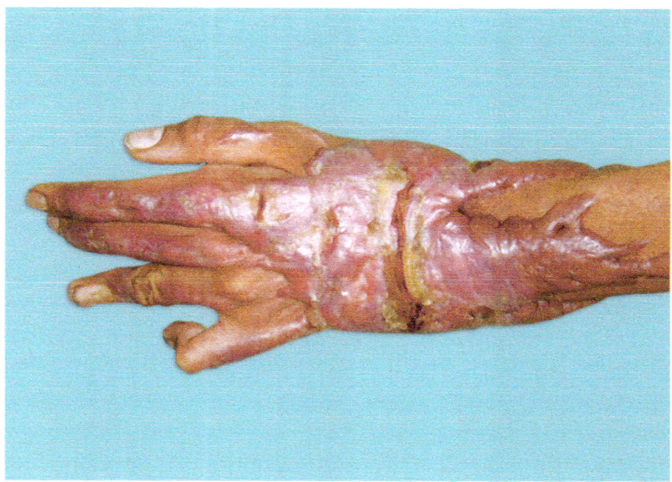

FIG. 14: Post-burn hypertrophic scar over dorsum of hand and distal forearm leading to contracture at wrist and fingers with deformity of fingers.

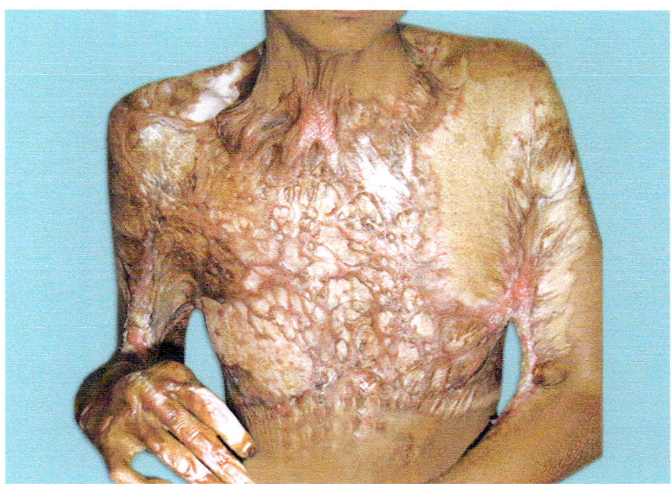

FIG. 15: Hypertrophic scarring over chest causing contracture of neck and both axilla.

Joint contractures due to destruction of skin are very frequent specially when present over joints. Secondary contractures cause shortening of musculotendinous units and neurovascular bundles and tissues around a joint leading to decreased range of movement. Primary arthro-osseous contractures result from direct deep fourth degree burns over a joint, leading to severe and irreversible processes. Contractures can occur at any joint of the body. This joint dysfunction can also be a result of immobilization from burn injury. A contracture is different from spasticity, but they are often related. Spasticity is an abnormal increase in muscle tone. This can worsen the development of contractures.

SUMMARY

Skin is the largest organ in the human body forming its outer protective covering like a shield. When it is damaged in the case of a burn patient, it alters even the internal milieu. Therefore, it is important to restore its structure and function as soon as possible by conservative and surgical means. In order to achieve this goal, it is essential to understand the various biological processes which tend to heal the skin wounds and how they can be hastened. The wound healing response is by and large predictable with some degree of variability. Sometimes, the healing processes go haywire as is evident from development of HTS and keloids. Newer modalities are being explored to maximize the rate of wound healing and minimizing the scar.

Webster states "The great ignominy of the plastic surgeon is his inability to remove a scar without leaving another one. The best we can do is to occasionally improve on another surgeon's scar while indeed he may be improving on several of ours."

BIBLIOGRAPHY

1. Aarabi S, Longaker MT, Gurtner G.C. Hypertrophic scar formation following burns and trauma: new approaches to treatment. PLoS med. 2007;4(9):e234.
2. Abazari M, Ghaffari A, Rashidzadeh H, Badeleh SM, Maleki Y. A Systematic Review on Classification, Identification, and Healing Process of Burn Wound Healing. int j lower extrem wounds. 2002;21(1):18-30.
3. Abdullahi A, Jeschke MG. Nutrition and anabolic pharmacotherapies in the care of burn patients. Nutr clin pract: official pub Am Soc Parent Enteral Nutr. 2014;29(5):621-30.
4. Amini-Nik S, Yousuf Y, Jeschke MG. Scar management in burn injuries using drug delivery and molecular signaling: current treatments and future directions. Advan drug deliv rev. 2018;123:135-54.
5. Babu M, Wells A. Dermal-epidermal communication in wound healing. Wounds. 2001;13(5):183-9.
6. Badylak SF. Regenerative medicine and developmental biology: the role of the extracellular matrix. Anat Rec B New Anat. 2005;287(1):36-41.
7. Bhar B, Chouhan D, Pai N, Mandal BB. Harnessing multifaceted next-generation technologies for improved skin wound healing. ACS Applied Bio Materials. 2021;4(11):7738-63.
8. Chalain TMB, Tang C, Thonson HG. Burn area color changes after superficial burns in childhood: can they be predicted? J Burn Care Rehabil. 1998;19:39-49.
9. Clarke J. Burns. Br Med Bullet. 1999;55(4):885-94.
10. De-Souza DA, Greene LJ. Pharmacological nutrition after burn injury. J Nutr. 1998;128(5):797-803.
11. Edgar DW, Homer L, Phillips M, Gurfinkel R, Rea, S, Wood FM. The influence of advancing age on quality of life and rate of recovery after treatment for burn. Burns: j Int Soc Burn Injur. 2013;39(6):1067-72.
12. Ferguson MW, O'Kane S. Scar-free healing: From embryonic mechanisms to adult therapeutic intervention. Philosoph Transact Royal Soc B: Biol Sci. 2004;359(1445):839-50.
13. Gillitzer R, Goebeler M. Chemokines in cutaneous wound healing. J Leukocyte Biol. 2001;69(4):513-21.
14. Greaves MW, Vella Briffa D. UV-A and the skin. Br J Dermatol. 1985;105 477-82.
15. Gupta A, Kowalczuk M, Heaselgrave W, Britland ST, Martin C, Radecka I. The production and application of hydrogels for wound management: A review." Eur Polymer J. 2018;111(2019):134-51.
16. Gurtner GC, Werner S, Barrandon Y, Longaker MT. Wound repair and regeneration. Nature. 2008;453(7193):314-21.
17. Hall C, Hardin C, Corkins CJ, Jiwani AZ, Fletcher J, Carlsson A, et al. Pathophysiologic Mechanisms and Current Treatments for Cutaneous Sequelae of Burn Wounds. Comprehen Physiol. 2017;8(1):371-405.
18. Hantash BM, Zhao L, Knowles JA, Lorenz HP. Adult and fetal wound healing. Front Biosci. 2008;13:51-61.
19. Jeschke MG, van Baar ME, Choudhry MA, Chung KK, Gibran NS, Logsetty S. Burn injury. Nat rev Dis primers. 2020;6(1):11.
20. Kahn AM, Cohen MJ, Kaplan L. Treatment for depigmentation resulting from burn injuries. J burn care rehabil. 1991;12(5):468-73.
21. Kantak NA, Mistry R, Varon DE, Halvorson EG. Negative Pressure Wound Therapy for Burns. Clin plast surg. 2017;44(3):671-7.
22. Kim H, Shin S, Han D. Review of History of Basic Principles of Burn Wound Management. Medicina (Kaunas, Lithuania). 2022;58(3):400.
23. Kulp GA, Tilton RG, Herndon DN, Jeschke MG. Hyperglycemia exacerbates burn-induced liver inflammation via noncanonical nuclear factor-κB pathway activation. Molecul med. (Cambridge, Mass). 2012;18(1):948-56.
24. Kumaresan PV, Babu RM, Gupta PD. Ultrastructural studies of keloids. Biomed Letters. 1998;58:41-50.
25. Latha B, Babu M. The involvement of free radicals in burn injury: a review. Burns: j Int Soc Burn Injur. 2001;27(4):309-317.
26. Leventhal D, Furr M, Reiter D. Treatment of keloids and HTS: A meta-analysis and review of the literature. Arch Facial Plast Surg. 2006;8(6):362-8.
27. Markiewicz-Gospodarek A, Kozioł M, Tobiasz M, Baj J, Radzikowska-Büchner E, Przekora A. Burn wound healing: clinical complications, medical care, treatment, and dressing types: the current state of knowledge for clinical practice. Int j environ res pub health. 2022;19(3)1338.
28. Martin P. Wound healing--Aiming for perfect skin regeneration. Science. 1997;276(5309):75-81.

29. Meenakshi J, Jayaraman V, Amakrishnan KMR, Babu M. Keloids and HTS: A review. Indian J Plast Surg. 2005;38(2):175-9.
30. Meenakshi J, Jayaraman V, Ramakrishnan KM, Babu M. Ultrastructural differentiation of abnormal scars. Ann Burn Fire Disaster. 2005;28(2):83-8.
31. Merchant N, Boudana D, Willoughby L, Lin J, Rehou S, Shahrokhi S, Jeschke MG. Management of adult patients with buttock and perineal burns: The Ross Tilley Burn Centre experience. j trauma acute care surg. 2014;77(4):640-8.
32. Morgan JE, Gilchrest B, Golwyn RM. Skin pigmentation: Current concepts and relevance to Plastic surgery. Plast Reconstruct Surg. 1975;56:617-28.
33. Nurden AT, Nurden P, Sanchez M, Andia I, Anitua E. Platelets and wound healing. Front Biosci. 2008;13(5):3532-48.
34. Okuno R, Ito Y, Eid N, Otsuki Y, Kondo Y, Ueda K. Upregulation of autophagy and glycolysis markers in keloid hypoxic-zone fibroblasts: Morphological characteristics and implications. Histol histopathol. 2018;33(10):1075-87.
35. Oryan A, Alemzadeh E, Mohammadi AA, Moshiri A. Healing potential of injectable Aloe vera hydrogel loaded by adipose-derived stem cell in skin tissue-engineering in a rat burn wound model. Cell tissue res. 2019;377(2):215-27.
36. Papini R. Management of burn injuries of various depths. BMJ. 2004;329(7458):158-60.
37. Quinn KJ. Silicone gel in scar treatment. Burns. 1987;13:533-40.
38. Ramakrishnan M, Prathiba V, Sridhar Rao K, Jayaraman V, Babu M, Gupta PD. Expression of Keratin in Postburn Scars and Keloids. Ann Mediterranean Burns Club Burns Fire Disast. 1995;220-3.
39. Siahaan RC, Sitorus M, Mulia R Gea S. In Vitro Investigation of Bacterial Cellulose/Turmeric Extract (BC-TE) Nanocomposite for Burn Wound Dressing. 2020;297-300.
40. Tredget EE, Levi B, Donelan MB. Biology and principles of scar management and burn reconstruction. Surg Clin North Am. 2014;94(4):793-815.
41. Tsukada S. The melanocytes and melanin in human skin autografts. Plast Reconst Surg. 1974;53:200-7.
42. Tyack ZF, Pegg S, Zirvani J. Post burn dyspigmentation: Its assessment, management, and relationship to scarring. A review of the literature. J Burn Care Rehabil. 1997;18:435-40.
43. Van Zuijlen PPM, Gardien KLM, Jaspers MEH, Bos EJ, Baas DC, Van Trier AJ.M, et al. Tissue engineering in burn scar reconstruction. Burns trauma. 2015;3:18.
44. Wang M, Xu X, Lei X, Tan J, Xie H. Mesenchymal stem cell-based therapy for burn wound healing. Burns trauma. 2021;9:tkab002.
45. Wang W, Lu KJ, Yu CH, Huang QL, Du YZ. Nano-drug delivery systems in wound treatment and skin regeneration. J nanobiotechnol. 2019;17(1):1-15.
46. Werner S, Kreig T, Smola H. Keratinocyte-fibroblast interactions in wound healing. J Investig Dermatol. 2007;127(5):998-1008.
47. Yao Y, Zhang A, Yuan C, Chen X, Liu Y. Recent trends on burn wound care: Hydrogel dressings and scaffolds. Biomaterials Sci. 2021;9(13):4523-40.

CHAPTER

7

Immunological Responses to Burn Injury

Shankar Sriniwasan, Suvashis Dash

INTRODUCTION

Tissue injury brought on by heat, electricity, friction, chemicals, or radiation can lead to burns. Burns are classified as superficial, superficial partial-thickness, deep partial-thickness, and full-thickness injuries, depending on the depth of the damage. Still deeper burns can involve subcutaneous tissue, muscle and even bone.[1] Age and underlying systemic disorders, in addition to the size, depth, and location of the damage, all influence how severe the burn is. While extensive burns, which are defined as those that impact more than 20% of the total body surface area (TBSA), typically require special care, superficial minor burns typically heal rather well. Additionally, the larger burns are more likely to result in consequences like sepsis and infections.[2]

Burn causes inflammation, and the innate immune response and its cells are stimulated by the inflammatory reaction once it is triggered, protecting the damaged area from infections. Moreover, inflammatory cells eliminate debris and dead cells, making it possible for fibroblasts and keratinocytes to start tissue repair **(Flowchart 1)**.

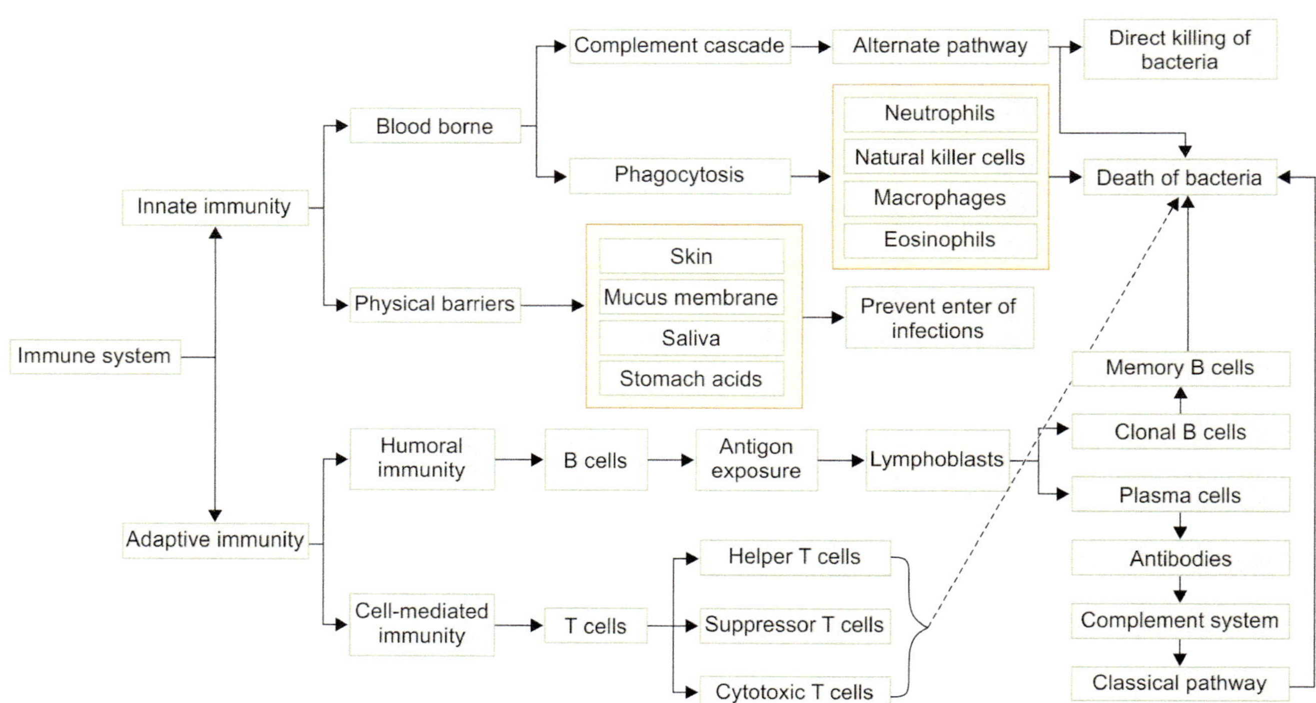

FLOWCHART 1: Basic outline of the immune system.

Alteration of host defense mechanisms in thermal injury is a complex interaction of nutrition, hypermetabolism, and immunological alteration leading to a complex tango of events which, to date, is an unresolved problem.[3]

INNATE IMMUNITY

Barriers: Skin and mucosa are important defense mechanisms against microbiological invasion. Any breach of this barrier is a harbinger for infection and its attendant complications. Any organism which gains entry must first contend with local conditions at the point of entry. Vasoactive amines, such as histamine and serotonin, kinin polypeptides, and various other mediators, initiate a local inflammatory response. They cause constriction of venular sphincters and dilatation of capillaries, resulting in increased capillary permeability. Thus, fluid and fibrinogen leave the dilated vessels and create a fibrin network which localizes bacteria. Leucotaxis is also aided by the kinin system.

Serum has two classes of protein:

1. Beta lysine which is lethal to gram-positive organisms
2. A group of proteins called complement which acts against gram-negative organisms

If local mechanisms do not stem the infection, the microorganisms are transported to the lymph nodes by the lymphatics where macrophages phagocytose the organisms. The specific immune responses are now called into play at this location by the lymphocytes.[3,4]

ADAPTIVE IMMUNITY

Adaptive immunity can be discussed under two subdivisions: Cell-mediated and humoral. The lymphocyte is the key cell in the initiation of specific immune response. It is the only cell capable of recognizing an antigen as foreign and initiating specific mechanisms for its disposal. Lymphocytes form two response systems:

1. T cell, associated with cell-mediated immunity (CMI)
2. B cell, associated with humoral or antibody-mediated immunity

Both T and B lymphocytes arise from a common bone marrow stem cell. On maturity, the T and B lymphocytes seed the peripheral lymphoid organs. It must be emphasized here that there is a complex interaction between these systems and that any simplified description is only to aid in the understanding of this complex process.

Cell-mediated Immunity

Stimulation of CMI causes the T lymphocytes to undergo blast transformation and proliferate. T-cell cooperation is needed for B-cell responses to occur. T cells also secrete a variety of lymphokines which regulate immune responses. Lymphokines also activate macrophages to increase microbicidal activity. Altered CMI following burns has been well studied and documented. This is evidenced by the prolonged survival of allografts in extensively burnt patients. There is a decrease in total counts and an increase in suppressor T cells (lymphocytes also have a depressed responsiveness owing to the generation of a subpopulation of T cells called suppressor T cells).[3,4]

Humoral Immunity

The hallmark of humoral immunity is the production of antibodies by the B lymphocytes. Antibodies which have significant activity against microorganisms are immunoglobulin G (IgG), IgM, and IgA.

All immunoglobulins are decreased in quantity during the 1st week post burn and return to normal levels during the 2nd week after the injury. The decrease in IgG levels is more than IgM or IgA. The initial decrease is followed by higher-than-normal concentrations owing to antigenization, which burn patients are subjected to during their clinical course. The serum IgM level is elevated owing to widespread fungal infection in these patients.

Complement system: It is a complex integrated network of serum proteins that bridges both specific and nonspecific immunity. On activation, they mediate inflammation and tissue damage and facilitate phagocytosis. Edema formation in injured tissue is complement-dependent. Complement components C3a and C5a facilitate serotonin and histamine release which cause vasodilatation and thus edema.[5,6]

A coordinated immunoinflammatory response requires the regulation of many cell types achieved by the actions of soluble protein (cytokine) and lipid or peptide (autacoid) mediators released by macrophages, neutrophils, lymphocytes, platelets, and endothelium. Some cytokines, such as tumor necrosis factor alpha (TNF-α), interleukin-1 (IL-1), and IL-8, have pro-inflammatory actions while IL-4, IL-10, and IL-13 have counter regulatory activities. Some cytokines (e.g., IL-1) are released early while IL-6 and IL-8 appear later in the pathological continuum.[6-8]

Cytokines and autacoids regulate the amplitude and duration of the immune response. They have multiple effects on cell differentiation and there is considerable overlap in their actions. To attempt to control and localize an inflammatory process, both pro- and anti-inflammatory mediators are released simultaneously. A balance between these two competing mechanisms is critical if homeostasis is to be maintained.[9] Their often-compartmentalized production results in serum concentrations which do not reflect accurately their local physiological levels. Quite aptly, Cavaillon et al. have described serum cytokine concentrations as being tip of the iceberg.[10]

IMMUNOMODULATORY THERAPIES

The treatment of severe sepsis and septic shock has centered around the eradication of established infection with appropriate surgical interventions and antibiotics along with intensive organ support. With the realization that the pathological effects of sepsis can result from the direct actions of microorganisms and their toxins and indirectly from the host response, interest has been sparked off in newer immunomodulatory therapies. These therapies have attempted to attenuate the actions of bacterial toxins, limit host inflammatory response, or reduce tissue damage resulting from established inflammatory processes. Anticytokine therapies have attempted to inhibit pro-inflammatory or enhance anti-inflammatory responses. In all this, a delicate balance needs to be achieved between inhibition of an excessive response and ablation of essential host defenses. Derangement of either can lead to systemic sepsis and death.[11,12]

Endotoxin

Endotoxin or lipopolysaccharide (LPS) is found within the external membrane of the cell wall of gram-negative bacteria and is released from growing and damaged microorganisms. LPS binds to many serum carrier molecules, the most important of which is lipopolysaccharide-binding protein (LBP). The LPS–LBP complex interacts with macrophages via the CD14 cell-surface receptor. LPS is a potent stimulator of cytokine production. Administration of endotoxin to healthy human volunteers produced clinical features of sepsis.

Antiendotoxin Therapies

In early studies, polyclonal human antisera with high levels of anti-LPS antibodies were shown to reduce the mortality arising from gram-negative sepsis. With technological advances came anti-LPS monoclonal antibodies (e.g., HA-1A and E5). Despite encouraging animal study reports, large, random, controlled trials in humans have been disappointing.[13,14]

Tumor Necrosis Factor Alpha (TNF-α)

TNF-α is a polypeptide produced predominantly by the cells of the reticuloendothelial system. It has a short half-life and a pivotal role in the expression of sepsis. It acts directly on cells and stimulates the release of other mediators of inflammation.

Anti-TNF-α Therapies

Anti-TNF-α monoclonal antibodies are some of the most promising therapeutic modalities available. Unfortunately, this did not bear out in some large-scale studies. Early measure of TNF-α/IL-10 plasma post burn injury is inversely related to burn size and the injury severity scores.[15]

Interleukins

The interleukins are a class of cytokines produced by many cell types. IL-1 and IL-8 have pro-inflammatory action, while IL-4 and IL-10 have anti-inflammatory actions. IL-6 is regarded as the best available serum marker of the severity of inflammation. IL-1 is a key mediator in the immuno-inflammatory cascade, interacting closely with other cytokines, particularly TNF-α.[6,7,10]

Anti-IL-1 Therapies

Interleukin-1 receptor antagonist (IL-1Ra) is the most extensively investigated therapy. Unfortunately, as with other therapies, it has not been found to be effective clinically.[16]

Other Potential Immunomodulatory Therapies

The autacoids are important mediators in the immunoinflammatory cascade and include arachidonic acid derivatives—prostacyclin, thromboxane A2, prostaglandins (particularly PGE2), and leukotrienes.

- Cyclooxygenase (COX) is an enzyme central to the production of these derivatives, and COX inhibitors appear to have some benefits in septic models. Ibuprofen was tried but it conferred no survival advantage.[17]
- Selective thromboxane A2 (TXA2) inhibition may be preferable to nonselective COX inhibition as prostacyclin synthesis would be maintained. The azole antifungal agent ketoconazole is a selective thromboxane synthetase inhibitor and a reduction in mortality has been observed in a small placebo-controlled trial.[18]
- Platelet-activating factor (PAF) is a proinflammatory mediator produced by the endothelium, neutrophils, and platelets. Treatment with the naturally occurring PAF antagonist, BN 52021, has produced encouraging results.[19]
- Bradykinin is a potent proinflammatory mediator that is a potent stimulator of other autacoids and nitric oxide. The bradykinin antagonist CP-0127 has been tried and shown to be useful in a small population of patients with gram-negative infection.[20]

- Nitric oxide synthetase inhibition[21]
- *Fungal glycans*: They increase macrophage microbicidal activity and induce monokine release, e.g., glucan.[22]
- Thymic extracts, e.g., thymopentin (TP-5), are licensed for use and work by their ability to activate T-cell population. They decrease prostaglandin E2 production. PGE2 is an immunosuppressant and inhibits T-cell activation.[23]
- Granulocyte colony-stimulating factor has been shown to have benefit.[24]
- Decreasing bacterial translocation following burns can be achieved by giving prostaglandin analogs, e.g., misoprostol, enisoprost.[24,25]
- *Lipopolysaccharide antagonist*: Polymyxin B. It absorbs LPS and prevents endotoxemia.[26]
- Free radical scavengers like superoxide dismutase improve survival in animal models.[27]
- Interferon gamma (IFN-γ) enhances macrophages' phagocytic and bactericidal abilities, aiding in pathogen elimination in septic patients. A recent study showed that IFN-γ treatment upregulated monocytic human leukocyte antigen-DR (mHLA-DR) expression and increased monocyte TNF-α secretion, proving its efficacy in treating sepsis. However, its clinical safety remains a concern.[28]

The complexities of the immunoinflammatory cascade are such that pharmacological intervention has proved difficult and cumbersome, not to mention that it is prohibitively expensive and beyond the reach of the common man. Despite encouraging results from animal studies, no therapy has been shown to produce an unequivocal reduction in mortality in clinical sepsis trials. It is unlikely that any single agent will do the trick and the early use of immunostimulants followed by immunosuppressants later may prove to be the most useful approach. It is nevertheless certain that the benefits are likely to be small and unlikely to be realized in the absence of optimal resuscitation, surgery, antibiotics, and intensive care therapy.

NUTRITIONAL IMMUNOMODULATION

Probiotics

As a local defense barrier, the gut mucosal layer stops endotoxins and germs from penetrating into the extraintestinal environment. Normal mesenteric blood flow, which is disrupted by physiological stress after burn injuries, is necessary for the preservation of gut health. Postburn blood flow is diverted to the area of injury and increases in oxygen consumption. This leads to hypoxemia and the generation of free radicals, which have an adverse effect on various tissues, including the gastrointestinal (GI) tract.[30,31] When splenic perfusion decreases, inflammatory factors are released from the digestive system, disrupting cell function and activating neutrophils and other proinflammatory cells. This leads to GI ischemia, and the stressful digestive system plays a role as a proinflammatory source and causes the innate immune system's intestinal barrier to temporarily weaken, which in turn causes bacterial immigration to extraluminal space **(Fig. 1)**.[32]

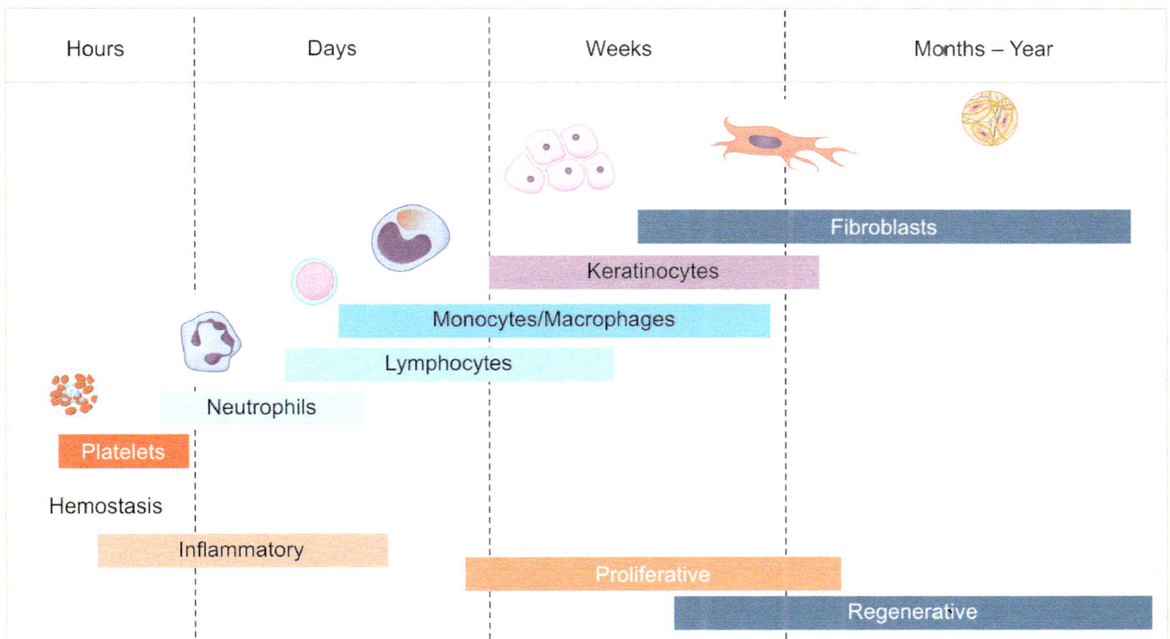

FIG. 1: Immune response following burn injury.

Lactobacillus acidophilus and *Lactobacillus casei* that colonize the small intestine of humans and prevent the growth of harmful microbes by producing organic acids, cytokines, and bactericidal substances are the major strains of probiotics. Immune-stimulating mechanisms associated with probiotics include an increase in macrophages and natural killer cells, the prevention of pathogens attaching to intestinal cells, and the reduction of the inflammatory response brought on by the pathogen.[33,34]

Many researches support adding external gut flora or probiotics to maintain intestinal barrier integrity.[33,34] Probiotics are live microorganisms that prevent bacterial growth by residing in the host intestine **(Fig. 2)**. They activate intestinal epithelium, toll-like receptor 2 (TLR2) and enhance phagocytosis.[35] Probiotics affect the immune system by producing cytokines that improve the body's response to pathogens, including activation of natural killer cells, increased phagocytic capacity of polymorphonuclear cells, and rapid production of specific antibodies and immunoglobulins against pathogenic bacteria.[36,37]

Immunonutrition

The main causes of death in burn sepsis are multiple organ dysfunction.[36] In burn patients, loss of the epidermal barrier, suppression of normal host defenses, and severe hypermetabolism occur. Immunonutrition is likely to be beneficial in such conditions. It has been found to improve the immune function in a number of animal models and humans,[38,39] but its impact on mortality and other clinically significant outcomes is not clearly known. The use of immunonutrition in critically sick patients has been evaluated in several studies, none of which was able to show any effect on a decrease in mortality. Different types of immunonutrition, omega-3 fatty acids (fish oil), branched-chain amino acids (BCAAs) glutamine, arginine, and nucleotides are used **(Fig. 3)**.[40,41]

Omega-3 Fatty Acids

Omega-3 fatty acids have anti-inflammatory, antiarrhythmic, immunomodulating, and cardiovascular benefits. Supplementing critically ill patients with omega-3 fatty acids can reduce energy expenditure, length of stay, and mortality. In burns, inadequate nutrition and infectious complications can prolong hospital stay, and cause organ dysfunction.[42]

It is seen that supplementing critically ill patients with acute respiratory distress syndrome with omega-3 fatty acids primarily from fish oil, specifically docosahexaenoic acid (DHA) and eicosapentaenoic acid (EPA) decreases energy expenditure, length of stay, time spent on ventilation, and mortality without significantly harming the patients.[43,44] These fatty acids also have been found to reduce inflammation and immunosuppressive metabolites. A study revealed that there is no significant difference in the mortality or infection rates, but a reduction in hospital stay. Omega-3 fatty acids can prevent

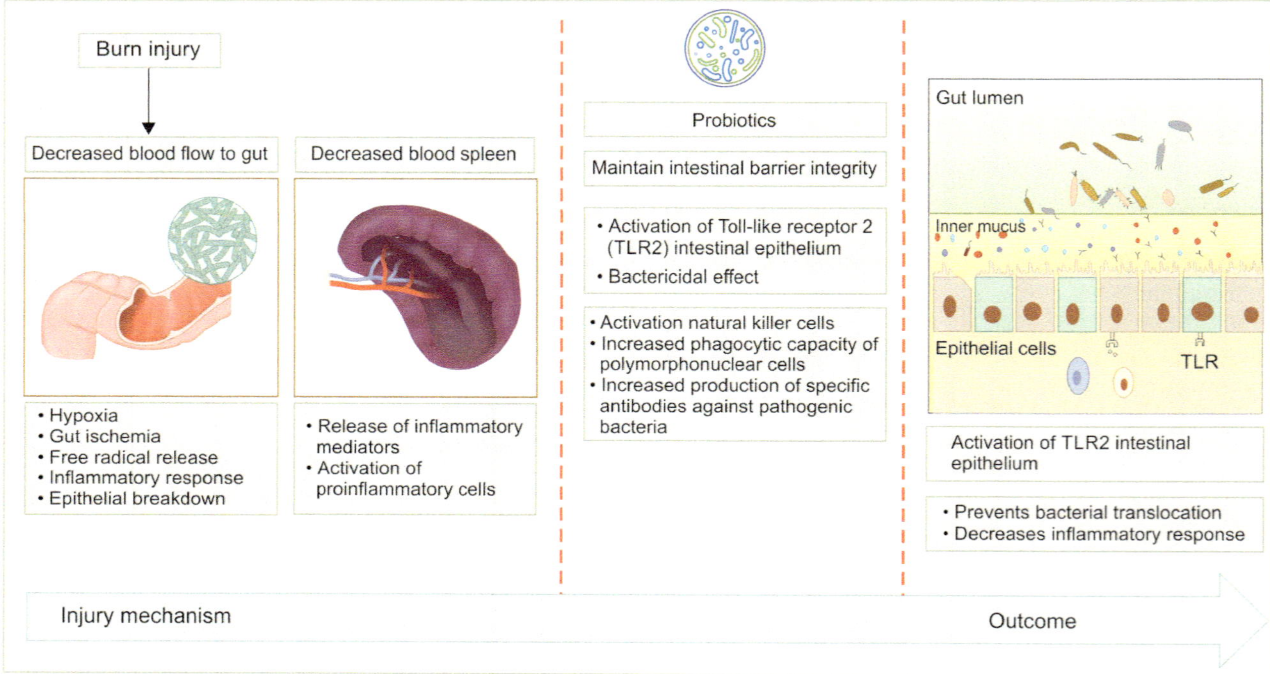

FIG. 2: Mechanism of probiotics in burn injury inflammation mitigation.

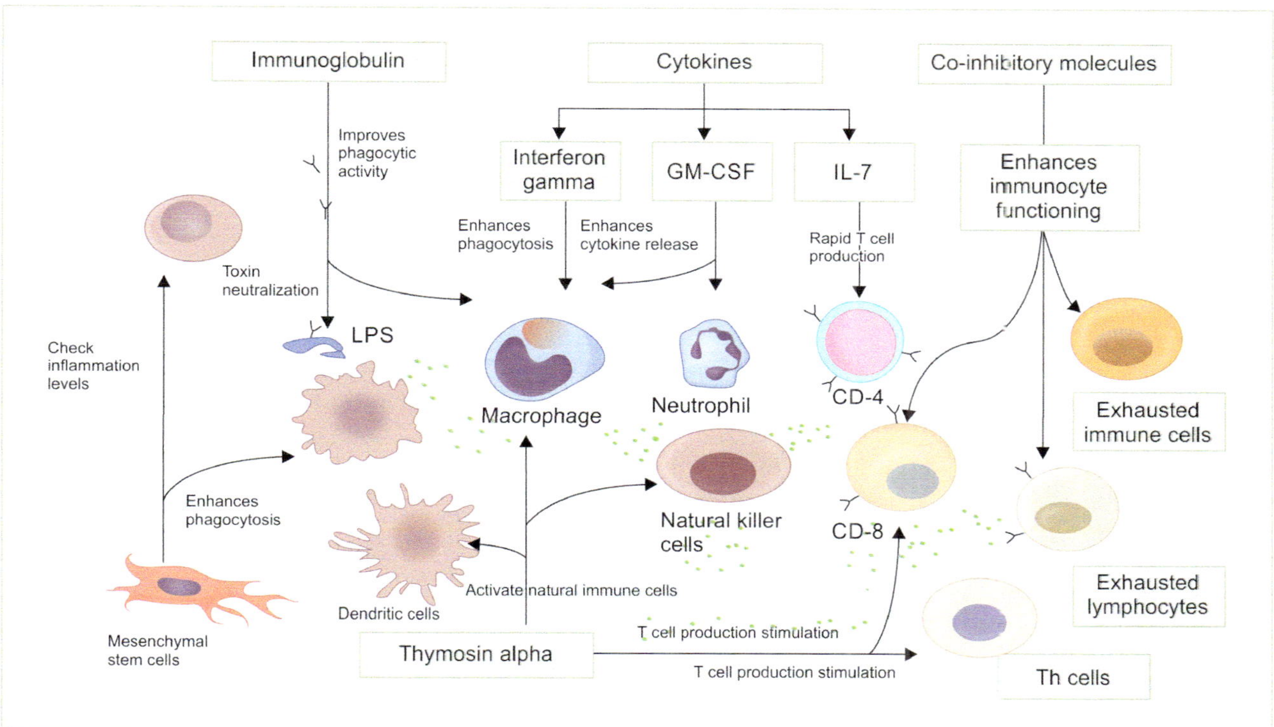

FIG. 3: Modes of action of different classes of immunotherapy agents.[29]
(GM-CSF: granulocyte macrophage-colony-stimulating factor; IL-7: interleukin-7; LPS: lipopolysaccharide; Th cells: T helper cells)

episodes of infection and delay the deterioration of muscles after severe burns.[45,46] However, a meta-analysis did not find benefit of omega-3 support in reducing the various complications, mortality, and length of stay in burn patients.[45] In addition, according to the latest European Society for Clinical Nutrition and Metabolism (ESPEN) recommendations, lipid contents of nutrition regimens should be kept to less than 35% of energy requirements.

Glutamine

Glutamine serves as the primary carrier of nitrogen in the body and is considered an amino acid that becomes essential under certain conditions. It plays a crucial role as a source of energy for immune cells and cells lining the intestines, while also serving as a precursor for glutathione, an important antioxidant.[47] Among immunomodulating agents used in burn cases, glutamine has been most extensively researched.[47,48] Administering glutamine through enteral feeding resulted in significant reductions in both length of hospital stay and mortality rates compared to an isonitrogenous control. Other amino acids did not demonstrate significant effects on mortality rates, length of hospital stay, or infection rates.[49]

Immunonutrient Precursor (Ornithine α-ketoglutarate)

Ornithine α-ketoglutarate (OKG) is a precursor to arginine and glutamine. It has demonstrated anabolic effect by release of growth hormone and insulin, leading to trophic alterations. However, studies failed to show significant positive effects of OKG on mortality and length of stay compared to isonitrogenous controls.[50,51] One prospective, double-blinded study found that supplementing with two boluses of ornithine α-ketoglutarate (10 g) for 3 weeks improved wound healing.[52] There is no conclusive data about this agent's effect on patient outcomes or the ideal length of dosing. Recent ESPEN recommendations strongly encourage using it as an immunomodulator.[51]

Nucleotides

The primary source of nucleotides is endogenous generation; however, evidence suggests that exogenous supplies are necessary for intestinal mucosal growth, immunological competence, and recovery. Nucleotides are essential biological molecules for biochemical reactions, synthesis, and recovery in an injury state. Nucleotides are conditionally essential for optimal function and cell proliferation. Studies show improved clinical outcomes

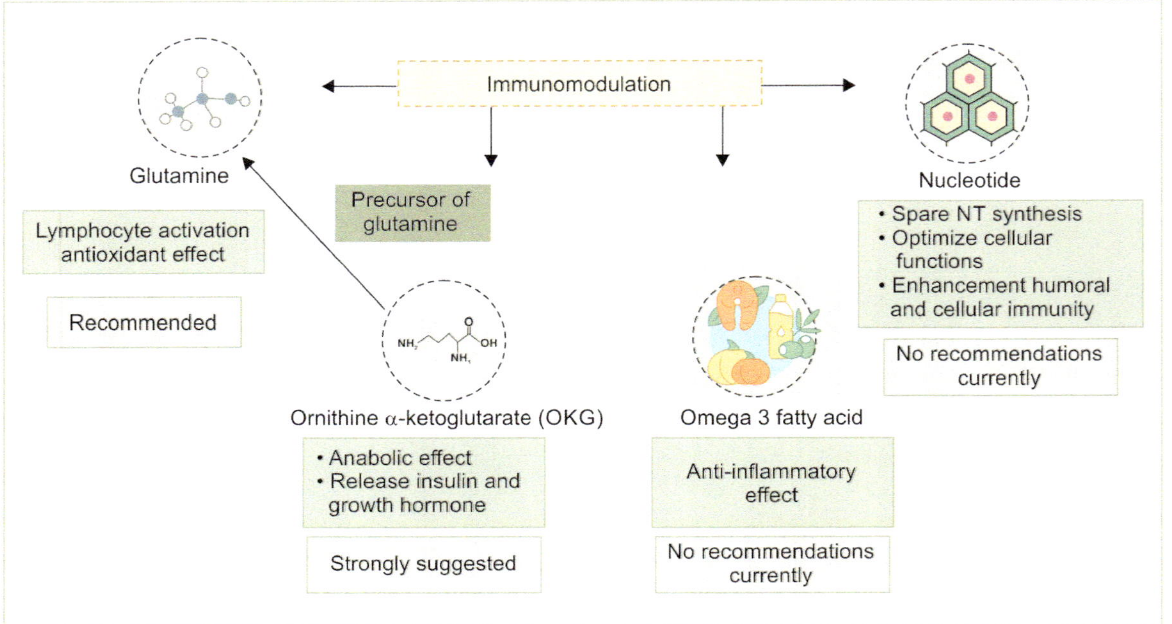

FIG. 4: Different classes of immunomodulators used in critically ill patients and burns.
(NT: nucleotide; OKG: ornithine α-ketoglutarate)

when combined with other nutrients. Nucleotides are usually absent in medical nutrition products except for immune-modulating formulations.[53-55]

Combined Immunonutrients

Combined immunonutrient regimens have been investigated with the rationale for combining their supplementary mechanism on immunomodulation or providing muscle fuel and reducing sepsis. But, studies have failed to report a clear impact on mortality or length of stay versus isonitrogenous controls.[56,57] There was also no change in incidence of burn wound infection. However, one study showed some effect with a reasonable positive impact on burn wound infection rates and length of stay.[57] This formula, with high-protein, low-fat, and low-linoleic acid content, was supplemented with omega-3 fatty acids, arginine, cysteine, histidine, vitamin A, zinc, and ascorbic acid. As there is no possibility of determining which agent and what dose of that agent led to improved outcomes, the uncertainty remains **(Fig. 4)**.

IMMUNOTHERAPY (FIG. 5)

There is a decrease in serum levels of gamma globulin in burned children. The levels return to normal in 7–9 days. The consensus is that there is a marked drop in IgG levels immediately post burn which gradually returns to normal approximately 2 weeks after the insult. The severity of suppression of IgG is related to burn size, and the degree of depletion of IgG can be correlated with mortality from sepsis. IgG concentrations under 300 mg% within a day or two of admission carry a very poor prognosis. An adequate concentration of IgG is critical to the outcome.[58]

It is reasonable to:

- Stimulate production by vaccination
- Increase serum concentration by passive immunization
- Combination of the above

Active early attempts centered on the development of vaccines against *Pseudomonas aeruginosa*. This is not in widespread use today because the incidence of life-threatening infections due to *Pseudomonas* infection has fallen and for the vaccine to be effective, it is necessary to vaccinate the patient several days before infection becomes a threat to get sufficient antibody levels in the serum. This luxury of time is often not available.[23,59]

Passive immunization: It holds a lot of promise. It is attractive because the product is immediately available and effective at the time of administration. Cutter® IVIg was first tried in the US and was successful. It was 90% IgG fractionated from a pool of donors. It had excellent antibody titers against all types of *P. aeruginosa* along with useful titers against streptococci, *Escherichia coli*, *Staphylococcus aureus*, and some viruses too.[60,61]

Pentaglobin®, that is, IgM-enriched intravenous immunoglobulins, show antibacterial, antitoxic, anti-inflammatory, and immune-modulating activities. Pentaglobin embodies natural principles of physiological

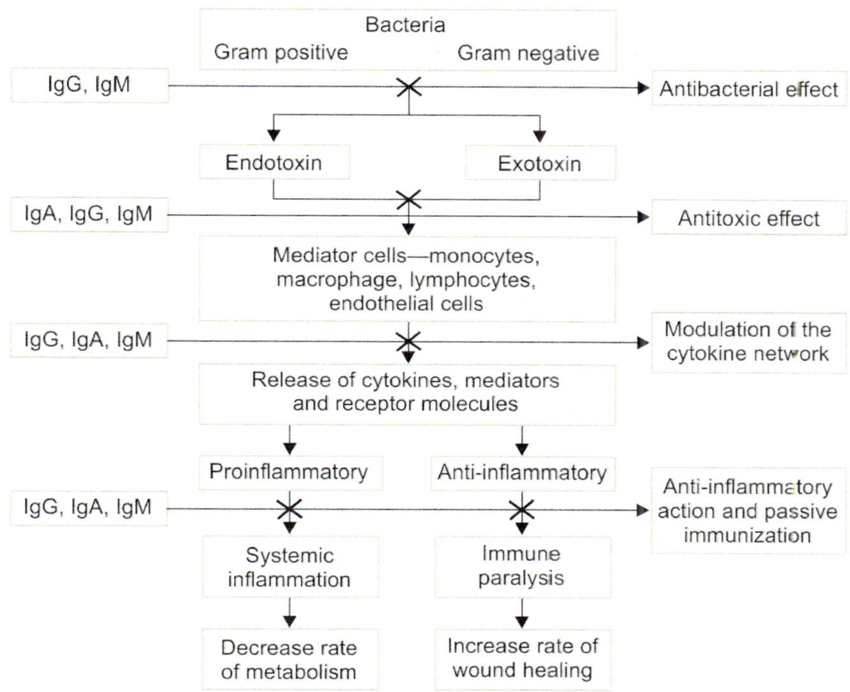

FIG. 5: Rationale for immunotherapy with IV immunoglobulins

defense mechanisms and presents a rational basis for the therapy of sepsis. Hence, it reduces the rate of metabolism and energy requirement.[62,63]

SUMMARY

Active vaccination is not practical because of the changing spectrum of pathogenic microorganisms in burn patients. Passive immunization holds a lot of promise. A high titer, polyvalent immunoglobulin product that offers protection against gram-negative organisms (other than *Pseudomonas*) is desirable. A combination of topical and systemic antibiotics, better nutrition, and immunomodulatory methods will play a decisive role in the management of burn patients in the foreseeable future.[64]

REFERENCES

1. American Burn Association. National Burn Repository 2019 Update, Report of data from 2009–2018. ameriburn.site-ym.com https://ameriburn.site-ym.com/store/ViewProduct.aspx?id=14191872 (2019).
2. Nguyen CM, Chandler R, Ratanshi I, Logsetty S. In: Jeschke MG, Kamolz L.-P, Sjöberg F, Wolf SE (Eds). Handbook of Burns. New York: Springer International Publishing; 2020. pp. 529-47.
3. Stanojcic M, Abdullahi A, Rehou S, Parousis A, Jeschke MG. Pathophysiological response to burn injury in adults. Ann Surg. 2018;267:576-84.
4. Burgess M, Valdera F, Varon D, Kankuri E, Nuutila K. The immune and regenerative response to burn injury. Cells. 2022;11(19):3073.
5. el-Lati SG, Dahinden CA, Church MK. Complement peptides C3a- and C5a-induced mediator release from dissociated human skin mast cells. J Invest Dermatol. 1994;102(5):803-6.
6. Jawa RS, Anillo S, Huntoon K, Baumann H, Kulaylat M. Analytic review: Interleukin-6 in surgery, trauma, and critical care: Part I: Basic science. J Intensive Care Med. 2011;26(1):3-12.
7. Tilg H, Dinarello CA, Mier JW. IL-6 and APPs: Anti-inflammatory and immunosuppressive mediators. Immunol Today. 1997;18(9):428-32.
8. Duell BL, Tan CK, Carey AJ, Wu F, Cripps AW, Ulett GC, Recent insights into microbial triggers of interleukin-10 production in the host and the impact on infectious disease pathogenesis. FEMS Immunol Med Microbiol. 2012;64(3):295-313.
9. Rowan MP, Cancio LC, Elster EA, Burmeister DM, Rose LF, Natesan S, et al. Burn wound healing and treatment: Review and advancements. Crit. Care. 2015;19:243.
10. Cavaillon JM, Adib-Conquy M, Fitting C, Adrie C, Payen D. Cytokine cascade in sepsis. Scandinavian J Infect Dis. 2003;35(9):535-44.

11. Finnerty CC, Herndon DN, Chinkes DL, Jeschke MG. Serum cytokine differences in severely burned children with and without sepsis. Shock. 2007;27:4-9.
12. Bascones-Martinez A, Mattila R, Gomez-Font R, Meurman JH. Immunomodulatory drugs: Oral and systemic adverse effects. Med Oral Patol Oral Cir Bucal. 2014;19(1):e24-31.
13. Wright SD, Ramos RA, Tobias PS, Ulevitch RJ, Mathison JC. CD14, a receptor for complexes of lipopolysaccharide (LPS) and LPS binding protein. Science. 1990;249(4975):1431-3.
14. Agramonte-Hevia J, González-Arenas A, Barrera D, Velasco-Velázquez M. Gram-negative bacteria and phagocytic cell interaction mediated by complement receptor 3, FEMS Immunol Med Microbiol. 2002;34:255-66.
15. Tsurumi A, Que YA, Ryan CM, Tompkins RG, Rahme LG. TNF-α/IL-10 ratio correlates with burn severity and may serve as a risk predictor of increased susceptibility to infections. Front Public Health. 2016;4:216.
16. Dinarello CA. Anti-cytokine therapies in response to systemic infection. J Investig Dermatol Symp Proc. 2001;6(3):244-50.
17. Aronoff DM. Cyclooxygenase inhibition in sepsis: Is there life after death? Mediators Inflamm. 2012;2012:696897.
18. Yu M, Tomasa G. A double-blind, prospective, randomized trial of ketoconazole, a thromboxane synthetase inhibitor, in the prophylaxis of the adult respiratory distress syndrome. Critical Care Med. 1993;21(11):1635-41.
19. Upton JE, Grunebaum E, Sussman G, Vadas P. Platelet activating factor (PAF): A mediator of inflammation. Biofactors. 2022;48(6):1189-202.
20. Maeda H, Akaike T, Wu J, Noguchi Y, Sakata Y. Bradykinin and nitric oxide in infectious disease and cancer. Immunopharmacology. 1996;33(1-3):222-30.
21. Bath PM, Coleman CM, Gordon AL, Lim WS, Webb AJ. Nitric oxide for the prevention and treatment of viral, bacterial, protozoal and fungal infections. F1000Research. 2021;10:536.
22. Barreto-Bergter E, Figueiredo RT. Fungal glycans and the innate immune recognition. Front Cellular Infect Microbiol. 2014;4:145.
23. Amirghofran Z, Ahmadi H, Karimi MH. Immunomodulatory activity of the water extract of Thymus vulgaris, Thymus daenensis, and Zataria multiflora on dendritic cells and T cells responses. J Immunoassay Immunochem. 2012;33(4):388-402.
24. Dale DC, Liles WC, Summer WR, Nelson S. Granulocyte colony-stimulating factor: Role and relationships in infectious diseases. J Infect Dis. 1995;172(4):1061-75.
25. Martínez-Colón GJ, Moore BB. Prostaglandin E2 as a regulator of immunity to pathogens. Pharmacol Ther. 2018;185:135-46.
26. Lynn WA, Golenbock DT. Lipopolysaccharide antagonists. Immunology Today. 1992;13(7):271-6.
27. Akaike T, Suga M, Maeda H. Free radicals in viral pathogenesis: Molecular mechanisms involving superoxide and NO. Proc Soc Exp Biol Med. 1998;217(1):64-73.
28. Döcke WD, Randow F, Syrbe U, Krausch D, Asadullah K, Reinke P, et al. Monocyte deactivation in septic patients: Restoration by IFN-gamma treatment. Nat Med. 1997;3(6):678-81.
29. Liu D, Huang SY, Sun JH, Zhang HC, Cai QL, Gao C, et al. Sepsis-induced immunosuppression: Mechanisms, diagnosis and current treatment options. Military Med Res. 2022;9:56.
30. Koren L, Gurfinkel R, Glezinger R, Perry ZH, Lev-Ari S, Rosenberg L. The effect of Lactobacillus bacteria supplement on sepsis and its complications in patients with acute burns. Burns. 2007;33(5):594-8.
31. Petrof EO, Dhaliwal R, Manzanares W, Johnstone J, Cook D, Heyland DK. Probiotics in the critically ill: A systematic review of the randomized trial evidence. Crit Care Med. 2012;40(12):3290-302.
32. Magnotti LJ, Deitch EA. Burns, bacterial translocation, gut barrier function, and failure. J Burn Care Rehabil. 2005; 26(5):383-91.
33. Putra O, Pebrianton H, Suharjono S, Iswinarno I, Rahayu D. (eds), The Role of Probiotics in Inflammatory Responses of Critically-Ill Burn Patients (A Randomized Clinical Trial). Health Science International Conference (HSIC 2017). Amsterdam: Atlantis Press; 2017.
34. Jamalifar H, Rahimi H, Samadi N, Shahverdi A, Sharifian Z, Hosseini F, et al. Antimicrobial activity of different Lactobacillus species against multi-drug resistant clinical isolates of *Pseudomonas aeruginosa*. Iran J Microbiol. 2011;3(1):21-5.
35. Eslami M, Bahar A, Keikha M, Karbalaei M, Kobyliak NM, Yousefi B. Probiotics function and modulation of the immune system in allergic diseases. Allergol Immunopathol. 2020;48(6):771-88.
36. Jebur MSh. Therapeutic efficacy of Lactobacillus acidophilus against bacterial isolates from burn wounds. N Am J Med Sci. 2010;2(12):586-91.
37. Sharma BR, Harish D, Singh VP, Bangar S. Septicemia as a cause of death in burns: An autopsy study. Burns. 2006;32(5):545-9.
38. Preiser JC, Wernerman J. Glutamine, a life-saving nutrient, but why?. Crit Care Med. 2003;31(10):2555-6.
39. Windle EM. Glutamine supplementation in critical illness: Evidence, recommendations, and implications for clinical practice in burn care. J Burn Care Res. 2006;27(6):764-72.
40. Heyland DK, Novak F, Drover JW, Jain M, Su X, Suchner U. Should immunonutrition become routine in critically ill patients? A systematic review of the evidence. JAMA. 2001;286(8):944-53.
41. Tan HB, Danilla S, Murray A, Serra R, El Dib R, Henderson TO, et al. Immunonutrition as an adjuvant therapy for burns. Cochrane Database Syst Rev. 2014;2014(12):CD007174.
42. Mi L, Shi JX, Xu HZ, Jin ZM, Shao BR, Wang ZJ, et al. The changes in arachidonic acid metabolic state after burns and their significance. Chin J Plastic Surg Burns. 1993;9(3):189-92.
43. Mi L, Shi JX, Xu WS, Xu HZ. The effects of fat intake on immunomodulation in burned patients. Chin J Plastic Surg Burns. 1992;8(4):257-60.
44. Zhou YY, Wang Y, Wang L, Jiang H. The efficacy of omega-3 polyunsaturated fatty acids for severe burn patients: A systematic review and trial sequential meta-analysis of randomized controlled trials. Clin Nutr ESPEN. 2024;59:126-34.
45. Wibbenmeyer LA, Mitchell MA, Newel IM, Faucher LD, Amelon MJ, Ruffin TO, et al. Effect of a fish oil and arginine-fortified diet in thermally injured patients J Burn Care Res. 2006;27:694-702.
46. Siritientong T, Thet D, Buangbon M, Nokehoon P, Leelakanok N, Methaneethorn J, et al. Nutritional support with omega-3 fatty acids in burn patients: A systematic review with meta-analysis of randomized controlled trials. Nutrients. 2022;14(14):2874.
47. Wischmeyer PE. The glutamine story: Where are we now? Curr Opin Crit Care. 2006;12(2):142-8.
48. Zhou YP, Jiang ZM, Sun YH, He GZ, Hong S. The effects of supplemental glutamine dipeptide on gut integrity and clinical outcome after major escharectomy in severe burns: A randomized, double-blind, controlled clinical trial. Clin Nutr. 2004;(Suppl 1):55-60.
49. Garrel D, Patenaude J, Nedelec B, Samson L, Dorais J, Champoux J, et al. Decreased mortality and infectious morbidity in

adult burn patients given enteral glutamine supplements: A prospective, controlled, randomized clinical trial. Crit Care Med. 2003;31(10):2444-9.

50. Donati L, Ziegler F, Pongelli G, Signorini MS. Nutritional and clinical efficacy of ornithine alpha-ketoglutarate in severe burn patients. Clin Nutr. 1999;18(5):307-11.
51. Rousseau AF, Losser MR, Ichai C, Berger MM. ESPEN endorsed recommendations: Nutritional therapy in major burns. Clinical Nutr. 2013;32(4):497-502.
52. Coudray-Lucas C, Bever H, Cynober L, Bandt JP, Carsin H, Coudray-Lucas C, et al. Ornithine alpha-ketoglutarate improves wound healing in severe burn patients: Aa prospective randomized double-blind trial versus isonitrogenous controls. Crit Care Med. 2000;28(6):1772-6.
53. Hess JR, Greenberg NA. The role of nucleotides in the immune and gastrointestinal systems: Potential clinical applications. Nutr Clin Pract. 2012;27(2):281-94.
54. Gil A. Modulation of the immune response mediated by dietary nucleotides. Eur J Clin Nutr. 2002;56(Suppl 3):S1-4.
55. Toledo J, Danilla S, Leniz P, Pineros J, Fernandez A, Roldan P, et al. Early immunonutrition in moderately burned patients: A prospective, double masked, randomized controlled trial. Burns. 2007;33(1 Suppl):s61-s62.
56. Saffle JR, Wiebke G, Jennings K, Morris SE, Barton RG, Saffle JR, et al. Randomized trial of immune-enhancing enteral nutrition in burn patients. J Trauma-Injury Infect Crit Care. 1997;42(5): 793-802.
57. Gottschlich MM, Jenkins M, Warden GD, Baumer T, Havens P, Snook JT, et al. Differential effects of three enteral dietary regimens on selected outcome variables in burn patients. [see comment]. J Parenter Enteral Nutr. 1990;14(3):225-36.
58. Kuzin MI, Sologub VK, Kolker II, Stanislavsky ES, Grishina IA, Panova Y, et al. Actual problems of immunoprophylactic and immunotherapy of burn infection. Burns. 1983;10(1):34-40.
59. Moldawer LL, Hotchkiss R. Immunotherapy: It is not just for cancer anymore. J Leukocyte Biol. 2018;103(1):9-11.
60. Holder IA. Pseudomonas vaccination and immunotherapy: An overview. J Burn Care Rehabil. 2001;22(5):311-20.
61. Ionescu A, Meitert E, Vasiliu S, Meitert T, Milicescu S, Sima F, et al. The immunoprophylaxis and immunotherapy of Pseudomonas infections in burns with polyvalent *Pseudomonas aeruginosa* corpuscular vaccine. Arch Roum Pathol Exp Microbiol. 1979;38(3/4):317-29.
62. Karlov VA, Belotskiĭ SM, Alekseev AA, Gutsu EV, Dikovskaia ES, Filiukova OB, et al. Immunokorrektsiia pentaglobinom pri ranevoĭ infektsii i ozhogovoĭ bolezni [Immunocorrection with pentaglobin in wound infection and burn disease]. Antibiot Khimioter. 1991;36(5):42-5.
63. Herek O, Ozturk H, Ozyurt M, Albay A, Cetinkursun S. Effects of treatment with immunoglobulin on bacterial translocation in burn wound infection. Ann Burns Fire Disasters. 2000;13(1):13-7.
64. Boldeanu L, Boldeanu MV, Bogdan M, Meca AD, Coman CG, Buca BR, et al. Immunological approaches and therapy in burns (Review). Exp Ther Med. 2020;20(3):2361-7.

CHAPTER 8

The Immunobiology of Skin Transplant: Rejection and Acceptance

Rakesh Kain, Archana Sinha

INTRODUCTION

Attempts at skin transplantation have been recorded over the centuries, often in graphic detail. The earliest reports of transplantation in humans included several miracles. One of best-known examples is the 13th century story of Cosmos and Damian. They were Christian Arab saints who were martyred around 300 AD and were reputed to have successfully replaced the diseased leg of sexton with that from a moor who had died several days earlier. India was the original home of this practice while Europe greatly altered it.[1]

All cells and tissue that the immune system recognizes as alien are identified and targeted for destruction. Because of their inability to express foreign antigens capable of triggering an immune response, only tissues from genetically identical donors are excluded. Change in a single amino acid in a major histocompatibility complex (MHC) can cause the skin transplant rejection in a mouse, even though it is the smallest difference that can occur. Genetic differences between the donor and the recipient can be used to determine the transplantation barrier. Generally speaking, there are both antigen specific and nonspecific responses including antibody mediated, T-cell mediated and inflammatory reactions.

Reducing the antigenic difference between the donor and the recipient, avoiding transplanting into a sensitized recipient, or use of immunosuppressive medications on the patient are the various methods to lessen transplant rejection. Understanding how the immune system reacts to transplanted tissue allows the use of currently available drugs and it can also aid in the development of novel products or protocols for use in future.

THE SCIENTIFIC BASIS OF TRANSPLANTATION

The 1950s saw the start of the contemporary transplantation era. But, the decade that preceded it was pivotal for transplantation because it was then that Peter Medawar and associates demonstrated that the rejection of a tissue allograft resulted from the recipient's immune response, and from a nonspecified inflammatory reaction.[2]

In order to investigate skin grafting at the burns unit at Glasgow Royal Infirmary, Medawar came to Glasgow with funding provided by the Medical Research Council. He collaborated with renowned plastic surgeon Tom Gibson, who had a keen interest in researching skin transplant rejection.

A young woman suffered from severe burns due to fall onto an open gas fire was admitted to the hospital shortly after Medawar arrived. Gibson used several little pinch skin grafts from her brother to treat the women's wounds. Medawar removed the biopsies of the skin grafts' for histological analysis in order to investigate their fate.[3] The grafts were destroyed as anticipated after a few days, and they perished even faster when a second set from the same donor was applied 2 weeks later. This so-called "second set" occurrence was interpreted as unmistakable proof that actively acquired immunity, rather than a generalized inflammatory response, was the cause of the rejection response. These results were published by Medawar and Gibson (1944).[4] They came to the conclusion that rejection was caused by an antibody that had not yet been identified.

It was now widely acknowledged that immunological pathways caused graft rejection, regardless of whether cellular immunity or antibodies played the role. It was believed that immunological rejection would inevitably occur, and that there was presently no proven method to stop rejection. The efforts to overcome graft rejection have yielded, at most, only patchy results.

Behavior of Transplanted Tissue

It is crucial to remember that the transplanted reacts to the surroundings in the recipient and does not remain an inactive organ. It generates a variety of cytokines as well as other substances and modifies the expression of cell surface. It reacts in this way to both immunological attack and physiological stress. The graft's normal tissue responses increase it's immunogenicity and antigenicity which affects the survival and function of transplant.

TRANSPLANTATION AND GENETIC BARRIERS

One way to conceptualize the degree of antigenic diversity between donor and recipient is in terms of individual genetic differences. Transplanted tissue contains a wide variety of chemicals that the recipient's immune system identifies as alien. Among them are the blood group antigens against which antibodies have already been produced. Then, recipient T-cell receptors may directly recognize MHC molecules. Moreover, every protein in the transplanted tissue has the ability to break down into peptides, which might cause the recipient's cells to react **(Table 1)**.

THE IMMUNOGENIC ELEMENTS

Numerous distinct immunogenic molecules, some of which may be the graft's functioning cells, are present in donor tissue. The recipient's immune system identifies these molecules as alien substances. Collectively, they perform one or more distinct tasks. Typically, these cells exhibit only a minimal level of immunogenic response in recipient organ. Among them is the blood group antigen, against which antibodies have already been produced. The MHC molecule is another, which recipient T cell receptors may be able to detect directly. The vasculature of whole of the body is lined with endothelial cells. While the endothelium is normally dormant, it can get stimulated in a number of ways, including cytokines and interactions between cells. Selectins and integrins are two types of adhesion molecules found in the endothelium. Interferon (IFN)-γ, a cytokine, and tumor necrosis factor (TNF)-α cause endothelial cells to produce adhesion molecules differently and to express more MHC-1 and MHC-2 antigens. Endothelium is therefore highly antigenic, especially following activation.[5]

THE MECHANISM OF GRAFT REJECTION

There are two types of immune systems which work together. One is an innate immune system that provides a basic phagocytic and inflammatory defence against bacteria and other organisms. It consists of cells of monocyte and granulocyte origins, macrophages, neutrophils, and eosinophils, together with complement components. Other is "adaptive immune" system where two distinct classes of lymphocytes gets activated. Bone marrow is the source of B cells, which produce antibodies against antigens.[6]Although they originate in the bone marrow, the T cells go through the thymus before being able to identify antigen peptide fragments on the surface of antigen-presenting cells that have high MHC positivity. Once activated, B and T cells can be reactivated more easily, resulting in a larger and faster response when exposed to the same antigen again **(Fig. 1)**.[1]

The immune system operates by importing a vast armamentarium to the site of inflammation. The number of possible reactions and combinations of immunological components that come into play to destroy a transplant has led to some difficulty in understanding the process fully.

TABLE 1: Genetic relation affecting outcome of transplant.

Transplant	Donor–patient relationship	Outcome of transplant
Autograft	Same individual	No foreign antigen, therefore, no rejection
Isograft	Genetically identical donor and recipient (monozygotic twin)	No foreign antigen, therefore, no rejection
Allograft	Genetically different individuals of same species (the usual clinical situation)	• Recognition mainly of mismatched donor MHC antigens • Vigorous rejection without MHC matching and immunosuppression
Xenograft	Different species (e.g., pig to human)	The more the evolutionary distance between two species, stronger the cellular rejection reaction; in certain species combinations, preformed antibodies cause hyperacute rejection

(MHC: major histocompatibility complex)

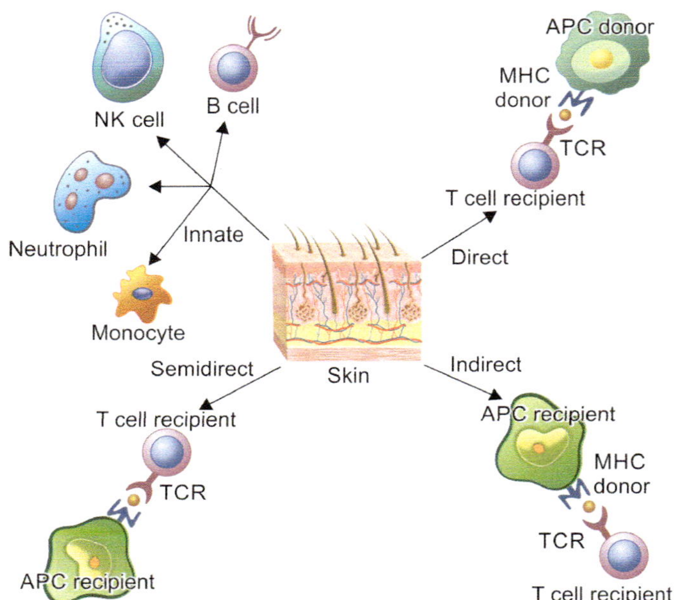

FIG. 1: Allorecognition pathways—direct pathway is the process whereby the donor's major histocompatibility complex (MHC) molecules on antigen presenting cells (APCs) are recognized by the T cells receptors (TCRs) of recipient's T cells. Indirect pathway recognizes the processed peptide presented by recipient's MHC on APCs. Semi-direct pathway is where T-cell activation occurs by transfer of the donor's MHC onto the recipient's APCs.
(NK: natural killer)

The Recipient in the Graft

Cells must move from the bloodstream into the transplanted tissue during the rejection process. The adhesion molecules like E-selectin, P-selectin, etc., are expressed by the endothelium on the surface immediately after encountering agonists such as histamine and thrombin are applied. Leukocytes slow down and roll over the surface of the endothelial cells as a result, and integrin adhesion molecules are then activated. Leukocytes adhere firmly to endothelial cells by this and other methods, causing the cells to flatten against the vessel wall.

SKIN ALLOGRAFT REJECTION AND ACCEPTANCE

Skin is a strongly antigenic organ due to "skin specific antigen", an antigen presented by the skin graft after it is transplanted. Hence, it is subject to rejection.

The obvious alternative to split skin autograft and the problem of limited availability of donor sites is skin allograft. Though cultured keratinocytes can be used as substitutes for skin allografts, the facility and infrastructure for skin culture is not available in many of the developing countries. For such places, the only skin substitute that can be used in extensive burns where enough donor areas are not available, is allograft, taken from the burned patients' close relatives, particularly mother, father or siblings. However, all allografts from random donors start getting rejected in about 2 weeks' time. Even those obtained from parents start getting rejected in about 3 weeks if patient is not severely immunocompromised. Rejection of full thickness skin allograft by immunocompetent individuals is such a consistent and reproducible phenomenon that it has been the central model for the study of immunologically mediated tissue destruction in vivo since the work done by Medawar (Gibson and Medawar,[7] 1943). The only documented permanent coverage with skin allograft in humans has been in identical siblings (Converse and Duchet,[8] 1947; Stranc,[9] 1966; Caruso et al.,[10] 1996). It has been demonstrated that the sole benefit of employing allogeneic material is the prompt restoration of skin barrier function in terms of a biological dressing.[11]

Revascularization of skin-graft is the basis for the beginning of graft acceptance or rejection. The vascularization of graft begins immediately after a graft is applied to the host bed, be it an autograft or an allograft. By 6 hours, only the plasmatic imbibition nourishes the graft, although the host endothelium starts to proliferate. By 9 hours, inflammatory cells invade the graft. By 12 hours, the host endothelium penetrates the fibrin interface between graft and host and small communications start forming between graft and host vessels. This is called inosculation. By 24 hours, the host vessels grow into the graft and vascular communications are well established by 48 hours. By 4 days, the arterial end of the capillaries is open and slow arterial flow from the host to the graft begins. The circulatory outflow from the graft to the host (from the venous end of capillaries) starts around the 7th day and this brings the donors' antigens into the host circulation in case of allograft. The host then produces antibodies against the graft. By 10th day, this starts the rejection phenomenon and the process of rejection becomes clinically evident by the 14th day in the form of maceration of the graft. In fact, there are two types of reactions which take place following allograft transplant. The first is cellular reaction which is local and the evidence for the failure of homograft is found within the graft themselves or their immediate surroundings. The second reaction is humoral reaction which is systemic in nature and follows a general pattern of antigen-antibody reaction. Corollary to this is that if homograft is applied and removed before venous return is established, i.e., 7th day and then reapplied to the same or different area, it can survive for another 14 days till it is rejected again. Clinically hemorrhage, necrosis, or epidermolysis indicates graft rejection. The infiltrating immune cells and their ratio to each other, the structural correspondence of tissue anatomy, and the histological evidence of local artery damage are histopathological hallmarks of rejection.[12-14]

White graft rejection: When homograft is applied to a burn patient for a second time from the same donor, it is seen that it stays white and does not turn pink as no circulation is established in this graft and, therefore, it does not take as in normal circumstances. The explanation for this is that once a homograft is applied to the host for the first time, antibodies are formed against the homograft and they stay in the host circulation from that time onward. On second application of the same homograft, it is immediately rejected by the host and does not take at all. In other words, the graft remains white. This is called "white rejection", also called "second set rejection".

In case of major burns, the immunocompromised state of the patient can delay rejection of allografts for several weeks.

Allograft skin is used as a biological dressing in the management of severely burned patient. Thus, widely meshed (>1:6) split skin autograft is interleaved with allograft either by overlaying (Alexander et al,[15] 1981; Phipps and Clarke,[16] 1991) or insertion of allograft in holes cut in autograft sheets (Yang et al.,[17] 1979). Except for an isolated case report (Takiuchi et al.,[18] 1982) allografts do not survive in the long term, the rejection always occurring before 3 months and often within the first 3 weeks of transplantation. Attempts to modify this outcome with general immunosuppression were made (Burke et al.[19,20] 1974 and 1976) but encountered the serious complication of sepsis as a result of immunodeficiency.[17]

Experimental studies in animal model showed that skin allograft survival was prolonged by cyclosporine (Borel and Meszaros,[21] 1976; Black et al,[22] 1988). However, the actual fate of the allograft in many of these studies is not clear. In 1989, Frame et al.[23] treated patients with cyclosporin after allografting. The allografts survived during drug treatment but were rejected after cessation of therapy.[1]

Thus, allogenic skin grafts are useful for treating patients with extensive burns, but they come with a number of restrictions and drawbacks, the most common of which being early or delayed rejection.

TYPES OF REJECTION

According to time interval and host response against graft, the rejection can be classified into four categories:

1. *Hyperacute rejection*: It occurs after few minutes to several hours after transplantation. Preformed anti-donor antibodies cause complement fixation and thrombosis in the graft vasculature. Preexisting antibodies rarely cause hyperacute rejection in skin transplants because they are not primary vascularized grafts.[24]
2. *Accelerated acute rejection (1–4 days)*: This happens when the recipient's T-cells have been exposed to foreign cells and tissues earlier, immunizing them against the donor's antigens (presensitized T cells, also known as "second set" rejection).
3. *Acute rejection (days to weeks)*: It happens when graft rejection occurs in several weeks to months. The initial 3 months period after transplantation is at maximal risk of rejection. The primary immunological response is T-cell activation. These cells fall into two subtypes: (1) CD-8 positive cells, also known as cytotoxic cells (Tc), and (2) CD-4 positive cells, also known as helper cells (Th). While CD-8 cells produce a variety of cytokines, CD-4 cells may be cytotoxic.
4. *Chronic rejection*: Following transplantation, chronic rejection typically manifests itself months to years later. In light of the concurrent nature of other processes, defining chronic rejection can be challenging. The immune processes responsible for chronic graft failure involve subacute cell-mediated injury and the binding of antidonor antibodies. The parenchyma and the vasculature are the areas that are damaged. The immune processes behind graft vasculopathy persist, presumably due to the release of growth factors within the transplant, and include hypertension, hyperlipidemia, and cytomegalovirus (CMV) infection.

GRAFT-VERSUS-HOST DISEASE

Transplantation between genetically nonidentical individuals is, at present, constrained by two major immunological responses. First is graft rejection and second is graft-versus-host disease (GVHD).[25]

In a burn patient whose immunity is very low, e.g., if the patient is in sepsis, even if homografts are applied repeatedly to the host's raw areas, no antibodies are formed against the graft by the host because of diminished immunological response. Therefore, the graft is not rejected.[26] Instead, gradually the homografts antigens start becoming stronger and they mount an immune response against the host. The host's antigens become foreign to the homograft and the homograft starts forming antibodies which destroy the host cells. This is called GVHD or "Runting syndrome" **(Figs. 2A to C)**. Patient may manifest with anemia, weight loss, fever, edema, ulceration, loss of hair, and splenomegaly.[27]

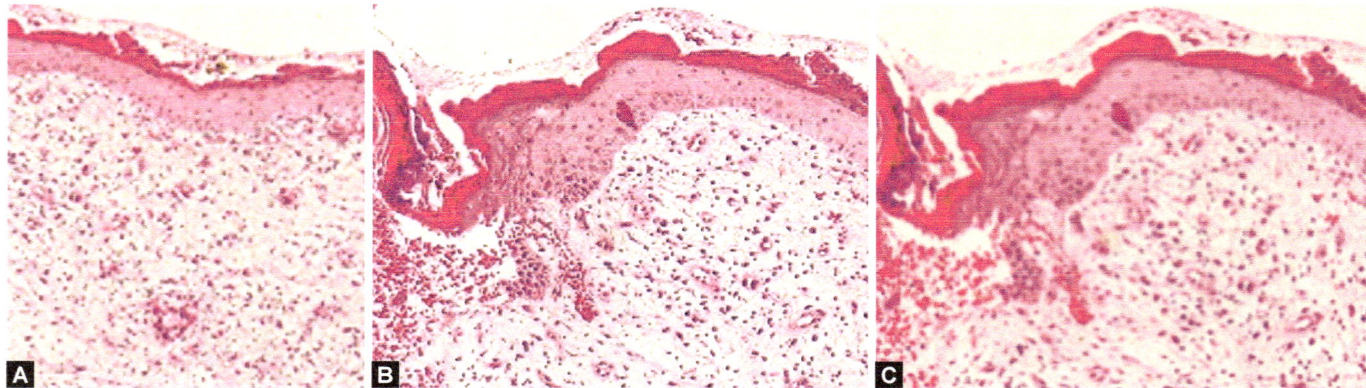

FIGS. 2A TO C: Histopathological picture of graft-versus-host disease (GVHD). (A) Crusting in stratum corneum and lymphocytic exocytosis along with perivascular mononuclear inflammatory infiltrate (10×, H&E). (B) Papillary dermal edema and hemorrhage (10×, H&E). (C) Dyskeratotic keratinocytes with perivascular and interstitial eosinophilic infiltrate (40×, H&E).

Courtesy: Department of Pathology, Vardhman Mahavir Medical College (VMMC) and Safdarjung Hospital, New Delhi.

Acute GVHD is characterized by a distinctive syndrome comprising dermatitis, hepatitis, and enteritis. The severity of disease is defined by a grading scheme from 0 to 5.

- 0 and 1 are mild diseases.
- 2 is moderate.
- 3 and 4 are severe and/or life-threatening and 5 is life-threatening.

Even with optimal immunosuppression, patient shows significant morbidity and mortality. In the long term after skin transplantation, after 100 days, a different form of GVHD may emerge even though initially it may have been considered as successful graft "take". This is considered as autoimmune phenomenon with relative immunodeficiency (Herman Waldman,[26] 1995). Experimental work in animal models shows that both forms of GVHD can be caused by both CD4 and CD8 cells.

Treatment for Graft-versus-host Disease

- *Ultraviolet A1 (UVA-1) phototherapy*: Clinical responses of sclerotic skin to UV-A1 phototherapy were modest cause of UV-A1—induced skin darkening, which is photo-protective and attenuates antifibrotic responses.
- *Low-dose methotrexate*: Methotrexate (MTX) appears to be a well-tolerated, inexpensive, and possibly steroid-sparing agent that is worthy of further evaluation in GVHD.
- Extracorporeal photochemotherapy (ECP), considered as an effective treatment for patients with erythrodermic cutaneous T-cell lymphoma, has recently been used successfully in the treatment of GVHD and prospective trials for treatment of chronic GVHD.
- Anti-inflammatory proteins in combination with steroids.

Approaches to Delay Alloskin Graft Immune Rejection

The use of allogenic skin grafts in extensive burn patients is limited as they are prone to rejection by triggering host immune response. In addition, systemic immunosuppressive drugs used in organ transplant cannot effectively prevent skin graft rejection. Their use in already immunologically compromised host can significantly increase the risk of infection. Pretreatment of skin allograft is an alternative to decrease the immunogenicity and delay rejection. This may be achieved by following:

- *Preservation of allogenic skin homograft in glycerol*: Langerhans (LC) cells in the glycerol treated graft cannot migrate out via lymphatic vessels to the draining nodes to activate alloreactive T cells, rendering them to be less immunogenic than cryopreserved grafts. However, induction of rejection response via indirect route is possible. In glycerol-treated allografts, rejection is delayed for up to 9 days.[28-31]
- *Depletion of donor-dendritic cells (DCs)*: The majority of DC-based measures try to prevent donor-derived dendritic and Langerhans cells (LC) from presenting antigens (DC).
    - Gliotoxin and epipolythiodioxopiperazine (ETP) immunosuppressive mycotoxin treatment decreases epidermal LCs.[32]
    - 10-dimethyl-1,2-benzanthracene (DMBA), which has been employed in the past, works by removing class II MHC antigens from the graft and LCs as a result. Its application in human transplant is not feasible due to its severe carcinogenic properties.[33]
    - By modifying the activity of DCs,[34] norcantharidin (NCTD, $C_8H_8O_4$), which is often used to enhance hematopoiesis, lengthens the time it takes for a transplant to get rejected.

  - Photodynamic therapy (PDT) uses methyl aminolevulinic acid (MLA) and aminolevulinic acid (ALA), two light-sensitive medicines, as photosensitizing agents. The medications are activated by nonthermal light.[35]
  - Short wavelength UVC can also successfully eliminate LCs in the graft prolonging its survival.[36]
- *Preventing oxidative damage*: Inflammatory cells infiltrating the graft produce reactive oxygen species (ROS) damaging the cell membranes accelerating the graft rejection. Antioxidant therapy such as Salen-Mn can prolong graft survival by preventing inflammation.[37]

Tissue Engineering for Skin Reconstruction

Skin replacements created by bioengineering can be a useful alternative to autograft or allograft. From the use of single skin cells or biologic scaffolds to the combination of cells and scaffolds for the treatment and repair of burns and chronic skin ulcers, tissue engineering of biologic skin substitutes has advanced significantly. The immunogenicity of skin allotransplantation and the lack of autologous split-thickness skin graft may be addressed by tissue-engineered skin substitutes.

CULTURED KERATINOCYTES ALLOGRAFT

Autogenous cultured keratinocytes normally take 3–4 weeks to grow a thin sheet of skin. Cultured allograft keratinocytes can overcome this problem and raise the prospect of banks of frozen skin readily available for transplantation. However, there are the disadvantages of high production costs, time consuming which limits its widespread use.[38] A consideration of how alloantigens are recognized in the skin suggests that cultured keratinocytes can survive without rejection.[39]

In the skin, the LC is the dendritic cell and the immunogenicity of skin allograft correlates directly with the density of the LCs,[40] which they contain functionally. However, LCs are complex because the efficiency with which they process and present antigen and activate T cell depends upon their location and differentiation.[40,41] LCs in the epidermis encounter antigen, which is then processed and displayed in association with MHC class 1 or 2.[42] LCs then migrate to lymph node and mature to a cocktail of cytokine signals. In the lymph node, the MHC antigen complex displayed at the LC plasma membrane is presented to any T cell reactive to the original antigen. In skin allograft responses, the evidence is that host T cells are activated by donor LCs which migrate from the graft to the draining lymph node. Thus, if the afferent lymphatics are severed, graft rejection is either abrogated (Barker and Billingham,[43] 1968) or delayed (Tilney and Gowans,[44] 1970).

Langerhans cells are nonadherent in vitro and are eliminated from primary keratinocyte culture within 7 days as a consequence of change in medium (Morhenn et al.,[45] 1982; Hammond et al.,[46] 1987). Cultured keratinocyte does not constitutively express MHC class 2 glycoproteins or the costimulatory molecules CD80 and CD86 (Nickoloff and Turka,[47] 1994) and fail to stimulate autologous lymphocyte in mixed lymphocyte reactions.

There is very little clinical or histological evidence for acute rejection of cultured keratinocyte allografts on ulcers or wounds.[17,48,49] Aubock et al.[50] (1988) used cultured allograft to partially cover tangentially excised third-degree burns and split thickness donor site. These grafts were rejected after 14 days, about 4–5 days longer than that reported for split thickness allograft. Histologically, rejection was accompanied by a mononuclear cell infiltration and vacuolation and necrosis of grafted epithelium.[17,39,42,51,52] Allogenic keratinocytes, despite having obvious disadvantages, present as a promising tool which can be further modified by immunomodulation. Viral transfection of keratinocytes represents an efficient method.[53-55]

Vogt et al. showed that in a pig model, transplanting retrovirally transfected keratinocytes resulted in epidermal regeneration and the production of growth hormones and β-galactosidase.[56]

Nevertheless, there are still a lot of restrictions on genetically modified keratinocytes since they can trigger an uncontrollable immune response and only permit the transfer of small genes. In conclusion, genetically altered keratinocytes may establish the basis for a skin substitute that is both broadly applicable and immunologically compatible.[57,58]

THREE-DIMENSIONAL BIOPRINTING

Three-dimensional (3D) bioprinting is another possible method for creating skin tissue. The process entails arranging scaffolds and cells in many configurations, potentially resulting in an exact replication of human skin.[59] Shape retention, flexibility, and reproducibility are some of its benefits. There are currently tissue-engineered multilayered skin grafts available;[60] however, these often deteriorate with time. Stable engraftment is hindered by the typical absence of dermal vasculature in tissue-engineered skin grafts. It may be encouraged by creating a bilayered replacement dermal vasculature.[61]

Also, human vascular cells can provide angiocrine factors promoting healing.[62] Significant advances have been made in the field of tissue bioengineering but still skin microvasculature is complex and very difficult to replicate. Till date, the lowest diameter reported of a 3D bioprinted perfused vessel in a skin construct is 80 μm,[63] while the size of skin microvasculature at the superficial horizontal plexus level is <26 μm.[64]

Bioprinting methods such as microextrusion, inkjet, and laser-assisted printing are being currently explored for development of complex synthetic skin models.[65,66] Incorporating pigment producing melanocytes and immune cells in the tissue-engineered skin graft is also under research.[67,68]

Although 3D bioprinting shows promising results so far, further research is needed to overcome the disadvantages such as optimal cell and scaffold combinations, vascularity, and production costs.[69]

THE PRESENT AND FUTURE OF SKIN ALLOGRAFT

The several mechanisms underlying allograft rejection are now well understood. The dream of homologous skin graft becoming accepted by the host forever may be fulfilled in future. In contrast to the transplantation of other organs, skin has the lowest morbidity rate when it comes to live donors and is easily accessible in the patient.[9,14,32,33] Moreover, skin homografts can be obtained from live as well as cadaveric donors.

It is not appropriate to use prolonged immunosuppression to extend the survival of skin allografts. An effective method of lowering rejection would be to immunomodulate allogenic grafts instead.

A skin substitute that is immunologically compatible and widely accepted can be produced using autologous or genetically modified allogenic cultured keratinocytes.[70]

According to Deuse et al.,[71] hypoimmunogenic skin grafts created with universal cells can supply universal, readily available transplantable skin substitutes with minimal immunogenicity.

SUMMARY

Despite intensive efforts, it has not yet been possible to create a skin substitute that is fully developed, universally applicable, immunologically compatible, and capable of providing an aesthetically pleasing result. Consequently, forward-looking research is focusing on the immunological modification of allogeneic skin grafts. The long-term goal remains to create an off-the-shelf, transplantable skin substitute with high biological functionality and reduced immunogenicity. However, achieving this goal will require extensive research efforts to generate further results.

REFERENCES

1. Hutchinson Ian V. The immunobiology of transplant rejection and acceptance. In: Hakim NS, Danovitch GM (Eds). Transplantation Surgery, Springer Specialist Surgery Series. London: Springer; 2001. pp. 55-72.
2. Waldmann H, Polliak A, Hale G, Or R, Cividalli G, Weiss L, et al. Elimination of graft versus host disease by in-vitro depletion alloreactive lymphocytes monoclonal rat antihuman lymphocyte antibody (CAMPATH-1). Lancet. 1984;2:483-6.
3. Bradley Andrew J, Hamilton David N. Organ transplantation: an historical perspective. Transplant Surg. 1990:1-5.
4. Medawar PB. The behavior and fate of skin autografts and skin homografts in rabbits. J Anatomy. 1944;78:176-99.
5. Andrew BJ, Hamilton David NH. Organ transplantation: a historical perspective. Transplant surg. 1990:1-6.
6. Pedersen NC, Moris B. The role of the lymphatic system in the rejection of homograft: a study of lymph from renal transplant. J Exp Med. 1970;131:936.
7. Gibson T, Medawar PB. The fate of skin homograft in man. J Anat. 1943;77:299.
8. Converse JM, Duchet G. Successful homologous skin grafting in a war burn using an identical twin as a donor. Plast Reconst Surg. 1947;2:342-4.
9. Stranc ML. Skin Allograft survival in a severely burned triplet; study of triplet zygotic type. Plast Reconstr Surg. 1966;37: 280-90.
10. Caruso DM, Gregory MW, Schiller WR. The use of skin from a monozygotic twin combined with cultured epithelial autografts as coverage for a large surface area burns: a case report and review of the literature. J Burn care rehabil. 1996;17:432-4.
11. Horch R, Stark GB, Kopp J, Spilker G. Cologne Burn Centre experiences with glycerol-preserved allogeneic skin: Part I: Clinical experiences and histological findings (overgraft and sandwich technique). Burns. 1994;20:S23-6.
12. Krenzien F, Keshi E, Splith K, Griesel S, Kamali K, Sauer IM, et al. Diagnostic Biomarkers to Diagnose Acute Allograft Rejection After Liver Transplantation: Systematic Review and Meta-Analysis of Diagnostic Accuracy Studies. Front Immunol. 2019;10:758.
13. Von Visger J, Cassol C, Nori U, Franco-Ahumada G, Nadasdy T, Satoskar AA. Complete biopsy-proven resolution of deposits in recurrent proliferative glomerulonephritis with monoclonal IgG deposits (PGNMIGD) following rituximab treatment in renal allograft. BMC Nephrol. 2019;20:53.
14. Jang JK, Kim KW, Choi SH, Jeong SY, Kim JH, Yu ES, et al. CT of acute rejection after liver transplantation: A matched case–control study. Eur Radiol. 2019;29:3736-45.
15. Alexander JW, MacMillan BG, Law E, Kittur DS. Treatment of severe burns with widely meshed skin autografts and meshed skin allograft overlay. J Trauma 1981;21:433-8.
16. Phipps AR, Clarke JA. The use of intermingled auto graft and parental allograft skin in the treatment of major burns in children. Br J Plast Surg. 1991;44:608-11.
17. Yang CC, Shih TS, Chu TA, Hsu WS, Kuo SY, Chao YF. The intermingled transplantation of autografts and homografts in severe burns. Burns. 1980;6:141-5.
18. Takiuchi L, Higuchi D, Sei Y, Nakajima T. Histological identification of prolonged survival of a skin Allograft on an extensively burned patient. Burns. 1982;8:164-7.

19. Burke JF, May JW Jr, Albright N, Quinby WC, Russell PS. Temporary skin transplantation and immunosuppression for extensive burns. N Eng J Med. 1974;290:269-71.
20. Burke JF, Quinby WC JR, Bondoc CC. Primary excision and prompt grafting as routine therapy for the treatment of thermal burns in children. Surg Clin North Am. 1976;56:477-94.
21. Borel JF, Feurer C, Gubler HU, Stahelin H. Biological effects of cyclosporine A: A new antilymphocytic agent. Agents Actions. 1976;6:468-75.
22. Black KS, Hewitt CW, Smelser S, Yearsley S, Bazzo DE, Achauer BM. Cyclosporine and skin allografts for the treatment of thermal injury. Transplantation. II. Development of an experimental massive third-degree burn model demonstrating extensive graft survival. 1988;45:13-6.
23. Frame JD, Sanders R, Goodacre TEE, Morgan BDG. The fate of meshed allograft skin in burned patients using cyclosporine immunosuppression. Br J Plast Surg. 1989;42:27-34.
24. Colletti LM, Johnson KJ, Kunkel RG, Merion RM. Mechanisms of hyperacute rejection in porcine liver transplantation. Antibody mediated endothelial injury. Transplantation. 1994;57:1357-63.
25. Codner MA, Shuster BA, Steinman RM, Harper AD, LaTrenta GS, Hoffman LA. Migration of donor leukocytes from limb allografts into host lymphoid tissues. Ann Plastic surg. 1990;25:353-9.
26. Delves Peter J, Roitt Ivan M. Graft Vs Host Diesease. in: Delves PJ, Roitt IM (Eds). Encyclopedia of Immunology, 2nd edition, vol. 2. United States: Academic Press Ltd. (Harcourt Brace and Co. Publishers); 1998. pp. 1015-20.
27. Lapidot T, Singer TS, Salomon O, Terenzi A, Schwartz E, Reisner Y. Booster irradiation to the spleen following total body irradiation. A new immunosuppressive approach for allogenic bone marrow transplantation. J Immunol. 1988;141:2619-24.
28. Van Baare J, Buitenwerf J, Hoekstra MJ, du Pont JS. Virucidal effect of glycerol as used in donor skin preservation. Burns. 1994;20:S77-80.
29. De Backere AJC. Euro Skin Bank: large scale skin-banking in Europe based on glycerol-preservation of donor skin. Burns. 1994;20:S4-9.
30. Van Baare J, Ligtvoet EEJ, Middelkoop E. Microbiological evaluation of glycerolized cadaveric donor skin. Transplantation. 1998;65:966-70.
31. Richters CD, Hoekstra MJ, Van Baare J, Du Pont JS, Kamperdijk EWA. Morphology of glycerol-preserved human cadaver skin. Burns. 1996;22:113-6.
32. McMinn PC, Halliday GM, Muller HK. Effects of gliotoxin on Langerhans' cell function: contact hypersensitivity responses and skin graft survival. Immunology. 1990;71:46-51.
33. Halliday GM, Muller HK. Induction of tolerance via skin depleted of Langerhans cells by a chemical carcinogen. Cell Immunol. 1986;99:220-7.
34. Hsieh CH, Liao HF, Kuo CD, Huang YC, Shueng PW, Hsu YP, et al. Norcantharidin modulates development of dendritic cells and prolongs skin allograft survival. Transplantation. 2011;92:848-57.
35. Obochi MO, Ratkay LG, Levy JG. Prolonged skin allograft survival after photodynamic therapy associated with modification of donor skin antigenicity. Transplantation. 1997;63:810-7.
36. Lee CH, Wu SB, Hong CH, Yu HS, Wei YH. Molecular mechanisms of UV-induced apoptosis and its effects on skin residential cells: the implication in UV-based phototherapy. Int J Mol Sci. 2013;14:6414-35.
37. Tocco G, Illigens BM, Malfroy B, Benichou G. Prolongation of alloskin graft survival by catalytic scavengers of reactive oxygen species. Cell Immunol. 2006;241:59-65.
38. Kogan S, Halsey J, Agag RL. Biologics in Acute Burn Injury. Ann Plast Surg. 2019;83:26-33.
39. Kries RW, Hoekstra MJ, Mackie DP, Vloemans AF, Hermans RP. Historical appraisal of the use of skin Allograft in the treatment of extensive full skin thickness burns at the red cross hospital burn center, Beverwijk, Netherlands. Burns. 1992;18:S19-22.
40. Larsen CP, Barker H, Morris PJ, Austyn JM. failure of mature dendritic cells of the host to migrate from the blood in to cardiac or skin allografts. Transplantation. 1990;50:294-301.
41. Larsen CP, Steinman RM, Witmer-Pack M, Hankins DF, Morris PJ, Austyn JM. Migration and maturation of Langerhans cells in skin transplants and explants. J Exp Med. 1990;172:1483-93.
42. Hefton JM, Madden MR, Finkelstein J, Shires GT. Grafting of burn patients with Allograft of cultured epidermal cells. Lancet. 1983;2:428-32.
43. Barker CF, Billingham RE. The role of afferent lymphatics in the rejection of skin allografts. J exp med. 1968;128:197-220.
44. Tilney NL, Gowans JL. The sensitization of rats by allografts transplanted to a lymphatic pedicle. J exp med. 1970;133: 951-62.
45. Morhenn VB, Benike CJ, Cox AJ, Charron DJ, Engleman EG. Cultured human epidermal cells do not synthetize HLA-DR. J invest Dermatol. 1982;78:32-7.
46. Hammond EJ, Stanley MA Munro AJ. Prolonged survival of cultured keratinocyte allografts in the immunosuppressed mouse. Transplantation. 1987;44:106-12.
47. Nickoloff BJ, Nestle FO, Zheng XG, Turka LA. T lymphocytes in skin lesions of psoriasis and mycosis fungoides express B7-1: a ligand for CD28. Blood. 1994;83:2580-6.
48. Sakabu SA, Hansborough JE, Cooper ML, Greenleaf G. Cyclosporine A for prolonging Allograft survival in patients with massive burns. J Burn care Rehabil. 1990;11:410-8.
49. Sawada Y. Survival of an extensively burned child following use of fragments of autograft skin overlain with meshed autograft skin. Burns Incl Therm Inj. 1985;11:429-33.
50. Auböck J, Irschick E, Romani N, Kompatscher P, Höpfl R, Herold M, et al. Rejection after a slightly prolonged survival time of Langerhans cells free allogenic cultured epidermis used for wound coverage in humans. Transplantation. 1988;45:730-7.
51. Teepe RGC, Kreis RW, Koeburgge EJ, Kempenaar JA, Vloemans AF, Hermans RP, et al. The use of cultured autologous epidermis in the treatment of extensive burn wounds. J Trauma. 1990b; 30:269-75.
52. Wu J, Barisoni D, Armato U. An investigation in to the mechanism by which human dermis does not significantly contribute to the rejection of allo-skin graft. Burns. 1995;21:11-6.
53. Garlick JA, Katz AB, Fenjves ES, Taichman LB. Retrovirus-mediated transduction of cultured epidermal keratinocytes. J. Invest Dermatol. 1991;97:824-9.
54. Braun-Falco M, Doenecke A, Smola H, Hallek M. Efficient gene transfer into human keratinocytes with recombinant adeno-associated virus vectors. Gene Ther. 1999;6:432-41.
55. Chen M, Li W, Fan J, Kasahara N, Woodley D. An efficient gene transduction system for studying gene function in primary human dermal fibroblasts and epidermal keratinocytes. Clin Exp Dermatol. 2003;28:193-9.

56. Vogt PM, Thompsont S, Andree C, Liu P, Breuing K, Hatzis D, et al. Genetically modified keratinocytes transplanted to wounds reconstitute the epidermis. Proc Natl Acad Sci USA. 1994;91:9307-931.
57. David RM, Doherty AT. Viral Vectors: The Road to Reducing Genotoxicity. Toxicol Sci. 2017;155:315-25.
58. Collins DE, Reuter JD, Rush HG, Villano JS. Viral Vector Biosafety in Laboratory Animal Research. Comp Med. 2017;67:215-21.
59. Tarassoli SP, Jessop ZM, Al-Sabah A, Gao N, Whitaker S, Doak S, et al. Skin tissue engineering using 3D bioprinting: An evolving research field. J Plast Reconstr Aesthetic Surg. 2018;71:615-23.
60. Zaulyanov L, Kirsner RS. A review of a bi-layered living cell treatment (Apligraf) in the treatment of venous leg ulcers and diabetic foot ulcers. Clin Interv Aging. 2007;2:93.
61. Shepherd BR, Enis DR, Wang F, Suarez Y, Pober JS, Schechner JS. Vascularization and engraftment of a human skin substitute using circulating progenitor cell-derived endothelial cells. FASEB J. 2006;20:1739.
62. Tonnesen MG, Feng X, Clark RAF. Angiogenesis in wound healing. J Invest Dermatol Symp Proc. 2000;5:40.
63. Abaci HE, Guo Z, Coffman A, Gillette B, Lee WH, Sia SK, et al. Human skin constructs with spatially controlled vasculature using primary and iPSC derived endothelial cells. Adv Healthcare Mater. 2016;5:1800-7.
64. Braverman IM, Sibley J. Ultrastructural and three-dimensional analysis of the contractile cells of the cutaneous microvasculature. J Invest Dermatol. 1990;95:90-6.
65. Derr K, Zou J, Luo K, Song MJ, Sittampalam GS, Zhou C, et al. Fully three-dimensional bioprinted skin equivalent constructs with validated morphology and barrier function. Tissue Eng Part C Methods. 2019;25:334-43.
66. Pourchet LJ, Thepot A, Albouy M, Courtial EJ, Boher A, Blum LJ, et al. Human skin 3D bioprinting using scaffold-free approach. Adv Healthcare Mater. 2016;6:1601101.
67. Min D, Lee W, Bae IH, Lee TR, Croce P, Yoo SS. Bioprinting of biomimetic skin containing melanocytes. Exp Dermatol. 2018;27:453-9.
68. Vidal Yucha SE, Tamamoto KA, Nguyen H, Cairns DM, Kaplan DL. Human skin equivalents demonstrate need for neuro-immuno-cutaneous system. Adv Biosyst. 2019;3:1800283.
69. Vijayavenkataraman S, Lu WF, Fuh JYH. 3D bioprinting of skin: A state-of-the-art review on modelling, materials, and processes. Biofabrication. 2016;8:032001.
70. Eming SA, Krieg T, Davidson JM. RETRACTED: Gene therapy and wound healing. Clin Dermatol. 2007;25:79-92.
71. Deuse T, Hu X, Gravina A, Wang D, Tediashvili G, De C, et al. Hypoimmunogenic derivatives of induced pluripotent stem cells evade immune rejection in fully immunocompetent allogeneic recipients. Nat Biotechnol. 2019;37:252-8.

CHAPTER

9

Microbiology in Burns

Deepthi Nair, Rojaleen Das

INTRODUCTION

Burn injuries continue to be a prevalent and devastating form of trauma. These patients require immediate and effective care in order to minimize morbidity and mortality. Invasive infection is now the chief reason for death and morbidity after burn injury, being responsible for 51% of the deaths.[1]

Because of developments in contemporary medical care during the past few decades, the survival rates for burn patients have significantly increased. Improvements in fluid treatment, nutrition, burn wound care, respiratory care, and infection control procedures have all been credited with better result. Consequently, in the last 40 years, the number of burn-related mortality has decreased by half.[1-3] In patients with burns involving >40% of the total body surface area (TBSA), sepsis from burn site infection and other infectious consequences continue to account for 75% of all deaths. These complications are greatly exacerbated by inhalation injuries.[4-6]

Burn wound infections have been enigmatic in terms of diagnosis. Multiple factors contribute toward this fact, which include recognition of colonization versus true infection, numerous/multiple pathogens/colonizers, confounding symptoms and signs, poor sampling methods, and difficult microbiological techniques.[7] Several workers have published papers on evaluating the most accurate and reproducible methods for diagnosing wound infections. Chronic burn wounds contain a large number of bacteria inherent within them. The numbers of bacteria which constitute infection in an ordinary acute surgical wound (i.e., > or = 10^5 microorganisms/g of tissue) are not valid in burn wounds. Direct correlation with quantitative count is no more seen to be a foolproof method. Burn wound colonization may be diagnosed when bacteria are present at low concentrations [<10^5 colony-forming units (CFU)] on the wound surface. No surrounding erythema or cellulitis is evident, but deterioration of the wound surface can be observed.

Deep fluid culture correlated with histopathology examination and clinical signs and symptoms in immunocompromised patients like burns has been found to be more useful than quantitative counts alone. Despite levels of microorganisms as great as 10^8/g of burned tissue, these burn wounds go on to heal adequately.[8-10] The presence of cellulitis is the foundation of the clinical diagnosis. Burn wound cellulitis can be observed when the area of erythema extends beyond what would be expected for the injury alone.

Burn wounds often are polymicrobial, contain three or more microorganisms, both gram-positive and gram-negative bacteria, as well as aerobic and anaerobic species. They often contain fungal flora, especially in long-standing wounds where multiple broad-spectrum antibiotics have been given. This cohabitation of flora with the resultant competition for nutrients and space is thought to decrease their virulence and ability to harm tissues.[8,11] Due to differences in the way acute and chronic wounds respond to diverse numbers of microorganisms, emphasis is currently being placed on clinical signs and symptoms as compared to actual numbers of microorganisms in a wound. Microorganisms invade the burn eschar over time, leading to burn wound infection and progressing to burn wound sepsis. The use of systemic antibiotics, effective topical treatments, and early burn wound excision with closure have all decreased the incidence of burn wound sepsis. Along with the classical signs of infection (erythema, edema, heat, purulent exudates, and pain), there are a few more criteria which have been included, namely serous exudates with concurrent inflammation, delayed healing, discoloration of granulation tissue, friable granulation tissue, pocketing at the base of the wound, foul odor, and wound breakdown. As the patient is being monitored, the symptom of increasing pain and dehiscence of wound is a good predictor of infection.[11,12] There are several sequelae of burn wound infection which include cellulitis, conversion of a second-degree burn to full-thickness third-degree burn, septicemia, gas gangrene, graft failure, delayed healing, scarring, etc.[13]

PATHOGENESIS OF WOUND INFECTION AND IMMUNOLOGY OF SKIN

The body site, the patient's age, sex, and other factors all affect how thick the epidermis and dermis are. Deeper burn injuries occur because the dermal layer of the skin is thinner in newborns, young children, and elderly. Because the shafts of appendages are lined with epithelial cells, the dermis has the ability to generate new epithelial cells to replace those lost from the epidermis. Both layers of the skin contain nerve endings and the dermal connective tissue offers the skin's remodeling a stable structural foundation.[3] Thermal injuries weaken an individual's immune system. This was demonstrated by the fact that these patients' homografts thrive for a longer time.[14,15] Innate and adaptive immune responses include the two categories of host defenses.

The first line of defense that comes into play as soon as the skin is broken by a burn wound is the innate immune response.[16] The systemic aspect of immunity is also activated when the wound is deep, encompasses huge areas, or affects vital organ systems. A wide range of presentations are caused by the reaction of body to burn injury and major side effects such severe sepsis, multiple-organ dysfunction syndrome (MODS), and systemic inflammatory response syndrome (SIRS) can increase morbidity and death.[17]

Unfortunately, because of the pathophysiology of burns, definitions developed by the American College of Chest Physicians and Society of Critical Care Medicine for SIRS, sepsis, severe sepsis, and septic shock inadequately describe the septic responses of the burn patient. Large burns, those covering >20% of the TBSA, compromise the barrier function of the skin that prevents entry of microorganisms, triggering a prolonged, constant exposure to host immune response mediators that is not observed in other critical illnesses. The profound biphasic immune response, described as hyperinflammation, followed by severe immunodepression, has a clinical presentation that mimics SIRS, sepsis, and the already mentioned states. This finding led to a consensus conference in 2007 by members of the American Burn Association, who determined the definition of sepsis for burn patients that is used today.[18] The group also adjudicated that the terms and clinical descriptions of SIRS, severe sepsis, and septic shock were not useful for the burn.

Sepsis is a change in the burn patient that triggers the concern for infection. It is a presumptive diagnosis where antibiotics are usually started and a search for a cause of infection should be initiated. However, there is need for clinical interpretation and the diagnosis needs to be with the discovery of an infection.[19,20] The definition is age dependent with adjustments necessary for children.

MICROBIAL ETIOLOGY

The patient's gastrointestinal system, upper respiratory tract, and skin are the sources of the endogenous microorganisms colonizing the burn wound.[21] The typical microbiota of the vagina, mouth, and stomach is rich and varied. Additionally, a patient's skin surface may come into contact with microorganisms through water, food, air, contaminated external environmental surfaces, and the hands of healthcare personnel.[22] Colonization is made possible by slowly healing wounds that expose devitalized tissue over time. Gram-positive bacteria from the patient's external environment or endogenous skin flora are the first to cause problems after an injury.[23] In the initial days following damage, endogenous gram-negative bacteria (GNB) from the patient's gut flora also quickly colonize the burn wound surface.[24]

Numerous different endogenous anaerobic bacteria can colonize wounds that have a suitably hypoxic environment. Anaerobic bacterial cultures are either absent or very minimal in the majority of published research. However, anaerobes are discovered in significant quantities when wounds are examined using the proper microbiological procedures. Anaerobes have been referred to as "invisible villains" and "the secret pathogens." Yeast and fungal colonization of wounds typically happens later as a result of broad-spectrum antibiotic therapy.[25]

Antimicrobial medications tend to be less effective against microorganisms originating from the patient's normal flora than against those transmitted from the hospital environment.[26] The most frequent bacteria that colonize and infect burn wounds are listed in **Table 1 and Box 1**. Group A, beta-hemolytic *streptococci*, or *Streptococcus pyogenes*, were the most common pathogen associated with burn wound infections and a leading cause of mortality until the discovery of antibiotics. When Penicillin G was developed in the 1950s, *Staphylococcus aureus (S. aureus)* "wiped out" the *streptococci*. *Staphylococcus aureus* is still a frequent cause of early burn wound infection today. One of the main causes of burn wound infection is *Pseudomonas aeruginosa*

TABLE 1: Invasive microbial infection in burn wound.

Group	Species
Gram-positive organisms	• *Staphylococcus aureus* • Methicillin-resistant *Staphylococcus aureus* • Coagulase-negative *Staphylococcus aureus* • *Enterococcus* species • Vancomycin-resistant *Enterococcus*
Gram-negative organisms	• *Pseudomonas aeruginosa* • *Escherichia coli* • *Klebsiella pneumoniae* • *Serratia marcescens* • *Enterobacter* species • *Proteus* species • *Acinetobacter* species • *Bacteroides* species
Fungi	• *Candida* species • *Aspergillus* species • *Rhizopus* species • *Mucor* species
Virus	• Herpes simplex virus • Cytomegalovirus • Varicella zoster virus

(*P. aeruginosa*), which originates from the patient's surroundings or from their own endogenous gut flora.

The prevalence of uncommon infectious diseases has been gradually rising **(Box 1)**.[27] Anaerobic bacterial infections are less prevalent, although they usually result from electrical burns or from using open wound dressings instead of occlusive dressings.[28] Antimicrobial resistance has emerged globally in a wide range of bacterial and fungal infections, especially nosocomial isolates, which restricts the therapeutic choices available for efficient treatment.[29] As serious pathogens, methicillin-resistant *S. aureus* (*MRSA*), vancomycin-resistant *Enterococci* (*VRE*), and multiple resistant GNB with various beta-lactamase types—such as extended spectrum, AmpC, and metallo-beta—have been identified in hospitalized patients.[26]

Due to the use of broad-spectrum topical and systemic treatments when infection emerges in the burned patient, fungal infections—particularly *Candida* species—have grown in importance as opportunistic pathogens and have shown growing degrees of resistance to antifungal drugs.[30]

QUANTITATIVE MICROBIOLOGY: SIGNIFICANCE OF MICROBIAL NUMBERS

Bendy et al.[10] swabbed decubitus ulcers and found that a bacterial load of 10^6 CFU/mL of wound fluid slowed

BOX 1 Microflora of wounds.

Aerobic and facultative microorganisms found and the type of wound (A—acute and C—chronic)

Gram-positive:
- Coagulase-negative *staphylococci* A, C
- *Staphylococcus aureus* A, C
- Beta-hemolytic *Streptococcus* (group C) A, Beta-hemolytic *Streptococcus* (group G) C
- *Streptococcus* species (fecal) A
- *Streptococcus* species (viridans) A, C
- *Streptococcus intermedius* C
- *Corynebacterium xerosis* C, *Corynebacterium* species A, C
- *Micrococcus* species C
- *Bacillus* species A

Gram-negative:
- *Escherichia coli* A, C; *Escherichia hermannii* A
- *Serratia liquefaciens* C
- *Klebsiella pneumoniae* A, C; *Klebsiella oxytoca* A, C
- *Enterobacter cloacae* A, C; *Enterobacter aerogenes* C
- *Citrobacter freundii* C
- *Proteus mirabilis* A, C; *Proteus vulgaris* C
- *Providencia stuartii* A
- *Morganella morganii* C
- *Acinetobacter calcoaceticus* A, C
- *Pseudomonas aeruginosa* A, C
- *Stenotrophomonas maltophilia* A

Anaerobic and facultative anaerobic microorganisms isolated from acute and chronic wounds of varied etiology:
- *Clostridium limosum* A; *Clostridium bifermentans* A; *Clostridium difficile* C; *Clostridium sporogenes* A, C; *Clostridium ramosum* C; *Clostridium tertium* A; *Clostridium histolyticum* A, C; *Clostridium septicum* A; *Clostridium barati* C; *Clostridium clostridioforme* A, C; *Clostridium perfringens* A, C; *Clostridium cadaveris* A, C
- *Peptostreptococcus asaccharolyticus* A, C; *Peptostreptococcus anaerobius* A, C; *Peptostreptococcus* species A, C; *Peptostreptococcus micros* A, C; *Peptostreptococcus prevotii* A, C; *Peptostreptococcus magnus* A, C; *Peptostreptococcus indolicus* C
- *Bacteroides thetaiotaomicron* C; *Bacteroides caccae* C; *Bacteroides capillosus* C; Bacteroides stercoris C; *Bacteroides fragilis* A, C; *Bacteroides uniformis* A, C; *Bacteroides ovatus* A; *Bacteroides ureolyticus* A, C
- *Prevotella oralis* A, C; *Prevotella oris* A, C; *Prevotella* disiens A; *Prevotella bivia* C; *Prevotella buccae* C; *Prevotella* species A; *Prevotella corporis* A, C; *Prevotella intermedia* A; *Prevotella melaninogenica* C
- *Porphyromonas asaccharolytica* A, C
- *Propionibacterium acnes* A, C
- *Sphingobacterium multivorum* C
- *Eubacterium limosum* C
- *Fusobacterium necrophorum* C
- *Veillonella* species A

Fungi:
- *Candida parapsilosis* A
- *Candida krusei* A

healing. This finding highlighted the clinical significance of the microbial load in delaying wound healing. Subsequent tissue biopsy specimens were shown to be better specimens.[31,32] Quantitative cultivation of tissue biopsy specimens is labor intensive for the microbiology laboratory and has no bearing on expediting the treatment of burn wounds. A fast Gram stain has been found to be a reliable indicator of a microbial load of 10^5 CFU/g of tissue if a single microbe was observed on the prepared slide.[33,34] More recently, it has been shown that quantitative tissue cultures are a more accurate predictor of the chance of wound infection than swab cultures and that a critical quantity of bacteria of $>10^4$ CFU/g of tissue must be reached to produce infection in wounds. Some writers rank histopathology as the most important approach since it shows actual invasion.[35] Surface imprinting with a velvet pad is another method that has been used. Dermabrasion has also been employed as a sample technique.

Deep-tissue biopsy procedures and quantitative research based on surface sampling techniques have been the two most widely used approaches. There has been debate on the usefulness of superficial cultures in the evaluation of wounds. It has been suggested that while biopsied tissue may produce a sizable number of bacteria, purulent wound fluid may not grow any microbes.[36] Furthermore, it has been suggested that a variety of aerobic and anaerobic microbes are likely to be present in superficial tissue, some of which may infiltrate deeper tissue. It is quite unlikely that deeper tissue may be "infected," while the superficial tissue is "sterile." Microorganisms colonize most wounds and inadequate microbiological technique is more likely to be the cause of the failure to isolate them.

According to some authors quantitative bacteriology does not provide greater information than that obtained from surface swabs. Infact swabs yielding more than 30 CFU definitely indicate a tissue count of 10^5 FU/g. It is controversial whether tissue biopsies, which are invasive, possibly unpleasant for the patient, and nonroutine—requiring professional manipulation and adding to the microbiology laboratory's workload—are necessary to quantify microorganisms. Tissue biopsies continue to play an important role in the identification of fungi, anaerobes, and other relatively uncommon infections.[37]

SIGNIFICANCE OF SPECIFIC MICROORGANISMS

Numerous studies have been conducted on the effects of particular microbes on the development and healing of burn wounds. It is only possible to confirm the existence of microorganisms and their identity as the causative agent of infection or delayed healing if they exist as a pure monomicrobial flora. Aerobes and anaerobes are both involved in the polymicrobial etiology of burn wounds. Polymicrobially infected wounds cannot be used to distinguish between pathogenic and nonpathogenic species and the existence of a pathogen in a mixed-culture infection does not always indicate that specific microbe as the cause of the illness. In wounds that are polymicrobially infected, the diagnosis of infection should be made primarily on the basis of clinical indicators, such as fever, erythema, edema, heat, and pain; microbiological results can be useful, but they are sometimes deceptive. However, microbiological data may need to be prioritized more when clinical signs of illness are less obvious. Aerobic pathogens, including GNB, *P. aeruginosa, and S. aureus,* have been commonly identified as the source of infection and delayed wound healing. Because of its high incidence and tendency toward more severe consequences, *S. aureus* is thought to be the most problematic bacterium in burn wound infections.[38,39]

At a conference of the European Tissue Repair Society and the European Wound Management Association, it was decided that the presence of *P. aeruginosa* or beta-hemolytic (group A) *streptococci* in a chronic wound was an urgent sign that antibiotic therapy needs to be started.[40,41] Long-term burn wounds create a symbiotic ecosystem, as evidenced by the coexistence of aerobic and anaerobic microbes. Anaerobic bacteria grow more readily when oxygen-consuming aerobic bacteria cause tissue hypoxia and a decrease in redox potential. Similarly, certain nutrients produced by one bacterium may promote the growth of fastidious and potentially pathogenic cohabiting microorganisms.[42]

As a result, *Prevotella melaninogenica* (*P. melaninogenica*) grows more readily in vitro when *S. aureus* is present. This is because *P. melaninogenica* is more harmful when vitamin K is present. By supplying succinate, a crucial growth factor, *Klebsiella pneumoniae* (*K. pneumoniae*) has been shown to play a key role in increasing the virulence of *P. melaninogenica*. Additionally, certain anaerobes have the ability to reduce the function of host immune cells, which gives them and other coexisting microorganisms a competitive edge. *P. melaninogenica* only displayed antiphagocytic activity when hemin and vitamin K, which are supplied by bacteria such as *S. aureus*, were present. Moreover, succinate prevents *S. aureus* and *Escherichia coli* (*E. coli*) from phagocytosing and moving about.

It is theoretically more harmful to have both *S. aureus* and a pigmenting gram-negative anaerobe in a wound than it is to have the same amount of *S. aureus* by itself. Because this will decide whether pathogenic interactions are likely to occur, the makeup of the polymicrobial wound flora is likely to be more significant than the presence of particular pathogens. The immune response in managing wound microflora is another essential component of wound healing that should not be undervalued. In addition to debilitating illnesses such as diabetes mellitus, chronic granulomatous disease, other immune deficiencies, and bacteria, factors including tissue necrosis, hypoxia, and ischemia also hinder immune cell activation in a wound. Addressing the issue of burn wound infection requires evaluating the host and microbial components together, in addition to the patient's symptomatology and clinical indications.

BIOLOGICAL ANALYSIS OF WOUNDS

There is not much agreement on the following topics: When and how a sample should be collected, how to send a specimen to the laboratory, and what analyses should be ordered. There is further confusion since medical professionals frequently believe that a microbiological report can definitely determine whether a wound is infected[43] and because receiving an antibiogram for a specific pathogen can frequently be deceptive and lead to needless therapy. Nevertheless, as mentioned earlier in this chapter, it is still imperative that the burn wounds be evaluated clinically, microbiologically, and histopathologically. The data generated is crucial for hospital infection control as it can forecast internal spread and progression of infections.

Wound-sampling Methods

In general, samples of wound tissue or fluid can be used to examine the quantitative and qualitative microbiology of wounds. Tissue biopsies are typically carried out and the fluid is swabbed.

Wound Tissue Sampling

The most effective technique for identifying the microbial load and the presence of invasive pathogens is the acquisition of a deep tissue biopsy after initial debridement and cleaning of superficial debris. Following aseptic tissue extraction, the tissue is homogenized, weighed, serially diluted, and plated onto both selective and nonselective media. After that, they are cultured in both aerobic and anaerobic environments to yield both quantitative and qualitative data. The microbial composition of superficial, devitalized tissue extracted by curettage may also be examined. An additional method—dermabrasion—is a less intrusive procedure than a biopsy.[44] It is recommended to collect and send for workup multiple samples from various locations of the burn wound.

Two parallel incisions in the skin, each measuring 1–2 cm in length and 1.5 cm apart, are made to extract a piece of the underlying fat after the wound has been cleaned with isopropyl alcohol. A 3 mm punch biopsy technique can provide biopsies weighing between 0.02 and 0.5 g. This method requires a lot of technical skill. Histopathological analysis can identify bacteria and fungi [periodic acid Schiff (PAS) and Gomori methenamine silver (GMS)]; however, cultures are required to confirm the diagnosis and provide pathogen sensitivity. Viruses that are linked to wounds, such as the herpes simplex virus (HSV) (Giemsa), are isolated by identifying inclusions on light or electron microscopy. Additionally, histology provides guidance for burn wound stages.[45,46]

The various stages of burn wound infection are as follows:

1. Stage I—colonization:
   a. Superficial—microorganisms present only on burn wound surface
   b. Penetrating—variable depth of microbial penetration of eschar
   c. Proliferating—variable level of microbial proliferation at nonviable-viable tissue interface (subeschar space)
2. Stage II—invasion:
   a. Microinvasion—microorganisms present in viable tissue immediately subjacent to subeschar space
3. Stage III—deep invasion:
   a. Penetration of microorganisms to variable depth and expanse within viable subcutaneous tissues
   b. *Microvascular involvement*: Microorganisms within small blood vessels and lymphatics (thrombosis of vessels is common)

Wound Fluid Sampling

Cotton-tipped swabs are used to capture samples of superficial wound fluid and tissue debris. When there is a significant amount of burn wound fluid present, needle aspiration sample may be used. This works better than swabbing. For sampling deeper pockets of fluid, the syringe technique might be employed. As long as the procedure is applied with strict asepsis, samples can be recovered with little to no external contamination. Irrigating the pus-filled cavity with sterile saline and gently rubbing it can help provide fluid for aspiration.

Since an alginate-tipped swab will dissolve and release all associated bacteria when transferred to an appropriate diluent, it can also be utilized to perform a fully quantitative analysis. The usefulness of the swab sample technique and the necessity of cleaning a wound before swabbing remains disputed despite its widespread use. For the purpose of microbiological examination, a range of additional methods have also been employed, such as cylinder scrubbing, filter paper discs, and dry and presoaked velvet pads. Since every sampling technique is said to offer advantages the question of what kind of sample is necessary to get the most useful data remains open for discussion and disagreement.[40,44,47] A microbiology laboratory's output can also lead to incorrect interpretations and unsuitable therapy. Without a doubt, the gold standard for conclusive evidence regarding microbes is tissue biopsy or excision. The best use of this procedure is to know when skin grafting and surgical wound closure are the best options.[48] The usefulness of a single biopsy sample is questionable, especially in cases of chronic wounds.

Purulent fluid aspirates are good indicators of a wound infection. Although the purpose of superficial swab samples has been hotly contested, for the majority of wounds, the process is straightforward, affordable, noninvasive, and practical. The argument against swab sampling is that the organisms of deeper tissue are not reflected in the superficial colonizers and the presence of harmful bacteria is not correlated with future cultures.[47] The swab collection process needs to be done carefully because if it is done before the wound has been cleaned or any devitalized superficial material has been removed, the ensuing culture will only include superficial colonizers and will yield inaccurate results. The patient should be treated empirically and vital tissue must be sampled or no specimen should be collected at all.[49]

According to a different theory, any flora found in deeper tissues is probably also present in the superficial detritus because endogenous microbes contaminate most wounds. Consequently, there are justifications for the practical application of the swab sample technique. Perhaps, it can be proposed for routine management that samples for microbiological examination should only be taken from wounds that are clinically infected or that show no clinical evidence of infection but are worsening or have a history of failing to heal. However, indiscriminate and improper wound swabbing wastes money and labor resources needlessly. When collecting a wound sample for microorganism analysis, it is crucial to take into account the method and dosage of antimicrobial therapy.

While systemic antibiotic therapy is more likely to affect the microflora of deep tissues, topical antimicrobial drugs will likely have a major impact on the microbial isolation from swab samples. In conclusion, superficial swabbing is a reasonable and easy way to evaluate the microbiota of wounds that are not healing or are clinically infected. A useful indicator of the microbial load will come from semiquantitative analysis and a difficult but informative qualitative study will show the diversity of microorganisms and potential for microbial synergy. Requesting aerobic and anaerobic microbiological studies is a crucial step in gathering the data needed to determine the best course of systemic treatment.

Sample Transport

It is crucial that the specimen be delivered to the laboratory as soon as possible. This is especially true for swabs, which have a tendency to dry up. In these situations, aspirates of purulent fluid and tissue samples are preferred over swabs because they preserve the damp and condensed environment necessary to support microbial survival. If the culture is not started within an hour or two of the sampling, prereduced commercial transport medium can be utilized. This provides an affordable and efficient way to support the growth of both anaerobic and aerobic bacteria. Microorganisms on cotton swabs require a prereduced, nonnutritive transport medium to remain viable since swab samples are vulnerable to desiccation and oxygen exposure.

The majority of microorganisms are viable at room temperature or at 25°C; temperatures higher or lower than this may impede or kill particular flora.

Processing of Wound Specimens

A clinical description of the burn wound must be sent with the specimen when it arrives at the laboratory. Details about the kind and severity of the wound, the location of the wound, clinical infection symptoms, necrosis, related bad odor, and antibiotic treatment—all these play a major role in helping the microbiologist choose the right tests and interpret laboratory data in an accurate manner. Additionally, giving microbiologists information on the use of antibiotics now may help them identify which antimicrobials are no longer as effective against certain microbes. When employing manual procedures, findings for microbial culture and antibiotic sensitivity are typically generated in 48–72 hours (but they occasionally take much longer).[50]

Numerous quick investigations need to be taken into account. Since Gram's stain has been around for more than a century, it is still the most significant stain in microbiology. Direct Gram staining of swabs, pus, or biopsies is one of the most practical and efficient quick tests in the microbiology.[51] It is frequently employed as a quick method to direct antibiotic therapy for illnesses that pose a serious risk to life **(Figs. 1 and 2)**. Furthermore, it has been demonstrated that the presence of microorganisms in a Gram-stained smear made from a wound swab consistently represents a microbial load of more than 10^6 organisms isolated from open burn wounds using a quantitative swab technique. Gram stain-based

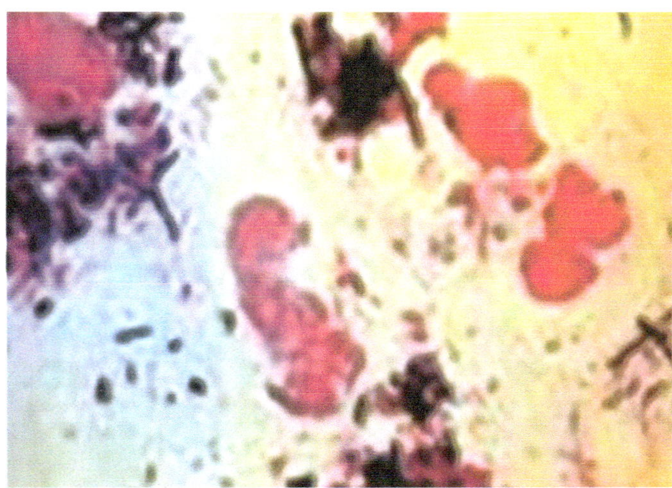

FIG. 1: Gram stain of pus from wound showing polymorphs and gram-positive and gram-negative bacteria.

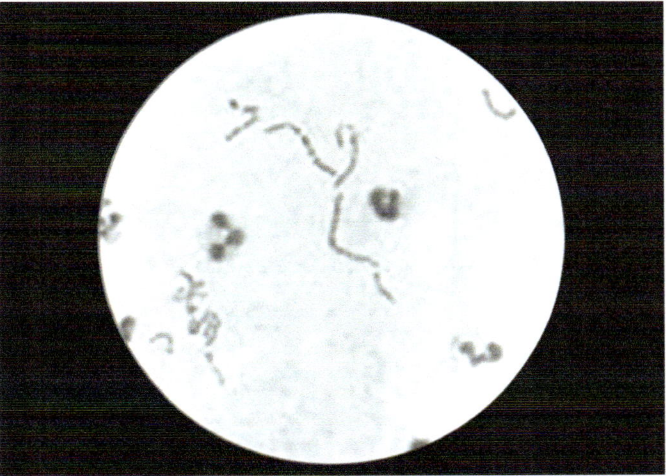

FIG. 2: Pus cells with *streptococci* in chains.

speciation is limited to gram-positive spore-forming anaerobes such as *Clostridium perfringens*.

The ability to distinguish between a contaminant, colonizer, and actual pathogen makes the Gram stain an inconclusive diagnostic technique. Its application in assessing samples at risk of skin/mucosal microflora contamination has been stated to be too unreliable to help in antibiotic selection. To quickly evaluate the microbial burden, tissue biopsy specimen homogenate stained with Gram stain is frequently utilized.[52,53] The coexistence of bacteria and leukocytes is probably a reliable sign of infection.[54] Nevertheless, Gram stain is still a fast, standardized, affordable, and dependable way to identify wound infections, especially when dealing with a single pathogen.

Other stains which have potential in assessing burn wounds are the fungal stains. Potassium hydroxide (KOH) is used to dissolve keratin and highlight fungal elements in wet smears. It has a great role to play in nail, hair, and skin samples, although the role in burn wounds is limited. Lactophenol cotton blue preparation is an excellent and cheap stain used for staining and fixing fungal elements which are very clearly delineated using this method. Histopathological tissue can be fixed and stained with PAS base which specifically stains and demarcates the only fungal tissue. More expensive stains as the fluorescent Calcofluor white stain, immunoperoxidase, and other immunohistochemical stains are used in specialized setup. Giemsa has been used successfully to demonstrate inclusion bodies of viruses such as herpes and in mycology.

Culture and Sensitivity of Wound Specimens

Typically, nonselective and selective media are used in routine isolation analysis of wound specimens to cultivate aerobic and anaerobic bacteria and yeasts **(Fig. 3)**. Anaerobic bacteria must also be suspected if a material is purulent and/or malodorous; yet anaerobic microbiology is frequently left out of a standard study. After the cultures are incubated for 24–48 hours under aerobic or anaerobic conditions, qualitative and semiquantitative evaluations are often conducted. As probable aerobic pathogens, *S. aureus*, *P. aeruginosa*, and beta-hemolytic *streptococci* are typically identified, and their proliferation is frequently described as mild to profuse.[55] Anaerobes, with the possible exception of *Clostridium* species, are likely to be described as "mixed" with aerobic microflora if they are examined.

The aerobic pathogens are the ones for which antibiograms are most commonly conducted, especially if they are cultivated in large quantities with little coexisting microflora. Anaerobes should be suspected and looked into if aerobes are absent, but the wound is reported to be clinically infected. On selective culture media, many endogenous anaerobic bacteria take 2–5 days to grow. Nonetheless, the fastidious anaerobes frequently develop more quickly in mixed aerobic–anaerobic cultures **(Fig. 4)** that represent polymicrobial wounds because of the availability of critical growth factors supplied by cohabiting facultative bacteria. The following standards provide broad parameters for evaluating burn wound microscopy and culture.

- Gram staining needs to be done every time. A single bacterial morphology and a large number of leukocytes can be used to identify the likely culprit early on.
- In order to grow aerobic, anaerobic, and fungal micro-organisms, wound specimens should be cultured.

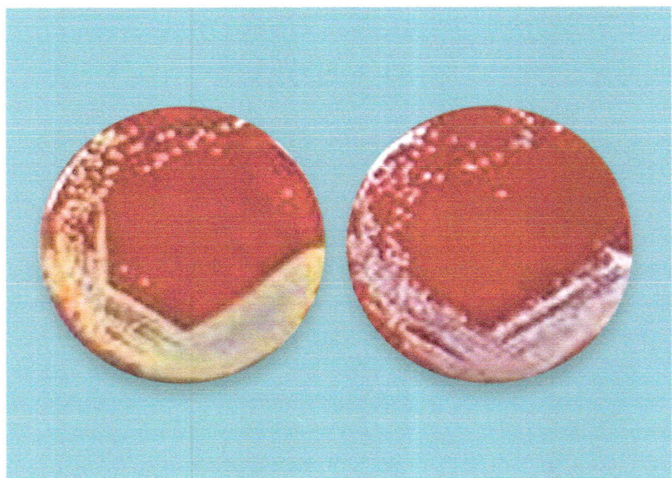

FIG. 3: Blood agar plates showing growth of *Staphylococcus aureus.*

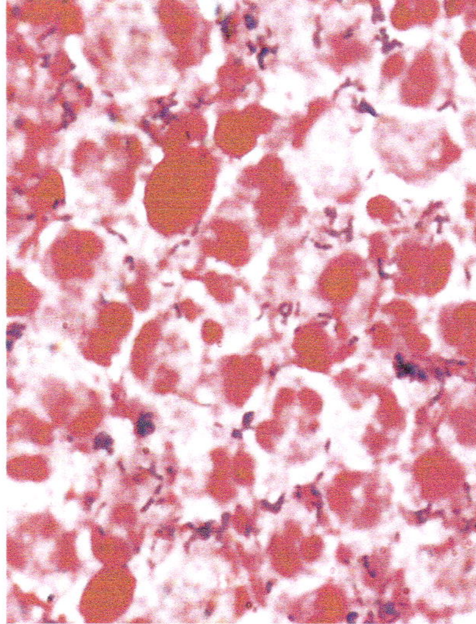

FIG. 4: Mixed aerobic and anaerobic flora in burn.

- For the isolation, at least one selective and one nonselective culture medium ought to be utilized.
- An antibiogram should be carried out if one microorganism is obviously prevalent (i.e., in pure culture or in abundance with little to no interaction of other bacteria).
- Antibiograms on common bacteria in mixed cultures ought to be carried out as well, especially if a significant number of leukocytes is seen in the specimen's initial Gram stain.

The specific pattern of microbial colonization of burn wounds, time-related changes in the predominant microbial flora of the wound in individual patients, the antimicrobial susceptibility profiles of microorganisms implicated in infections within a specific time period, and trends in the nosocomial spread of these pathogens should all be routinely determined and tracked by burn centers. To get these data, several burn centers use a laboratory microbiologic monitoring approach that involves routinely sampling burn wounds and other anatomic areas.[7]

The microorganisms found in a complex biofilm surrounding a burn lesion differ from their in vitro planktonic or free living counterparts in terms of their physiology and metabolism. As of now, there are no established guidelines for routinely evaluating microorganisms that are a member of a biofilm for antibiotic susceptibility. The modified broth microdilution plate approach can yield a precise outcome. In burn units, infection control protocol must be optimized. The most important requirements are to adhere to stringent infection control procedures, such as physical isolation in a separate room, wearing gowns and gloves while interacting with patients, washing your hands both before and after each visit, and using the proper empirical antibiotic therapy. These have a major role in lowering the frequency of infections caused by bacteria resistant to antibiotics. In addition to supporting efforts to lessen the burden of illness caused by antibiotic-resistant organisms, an institutional policy governing the appropriate selection and use of antimicrobials for the treatment of infections in burn patients may also help to minimize hospital expenses, length of stay, and side effects associated with these agents.

Reporting of Microbiological Results

When it comes to delivering information on wounds that are failing to heal or are deteriorating, the laboratory is essential. The following pathogens or groups of microorganisms should be routinely detected and reported by the microbiology laboratory (providing antibiograms when necessary): *S. aureus, P. aeruginosa*, beta-hemolytic *streptococci, coliform bacteria*, pigmented gram-negative anaerobes (*Prevotella* and *Porphyromonas* species), nonpigmented gram-negative anaerobes (mainly Bacteroides, *Prevotella*, and *Fusobacterium* species), *Peptostreptococcus* species, *and Clostridium* species. It is necessary to look for fungal species such as *Aspergillus*, *Penicillium*, *Mucor*, and *Candida* species in patients receiving broad-spectrum antibiotic therapy for chronic burn wounds.

The results of microbiological investigations (e.g., Gram stain, culture, and antibiograms) must be interpreted in conjunction with the clinical information provided by the burn surgeon (e.g., wound type, location, condition, signs of infection, and sampling method). Based on the clinical presentation, the medical microbiologist may have to evaluate the relevance of a specific wound pathogen. In conclusion, constant communication between the microbiologist and the clinician is necessary so that:

- Only burn wounds that exhibit clinical signs of infection or that are not healing are sampled in order to maximize the potential benefits of a microbiological investigation.
- The microbiologist is well versed with the wound's clinical appearance, when the laboratory forms are filled with adequate clinical information.
- The wound sample technique must be known to the microbiologist.
- The microbiologist is conscious of the surgeons requirements and the urgency of the results.
- The practitioner comprehends the reasoning behind the recommendations made by the microbiologist, such as the fact that if there are no inflammatory cells visible in the Gram stain and no clinical signs of infection, the reporting of a mixed culture and an antibiogram for a bacterium isolated from a mixed culture may not be provided. In addition to providing the patient with the proper care, constant dialogue between the clinician and microbiologist in the management of burn wound complications undoubtedly saves a large amount of money and time (medical, nursing, and microbiological).

OTHER MICROBIOLOGICAL METHODS

Blood cultures: A vital component in diagnosing sepsis episodes is blood culture. Before the temperature rises, it is the ideal moment to collect the specimen. The body rids the bloodstream of microbes when the temperature rises above 39.5°C. Over 39.5°C, as most bacteria cannot survive for an extended period of time. It is important to take precautions to keep the blood culture vial sterile. Before collecting the specimen, the collection site needs to be carefully and aseptically cleaned. On the request sheet, suitable remarks should be given if the site is through a hazardous region.

It can be challenging to differentiate the diagnosis of sepsis in burn patients from the typical hyperdynamic, hyperthermic, and hypermetabolic postburn condition. Blood cultures typically yield negative results. Spikes in fever are not correlated with the severity of infection.

Clinical diagnosis of sepsis is made by satisfying at least three of the following criteria:

1. Burn wound infection (>10^5 organisms/g tissue) with histologic or clinical evidence of invasion
2. Thrombocytopenia (<50,000) or falling rapidly
3. Leukocytosis or leukopenia (>20,000 or <3,000)
4. Unexplained hypoxia, acidosis, or hyper/hypoglycemia
5. Prolonged paralytic ileus
6. Hyper/hypothermia (>39°C or <36.5°C)
7. Positive blood cultures
8. Documented catheter or pulmonary infection
9. Altered mental status
10. Progressive renal failure or pulmonary dysfunction

Urinary tract infection (UTI)—if suspected to be cause of sepsis, urine must be collected aseptically. On the request slip, appropriate remarks should be written (e.g., temperature 39.8°C, clean catch, suprapubic, etc.).

Respiratory infection: Bronchial washings are necessary to determine the etiologic agent or infection if a respiratory infection is suspected or proven by clinical signs or an X-ray. Nevertheless, the organisms recovered from lung abscesses are more closely connected with organisms from the wound than with the organisms isolated from sputum specimens, according to recent mortality research.

AUTOMATION IN CULTURE AND SENSITIVITY

Cultivation of the fluid or macerated tissue sample using rapid systems of isolation, such as BacT Alert 3D, BACTEC (for pyogenic bacteria), and TREK/ESP systems, can greatly hasten (6–24 hours) the isolation of pathogens but have a limited role to play in mixed flora. However, quantifying the samples has not been standardized using these systems. They also are unable to process swabs, velvet pads, filter paper, etc. Fluid, pus, or homogenized tissue is an appropriate sample for these systems. Their prohibitive cost precludes their use in routine and also in surveillance. These automated machines have a critical role to play in blood cultures in burn wound septicemias.[7]

These days, the majority of laboratories regularly identify and test the bacteria's susceptibility using an automated technique. These are comparable to products such as Dade Behring's Microscan in Deerfield, IL; Phoenix from Becton Dickinson in Franklin Lakes, NJ; and VITEK from bioMérieux in Durham, NC. These need to be used in conjunction with agar dilution for the confirmation of certain automated system's susceptibility results and disc diffusion for screening and E-test. This is especially true when uncommon multidrug-resistant organisms (MDRO) are found, such as multidrug-resistant (MDR) *Acinetobacter* species, MDR *Pseudomonas* species, VRE, and Vancomycin-intermediate or -resistant *S. aureus* (VISA/VRSA).

There is little information available regarding the ability of systemically administered antibiotics to penetrate the devascularized burn eschar and the majority of antimicrobial drugs have not been the subject of controlled clinical efficacy trials in the treatment of burn wound infections.[56] Therefore, burn victims may not respond clinically if their infection is caused by bacterial strains that seem to be responsive to a specific antimicrobial drug in vitro. Aside from these, there are currently no published standard procedures that enable clinical microbiology laboratories to regularly test isolates from burn wounds for antibiotic sensitivity against widely used topical antimicrobial drugs.

Polymerase Chain Reaction

The role of molecular tests in rapid diagnosis of infective conditions has been very well elucidated for slow-growing and difficult-to-grow pathogens. Its role in certain infective diseases such as tuberculosis and meningitis is noncontroversial. Detection of role of viral infections of burn wounds has been possible with this technique. Using polymerase chain reaction (PCR)-based virus detection and immunohistochemical staining, burn wound infection with HSV-1 can be identified.[36]

Attempts have been made to identify and quantify *P. aeruginosa* in wound biopsy samples using real-time PCR. This technique yielded a lower detection limit of 10^3 CFU/g of tissue or a few copies per reaction, and a linear quantitative detection range of 7 logs. The duration between sample collection and outcome was under 60 minutes. This technique may enable early and customized treatment by enabling the quick quantitative identification of infections in burn patients.[57] Antibiotic susceptibility testing on the various species of bacteria present in a particular sample still requires bacterial tissue biopsy culture, even though molecular techniques provide quick quantification of individual organisms.

Molecular studies to identify the mutational type can significantly help in the quick identification of resistance if a prominent resistotype is anticipated. For burn surgeons, emerging patterns of antibiotic resistance in bacterial infections that cause burn wounds provide a significant treatment challenge. Infections of the burn wound and other anatomic sites in patients with major thermal injury have been linked to antibiotic-resistant organisms such as *MRSA*, *VRE*, and multiple-resistant gram-negative rods such as *P. aeruginosa*, *Acinetobacter* species, and various members of the *Enterobacteriaceae* family. Occasionally, these infections manifest as nosocomial outbreaks. The use of molecular biology in epidemiological typing of isolates through the use of Pulse Field Gel Electrophoresis (PFGE), MultiLocus Strain Typing (MLST), and restriction fragment length polymorphisms (RFLP) allows for the quick identification of changes that result in resistance. Multilocus strain typing, etc. will definitely play an enormous role in the future in burn microbiology.[7]

Gas Liquid Chromatography

This is especially helpful when anaerobic bacteria are present. Direct gas liquid chromatography (GLC) analysis on the material can be used to quickly determine the presence of potentially harmful anaerobic bacteria because these microorganisms can be identified by the fatty acids that are created as byproducts of metabolism. However, purulent drainage from contained abscesses is typically the only specimen type that can benefit from this kind of research. The expenses and skill required to operate such equipment have made GLC a useful technique for quickly identifying anaerobic bacteria in clinical specimens, unfeasible as a standard practice in microbiology laboratories.

ANTIBACTERIAL THERAPY

Burn wound progression is complex and caused by additive effects of inadequate tissue perfusion, free radical damage, and systemic alterations in the cytokine milieu of burn patients, leading to protein denaturation and necrosis. The current mainstays of treatment include adequate fluid resuscitation, nutritional support, and local wound care with an emphasis on topical antimicrobial agents and dressings.

Topical Therapy

Topical therapy is used to prevent and treat infections or used as an adjunct to surgical treatment and systemic antibiotics. Systemic antimicrobial agents should be directed at the underlying pathogen recovered from culture or determined empirically from the treating burn unit's antibiogram, while culture results are pending. Antifungal agents may also be used; however, pathogen identification is necessary in order to determine the ideal antifungal agent. The goal of wound treatment should be to completely remove devitalized tissue as soon as possible. A variety of topical medications are available for the microbial control of the burn wound. These medications include fusidic acid, bacitracin, neomycin, polymyxin B, 0.5% silver nitrate, bacitracin/polymyxin B, mupirocin, and mycostatin. Every agent has pros and cons and none is completely effective. Nearly all substances have an impact on wound healing and raise metabolic rate. The antimicrobial properties, adverse event profiles, and penetration of eschars of these different agents vary.

- *Bacitracin*: It is an antibiotic ointment that is effective against a variety of gram-positive bacteria.

MRSA and certain intestinal bacteria are particularly susceptible to the enhanced activity of mupirocin (Bactroban) against gram-positive bacteria. It is often used as a topical treatment for minor burns and skin wounds.

- *Neomycin*: It is another topical antibiotic commonly found in combination with other antibiotics such as polymyxin B and bacitracin in over-the-counter ointments.
- *Polymyxin B*: Often combined with other antibiotics, polymyxin B is effective against GNB and is used topically.
- *Fusidic acid*: This antibiotic is effective against a range of bacteria, including *S. aureus*. It is used topically in some regions for the treatment of skin infections.
- *Silver Sulphadiazine*: For burn patients, 1% cream is the most often utilized topical antibacterial treatment. It has a wide range of antibacterial coverage, including gram-positive bacteria, the majority of GNB, and some kinds of yeast. Its antimicrobial characteristics are obtained from the dual processes of its silver and sulfa moieties (functional components). Certain GNB do have plasmid-mediated resistance, such as certain *Pseudomonas* species. Silver sulfadiazine inhibits fibroblast contraction but prevents epithelialization, in contrast to mafenide or silver nitrate.
- *Mafenide Acetate*: One of the first proven topical antibacterial medicines is mafenide acetate 11.1% cream (Sulfamylon®, for example). Mafenide has diminished antifungal qualities but a wide range of antibacterial activity, including the ability to combat *Enterococci* and *Pseudomonas* resistant to silver sulfadiazine. Its precise mode of action is unclear but believed to be connected to its sulfa- moiety, which is soluble in water. Fibroblasts and epithelial cells are poisoned by mafenide cream. In contrast to other topical medications, mafenide penetrates the eschar quite well. Mafenide is therefore frequently applied to electrical burns, filthy or infected burn wounds, and damaged ears in order to prevent chondritis.
- Mycostatin ointment or powder in conjunction with other topical treatments lowers the occurrence of fungal infections in individuals with severe burns (>40% body surface area). Mafenide and mycostatin, however, should not be mixed together as both become inactive. Moreover, oral mycostatin (5–15 mL) administered three times a day decreases the overgrowth of alimentary fungi. The incidence of *Candida* septicemia in our patients has significantly lowered with this regimen.

Systemic Antibiotic Use and its Guidelines

Antibiotics are indicated when there is evidence of pneumonia (common in inhalational burn injuries) and when there is evidence of sepsis. Large burn wounds also often warrant the need for antibiotic use systemically. Specific choice of antibiotics depends on the local surveillance information and knowledge of antibiotic resistance pattern. Antibiotic prophylaxis has also been used in burn surgery at the time of wound manipulation, but few studies have supported the use of systemic antibiotics during acute burn surgery. In the prophylaxis of wound infections following surgery for minor-to-severe burns, antibiotics do not seem to be helpful. In patients with burns exceeding 40% TBSA, surgical intervention has been suggested by a few studies. In these cases, antimicrobial therapy should target the pathogen that was recovered on culture if an infection is found. Empirical therapy is started immediately when there is indication of sepsis or an invasive infection. To help guide empirical treatment, the antibiogram of burn facility needs to be established.

There is currently no consensus on optimal empirical treatment and recommendations for empirical therapy are based on the following criteria:

- Extent and depth of the burn wound
- Age, state of hydration, creatinine clearance, and serum protein levels of patient
- Presence of sepsis
- Length of time since the burn was sustained
- Prior administration of antibiotics
- The likely pathogens encountered in the burn unit (pathogens vary somewhat from center to center, but useful information can be obtained from surveillance cultures)
- It is important to remember that in burn patients, the pharmacokinetics of many antibiotics are often altered and some patients may experience periods during which subtherapeutic concentrations extend beyond the postantibiotic effect unless the dosing regimens are altered appropriately.[58]
- Discolored areas of the wound that are black or brown are local indicators of an invasive wound infection.
- Quick separation of eschar
- Wounds converting to full thickness
- Periwound erythema spreading
- Punctate hemorrhagic subeschar lesions
- Violent or black lesions in unburned tissue (ecthyma gangrenosum)

The culture and sensitivity report can be used as a basis for future modifications to the initial empirical therapy.

These patients' prolonged stay in the burn unit frequently result in the nosocomial resident microflora, which is typically resistant to multiple drugs, colonizing the area. Maintaining sterility in a burn wound is not practically possible. Skin graft survival rates exceed 90% when bacterial counts of less than 10^3 organisms/g are present, as they are often noninvasive. Specific antimicrobial treatment is always guided by bacterial cultures from wound, sputum and urine.

Replace beta-lactam antibiotic if allergy with clindamycin or macrolide antibiotic through regular triweekly sputum, urine, and wound cultures as a means of bacterial surveillance. Furthermore, punch biopsies are taken at every 18% BSA of burn in order to monitor the wound till it closes. Within 48 hours, the identification of the organism and its antibiotic sensitivity in vitro should be available. It is also possible to assess susceptibilities to topical antimicrobials using agar diffusion experiments. A modification in topical treatment is recommended if quantitative biopsies show a microbial density of more than 10^3 organisms/g. Bacterial counts of 10^5 indicate the presence of a deteriorating wound infection, which should be investigated further with a fast histological investigation and Gram stain. At this stage, the wound needs to be debrided and systemic antibiotics given.

Empirical antibiotic therapy for burn wound infections is initiated based on clinical judgment before specific information about the causative microorganisms is available. The choice of empirical antibiotics should cover a broad spectrum of potential pathogens commonly associated with burn wound infections. However, specific guidelines can vary and healthcare providers should consider local resistance patterns and individual patient factors. Following is a general outline of empirical antibiotic guidelines for burn wound infections:

- *First-line empirical antibiotics*:
    - Ceftriaxone or cefotaxime: These are third-generation cephalosporins with broad-spectrum activity against gram-positive and GNB.
    - Piperacillin-tazobactam: This combination provides coverage against a broader range of organisms, including many GNB and some gram-positive bacteria.
- *Consideration for severe infections or risk factors*:
    - For more severe infections or in cases where there is a higher risk of MDRO, healthcare providers may consider combining antibiotics, such as:
        - *Vancomycin*: Effective against gram-positive bacteria, including *MRSA*
        - *Ciprofloxacin or levofloxacin*: Fluoroquinolones that provide coverage against GNB
        - *Aminoglycosides* (e.g., gentamicin): Active against many GNB
- *Adjustment based on local resistance patterns*:
    - Empirical antibiotic choices should be adjusted based on local resistance patterns and the results of microbial cultures and sensitivity testing.
- *Consideration for fungal infections*:
    - In some cases, especially in immunocompromised patients or if there is a suspicion of fungal infection, antifungal agents such as fluconazole or an echinocandin may be added.

It is important to note that these are general guidelines and the specific choice of antibiotics should be tailored to individual cases. Additionally, the duration of empirical therapy should be based on clinical response and the results of microbial cultures.

Antibiotics for Deep Infections

Systemic antibiotics that are appropriate are given as required. The following definitions should serve as the foundation for the proper use of antibiotics: *Prophylaxis*—a precautionary or preventive measure intended to maintain health and stop the spread of illness. *Perioperative*—prophylaxis is another term for this. It is the use of systemic antibiotics before, during, and after any kind of surgical procedure. Depending on the surgical technique, the administration window should be brief and restricted to one to three doses. *Therapeutic*—the use of antibiotics to treat infections falls under this category. The course of treatment may extend for a few days, depending on the infection.

Systemic antibiotic treatment for burn wound sepsis is continued for at least 72 hours after evidence of sepsis has resolved. If the wounds appear clean, other sources such as the lungs, kidneys, and peripheral veins should be suspected as the primary source of infection. The commonly used agents in several situations are vancomycin, imipenem, timentin, or ceftazidime for coverage against the usual strains of *S aureus* and *P. aeruginosa* prevalent in the burns unit. Routine perioperative antibiotics should also take ward-endogenous organisms into account. Postoperative antibiotics are continued until quantitative excisional wound biopsies from surgery are identified.

Suggested regimen[59,60]

- For patients with burns of 2 weeks' duration and/or who are colonized with MDR gram-negative bacilli seek advice from a clinical microbiologist.
- Modify therapy, if appropriate, in the light of culture and susceptibility test results (blood culture and burn wound surveillance cultures).
- *Duration of treatment*: 5 days—if a significant pathogen is isolated from blood cultures or the burn wound

and 3 days—if a pathogen is not isolated from blood cultures or the burn wound. As there is no or only limited margin for error in patients who are severely ill with suspected infection within 5 days of sustaining a burn, broad-spectrum cover, with an agent such as cefuroxime, should be administered if an aerobic gram-negative bacillus cannot be excluded.

- It is important to remember that in burn patients, the pharmacokinetics of many antibiotics are often altered and some patients may experience periods during which subtherapeutic concentrations extend beyond the postantibiotic effect unless the dosing regimens are altered appropriately.
- Tetanus immunization is important (neonates, the elderly, or the debilitated may require immunoglobulin).
- In case of MDRO, immediate intimation should be given to the infection control personnel and advice from them may be gathered. MDRO include *MRSA*, VRE, ESBL producing GNB, and MDR. *Pseudomonas* and MDR *Acinetobacter* and recently, pan drug-resistant *Pseudomonas* and *Acinetobacter* which are resistant to almost all the known antibiotics.
- *S. aureus* tends to remain localized to the wound. If patient becomes toxic consider toxic shock syndrome (TSS).
- *Candida* species remain localized but rarely do invade. Always prove invasion with this pathogen.
- Pneumonia is the most prevalent of complications with high mortality. *S. aureus* is most commonly implicated. Septic thrombophlebitis is also frequently seen.
- Daptomycin [4 mg/kg intravenous (IV) q24h] can be used instead of vancomycin.

Antibiotics for burn wound sepsis where MDRO are seen.[58,59]

- Vancomycin (1 g IV q12h) + amikacin (10 mg/kg loading then 7.5 mg/kg IV q12h) + piperacillin 4 g IV q4h) (give half q24h piperacillin dose in subeshcar tissue and surgical removal of eschar in 12 hours).
- For resistant bacteria, piperacillin + tazobactam may be used instead of piperacillin.
- For ESBL producing GNB, imipenem or meropenem can replace piperacillin-tazobactam combination).

Other suggested regimens:[61]

- *Pseudomonas* species—tobramycin/amikacin or aztreonam + piperacillin/ceftazidime/cefoperazone or cefepime or quinolones
- Resistant GNB—gentamicin or aztreonam or amikacin + piperacillin or mezlocillin or third-generation cephalosporin or cefepime. Quinolones or trimethoprim-sulfamethoxazole combination may be kept as reserve in resistant but non-ESBL GNB infections.
- In ESBL or AmpC producing GNB infections, metallo-beta-lactams—imipenem and meropenem *must be used*. Other group of antimicrobials may be combined if proven as sensitive and no deleterious effect of combination is seen.

Suggested groups of antibiotics *to be tested/applied in the microbiology laboratory* for nosocomial isolates as primary, primary but selective use, and supplemental or reserved use for each major group of bacteria.[62]

- *Enterobacteriaceae* (*Klebsiella* species, *E. coli*, *Proteus* species, etc.):
  - Primary—ampicillin, cefazolin, cephalothin, gentamicin, and tobramycin
  - Primary but selective use—cefuroxime, cefepime, cefotaxime, ceftriaxone, cefoxitin, piperacillin, amoxicillin-clavulanate, ampicillin-sulbactam, piperacillin-tazobactam, ticarcillin-clavulanate, amikacin, ciprofloxacin, meropenem, and imipenem
  - Reserve—aztreonam, ceftazidime, chloramphenicol, tetracycline, newer agents, and agents under trial
- *Pseudomonas* species:
  - Primary—ceftazidime, gentamicin, tobramycin, and piperacillin
  - Primary but selective use—amikacin, aztreonam, cefepime, piperacillin—tazobactam, ticarcillin, imipenem, meropenem, and ciprofloxacin
- *Staphylococcus* species:
  - Primary—oxacillin (group representative of beta-lactams drugs and resistance to this eliminates the whole group including even metallo-beta-lactams such as imipenem and meropenem), penicillin, erythromycin/azithromycin/clarithromycin, and trimethoprim—sulfamethoxazole.
  - Primary but selective use—vancomycin, teicoplanin, daptomycin, linezolid, doxycycline/tetracycline, rifampicin (rifampicin should bever be used alone in therapy).
  - Reserve—ciprofloxacin or ofloxacin or levofloxacin, moxifloxacin, Synercid (quinupristin and dalfopristin combination), and gentamicin.
- *Enterococcus* species:
  - Primary—ampicillin and penicillin
  - Primary but selective use—vancomycin, daptomycin, linezolid, and Synercid
  - Reserve—high-level gentamicin and streptomycin
- *Acinetobacter* species:
  - Primary—ceftazidime, ampicillin-sulbactam, imipenem, meropenem, gentamicin, and tobramycin

    - Primary but selective use—cefepime, cefotaxime, ceftriaxone, piperacillin, piperacillin-tazobactam, ticarcillin-clavulanate, trimethoprim-sulfamethoxazole.
    - Reserve—colistin, polymyxin B (to be used in highly resistant MDR *Acinetobacter* and *Pseudomonas* species)
- *Burkholderia* species:
    - Primary—trimethoprim-sulfamethoxazole
    - Primary but selective use—ceftazidime, minocycline, and meropenem
- *Stenotrophomonas* species:
    - Primary—trimethoprim-sulfamethoxazole
    - Primary but selective use—levofloxacin and minocycline

The oral antibiotics (usually tested in the primary category for each group of bacteria) included in the abovementioned list are more for mild burn wounds and infections which do not warrant parenteral antibiotics. This in the case of burn wounds can be omitted altogether and topical agents can be used instead of oral agents, the choice of which lies in the clinician's experience.

The selective-use category of antibiotics is primarily parenteral and is advocated for serious infections such as the burn wound septicemias and other deep infections related to burn wounds **(Table 2)**. For polymicrobial infections and infections in multiple sites also, a combination of antimicrobials is advocated as has been suggested previously in this chapter. Reserve drugs are used in special situations where highly drug-resistant pathogens are expected.

TABLE 2: New antibiotics and older antibiotics with new indications or treatment options.[63,64]

Antibiotic	Drug class	Initial development period	Antibacterial spectrum	Limitations/adverse effects or new issues	Current status
Newer agents: Gemifloxacin, Garenoxacin, Sitafloxacin, Delafloxacin	Fluoroquinolone	Early 1960s	Variety of gram-positives (not *VRE*, *MRSA*) and gram-negatives	• Resistance already established in some places due to widespread ciprofloxacin use • Role uncertain, given availability of older agents	Garenoxacin development halted
Ramoplanin	Glyco peptides	Early 1980s	Gram-positives, including *VRE*	Not absorbed orally—used for temporary suppression of fecal *VRE* colonization	Not US FDA approved in phase III trials
Daptomycin	Lipopeptide	Late 1980s	Gram-positives: *VRE*, *MRSA*, and *SA*-RVS	Myalgia at high doses	US FDA approved
Linezolid, tedizolid	Oxazolidinone	Late 1980s	Gram-positives: *VRE* and *MRSA*, *SA*-RVS, some *Mycobacteria* species, *Nocardia* species	Hematological toxicity, especially thrombocytopenia; peripheral neuropathy (rare)	US FDA approved
Quinupristin, dalfopristin	Streptogramin	Early 1990s	Gram-positives: VRE (not *Enterococcus faecalis*), *MRSA*, *SA*-RVS	Infusion site pain, arthralgia, and myalgia	US FDA approved
Oritavancin, dalbavancin	Novel glycopeptides	Late 1990s	Gram-positives: *VRE* (oritavancin only), *MRSA*, *SA*-RVS	Toxicity uncertain	US FDA approved
Telithromycin, cethromycin	Ketolide (related to macrolides)	Late 1990s	Typical and atypical respiratory pathogens, including *Mycoplasma* and *Chlamydia* species	Hepatotoxicity, blurred vision, QT changes on ECG	US FDA approved
Tigecycline	Glycylcycline (semisynthetic derivative of minocycline)	Late 1990s	Gram-positives: *VRE*, *MRSA*, *SA*-RVS; some gram-negatives	Nausea, vomiting, and headaches	US FDA approved

Continued

Continued

Antibiotic	Drug class	Initial development period	Antibacterial spectrum	Limitations/adverse effects or new issues	Current status
Older agents penicillin G	β-Lactam	Late 1930s	Gram-positives: *Streptococci, Enterococci, Clostridium, Listeria* species	Continuous infusion provides high serum levels for intermediate-resistant strains (e.g., some *VRE*). Suitable for hospital-in-the-home treatment in some cases	
Colistin, polymyxin B	Cationic peptides	1950s	Gram-negatives, including *Pseudomonas aeruginosa, Acinetobacter baumannii, Klebsiella pneumoniae*	Renal toxicity, neurotoxicity	
Amphotericin B	Polyene	Late 1950s	Most fungi	Preliminary data suggest that continuous infusion may reduce renal toxicity and hence, reduce the need to switch to newer, more expensive liposomal analogs	
Gentamicin	Aminoglycoside	Early 1960s	Many gram-negatives	Meta-analyses suggest a once-daily dose of 4–6 mg/kg daily† is associated with reduced renal and ototoxicity, but efficacy is similar to multidose regimens	
Ceftaroline	Fifth-generation cephalosporin	Early 2000s	Both gram-positive and some gram-negative bacteria	Hemolytic anemia, stomach pains, bleeding gums, chills, dark urine, difficulty with breathing, fever, general body swelling, headache, loss of appetite, nausea or vomiting, nosebleeds, pale skin, sore throat, unusual tiredness or weakness, or yellowing of the eyes or skin	

(ECG: electrocardiogram; FDA: Food and Drug Administration; *MRSA*: methicillin-resistant *Staphylococcus aureus*; SA-RVS: *Staphylococcus aureus* with reduced vancomycin susceptibility; VRE: vancomycin-resistant *Enterococci*)

† Recommended dose for an adult with normal renal function.

A brief mention of some of the newer agents available for use in the various subcategories of bacteria observed in the nosocomial setting is enlisted further. However, this is an ever-expanding field and even at the time of publication of this document, several more agents will have been tried and tested for human use.

Multidrug-resistant bacteria for which there are currently few available treatment options.

Gram-negatives:

- *Acinetobacter baumannii*
- *P. aeruginosa*
- *Stenotrophomonas maltophilia*
- ESBL and very rare metallo-beta-lactamase (MBL) *K. pneumoniae*

Gram-positives:

- *MRSA*
- Vancomycin-intermediate or -resistant *S. aureus*
- *S. aureus* with reduced susceptibility to vancomycin and/or linezolid
- Methicillin-resistant coagulase-negative *staphylococci*
- *VRE*

FUNGAL INFECTIONS

In patients with significant burns and severely compromised immune systems, invasive burn wound infections caused by *Candida* species, *Aspergillus* species, and other opportunistic fungi (such as *Alternaria* species, *Fusarium* species, *Rhizopus* species, and *Mucor* species) are significant emerging causes of late-onset morbidity and mortality.[64] Children who have burn injuries are especially vulnerable to fungal infections that affect the burn area. Colonization of burn wound with fungi from the surrounding environment and/or in the case of *Candida* species from the patient's own gastrointestinal or upper respiratory tract flora typically arises after the 2nd week of thermal injury.[65]

Aspergillus and *Candida* species are the most common causes of infections, which typically manifest as a darkening of the burn wound region that resembles ecthyma gangrenosum.[66] Even though they are extremely uncommon, burn wound infections caused by zygomycetes such as *Rhizopus* and *Mucor* are significant because of their extraordinary capacity to spread quickly across fascial tissue planes, enter the vasculature, and are linked to a very high death rate. The most reliable method for diagnosing fungal infections in burn wounds is to examine tissue samples from the burns histologically and culture the biopsy sample. Aggressive, extensive surgical removal of the afflicted regions of the burn wound prior to the onset of deep invasion in conjunction with systemic antifungal medications may lead to an improved chance of survival.[66] When combined with the best possible local wound care, using an isolation room with laminar airflow appears to reduce the risk of both local and systemic fungal infections. By using an antifungal cream such as nystatin or clotrimazole topically, burn wound infections, and septicemia may be prevented.[65] Because the expanding arsenal of antifungal drugs has variable efficacy, culture samples are required to identify the infecting genus and species if histology reveals a fungal aetiology.[67] Previously, amphotericin B was the recommended treatment; however in some institutions, infections with *Fusarium* species and *Aspergillus terreus*, which are inherently resistant to amphotericin B, have become more common.[68] Voriconazole is frequently used in these situations. Posaconazole is a novel agent with potential for wider antifungal activity; however, its availability is restricted to oral formulations.[69] If an invasive *Candida* species is confirmed, treatment with ketoconazoles or amphotericin B may be started. Although significantly more costly, liposomal amphotericin B has a greater absorbance and efficacy, as well as fewer side effects.[70] Another novel antifungal on the horizon that is showing promising results in the treatment of resistant aspergillosis and candidiasis is caspofungin, an echinocandin.

VIRAL INFECTIONS

Herpes group of viruses, mainly varicella-zoster virus and HSV but also less frequently cytomegalovirus are becoming more and more recognized as causes of wound infections in patients with thermal injuries.[71] These infections can result from exogenous reinfection in patients who have already been infected, reactivation of a dormant virus, or original viral infection. HSV burn wound infections usually affect healing or recently healed partial-thickness burns, especially those in the nasolabial area.[72] They can also affect skin graft donor sites. In contrast, cytomegalovirus (CMV) burn wound infections usually involve full-thickness burns. HSV can cause clusters of tiny vesicles, also known as vesiculopustules, inside or around the burn wound's edges. These appear 2–6 weeks after the burn injury.

Burn wound herpes virus infections often resolve on their own, while they can sometimes spread throughout the body. The most reliable methods for making a diagnosis are histological analysis or culture of biopsy material from burn wounds.

COMPLICATIONS

- Bloodstream infections, pneumonia, and other systemic infections are frequently caused by germs that originate from burn wound infections.
- MODS, SIRS, and even death may result from them.

SUMMARY

Burn care is a multisystem approach that necessitates the involvement of multiple healthcare providers. Such infections require lengthy treatment, which raises the possibility of consequences, including iatrogenic events. Therefore, ongoing diligence is required. It is advisable to discuss with an infectious disease specialist if there are bacteria that are resistant to drugs. With an increase in the percentage of TBSA burned, the basal metabolic rate rises. Enteral feedings ought to be initiated early.

Preventing the nosocomial spread of MDR pathogens is a major priority while a patient is in the hospital, particularly if they have a higher than average percentage of TBSA burns (about 30%) or if they are known to have MDR bacteria colonized, such as *MRSA*, *VRE* species, or GNB that are known to become resistant (such as *Pseudomonas*, *Klebsiella*, and *Acinetobacter* species). Handwashing practices ought to be strictly enforced. All patients with burn injuries should get standard precautionary measures. If at all feasible, patients should be handled in single rooms while using contact precautions. When it is anticipated that you will come in touch with contaminated material or open wounds, wear gloves and a gown. The use of caps and masks should be determined by the presence of microorganisms resistant to many drugs.

The potential of spreading MDR germs makes patient transfers between hospitals highly risky and require aggressive infection control measures. A multidisciplinary team of surgeons, nurses, infection control specialists, and infectious disease doctors works to avoid burn wound infections. Improving the morbidity and death rates related to burns requires a focus on early wound care, infection control procedures, and long-term rehabilitative treatment. Early removal of burned tissue, prompt closure, and stringent observance of infection control procedures are necessary to mitigate poor outcomes.

REFERENCES

1. Norbury W, Herndon DN, Tanksley J, Jeschke MG, Finnerty CC; Scientific Study Committee of the Surgical Infection Society. Infection in burns. Surg Infect. 2016;17(2):250-5.
2. American Burn Association. (2000). Burn Incidence Fact Sheet. [online] Available from https://ameriburn.org/resources/burn-incidence-fact-sheet/ [Last accessed May, 2024].
3. Lionelli GT, Pickus EJ, Beckum OK, Decoursey RL, Korentager RA. A three decade analysis of factors affecting burn mortality in the elderly. Burns. 2005;31:958-63.
4. Roth JJ, Hughes WB (Eds). The Essential Burn Unit Handbook. St. Louis, Mo: Quality Medical Publishing; 2004.
5. Atiyeh BS, Gunn SW, Hayek SN. State of the art in burn treatment. World J Surg. 2005;29:131-48.
6. Bang RL, Sharma PN, Sanyal SC, Najjadah IA. Septicaemia after burn injury: a comparative study. Burns. 2002;28:746-51.
7. Fitzwater J, Purdue GF, Hunt JL, O'Keefe GE. The risk factors and time course of sepsis and organ dysfunction after burn trauma. J Trauma. 2003;54:959-66.
8. Church D, Elsayed S, Reid O, Winston B, Lindsay R. Burn Wound Infections. Clin Microbiol Rev. 2006;19(2):403-34.
9. Smolle C, Cambiaso-Daniel J, Forbes AA, Wurzer P, Hundeshagen G, Branski LK, et al. Recent trends in burn epidemiology worldwide: a systematic review. Burns. 2017;43(2):249-57.
10. Bendy RH, Nuccio PA, Wolfe E, Collins B, Tamburro C, Glass W, et al. Relationship of quantitative wound bacterial counts to healing decubiti: Effects of gentamicin. Antimicrob Agents Chemother (Bethesda). 1964;4:147-55.
11. Lookingbill DP, Miller SH, Knowles RC. Bacteriology of leg ulcers. Arch Derm. 1978;114:1765-8.
12. Teplitz C, Davis D, Mason AD, Moncrief JA. Pseudomonas burn wound sepsis. I: Pathogenesis of experimental burn wound sepsis. J Surg Res. 1964;4:200-16.
13. Dow G, Browne A, Sibbald RG. Infection in chronic wounds: Controversies in diagnosis and treatment. Ostomy Wound Manag. 1999;45:23-40.
14. Gardner SE, Frantz RA, Troia C, Eastman S, MacDonald M, Buresh K, et al. A tool to assess clinical signs and symptoms of localized infection in chronic wounds: Development and reliability. Ostomy Wound Manag. 2001;47:40-7.
15. Andrews JM. BSAC standardized disc susceptibility testing method (version 5). Journal of antimicrobial chemotherapy. 2006;58(3):511-29.
16. Wolfe JH, Wu AV, O'Connor NE, Saporoschetz I, Mannick JA. Anergy, immunosuppressive serum and impaired lymphocyte blastogenesis in burn patients. Arch Surg. 1982;117:1266-71.
17. Schwacha MG, Holland LT, Chaudry IH, Messina JL. Genetic variability in the immune-inflammatory response after major burn injury. Shock. 2005;23:123-8.
18. Steinstraesser L, Oezdogan Y, Wang SC, Steinau HU. Host defense peptides in burns. Burns. 2004;30:619-27.
19. Bone RC. Immunologic dissonance: a continuing evolution in our understanding of the systemic inflammatory response syndrome (SIRS) and the multiple organ dysfunction syndrome (MODS). Ann Intern Med. 1996;125:680-7.
20. Gibran NS, Heimbach DM. Current status of burn wound pathophysiology. Clin Plast Surg. 2000;27:11-22.
21. Lu J, Yang M, Zhan M, Xu X, Yue J, Xu T. Antibiotics for treating infected burn wounds. Cochrane database Syst Rev. 2017;2017(7):CD012084.
22. Heimbach DM, Mann R, Engrav L. Evaluation of the burn wound management decisions. In: Herndon DN (Ed). Total Burn Care. London, England: Saunders; 2002. pp. 101-8.
23. Santaniello JM, Luchette FA, Esposito TJ, Gunawan H, Reed RL, Davis KA, et al. Ten year experience of burn, trauma, and combined burn/trauma injuries comparing outcomes. J Trauma. 2004;57:696-700.
24. Sheridan RL. Evaluating and managing burn wounds. Dermatol Nurs. 2000;12:17-8.
25. Erol S, Altoparlak U, Akcay MN, Celebi F, Parlak M. Changes of microbial flora and wound colonization in burned patients. Burns. 2004;30:357-61.
26. Weber JM, Sheridan RL, Schulz JT, Tompkins RG, Ryan CM. Effectiveness of bacteria-controlled nursing units in preventing cross-colonization with resistant bacteria in severely burned children. Infect Control Hosp Epidemiol. 2002;23:549-51.
27. Ekenna O, Sherertz RJ, Bingham H. Natural history of bloodstream infections in a burn patient population: the importance of candidemia. Am J Infect Control. 1993;21:189-95.
28. Rennie RP, Jones RN, Mutnick AH. Occurrence and antimicrobial susceptibility patterns of pathogens isolated from skin and soft tissue infections: report from the SENTRY Antimicrobial Surveillance Program (United States and Canada, 2000). Diagn Microbiol Infect Dis. 2003;45:287-93.
29. Ramzy PI, Wolf SE, Irtun O, Hart DW, Thompson JC, Herndon DN. Gut epithelial apoptosis after severe burn: effects of gut hypoperfusion. J Am Coll Surg. 2000;190:281-7.
30. Altoparlak U, Erol S, Akcay MN, Celebi F, Kadanali A. The time-related changes of antimicrobial resistance patterns and predominant bacterial profiles of burn wounds and body flora of burned patients. Burns. 2004;30:660-4.
31. Agbenorku P, Amankwa R, Agbenorku M, Asare NY. The burns menace: antibiotics for the fight against burns bacterial infection, a systemic review. Surgical Science. 2016;7(12):532-8.
32. Agnihotri N, Gupta V, Joshi RM. Aerobic bacterial isolates from burn wound infections and their antibiograms—a five-year study. Burns. 2004;30:241-3.

33. Murray PM, Finegold SM. Anaerobes in burn-wound infections. Rev Infect Dis. 1984;6(Suppl 1):S184-6.
34. Baddley JW, Moser SA. Emerging fungal resistance. Clin Lab Med. 2004;24:721-35.
35. Robson MC, Heggers JP. Delayed wound closures based on bacterial counts. J Surg Oncol. 1970;2:379-83.
36. Heggers JP, Robson MC, Doran ET. Quantitative assessment of bacterial contamination of open wounds by a slide technique. Trans R Soc Trop Med Hyg. 1969;63:532-4.
37. Levine NS, Lindberg RB, Mason AD Jr, Pruitt BA Jr. The quantitative swab culture and smear: a quick, simple method for determining the number of viable aerobic bacteria on open wounds. Journal of Trauma and Acute Care Surgery. 1976;16(2):89-94.
38. Breidenbach WC, Trager S. Quantitative culture technique and infection in complex wounds of the extremities closed with free flaps. Plast Reconstr Surg. 1995;95:860-5.
39. Pruitt BA, McManus AT, Kim SH, Goodwin CW. Burn wound infections: Current status. World J Surg. 1998;22:135-5.
40. Robson MC. Wound infection. A failure of wound healing caused by an imbalance of bacteria. Surg Clin North Am. 1997;77:637-50.
41. Lawrence JC. The bacteriology of burns. J Hosp Infect. 1985;6:3-17.
42. PG B. The anaerobic and aerobic microbiology of wounds: a review. Wounds. 1998;10:170-8.
43. Bowler PG. The prevalence and significance of anaerobic bacteria in wounds. M Phil thesis. Cardiff, United Kingdom: University of Wales College of Medicine; 1999.
44. Bowler PG, Duerden I, Armstrong G. Wound Microbiology and Associated Approaches to Wound Management. Clin Microbiol Rev. 2001;14(2):244-69.
45. Armstrong DG, Athanasiou KA. The edge effect: how and why wounds grow in size and depth. Clin Pediatr Med Surg. 1998;15:105-8.
46. Mayrand D, McBride BC. Ecological relationships of bacteria involved in a simple, mixed anaerobic infection. Infect Immun. 1980;27:44-50.
47. Neil JA, Munro CL. A comparison of two culturing methods for chronic wounds. Ostomy Wound Manag. 1997;43:20-30.
48. Pallua N, Fuchs PC, Hafemann B, Völpel U, Noah M, Lütticken R. A new technique for quantitative bacterial assessment on burn wounds by modified dermabrasion. J Hosp Infect. 1999;42:329-37.
49. Kasten KR, Makley AT, Kagan RJ. Update on the critical care management of severe burns. J Intensive Care Med. 2011;26(4):223-36.
50. Latenser BA, Miller SF, Bessey PQ, Browning SM, Caruso DM, Gomez M, et al. National Burn Repository 2006: a ten-year review. J Burn Care Res. 2007;28(5):635-58.
51. Perry CR, Pearson RL, Miller GA. Accuracy of cultures of material from swabbing of the superficial aspect of the wound and needle biopsy in the preoperative assessment of osteomyelitis. J Bone Joint Surg. 1991;73A:745-9.
52. Robson MC. Lessons gleaned from the sport of wound watching. Wound Rep Regen. 1999;7:2-6.
53. Papasian CJ, Kragel PJ. The microbiology laboratory's role in life-threatening infections. Crit Care Nurs Q. 1997;20:44-59.
54. Vindenes H, Bjerknes R. Microbial colonisation of large wounds. Burns. 1995;21:575-9.
55. Popescu A, Doyle RJ. The Gram stain after more than a century. Biotechnol Histochem. 1996;71:145-51.
56. Hussey MJ, Levy ES, Pombar X, Meyer P, Strassner HT. Evaluating rapid diagnostic tests of intra-amniotic infection: Gram stain, amniotic fluid glucose level, and amniotic fluid to serum glucose level ratio. Am J Obstet Gynecol. 1998;179:650-6.
57. Meislin HW, McGehee MD, Rosen P. Management and microbiology of cutaneous abscesses. JACEP. 1978;7:186-91.
58. Brook I, Randolph JG. Aerobic and anaerobic bacterial flora of burns in children. J Trauma. 1981;21:313-8.
59. Zhou L, Zhang K, Sun T. Clinical investigation of burn wound infection with type I herpes simplex virus. Zhonghua Shao Shang Za Zhi. 2001;17(2):105-7.
60. Pirnay J-P, De Vos D, Duinslaeger L, Reper P, Vandenvelde C, Cornelis P, et al. Quantitation of Pseudomonas aeruginosa in wound biopsy samples: from bacterial culture to rapid 'real-time' polymerase chain reaction. Crit Care. 2000;4(4):255-62.
61. Murphy KD, Lee JO, Herndon DN. Current pharmacotherapy for the treatment of severe burns. Expert Opin Pharmacother. 2003;4:369-84.
62. Masterton RG, Galloway A, French G, Street M, Armstrong J, Brown E, et al. Guidelines for the management of hospital-acquired pneumonia in the UK: report of the working party on hospital-acquired pneumonia of the British Society for Antimicrobial Chemotherapy. Journal of Antimicrobial Chemotherapy. 2008;62(1):5-34.
63. Avni T, Levcovich A, Ad-El DD, Leibovici L, Paul M. Prophylactic antibiotics for burns patients: systematic review and meta-analysis. BMJ. 2010;340:c241.
64. Kelly EJ, Oliver MA, Carney BC, Shupp JW. Infection and burn injury. European Burn Journal. 2022;3(1):165-79.
65. Casapao AM, Davis SL, Barr VO, Klinker KP, Goff DA, Barber KE, et al. Large retrospective evaluation of the effectiveness and safety of ceftaroline fosamil therapy. Antimicrob Agents Chemother. 2014;58(5):2541-6.
66. Sanford JP. Skin infections, burn wound infection and burn wound sepsis. In: Gilbert DN, Moellering RC Jr, Eliopoulos GM, Sande MA (Eds). The Sanford Guide to Antimicrobial Therapy, 38th edition. Northwestern University: Antimicrobial Therapy; 2008. p. 48.
67. Meyers BR (Ed). Skin and soft tissue infections—burn wound infection and sepsis. Antimicrobial Therapy Guide, 12th edition. Newton, Pennsylvania, USA: Antimicrobial Prescribing Inc.; 2003. p. 140.
68. Clinical & Laboratory Standards Institute, 14th Edition. (2024). Performance Standards for antimicrobial susceptibility testing [M100-S18].
69. Patrick G, Charles P, Grayson ML. The dearth of new antibiotic development: why we should be worried and what we can do about it. MJA. 2004;181(10):549-53.
70. Burdge JJ, Rea F, Ayers L. Non-candidal, fungal infections of the burn wound. J Burn Care Rehabil. 1988;9:599-601.
71. Becker WK, Cioffi WG Jr, McManus AT, Kim SH, McManus WF, Mason AD, et al. Fungal burn wound infection. A 10-year experience. Arch Surg. 1991;126:44-8.
72. Tang D, Wang W. Successful cure of an extensive burn injury complicated with mucor wound sepsis. Burns. 1998;24:72-3.

SECTION

2

Early Care in Burns

CHAPTER 10

Initial Evaluation and Resuscitation of Burn Patient

Madhuri Gore, Suvashis Dash

INTRODUCTION

The initial goal of burn management is to achieve wound closure at the earliest. The efforts in this direction must begin at the first interaction between the victim and the healthcare worker. The decision regarding the need for admission to burn unit or management on outpatient basis should be protocol-based to minimize errors. Burns pose a significant burden on global health morbidity and mortality, especially in the low- and middle-income countries.[1,2]

The plan of management of patients with large burns that require inpatient care is usually determined by the severity of the alterations in physiology due to the burn injury. These patients require a coordinated approach that involves a specialized team.[3,4] Hospitalization is divided into four general phases:

1. Initial evaluation and resuscitation
2. Initial wound excision and biologic closure
3. Definitive wound closure
4. Rehabilitation and reconstruction

An orderly and systematic initial evaluation is valuable for delivery of comprehensive care. The early management extends from first aid at site to complete resuscitation of the patient forming the emergency burn care pathway and remains the chief determinant of outcome, especially in a patient with major burn **(Flowchart 1)**.

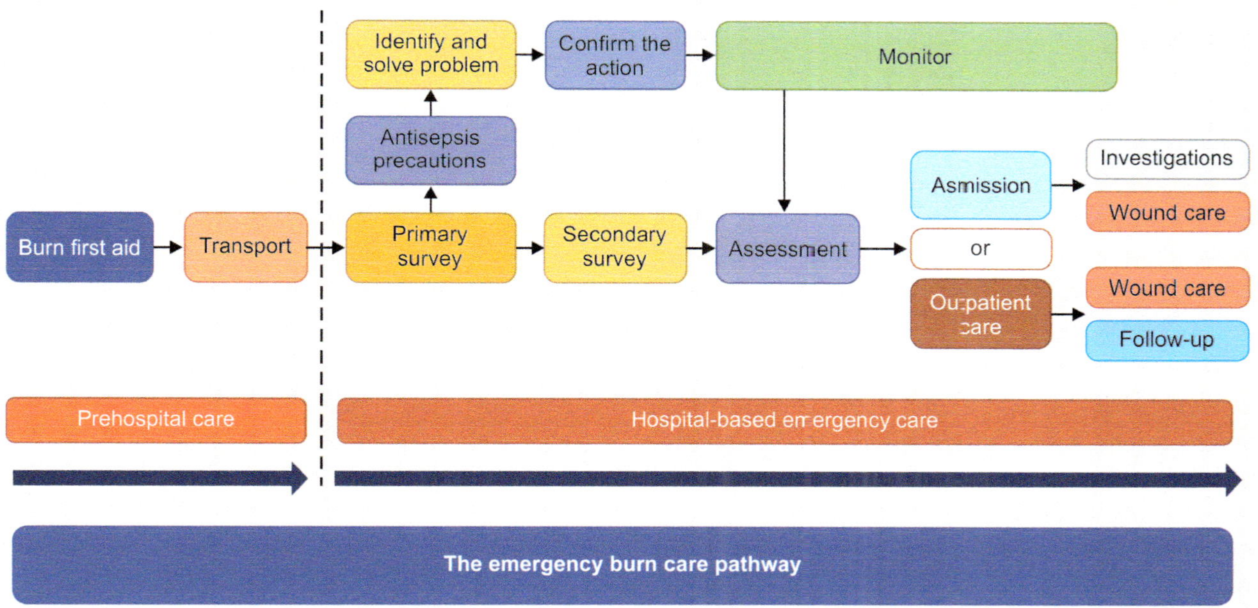

FLOWCHART 1: The emergency burn care pathway. It starts with prehospital care, followed by hospital-based care.

FIRST AID: THERMAL BURNS

First aid to a burn patient is generally provided by the relatives, friends, and other persons present at the site of burn accident. A specialist burn surgeon is not present at the site. However, the role of a burn specialist in carrying out first aid in burns is to educate the masses about the basics of burn injuries and do's and don'ts. Media has a great role to play in dissemination of this knowledge. This information should also be given to school children in their curriculum. All police and fire brigade personnel, etc., should receive this training as part of their induction into service as they may be required to provide first aid to victims of burn disasters. Some of the points mentioned below may be possible only in the nearest medical facility.[5-7]

Management on Site [7-9]

First, make the scene safe for the rescuer.

- If an individual is actually in flames, instruct the victim to STOP, DROP, and ROLL. Douse the fire with water or sand.
- Switch off the mains in the event of electric burns.
- *Check for signs of circulation, breathing, coughing, or movement.* If there is no breathing or other sign of circulation, begin cardiopulmonary resuscitation (CPR).
- *Cool the burn*: Immerse affected extremity in bucket full of tap water till burning sensation disappears OR hold the burnt part under running tap water till the burning pain disappears OR apply cold compresses on the burnt area.
- *Do not use ice* as this can cause cold injury and further damage to skin.
- *Do not* immerse severe large burns in cold water.
- Doing so can lead to hypothermia.
- *Do not* remove clothes that are adherent to wounds.
- *Do not* apply any local agent on the wound (especially colorful agents like gentian violet, mercurochrome, "*ratanjot*", etc.), as this interferes with the evaluation of burn depth and extent.
- Do not break the blisters. Broken blisters are more vulnerable to infection.
- *Cover the area of the burn, this reduces the pain.* Use a clean cloth. Sterile polyethylene drape is very useful for covering the burnt area as it is nonadherent and helps to avoid hypothermia. Do not use fluffy cotton wool as it irritates the burn wound.
- If the patient is conscious, give salt-sugar solution to the patient orally in case of minor or moderate burns. Avoid giving anything orally to extensively burned patient.
- Shift patient to appropriate facility for management **(Box 1)**.

BOX 1 Key points in first aid.

- Stop the burning process
- Maintain airway
- If a burnt patient is unconscious, think of smoke inhalation and/or associated head injury
- If a burnt patient is breathless, think of inhalation injury, chest trauma and/or aspiration
- If a burnt patient is in shock early after the incident, think of associated chest or abdominal trauma causing blood loss or spinal trauma
- Shift the patient to appropriate burn care facility

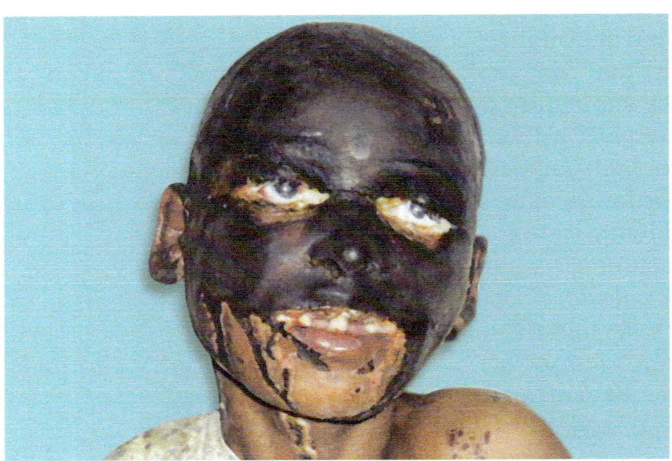

FIG. 1: Chemical burns of face involving the eyes, nose, and mouth.

FIRST AID: CHEMICAL BURNS[10,11]

Chemical burn injuries are not hyperthermic but are due to tissue reactions to noxious substances, including oxidizing agents, reducing agents, corrosives, protoplasmic poisons desiccants, and vesicants **(Fig. 1)**.

- *Remove the cause of the burn* by flushing the chemicals off the skin surface with cool, running water for 15 minutes or more. Clothes soaked in chemical should be removed. Deep alkali burns should be irrigated for 24 hours. Water is preferable for irrigation of mucosal surfaces or eyes. Dilution of the chemical is of paramount importance and not neutralization. Neutralization can produce exothermic damage as well. If the burning chemical is a powder-like substance such as lime, brush it off the skin before flushing.
- Initial *copious hydrotherapy* is indicated for all chemical burns except those caused by dry-lime, phenol, concentrated sulfuric acid, sodium metal, and muriatic acid; they are either not miscible with water or react with water exothermically.
- *Antidotes* are helpful for burns from hydrofluoric acid (HFA), phenol, and white phosphorus.

Hydrofluoric acid causes liquefaction necrosis of the subcutaneous tissue and can penetrate to bone. Systemic complications of HFA toxicity include hypocalcemia and pulmonary edema. HFA wounds should be covered with a 10% calcium gluconate solution mixed to a slurry with a ointment or infiltrated if the burn is excruciatingly painful.

Phenol is an acidic alcohol that produces local coagulation and systemic toxicity in large doses, including fatal arrhythmias. Acute phenol burns are treated topically by irrigation with polyethylene glycol solution.

White phosphorus is contained in grenades and antipersonnel mines. Once particles are embedded in skin, white phosphorus causes burn by both chemical and thermal reactions, as particles are spontaneously ignited with prolonged exposure to air. Patients should be submersed in water until embedded particles can be surgically debrided. The skin is washed with a solution of 5% sodium bicarbonate, 3% copper sulfate, and 1% hydroxy-cellulose to blacken the particles and aid earlier identification. Prolonged exposure to copper sulfate solution can induce coagulopathies.

- *Remove clothing or jewelry* that has been contaminated by the chemical.
- *Cover* the burned area loosely with a dry, clean cloth.
- Patient with even *a minor chemical burn* on the eye, hands, feet, face, groin or buttocks, or over a major joint should be treated at a burn center.

FIRST AID: ELECTRICAL BURNS[6,12]

High-voltage electrical injuries are classified as major burns due to associated massive tissue damage. On average, high-voltage cutaneous involvement is only 10–15% body surface area (BSA), but this visible injury is only a small portion of the overall tissue destruction **(Fig. 2)**. The human body serves as a volume conductor to electricity. Current flow is, therefore, concentrated in the extremities by their narrowing. Since bone has the highest resistance to electrical current, conduction through bone produces the greatest amount of heat. For this reason, damage to muscle by electricity is greatest at tendinous attachments and periosteal regions. Massive muscle destruction causes myoglobinuria. Precipitation of myoglobin in the renal tubules can produce acute tubular necrosis and acute renal failure. In addition, high-voltage electrical burns are commonly associated with dislocations, fractures, vertebral injuries, myocardial damage, neurological sequelae, and intra-abdominal injuries due to concomitant trauma. The most common cause of early mortality is cardiopulmonary arrest due to fibrillation. While helping someone with an electrical burn and waiting for medical help, following steps are recommended:

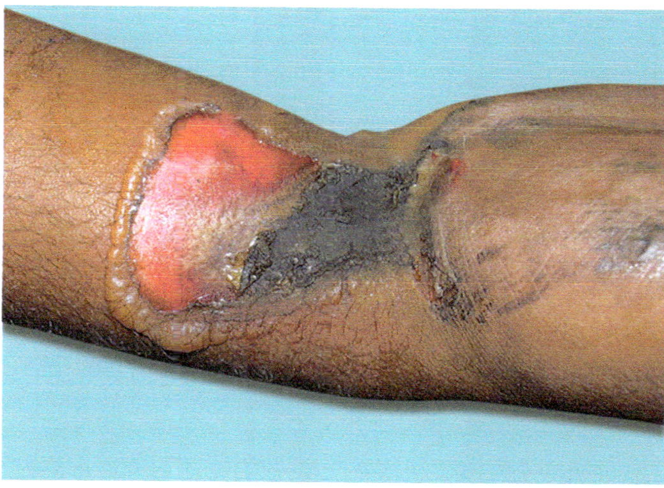

FIG. 2: Electrical burns involving wrist—even though external injury appears to be a minor burn but the underlying tissue destruction is extensive involving muscles, nerves, vessels, and bone.

- *Look first, do not touch.* The victim may still be in contact with the electrical source. Touching the person may allow the current to pass through the rescuer.
- *Turn off the source of electricity if possible.* If this is not possible, move the source away from the injured person using a nonconducting object made of cardboard, plastic, or wood.
- *Check for signs of circulation, breathing, coughing, or movement.* If absent, begin CPR immediately.
- *Prevent shock.* Lay the person down with the head slightly lower than the trunk and the legs elevated.
- *Cover the affected areas.* If the person is breathing, cover all burned areas with a clean cloth. Do not use a blanket or towel. Loose fibers can stick to the burns.

TRANSPORTATION

Almost all burn patients in India are transported, at least initially, by the relatives of the victim to the nearest medical facility. Only an extremely small number of them have inhalational injury significant enough so as to require immediate control of airway and intubation or oxygen therapy to avoid complications and death. The burn patients, as opposed to the multiple trauma patients with active blood loss, are unlikely to develop shock or airway obstruction in the first 1 hour or so postburn. Commonly, it is only during disasters with a number of casualties occurring together that the ambulances are rushed to the site and/or the police/fire brigade personnel transport the victims. In such situations only, there is a possibility of intravenous (IV) fluid being started or oxygen being administered to patients on site and continued during transportation. In the large cities where specialized burn centers are available, the patient may be transported directly to it. Otherwise, they are transported to the nearest medical facility. Here, the initial treatment is started, and then transfer to a burn facility is considered.[13,14]

The procedures that should be performed in the prehospital setting (on site) by trained paramedics before and during transportation to the initial medical facility or from the latter by medical personnel before a long transportation to a specialized burn care center are:

- *Check airway:* If deep facial burns are present and/or there is a history of smoke exposure with obtundation or stridor or other symptoms of impaired airway—*intubate* **(Fig. 3)**
- *Initiate high-flow oxygen therapy* if history of smoke exposure is present, to treat carbon monoxide toxicity.
- *Check for other injuries* especially to chest (rib fractures, pneumothorax, etc.) **(Fig. 4)** due to other trauma suffered in the accident.
- *Assess hemodynamic* stability and perfusion by looking for evidence of impending burn shock.
- *Start intravenous infusion:* If burn size is greater than 15% of total body surface or if there are other injuries, infuse Ringer's lactated (RL) solution.

The rate of fluid infusion depends on total body surface area (TBSA) burned and is as follows:

- Body surface area:
    - 15–25% TBSA burn = 500 mL/h
    - 25–50% TBSA burn = 750 mL/h
    - >50% TBSA burn = 1 L/h

The transport vehicle should have adequate supply of crystalloids as well as colloids needed for resuscitation.

- *Assess depth and size of burn while* keeping the patient warm (remove wet clothes). Cover patient with clean sheet to conserve heat.
- *High tension (>1,000 volts) injury*—Look for cardiac abnormalities, entrance and exit sites, and other injuries.
- *Remove any constricting objects* (rings, bangles, etc.)
- *Information to receiving center:* Pretransport information and coordination with burn center are integral aspects of prehospital care. Paramedics and emergency medical technicians (EMTs) are trained to stabilize patients, administer medications, and perform life-saving procedures during transportation. Information sent for transfer from the initial medical facility to a burn unit or higher center should include:
    - Neurologic status
    - Smoke exposure and airway status
    - Hemodynamic stability
    - Approximate size, depth, and areas involved in burn

Ambulances, equipped with advanced life-support systems and skilled personnel, are the primary mode of transportation for patients requiring urgent medical attention. These vehicles serve as mobile healthcare units, capable of providing critical interventions on the way to the hospital. Specifically, for the purpose of burns, availability of dressing materials and prevention of hypothermia is important. The ambulance used for transporting the victim should have all the resuscitation equipment and a competent team of qualified doctor and nurse/paramedics. Safety during transfer is more important than speed. The transport should be by the fastest mode available. Helicopter and specialized

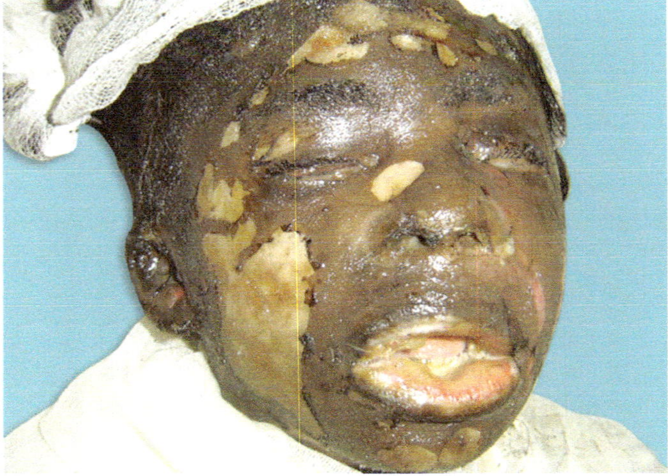

FIG. 3: Facial burns with inhalation injury of the patient—eyebrow and eyelashes singed, facial burns with perioral swelling, with shoots in external nasal opening.

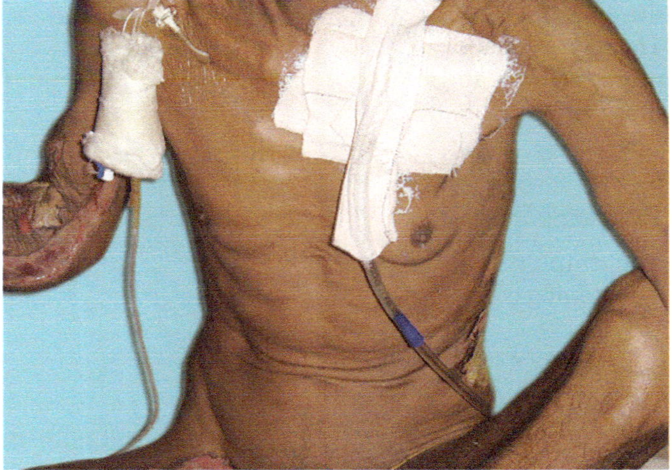

FIG. 4: Chest tube drainage in situ for pneumothorax because of fractured ribs following a fall from height due to electric injury.

BOX 2 Key points during transportation.

- Assess airway. Intubate if necessary
- Secure two large bore intravenous lines for > 20% burn extent
- Start intravenous Ringer's Lactate (RL) infusion at desired rate.
- Insert nasogastric tube
- Introduce urethral catheter to monitor urine output during transport
- Apply topical agent. Wrap in sterile clean drape. Avoid hypothermia
- Carry resuscitation equipment and develop competence to use it
- Intimate receiving center
- Provide information about patient's condition, treatment given, and actual incident

transport units further enhance the capacity to reach remote or inaccessible locations promptly.[13,14]

It must be remembered that initial treatment of an extensively burnt patient has to do more with care of airway, breathing and circulation, and resuscitation with IV fluids which comes in the domain of every qualified medical practitioner than the wound itself, which has to be simply protected from further contamination. This much treatment is presently available in almost all parts of the country. Hence, the practice of transporting the patient in great hurry to a higher center without providing simple care should be discouraged **(Box 2)**.

EARLY MANAGEMENT OF MAJOR BURNS

The burn wound should never take precedence over potential life-threatening conditions. As described by the American College of Surgeons (ACS) Committee on Trauma, evaluation of the burn patient is organized into a primary survey and a secondary survey using modification of the methodology of Advanced Trauma Life Support Course.[15]

Primary Survey

The emphasis is on detection and treatment of life-threatening conditions.

A: Airway Patency

Heat affects primarily the oral and nasal cavity and supraglottic area of the pharynx and causes edema and mechanical upper airway obstruction. The gas, particle, and chemical components of the smoke affect primarily the airway mucosa and cause the actual chemical burn. The initial smoke injury occurs shortly after exposure within 30 minutes to 1 hour, but the ensuing intense inflammatory reaction evolves over a period of hours to days resulting in lung damage. The initial edema usually wears off within a day or two and is evident by air leak by the sides of the endotracheal tube. Inhalation injury should be suspected in all the following situations **(Figs. 5 and 6)**.[16]

- Individuals who sustained injury in a closed space
- Patients with extensive burns or with burns on the face
- Patients who were unconscious at the time of injury
- Patients with singed nasal and facial hair, hoarseness, or wheezing
- Patients who are coughing up carbonaceous sputum
- Explosions with burns to head and torso
- Carboxyhemoglobin level > 10%

Pulmonary injury is known to result in substantially increased burn mortality and morbidity. When indicated, early intubation and positive pressure ventilation have been shown to improve outcome **(Flowchart 2)**. A number of techniques have been used to assess the degree of supraglottic and subglottic injury and to determine the need for endotracheal intubation. Fiberoptic bronchoscopy or laryngoscopy and virtual bronchoscopy can reveal physical evidence of mucosal injury. In the author's experience, in patients with clinical suspicion of inhalation injury, fiberoptic bronchoscopy confirmed the suspicion in 93% of patients. Hence, in the absence of diagnostic modalities, high index of suspicion should guide the management.[17-19]

As the injury process is progressive during the first 18–24 hours, initial appearance does not accurately predict the severity of subsequent airway compromise. With increase in edema, it becomes much more difficult to secure an airway. This can be a particular problem in small children. Endotracheal intubation is, thus, preferably performed on admission, before severe edema develops. On the other hand, unnecessary intubation and sedation can worsen a patient's condition. The decision to intubate should be made carefully by an experienced clinician.[17,19]

Definite indications for endotracheal intubation are:

- *Deep facial burns:* Especially of the mouth and oropharynx; development of edema may impair patency in the near future
- Massive body burns, especially in the presence of circumferential chest burns, as ventilatory support is needed
- Severe inhalation injury

A patient with inhalation injury can be closely monitored for upper airway obstruction without a tube, preferably with the head elevated at 30°, only if intubation

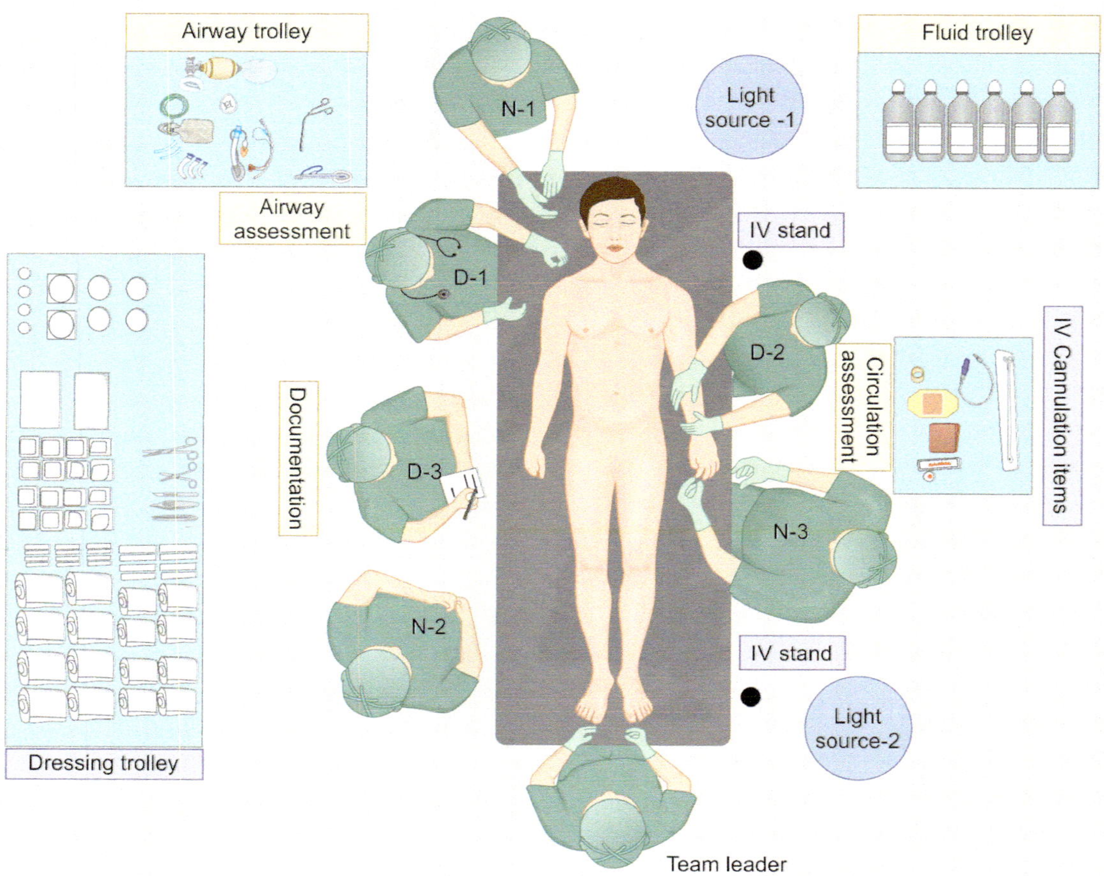

FIG. 5: Primary survey assessment and position of the team and equipment in an ideal setup.

Note: D: Doctor; N: nurse—manpower may change as per availability.

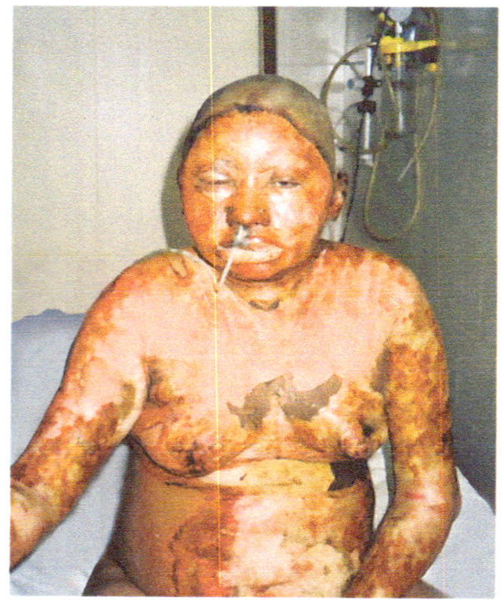

FIG. 6: Burn distribution suggestive of inhalation injury.

Courtesy: Dr Madhuri Gore.

will be technically possible later. However, if anatomic distortion from face and neck burns is increasing to a point where safe intubation might soon be precluded, the procedure is carried out immediately. If edema distorts the anatomy, intubation using fiberoptic bronchoscope should be resorted to by an experienced clinician. *Prolonged and multiple attempts at intubation can further aggravate the hypoxia and may precipitate cardiac arrest.* So, in the absence of expertise, the option of a tracheostomy should be exercised even if the incision has to be made through burnt skin **(Fig. 7)**.

Once a definitive airway is secured, continuous administration of humidified oxygen is indicated to maintain adequate oxygenation as well as to assist in clearing the airway of inspissated products of combustion. If the patient's hemodynamic condition tolerates, elevation of the head end of the bed by 30° is helpful in reducing neck and chest wall edema. The early addition of bronchodilators, usually by aerosol, is especially advantageous in managing the bronchospasm seen after chemical injury. Nebulization with heparin + saline helps in limiting the alveolar damage. After a secure airway is established, the need for ventilatory support is assessed. Blood gases are often misleading as far as saturation is concerned as the carboxyhemoglobin is the confounding

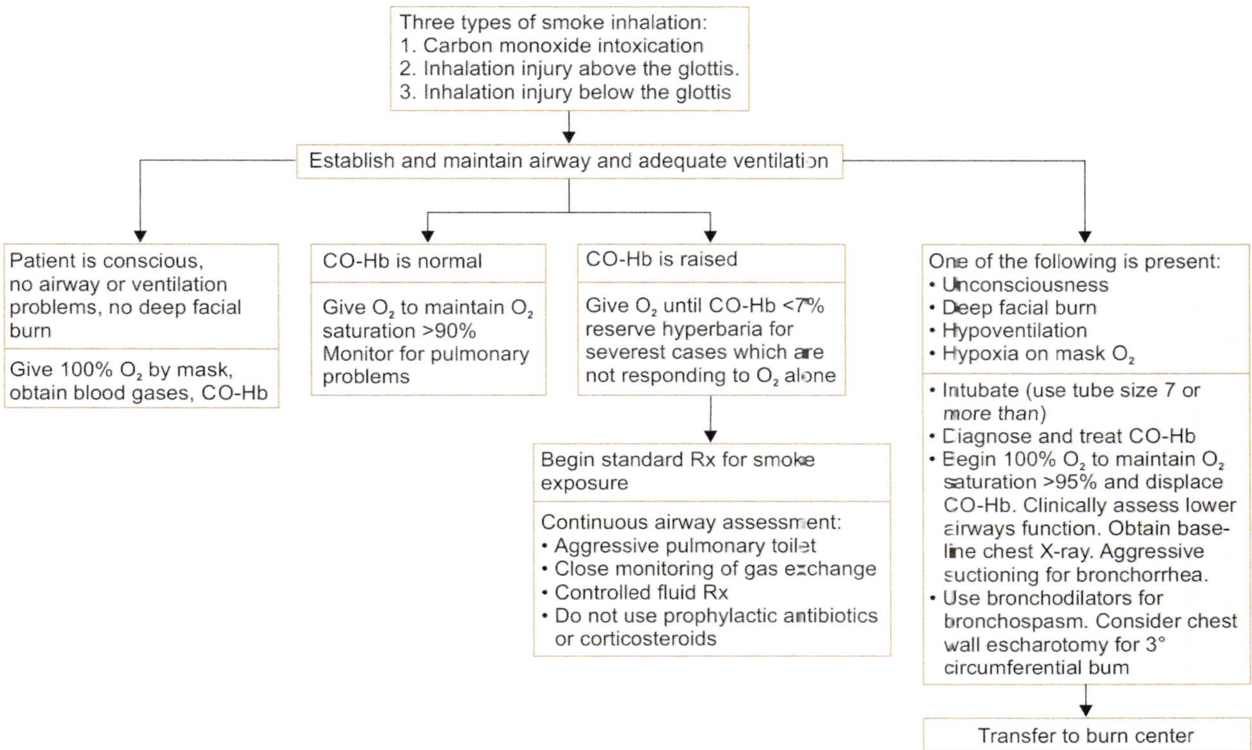

FLOWCHART 2: Algorithm for management of smoke inhalation.
(CO-Hb: carboxyhemoglobin; O_2: oxygen; Rx: prescription)

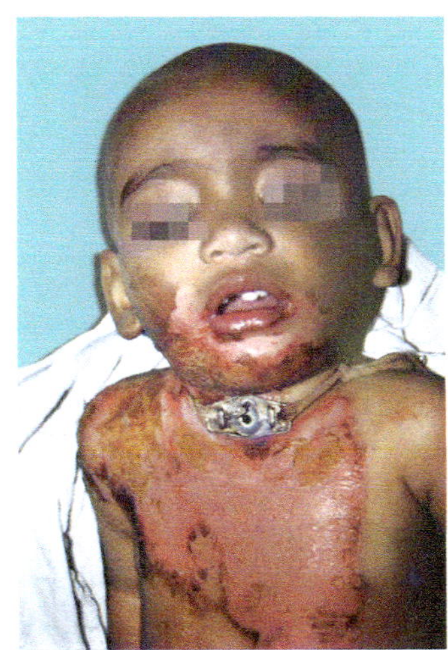

FIG. 7: Tracheostomy for laryngeal edema due to smoke inhalation.

factor. The pH and bicarbonates can, however, guide therapy.

B: Breathing

Breathing is evaluated for depth of respiration and effort.[16] Detection of wheezing or rales suggests either inhalation injury with bronchospasm or aspiration of gastric contents. In a patient with burn, the respiratory effort and hence the gas exchange may be inadequate due to:

- *Mechanical restriction of breathing*: Deep dermal or full-thickness circumferential burns of the chest can limit chest excursion and prevent adequate ventilation. This may require escharotomies.
- *Blast injury:* If there has been an explosion, blast lung can complicate ventilation. Penetrating injuries can cause tension in pneumothorax and the blast itself can cause lung contusions and alveolar trauma and lead to adult respiratory distress syndrome.
- *Smoke inhalation*: The products of combustion, though cooled by the time they reach the lungs, act as direct irritants to the lungs, leading to bronchospasm, inflammation, and bronchorrhea. Patients may need a period of ventilation, as this allows adequate oxygenation and permits regular lung toilet.
- *Carboxyhemoglobin*: Carbon monoxide binds to deoxyhemoglobin with 40 times the affinity of oxygen. It also binds to intracellular proteins, particularly the cytochrome oxidase pathway. These two effects lead to intracellular and extracellular hypoxia. *Pulse oximetry cannot differentiate between oxyhemoglobin and carboxyhemoglobin and may, therefore, give normal results.* However, blood gas analysis can reveal

metabolic acidosis and raised carboxyhemoglobin levels but may not show hypoxia. Treatment is with 100% oxygen, which displaces carbon monoxide from bound proteins six times faster than atmospheric oxygen. Patients with carboxyhemoglobin levels greater than 25–30% should be ventilated. It takes longer to shift the carbon monoxide from the cytochrome oxidase pathway than from hemoglobin. Hence, oxygen therapy should be continued until the metabolic acidosis has been corrected.

C: Circulatory

Circulatory status is evaluated with pulse rate and blood pressure and when indicated venous access is established with two wide-bore IV lines in upper limbs in unburnt area. Initial fluid of choice is crystalloid, preferably RL. Colloids should be considered in patients not responding to crystalloids. *Profound hypovolemia is not the normal initial response to a burn.* If a patient is hypotensive then it may be due to delayed presentation, cardiogenic dysfunction, or an occult source of blood loss (chest, abdomen, or pelvis). In patients with circumferential deep-partial or full-thickness burns of extremities and electrical injury, assessment of distal circulation is mandatory for detection. The circulatory compromise can occur later as edema develops after initiation of fluid resuscitation. On securing vascular access, blood samples should be collected and sent for blood counts, packed cell volume, estimating urea and electrolytes, blood group, and clotting profile. The resuscitation regimen should be determined as per centers' protocol and begun. A urinary catheter is mandatory to monitor urine output in all adults with burns covering >20% of TBSA. Urine output in children can be monitored with external catchment devices or by weighing nappies provided the injury is <20% of TBSA. In children, the intraosseous route can be used for fluid administration if IV access cannot be obtained but should be replaced by IV lines as soon as possible.[16,20]

D: Neurological Disability

All patients should be assessed for responsiveness with the Glasgow Coma scale; they may be confused because of hypoxia or hypovolemia.[16,17,20]

E: Exposure with Environment Control

Whole of the patient should be examined (including the back) to get an accurate estimate of the burn area and to check for any concomitant injuries. Burn patients, especially children, easily become hypothermic. This may lead to hypoperfusion and deepening of burn wounds. Patients should be covered and warmed as soon as possible.[20]

Secondary Survey

Burn patients should undergo a burn-specific secondary survey, which should be done rapidly in systematic manner only after the primary survey is completed, and patient is stabilized. This includes history, for determination of the mechanism of injury, a complete head-to-toe examination, the consideration of the possibility of abuse, and a detailed assessment of the burn wound. Details regarding circumstances of the burn, for example, duration and mode of burning, open or closed spaces, contact with smoke and chemicals, etc., should be obtained from bystanders or rescuers. The purpose of secondary survey is to identify significant injuries and obtain a definitive diagnosis of all injuries produced by the burn injury. The burn wounds are thoroughly assessed in secondary survey, to estimate the extent and depth of burns. Circumferential burns of limbs are noted, and peripheral circulation must be repeatedly examined for any compromise due to edema and development of eschar.[20,21]

History: **The history of a burn injury can give valuable information about the nature and extent of the burn, the** likelihood of inhalational injury, the time of burn, the depth of burn, and probability of other injuries. The exact mechanism of injury and any prehospital treatment must be recorded. A quick history of Allergies, Medications, Past medical history including vaccinations, Last oral intake, and Events of injury (A.M.P.L.E) must be obtained. A complete head-to-toe examination, including a second review of airway and lungs and level of consciousness follows **(Table 1)**.

Patients' smoking habits should be determined as these may affect blood gas analysis. Development of edema after initiation of fluid resuscitation may hamper the patient's ability to vocalize. Hence, detailed history should be obtained from the patient at the initial assessment. After completing initial assessment and initiation of resuscitation, the complete extent and depth of burn wound should be evaluated.

ADMISSION CRITERIA

Burn Surface Area Assessment

An accurate estimate of the size of the burn is important for treatment and transfer decisions. The size or extent of the burn can be estimated in a number of ways. When calculating burn area, erythema should not be included. This may take a few hours to fade, so some overestimation is inevitable if the burn is estimated acutely.[22]

- *Wallace's "Rule of 9"* is a quick and practical way of estimating the surface area affected by burn. The adult

TABLE 1: Points to be considered in a head-to-toe examination.

Parts	Examination points
Head	Scalp burns, hematoma, and skull and facial fractures
Ear	Ear burns and blisters
Eye	Corneal burns and ocular hypertension
Neck	Circumferential burns, any missed neck injury, and contusion
Chest	Re-evaluate the lung window, auscultation, and rib fracture
Abdomen	Feel of abdomen, distention, and abdominal compartment syndrome
Perineum	Any injury and bleeding per rectum
Pelvis	Pelvic compression
Back	Examination of back and spine
Extremities	Capillary refill, injury, circumferential burns, and bony deformity
Neurological	Glasgow Coma scale or AVPU

(AVPU: alert, verbose, pain response, unconscious)

body configuration is divided into anatomic regions that represent 9% or multiples of 9% of the TBSA **(Fig. 8)**.

- Head and neck = 9%
- Front of trunk = 18%
- Back of trunk = 18%
- Upper limb each = 9%
- Lower limb each = 18%
- Perineum and external genitalia = 1%

Body surface area proportions differ considerably for children. Using "Rule of 9" for a child can lead to wrong estimation of the extent, and hence improper fluid resuscitation. For patients younger than 15 years, a more precise method of burn size estimation must be used.[23,24]

- *Lund and Browder's chart:* Perhaps, the most accurate method is the age-specific Lund and Browder's chart **(Table 2)** that compensates for the changes in body proportions with growth. The burn area is drawn on a cartoon figure and an associated age-specific table is used to calculate the body surface area involved. This provides more accurate distribution of body surface area and is especially valuable for burnt children. For a burn unit, adoption of this burn extent estimation chart is advisable. Its use also facilitates comparison of data from different units.[25]
- *Palmar surface:* The surface area of an individual's palm (including fingers) is roughly 0.8% of TBSA, though it is taken as 1% for all practical purposes **(Fig. 9)**. Palmar surface area can be used to estimate

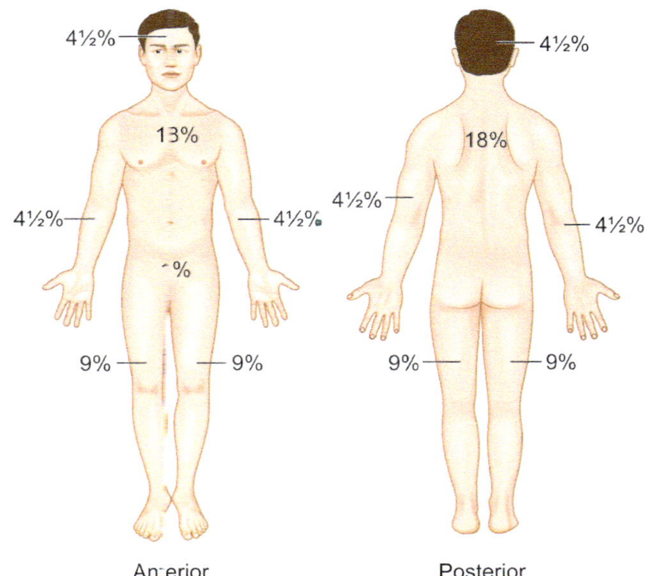

FIG. 8: Wallace's rule of 9 showing distribution of different anatomic region in terms of percentage of total body surface area.

relatively small burns (< 15% of TBSA) or very large burns (> 85%, when unburnt skin is counted) or areas of irregular or nonconfluent burns.[26,27]

While assessing the extent of burn, it is important that the entire body surface is exposed and assessed. The environment should be kept warm, and hypothermia should be avoided. Burns of the pigmented skin can be difficult to assess and it may be necessary to remove all the loose epidermal layers to unveil the exact burn size.

BURN UNIT REFERRAL

To standardize the treatment categorization, the American Burn Association has identified three treatment categories for burn patients: Major, moderate, and minor burn injuries **(Table 3)**.[28]

Major burn injuries: This group includes partial-thickness burns with greater than 25% TBSA in adults (20% in children); all full-thickness burns with a TBSA of 10% or greater; all burns involving hands, face, eyes, ears, feet, and perineum; all inhalation injuries; electrical burns of any extent; complicated burn injuries involving fractures or other major trauma; and all poor-risk patients **(Fig. 10)**. Major burn patients should be transported to a burn center. The choice of a hospital depends on distance and time, the patient's burn complications (respiratory condition and shock), and availability of bed. The American Burn Association emphasizes the importance of direct communication and transfer agreements among hospitals. This system is highly desirable though nonexistent in India at present. If the seriousness of the patient's injury dictates

TABLE 2: Lund and Browder chart for estimating area of burns.

Area	Birth to 1 year	1–4 years	5–9 years	10–14 years	15 years	Adult	2nd*	3rd*	Total body surface area
Head	19	17	13	11	9	7			
Neck	2	2	2	2	2	2			
Anterior trunk	13	13	13	13	13	13			
Posterior trunk	13	13	13	13	13	13			
Right buttock	2.5	2.5	2.5	2.5	2.5	2.5			
Left buttock	2.5	2.5	2.5	2.5	2.5	2.5			
Genitalia	1	1	1	1	1	1			
Right upper arm	4	4	4	4	4	4			
Left upper arm	4	4	4	4	4	4			
Right lower arm	3	3	3	3	3	3			
Left lower arm	3	3	3	3	3	3			
Right hand	2.5	2.5	2.5	2.5	2.5	2.5			
Left hand	2.5	2.5	2.5	2.5	2.5	2.5			
Right thigh	5.5	6.5	8	8.5	9	9.5			
Left thigh	5.5	6.5	8	8.5	9	9.5			
Right leg	5	5	5.5	6	6.5	7			
Left leg	5	5	5.5	6	6.5	7			
Right foot	3.5	3.5	3.5	3.5	3.5	3.5			
Left foot	3.5	3.5	3.5	3.5	3.5	3.5			
Total	100	100	100	100	100	100			

Note: The figures can be colored in red for full-thickness burns (3rd*) and blue for partial-thickness burns (2nd*).

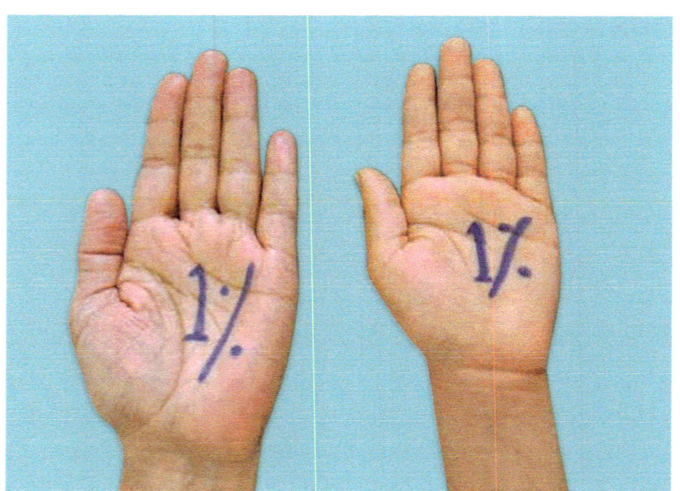

FIG. 9: Palmar surface of hand with fingers closed representing 1% of body surface area in adult (left) and child (right).

transportation to the closest emergency department of a hospital, then subsequent transfer to a burn center should be arranged after cardiopulmonary stabilization and IV fluid therapy for shock.[29,30]

Moderate, uncomplicated burn injuries: This second group includes partial-thickness burns of 15–25% TBSA in adults (10–20% in children); full-thickness burns of < 10% TBSA; and burns that do not involve eyes, ears, face, hands, feet or perineum. Excluded from the group are electrical injuries, complicated injuries (fractures), inhalation injuries, and all poor-risk patients (elderly patients and patients with an intercurrent disease). Most of the patients in this group should receive emergency care at the site of the injury and be transported directly either to a hospital where burn care expertise is available or to a hospital with a burn center.[28]

TABLE 3: American Burn Association's grading system for burn severity and disposition of patients.[28]

	Types of burn		
	Minor	**Moderate**	**Major**
Criteria	< 10% TBSA burn in adults < 5% TBSA burn in young or old < 2% full-thickness burn	10–20% TBSA burn in adult 5–10% TBSA burn in young or old 2–5% full-thickness burn Excluding High-voltage injury Suspected inhalation injury Circumferential burn Concomitant medical problem predisposing the patient to infection (e.g., diabetes and sickle cell disease)	> 20% TBSA burn in adult > 10% TBSA burn in young or old > 5% full-thickness burn High-voltage burn Known inhalation injury Any significant burn to face, eyes, ears, genitalia or joints Significant associated injuries (e.g., fracture and other major trauma)
Disposition	Outpatient management	Hospital admission	Referral to burn center

Note: Young = patient younger than 10 years of age; adult = patient 10–50 years of age; old = patient older than 50 years of age.

(TBSA: total body surface area)

Source: Adapted from Hospital and prehospital resources for optimal care of patients with burn injury: Guidelines for development and operation of burn centers. American Burn Association. J Burn Care Rehabil. 1990;11(2):98-104.

With additional information form Hartford CE. Care of outpatient burns. In: Herndon DN (Ed). Total Burn Care. Philadelphia: Saunders; 1996. pp. 71-80.

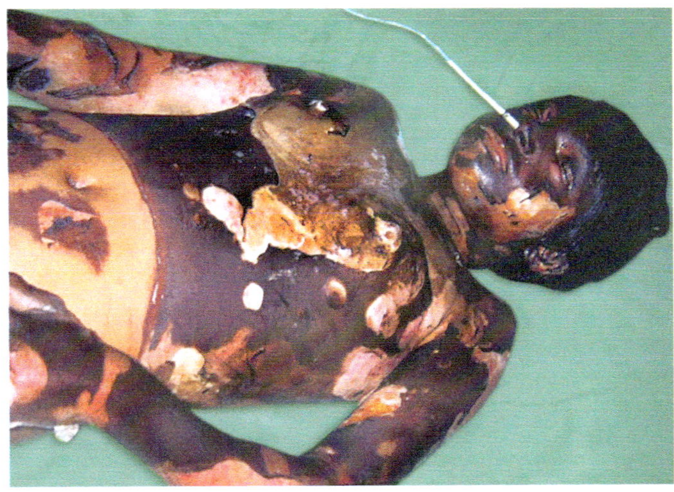

FIG. 10: Major burn injury.

Minor burn injuries: The third group includes partial-thickness burns with a TBSA of < 15% in adults (10% in children); full-thickness burns with a TBSA of < 2%; and burns not involving eyes, ears, face, hands, feet or perineum. It excludes electrical injuries, inhalation injuries, fractures, and all poor-risk patients. The patients in this group may be transported to a hospital emergency department where definitive care begins.[27,28]

In Indian setting, it is highly desirable to provide treatment to patients with moderate and minor burns in a Level 2 hospital with support from burn unit at Level 1 (tertiary care) hospital whenever necessary. This can control the patient load in the few burn centers available, and hence help improve the quality of care.

Burn Unit Admission Criteria[31]

A burn unit may treat adults or children or both.

Burn injuries that should be treated at a burn unit in developing countries include the following:

- Partial-thickness burns > 15% TBSA
- Burns that involve the face, hands, feet, genitalia, perineum, or major joints
- Full-thickness burns in any age group
- Electrical burns, including lightning injury
- Chemical burns
- Inhalation injury
- Burn injury in patients with pre-existing medical disorders that may complicate management, prolong recovery, or affect mortality
- Any patient with burns and concomitant trauma (such as fractures) **(Fig. 11)** in which the burn injury poses the greatest risk of morbidity or mortality. In such cases, if the trauma poses the greater immediate risk, the patient may be initially stabilized in a trauma center before being transferred to a burn unit. Physician judgment is necessary in such situations and should be in concert with the triage protocols.
- Burned children in hospitals without qualified personnel or equipment for the care of children
- Burn injury in patients who require special social, emotional, or long-term rehabilitative intervention

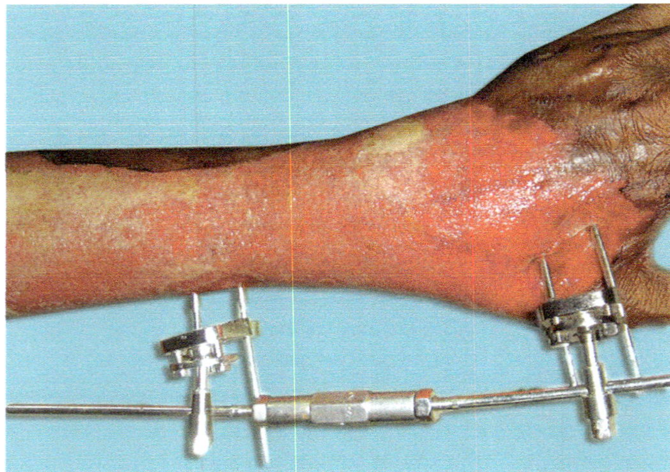

FIG. 11: Fracture of the lower end of radius, along with burns in the forearm and hand, due to a fall after sustaining electric burns.

Selection for outpatient care: Outpatient management is best coordinated with the burn unit's team of doctors, nurses, and therapists because their expertise may facilitate attaining optimal outpatient results. Several factors are relevant to a decision regarding outpatient care. No question of airway compromise should exist. The wound must be small enough so that IV fluid resuscitation is not required. The patient must be capable of oral intake of an adequate amount of fluids. Burns on the face, ears, hands, genitals, or feet should be initially managed in an inpatient setting. The patient and his/her family must be able to comply with an outpatient care plan. An adult caregiver must be present with a child being managed in an outpatient setting. A family member must be available to perform necessary wound cleansing, inspection, and dressing applications because most patients cannot do these themselves. The family must have adequate transportation to return for follow-up visits and unexpected emergency visits. Specific conditions that mandate an early return should be detailed. Particularly important are pain and anxiety associated with wound care to the degree that wound care is compromised. This can be suspected if the wound shows signs of infection or appears deeper than appreciated at the time of the initial examination. In such a situation the patient should be admitted. If abuse is suspected, outpatient management is contraindicated. If on initial examination surgery is clearly needed for a full-thickness burnt area, the patient should be admitted. Despite all these stipulations, most patients with small burns can be successfully managed in an outpatient setting.[6]

OUTPATIENT WOUND CARE STRATEGIES[6,32]

The components of outpatient burn care include:

- Patient and family teaching
- Wound cleansing
- Choice of topical agent or membrane dressing
- Pain control
- Early return instructions
- Follow-up clinic visits
- Long-term follow-up

Wound cleansing and dressing techniques must be taught to whosoever will be doing the dressing changes. Documenting this teaching is ideal.

INPATIENT MANAGEMENT

According to American Burn Association, a major burn is defined as a burn covering 20% or more of TBSA in adults (>10% for children), and all these patients require admission in burns unit.[28] Rapid assessment is vital. The general approach to a major burn can be extrapolated to managing any burn. Once the initial resuscitation is done the wound coverage need to be planned as per the protocol of the burn center.

Fluid Therapy (See Appendix 1.1)

Fluid losses from the injury must be replaced to maintain homeostasis. The main aim of resuscitation is to maintain tissue perfusion to the zone of stasis and so prevent the deepening of burn. This is not easy, as too little fluid can cause hypoperfusion whereas too much may lead to edema causing tissue hypoxia. Burns covering >15% of TBSA in adults and >10% in children warrant formal resuscitation as physiological compensatory mechanisms may not be adequate to combat the fluid loss. There is no ideal resuscitation regimen and many are in use. All the fluid formulas are only guidelines, and their success depends on adjusting the amount of resuscitation fluid against monitored physiological parameters. The greatest amount of fluid loss in burn patients is in the first 24 hours after injury. For the first 8–12 hours, there is a general shift of fluid from the intravascular to interstitial fluid compartments.[27] This means that any fluid given during this time will rapidly leave the intravascular compartment. Colloids have no advantage over crystalloids in maintaining circulatory volume in this situation. Fast fluid boluses probably have little benefit, as a rapid rise in intravascular hydrostatic pressure will just drive more fluid out of the circulation. However, much

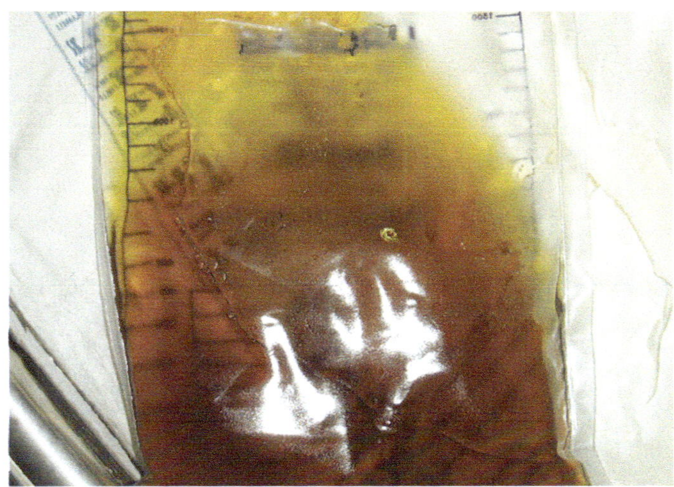

FIG. 12: Brownish urine suggestive of myoglobinuria.

protein is lost through the burn wound, so there is a need to replace this oncotic loss. Some resuscitation regimens introduce colloid after the first 8 hours, when the loss of fluid from the intravascular space is decreasing. The following facts need to be considered while planning fluid resuscitation.[33,34]

- Burn patients may have substantially higher fluid requirements than other trauma patients depending on the surface area involved.
- Fluid needs to be titrated to maintain adequate output, and special care needs to be taken when myoglobinuria is present **(Fig. 12)**.
- The greatest loss of fluids occurs in the first 48 hours.
- The fluid should be administered at constant drip rate and surges should be avoided. If indicated, aliquots of 250 mL of RL may be administered.
- The fluid volume for each patient should be adjusted according to urine output (30–35 mL per hour minimum) and hematocrit (32%). Insert urinary catheter.
- In children, provision for the daily maintenance requirement (weight or surface area-based formula) on top of the calculated amount should be made if Parkland formula is being used.
- Sodium salt solutions (crystalloids) are the essential components of fluid resuscitation.
- The most appropriate fluid is RL because its composition is the closest to that of extracellular fluid. Also, lactate is a source of base due to its conversion to bicarbonate in the liver.
- Fluids should be free of glucose (exception being small children), since glucose intolerance is characteristically present due to high circulating levels of stress hormones.

TABLE 4: Resuscitation formulas (adult) for first 24 hours.

Formula	Crystalloids	Colloids	Daily need
Parkland	4 mL/kg/% TBSA burn	None	None
Brooke (modified)	2 mL/kg/% TBSA burn	None	2.0 L
Galveston	5 L/m^2 burned area	None	1.5 L/m^2 BSA
Safdarjung formula	2 mL/kg/% TBSA burn + DNS maintenance fluid	None	As per weight

(BSA: body surface area; DNS: dextrose normal saline; TBSA: total body surface area)

- The time frame of fluid resuscitation is to be calculated from the time of burn and NOT from the time of initiation of therapy.

  The resuscitation formulae most commonly used for fluid calculation are the Parkland formula, a pure crystalloid formula (4 mL × % burnt area × body weight in kg), modified Parkland's formula or modified Brooke's formula **(Table 4)**. The calculated volume is then given at different rates:[35,36]
  - *First 8 hours:* Half of total to be given.
  - *Next 16 hours:* Half of total to be given.
  - *Next 24 hours:* Half of total given on first day

Any fluid already given should be deducted from the calculated requirement. RL solution without dextrose is the fluid of choice except in children under 2 years, who should receive 5% dextrose RL.[37] Early work by Baxter and by Shires established the basis for modern protocols for fluid resuscitation.[38] They showed that edema fluid in burn wounds is isotonic and contains same amount of protein as plasma and the greatest loss of fluid is into the interstitial fluid compartment. It led to successful clinical trial of Parkland formula.

Modified Brooke's is another popular formula used by various burn centers around the world. As per this formula, the fluid requirement in the first 24 hours in acute burn is 2 mL/kg body weight/% of burn surface area along with daily maintenance fluid for adults. This formula also uses crystalloid, in the form of RL. The total calculated fluid is administered in two halves like in Parkland formula. Then, the flow rate is adjusted as per the urine output with target of 0.5–1 mL/kg/h.[39,40]

Safdarjung formula (used in Safdarjung Hospital Burn Center, New Delhi): This formula is a modified version of Brooke's formula. As per this formula, the fluid requirement in the first 24 hours in acute burn is 2 mL/kg body weight/% of burn surface area. Along with this, 2,500 mL maintenance fluid in the form of 5% dextrose normal saline (DNS) (for a 50 kg patient,

50 mL/kg/day is taken) is infused. The total calculated amount is divided into two halves, one half is infused over first 8 hours, the second half is infused over the next 16 hours. Patients resuscitated with this formula have been shown to have less hyponatremia and the dextrose provides additional calories. Calculation of maintenance fluid is done by 4-2-1 method for pediatric patients. Maintenance fluid calculation is done by considering 4 mL/kg/h for initial weight of 0–10 kg; for next 10–20 kg, 2 mL/kg/h is taken; and remaining weight (>20 kg) is calculated as 1 mL/kg/h DNS. Rate to be adjusted to prevent fluid overload.[41]

Colloid use is controversial. Some units introduce colloid after 8 hours, as the capillary leak begins to shut down, whereas others wait until 24 hours. Fresh frozen plasma is often used in children and albumin or synthetic high molecular weight starches are used in adults. Generally, at the end of 24 hours, colloid infusion is begun at a rate of 0.5 mL × TBSA (%) × body weight (kg) besides maintenance crystalloid (usually dextrose-saline) infusion. The endpoint to aim for is a urine output of 0.5–1.0 mL/kg/h in adults and 1.0–1.5 mL/kg/h in children. High-tension electrical injuries require substantially more fluid (up to 9 mL × % burn area × kg body weight) in the first 24 hours and a higher urine output (1.5–2 mL/kg/h). Inhalational injuries also require more fluid.[27]

The above regimens are merely guidelines to the probable amount of fluid required. This should be continuously adjusted according to urine output and other physiological parameters (pulse, blood pressure, and respiratory rate). Investigations at intervals of 4–6 hours are mandatory for monitoring a patient's resuscitation status. These include packed cell volume, plasma sodium, base excess, and lactate.[33,34]

The debate on the choice of resuscitation fluid has been going on. Different fluids are expected to cause varying degrees of plasma volume expansion **(Table 5)**. However, it was shown that changes in plasma volume were not related to the type of resuscitation fluid in the first 24 hours, concluding that colloid solutions should not be used during this period until capillary permeability returns to near normal. Others have argued that normal capillary permeability is restored somewhat earlier (6–8 hours after burn) and colloids can be started earlier.[42,43] Moncrief and Pruitt studied hemodynamic effects of fluid resuscitation in burns culminating in Brooke's formula, which recommended use of 0.5 mL of colloid/% of burn/kg body weight and has now been modified to all crystalloid resuscitation in first 24 hours. Efforts to avoid wrong calculation of resuscitation fluid have led to usage of Burns wheel, Palmtop computer, and Resuscitation Burn Card, etc., at some burn centers.[44-46] There is continuing debate over the merits of colloid versus crystalloids for the resuscitation of major burns.[47] The crystalloid resuscitation is widely accepted. Hypertonic saline solution has theoretical advantage and has been shown to decrease net fluid intake and decrease edema.[48,49] No significant difference was found in volume requirement or weight gain in patients over 20% TBSA burns, randomized on hypertonic saline or RL solution for resuscitation.[50] Some have found an increase in renal failure with hypertonic saline.[51] According to Berger et al, Hypertonic saline solutions, whether with dextran or not, have shown no advantage over the classic RL solution.[52] When using hypertonic saline, care must be taken to avoid serum sodium concentration greater than 160 mEq/dL.[53] Some burns unit use a modified hypertonic solution of sodium bicarbonate added to lactated Ringer's solution with success.[54] Some studies favor administration of protein-based colloids during the resuscitation period for major burns, starting in the early period after injury. These studies claim more beneficial effect than potential side-effects.[55] The results with albumin are varied. Some studies show that use of albumin does not reduce mortality when

TABLE 5: Preload expanding properties of standard fluids.

Fluid	Osmolarity (mOms/L)	Colloid osmotic pressure	pH	Distribution space	Ratio of fluid infused to intravascular expansion
5% dextrose	250	0	4	Total body water	8:1
Normal saline	308	0	5	Extracellular	3:1
Ringer's lactate solution	270	0	6.5	Extracellular	3:1
Hypertonic lactated saline (250 mEq Na^+/L)	450	0	6–7	Extracellular expansion by fluid shifts from cells	<3:1*
6% albumin	250	20–24	6–7	Intravascular	1:1
Dextran 70	300–303	20–40+	6–7	Intravascular expansion by fluid shift	<1:1

*Depends on tonicity of fluid and plasma osmolarity.

compared with crystalloids,[56,57] while other claims higher mortality rate with liberal use of albumin.[52] According to Cochran et al., there was no increase in mortality with albumin.[58] There was no reduction in multiple organ dysfunction score with albumin.[59]

According to Berger et al., artificial colloids, particularly gelatine, remain a useful tool in patients with major burns and hemodynamic instability and can be given as early as 6 hours after injury.[52] Chen et al., studied utility of hydroxyethyl starch in burns resuscitation and claimed that it can partially substitute plasma and be used in fluid resuscitation, but plasma protein replenishment should be emphasized.[60] The use of composite sodium lactate and sorbitol (CISS) in resuscitation fluid during shock stage of the patients with major burns can be beneficial to the replenishment of blood volume, control of shock, promotion of diuresis, subsidence of edema, and can also provide electrolytes and energy, without the influence on the level of blood glucose.[61] Some found no added advantage with fresh frozen plasma and recommended its use only for specific coagulation disorders while according to others, it is useful for resuscitation of burns.[58] High dose (66 mg/kg/h) IV ascorbic acid (vitamin C) in early phase of fluid resuscitation has been found to be advantageous.[62,63] This group showed reduced weight gain, wound edema, improved oxygenation and reduced requirement of resuscitation fluid volume.[63]

The ideal burn resuscitation formula does not exist. Whichever formula is used, patients must be monitored closely, and the fluid resuscitation is individualized according to the response. Patients with delay in resuscitation, associated trauma, inhalation injury, or alcohol abuse may require greater than predicted quantity of fluid. The goal is to maintain urine output in the range of 0.5–1 mL/kg/h for adults and 1–1.5 mL/kg/h in children. In patients with fluid requirements greater than 150% of that predicted by formula, the addition of colloid at 12 hours can reduce total fluid requirements and burn edema. Early placement of pulmonary artery catheters can be useful in patients with known myocardial dysfunction, age greater than 65 years, severe inhalation injury, or fluid requirements greater than 150% of that predicted by formula.[64] Gastrointestinal fluid resuscitation by oral and rectal route has been tried for burn patients in peripheral areas.[65]

For burned children, the commonly used formulae are modified to account for changes in surface area to mass ratios. These changes are necessary because a child with a burn requires more resuscitation fluid per kilogram as compared to an adult (See **Appendix 1.2**).[66]

In the Galveston formula the daily fluid requirement for a child with burn is augmented to 2 L/m^2 of TBSA against 1.5 L/m^2 for an adult.

Intravenous Access

A peripheral vein catheter through unburnt skin is the preferred route for fluid administration. A central line or pulmonary artery line is only occasionally required to monitor the patient during the initial resuscitation period and is removed as soon as possible. The possibilities for IV access are as follows.

Choices for venous access:
- *First choice:* Peripheral vein; unburnt area
- *Second choice:* Central vein; unburnt area
- *Third choice:* Peripheral vein; burnt area
- *Worst choice:* Central vein; burnt area

Monitoring lines are required primarily for the elderly patients or patients with severe heart disease. A high complication rate has been reported with central catheters in burn patients as a result of infection.

Common Pitfalls in Initial Fluid Resuscitation

- *Initial under resuscitation:* The largest fluid shifts occur in the first several hours postburn. Initial crystalloid infusion based on a formula will often be inadequate. If shock state is present due to delay in initiation of resuscitation, more volume of fluid is needed for resuscitation. A volume expander such as a nonprotein colloid or protein solution or hypertonic saline can be very useful along with isotonic crystalloid for successful resuscitation.[42,43]
- *Initial over resuscitation:* Aggressive fluid infusion is now frequently initiated in most emergency rooms with placement of large bore lines. The practice of "wide-open" fluid infusion during early assessment and transport regardless of hemodynamic response is to be avoided. The excess fluid cannot be compensated for by decreasing infusion rate in subsequent hours because the extra fluid is already out of the vascular space.

  Pruitt coined the term "fluid creep". This phenomenon occurs when there is excessive fluid accumulated in the body during resuscitation.[66] The prevalence of fluid creep varies from 30–90%. The fluid creep increases in patients with large areas, receiving only crystalloids. Other precipitating factor is opioid use. In the initial period, the leaky capillaries allow the fluid to shift to the third space, and a decrease in oncotic pressure. The imbalance does not reverse even if the capillary permeability changes. So, the continuous accumulation of the fluid leads to fluid creep, which is popularly called "fluid begets fluid".[67] The adverse effects due to fluid creep are abdominal compartment syndrome, intra-abdominal hypertension, pulmonary edema, cerebral edema, and ocular hypertension.[68] Prevention of fluid creep should be done by use of a protocolized formula and keeping a tab on input and use of colloids. The management of fluid creep is done by colloid rescue, hypertonic saline, high-dose vitamin C, and rarely plasmapheresis.[69]

- *Striving for ideal numbers:* It is quite possible to achieve ideal numbers (pulse < 120 beats/min, blood pressure > 100 mm Hg, and urine output 0.5–1 mL/kg body weight/h) in a young patient with a moderate-sized uncomplicated burn. In a massive burn (> 60% TBSA), especially in the presence of inhalation injury or in the elderly, attempts at pushing fluids beyond reasonable amounts to achieve "ideal numbers" only accentuate edema-induced complications. Adequate perfusion is not the same as "ideal numbers". While planning the treatment, possibility of pulmonary and chest wall edema-induced complications needs to be considered.[42]
- *Consideration of fluid alone for treatment of impaired perfusion:* Hypovolemia from burn-induced fluid and protein shifts is the predominant cause of hypoperfusion and fluid infusion is the treatment. However, two other processes must be considered. The first is impaired cardiac output due to an increasing mean airway pressure, particularly from a noncompliant chest wall burn. Ventilator adjustments, chest wall escharotomy, elevation of the headend of the bed to decrease chest edema, and the use of an agent, such as low-dose dopamine, to assist fluids can be very helpful in maintaining perfusion. Secondly, cardiac depression from a deep body burn is well described, particularly in the elderly. Supplementation of fluids, both crystalloid, and colloid, with a beta agonist can help reverse a downward course reflected by continually increasing fluid requirements and decreasing perfusion.[70,71]
- *Use of urine output alone as monitor for volume restoration:* Although usually a reliable indicator of renal perfusion, factors such as high plasma alcohol or glucose levels often lead to an inappropriately high urine output relative to the status of tissue perfusion. The value of the urine output must be considered to be unreliable under these circumstances.[43]
- *Failure to secure IV lines:* As edema develops, the IV catheter may slip out of the vein into the surrounding tissue. Not only does this lead to transient hypovolemia, but finding a new site when edema is present can be extremely difficult. A solution is to secure the IV line with sutures.

Monitoring of Resuscitation

In a burn patient, no single monitor of perfusion can be a completely reliable indicator of tissue oxygenation (perfusion). Therefore, several standard hemodynamic monitors and laboratory tests should be utilized.[42,43]

Physiologic Measurements

- *Oxygenation:* Use of a pulse oximeter is standard for a major burn.
- *Baseline body weight:* The baseline weight is used to estimate the initial fluid replacement and can be obtained by history or be estimated.
- *Arterial pressure:* The increased sympathetic tone characteristic of this early period makes arterial pressure an insensitive measure of volume status. However, a minimal level of perfusion pressure (> 80 mm Hg) must be maintained. Thus, blood pressure monitoring is necessary.

  An arterial line may be required if:
  - Patient is hemodynamically unstable.
  - Extremities are burned and sphygmomanometer pressure cannot be obtained manually.
  - If frequent blood gas analyses are required.

  The arterial catheter should be placed through unburnt skin and should be removed as soon as possible.
- *Pulse rate:* Tachycardia is inevitable in early postburn period due to hypovolemia and catecholamine release from tissue trauma and pain. The degree of tachycardia can be very useful for determining adequacy of volume replacement. The exception would be an elderly or the patient with pre-existing heart disease in which the heart rate cannot increase in proportion to the stimulus. In most patients, *a pulse rate of < 120 beats/minute usually indicates adequate volume while > 130 beats/minute usually indicates more fluid is needed.*
- *Urine output:* The status of renal blood flow is usually an accurate reflection of the adequacy of systemic perfusion during this early phase of injury. A urine output of 0.5–1 mL/kg body weight/hour normally reflects adequate renal blood flow, assuming there are no factors such as alcohol, hyperglycemia, or mannitol that alter the relationship between renal blood flow and urine output.
- *Intake–Output:* What goes in and what comes out should be carefully tabulated. Intake may far exceed output during this phase as edema develops.
- *Blood gases:* The monitoring of arterial oxygen and carbon dioxide tension is required to judge the adequacy of ventilation. The measurement of pH and acid–base balance is extremely useful for the assessment of tissue oxygenation. A base deficit during this phase usually reflects impaired tissue oxygenation due to hypovolemia or carbon monoxide toxicity (also cyanide).

- *Electrocardiographic monitoring:* Arrhythmias are not common in young patients as long as oxygenation is adequate. They become a major concern in patients older than 45 years as a result of the response to burn stress. Electrocardiograph (ECG) monitoring is also indicated in patients with electrical injury.
- *Body temperature:* The burn patient is very prone to hypothermia during this early period, especially with infusion of cold fluids. A decrease in temperature can lead to further hemodynamic instability and impaired perfusion.
- *Central venous pressure (CVP):* The CVP in a large burn at this stage is usually low, 0–5 cmH_2O, even with adequate fluid resuscitation. Therefore, it can be very dangerous to use an arbitrary value of CVP as an endpoint of resuscitation. Too much or too little fluid can be infused based on an arbitrary value.
- *Pulmonary artery wedge pressure:* The majority of young patients, even with massive burns, do not require the use of these measurements for initial resuscitation. A selected group of patients can benefit from this measurement. These include:
  - Elderly or patients with pre-existent heart disease with large burn or smoke inhalation.
  - Young patient with massive burn who is not maintaining perfusion despite fluid intake well more than predicted.
- Cardiac output and mixed venous oxygen tension: The primary objective of fluid management is to maintain adequate tissue oxygen delivery. The direct measurement of cardiac output (cardiac index) can assist in the determination of oxygen delivery. A cardiac index in excess of 2.5 $L/min/m^2$ is considered normal for an uninjured person. The value for mixed venous oxygen tension (PvO_2), however, can greatly assist in this determination.

Association of mixed venous gas:

- $PvO_2 > 35$ *mm Hg*: Oxygen delivery adequate
- $PvO_2 > 30–35$ *mm Hg*: Oxygen delivery marginal
- $PvO_2 < 30$ *mm Hg*: Oxygen delivery inadequate

Laboratory Measurements (See Appendices 1.3–1.7)

- *Hemoglobin and hematocrit:* Baseline hematocrit and hemoglobin are useful for monitoring although changes in their values may not accurately reflect changes in blood volume due to the selective loss of the plasma component of blood **(Table 6)**.
- *White blood cell (WBC):* Initial WBC counts may be high, normal, or low depending on the magnitude of the stress response and white cell sequestration into the burn. Low WBC count in association with inhalation injury is indicative of poor prognosis.

TABLE 6: Hematocrit changes after a large burn.

Findings	Causes
Hematocrit increased	Plasma volume decreases while circulating red blood cell volume remains relatively constant
Hematocrit normal	• Normalization of blood volume has occurred • Decrease in both plasma and red blood cell volume, the latter from, e.g., hemolysis
Hematocrit decreased	• Hemolysis from prolonged heat exposure, with only plasma volume replacement Major loss of blood from nonburn injury with only plasma volume replacement • Pre-existing anemia and hypervolemia (unlikely)

- *Electrolytes:* Since the initial losses are primarily plasma, the sodium (Na^+), chloride (Cl^-), and potassium (K+) ions values remain relatively constant despite hypovolemia and vary mainly as a result of the type of resuscitation fluid used. K^+ increases in case of severe hemolysis or renal impairment. The bicarbonate (HCO_3) content varies depending on the status of perfusion and acid–base balance.
- *Creatinine and blood urea nitrogen:* Baseline values are helpful to define normal status.
- *Plasma proteins:* A marked decrease in plasma proteins occurs early postburn.
- *Plasma myoglobin:* The plasma value of myoglobin is obtained in very deep burns, especially electrical burns. Myoglobin, released from deeply injured muscles, affects renal function. A higher urine output should be maintained to a minimum of 2 mL/kg/h.
- *Prothrombin time, Partial thromboplastin time, and platelets:* Initial values during this period is useful for determining whether clotting factors may be needed. It is not common to have the need for replacing clotting factors and platelets during the first 36-hour period unless a prolonged shock state has initiated disseminated intravascular coagulation or pre-existing liver or hematologic disease is present.

Imaging

- *Chest radiograph:* An initial chest radiograph obtained in all patients with inhalation injury usually does not show many changes. Development of acute respiratory distress syndrome (ARDS) will be seen in 48 hours postinsult.
- *Point of care ultrasonography (POCUS):* Lung ultrasound and inferior vena cava diameter are usually used as markers. Fluid overload is easily detected by POCUS as extravascular lung fluid accurately before development of any clinical symptoms. But these need skilled person to evaluate.[72,73]

Initial Management of Burn Wound

After ensuring airway patency, adequacy of respiration, and initiation of fluid resuscitation attention is directed to complete evaluation of the extent and depth of the burn wound. Till such time, care should be taken to avoid hypothermia due to exposure. Based on the depth of involvement, the burn wound is classified into *superficial, superficial partial-thickness, deep partial-thickness,* and *full-thickness burn* **(Figs. 13 to 17)**. Burn depth has an impact on healing time, the need for hospitalization, surgical intervention, and the potential for scar development. Although accurate classification is not always possible initially, the causes and physical characteristics of burns are helpful in categorizing their depth **(Table 7)**. Use of light amplification by stimulated emission of radiation (LASER), vital dye, ultrasound, or thermography for estimation of burn depth is expensive and cumbersome.[15] Visual estimation by experienced eyes is the most practical approach.

Recently, it has been proposed that objective assessment of burns wound depth have increased accuracy especially for the purpose of telemedicine **(Table 8)**.[74-80]

Other methods of assessment of burn depth are given in **Table 8**.

Wound care: For an acute burn which is to be transferred to a burn center, cling film is an ideal dressing as it protects the wound, reduces heat and evaporative losses, controls pain, and does not alter the wound appearance.[17] This permits accurate evaluation by the burn team later.

For inpatients, the protocol followed at the author's unit is as follows:

- *Partial-thickness burn wound:* Wounds are cleaned with 0.5% chlorhexidine solution and normal saline.

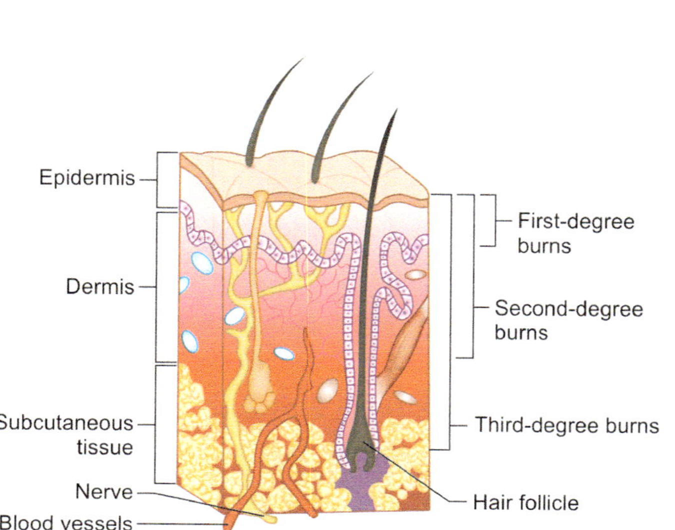

FIG. 13: Line diagram showing depth of burn injury.

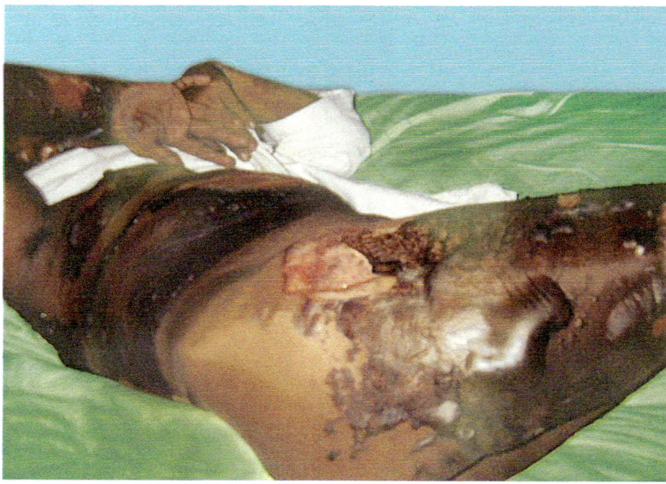

FIG. 14: Superficial partial-thickness burn with blister.

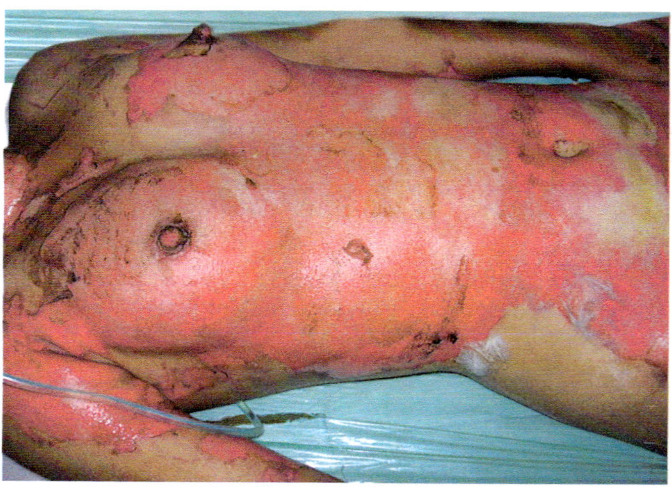

FIG. 15: Superficial partial-thickness burn after debridement of dead skin.

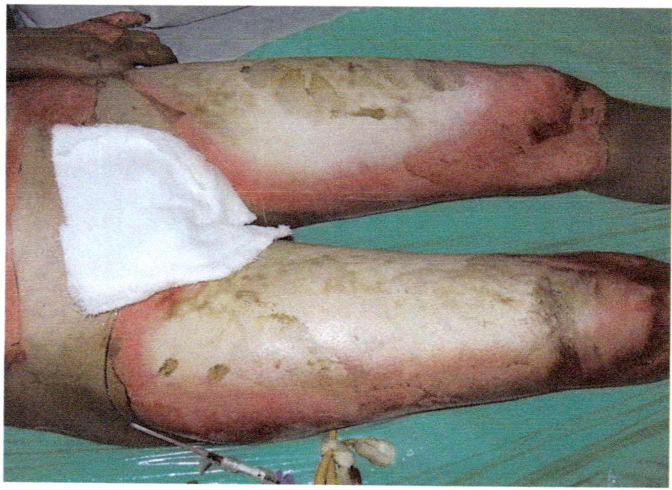

FIG. 16: Deep partial-thickness burn.

Blisters are deroofed and loose skin is removed for ease of dressing, except for palmar blisters (painful), unless these are large enough to restrict movement. Wounds over face and hands and all burns in children are covered with collagen sheets if the patient is received within 6 hours of burn injury **(Fig. 18)**. Once collagen is firmly adherent, secondary dressings are not needed. The author previously used banana leaf dressing with 1% silver sulfadiazine (SSD) for dressing of all other partial-thickness wounds.[81] This is covered with sterile Gamgee cotton pads and bandaged firmly **(Fig. 19)**.[82,83]

- *Full-thickness burn wounds:* In the author's unit, if early excision is planned, full-thickness burn wounds receive exposure treatment with application of povidone-iodine ointment two or three times a day after cleaning of the wound with 0.5% chlorhexidine solution. If early excision is not feasible, the wounds are dressed with banana leaf dressing with povidone-iodine ointment as the topical agent. At most other places the wounds are dressed with 1% SSD.[82,83]
- *Infected wounds:* Exposure treatment with povidone-iodine cream is used in the authors' unit. Many other units prefer closed dressing with antimicrobial agent as per organism grown.

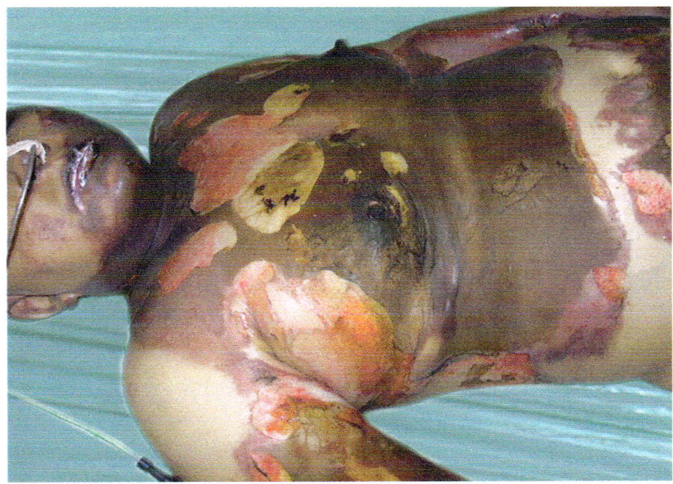

FIG. 17: Full-thickness burn.

TABLE 8: Modern methods of objective assessment of burns wound depths.

Methods	Features
LASER Doppler flowmetry	This has good accuracy for depth determination among superficial and deep burns
LASER Doppler imaging	Very high accuracy, it combines use of LASER doppler and scanning technology
Nera infrared spectroscopy	The infrared spectroscope scans the burnt area to differentiate between superficial and deep burns
Optical coherence tomography	It measures the reflected light from collagen to determine the depth of burn wound
Orthogonal polarization spectral	This method uses polarized light to study the microcirculation pattern in the tissue to determine the burn depth
Thermal imaging	It uses surface temperature of the wound as a guide to know the depth of burn. This is easy and fast to use but less reliable clinically
Vital dyes—fluorescein, and indocyanine green	They help in superficial burns, but are less predictable for deep burns

(LASER: light amplification by stimulated emission of radiation)

TABLE 7: Clinical classification of burns.

Burns	Involvement	Features	Depth
First-degree (Sunburn)	Epidermis	Erythema only Heals in <5 days	Partial-thickness
Second-degree			
Superficial dermal or superficial partial-thickness	Epidermis and papillary dermis	Extremely painful Blister formation. Wet, glistening pink Heals in 10–15 days.	Partial-thickness
Deep dermal or deep partial-thickness	Epidermis, papillary dermis, and part of reticular dermis	Less painful, waxy white appearance. Heals in 3–5 weeks	Partial-thickness
Third degree	Entire thickness of skin	Painless, inelastic, translucent, parchment like eschar with visible thrombosed veins	Full-thickness
Fourth degree	Skin, subcutaneous tissue, muscle, carbonization of limb or gangrene	Require skin grafting. Thick eschar to gangrene	Full-thickness

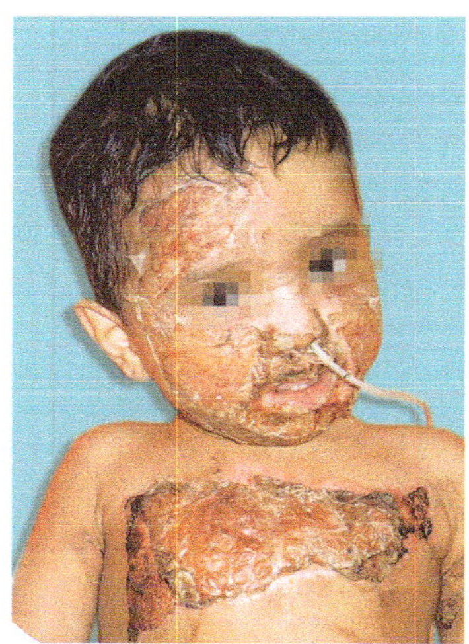

FIG. 18: Superficial partial-thickness burn with collagen application.

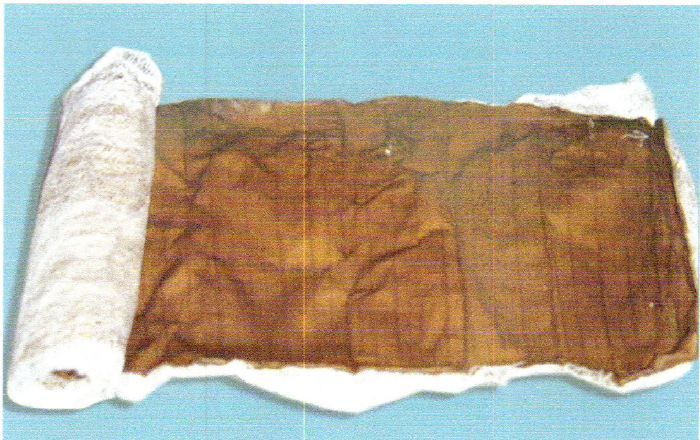

FIG. 19: Autoclaved banana leaf dressing.

Early Surgical Management

Surgical procedures such as escharotomy may be needed early in patients with full-thickness circumferential burns of extremities or chest wall.

Impaired Chest Wall Compliance

Respiratory excursion can be markedly impaired by a circumferential deep partial or full-thickness burn of the chest wall. The loss of elasticity in the burns of the chest wall markedly increases the work of breathing. As more subeschar edema develops, significant respiratory effort is required just to maintain adequate gas exchange. Any process that compromises the necessary increase in inspiratory force and muscle activity, such as hypoxia, hypovolemia, pain, or sedation, accentuates the severity of lung dysfunction. Symptoms may not be clearly evident until edema development peaks at about 10–12 hours. The first clinical evidence of the chest wall restrictive defect is often labored breathing followed by a rapid respiratory deterioration, particularly in the patient who is not receiving ventilatory support. Clearance of secretions can be impaired due to the inability to generate a hyperinflation. In the combined chest burn and inhalation injury, it is very difficult to distinguish the degree of impairment in total lung compliance due to the increased airway edema and bronchospasm compared with that due to the impaired chest wall movement. An extremely deep burn results in tissue contraction due to desiccation, making the chest wall tight even before edema develops.

Patient with *noncircumferential* full-thickness or partial-thickness burn is monitored closely for evidence of respiratory restriction. Escharotomies are usually not required in a partial-thickness burn unless the edema is so massive that the burned skin is tight. For *circumferential* full-thickness burn, chest wall escharotomy is performed early. Even with an escharotomy, the restrictive process can be of such magnitude that hypoventilation is clearly evident. In these patients, endotracheal intubation and positive-pressure ventilation should be initiated before obvious pulmonary deterioration.

Impaired distal perfusion and need for escharotomy: A full-thickness burn tissue has complete loss of elasticity. Hence, as subeschar edema develops under the burnt tissue, the tissue pressure increases. Fluid resuscitation leads to the development of burn wound edema and further swelling of the tissue beneath this inelastic burnt tissue. With circumferential full-thickness burn of extremity, this increase in tissue pressure initially decreases the venous return. This further augments the tissue pressure and leads to impairment of arterial flow causing ischemia **(Fig. 20)**. Initially, limbs at risk should be elevated and observed. Perfusion to the distal extremity should be closely monitored. Pain and color are unreliable indicators of perfusion in the presence of a burn.[27] A warm extremity invariably indicates good flow, but cool skin does not always indicate that the problem is due to proximal constriction. Hypovolemia may as well be the cause. Use of simple handheld Doppler equipment provides valuable information about perfusion. Evidence of ischemia mandates escharotomy **(Flowchart 3)**. Both of these situations require division of the burn eschar. Only the burnt tissue is divided, not any underlying fascia, differentiating this procedure from a fasciotomy. Unless decreased blood flow is evident in the accident and emergency department, the escharotomy should be performed in the burn center after quick transfer. In general, finger escharotomies should be performed in a burn center only because of the associated potential morbidity.

Principles of Escharotomy

- The escharotomy incisions should be located as shown in **(Fig. 21)**. Incisions are made along the midlateral or medial aspects of the limbs, avoiding any underlying structures. For the chest, longitudinal incisions are made at each midaxillary line to the subcostal region. The lines are joined up by a chevron incision running parallel to the subcostal margin.[3] This creates a mobile breastplate that moves with ventilation.
- Anesthesia is not required as the full-thickness burn is insensate.
- The procedure should preferably be performed in an operation theater but can be performed bedside with all aseptic precautions.
- The incision should be deep enough to allow separation of the edges, permitting bulging of viable tissue.
- Pain and significant bleeding are indicative of excessively deep incision.
- Escharotomy must extend completely through the length of burnt tissue crossing the joints till healthy skin is reached.
- Escharotomies are best done with electrocautery, as they tend to bleed. Use of microcrystalline collagen to pack the incision site can help control punctate

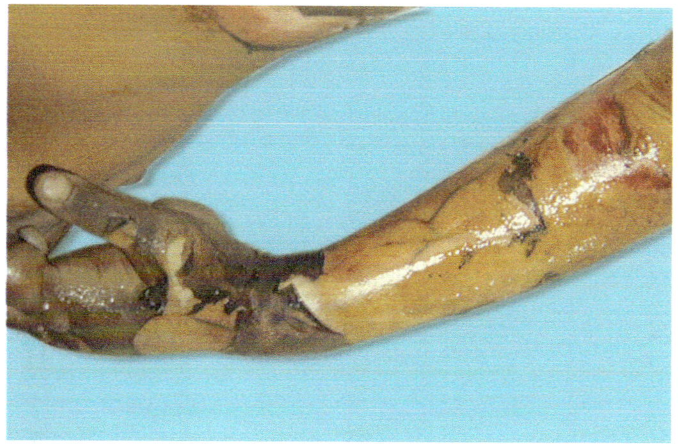

FIG. 20: Circumferential full-thickness burn of forearm leading to ischemic damage to hand.

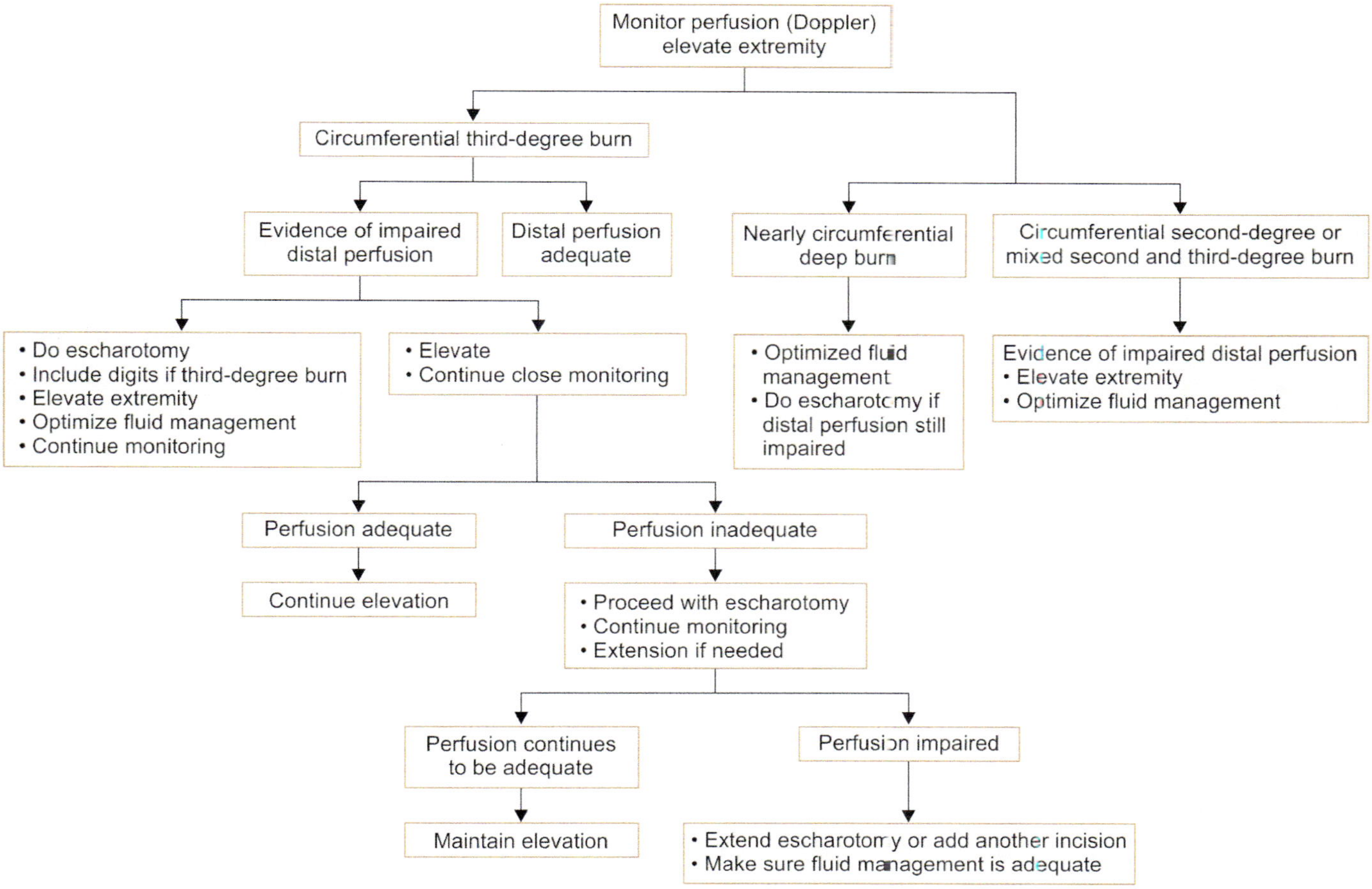

Monitor perfusion (Doppler) elevate extremity

- Circumferential third-degree burn
  - Evidence of impaired distal perfusion
    - • Do escharotomy • Include digits if third-degree burn • Elevate extremity • Optimize fluid management • Continue monitoring
  - Distal perfusion adequate
    - • Elevate • Continue close monitoring
      - Perfusion adequate → Continue elevation
      - Perfusion inadequate → • Proceed with escharotomy • Continue monitoring • Extension if needed
        - Perfusion continues to be adequate → Maintain elevation
        - Perfusion impaired → • Extend escharotomy or add another incision • Make sure fluid management is adequate
- Nearly circumferential deep burn
  - • Optimized fluid management • Do escharotomy if distal perfusion still impaired
- Circumferential second-degree or mixed second and third-degree burn
  - Evidence of impaired distal perfusion • Elevate extremity • Optimize fluid management

FLOWCHART 3: Algorithm for management of circumferential extremity burn.

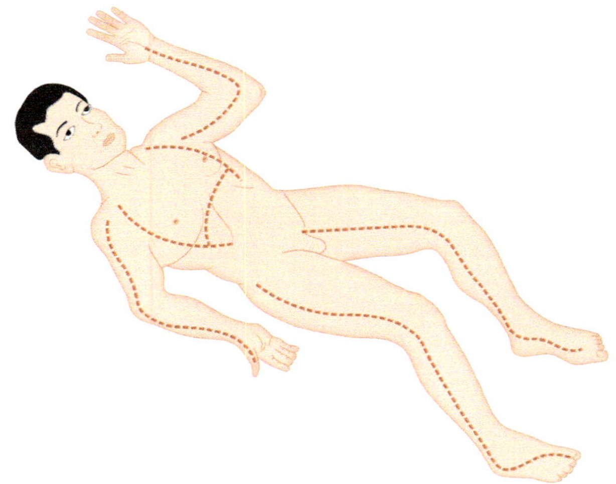

FIG. 21: Common sites for escharotomy.

BOX 3 **Key points for escharotomy and fasciotomy.**

- Remove constricting objects
- Immediate elevation of burned extremities
- Perform early escharotomies on circumferential full-thickness burn
- Consider early fasciotomies for electrical burns involving extremities
- Decreasing Doppler flow signal with adequate blood pressure or tissue pressure > 25 mm Hg means escharotomy/fasciotomy is needed
- Escharotomy is performed without anesthesia while fasciotomy requires regional anesthesia
- Escharotomy must extend completely through the burnt tissue
- Hemostasis is obtained with pressure, cautery, or micro-crystalline collagen

bleeding. Larger vessels usually require suture ligatures or cautery.
- Dressing should be applied using a topical agent and nonadherent wound cover.
- Monitoring of distal perfusion should be continued after escharotomy and if the impairment persists, existing escharotomies should be extended or additional escharotomies should be performed.

Fasciotomy

Treatment of the high-voltage electrical burn victim should include prompt initiation of aggressive fluid resuscitation and serial assessment of distal vascular integrity. Development of compartment syndromes should be anticipated. Deeper muscle groups sustain the greatest injury. Urgent surgical intervention for fasciotomies and muscle compartment explorations under regional or general anesthesia is often indicated. Intraoperative exploration, decompression, and debridement are an essential part of early treatment. Serial technetium-99m stannous pyrophosphate muscle scans have been shown to be useful in assisting determination of progressive muscle damage.[84] If fasciotomies are delayed, development of compartment syndrome and acute renal failure is imminent along with development of gangrene of the affected extremity **(Box 3)**.

Besides early fasciotomy, fluid resuscitation demands attention. If the urine is rose-pigmented from hemochromogens, the urine output should be maintained at 100–125 mL/h (1–2 mL/kg/h) in adults or twice the normal hourly rate in infants and young children, until gross pigment is cleared **(Figs. 22 and 23)**. The urine can be alkalinized by IV administration of sodium bicarbonate to prevent myoglobin precipitation. In severe injuries, IV mannitol (12.5 g in an adult) is given in addition to aggressive fluid replacement to promote an osmotic diuresis.[84] Early use of other diuretics is contraindicated.

INITIAL MANAGEMENT OF BURNS INVOLVING SPECIAL AREAS

The face, ears, hands, genitals, and feet have functional and cosmetic significance that far exceeds their size. Burns of these areas need special attention and this should be initiated early during the treatment.

- Face burns:
  - Suspect inhalation injury in patient with burns of face.
  - After proper cleansing, apply collagen sheet in a patient with superficial partial-thickness burns, if seen within 6 hours of injury.
  - Deep partial or full-thickness wounds may be treated by exposure with SSD cream smear or may be covered with face mask of nonadherent dressing and Gamgee cotton pads.
  - Keep 30° propped-up position. Insert Ryle's tube for feeding.
- Eye burns:
  - History of mode of burns and eye examination
  - Observe for singed eyelashes, eyebrows, eyelid edema, conjunctival lacerations, corneal opacity, any foreign body, pupil size, and reaction to light.
  - If chemical injury is suspected, irrigate the eye with normal saline 0.9% for 15–20 minutes.
  - Application of ophthalmic antibiotic ointment 6-hourly reduces risks of corneal drying and infection.
  - Cover the eye with eye shield and NOT with gauze and cotton pad.

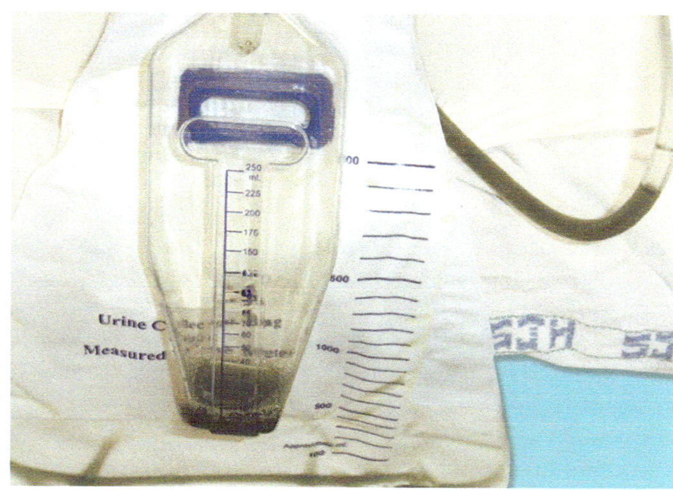

FIG. 22: Dark reddish black urine due to myoglobinuria suggestive of renal insult following electric burns with gangrenous changes in hand.

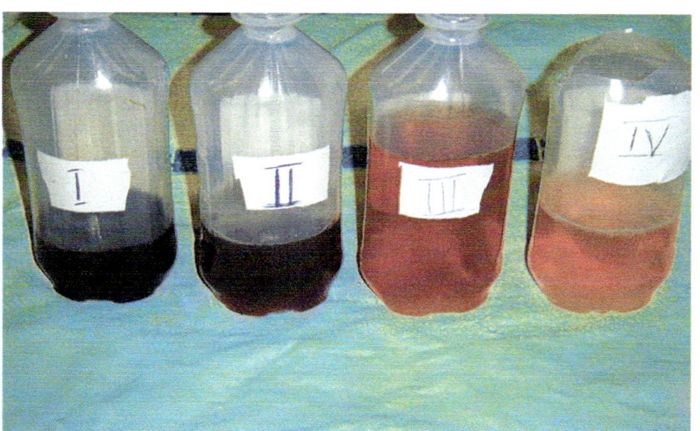

FIG. 23: Rapid fluid infusion with IV mannitol and sodium bicarbonate till urine gradually clears to its normal color—this prevents hemochromogens from blocking the renal tubules.

- Repeat examination daily to look for corneal ulcer, abscess, or other complications.
- In the event of corneal injury or with severe burns of the eyelids, an ophthalmologist's consultation should be obtained.
- Early tarsorrhaphy should be avoided as it increases lid deformity and prevents serial examinations of the corneal surface.

- Ear burns:
  - History of burn injury and examination of ear
  - Examine the auricle for edema, tenderness, and look for discharge from canal.
  - If blisters are present, puncture them and expel the fluid out but avoid removing any skin which is still firmly attached.

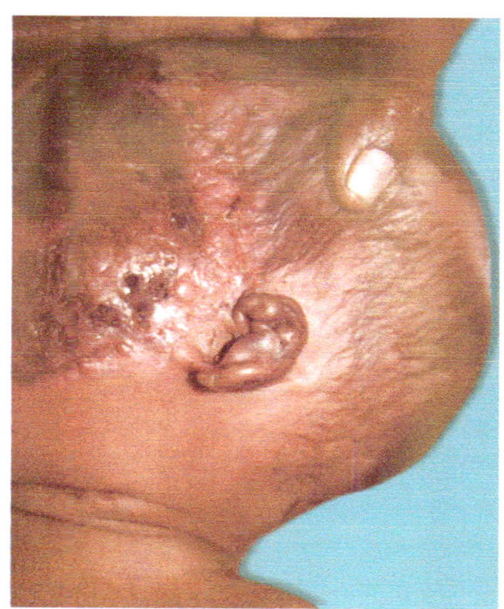

FIG. 24: Chondritis following ear burn.

  - Avoidance of any pressure on the burned auricle is essential (no pillows). Pressure is the biggest cofactor in the production of chondritis. **(Fig. 24)**.[85]
  - Apply paraffin gauze into the canal and apply povidone-iodine ointment on the burnt pinna. Wrap the ear with nonadherent dressing and Gamgee cotton pad and apply mastoid bandage gently.

    Most ear burns respond well to conservative treatment, although occasionally, immediate coverage of exposed cartilage with a temporoparietal fascial flap and skin graft may be required to salvage the pinna.

- Hand burns:
  - Hand burns assume a high priority from the onset of care.
  - During the first 24–48 hours, adequate blood flow must be ensured. The consistency, the temperature, and the presence of pulsatile flow detectable by Doppler ultrasonography monitoring of the digital pulp should be regularly performed. If any doubt exists, escharotomy or fasciotomy should be performed.
  - While dressing a hand burn, each finger should be wrapped individually with nonadherent tulle grass and web spaces should be separated. The hands should be splinted in a position of function: The metacarpophalangeal joints at 70–90°, the interphalangeal joints in extension, the first web space open, and the wrist at 20° of extension.[86]
  - The hands should be elevated to minimize edema and a therapist should perform range-of-motion exercises twice daily.

  - Deep dermal and full-thickness burns should undergo early excision and sheet autograft closure.
- Feet burns:
  - Feet burns require specific care; therefore, admit the patient with burns to feet (especially circumferential burns).
  - Assess the depth of the burns (**Fig. 25**). Strict limb elevation of the involved extremity is needed.
  - Look for capillary refill to assess vascularity.
  - Do escharotomy early to avoid gangrene of the distal part in patients with circumferential burns. Perform primary excision with skin grafting whenever possible.
  - Apply antimicrobial cream and paraffin gauze in web spaces.
  - Throughout the day, encourage the patient for active as well as passive physiotherapy of ankle joint to prevent early contracture formation.
- Perineal burns:
  - Admission of patient with perineal burns is necessary for specific care.
  - Assess extent and depth of the burns. Look for the skin loss and edema.
  - Perurethral catheterization is essential to avoid contamination by urine.
  - Apply a layer of Silverex ointment over burnt area and cover it with double layer of paraffin gauze and Gamgee or keep it exposed.
  - Administer appropriate antibiotic cover including anaerobic organisms, according to protocol.

PAIN MANAGEMENT

Burn injuries cause one of the most intense and prolonged pain. Burn pain is difficult to control because of its unique characteristics, its multiple components, and its changing patterns over time (**Box 4**).[87] Cleansing wounds, changing dressings, and providing physical therapy involve repeated manipulations of painful sites. The sometimes-excruciating pain, along with extreme intra- and inter-individual variability in severity, complicates the task of providing analgesia to burn patients.

Current research suggests that early vigorous analgesic intervention is crucial to prevent the adverse consequences of uncontrolled pain. For example, the burn patient who associates dressing changes with agonizing pain is difficult to treat, even with massive doses of opioids. Prompt, aggressive analgesia is critical to avert the cycle of pain, anxiety and more pain and to minimize adverse psychological effects of pain commonly encountered in burn patients.

Acetaminophen (paracetamol) or nonsteroidal anti-inflammatory drugs (NSAIDs) with opioids can be a basic treatment for burn pain.[87] Traditional analgesic regimens usually neglect or ignore the inflammatory component of burn pain, but it is extremely important, especially during early treatment. Traditional NSAIDs are not recommended in burn patients who are scheduled to undergo extensive excision and grafting procedures because their antiplatelet effects may increase blood loss. However, this class of drugs may help patients who require minimal skin grafts to reduce pain from superficial burn areas or at donor sites (normal skin areas where skin is harvested for grafting). Newer NSAIDs, the cyclooxygenase-2 (COX-2) inhibitors, offer analgesia with few side effects, including minimal inhibition of platelet function.[87] Although the effects of COX-2 inhibitors on wound healing remain to be demonstrated, such medications may constitute a major advance in the treatment of burn pain. These drugs can be introduced early during treatment to reduce peripheral and central sensitization, decrease opioid requirements, and reduce side effects.

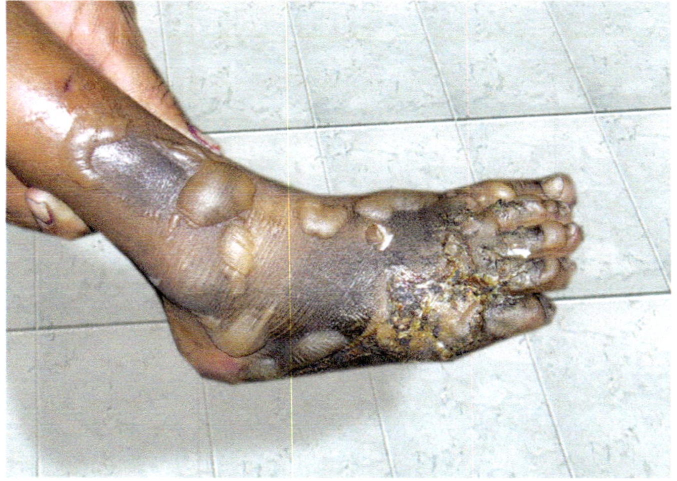

FIG. 25: Burns of foot.

BOX 4 Unique characteristics of burn pain.

- Three major components:
  i. *Background*: At rest in burned areas and at skin graft donor sites
  ii. *Breakthrough*: During simple activities such as changing position, turning in bed, or walking
  iii. *Procedural*: During wound care procedures that must be performed daily or even several times a day; can reach excruciating levels
- Is highly variable among patients and within each individual
- Can last for weeks or months
- Does not decline over time except toward the end of hospitalization

Closed dressing over the partial-thickness burns wounds contributes significantly to pain relief as the exposed nerve endings are protected from external stimuli. In patients with major burns (i.e., with > 25 % TBSA burns), analgesics should be administered by IV route during early management (i.e., 48–72 hours after injury) as absorption by intramuscular route is unpredictable and oral administration may not be possible. For minor burns, the pain medication may be administered by oral route.

The medications and their recommended dosages are as follows:

- *Morphine:* It should be administered only after resuscitation has been initiated and following precautions should be observed:
    - Do not give if patient is asleep. Do not give for sleep; give only for pain.
    - Do not give if patient is in shock or in sepsis.
    - Monitoring of ECG, pulse, respiration, and oxygen saturation is essential.
    - Do not give if respiratory rate is < 20 breaths/minute or oxygen saturation is < 95%.

In adults, patient-controlled analgesia (PCA) probably provides maximum pain relief. Morphine infusion is given intravenously using PCA pump with total dose 15 µg/kg/h as continuous infusion and can be combined with patient administered boluses.

Morphine can be administered 0.03 mg/kg every 4 hours intravenously after stabilizing the patient with resuscitation.

Oral morphine (0.1 mg/kg every 4 hours) can be given after 48–72 hours postburn. This can be used to provide relief from both background as well as procedural pain experienced during bath, dressing, or physiotherapy.

- *Buprenorphine:* An alternative for morphine, buprenorphine should be administered by observing same precautions as morphine. The dose is 300–600 µg slowly intravenously over 10–15 minutes every 6 hours for adults. It is not recommended for children under 6 months of age. For children, the recommended dose is 3–6 µg/kg of bodyweight, 6 hourly.
- *Butorphanol:* 1–4 mg every 3–4 hours, slowly intravenously
- *Pentazocine:* Pentazocine lactate 30 mg intravenously 3–4 hourly is recommended for adults. It is not recommended for children below 1 year of age. Above 1 year of age, the dose recommended is 0.5 mg/kg every 6 hours.

Besides the abovementioned opioids, the following NSAIDs can be used to provide effective pain relief.

- *Diclofenac:* 1 mg/kg intravenously 6 hourly as slow infusion
- *Tramadol:* 50–100 mg intravenously slowly or as infusion every 4–6 hours up to a maximum dose of 600 mg/day.
- *Ibuprofen:* IV ibuprofen is under investigation. The oral preparation can be used in children as well as adults in minor or moderate burns on admission and in major burns after the resuscitation is complete. The recommended dose is 10 mg/kg 4 hourly.
- *Paracetamol:* 15 mg/kg can be used orally for procedural pain relief.

Orally administered acetaminophen (15 mg/kg) and codeine can be combined along with opioids for effective pain relief in major burns.

Agents such as ketamine, propofol, fentanyl, alfentanyl, etc., should be used for controlling procedural pain under supervision of an anesthetist and after complete resuscitation in a patient with major burn.

Anxiolytics such as lorazepam or midazolam may be combined with opioids or NSAIDs especially for relief of procedural pain. The recommended dose is 0.03 mg/kg slow intravenously.

Adequate pain relief is an important but often neglected aspect of early management of burn. If attended to appropriately in the initial period, it contributes significantly to sustained compliance of the patient with various treatment procedures.

EARLY REHABILITATIVE CARE

Once the patient's survival has been assured, function and cosmesis become the biggest factors for subsequent quality of life. However, if efforts to achieve these goals are not begun early in the initial management, the ultimate outcome may be less than desirable despite successful resuscitation and burn wound closure. Rehabilitation of the burn patient should begin during the acute resuscitation period and continue until the patient's scars mature and occupation resumes. Rehabilitation plans are carried out principally by the occupational and physical therapists.

There are principles which must be applied soon after burn to ensure the earliest and optimal rehabilitation of the patient. Rehabilitative care should commence on the day of the injury and the goals of burn patients' rehabilitation are:

- To limit or prevent loss of motion.
- To prevent or minimize anatomic deformities.
- To prevent loss of lean muscle mass.
- To ensure return of the patient to work or normal activity as soon and as completely as possible.

Much consideration must be given to a program of rehabilitation for the burn patient and every patient needs an individually tailored plan of care. There are few principles for the rehabilitation of the burn patients:[86]

1. The program should start early, preferably on the day of injury.
2. A program of care should avoid prolonged periods of immobility and any body part that can move freely should be moved frequently.
3. Range-of-motion exercises should be started on the day of injury.
4. There should be a planned program of daily activity and rehabilitative care. The plan should be reviewed daily as rehabilitative needs change.

On admission, plans should consider the prevention of skin and muscle contracture and anatomic deformity. The institution of such plans should be individually tailored. Early standing and ambulation and participation in daily living activities are important and all extremities should be actively moved frequently throughout the day. Proper positioning is essential for the prevention of contractures. It has not been uncommon in the past for burned patients to develop contractures of both burned and nonburned joints. The incidence of contractures in healing patients has been significantly reduced through the use of frequent active or appropriate passive motion exercises and proper positioning. Burned patients and their families should be taught the importance of early active exercise and proper positioning during rest and sleep. Standing and ambulation should be instituted as soon as possible. Such exercise can reduce the loss of muscle mass and help stimulate the appetite. Frequent standing and ambulation also reduce the risks of pressure necrosis. Additionally, requiring the patient to get out of bed and sit in a chair for some part of the day increases respiratory tidal volumes and the patient's sense of normalcy. This provides a great psychological boost to the patient.

MEDICAL RECORDS

Most of the burn patients are medicolegal cases and are to be informed to the law enforcement authorities and meticulous medical records are of significant value in the court of law. Besides the routine record of history and clinical examination, the following information should be sought and entered in the medical records of the patient.

- Record the time of burn, exact incident, and people present at the site.
- Name and relation of person bringing the patient to hospital and providing information.
- Record details of prehospital treatment and comorbid conditions.
- Record the actual incident in notes and not just "scalds with hot tea" or "flame burns with kerosene".
- If the patient wishes to change the statement, record the new statement and place signature with name, date, and time. Inform the police constable on duty about the patient's wish to change statement.
- Inform the expected prognosis and patient's condition to the close relatives and record it on the case paper with the signature of the relative and name with date and time.
- The consultant should enter his/her observations and treatment decisions in the record in his/her own writing with signature, date, and time.
- Detailed orders including special instructions, wound management plan, and monitoring instructions should be recorded. Details of procedures performed during resuscitation and reports of investigations should be recorded

SUMMARY

- The early management of seriously burnt patients is similar to the management of other trauma victims. Life-threatening injuries must be treated first, followed by secondary survey. Airway, breathing, and circulation should be attended to on priority. High index of suspicion is required for inhalation injuries. Hypothermia should be avoided. If the burn surface area is greater than 15% in an adult and greater than 10% in a child, IV fluids should be administered to restore the circulating blood volume in order to maintain tissue perfusion and oxygenation.
- Sodium containing crystalloid is the fluid of choice and the most useful indicator of fluid resuscitation is hourly monitoring of urine output.
- Meticulous estimation of the extent and depth of burn is necessary for planning the wound management. Burns of special areas deserve attention. The rehabilitative measures should be initiated early.
- Completeness of medical records is highly desirable. Systematic initial evaluation, methodical application of basic surgical principles of resuscitation, and vigilant monitoring using simple clinical parameters leads to successful initial management of a burn patient and also lays the foundation for ultimate satisfactory outcome.

REFERENCES

1. Shah NR, Palackic A, Brondeel KC, Walters ET, Wolf SE. The Burn Wound. Surg Clin North Am. 2023;103(3):453-62.
2. Schoenbrunner A, Banda W, Gosman AA. Global burn care: Education and research. Clin Plast Surg. 2017;44(3):485-93.
3. American Burn Association. (2019). National Burn Repository 2019 Update: Report of data from 2009-2018. [online] Available from ameriburn.site-ym.com [Last accessed June, 2024).
4. Schaefer TJ, Nunez Lopez O. Burn resuscitation and management. In: StatPearls [Internet]. Treasure Island (FL): StatPearls Publishing; 2024. Available from: https://www.ncbi.nlm.nih.gov/books/NBK430795/ [Last accessed June, 2024],
5. Jeschke MG, van Baar ME, Choudhry MA, Chung KK, Gibran NS, Logsetty S. Burn injury. Nature Reviews Disease Primers. 2020;6(1):11.
6. Hudspith J, Rayatt S. First aid and treatment of minor burns. BMJ. 2004;328(7454):1487-9.
7. Harish V, Li Zhe, Maitz PKM. First aid is associated with improved outcomes in large body surface area burns. Burns. 2019;45(8).
8. Wood FM, Phillips M, Jovic T, Cassidy JT, Cameron P, Edgar DW; Steering Committee of the Burn Registry of Australia and New Zealand (BRANZ). Water First Aid is Beneficial in Humans Post-Burn: Evidence from a Bi-National Cohort Study. PLoS One. 2016;11(1):e0147259.
9. McLure M, Macneil F, Wood FM, Cuttle L, Eastwood K, Bray J, et al. A Rapid Review of Burns First Aid Guidelines: Is There Consistency Across International Guidelines? Cureus. 2021;13(6):e15779.
10. VanHoy TB, Metheny H, Patel BC. Chemical Burns. In: StatPearls [Internet]. Treasure Island (FL): StatPearls Publishing; 2024. [online] Available from: https://www.ncbi.nlm.nih.gov/books/NBK499888/ [Last accessed June, 2024].
11. Abston S, Blakeney P, Desai M, et al. Chemical burns. Resident Orientation Manual. Texas: Galveston Shriners Burn hospital and The University of Texas Medical Branch Blocker Burn Unit; 2000.
12. Bounds EJ, Khan M, Kok SJ. Electrical Burns. In: StatPearls [Internet]. Treasure Island (FL): StatPearls Publishing; 2024. [online] Available from: https://www.ncbi.nlm.nih.gov/books/NBK519514/[Last accessed June, 2024].
13. Dries DJ. Burn care: Before the burn center. Scand J Trauma Resusc Emerg Med. 2020;28(1):97.
14. Hughes A, Almeland SK, Leclerc T, Ogura T, Hayashi M, Mills JA, et al. Recommendations for burns care in mass casualty incidents: WHO Emergency Medical Teams Technical Working Group on Burns (WHO TWGB) 2017-2020. Burns. 2021;47(2):349-70.
15. Johnson RM, Richard R. Partial-Thickness Burns: Identification and Management. Adv Skin Wound Care. 2003;16(4):178-87.
16. American Burn Association. (2024). Advanced Burn Life Support. [online] Available from https://ameriburn.org/education/advanced-burn-life-support-abls/. [Last accessed June, 2024].
17. Hettiaratchy S, Papini R. Initial management of a major burn: I—overview. BMJ. 2004;328(7455):1555-57.
18. Thussu T, Tiwari VK, Suri JC, Sarabahi S. Inhalation score—A novel technique for assessing severity of inhalational burns in correlation to bronchoscopic findings. Ann Burns Fire Disasters. 2023;36(1):40-8
19. Gupta K, Mehrotra M, Kumar P, Gogia AR, Prasad A, Fisher JA. Smoke inhalation injury: Etiopathogenesis, diagnosis, and management. Indian J Crit Care Med. 2018;22(3):180-8.
20. Lang TC, Zhao R, Kim A, Wijewardena A, Vandervord J, Xue M, et al. A critical update of the assessment and acute management of patients with severe burns. Adv Wound Care (New Rochelle). 2019;8(12):607-33.
21. Zemaitis MR, Planas JH, Waseem M. Trauma Secondary Survey. In: StatPearls [Internet]. Treasure Island (FL): StatPearls Publishing; 2024 [online] Available from: https://www.ncbi.nlm.nih.gov/books/NBK441902/ [Last accessed June, 2024].
22. Giretzlehner M, Dirnberger J, Owen R, Haller HL, Lumenta DB, Kamolz LP. The determination of total burn surface area: How much difference? Burns. 2013;39(6):1107-13.
23. Smith JJ, Malyon AD, Scerri GV, Burge TS. A comparison of serial halving and the rule of nines as a pre-hospital assessment tool in burns. Br J Plast Surg. 2005;58(7):957-67.
24. Livingston EH, Lee S. Percentage of burned body surface area determination in obese and nonobese patients. J Surg Res. 2000;91(2):106-10.
25. Lund CC, Browder NN. The estimate of areas of burns. Surg Gynecol Obs. 1944;79:352-8.
26. Mance M, Prutki M, Dujmovic A, Miloševic M, Vrbanovic-Mijatovic V, Mijatovic D. Changes in total body surface area and the distribution of skin surfaces in relation to body mass index. Burns. 2020;46(4):868-75.
27. Hettiaratchy S, Papini R. Initial management of a major burn: II—assessment and resuscitation. BMJ. 2004;329(7457):101-3.
28. Hospital and prehospital resources for optimal care of patients with burn injury: Guidelines for development and operation of burn centers. American Burn Association. J Burn Care Rehabil. 1990;11:98-104.
29. Brekke RL, Almeland SK, Hufthammer KO, Hansson E. Agreement of clinical assessment of burn size and burn depth between referring hospitals and burn centres: A systematic review. Burns. 2023;49(3):493-515.
30. Freiburg C, Igneri P, Sartorelli K, Rogers F. Effects of differences in percent total body surface area estimation on fluid resuscitation of transferred burn patients. J. Burn Care Res. 2007;28:42-8.
31. American Burn Association. 2024. Guidelines for Burn Patient Referral. [online] Available from https://ameriburn.org/resources/burnreferral/ [Last accessed on June, 2024].
32. Sheridan RL. Burns. Crit Care Med. 2002;30(11 Suppl):S500-14.
33. American Burn Association. Shock and fluid resuscitation. In: Advanced Burn Life Support Course, Provider Manual. Chicago: American Burn Association; 2018. pp. 31-8.
34. Vivó C, Galeiras R, del Caz MDP. Initial evaluation and management of the critical burn patient. Med Intensiva. 2016;40(1):49-59.
35. Guilabert P, Usúa G, Martín N, Abarca L, Barret JP, Colomina MJ. Fluid resuscitation management in patients with burns: Update. Br J Anaesth. 2016;117(3):284-96.
36. Baxter CR, Shires T. Physiological response to crystalloid resuscitation of severe burns. Ann N Y Acad Sci. 1968;150(3):874-94
37. Wolf SE, Herndon DN. Burns and radiation injuries. In: Moore EE, Feliciano DV, Mattox KL (Eds). Trauma, 5th edition. United States: McGraw-Hill, 2004. pp. 201-26.

38. Baxter CR. Fluid volume and electrolyte changes in the early post- burn period. Clin Plast Surg. 1974;1(4):693-703.
39. Zodda D. Calculated decisions: Parkland formula for burns. Pediatr Emerg Med Pract. 2018;15(Suppl 4):1-2.
40. Zodda D. Calculated decisions: Parkland formula for burns. Emerg Med Pract. 2018;20(Suppl 2):S1-2.
41. Bedi MK, Sarabahi S, Agrawal K. New fluid therapy protocol in acute burn from a tertiary burn care centre. Burns. 2019;45(2):335-40.
42. Greenhalgh DG, Cartotto R, Taylor SL, Fine JR, Lewis GM, Smith DJ Jr. Burn Resuscitation Practices in North America: Results of the Acute Burn Resuscitation Multicenter Prospective Trial (ABRUPT). Ann Surg. 2023;277(3):512-9.
43. Tricklebank S. Modern trends in fluid therapy for burns. Burns. 2009;35(6):757-67.
44. Milner SM, Hodgetts TJ, Rylah LT. The Burns Calculator: A simple proposed guide for fluid resuscitation. Lancet. 1993;342: 1089-91.
45. Milner SM, Christophers SM. Palm-top computer application for fluid resuscitation in Burns. Plast Reconstructive Surgery. 2001;108(6):1838-9.
46. Malic CC, Karoo ROS, Austin O, Phipps A. Resusitation Burn Card-A useful tool for burn injury assessment. Burns. 2007;33(2):195-9.
47. Hemington-Gorse SJ. Colloid or crystalloid for resuscitation of major burns. J Wound Care. 2005;14(6):256-8.
48. Demling RH, Gunther RA, Haines B, Kramer G. Burn edema. Part 2: Complications, prevention and treatment. J Burn Care Rehab. 1982;3:199-206.
49. Monafo WW. The treatment of burn shock by the intravenous and oral administration hypertonic lactated saline solution. J Trauma. 1970;10(7):575-86.
50. Gunn ML, Hansbrough JF, Davis JW, Frust SR, Field TO. Prospective randomized trial of hypertonic sodium lactate versus lactated Ringer's solution for burn shock resuscitation. J Trauma. 1989;29:1261-7.
51. Huang PP, Stucky FS, Dimick AR, Treat RC, Bessey PQ, Rue LW. Hypertonic sodium resuscitation is associated with renal failure and death. Ann Surg. 1995;221(5):543-54.
52. Berger MM, Bernath MA, Chioléro RL. Resuscitation, anaesthesia, and analgesia of the burned patient. Curr opin Anaesthesiol. 2001;14(4):431-5.
53. Warden GD. Fluid resuscitation and early management. In: Herndon DN (Ed). Total Burn Care. Philadelphia: Saunders; 2007. pp. 53-60.
54. Du GB, Slater H, Goldfarb IW. Influence of different resuscitation regimens on acute weight gain in extensively burned patients. Burns. 1991;17(2):147-50.
55. Fodor L, Fodor A, Ramon Y, Shoshani O, Rissin Y, Ullmann Y. Controversies in fluid resuscitation for burn management: Literature review and our experience. Injury. 2006;37(5):374-9.
56. Alderson P, Bunn F, Lefebure C, Li WP, Li L, Roberts I, et al. Human albumin solution for resuscitation and volume expansion in critically ill patients. Cochrane Database Syst Rev. 2004;18(4):CD001208.
57. Liberati A, Moja L, Moschetti I, Gensini GF, Gusinu R. Human albumin solution for resuscitation and volume expansion in critically ill patients. Intern Emerg Med. 2006;1(3):243-5.
58. Cochran A, Morris SE, Edelman LS, Saffle JR. Burn patient characteristics and outcomes following resuscitation with albumin. Burns. 2007;33(1):25-30.
59. Cooper AB, Cohn SM, Zhang HS, Hanna K, Stewart TE, Slutsky AS; ALBUR Investigators. Five percent albumin for adult burn shock resuscitation: Lack of effect on daily multiple organ dysfunction score. Transfusion. 2006;46(1):80-9.
60. Chen J, Han CM, Xia SC, Tang ZJ, Su SJ. Evaluation of effectiveness and safety of a new hydroxyethyl starch used in resuscitation of burn shock. Zhonghua Shao Shang Za Zhi. 2006;22(5):333-6.
61. Zeng JZ, Huang XY, Yang XH, Lei SR, Xiao MZ, Xie TH, et al. The use of composite sodium lactate and sorbitol composition in fluid resuscitation for Shock in patients with major burn. Zhonghua Shao Shang Za Zhi. 2005;21(5):336-8.
62. Sakurai M, Tanaka H, Mastuda T, Goya T, Shimazaki S, Matsuda H. Reduced resuscitation fluid volume for second degree experimental burns with delayed initiation of vitamin C therapy (beginning 6 hours after injury). J Surg Res. 1997;73(1):24-7.
63. Tanaka H, Mastuda T, Miyangatani Y, Yukioka T, Matsuda H, Shimazaki S. Reduction of resuscitation fluid volumes in severely burned patients using ascorbic acid administration: A randomized prospective study. Arch Surg. 2000;135(3):326-31.
64. Yowler CJ, Fratianne RB. Current status of burn resuscitation. Clin Plast Surg. 2000;27(1):1-10.
65. Cancio LC, Kramer GC, Hoskins SL. Gastrointestinal fluid resuscitation of thermally injured patients. J Burn Care Res. 2006;27(5):561-9.
66. Pruitt BA Jr. Protection from excessive resuscitation: "Pushing the pendulum back". J Trauma. 2000;49(3):567-8.
67. Saffle JIL. The phenomenon of "fluid creep" in acute burn resuscitation. J Burn Care Res. 2007;28(3):382-95.
68. Baxter CR. Problems and complications of burn shock resuscitation. Surg Clin North Am. 1978;58(6):1313-22.
69. Saffle JR. Fluid creep and over-resuscitation. Crit Care Clin. 2016;32(4):587-98.
70. Comish P, Walsh M, Castillo-Angeles M, Kuhlenschmidt K, Carlson D, Arnoldo B, et al. Adoption of rescue colloid during burn resuscitation decreases fluid administered and restores end-organ perfusion. Burns. 2021;47(8):1844-50.
71. Lawrence A, Faraklas I, Watkins H, Allen A, Cochran A, Morris S. et al. Colloid administration normalizes resuscitation ratio and ameliorates fluid creep. J Burn Care Res. 2010;31(1):40-7.
72. Lichtenstein DA, Mezière GA. Relevance of lung ultrasound in the diagnosis of acute respiratory failure: The BLUE protocol. Chest. 2008;134(1):117-25.
73. Lichtenstein DA, Mezière GA, Lagoueyte JF, Biderman P, Goldstein I, Gepner A. A-lines and B-lines: Lung ultrasound as a bedside tool for predicting pulmonary artery occlusion pressure in the critically ill. Chest. 2009;136(4):1014-20.
74. Tsunoi Y, Sato N, Nishidate I, Ichihashi F, Saitoh D, Sato S. Burn depth assessment by dual-wavelength light emitting diodes-excited photoacoustic imaging in rats. Wound Repair Regen. 2023;31(1):69-76.
75. Promny D, Billner M, Reichert B. [Objective burn depth assessment of hand burns]. Handchir Mikrochir Plast Chir. 2019;51(5):362-6.
76. Claes KEY, Hoeksema H, Vyncke T, Verbelen J, De Coninck P, De Decker I, et al. Evidence based burn depth assessment using laser-based technologies: Where do we stand? J Burn Care Res. 2021;42(3):513-25.
77. Shin JY, Yi HS. Diagnostic accuracy of laser Doppler imaging in burn depth assessment: Systematic review and meta-analysis. Burns. 2016;42(7):1369-76.

78. Heimbach D, Engrav L, Grube B, Marvin J. Burn depth: A review. World J Surg. 1992;16(1):10-5.
79. McUmber H, Dabek RJ, Bojovic B, Driscoll DN. Burn depth analysis using indocyanine green fluorescence: A review. J Burn Care Res. 2019;40(4):513-6.
80. Simmons JD, Kahn SA, Vickers AL, Crockett ES, Whitehead JD, Krecker AK, et al. Early assessment of burn depth with far infrared time-lapse thermography. J Am Coll Surg. 2018;226(4): 687-93.
81. Gore MA, Akolekar D. Evaluation of banana leaf dressing for partial thickness burn wounds. Burns. 2003;29(5):487-92.
82. Norman G, Christie J, Liu Z, Westby MJ, Jefferies JM, Hudson T, et al. Antiseptics for burns. Cochrane Database Syst Rev. 2017;7(7):CD011821.
83. Wasiak J, Cleland H, Campbell F, Spinks A. Dressings for superficial and partial thickness burns. Cochrane Database Syst Rev. 2013;2013(3):CD002106.
84. Abston S, Blakeney P, Desai M, Edgar P, Heggers J, Herndon D, et al. Electrical injuries. Resident Orientation Manual. Texas: Galveston Shriners Burn hospital and The University of Texas Medical Branch Blocker Burn Unit; 2000.
85. Sarabahi S. Management of ear burns. Indian Journal of Burns. 2012;20(1):11-7.
86. Young AW, Dewey WS, King BT. Rehabilitation of burn injuries: an update. Physical Medicine and Rehabilitation Clinics. 2019;30(1):111-32.
87. Richardson P, Mustard L. The management of pain in the burns unit. Burns. 2009;35(7):921-36.

CHAPTER

11

Respiratory Tract Injury in Burns

JC Suri, MK Sen, Thakur Thussu

INTRODUCTION

Injury to respiratory tract due to burns was little appreciated prior to 1940s. A pivotal point in the understanding of pulmonary injury in burn patients happened to be the famous "Boston night-club fire" in 1942. Between 1945 and 1975, several innovations took place, which went a long way to recognize the respiratory injuries and treat these patients in a better and scientific way. Management has changed over the ensuing decades greatly and survival has become more likely.[1]

Injury to the respiratory tract in a patient with burns can occur in several ways. Firstly, there may be respiratory tract involvement in pure thermal injuries. Second, there can be nonthermal involvement of the respiratory tract due to inhalation of either asphyxiant gases [such as carbon monoxide (CO) and cyanide] or irritant gases (such as chlorine, ammonia, and oxides of sulfur and nitrogen).[2] Anoxia is a very important mode of injury in respiratory tract involvement due to inhalation. Inhalation injuries are reported in 19–28% of all burn patients. On the other hand, the incidence may rise to very high in victims who die.[3-5]

PATHOGENESIS

The principal effects of inhalation injury include asphyxia and direct respiratory tract injury. Asphyxia can result from hypoxia or intoxication by CO or cyanide. These factors can affect the patient either alone or in combination. Direct injury to the respiratory tract can involve the airway or the alveolar-capillary membrane. Involvement of the airway results in upper airway obstruction, tracheobronchitis, bronchiolitis, or atelectasis. The larynx is exposed to the most intense thermal damage, and also to maximal concentration of chemical in inhalational injury.[2,3] On the other hand, alveolar-capillary membrane injury can result in pulmonary edema due to high permeability of the membrane. Inhalation injury has now become one of the most important causes of death in burn patients. The mortality from smoke inhalation alone is low (0–11%). However, in combination with cutaneous burns, it may be fatal in 30–90% of patients. It has been recently reported that the presence of inhalation injury increases burn mortality by 20% and that inhalation injury predisposes to pneumonia. Pneumonia has been shown to independently increase burn mortality by 40% and the combination of inhalation injury and pneumonia leads to a 60% increase in deaths.[2,6]

Cutaneous burns can result in pulmonary dysfunction, chest wall restriction (e.g., circumferential neck and chest burns) or upper airway compression. Quite often, a combination of smoke inhalation injury and cutaneous burns coexist in the same patient. When considered together with total body surface area (TBSA) burned, the respiratory sequential organ failure assessment (SOFA) scores can dynamically assess the severity of the patient's lung injury status.[3,4]

Other comorbid respiratory complications in a patient with burns include concomitant chest trauma and exacerbations in a preexisting cardiopulmonary disease such as cardiogenic pulmonary edema or chronic obstructive pulmonary disease (COPD). There may be a variety of nosocomial/iatrogenic problems in such patients. They include hydrostatic pulmonary edema (due to overenthusiastic fluid resuscitation), pneumonia (aerogenous or hematogenous), sepsis-related permeability edema [acute respiratory distress syndrome (ARDS)], drug-induced conditions (hypoventilation due to morphine or hyperventilation due to mafenide), pulmonary embolism and complications due to artificial airways and aspiration. Hyperglycemia in burn patients can lead to increased incidence of infections, including pneumonia.[4,6]

Direct injury to respiratory epithelium and alveolar macrophages by chemicals like aldehyde that are present in smoke can trigger inflammation. This occurs due to release of chemotactic factors as well as activation of phospholipase. The various chemotactic factors lead to priming of neutrophils; entrapment of these primed neutrophils in the pulmonary vasculature, in turn, leads to their activation and degranulation, resulting in release of proteolytic enzymes and oxygen radicals which cause lung edema.[7] Activation of phospholipase, on the other hand, results in formation of prostaglandins (thromboxane A_2) leading to bronchoconstriction, hypoxic pulmonary vasoconstriction, and lung damage. Airway obstruction and ventilation-perfusion mismatch also occur.[8]

The pathological alterations induced by inhalation injury on lung host defenses include mucosal burns, laryngeal obstruction, tracheobronchitis, paralysis of mucociliary apparatus, bronchorrhea, mucosal sloughing, bronchospasm, airway edema, atelectasis, phagocyte dysfunction, alveolitis, and a decrease in pulmonary surfactant levels. The potential immunosuppressive mediators following thermal burns usually include bacterial endotoxin, prostaglandin (PGE2), endogenous glucocorticoids, cytokines [tumor necrosis factor alpha (TNF-α)], interleukins, and interferon, histamine, immune complexes, neuropeptides, autoantibodies, and suppressor peptides. After burn and inhalation injury, the microbiota in the airway is altered in patients with a partial pressure of oxygen in arterial blood/fraction of inspiratory oxygen (PaO_2/FiO_2) ratio < 300 very early.[7,8]

Thus, a plethora of pathological effects of burn injury occurs on the host defenses. They can result from depression in cell-mediated immunity, activation (and subsequent depletion) of the complement system, suppression of phagocyte functions (macrophage and neutrophil), release of immunosuppressive mediators, increased consumption of immunoglobulins, depletion of fibronectin and serum opsonic activity, and an increase in T-suppressor cell activity.[8]

Pathophysiology of Lung Parenchymal Damage by Smoke Inhalation

Incomplete products of combustion present, for instance, in burning cotton, aldehydes and oxides of sulfur and nitrogen, hydrochloric acid and CO, etc., are all responsible for damage to lung parenchyma.[9,10] Upper airway damage, on the other hand, is mainly due to direct thermal injury and chemical irritation.

A gradually progressive edema of the tracheobronchial mucosa takes place over the initial 24 hours. In the tracheobronchial mucosa, areas of de-epithelialization are demonstrable; in the lower respiratory tract focal areas of congestion and edema alternating with areas of collapse and pneumonia are seen. Lesions in the airway range from superficial desquamation of epithelium to focal necrosis and formation of pseudomembranes comprising mucus, cellular debris, fibrinous exudates, polymorphonuclear leukocytes and clumps of bacteria. Tracheobronchial casts can ultimately lead to respiratory obstruction. A significant decrease in pulmonary compliance takes place due to increase in extravascular lung water and pulmonary lymph flow.[8,9]

Inactivation of surfactant results from inhalation injury, leading to extensive microatelectasis. Microvascular injury with increased fluid flux into interstitium and alveolar space, resulting in profound hypoxemia and ARDS can also ensue.

CLINICAL FEATURES AND DIAGNOSIS

The general impact of respiratory complications of smoke inhalation (airway injury, parenchymal injury, and late-onset problems) is significantly higher in cases who have concomitant cutaneous burns (**Table 1**).

Fiberoptic bronchoscopy (FOB) helps to confirm the diagnosis of inhalational injury and contributes to the precise assessment of severity of injury and its categorization. Critical upper airway obstruction due to direct thermal injury, diffuse capillary leak, increased

TABLE 1: Presenting symptoms and signs of inhalation injury

	Relative frequency (%)
Dyspnea	3–17
Hoarseness	13–61
Throat pain	10–13
Chest pain	32–41
Cough	9–76
Hemoptysis	6–18
Carbonaceous sputum	9–80
Cyanosis	6–15
Tachypnea	25–80
Stridor	5–33
Wheezing	13–47
Rhonchi	23–52
Crackles	23–35

resuscitation fluids used in these patients, and hot fluid aspiration is a catastrophic event that can be averted if timely bronchoscopic grading and assisted intubation is performed.[11] Secondly, if airway burns are suspected and objectively diagnosed early, volume of resuscitation fluids can be adjusted. Patients with airway burns have 40–50% excess demand of fluids for resuscitation. Prognostically also significant correlation exists between inhalation injury and mortality.[12] FOB is considered the gold standard for diagnosis of airway injury.[13] Its advantages include ease of doing and learning, objective assessment of airway injury, therapeutic interventions such as FOB-assisted intubation, bronchoalveolar lavage (BAL) and removal of debris, and mucous plugs from the airways. BAL fluid can be assessed for leukocyte differentiation, cell morphology, and culture sensitivity **(Figs. 1 and 2)**. Neutrophilia in BAL fluid is associated with longer hospital stay and need for ventilation.[14] Other features on BAL fluid analysis indicating worse prognosis are increased number of bronchial epithelial cells[15] and elevated IL-10 levels. **Box 1** explains the Abbreviated Injury Score (AIS) which is widely used to grade airway burns **(Figs. 3 to 6)** and **Box 2** describes the procedure. FOB should be an integral part of all burn centers as far as possible. Limitations of FOB includes its inability to assess distal airways and lack of availability of FOB at most of the places especially in burn centers of developing countries is another problem. Differences in individual host responses to inflammatory process and characteristics of inhaled gases also cause discordance between bronchoscopic appearance and actual severity of injury. Therefore, it is pertinent to continuously assess clinically and correlate it with bronchoscopic findings.[13]

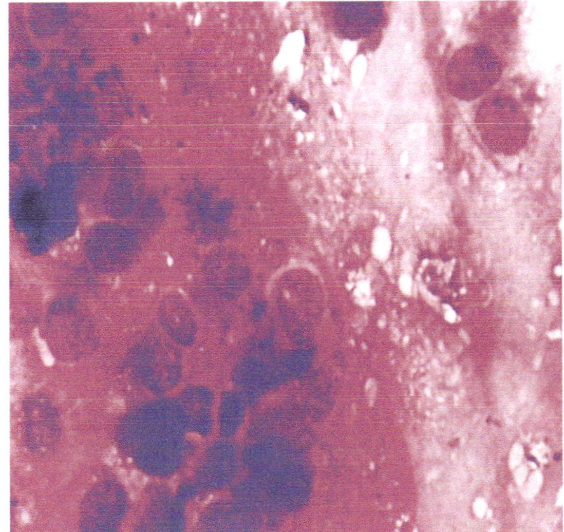

FIG. 2: Giemsa stained bronchoalveolar lavage (BAL) fluid smear showing mucin and epithelial cells (400 ×).

BOX 1 Abbreviated injury score for grading of inhalation burns.

- *G0*: No injury
- *G1*: Mild injury, patchy areas of erythema only
- *G2*: Moderate injury, moderate edema and erythema, carbonaceous deposits
- *G3*: Severe injury, severe inflammation with friability, copious soot particles with ulceration, bronchorrhea, and bronchial obstruction
- *G4*: Massive injury, mucosal sloughing, ulceration, and endoluminal obstruction

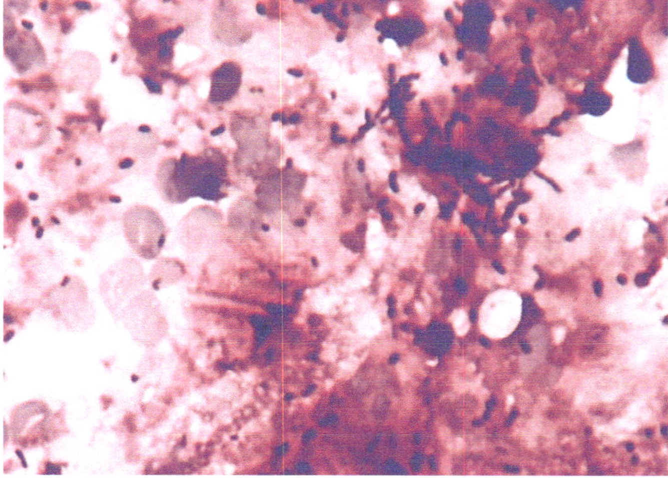

FIG. 1: Infected bronchoalveolar lavage fluid showing bacilli.

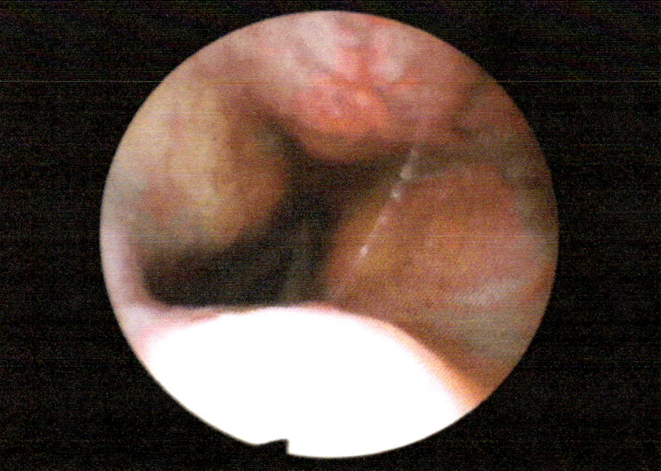

FIG. 3: Vocal cord edema on fiberoptic bronchoscopy (FOB).

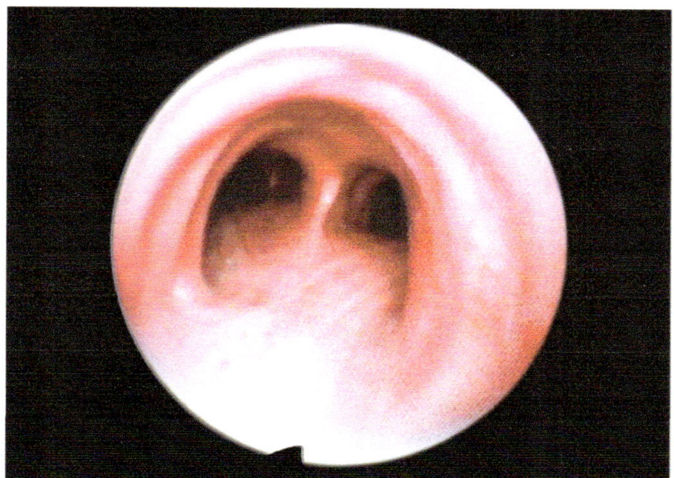

FIG. 4: Mild mucosal hyperemia and edema on bronchoscopy. Indistinct tracheal rings and blunting of carina can be seen. Grade 1 [abbreviated injury score (AIS)].

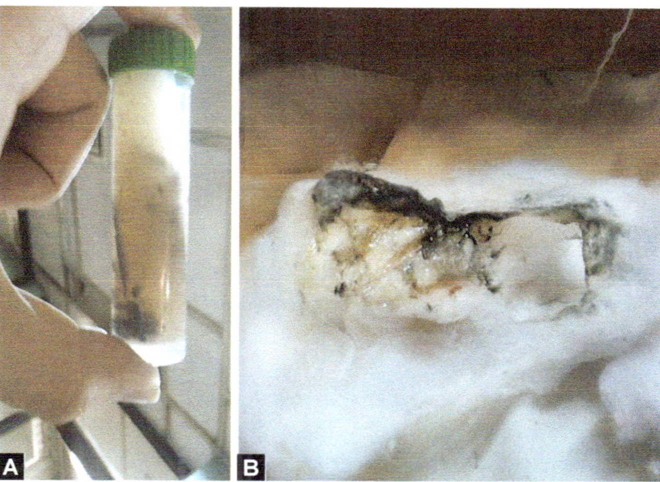

FIGS. 6A AND B: Bronchoalveolar lavage (BAL) fluid from a patient with inhalation injury containing carbonaceous material.

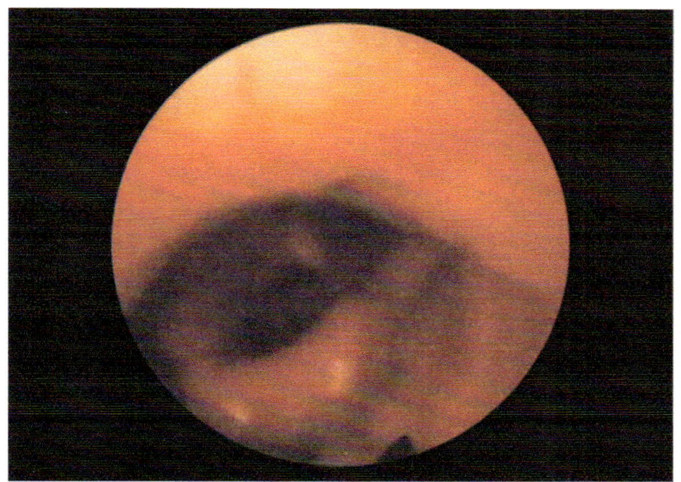

FIG. 5: Moderate injury, moderate edema, and erythema with carbonaceous deposits as seen on FOB—Grade 2 [abbreviated injury score (AIS)].

BOX 2 Conduct of fiberoptic bronchoscopy (FOB).

- Initial assessment to be performed within 72 hours of burns
- Detailed informed consent including possibility of intubation:
  - NPO for 2 hours
  - Nostrils packed with 4% lidocaine for 10 minutes prior to the procedure
  - 10% lidocaine to be sprayed on the posterior pharyngeal wall 2–3 minutes before introducing the scope
  - Endotracheal tube to be mounted on the scope in case immediate intubation is needed
  - Assessment done till both principal bronchi and scoring is recorded
  - Therapeutic maneuvers like removal of mucous plugs, lavage, biopsy, or endotracheal intubation performed as per requirement

Rigid laryngoscopy and flexible nasopharyngoscopy are also helpful. In addition, repeated bronchoscopies with lavage can also be done to help in cleaning mucosal plugs. Chest skiagrams are of minimal help in the initial period.[16,17]

Xenon lung scans can evaluate alveolar air trapping. Simultaneous thermal and dye dilution methods can be used to assess extravascular lung water and determine parenchymal fluid levels. Measurements of serum carboxyhemoglobin (COHb) levels are of immense importance.[16,17]

A battery of diagnostic tests is therefore judiciously utilized in the management of patients with involvement of respiratory system. They include objective measurement of asphyxiants in the blood (COHb and cyanide), arterial blood gases (ABGs), chest roentgenogram, endoscopic examination (laryngoscopy, nasopharyngoscopy, and bronchoscopy), radionuclide scanning, and pulmonary function tests (spirometry).[18]

Respiratory Complications of Smoke Inhalations

Common clinical presentations vary from patient to patient and depend to a large extent on the degree of burns. At one end of the spectrum are patients with smoke exposure without overt respiratory dysfunction and no respiratory injury with normal objective tests. There may be subclinical injury with normal/abnormal objective tests. Various grades of clinically overt respiratory dysfunction can be present. At the other end, there may be cardiopulmonary arrest or asphyxiant death at the scene of exposure. The various symptoms and signs include dyspnea, hoarseness, throat pain, chest pain, cough, hemoptysis, production of carbonaceous sputum, cyanosis, tachypnea, stridor, wheezing, rhonchi, and crackles.[17]

In less severe cases, there is an evidence of airway obstruction and decreased pulmonary compliance on pulmonary function testing. After several days of injury, endobronchial debris can lead to small airway obstruction and atelectasis.

Pulmonary edema is a sinister end result that can result from multiple causes. ARDS is a common case scenario in a large majority of burn-patients undergoing treatment in tertiary care hospitals **(Table 2)**. Common risk factors associated with the occurrence of ARDS include sepsis syndrome with or without shock, severe trauma (thoracic or extrathoracic), pneumonia (bacterial and viral), aspiration of gastric contents, disseminated intravascular coagulation (DIC), and near drowning. Occasionally, it may be associated with fluid overload, smoke or toxic gas inhalation, extensive surface burns, fat embolization, anaphylactic reaction to drugs and blood, neurogenic injury, toxic drugs, and poisons. It is characterized by tachypnea, refractory hypoxemia, diffuse pulmonary infiltrates, and reduced lung compliance. Over the last decade, several studies have suggested that survival rates for patients with varying severity of ARDS may have improved. The diagnosis of ARDS becomes highly probable in the presence of the following features—tachypnea, $PaO_2/FiO_2 < 300$, $SpO_2/FiO_2 < 315$, presence of known common risk factors, diffuse pulmonary infiltrates on chest X-ray and reduced lung compliance. Hematological disturbances (such as coagulopathy, DIC, and thrombocytopenia), multiorgan failure, ratio of BAL fluid protein to serum protein being >0.8 and a characteristic pathology are also typical of ARDS.[18,19]

TABLE 2: Diagnosis of ARDS.

High probability	Moderate probability
Tachypnea	Tachypnea
• $PaO_2/FiO_2 < 300$ • $SpO_2/FiO_2 < 315$	PaO_2/FiO_2 300–350
Known common risk factors	Uncommon risk factors
Diffuse pulmonary infiltrates	Bilateral lung parenchymal opacities confirmed by chest radiograph, thoracic CT, or thoracic ultrasound with a well-trained operator
Reduced compliance	Near—normal compliance
Pulmonary hypertension	Normal pulmonary resistance
Coagulopathy (thrombocytopenia and DIC)	Normal coagulation or only thrombocytopenia
Multiorgan failure	Only pulmonary involvement
High bronchoalveolar lavage (BAL)/serum total protein ratios > 0.8	BAL/serum total protein < 0.6
Large protein molecules found in BAL > 70A	BAL molecular protein radii < 70A
Characteristic pathology	No pathology specimen available

(ARDS: acute respiratory distress syndrome; DIC: disseminated intravascular coagulation; FiO_2: fraction of inspired oxygen; PaO_2: partial pressure of oxygen; SpO_2: peripheral oxygen saturation)

Smoke inhalation injury has been clinically graded on the basis of bronchoscopic criteria as follows.[19,20]

Grade Features

0: No signs or symptoms referable to the respiratory tract. Absence of carbonaceous deposits, erythema, bronchorrhea, or obstruction (no injury)

1: Signs and symptoms limited to the upper respiratory passages, including mild laryngitis. Minor or patchy areas of erythema, carbonaceous deposits in peripheral or distal bronchi (mild injury)

2: Evidence of involvement of the trachea and bronchi or abnormal signs in the lungs other than those of frank consolidation. Moderate degree of carbonaceous deposits, erythema, bronchorrhea, with or without compromise of bronchi (moderate injury)

3: Dyspnea, cyanosis, wheezing, or transient stridor or frank signs of consolidation. Severe inflammation with friability, copious carbonaceous deposits, bronchorrhea, and bronchial obstruction (severe injury)

4: Evidence of extensive pulmonary involvement or of obstruction to the airways necessitating tracheostomy or resulting in severe asphyxia. Evidence of mucosal sloughing, necrosis, and endoluminal obstruction (massive injury)

Major risk factors include house fires, explosions, and other disasters. Direct thermal damage due to flame, liquid, or steam inhalation is rare. Thus, the spectrum and time course of respiratory problems require special attention in all patients. Classical clinical predictors should be watchfully monitored and they include exposure characteristics (like closed-space setting, entrapment, unconsciousness, and known inhaled toxin), respiratory signs and symptoms, presence of facial and cervical burns, and production of carbonaceous sputum **(Figs. 7 and 8)**.

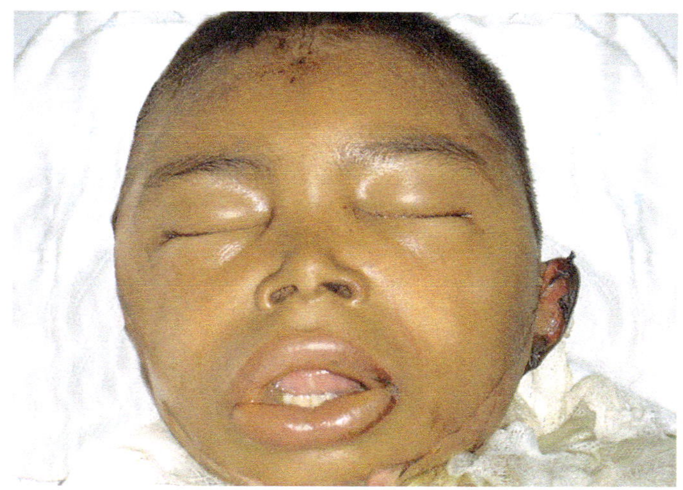

FIG. 7: Case with minimal burns of face but with signs of inhalation injury.

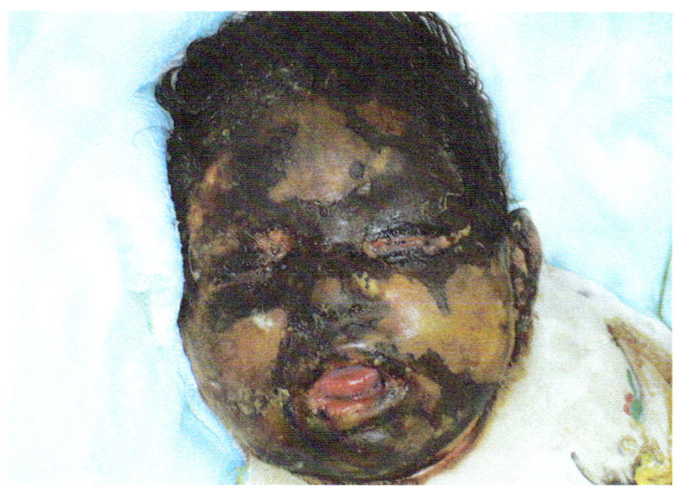

FIG. 8: A 3-year-old child with deep burns of entire face with evidence of inhalational injury.

Asphyxia manifests as altered sensorium, coma, nausea, and vomiting; upper airway obstruction as stridor, hoarseness, dyspnea, sore throat, painful swallowing, respiratory area burns, and pharyngeal edema/erythema; lower airway obstruction as dyspnea, tachypnea, wheezing, carbonaceous sputum, and parenchymal injury as dyspnea, tachypnea, and crackles. Resuscitative measures for cardiopulmonary arrest—successful cardiopulmonary resuscitation (CPR) (grade V); supportive measures for clinically obvious established respiratory dysfunction (grade II to IV) and accurate triage for exposure history [possible delayed-onset dysfunction (grade I)] should be promptly taken.

MANAGEMENT

Management of Inhalation Injury in Patients without Cutaneous Burns

The management of inhalation injury in patients without burns begins with a good history and examination of the accident scene.[21] Circumstances of inhalation should be examined (history of suicidal attempt); closed spaces (e.g., building and automobiles) result in more frequent and severe respiratory abnormalities. The severity of inhalation injury is also directly related to the duration of exposure. The lungs can be an efficient means for the absorption of inhaled toxicants, resulting in airway and pulmonary injury or systemic toxicity. The type of smoke inhaled is also an extremely important factor. Exposure to smoke from polyurethane foam results in severe parenchymal injury. Time elapsed between initial resuscitation and arrival at hospital and presence of comorbid disease(s) [COPD, coronary artery disease (CAD), etc.] are also important determinants of severity of diseases. A history of closed space fire, production of carbonaceous sputum, facial burn, singed nasal hair, perioral burn, hoarseness, and stridor or pharyngeal edema are important pointers to upper airway injury **(Fig. 7)**.[16,17]

Airway maintenance is of prime importance. Early intubation is indicated in case upper airway burn is present. Airway edema increases over 12–18 hours. Nebulization with bronchodilators, heparin (10,000 units in 3 mL N-Saline every 4 hours), and N-acetylcysteine (3–5 mL of 20% solution every 4 hours) is also very useful steps. Indications for endotracheal intubation include inability to protect airway respiratory distress, hoarseness/stridor, dyspnea, third degree facial burns, CO poisoning, and edema of supraglottic structures.[22]

The management of respiratory burns has two primary components, namely, (1) bronchial hygiene therapy and (2) mechanical ventilation.

The thrust areas of bronchial-hygiene therapy are as follows:[23]

- Oxygenation of the patient with humidified oxygen so as to maintain $SpO_2 > 90\%$ **(Fig. 9)**. Recent evidence has also highlighted the role of heated and humidified oxygen therapy with high flow nasal canula (HHHFNC) in hypoxic patents with smoke inhalation injury.
- *Therapeutic coughing*: Either voluntary or induced by placing index and middle fingers over sternal notch.
- Deep breathing exercises every 2 hours
- Therapeutic posturing and chest physiotherapy every 4 hours
- Turning the patient side-to-side every 2 hours

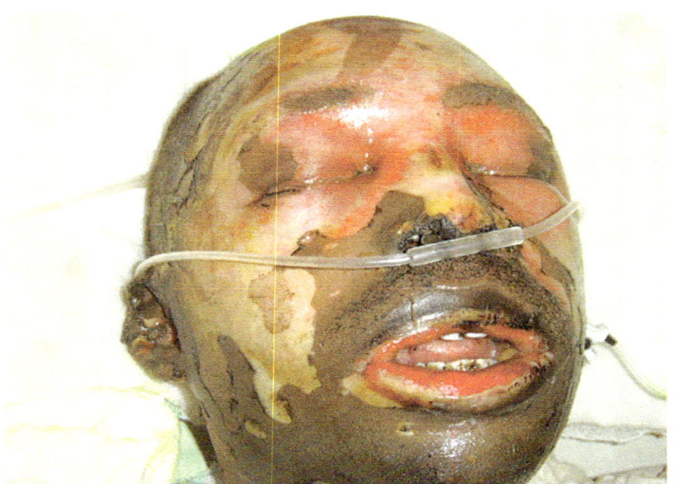

FIG. 9: Patient with facial burns with element of upper airway injury requiring only oxygenation by nasal prongs.

FIG. 10: X-ray chest showing acute respiratory distress syndrome (ARDS).

- Aerosolization of 3 mL of 20% N-acetylcysteine every 4 hours with a bronchodilator
- Aerosolizing 5,000 units of heparin with 3 mL of normal saline every 4 hours
- Nasotracheal suctioning as and when required
- Encouragement of early ambulation by postburn day 5
- Culture of endotracheal secretions thrice a week
- Therapeutic bronchoscopy

Therapeutic Bronchoscopy

Utility of early bronchoscopy in inhalational burns is well established. Serial bronchoscopic examinations offer additional therapeutic options and therefore are increasingly becoming inherent to protocols of burn management. Apart from visualizing the airway as discussed earlier, thick mucus plugs can be removed bronchoscopically. These plugs, which are formed as a result of desquamation of respiratory epithelium, obstruct the airway distal to it leading to atelectasis and pneumonia. Secondly, serial bronchoscopic washings remove slough and pseudomembranes thereby blunting the inflammatory cascade. BAL fluid can be assessed microscopically, biochemically as well as sent for culture and sensitivity as discussed earlier **(Figs. 1, 2, and 6)**.

Mechanical Ventilation[24,25]

Mechanical ventilation is mainly initiated in the scenario of acute refractory hypoxemia as seen in cases of ARDS **(Fig. 10)**. Several modes of ventilation are available to the clinician. The mode used should be the one which is able to support oxygenation and ventilation. Additionally, the clinician should also be experienced in its use.

The ARDS Network study conducted by the National Heart, Lung, and Blood Institute of US (NHLBI) recommends the use of low tidal volumes of 6 mL/kg of predicted bodyweight and a plateau pressure of 30 cmH_2O or less while using the volume-assist mode. If the patient becomes obstructed due to fibrin casts and develops an acute hypercapnia and hypoxia, pulmonary toilet should be done and change over to higher tidal volumes is considered. Initial flow rates of 40–100 L/min, inspiratory/expiratory (I: E) ratio of 1:1–1:3 and FiO_2 of 1.0 may be sufficient. Positive end-expiratory pressure (PEEP) is applied to recruit lung units, elevate mean airway pressure, and improve oxygenation. The level of PEEP varies with the disease process. Pressure-volume curves help in determining the optimal level of PEEP. The optimal level of PEEP is the one that results in the lowering of pulmonary shunt, improvement in arterial oxygenation, only a small change in cardiac output, A-V oxygen content differences, or mixed venous oxygen tension.

The various modes of ventilation available are as follows:

- Control mode, where the ventilator cycles automatically at a rate selected by the operator
- Assist-control mode, where the ventilator only assists every spontaneous breathing effort of the patient; a back-up control rate is set. Also set are tidal volume, inspiratory flow rate, flow waveform, sensitivity, and control rate.
- Synchronized intermittent mandatory ventilation (SIMV), where a preset number of ventilator-delivered mandatory breaths with preset tidal volume are delivered along with the facility of intermittent spontaneous breaths. It is usually a weaning mode.

- Pressure control mode, where a ventilator breath of constant pressure (pressure limited, time-cycled, and pressure triggered) is delivered. The inspiratory time, pressure limit, and back up rate are preset by the operator. Tidal volume is dependent on compliance of chest and airway resistance. This mode can be used in ARDS.
- Pressure support mode, is a pressure targeted, flow-cycled, and patient triggered breath. The patient must have an intact respiratory drive. It is a useful weaning mode.

Newer Modes of Mechanical Ventilation

- *High-frequency percussive ventilation (HFPV)*: It provides ventilation at low mean airway pressure and supports the lung-protective strategy of ventilation to reduce barotraumas. Subtidal volumes are delivered in a progressive stepwise fashion until a preset oscillatory equilibrium is reached and exhalation is passive.[12] A high-frequency time-cycled pressure ventilator [volume diffusive respirator (VDR) ventilator] is used. The pulsatile flow rate is set at 20 cmH_2O peak inspiratory pressure (PIP); the pulse frequency (high rate) set at 500–600. The low respiratory rate is set at 15–20 and demand PEEP on 3 cmH_2O. The I:E ratio (inspiration to expiration ratio) is set at 2:1. Settings of the ventilator can be adjusted later, based on clinical and ABG parameters.
- *Inverse ratio ventilation*: It involves the setting up of I:E ratio > 1:1. It maintains a high mean airway pressure and high peak alveolar pressure; it prolongs inspiratory time to allow for recruitment of lung units in dependent areas of chest. Time-constant sedation and paralysis are always required for this mode.
- *Airway pressure release ventilation (APRV)*: It is a pressure-regulated mode of ventilatory support which allows for time-cycled decreases in pressure to facilitate elimination of CO_2.

Alveolar dead space, that can be easily assessed by $PaCO_2$ and end-tidal CO_2, may be useful in assessment of inhalational injury, its prognosis, and response to treatment.

Weaning and Discontinuation of Mechanical Ventilation

Attempts should be made to remove the patient from mechanical ventilation as early as possible. The criteria that should be followed before any such attempt is made are as follows:

- Reversal of underlying cause of respiratory failure, namely improvement in respiratory burn/sepsis.
- Adequate oxygenation as evidenced by PaO_2/FiO_2 > 200–250, PEEP requirement ≤ 5–8 cmH_2O, $FiO_2 \leq 0.4$–0.5 and pH > 7.25.
- Hemodynamic stability or low-dose vasopressor requirement
- Presence of spontaneous inspiratory effort

A spontaneous breathing trial with T-tube breathing for 30 minutes or pressure-support/continuous positive airway pressure (CPAP) of 1 hour should be administered. Respiratory mechanics should be assessed.

- Respiratory rate < 24 in adults
- Spontaneous tidal volume > 4 mL/kg
- Expired minute volume < 15 L/min
- Negative inspiratory force > 30 cmH_2O
- Audible leak around endotracheal balloon cuff

Racemic epinephrine aerosolization can help in alleviating any inspiratory stridor that may be present following extubation (due to mucosal edema).

Late Complications of Inhalational Injury

- Tracheal stenosis due to tracheitis, tracheal ulceration, and tracheal granuloma formation. It occurs in the region of the endotracheal cuff (subglottic region). It is best prevented by paying attention to tracheal tube-cuff pressure, particularly in the background of hypotension.
- Obstructive/restrictive lung disease is occasionally observed following inhalation injury.

Spirometry, cardiopulmonary exercise testing, and rehabilitation are important aspects in the after-care of these patients.

Carbon Monoxide Poisoning

Carbon monoxide is the most common gas liberated during fires. It is colorless, tasteless, and has an affinity for hemoglobin that is 200 times that of oxygen. It causes reversible displacement of oxygen on the hemoglobin molecule. It interacts with the myoglobin of cardiac muscle and with mitochondrial cytochrome 3 oxidase complex leading to additional effects on cellular oxygen metabolism and organ function. When combined with hemoglobin (COHb), it results in impaired oxygen delivery to the tissues and a decrease in mixed venous oxygen content. Clinical features may result from mild headache and confusion in lower degrees of exposure to coma, seizures, and death in severe cases **(Table 3)**. In a case of blood COHb level of 5–10%, the symptoms include mild headache and confusion. Throbbing headache, blurred vision, and flushing of the skin occur when it rises to 11–20% while at a level of 21–30%, the clinical manifestations include disorientation, nausea,

TABLE 3: Signs and symptoms of carbon monoxide (CO) intoxication.

Carboxyhemoglobin level (in %)	Clinical manifestations
5–10	Mild headache, confusion
11–20	Throbbing headache, blurred vision, and flushing of the skin
21–30	Disorientation, nausea, and impaired manual dexterity
31–40	Irritability, dizziness, vomiting, and syncope
41–50	Tachypnea and tachycardia
50 and above	Coma, seizures, respiratory failure, and death

and impaired manual dexterity. Irritability, dizziness, vomiting, and syncope occur when the levels rise to 31–40%. In case the levels go to beyond 50%, coma, seizures, respiratory failure, and death may ensue.[26,27]

The elimination of CO is dependent on the level of oxygen in blood (FiO_2) and the law of mass action. It occurs in two phases—(1) a rapid distribution to other tissues and (2) a slower excretion phase. The elimination half-life of CO while breathing room air is 250 minutes; at 100% oxygen, it is 40 minutes while at 2 atmospheres hyperbaric oxygen (HBO), it is 30 minutes. At 2.5 atmospheres HBO, the dissolved oxygen content of plasma alone (> 5 mL/100 mL) is sufficient to meet the basal body oxygen requirements. The various neuropsychiatric sequelae of CO poisoning include Parkinsonism, cortical blindness, temporospatial disorientation, deafness, memory changes, mental retardation and frank psychosis.

Patients with mild-to-moderate exposure (COHb < 30%, no coma, and no neurologic findings) are probably treated adequately with 100% oxygen. A patient who is comatose on admission, has a COHb level of > 30% or has an existing neurologic deficit, and is at risk for permanent damage and a HBO chamber, if readily available, may benefit from a dive. The patient with associated problems [burns > 40% of body surface area (BSA), other injuries, or airway compromise] should be considered for hyperbaric treatment only if there is no risk to life endangered by the delay in treatment of the other problems. HBO therapy can, at times, be associated with several complications. They include barotrauma to ears, aspiration, seizure, hypocalcemia, oliguria, metabolic acidosis, respiratory acidosis, dysrhythmias, and rarely cardiac arrest. Indications for HBO include altered mental status, loss of consciousness/cardiac arrest at scene, focal neurological deficits, seizures, syncope, ischemic chest pain, ECG changes, new dysrhythmias, COHb > 25%, COHb > 15% with cardiovascular/cerebrovascular disease, pregnancy with COHb > 10% or with signs of fetal distress.

Cyanide Poisoning

Cyanide (CN) poisoning is usually seen with burning of polyurethane in the construction and furniture industries. It acts by inhibiting the final step of oxidative phosphorylation by binding the cytochrome AA3 complex resulting in lactic acidosis and cellular asphyxia. Exposure to cyanide results in altered level of consciousness, dizziness, headache, tachycardia, and tachypnea. Blood levels of CN should be measured and lethal levels range between 1.0–3.0 mg/L. Any patient with positive clinical criteria or blood CN levels > 0.20 mg/L should be treated. Cyanide is normally detoxified primarily by hepatic rhodanese and requires sulfate as a substrate. Treatment includes the following measures (3-step CN antidote package). Amyl nitrite is given by inhalation for 15–30 seconds each minute. Sodium nitrite (300 mg in 10 mL) is injected over 2–4 minutes with careful monitoring of blood pressure. These two steps produce methemoglobin (MetHb), which combines with cytochrome-bound-CN to yield cyano-MetHb. Sodium nitrite injection is given to keep MetHb levels below 40%. Finally, sodium thiosulfate (12.5 g in 50 mL of 50% dextrose) is injected over a 10-minute period. Vitamin B12 (hydroxocobalamin) 400 µg/kg intravenously is given to produce inactive cyanocobalamin. Cyanide shunted to these minor pathways must eventually be detoxified by rhodonase.[28,29]

Airway obstruction associated with inhalation injury must be treated with inhaled β_2-agonists (salbutamol and terbutaline), racemic epinephrine, aminophylline (0.5–0.9 mg/kg/h as infusion), and anticholinergic drugs (ipratropium bromide). The incidence of proximal airway edema on the modern battlefield is likely to increase with the advent of enhanced blast and thermobaric weapons systems. Current military medical doctrine suggests that soldiers who are at risk of airway closure from edema should have a surgical airway provided. Tracheal burns caused by thermal or chemical injuries are uncommon. They can be difficult to manage. Acutely, they are often life-threatening unless diagnosed quickly and managed properly. Tracheal burn injuries can lead to long-term stenosis, which requires specialized surgical techniques and chronic therapy, often with Montgomery T-tubes, for their proper management.

Impaired oxygenation: Impaired oxygenation due to other problems such as mechanical ventilation with PEEP, ventilatory strategies such as high-frequency oscillatory ventilation (HFOV), airway control, hypoventilation, overhydration (limitation of fluid intake), and airway secretions (bronchoscopic removal of secretions) should also be addressed simultaneously.[30]

Management of Inhalation Injury in Patients with Cutaneous Burns

Cutaneous burns affect pulmonary function by release of circulatory factors and intravascular hypoproteinemia. The degree of pulmonary dysfunction depends on effective care of the burn site (wound-care) for which these patients are primarily admitted under burn surgeons with active involvement of a pulmonologist. Basic principles of management are similar to those outlined in the section on care of inhalation injury without burns for which generally patients are admitted under pulmonologist/intensivist. Additional treatment of burn area is aimed at local wound care, and intravenous fluids are important measures.[13,19] The presence of facial and pharyngeal burns should raise the suspicion of upper airway injury. Early endotracheal intubation in such cases is desirable **(Figs. 11A and B)**. Tracheostomy can be performed to avoid permanent damage to upper airway or vocal cords **(Figs. 12A and B)**. Patient should be weaned off the ventilator and tracheostomy tube as early as is possible **(Fig. 13)**. Depolarizing muscle relaxants should be avoided. Stabilization of the endotracheal tube in patients with facial burns requires specialized skill. Controlled fluid management with close hemodynamic monitoring, mechanical ventilation with PEEP, and chest wall escharotomies for full-thickness thorax burns are other measures that may be helpful **(Fig. 14)**. Management of delayed sequelae includes the treatment of pneumonia and burn sepsis. A combination of inhalation and cutaneous burn injury leads to increased incidence of pneumonia (46%) due to local pulmonary changes

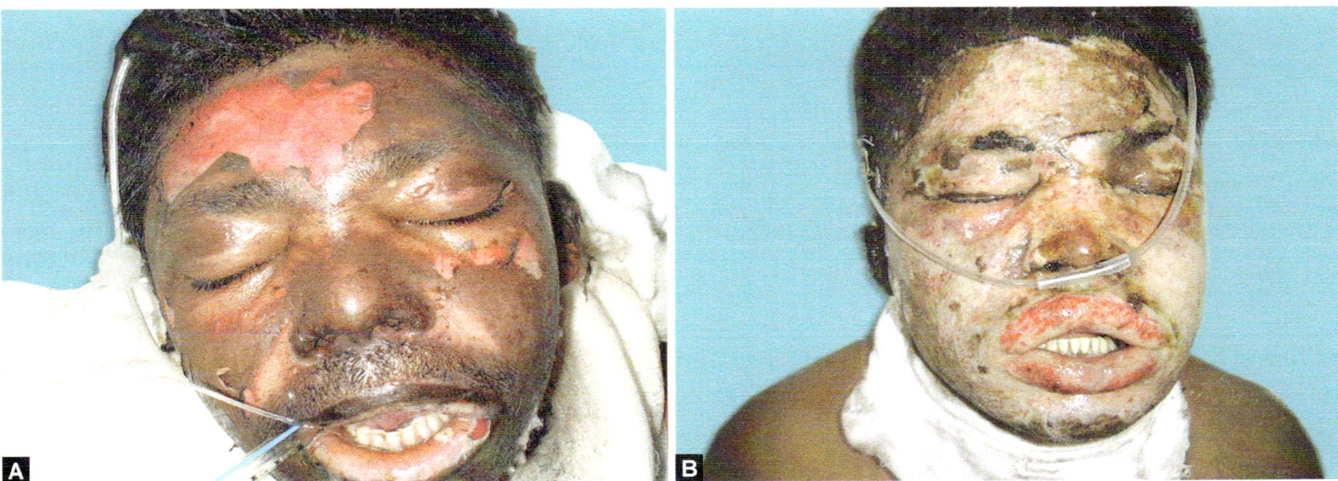

FIGS. 11A AND B: (A) Patient with facial burns with endotracheal tube in situ. (B) Same patient after 4 days of mechanical ventilation: Edema much reduced and patient extubated and then kept on nasal prongs only.

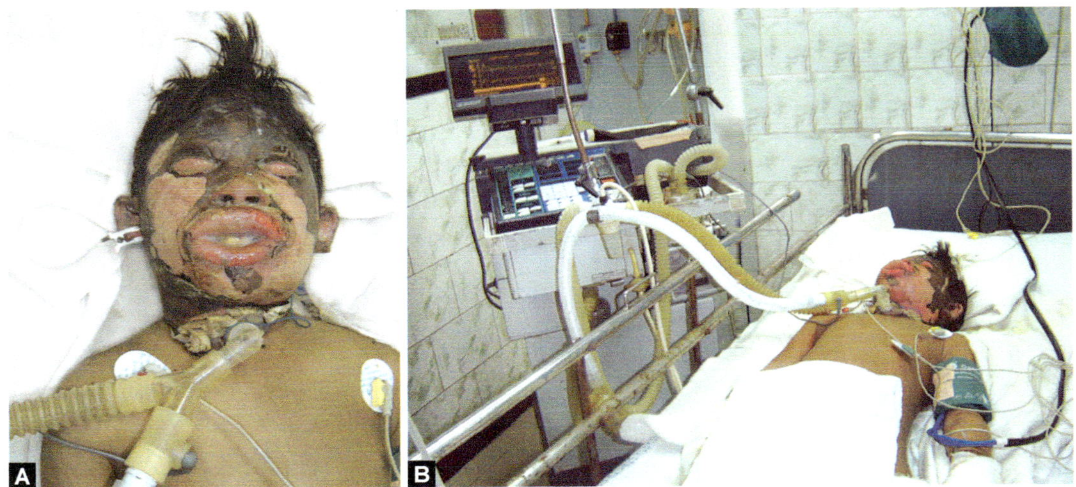

FIGS. 12A AND B: (A) Severe facial burns with inhalation injury—tracheostomy was done for ventilation. (B) Same patient on ventilator.

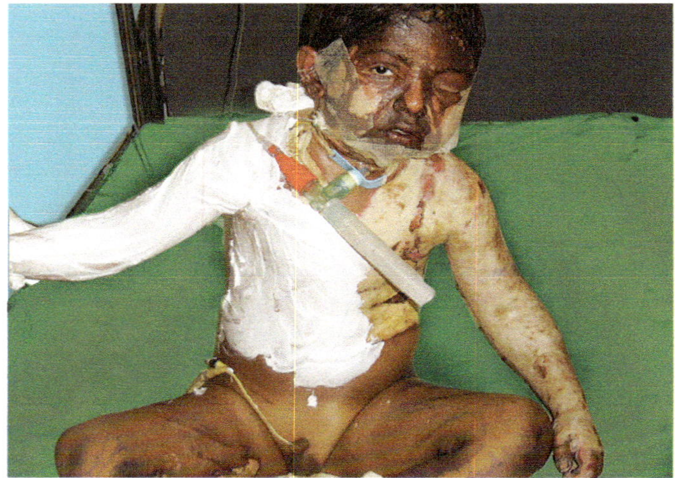

FIG. 13: Patient with tracheostomy, improved after mechanical ventilation and is being weaned off gradually.

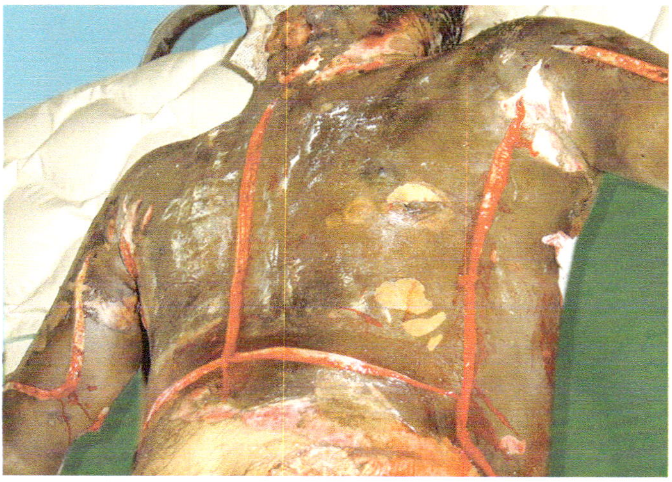

FIG. 14: Escharotomy incisions on chest in case of full-thickness circumferential chest burns.

and global immunosuppression. Enteral glutamine administration has been found to be helpful in burn patients.[31]

Preventive measures include meticulous wound care, pulmonary toilet, early removal of central lines and early extubation. Susceptible individuals (inhalation injury plus >20% BSA burn) should undergo the following additional measures—daily white blood cell (WBC) count, X-ray chest, and Gram's stain of sputum, sputum culture (every 3 days), early and effective treatment of burn wound (excision and grafting), etc.

Pneumonia usually develops during the second week after burn. It is evidenced by fever, sepsis, leukocytosis and

TABLE 4: Basic therapeutic priorities in patients with inhalation injury.

Respiratory problem	Response (s)
Asphyxia	Oxygenation, antidotes
Upper airway obstruction	Early, elective endotracheal intubation (rarely, tracheostomy)
Lower airway obstruction	
Mild	• Pulmonary toilet • Bronchodilators • Occasional therapeutic bronchoscopy
Severe (hypoventilatory failure)	Mechanical ventilation
Parenchymal injury	
Mild	Supplemental oxygen (e.g., low FiO_2 achievable by nasal prongs/mask)
Severe (with hypoxemic respiratory failure)	• Oxygenate [high FiO_2 (O_2 via ET tube)]: ○ Increase lung volume (CPAP and PEEP) ○ Minimize ongoing leak adjustments of resuscitative fluid volumes, composition, and infusion rates

(CPAP: continuous positive airway pressure; FiO_2: fraction of inspiratory oxygen; PEEP: positive end-expiratory pressure)

abnormal X-ray chest. Antibiotic use should be according to microbiological data. Pulmonary toilet and possible ventilatory support may be required. Development of ARDS is a sign of poor prognosis.

Basic therapeutic priorities in patients with inhalation injury are as follows **(Table 4)**.

Asphyxia is managed with oxygenation and specific antidotes; upper airway obstruction with early, elective endotracheal intubation (rarely, tracheostomy). Mild lower airway obstruction is managed with pulmonary toilet, bronchodilators, and occasional therapeutic bronchoscopy. In case of severe ventilatory failure, mechanical ventilation is instituted **(Fig. 12)**. Mild parenchymal injury is managed with supplemental oxygen (e.g., low FiO_2 achievable by nasal prongs/mask) and severe parenchymal injury (with hypoxemic respiratory failure) is managed with oxygen [high FiO_2 (O_2 via endotracheal tube)], increase in lung volume (CPAP and PEEP) and minimizing ongoing leak, adjustments of resuscitative fluid volumes, composition and infusion rates.[32,33]

SUMMARY

The salient points that need to be emphasized in the acute care of patients presenting with inhalation injury are as follows:

- Circumstances of the inhalation, e.g., history of a suicide attempt warrants careful patient observation and suggests early involvement of psychiatric personnel.
- The accident scene—inhalation injuries sustained in "closed spaces" (e.g., buildings and automobiles) result in severe respiratory abnormalities with greater frequency than those sustained in "open space".
- *Duration of exposure*: An estimation of the severity of inhalation injury can be made with this information.
- *Types of smoke involved (i.e., type of substrate burned)*: Very severe parenchymal lung injuries have been reported after exposure to polyvinylchloride smoke (plastics, plumbing, and electrical insulation), and polyurethane foam (furniture padding) smoke exposures, thus raising the index of suspicion for lower respiratory tract injury.
- *Time between initial resuscitation and hospital arrival*: Together with knowledge of CO elimination, half-life (largely based on estimates of the inspired O_2 fraction) and measured blood COHb level allows an estimate of peak COHb level. COHb levels have been shown to correlate with inhalation injury.
- *Patient's past medical history*: The presence of underlying bronchospastic lung disease, for example, may alter subsequent therapy.

The long-term prognosis of patients with inhalation injury is variable. Degree of recovery depends on the extent of pulmonary parenchymal injury and subsequent hypoxic damage to the organs. Residual reactive airway disease, bronchiectasis, bronchiolitis obliterans, and interstitial fibrosis may persist. Airway hyperreactivity generally improves over several months following inhalation injury. Cough, wheeze, and shortness of breath may, however persist even after mild inhalation injury.

REFERENCES

1. Stewart CL. The fire at Cocoanut Grove. J Burn Care Res. 2015;36(1):232-5.
2. Gupta K, Mehrotra M, Kumar P, Gogia AR, Prasad A, Fisher JA. Smoke Inhalation Injury: Etiopathogenesis, Diagnosis, and Management. Indian J Crit Care Med. 2018;22(3):180-8.
3. Shirani KZ, Pruitt BA Jr, Mason AD Jr. The influence of inhalation injury and pneumonia on burn mortality. Ann Surg. 1987;205(1):82-7.
4. Kadri SS, Miller AC, Hohmann S, Bonne S, Nielsen C, Wells C, et al. Risk factors for in-hospital mortality in smoke inhalation-associated acute lung injury: Data from 68 United States hospitals. Chest. 2016;150(6):1260-8.
5. Haponik EF. Clinical smoke inhalation injury: pulmonary effects. Occup Med. 1993;8:430-68.
6. MaCall JE, Cahill TJ. Respiratory care of the burn patient. J Burn Care Rehabil. 2005;26(3):2006.
7. Haponik EF, Munster AM. Clinical and Functional Assessment. In: Haponik EF, Munster AM (Eds). Smoke Inhalation and Burns. New York: McGraw-Hill Inc.; 1990. pp. 137-78.
8. Gueugniaud PY, Carsin H, Bertin-Maghit M, Petit P. Current advances in the initial management of major thermal burns. Intensive Care Med. 2000;26:848-56.
9. Miller K, Chang A. Acute inhalation injury. Emerg Med Clin North Am. 2003;21(2):533-57.
10. Haponik EF, Summer W. Respiratory complication in burned patients: Pathogenesis and spectrum of inhalation injury. J Crit Care. 1987;2:49
11. Thussu T, Tiwari VK, Suri JC, Sarabahi S. Inhalation score—A novel technique for assessing severity of inhalational burns in correlation to bronchoscopic findings. Ann Burns Fire Disasters. 2023;36(1):40-8.
12. Hassan Z, Wong JK, Bush J, Bayat A. Assessing the severity of inhalation injuries in adults. Burns. 2010;36:212-6.
13. Amin M, Shaarawy H, El-Rab EG. Role of fiberoptic bronchoscopy in management of smoke inhalation lung injury. Egyptian Journal of Chest Diseases and Tuberculosis. 2015;64:733-7.
14. Albright JM David CS, Bird MD, Ramirez L, Kim H, Burnham EI. The acute pulmonary response to the graded severity of smoke inhalation injury. Crit Care Med. 2012;40(4):1113-21.
15. Rabello E, Batista VF, Lago PM, Alvares RAG, Martinusso CA, Lapa e Silva JR. Bronchoalveolar lavage analysis in victims of severe facia burns. J Bras Pneumol. 2009;35(4):343-50.
16. Walker PF, Buehner MF, Wood LA, Boyer NL, Driscoll IR, Lundy JB, et al. Diagnosis and management of inhalation injury: an updated review. Crit Care. 2015;19:351.
17. American Burn Association. Inhalation injury: diagnosis. J Am Coll Surg. 2003;196:307-12.
18. Hassan Z, Wong JK, Bush J, Bayat A, Dunn KW. Assessing the severity of inhalation injuries in adults. Burns. 2010;36:212-6.
19. Woodson LC. Diagnosis and grading of inhalation injury. J Burn Care Res. 2009;30:143-5.
20. Endorf FW, Gamelli RL. Inhalation injury, pulmonary perturbations, and fluid resuscitation. J Burn Care Res. 2007;28:80-3.
21. Rabinowitz PM, Siegel MD. Acute inhalation injury. Clin Chest Med. 2002;23(4):707-15.
22. Davies J. In: Respiratory injury: smoke inhalation and burns. Haponik EF, Munster AM, editor. New York: McGraw Hill; 1990. Challenges for the future; p. 389
23. Chao KY, Lin YW, Chiang CE, Tseng CW. Respiratory Management in Smoke Inhalation Injury. J Burn Care Res. 2019;40(4):507-12.
24. Petrucci N, Iacovelli W. Lung protective ventilation strategy for the acute respiratory distress syndrome. Cochrane Database Syst Rev. 2007:CD003844.
25. Fitzpatrick JC, Cioffi Jr WG. Ventilatory support following burns and smoke-inhalation injury. Respir Care Clin N Am. 1997;3:21-49.

26. Weaver LK, Hopkins RO, Chan KJ, Churchill S, Elliott CG, Clemmer TP, et al. Hyperbaric oxygen for acute carbon monoxide poisoning. N Engl J Med. 2002;347:1057-67.
27. Weaver LK, Valentine KJ, Hopkins RO. Carbon monoxide poisoning: risk factors for cognitive sequelae and the role of hyperbaric oxygen. Am J Respir Crit Care Med. 2007;176:491-7.
28. Hall AH, Saiers J, Baud F. Which cyanide antidote? Crit Rev Toxicol. 2009;39:541-52.
29. O'Brien DJ, Walsh DW, Terriff CM, Hall AH. Empiric management of cyanide toxicity associated with smoke inhalation. Prehosp Disaster Med. 2011;26:374-82.
30. Latenser BA. Critical care of the burn patient: the first 48 hours. Crit Care Med. 2009;37:2819-26.
31. Garrel D, Patenaude J, Nedelec B, Samson L, Dorais J, Champoux J, et al. Decreased mortality and infectious morbidity in adult burn patients given enteral glutamine supplements: a prospective, controlled, randomized clinical trial. Crit Care Med. 2003;31:2444-9.
32. Mlcak RP, Suman OE, Herndon DN. Respiratory management of inhalation injury. Burns. 2007;33:2-13.
33. Dries DJ. Key questions in ventilator management of the burn-injury patient (Second of two parts) J Burn Care Res. 2009;30:211-20.

CHAPTER 12

Fluid, Electrolyte, and Acid–Base Disturbances in Burns

Sujata Sarabahi, Suvashis Dash, Rahul M

INTRODUCTION

A burn patient may experience electrolyte and acid-base disturbances at any point after the burn, and the severity of these disturbances is closely correlated with the patient's initial resuscitation care. Even in the most severe burns, prompt resuscitation has decreased the likelihood of oliguria leading to acute renal failure; as a result, hypovolemic shock is no longer the most common cause of burn-related deaths.[1]

HYPOVOLEMIA AND OLIGURIA

Hypovolemia following burns usually responds to fluid therapy. However, hypovolemia leading to oliguria may be seen in (1) extensively burned patients whose initial resuscitation has been delayed, (2) high-voltage electrical injury or associated crush injury leading to myoglobinuria which blocks renal tubules, and (3) burn patients with comorbidities. In these cases, the oliguria does not respond to fluid load alone and requires additional therapeutic intervention like colloid rescue or osmotic diuretic (mannitol).[2-4]

The literature advocates that the use of osmotic diuretic is indicated for electrical injury for flushing the renal tubules and avoiding precipitation of hemochromogens in the tubules. However, routine use of mannitol should be made with caution as it may cause deterioration of renal parameters.[4] The protocol followed at the senior author's institute is to start an initial loading dose of 25 g of mannitol followed by 12.5 g of mannitol, with 100 mEq sodium bicarbonate in 1 L of 0.45% normal saline (NS), at a rate of 2–10 mL/kg/h given till urinary output is adequate. The fluid therapy is guided by urine output, urine pH, and serum pH.[3,5,6] The downside of administering a diuretic is that urine output alone as a parameter for indicating the adequacy of fluid resuscitation loses its value.

Apart from the initial fluid loss following burns which is easily correctable, there is a continuous loss of watery exudates from the burned surface even in the convalescent period which needs to be replaced to prevent dehydration. The exact volume of fluid lost from the wounds which is to be replaced is difficult to estimate. By and large, in burns treated by the exposure method at normal room temperature, the daily evaporative and respiratory losses are calculated as 0.3 mL/cm^2 of body surface area burned.[7] The total body surface area is calculated from the formula of Du Bois and Du Bois as follows:[8]

$$\text{Area in cm}^2 = W^{0.425} \times H^{0.725} \times 71.84$$

(W = weight in kg and H = height in cm)

(The Du Bois nomogram is given in the appendix section of the book for easy calculations). Another formula given by Scott McDougal et al. is as follows:[9]

$$\text{Evaporative water loss in mL/h is} = (25 + \%\ \text{BSA burn}) \times \text{Total body surface area in m}^2$$

> **Hypovolemia**
> - Hypovolemia is mainly caused due to extensive burns with delayed resuscitation and in high-voltage electrical burns.
> - Monitoring of the patient is required to make individual modifications in fluid requirement.
> - Mannitol and sodium bicarbonate are to be used carefully in certain conditions.

These formulae provide a general guideline for resuscitation. When using them to estimate daily fluid requirements, one must consider the following factors as well: Whether the patient is having high temperature or tachypnea, the environmental temperature (controlled and optimum or uncontrolled and same as outside), urinary output, and whether closed or exposed technique for dressing wounds is used. Practically, if the wounds are dressed, the normal daily requirement (an average of 2.5–3.0 L/day for an adult) is added to the amount calculated by these formulae. Last but not the least, clinical monitoring of the burn patient and laboratory investigations are essential for individual modifications.

OVERHYDRATION

Large fluid infusions during the initial stage of resuscitation do not result in fluid overload because the majority is lost to extravascular space because of enhanced capillary permeability. The capillary permeability returns to normal 24–48 hours after burn which stops the further fluid loss and then reabsorption of significant volumes of this fluid that was seeped out begins, and the diuretic phase starts. Fluid excess can result in pulmonary edema, especially in elderly people and those who have pre-existing heart disease. Therefore, throughout the first postburn week, the patient's chest should be auscultated regularly. If the patient has a heart disease, pulmonary edema may be observed later during the healing process. Fluid restriction, the use of a diuretic, and sometimes intubation are used as treatments for this condition. On clinical examination, facial swelling will be seen even in patients with no burns in head and neck region.[10]

Fluid Creep

The phenomenon of fluid overloading, known as fluid creep and recognized as a landmark discovery in contemporary burn care, is caused by several factors, including the consensus Parkland formula that forbade the use of colloid, the impact of goal-directed resuscitation, and the overzealous crystalloid resuscitation performed on the scene.[2] Over-resuscitation of severely injured patient frequently leads to fluid overload and "resuscitation morbidity," including anasarca, orbital compartment syndrome, extremity compartment syndrome, and abdominal compartment syndrome (ACS), as well as pulmonary edema, necessitating a protracted and potentially challenging hospital stay. Many of these problems increase morbidity and death if not addressed quickly and properly. It is challenging to maintain the delicate balance between too little and too much fluid in burn patients while limiting hypoperfusion or fluid creep. This needs professionals with substantial burn experience. A reduction in the rate of fluid administration is necessary with rising urine output and clinical stability indicators. It is typically advised to reduce the intravenous fluid rate by 10% after 2 hours of acceptable urine output.[11,12]

HYPONATREMIA

The normal serum sodium level is 135–147 mEq/L and levels < 130 mEq/L are considered to be hyponatremia. This is the most common electrolyte imbalance seen in a burn patient and it can present at any stage. Early hyponatremia is seen following infusion of large amounts of Ringer lactate (RL; sodium concentration of 130 mEq/L) in the initial phase, which reduces the level of sodium in blood or when resuscitation is done orally with salt-free fluids in small burns. This can be managed simply by restricting fluid administration. A more severe hyponatremia is seen in pediatric burn patients resuscitated with hypotonic solutions or if overhydrated. The child may become apathetic or may show signs of cerebral irritation, convulsions, and hyperpyrexia. This can be corrected by withholding sodium-free fluids and giving sodium-containing fluids (hypertonic saline) and anticonvulsant medication. The dose of hypertonic saline can be calculated by the following formula:

$$\text{Sodium requirement in mEq/L} = (140 - \text{patient's sodium in mEq/L}) \times 60\% \text{ body weight in kg}$$

Half of this dose is given initially and response is observed followed by slow correction with the remaining amount. Serum electrolytes must be repeated every 4–6 hours to guide the further therapy with sodium. A further improvement can be done by promoting diuresis if the renal function is normal by giving a small dose of furosemide (the renal sodium loss may increase with this, but it will be lesser than the gain from the intravenous correction.

Hyponatremia

- Common causes include infusion of large amounts of RL, use of 0.5% silver nitrate and syndrome of inappropriate antidiuretic hormone (SIADH).
- This can be corrected by withholding sodium-free fluids and giving sodium-containing fluids (hypertonic saline) and symptomatic management.

The use of 0.5% silver nitrate as a topical antimicrobial agent can also increase sodium loss through eschar leading to hyponatremia.[13] Burn patients can develop hyponatremia as a manifestation of SIADH (syndrome of inappropriate antidiuretic hormone secretion) if all other causes have been excluded. Treatment of SIADH includes restriction of fluids and diuretics. Rarely, the burn may present with diabetes insipidus.[14]

Another treatable cause of hyponatremia in burn patients is the "sick cell syndrome" resulting from the inability of the red blood cells to exclude sodium because of receiving inadequate energy following an insufficient calorie intake by the patient. This leads to increased sodium concentration in the cells as well as increased hydrogen ions and water entering the cells whereas potassium is released from the cells into the extracellular space, thus resulting in intracellular edema and intracellular acidosis. This is manifested clinically by nonpitting edema, tachypnea, confusion, low serum sodium, and reversal of sodium/potassium ratio in urine.[15]

However, this condition is corrected by infusion of intravenous hypertonic glucose, potassium, insulin, or "GKI drip." This allows sodium and water to be released from the cells and potassium to enter the cells, thus restoring the homeostasis. Because of high incidence of insulin resistance, very high doses of soluble insulin (as high as 600 units of soluble insulin) may be required per day. On average, approximately 150 units of insulin and 600 g of glucose are required in 24 hours. This can be given in the following manner:[16]

25% glucose: 500 mL

Potassium chloride: 10 mEq

Plain insulin: 30 units
100 mL of this is given hourly in adults. In children, the dose is as follows:

- *9–10 years*: Approximately adult dose
- *5–9 years*: ½ to ¾ adult dose
- *2–5 years*: ¼ to ½ adult dose
- *<2 years*: ⅛ to ¼ adult dose

This is usually administered by an infusion pump. With this treatment, the serum sodium levels return to normal with increased excretion of sodium and water in urine with normal levels of nitrogen and potassium in urine.

HYPERNATREMIA

Following burns, hypernatremia (serum sodium > 150 mEq/L) occurs if a patient is dehydrated (if evaporative losses are not corrected), if an osmotic diuretic is given (in the form of mannitol or low-molecular-weight dextran), if there is sepsis, or rarely if there is diabetes insipidus-like syndrome (produced by excretion of large volumes of dilute urine). The reasons for dehydration can be increased water losses during burn sepsis by hyperventilation or hyperthermia and increased renal blood flow causing increased urinary water loss. This results in increased serum sodium levels. The management for this condition includes infusing sufficient fluids to replace water loss in the form of 5% dextrose over 48 hours.[17,18]

HYPOKALEMIA

Hypokalemia can occur in burns due to increased potassium losses (amounting to 100–200 mEq/L/day) following resuscitation with inadequate potassium replacement, sulfamylon dressings which cause kaliuresis, topical treatment with 0.5% silver nitrate soaks (which promotes transeschar potassium losses), or because of diarrhea (during burn sepsis or due to hyperosmolar feeding). A serum potassium level <3 mEq/L is life-threatening as it produces cardiac arrest. It is difficult to calculate accurately the degree of hypokalemia in relation to the extent of total body deficit. A fall in serum potassium from 4 to 3 mEq/L is usually associated with a total body deficit of 100–400 mEq; a larger deficit is required to lower the plasma potassium from 3 to 2 mEq/L. Therefore, although many rough guidelines exist for relating the deficit of potassium to the degree of hypokalemia, these are unreliable in an individual patient. Correction of the potassium deficit is mandatory. Therefore, daily serum potassium must be measured. In general, the oral route is the safest, and the intravenous route should be used when gastrointestinal problems limit the intake or absorption, in the presence of severe degree (<2.5 mEq/L) of hypokalemia with either respiratory muscle weakness or cardiac arrhythmias or when there is an anticipated shift of potassium into the intracellular fluid (recovery from diabetic ketoacidosis).

The most common replacement fluid is KCl, which is available as a concentrated solution (2 mEq/L) with an osmolality of 4,000 mOsmol/kg water. It must be diluted before infusion. When correcting hypokalemia, potassium should not be diluted in glucose-containing solutions as the glucose (via insulin) can lead to an initial lowering of the plasma potassium. Preferably, a large central vein should be used for infusion because of the irritant properties of hyperosmotic potassium solutions. When serum potassium is >2 mEq/L and no ECG abnormalities are present, potassium chloride is given as infusion at a rate of 10 mEq/h. When serum potassium is <2 mEq/L, ECG abnormality is present or in the presence of muscle weakness or paralysis, potassium chloride is infused at a rate of 40 mEq/h in saline. Offending drugs, e.g., diuretics, steroids, beta-agonists, gentamicin, ampicillin, penicillin, carbenicillin, ticarcillin, etc., should be discontinued.[18-20]

HYPERKALEMIA

Hyperkalemia is seen when acute renal failure occurs due to hemolysis and tissue destruction due to either extensive thermal injury (when inadequate resuscitation leads to acidosis) or high-voltage electrical injury. This is seen in the immediate postburn period. Later, if the patient goes into septicemia, the serum potassium levels may again be elevated following renal failure. Cardiac arrest may occur if serum potassium is >6 mEq/L.[18,19]

Hyperkalemia results in ECG abnormalities which include elevation of T waves, ST segment depression, and lengthening of the QRS segment. It is well known that administration of succinylcholine in a burn patient may cause sudden hyperkalemia which may be life-threatening, and this can happen any time in the acute period till months after sustaining burns. It is, therefore, essential to get serum potassium levels checked prior to getting any surgery done in a burn patient and use succinylcholine judiciously.

The standard treatment for correction of hyperkalemia is as follows:

- Calcium gluconate 10%, 10 mL over 2–5 minutes I/V. The onset of its action is in 1–3 minutes and the duration of action is 30–60 minutes. It may be repeated once if there is no response to the first dose.
- 10 units of regular insulin diluted in 500 mL of 10% dextrose at the rate of 150–200 mL/h. Its onset of action is within 20 minutes and the duration of action is 4–6 hours.
- IV salbutamol (4 µg/kg in 5 mL water) or salbutamol nebulization (2.5–5.0 mL) given over 15–20 minutes also lowers the potassium levels.
- Avoid drugs that predispose to hyperkalemia, for example, angiotensin-converting enzyme (ACE) inhibitors, beta-blockers, nonsteroidal anti-inflammatory drugs (NSAIDs), potassium-sparing diuretics, and heparin.

Hyperkalemia

- It occurs in acute renal failure due to extensive thermal or electrical injury.
- ECG abnormalities include elevation of T waves, ST segment depression, and lengthening of QRS segment.
- Start patient on anti-hyperkalemia measures and avoid use of drugs that predispose to hyperkalemia.

- Promote urinary potassium loss by loop diuretics.
- Potassium exchange resins
- Hemodialysis

HYPOCALCEMIA

Mild hypocalcemia (6–7 mg/dL) due to hypoalbuminemia and calcium sequestration in burned tissue may be seen in moderate burns (>30% TBSA). However, this may not manifest clinically. Depression of serum albumin by 1 g/dL lowers the total serum calcium concentration by approximately 1 mg/dL, though the ionized calcium is usually normal. Marked alkalosis also lowers serum calcium by increasing the protein binding. Severe hypocalcemia may result from either alkalosis in the shock stage or following the use of 0.5% silver nitrate soaks which may manifest clinically with cramps, facial nerve twitching, carpopedal spasms, tetany, Chvostek's sign, etc. This requires correction by intravenous calcium gluconate.

There is evidence that calcium administration in the critically ill may cause hypoxic cell damage, so calcium should be corrected in this setting only if the patient is symptomatic. Ionized calcium also should be determined to ascertain whether true hypocalcemia exists. When indicated, treatment of symptomatic hypocalcemia consists of 100–200 mg of elemental calcium (as 10% calcium gluconate) intravenously followed by a slow infusion of 0.5–2.0 mg/kg/h with frequent determination of total and ionized calcium levels as well as correction of underlying cause. It is crucial to ensure that hypomagnesemia is also corrected as this may potentiate the tendency to tetani and arrhythmias.[19,20]

HYPERCALCEMIA

Hypercalcemia is a rare problem in burn patients. Immobilization causes a mild elevation in calcium that is often symptomless, unlike the high rise seen in malignancy-related hypercalcemia.

HYPOMAGNESEMIA

Hypomagnesemia is rarely seen in burn patients if adequate nutrition is ensured. If the patient is on prolonged total parenteral nutrition (TPN) with inadequate magnesium supplements or if there are excess gastrointestinal and wound fluid losses, hypomagnesemia may manifest clinically with neurological signs, disorientation, neuromuscular irritability, seizures, and tetany. This can be corrected by intravenous magnesium chloride or magnesium sulfate. Magnesium is best retained when given slowly over several hours.

HYPOPHOSPHATEMIA

Hypophosphatemia with serum phosphorus levels < 1 mg/dL is observed in extensive burns that require a large amount of fluid for resuscitation leading to a dilutional effect and receiving large volumes of intravenous glucose solutions and antacid therapy. Therefore, it may be safer to monitor serum phosphorus levels as well. Phosphorus plays an important role in oxygen unloading from red cells, muscular activity, and neutrophil function. Enteral replacement of phosphorus is usually sufficient, although if levels are really low, intravenous sodium or potassium phosphate (0.08–0.16 mmoL/kg of sodium phosphate in 500 mL 0.45 NS over 6 hours) may be administered with caution only if phosphate is below 1.0 mg/dL.[19,20]

ACID–BASE BALANCE

A burn patient may have metabolic or respiratory acidosis or metabolic alkalosis.[21,22]

Metabolic Acidosis

Metabolic acidosis is usually seen in the early phase of extensive burns or in case the patient develops sick cell syndrome. It may even be seen on admission in the pediatric patients <2 years of age since their buffering capacity is less. Oliguria due to insufficient or delayed fluid resuscitation may elevate blood lactate levels to 2 mEq/L or more due to anaerobic metabolism. This condition is diagnosed by low arterial pH, in combination with low arterial PCO_2. It can be corrected by increasing fluid infusion and oxygen therapy for hypoxemia. If blood pH falls to below 7.1, it should be corrected by soda bicarbonate intravenously. However, in general, the underlying cause of the acidosis should be determined and appropriate treatment undertaken. Empirical bicarbonate therapy can be complicated by intracellular acidosis. The formula used for calculating the dose of soda bicarbonate is as follows:

$$\text{Base deficit} \times 0.3 \times \text{body weight (in kg)} = 8.4\%\ NaHCO_3\ \text{(in mL)}$$

Half of this dose is given immediately and 1 hour after this correction, arterial blood gas (ABG) is repeated and further correction is done according to the new pH value in order to keep the pH above 7.1.

It has been noticed that if plasma is used for treating burn shock, no early acidosis is seen because of alkalization[22,23] produced by the citrate in the transfused plasma. If saline or dextran alone is used for resuscitation, acidosis may occur and may require the addition of bicarbonate. It is essential to check this early metabolic acidosis as it predisposes to acute renal failure.[24]

Respiratory Acidosis

Except in individuals with an inhalational injury that causes pulmonary insufficiency, pulmonary edema, atelectasis, bronchopneumonia, or pulmonary thromboembolism with or without sepsis, it is rarely observed during the early postburn period. It is characterized by hypoxemia, low pH, and high pCO_2. In very severe cases, intubation and mechanical ventilation as well as antibiotics for treating sepsis are used as part of the treatment. The underlying cause of respiratory acidosis should be found and treated.[24,25]

Metabolic Alkalosis

Metabolic alkalosis can happen after severe burns and is linked to increased adrenocortical activity as well as a response to respiratory alkalosis brought on by elevated catecholamine excretion. Additionally, it comes after protracted hyperaldosteronism, hypokalemia, and protracted nasogastric suction brought on by paralytic ileus. In most cases, this necessitates fluid replacement and hypokalemia correction. To restore acid-base balance, the precipitating causes are removed and electrolyte deficits are corrected. When there is a volume and/or chloride deficit, adequate chloride must be given. Acetazolamide can aid in maintaining diuresis in the face of a metabolic alkalosis,[24,25] which is a carbonic anhydrase inhibitor with potassium supplement to increase urinary bicarbonate excretion. In fact, acetazolamide is frequently used in chloride-resistant metabolic alkalosis.

Metabolic acidosis
- It is usually seen in early phase of extensive burns.
- Condition is diagnosed by low arterial pH, in combination with low arterial pCO_2.
- It can be corrected by increasing fluid infusion and oxygen therapy for hypoxemia.

SUMMARY

Electrolyte imbalance and acid base disturbances are very commonly seen along with fluid loss following moderate to extensive acute burns. Timely resuscitation with the right kind of fluid can reduce the occurrence of electrolyte imbalances later on. If disturbances in electrolyte and pH are corrected in time it can help in reducing morbidity and mortality from burns to a great extent.

REFERENCES

1. Guilabert P, Usúa G, Martín N, Abarca L, Barret JP, Colomina MJ. Fluid resuscitation management in patients with burns: Update. Br J Anaesth. 2016;117(3):284-96.
2. Comish P, Walsh M, Castillo-Angeles M, Kuhlenschmidt K, Carlson D, Arnoldo B, et al. Adoption of rescue colloid during burn resuscitation decreases fluid administered and restores end-organ perfusion. Burns. 2021;47(8):1844-50.
3. Homsi E, Barreiro MF, Orlando JM, Higa EM. Prophylaxis of acute renal failure in patients with rhabdomyolysis. Ren Fail. 1997;19(2):283-8.
4. Culnan DM, Farner K, Bitz GH, Capek KD, Tu Y, Jimenez C, et al. Volume resuscitation in patients with high-voltage electrical injuries. Ann Plast Surg. 2018;80(3):S113-8.
5. Somagutta MR, Pagad S, Sridharan S, Nanthakumaran S, Arnold AA, May V, et al. Role of bicarbonates and mannitol in rhabdomyolysis: A comprehensive review. Cureus. 2020;12(8):e9742.
6. Brown CV, Rhee P, Chan L, Evans K, Demetriades D, Velmahos GC. Preventing renal failure in patients with rhabdomyolysis: Do bicarbonate and mannitol make a difference?. J Trauma Acute Care Surg. 2004;56(6):1191-6.
7. Davies JW, Lamke LO, Liljedahl SO. A guide to the rate of non-renal water loss from patients with burns. Br J Plast Surg. 1974;27(4):325-9.
8. Du Bois D, Du Bois E. Clinical calorimetry: A formula to estimate the approximate surface area if height and weight be known. Arch Intern Med. 1916;17:863.
9. McDougal WS, Slade CL, Pruitt BA Jr. Manual of Burns. New York: Springer; 2012.
10. Gibran NS, Heimbach DM. Current status of burn wound pathophysiology. Clin Plast Surg. 2000;27(1):11-22.
11. Atiyeh BS, Dibo SA, Ibrahim AE, Zgheib ER. Acute burn resuscitation and fluid creep: It is time for colloid rehabilitation. Ann Burns Fire Disasters. 2012;25(2):59.
12. Saffle JR. The phenomenon of "fluid creep" in acute burn resuscitation. J Burn Care Res. 2007;28(3):382-95.
13. Dai T, Huang YY, K Sharma S, T Hashmi J, B Kurup D, R Hamblin M. Topical antimicrobials for burn wound infections. Recent patents on anti-infective drug discovery. 2010;5(2):124-51.
14. Dash S, Ghosh S. Transient diabetes insipidus following thermal burn; a case report and literature review. Bull Emerg Trauma. 2017;5(4):311.
15. Koumpis E, Florentin M, Hatzimichael E, Liamis G. Hyponatremia in patients with hematologic diseases. J Clin Med. 2020;9(11):3721.
16. Cason JS. Treatment of Burns. London: Chapman and Hall; 1981:318-21.
17. Shrimanker I, Bhattarai S. Electrolytes. [Updated 2023 Jul 24]. In: StatPearls [Internet]. Treasure Island (FL): StatPearls Publishing; 2024.
18. Dilday J, Cameron C, Bell C. Acid-base, fluids, and electrolytes. In: Rodriguez CJ, Moore FD, Rhee PM (Eds). Surgical Critical Care and Emergency Surgery: Clinical Questions and Answers. New York: Wiley; 2022. pp. 145-54.
19. Whitmore SP, Gunnerson KJ. Acid-base and electrolyte disorders in emergency critical care. Emerg Department Crit Care. 2020:301-29.
20. Fencl V, Jabor A, Kazda A, Figge J. Diagnosis of metabolic acid–base disturbances in critically ill patients. Am J Respir Crit Care Med. 2000;162(6):2246-51.
21. Hamilton PK, Morgan NA, Connolly GM, Maxwell AP. Understanding acid-base disorders. Ulster Med J. 2017;86(3):161.
22. Reddi AS. Fluid, Electrolyte and Acid–Base Disorders: Clinical Evaluation and Management. Cham: Springer; 2018. pp. 391-401.
23. Kellum JA. Disorders of acid-base balance. Crit Care Med. 2007;35(11):2630-6.
24. Lanken PN. Intensive Care Unit Manual. Philadelphia: W. B Saunders Company; 2001. pp. 425-40.
25. Kaplan LJ, Frangos S. Clinical review: Acid–base abnormalities in the intensive care unit. Crit Care. 2004;9:1-6.

CHAPTER 13

Acute Renal Failure in Burns and its Management

Rajiv Kohli, Arun Goel, Aakanksha Goel

INTRODUCTION

The initial effects of a burn injury on the kidney and its functions are in response to circulatory and metabolic consequences, followed later by the effects of treatment and complications. Of all the viscera, kidney is the one that is most likely to be damaged by burns. This is because, after an extensive burn injury, there occurs a marked shift of intravascular fluid into the interstitial spaces all over the body, including the nonburnt sites, resulting in hypovolemia and decreased circulation. The levels of catecholamines, angiotensin II, and vasopressin are elevated.[1] These changes cause vasoconstriction and alteration of regional blood flow, especially in the kidney. This, in turn, decreases renal perfusion and urine output. Production of urine acts as a valuable indicator of function and indirectly of the blood flow to the kidney. Urinary specific gravity and osmolality increase. With timely and appropriate fluid and electrolyte replacement therapy, the hypovolemia is corrected and normal circulation is restored. Once the capillary permeability is restored, the fluid is withdrawn from the interstitial spaces back into the intravascular compartment, and diuresis occurs to remove this excess fluid. The renal function is also altered as a direct effect of the stress of burn trauma, in response to which the posterior pituitary releases antidiuretic hormone (ADH), and maximum reabsorption of water occurs. In addition to ADH, aldosterone is released from the adrenal cortex and maximum sodium is absorbed. Thus, under the influence of ADH and aldosterone, the kidney excretes an amount of urine just sufficient to handle the normal solute load, largely represented by urea.

If the resuscitation is delayed and/or inadequate, renal blood flow and glomerular filtration rate (GFR) decrease, which may ultimately lead to a prerenal form of acute renal failure (ARF). This may progress to intrinsic renal failure, which is usually caused by septicemia and nephrotoxic drugs. Renal failure may become part of the multiorgan dysfunction syndrome (MODS). In extensive third-degree burns, hemolysis occurs due to direct thermal damage to circulating erythrocytes with release of hemoglobin in large amounts into the circulation. In normal situations, this gets conjugated by haptoglobin and is transferred to the liver. In massive amounts, unconjugated free hemoglobin passes through glomeruli and is excreted in the urine, leading to degenerative changes in tubular cells and occlusion of renal tubules by the hemoglobin casts formed. Its combination with dehydration, acidosis, shock, and endotoxemia paves the way for renal failure. Free hemoglobin, absorbed by tubular epithelium, breaks into globin and heme. Heme causes tubular damage by producing oxygen-free radicals via iron ions.[2] In contact electrical burns, necrosis of muscles (rhabdomyolysis) releases intracellular components of the muscle (myoglobin, potassium, lactic acid, thromboplastin, creatine kinase, nucleic acids, phosphate, creatine, etc.) into the systemic circulation, leading to precipitation of myoglobin and blockage of renal tubules, again leading to renal failure. Severely burned patients with rhabdomyolysis are significantly more likely to develop renal failure (with a consequent greater risk of mortality) as compared to nonburned patients with rhabdomyolysis or severely burned patients without rhabdomyolysis. Renal replacement therapy (RRT) has been shown to be effective in removing myoglobin from the circulation.[3]

Acute renal failure or acute kidney injury (AKI), as it is known these days,[4] is one of the most devastating complications of burns with a high mortality rate. The term AKI has largely replaced ARF because of the recognition that smaller decrements in kidney function that do not result in overt organ failure are also of substantial clinical importance as they are also associated with increased morbidity and mortality. ARF and AKI are used interchangeably in this chapter. It has been said to affect from 0.5 to 30% of the patients admitted to a burn unit. The incidence depends not only on the severity of the burn injury but also on the definition of ARF used. Once ARF develops in a burn patient, the prognosis becomes remarkably unfavorable. They are likely to have an extended stay in the intensive care unit, with increased morbidity, mortality, and treatment costs. While renal function returns to normal in the majority of patients who survive, some do require long-term dialysis.[5] This fact has been recognized for over 60 years now, and most studies have reported a mortality rate of around 80% in those patients who require dialytic support. However, the prognostic importance of less severe forms of AKI, not requiring dialysis, is not well documented.[6]

DEFINING, QUANTIFYING, AND CLASSIFYING ACUTE RENAL FAILURE[7]

Acute renal failure is characterized by an abrupt and sustained fall in GFR, leading to accumulation of nitrogenous (clinically manifesting as a rise in urea and creatinine) and non-nitrogenous waste products. This potentially reversible condition is accompanied by metabolic disturbances such as metabolic acidosis and hyperkalemia, changes in the body's fluid balance, and effects on many other organ systems.

The two major functions of a healthy kidney are excretion of nitrogenous wastes and formation of urine. Creatinine is more specific in assessing renal function than blood urea nitrogen (BUN), but it corresponds only loosely to GFR. The same value of serum creatinine may correspond to different GFRs in two individuals with different body masses. However, a rise in serum creatinine values corresponds to a similar decline in GFR.

There is no universal definition of AKI.[8,9] Common criteria are either biochemical (rise in serum creatinine of 0.5 mg/dL or 50% from baseline), clinical (oliguria, urine output < 400 mL/day), or a combination of both. The acute dialysis quality initiative (ADQI) group[10,11] proposed the RIFLE system, classifying ARF into three severity categories (**R**isk of renal dysfunction, **I**njury to the kidney, and **F**ailure of renal function) and two clinical outcome categories (**L**oss of renal function and **E**nd-stage renal disease) **(Table 1)**.[10] Loss (persistent AKI) denotes the need for RRT for more than 4 weeks, whereas in end-stage renal disease (ESRD), the need is for longer than 3 months. The first use of RIFLE criteria in burn patients was reported by Lopes et al. in 2007, who reported an overall 35.7% rate of AKI, with 14.3% in class R, 8.7% in class I, and 12.7% in class F.[12]

In 2007, the Acute Kidney Injury Network (AKIN) proposed a modified version of the RIFLE system to increase its sensitivity and specificity.[8,13,14] The revised criteria were intended to simplify the definition and make it more clinically applicable. According to this modified version, there is "an abrupt (within 48 hours) reduction in kidney function with an absolute increase in serum creatinine of ≥ 0.3 mg/dL (≥ 26.4 μmol/L), a percentage increase in serum creatinine of ≥ 50% (1.5-fold from baseline), or a reduction in urine output (documented oliguria of < 0.5 mL/kg/h for > 6 hour)" **(Table 2)**.[13]

In 2010, taking into account the shortcomings of both above definitions, the Kidney Disease: Improving Global Outcomes (KDIGO) clinical practice guidelines established a consensus definition of AKI **(Table 3)**.[15-17]

Please note that the urine output criteria are the same for all the above three definitions.

Risk Factors for Renal Injury in Burns[18-22]

A number of risk factors have been found to be significantly associated with AKI in burn patients. Thus, older age is consistently associated with AKI. The kidneys of elderly people are more vulnerable to toxins derived from necrotic tissues and also from iatrogenic damage. Removing necrotic tissue as early as possible may reduce the production of toxins. Strategies to reduce

TABLE 1: RIFLE classification.[10]

	GFR criteria	Urine output criteria
Risk	Serum creatinine increased 1.5 times	< 0.5 mL/kg body weight/h for 6 hours
Injury	Serum creatinine increased 2 times	< 0.5 mL/kg body weight/h for 12 hours
Failure	Serum creatinine increased 3 times or creatinine = 4 mg%, when there was an acute rise of >0.5 mg	< 0.3 mL/kg body weight/h for 24 hours or anuria for 12 hours
Loss	Persistent acute renal failure, complete loss of kidney function for longer than 4 weeks	
End-stage renal disease (ESRD)	End stage renal disease for longer than 3 months	

TABLE 2: AKIN criteria.[13]

Stage	Serum creatinine	Urine output criteria
1	1.5–1.9 times baseline serum creatinine OR ≥ 0.3 mg/dL (≥ 26 µmol/L) increase in serum creatinine	< 0.5 mL/kg body weight/h for 6–12 hours
2	2.0–2.9 times initial/baseline serum creatinine	< 0.5 mL/kg body weight/h for ≥ 12 hours
3	≥ 3.0 times initial/baseline serum creatinine OR Increase in serum creatinine to ≥ 4.0 mg/dL (≥ 353.6 µmol/L) OR Initiation of renal replacement therapy OR, in patients < 18 years, decrease in eGFR to < 35 mL/min/1.73 m^2	< 0.3 mL/kg body weight/h for ≥ 24 hours OR Anuria for ≥ 12 hours

(eGFR: estimated glomerular filtration rate)

TABLE 3: KDIGO criteria.[15]

Stage	Serum creatinine	Urine output criteria
I	Increase to 1.5–1.9 times initial/baseline serum creatinine OR Increase in serum creatinine of ≥ 0.3 mg/dL (≥ 26.2 µmol/L) from the baseline	< 0.5 mL/kg body weight/h for 6–12 hours
II	Increase in serum creatinine to 2.0–2.9 times initial/baseline	< 0.5 mL/kg body weight/h for ≥ 12 hours
III	Increase in serum creatinine to a level ≥ 4.0 mg/dL (353.6 µmol/L) OR Initiation of renal replacement therapy	< 0.3 mL/kg body weight/h for ≥ 24 hours OR Anuria for ≥ 12 hours

medication-induced nephrotoxicity should also be taken. The greater the total body surface area (TBSA) burnt and the larger the full-thickness burn area out of the total, the greater the risk. AKI is more likely to occur with an associated inhalation injury, a higher Abbreviated Burn Severity Index (ABSI), and a Sequential Organ Failure Assessment (SOFA) score on admission. No association has been seen between the risk for AKI and serum creatinine or urine output at the time of admission. However, BUN at the time of admission is a significant risk factor. Gender, chemical burns, and BMI have not been found to be significant. Unfortunately, none of these factors can be altered by the burn surgeon.

CAUSES OF ACUTE RENAL FAILURE[23]

The reasons for AKI among patients with major burns are multifactorial. For long, a practically useful approach for the etiological diagnosis of ARF has been to divide the causes according to the likely source of renal injury. Thus, the causes can be: (1) prerenal, (2) renal, and (3) postrenal.

Prerenal

This form of AKI is considered to be, at least in initial phases, functional in nature; that is, the kidney malfunctions secondary to systemic factors that decrease renal perfusion, leading to a reduction in GFR. The causative systemic factors, if corrected rapidly, allow the renal function to return back to normal. However, in the presence of delayed or unsuccessful intervention, structural changes occur in the kidney, leading to a prolonged period required for recovery. Thus, there is a reversible increase in serum creatinine and BUN. The main causes in burned patients are acute hypovolemia and hypotension. This activates a number of neurohumoral vasoconstrictive systems to maintain them. Changes in preglomerular and postglomerular arteriolar resistance, mediated by prostaglandins and nitric oxide and activation of angiotensin II, enable renal blood flow and GFR to remain roughly constant across a wide range of mean arterial pressures. However, below a mean arterial pressure of 70 mm Hg, this autoregulation is impaired, and the GFR falls proportionately. Administration of drugs that interfere with autoregulation, like nonsteroidal anti-inflammatory drugs (NSAIDs) and angiotensin-converting enzyme (ACE) inhibitors, precipitates prerenal failure.[24]

Volume overload in AKI has been associated with worse outcomes. However, it is not clear whether AKI and worse outcomes are the consequence of severe disease (leading to worse outcomes) or whether fluid overload in itself is the reason for AKI and worse outcomes. The presumed pathophysiologic mechanisms of fluid overload being the cause of AKI include intra-abdominal hypertension (leading to decreased renal arteriolar and microcirculatory blood flow and also increased renal venous pressure) and abdominal compartment syndrome (ACS). ACS is characterized by a combination of increased intra-abdominal pressure and organ dysfunction, such as oliguria, respiratory insufficiency, or hemodynamic instability. The extent of gut edema and the amount of ascites, by increasing the volume of the abdominal cavity, might also be important contributing factors. Thus, the dictum should be "treat hypovolemia but prevent volume overload".[25]

Renal (Parenchymal or Intrinsic)

There is direct renal parenchymal damage and acute tubular necrosis (ATN), resulting from the continuation of the same pathophysiological processes that lead to prerenal hypoperfusion (ischemic ATN). The use of nephrotoxic drugs may also cause direct damage to the renal tubules (nephrotoxic ATN). Thus, timely stoppage of administration of the offending drug(s) is very important. Structural changes in the kidney can be seen on microscopy. Intrinsic renal failure is often multifactorial. The most common cause in burned patients is sepsis.[26,27] It is often accompanied by multiorgan dysfunction/failure.

Postrenal (Obstructed Urine Flow)

In burned patients, it is mainly the prerenal and the intrinsic renal failure that occur unless a patient with bladder neck obstruction due to an enlarged prostate or urinary calculous disease gets burnt to have an additional postobstructive failure.

EARLY AND LATE ACUTE KIDNEY INJURY[28]

Depending on the interval between the time of burn injury and the onset of ARF, two different forms of AKI have been described in burn patients. Early-onset and late-onset AKI have different etiologies. Burns affecting more than 20% of TBSA are likely to cause enough loss of extracellular fluid and albumin from plasma volume to produce shock and hypoalbuminemia. The ARF occurring in the first few days (within 5 days) after thermal injury is related to (1) a decrease in renal perfusion resulting from hypovolemia (due to fluid shifts from the intravascular compartment into the interstitial space and extensive fluid losses from the burnt areas, which may get accentuated by a delay in fluid resuscitation), (2) low cardiac output and systemic vasoconstriction during the resuscitation period, or (3) myoglobinuria with damage to tubular cells. Elevated levels of stress-related hormones, such as catecholamines, angiotensin, aldosterone, and vasopressin, have been implicated in the pathogenesis of this form of ARF. This form of ARF occurs less frequently than before because of the widespread availability of cheap intravenous electrolyte solutions and the aggressive fluid resuscitation performed nowadays in most burn units. However, this is still a life-threatening complication in patients with extensive deep burns and those with electrical burns.

The other form of ARF, developing at a later date (after 5 days), has a more complex pathogenesis. This form has been reported to be related to sepsis and MODS and very often proves fatal. While earlier, hypoperfusion and ischemia of the kidneys were thought to be the main causes of AKI in sepsis, there is now more data indicating that renal perfusion is not decreased in sepsis.[29] Instead, inflammation and apoptosis probably play an important role.[27,30] Burn patients experience an inflammatory response that is often more severe and lasts much longer as compared to other trauma cases. Systemic inflammatory response syndrome (SIRS) and pulmonary dysfunction have been found to be present in all patients with AKI, and they precede it. In a study of acute respiratory dysfunction in patients with major burns, acute respiratory distress syndrome (ARDS) was found to occur soon after the burn (usually within 3 days), and renal dysfunction was more common in patients with the most severe respiratory dysfunction.[31] MODS occurs more commonly in patients with inhalational injuries. Administration of nephrotoxic drugs like aminoglycosides, vancomycin, amphotericin B, etc., are also contributing factors in the development of late ARF.

DIAGNOSTIC APPROACH TO RENAL FAILURE

Acute kidney injury in a burn patient has no characteristic clinical findings. It needs to be anticipated/suspected based on the risk factors given above. Reduced urine output despite adequate fluid therapy infusions is usually the first sign of renal failure. Oliguria is a helpful sign, but neither specific nor sensitive. Measurement of blood urea, serum creatinine concentrations, and microscopic examination of urine are part of the basic investigations done for any burn requiring admission.

Serum Creatinine

In ARF, renal function is commonly monitored by daily estimations of serum creatinine. However, it has limitations as a marker of GFR in patients with ARF because its concentration depends not only on the urinary clearance of creatinine but also on the rate of production and the volume of distribution. Serum creatinine levels do not reflect the GFR accurately in the nonsteady-state condition of ARF.

Urine Volume

Acute anuria or severe oliguria is quite a specific clinical indicator of ARF. While prerenal forms of ARF are nearly always present with oliguria (< 400 mL/day in an adult), the renal and postrenal forms can be associated with any amount of urinary output, from almost nil to normal to polyuria. A severe ARF can coexist with a normal urinary output. The change in the amount of urine excreted precedes the biochemical alterations.

Urinary Indices

If the renal tubular function is intact, renal vasoconstriction during the initiation phase of ATN is associated with increased tubular reabsorption and the fractional excretion of sodium (FE_{Na}), i.e.,

$$\frac{\text{Urinary sodium} \times \text{plasma creatinine}}{\text{Plasma sodium} \times \text{urinary creatinine}} \times 100$$

should be < 1%. This physiological response is altered when the patient is administered diuretics in the form of furosemide or mannitol or has glucosuria. To differentiate between prerenal and renal forms of ARF, especially when the patient has received a diuretic, fractional excretion of urea is more specific and sensitive than that of sodium.

Other urinary indices are shown in **Table 4**.[32]

Biomarkers

A number of biomarkers have been proposed and are being studied for the early diagnosis of AKI. They are expected to detect "subclinical AKI" so that preventive measures can be taken early. Serum cystatin C and neutrophil gelatinase-associated lipocalin (NGAL) are the two biomarkers that have been shown to be early markers of renal injury. The levels of these markers change earlier than those of serum creatinine and also change with treatment and, thus help in monitoring the progress as well. These two biomarkers represent different aspects of renal injury, namely GFR by cystatin C and tubular stress or injury by NGAL.

TABLE 4: The most important urinary variables in the differential diagnosis between prerenal and renal forms of acute renal failure.

Urine analysis	Prerenal	Renal
Specific gravity of urine	> 1,020	1,010 approx
Osmolality (mOsm/kg H_2O) of urine	> 500	< 350
Urinary sodium concentration (mmol/L)	< 20	> 40
Fractional excretion of sodium (%)	< 1	> 2
Fractional excretion of urea (%)	< 35	> 35
Fractional excretion of uric acid (%)	< 7	> 15
Fractional excretion of lithium (%)	< 7	> 20
Low molecular weight proteins	Low	High
Brush border enzymes	Low	High
Ratio of urinary to plasma creatinine	> 40	< 20
Ratio of urinary to plasma osmolality	> 1.5	< 1.1
Urinary sediment	Hyaline and fine granular casts	Coarsely granular and cellular casts

Source: Adapted and modified from Lameire et al. (2005).[32]

Cystatin C is a protease inhibitor with a low molecular weight located in nucleated cells that is freely filtered through the glomeruli but not actively secreted (in contrast to creatinine). Its levels are increased even in the early stages with the impairment of GFR and are not affected by age, sex, or muscle mass.

Neutrophil gelatinase-associated lipocalin, a protein found in very low concentrations in the kidney, lung, stomach, colon, etc., and produced rapidly in the renal tubules in response to acute injury, can be easily detected in plasma and urine. Several studies have shown elevated cystatin C and NGAL levels to be associated with the development of AKI. However, there are conflicting reports. In one study, levels of serum creatinine, cystatin C, urine, and plasma NGAL were measured every 2 hours from admission to 48 hours in severely burned patients, and all four were found to be predictive of early AKI and early death at all points of time. The NGAL levels, however, were increased earlier after admission, while serum creatinine and cystatin C increased only 12 hours after admission.[33] Conversely, in another study, serum creatinine, cystatin C, and plasma NGAL were serially measured for a week, and it was found that serum creatinine and cystatin C identified patients at risk for AKI earlier than did NGAL.[19] Thus, more studies are needed to determine if cystatin C or NGAL can be a valuable tool for burn patients.

A pair of cell cycle arrest biomarkers, namely tissue inhibitor of metalloproteinases-2 (TIMP-2) and insulin-like growth factor-binding protein 7 (IGFBP7), are being studied to diagnose AKI.

PREVENTION OF ACUTE RENAL FAILURE

Several decades of extensive research at clinical and fundamental levels on the etiopathogenesis of AKI in thermal injury have shown that a burn injury complicated by renal failure has a greater overall morbidity and mortality. Hence, as is true for the burn injury itself, prevention of AKI should be the desired goal of every clinician. This will obviate the need for RRT and its associated complications and costs. While prevention is in every clinician's domain, once the failure sets in, a nephrologist must be called upon by the burn surgeon for appropriate and specialized management. One must remember the various risk factors associated with AKI and take appropriate steps. Various nonpharmacological and pharmacological strategies have been devised and used, apart from some novel therapies.

Nonpharmacological Strategies for Prevention of Acute Renal Failure

Fluids

An early and adequate fluid therapy is crucial in maintaining renal function in extensively burnt patients. Even a general practitioner, in a comparatively remote area, who sees the patient first should be able to start an intravenous drip and infuse fluids before the patient is transported to an appropriate burn care facility. Intravascular volume correction is the single most important factor in preventing renal failure. With the widespread availability of cheap intravenous fluids, the incidence of renal failure in burns due to hypovolemic causes has certainly come down over the decades. Various formulae, e.g., Parkland or Brooks, are available and used as guidelines. Once the patient is considered euvolemic, care must be taken to avoid fluid overload, and a maintenance regimen started, which takes account of renal and insensible losses, accounting for a positive balance of 500 mL/day. Hourly input should equal the previous hour's output plus 25 mL. This requires accurate observation and record-keeping by the nursing staff and reassessment by the doctors.

Nephrotoxin Exposure

Minimal nephrotoxin exposure is an important strategy to prevent ARF. Antibiotics like aminoglycosides, amphotericin B, vancomycin, etc., should be used carefully with regular monitoring of renal function, and if possible, serum levels of these drugs should also be monitored. It is important to avoid drugs like NSAIDs and ACE inhibitors during the prerenal phase of ARF.

Pharmacological Strategies for Prevention of Acute Renal Failure

Dopamine

Low-dose dopamine administration (1–3 µg/kg/min) to healthy individuals causes renal vasodilation with increased renal perfusion, natriuresis, and increased GFR. Because of these effects, it has been given as a prophylaxis for AKI. Recent studies, including large randomized controlled trials, have shown it to lack efficacy on renal outcome or overall mortality. The use of dopamine may also reduce splanchnic perfusion, depress respiration, suppress anterior pituitary hormone release and function, and worsen renal function in hypovolemic or normovolemic patients. Its routine use in ARF is not currently justified.

Diuretics

There is a theoretical rationale for the use of loop diuretics (e.g., furosemide) in ARF—inhibition of Na^+/ K^+/Cl^- pump in the thick ascending limb of the loop of Henle, with subsequent decrease in Na^+/K^+-ATPase activity, should reduce the oxygen requirement of these cells and thus their susceptibility to ischemic damage. It might also hasten recovery from AKI by washing out necrotic debris blocking the tubules and by inhibiting prostaglandin dehydrogenase, which reduces renovascular resistance and increases renal blood flow. However, there is scarce clinical data to support this, and recent studies have either correlated the use of diuretics with increased mortality or shown no benefit. It seems reasonable to use diuretics only in adequately resuscitated oliguric patients at a dose suitable to the degree of renal impairment (250 mg furosemide intravenous over 1 hour is a standard regimen) and to stop diuretics if oliguria persists. Converting oliguric to nonoliguric renal failure may help with fluid and electrolyte management, but it does not seem to affect the eventual need for dialysis or overall mortality and should not delay the start of RRT.

Other Novel Therapies

Various agents have been studied for potential use in the prevention of ATN, e.g., fenoldopam, atrial natriuretic peptide (ANP), theophylline, N-acetylcysteine, calcium-channel blockers, epidermal and insulin-like growth factors, scavengers of oxygen-free radicals and prostaglandins, erythropoietin, etc. None of these novel therapies have been proven to be effective or safe for humans with ARF.

MANAGEMENT OF ACUTE RENAL FAILURE

When a burn patient develops ARF and the kidneys can no longer maintain homeostasis with respect to load of metabolic acid and waste products, fluid, potassium, etc., a number of life-threatening complications frequently begin. Initially, management is based on supportive care, as there is no definitive pharmacological treatment. However, once this also fails, extracorporeal techniques for purification of blood, of which there are several ways (grouped under the common term RRT), need to be initiated before uremic complications emerge:

Supportive Treatment

The aim of supportive treatment of ARF in burns is to prevent further fall in renal function. It mainly consists of maintaining metabolism, taking care of life-threatening complications like hyperkalemia, pulmonary edema, metabolic acidosis, nutrition of the patient, and treatment of infections.

Fluid Balance

An accurate fluid balance should be maintained by daily measurements of body weight and input/output. In oliguric patients, daily fluid intake should be limited to 500 mL plus the previous day's urinary output unless there are signs of volume depletion/overload. Dietary sodium is restricted to 2 g/day. In the absence of hyperalimentation, an individual with ATN is expected to lose 0.3–0.5 kg body weight daily. If this expected weight loss does not occur or if there is weight gain, fluid therapy must be reassessed. Hyponatremia might necessitate stringent free water restrictions.

Acidosis

Severe metabolic acidosis (pH < 7.0) often occurs once ARF develops and arises through a variety of mechanisms related to both reduced renal function and the underlying cause of illness. Systemic acidosis impairs cardiac contractility, induces bradycardia, produces vasodilatation, and augments hyperkalemia. Reversing acidosis through the administration of sodium bicarbonate solution seems sensible, although there is very little evidence to show that it provides benefit. It can cause volume overload by increasing the sodium load. Hemodialysis or hemofiltration is usually required to treat severe acidosis in oligoanuric patients.

Hyperkalemia

Hyperkalemia is defined as serum potassium levels of > 5.5 mmol/L. Severe hyperkalemia (i.e., serum potassium > 6.5 mmol/L) is a medical emergency because of the risk of cardiac arrhythmias. Emergency treatment of hyperkalemia primarily dictated by changes in ECG includes the use of intravenous calcium, driving potassium into the cells with glucose and insulin, or nebulization with salbutamol. If these measures fail, emergency dialysis is indicated to save the patient's life. The treatment of hyperkalemia is summarized in **Table 5.**[34]

Pulmonary Edema

An oligoanuric patient with pulmonary edema resulting from fluid overload represents a clinical challenge. If significant ventilatory failure is present, supplementary oxygen, noninvasive ventilation or intubation and ventilation are to be started. Pharmacological treatment to offload the decompensated heart can be started in the form of intravenous opioids (diamorphine 2.5 mg) and intravenous infusion of nitrate (glyceryl trinitrate 50 mg in 50 mL of 0.9% saline at a rate of 2–20 mL/h, keeping the systolic blood pressure > 95 mm Hg) and attempts to provoke diuresis by furosemide 250 mg in 100 mL saline over 1 hour. If these measures fail, immediate hemodialysis or hemofiltration is to be done.

Nutritional Support

The goal of nutritional support is to preserve lean body mass, maintain immunocompetence, offer substrate for the acute inflammatory state, and help promote wound

TABLE 5: Summary of treatment strategies in hyperkalemia.[34]

Treatment	Immediacy of action	Reduction in K^+	Duration of action
10% calcium gluconate: 10–20 mL I/V over 2–5 minutes	1–3 minutes	Nil	30–60 minutes
Insulin/glucose 10 units plain insulin in 50 mL of 50% dextrose infused over 10–20 minutes	15–30 minutes	0.65–1.0 mmol/L	4–6 hours
Salbutamol (nebulized/intravenous) 10–20 mg via nebulizer or 0.5 mg IV	30 minutes	0.6–1.0 mmol/L	2–4 hours
Ion exchange resin 15 g three times a day orally	2–3 hours	0.5–1.0 mmol/g resin	4–6 hours
Hemodialysis	Immediate	< 1.5 mmol/L	When dialysis is ongoing

healing. It is an important part of the treatment of the burnt patient as a whole, with or without renal failure. As these patients are in a hypercatabolic state due to both burns and ARF, they are to be given a hypercaloric diet. This intake must be without excessive volume. Carbohydrate intake should be sufficient (>100 g/day) to avoid the breakdown of endogenous proteins for glucose. A combination of carbohydrates and lipids should be used. These patients also require enough protein of high quality. As far as possible, enteral feeding should be preferred over parenteral feeds. Fulfilling the nutritional requirement may not be possible without dialytic support.

Renal Replacement Therapy

In the last 25 years, RRT for the management of ARF has become routine.[35-37] There are three factors that need consideration:

1. Timing of the initiation of RRT
2. Selection of the specific modality of RRT
3. Dose or intensity of renal support

Timing of Initiation

The question of when to initiate renal replacement in renal failure has been debated since the time hemodialysis became available to clinicians. This is because of the benefits of earlier versus the risks of unnecessary treatment. There is no clarity as to what constitutes "early" as opposed to "late" therapy. With the technology for RRT becoming safer and treatment becoming routine, what was once considered "early" may now fall under "late" initiation of RRT.

The risks associated with RRT include catheter-related complications from insertion and infection and mechanical complications associated with the extracorporeal circuit (risk of severe blood loss, electrolyte disturbances, and hemodynamic compromise due to fluid and electrolyte shifts). Humoral and cellular mediators may be activated by exposure to extracorporeal circuits. Exposure of blood to bioincompatible surfaces of the circuit and recurrent episodes of dialysis-associated hypotension may delay recovery of the kidney function. Lastly, the financial implications of earlier initiation of treatment must also be considered.

Too soon is better than too late, and the treatment should be started before complications occur. In general, the indications for dialysis fall into three broad categories, namely (1) solute indications, e.g., marked azotemia; (2) volume indications, e.g., fluid overload; or (3) both. The following are the criteria for starting RRT: (1) Oliguria, with urine output <200 mL/12 hours; (2) anuria, with urine output <50 mL/12 hours; (3) hyperkalemia, serum potassium >6.5 mmol/L; (4) severe acidosis, pH <7; (5) azotemia, blood urea >200 mg/dL; (6) complications of severe uremia, namely encephalopathy, pericarditis, neuropathy, myopathy, etc.; (7) plasma sodium >155 mmol/L or <120 mmol/L; and (8) pulmonary edema.

Selection of the Specific Modality (Mode of RRT, Dialysis)[38]

As there are several techniques available, there is controversy about the selection of the best modality for a given patient. Dialysis is a process in which molecules from one solution (i.e., blood) diffuse across a semipermeable membrane into another solution (i.e., dialysate).[38] This membrane can be either biological (peritoneum) or artificial (hemodialysis or hemofiltration). This transfer of solute across the membrane is determined by the characteristics of the membrane and the solute concentration on the two sides. The movement of small-molecular-weight solutes from the blood to dialysate under the driving force of an electrochemical gradient is called diffusive clearance. Convective clearance (ultrafiltration), on the other hand, occurs when water is driven across the membrane by hydrostatic/osmotic forces. Solutes that can pass through the membrane pores move along with water (solute drag).

Vascular access: For hemodialysis, good vascular access is required to withdraw the blood from the patient, to be passed through a dialyzer and then returned. Effective vascular access can be in the form of placing one catheter in an artery and another in a vein. A double-lumen catheter can be placed in a central vein like the femoral, internal jugular, or subclavian, and blood can be withdrawn through one lumen and returned through the other with the help of a pump.

Anticoagulation: To avoid clotting in a dialysis membrane, circuit tubing, or at the vascular access, anticoagulants are generally required in patients undergoing dialysis. These are generally in the form of unfractionated heparins or low-molecular-weight heparins. Regional citrate anticoagulation or frequent saline flushing of the system is also used in patients in whom heparin cannot be used.

Types of dialysis modalities: Two types of dialysis modalities are available: (1) Intermittent therapy, extracorporeal dialysis, where the patient is treated for <24 hours, and (2) continuous therapy [(continuous renal replacement therapy (CRRT)], again an extracorporeal dialysis, where the patient is treated for 24 hours or more.[39] These modalities are detailed in **Table 6.**[38]

Which modality to be used?

Both the modalities have their advantages and disadvantages, as shown in **Table 7.**[34] Various studies have proved that both modalities are equally effective in treating such patients. Mortality rates are also similar

TABLE 6: Dialysis modalities for acute renal failure.

Intermittent therapies	Continuous therapies (CRRT)
Hemodialysis	Peritoneal dialysis
Hemofiltration	Ultrafiltration (SCUF)
Ultrafiltration	Hemofiltration (CAVH, CVVH)
EDD	• Hemodialysis (CAVHD, CVVHD) • Hemodiafiltration (CAVHDF, CVVHDF)
SLED	

(CAVH: continuous arteriovenous hemofiltration; CAVHD: continuous arteriovenous hemodialysis; CAVHDF: continuous arteriovenous hemodiafiltration; CVVH: continuous venovenous hemofiltration; CVVHD: continuous venovenous hemodialysis; CVVHDF: continuous venovenous hemodiafiltration; EDD: extended daily dialysis; SCUF: slow continuous ultrafiltration; SLED: slow low-efficiency dialysis)

Source: Adapted and modified from Abdeen and Mehta (2002).[38]

TABLE 7: Advantages and disadvantages of intermittent versus continuous renal replacement therapy.

	Intermittent hemodialysis	Continuous renal replacement therapy
Advantages	• Lower risk of systemic bleeding • More time available for diagnostic and therapeutic interventions • More suitable in severe hyperkalemia • Low cost	• Better hemodynamic stability • Fewer cardiac arrhythmias • Better pulmonary gas exchange • Better fluid control • Better biochemical control
Disadvantages	• Availability of dialysis staff • More difficult hemodynamic control • Inadequate dialysis dose • Inadequate fluid control • Inadequate nutritional support • Poor removal of inflammatory mediators	• Shorter stay in ICU • Good removal of inflammatory mediators • Can be done at bed side • Greater vascular access problem • Higher risk of systemic bleeding • Long term immobilization of patient • More filter problem • Higher cost

Source: Adapted and modified from Fry and Farrington (2006).[34]

for both modalities. The use of a particular modality depends upon the patient's condition, the availability of infrastructure at a particular center, the availability of trained manpower, and the experience of physicians and nurses in handling such patients. Peritoneal dialysis may not be possible in burn patients as the area may be burnt and the chances of infection are also greater.[40]

Intermittent therapies may be useful if more solute is to be removed, as in patients with sepsis. Intermittent therapy also leaves time for any surgical procedure(s) that might be required in such patients. If fluid removal is a major concern, continuous therapies are more useful, and a lot of fluid can be removed to help give the drugs and nutritional support to such patients. In hemodynamically unstable patients who have low blood pressure, continuous therapy is more useful. For burn patients, CVVHD or CVVH is the therapy of choice for most of the patients.[41,42]

Dose of Dialysis

This is how much dialysis has to be given to the patient. In ESRD, a KT/V of 1.2 per treatment is the acceptable minimum dose. Here K represents urea clearance, T is the time of dialysis, and V is the volume of urea distribution. Patients with ESRD have a relatively constant urea generation rate and are in a steady state. Patients with ARF tend to have a fluctuating body fluid composition and varying urea generation rates. These formulae may not always be correct. Nonetheless, three treatments per week with a KT/V of 1.2 seem good enough for ARF patients. Some studies have suggested that daily dialysis may be more useful for early recovery of these patients.

In CRRT, the dose of therapy is correlated with the effluent flow rate. There are studies comparing higher ultrafiltration rates with low ultrafiltration rates, but the results are conflicting. There is some consensus that ultrafiltration rates of 35 mL/kg/h show better results.

OUTCOME AND PROGNOSIS

The outcome of burn patients with AKI is poor. These patients require prolonged hospital stays, prolonged ICU treatment, greater need for ventilators, and prolonged stay on ventilators. Progressive renal injury, as suggested by RIFLE criteria, has poorer outcomes. Despite much progress in treatment modalities, mortality in a burn patient with ARF requiring renal replacement remains high, and in various studies, it is around 80%. The prognosis of severely burned patients with ARF has not improved for the last 50 years. It may be because of the fact that the burn patients developing ARF generally have multiorgan failure, resulting in high mortality. Early fluid resuscitation and the prevention of sepsis may reduce the incidence of acute renal dysfunction and mortality in burns.[43]

SUMMARY

Of all the viscera, kidney is most likely to be damaged in extensive burns because of a marked shift of intravascular fluid into the interstitial spaces all over the body resulting in hypovolemia and decreased circulation leading, in turn, to a decreased renal perfusion. ARF is one of the most devastating complication of burns with greatly increased morbidity and a high mortality rate. Over the last two decades, definition of ARF has been standardized. Depending upon the interval between the time of burn injury and the onset of ARF, two different forms of AKI, early onset and late onset having different etiologies, have been described in burn patients. Apart from measurement of blood urea, serum creatinine and examination of urine, a number of biomarkers have been isolated and studied to diagnose the problem early in subclinical state. Prevention of ARF is most important and it can be done even at a general practitioner level (first responder) by infusing electrolyte solutions available even in remote places. Once the patient reaches an appropriate medical facility, various nonpharmacological and drug therapies are available to minimize the renal damage and maintain normal renal function. Once, ARF sets in, RRT has to be instituted in association with a nephrologist who has various forms of dialysis therapies available at his disposal to select the most appropriate for the patient. Despite much progress in treatment modalities, mortality in patients requiring RRT remains as high as 80%. The prognosis has not improved in the last 50 years emphasizing the need for prevention of ARF.

REFERENCES

1. Aikawa N, Wakabayashi G, Ueda M, Shinozawa Y. Regulation of renal function in thermal injury. J Trauma. 1990;30(12 Suppl):S174-8.
2. Emara SS, Alzaylai AA. Renal failure in burn patients: A review. Ann Burns Fire Disasters. 2013;26(1):12-5.
3. Ko A, Song J, Golovko G, El Ayadi A, Ozhathil DK, Wermine K, et al. Higher risk of acute kidney injury and death with rhabdomyolysis in severely burned patients. Surgery. 2022;171(5):1412-6.
4. Bellomo R, Kellum JA, Ronco C. Acute kidney injury. Lancet. 2012;380(9843):756-66.
5. Mustonen KM, Vuola J. Acute renal failure in intensive care burn patients (ARF in burn patients). J Burn Care Res. 2008;29(1):227-37.
6. Coca SG, Bauling P, Schifftner T, Howard CS, Teitelbaum I, Parikh CR. Contribution of acute kidney injury toward morbidity and mortality in burns: A contemporary analysis. Am J Kidney Dis. 2007;49(4):517-23.
7. Thomas ME, Blaine C, Dawnay A, Devonald MA, Ftouh S, Laing C, et al. The definition of acute kidney injury and its use in practice. Kidney Int. 2015;87(1):62-73.
8. Lopes JA, Jorge S. The RIFLE and AKIN classifications for acute kidney injury: A critical and comprehensive review. Clin Kidney J. 2013;6(1):8-14.
9. Gameiro J, Fonseca JA, Outerelo C, Lopes JA. Acute kidney injury: From diagnosis to prevention and treatment strategies. J Clin Med. 2020;9(6):1704.
10. Bellomo R, Ronco C, Kellum JA, Mehta RL, Palevsky P; Acute Dialysis Quality Initiative Workgroup. Acute renal failure-definition, outcome measures, animal models, fluid therapy and information technology needs: The Second International Consensus Conference of the Acute Dialysis Quality Initiative (ADQI) Group. Crit Care. 2004;8(4):R204-12.
11. Bellomo R. Defining, quantifying, and classifying acute renal failure. Crit Care Clin. 2005;21(2):223-37.
12. Lopes JA, Jorge S, Neves FC, Caneira M, da Costa AG, Ferreira AC, et al. An assessment of the RIFLE criteria for acute renal failure in severely burned patients. Nephrol Dial Transplant. 2007;22(1):285.
13. Mehta RL, Kellum JA, Shah SV, Molitoris BA, Ronco C, Warnock DG, et al. Acute Kidney Injury Network: Report of an initiative to improve outcomes in acute kidney injury. Crit Care. 2007;11(2):R31.
14. Chung KK, Stewart IJ, Gisler C, Simmons JW, Aden JK, Tilley MA, et al. The Acute Kidney Injury Network (AKIN) criteria applied in burns. J Burn Care Res. 2012;33(4):483-90.
15. KDIGO Clinical Practice Guideline for Acute Kidney Injury. Section 2: AKI Definition. Kidney Int Suppl. 2012;2(1):19-36.
16. Clark A, Neyra JA, Madni T, Imran J, Phelan H, Arnoldo B, et al. Acute kidney injury after burn. Burns. 2017;43(5):898-908.
17. Murray PT, Mehta RL, Shaw A, Ronco C, Endre Z, Kellum JA, et al. Potential use of biomarkers in acute kidney injury: report and summary of recommendations from the 10th Acute Dialysis Quality Initiative consensus conference. Kidney Int. 2014;85(3):513-21.

18. Wu G, Xiao Y, Wang C, Hong X, Sun Y, Ma B, et al. Risk factors for acute kidney injury in patients with burn injury: A meta-analysis and systematic review. J Burn Care Res. 2017;38(5):271-82.
19. Rakkolainen I, Lindbohm JV, Vuola J. Factors associated with acute kidney injury in the Helsinki Burn Centre in 2006-2015. Scand J Trauma Resusc Emerg Med. 2018;26(1):105.
20. Kuvvet Yoldaş T, Atalay A, Balcı C, Demirağ K, Uyar M, Çankayalı İ. Acute kidney injury in burns in the intensive care unit: A retrospective research. Ulus Travma Acil Cerrahi Derg. 2023;29(3):321-6.
21. Folkestad T, Brurberg KG, Nordhuus KM, Tveiten CK, Guttormsen AB, Os I, et al. Acute kidney injury in burn patients admitted to the intensive care unit: A systematic review and meta-analysis. Crit Care. 2020;24(1):2.
22. Chen B, Zhao J, Zhang Z, Li G, Jiang H, Huang Y, et al. Clinical characteristics and risk factors for severe burns complicated by early acute kidney injury. Burns. 2020;46(5):1100-6.
23. Hilton R. Acute renal failure. BMJ. 2006;333(7572):786-90.
24. Pickkers P, Darmon M, Hoste E, Joannidis M, Legrand M, Ostermann M, et al. Acute kidney injury in the critically ill: An updated review on pathophysiology and management. Intensive Care Med. 2021;47(8):835-50.
25. Brusselaers N, Hoste EA. Acute kidney injury in patients with severe burn injury. In: Turner NN, Lameire N, Goldsmith DJ, Winearls CG, Himmelfarb J, Remuzzi G (Eds). Oxford Textbook of Clinical Nephrology, 4th edition. Oxford: Oxford University Press; 2016. pp. 2151-7 (Chapter 253).
26. Bellomo R, Wan L, Langenberg C, May C. Septic acute kidney injury: New concepts. Nephron Exp Nephrol. 2008;109(4):e95-e100.
27. Wan L, Bellomo R, Giantomassoa DD, Ronco C. The pathogenesis of septic acute renal failure. Curr Opin Crit Care. 2003;9:496-502.
28. Witkowski W, Kawecki M, Surowiecka-Pastewka A, Klimm W, Szamotulska K, Niemczyk S. Early and late acute kidney injury in severely burned patients. Med Sci Monit. 2016;22:3755-63.
29. Langenberg C, Wan L, Egi M, May CN, Bellomo R. Renal blood flow in experimental septic acute renal failure. Kidney Int. 2006;69(11):1996-2002.
30. Colpaert K, Hoste EA. Acute kidney injury in burns: A story of volume and inflammation. Crit Care. 2008;12(6):192.
31. Steinvall I, Bak Z, Sjoberg F. Acute kidney injury is common, parallels organ dysfunction or failure, and carries appreciable mortality in patients with major burns: A prospective exploratory cohort study. Crit Care. 2008;12(5):R124.
32. Lameire N, Van Biesen W, Vanholder R. Acute renal failure. Lancet. 2005;365(9457):417-30.
33. Yang HT, Yim H, Cho YS, Kym D, Hur J, Kim JH, et al. Assessment of biochemical markers in the early post-burn period for predicting acute kidney injury and mortality in patients with major burn injury: Comparison of serum creatinine, serum cystatin-C, plasma and urine neutrophil gelatinase-associated lipocalin. Crit Care. 2014;18(4):R151.
34. Fry AC, Farrington K. Management of acute renal failure. Postgrad Med J. 2006;82(964):106-16.
35. Alvarez G, Chrusch C, Hulme T, Posadas-Calleja JG. Renal replacement therapy: A practical update. Can J Anaesth. 2019;66(5):593-604.
36. Palevsky PM. Renal replacement therapy in acute kidney injury. Adv Chronic Kidney Dis. 2013;20(1):76-84.
37. Demsey D, Mordhorst A, Griesdale DEG, Papp A. Improved outcomes of renal injury following burn trauma. Burns. 2019;45(5):1024-30.
38. Abdeen O, Mehta RL. Dialysis modalities in the intensive care unit. Crit Care Clin. 2002;18(2):223-47.
39. Holm C, Hörbrand F, von Donnersmarck GH, Mühlbauer W. Acute renal failure in severely burned patients. Burns. 1999;25(2):171-8.
40. Ibrahim AE, Sarhane KA, Fagan SP, Goverman J. Renal dysfunction in burns: A review. Ann Burns Fire Dis. 2013;26(1):16-25.
41. Leblanc M, Thibeault Y, Quérin S. Continuous haemofiltration and haemodiafiltration for acute renal failure in severely burned patients. Burns. 1997;23(2):160-5.
42. Tremblay R, Ethier J, Quérin S, Béroniade V, Falardeau P, Leblanc M. Veno-venous continuous renal replacement therapy for burned patients with acute renal failure. Burns. 2000;26(7):638-43.
43. Chrysopoulo MT, Jeschke MG, Dziewulski P, Barrow RE, Herndon DN. Acute renal dysfunction in severely burned adults. J Trauma. 1999;46(1):141-4.

SECTION

3

Local Care of Burn Wound

CHAPTER

14

Burn Wound Management

Deepti Gupta, Sujata Sarabahi

INTRODUCTION

The survival of a moderate-to-extensively burnt patient depends on the successful management of the burn wound. A burn patient is always at risk as long as his/her wounds persist. There is a general consensus that burn wound infection is the primary cause of morbidity and mortality following an extensive burn injury. Hence, an early wound closure can eliminate not only the risk of infection but also the risk to life of the extensively burnt victim.

After the initial management and resuscitation of a burn patient is complete, the focus shifts to the management of the burn wound. This management requires a careful evaluation of the burn wound and it's nature.

MECHANISM OF WOUND HEALING

Superficial Dermal Burns

Superficial dermal burns involve the papillary layer of dermis and are typically pink and moist with intact hair **(Fig. 1)**. Sensations are retained as the sensory receptors in the deep dermis and hypodermis are spared.[1]

The remaining adnexal elements such as hair follicles, sweat glands, and sebaceous glands aid in re-epithelization of these wounds and such burns spontaneously heal over a period of 3 weeks **(Figs. 2A and B)**. Therefore, these wounds can be managed conservatively in the form of topical antimicrobial creams and dressings, to prevent infection, promote healing, and protect the fragile new epithelium.[2]

Deep Dermal Burns

Deep dermal burns involve the reticular layer and are dry and pearly (waxy) white in color. Hair can be easily pulled out **(Fig. 3)**. Some sensations may be present due to the sparing of sensory receptors in deeper layers of dermis and those in hypodermis.[1]

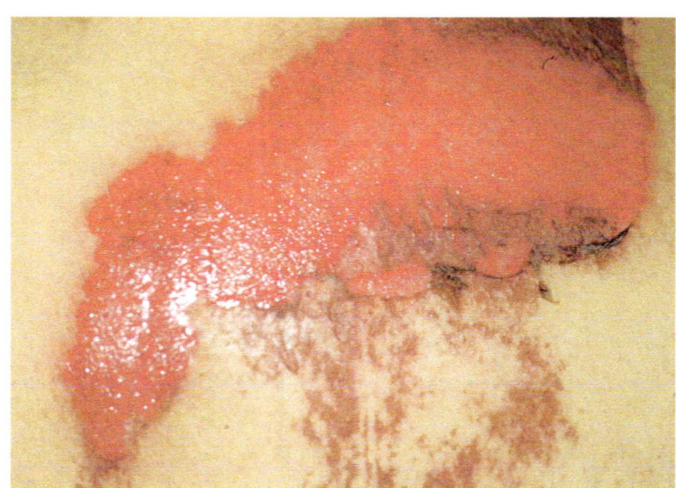

FIG. 1: Superficial dermal or superficial partial thickness burn with moist and red look.

Deeper a burn injury, greater is the loss of adnexal elements and only deeper parts of hair follicles or sweat glands survive. As the eschar separates, epithelial buds emerge from the site of these remaining epidermal appendages and from these tiny islands the neoepithelium proliferates over the wound surface **(Fig. 4)**. As this re-epithelialization is very slow, the healed skin shows hypertrophic scarring later. Superimposed bacterial infection can convert a partial-thickness wound into a full-thickness wound hampering the process of spontaneous healing. Thus, it is imperative to prevent this conversion by appropriate wound care.[2] The primary objective in treating a partial thickness burn injury is to provide an environment that inhibits microbial growth and at the same time promotes wound healing. Hypertrophic scarring can be prevented by early

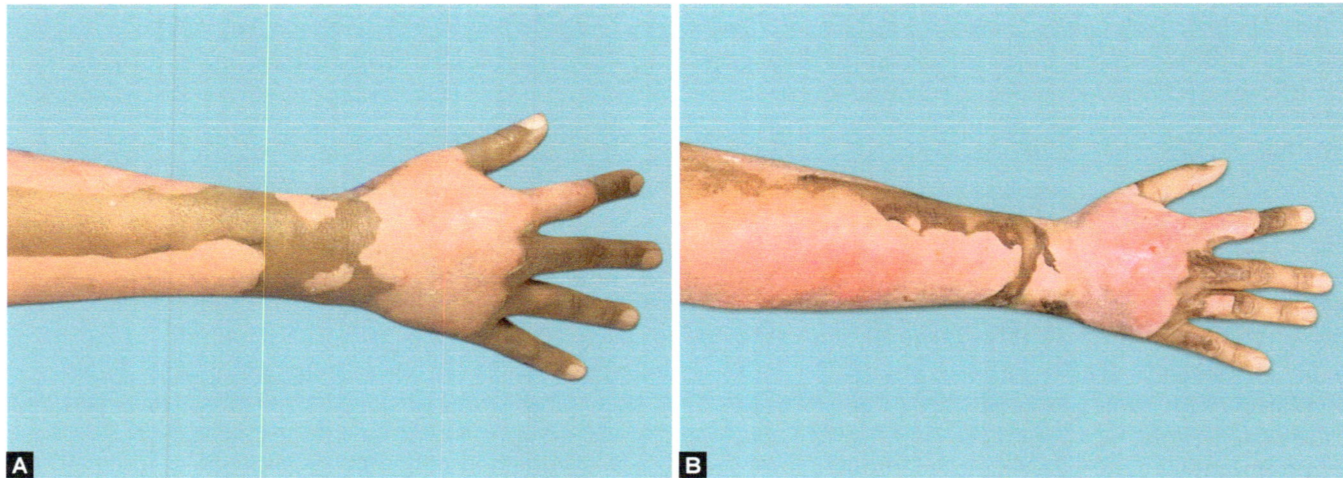

FIGS. 2A AND B: (A) Superficial partial thickness burn; (B) Closed dressing achieved complete healing in 10 days.

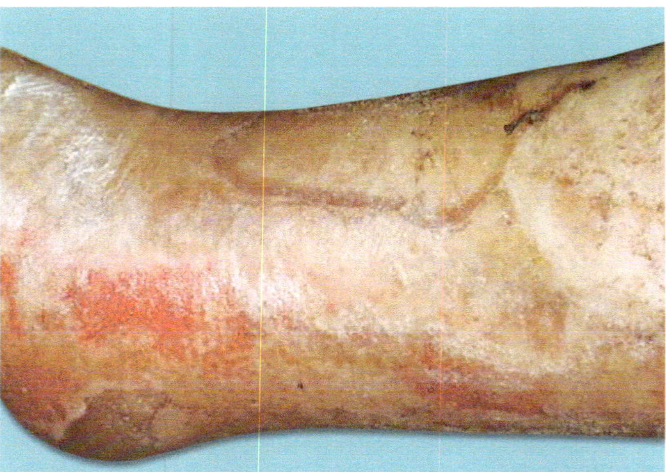

FIG. 3: Deep dermal burns with pearly white look.

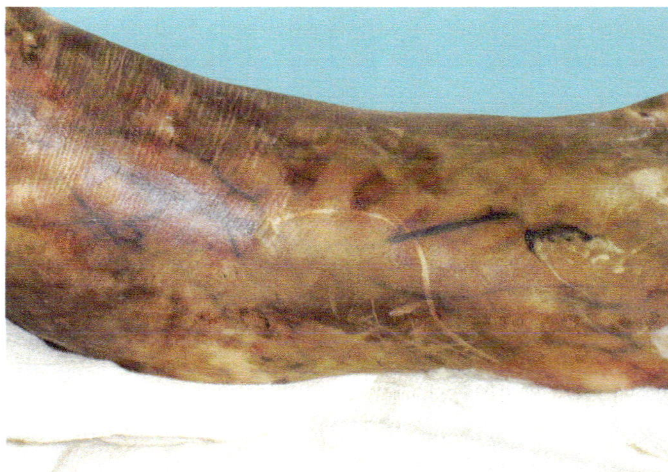

FIG. 5: Full thickness burns with charred look and thrombosed veins.

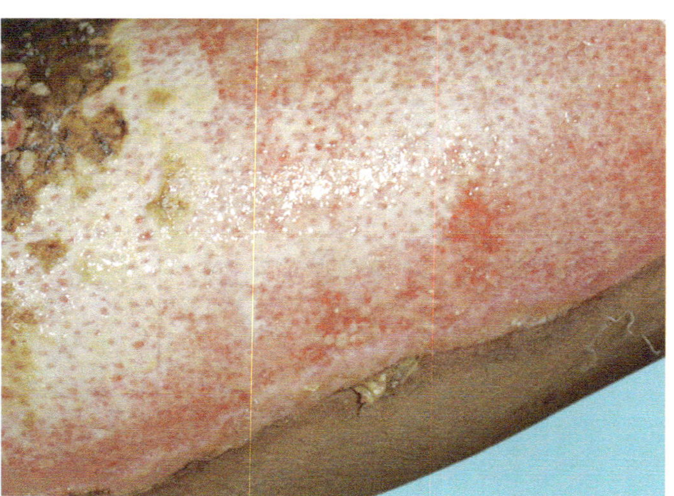

FIG. 4: Epithelialization occurring underneath the eschar, seen once the slough is removed.

tangential excision and resurfacing by skin grafts in such wounds.

Full-thickness Burns

Full-thickness burns **(Fig. 5)**, as the name indicates, involve the whole of epidermis and dermis and appear parchment-like with visible, thrombosed subcutaneous veins. Sensory receptors are completely destroyed resulting in insensate wounds. There are no chances of spontaneous healing as all epidermal elements are lost. In such burns, the dead tissues become dry, firm, and black resulting in eschar formation. Beneath this eschar, cellular and capillary activity in the underlying viable tissues produces a layer of red granulation tissue, which is exposed when the eschar separates. The granulation tissue is totally devoid of epithelial cells, so the healing of a burn raw area can take place only by epithelial migration from the normal surrounding epithelial edge and wound contraction. Initially, this ingrowth is rapid but only for a certain distance after which the cells stop growing. Over flexor aspects of joints or in areas where the skin is loose and contraction is possible, the wound closes on its own with the development of contractures **(Fig. 6)**. In areas where the underlying bone(s) prevent contraction, the granulation tissue remains as a non-healing wound till it is covered with a skin graft/flap **(Fig. 7)**. If these areas are not grafted at the earliest, they go on to develop chronic granulation tissue. Their vascularity reduces, the superficial layers of granulation tissue ooze serum that clots, and this is again invaded by inflammatory cells and capillaries to form fresh granulation tissue. As time passes, the deeper layers progressively mature into fibrous scar tissue with overlying thin granulations. Therefore, to avoid the formation of chronic granulation tissue and to prevent development of contractures, full-thickness wounds need early excision and resurfacing with a skin graft or early closure of raw areas if being managed conservatively.

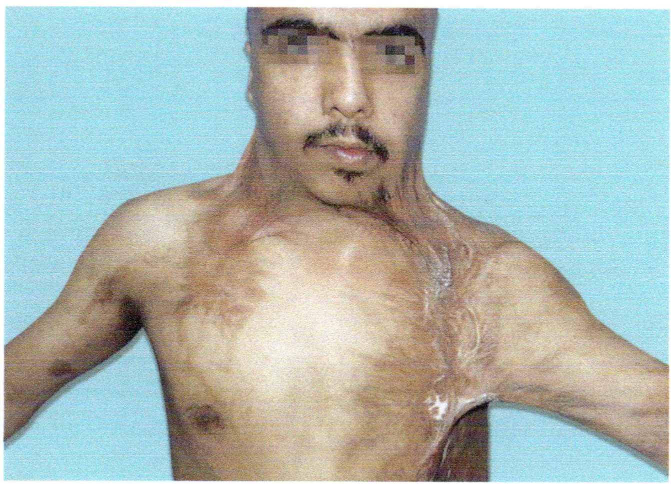

FIG. 6: Wound contraction in full thickness burns—if surgical intervention is not done the wound bed contracts leading to contracture of the neck and axilla.

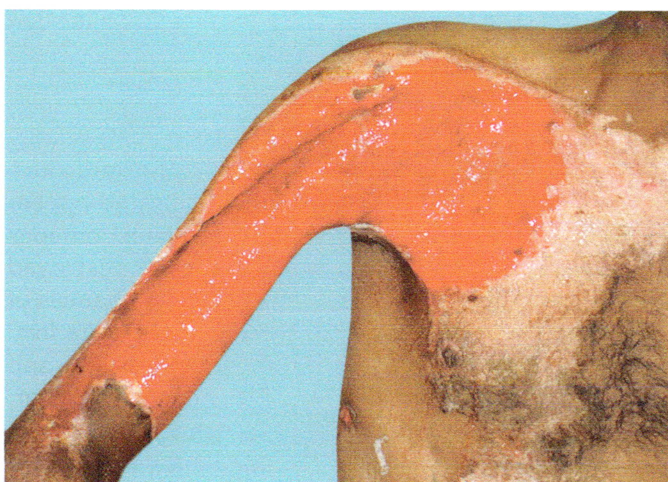

FIG. 7: Granulating wound—shows that epithelialization from the margins stops after a certain distance.

AIMS OF LOCAL BURN WOUND CARE

The basic aims of local burn wound care are:[3]

- Oxygenation of tissues
- Prevention of wound infection and sepsis
- Promotion of healing:
  - Prevention of damage to remaining viable epithelium
  - Prevention of damage to regenerating, delicate neoepithelium
  - Allowing free drainage of exudates from the wound and prevent them from coming in contact with the environment
- Early excision of dead tissue and resurfacing with skin grafts
- Encouragement of spontaneous slough separation in conservatively managed wounds
- Immobilization of the injured area to reduce pain

INITIAL CARE OF BURN WOUND

Once the resuscitation procedures have been initiated, the burnt area has to be evaluated in detail for its extent and depth. It is preferable to shift the patient to a specified dressing room where the wound can be managed with all aseptic precautions. This is important because immediately following burns the skin surface is sterile as all surface bacteria are killed by the heat. One should avoid introducing exogenous bacteria to the wound by all means in order to avoid burn wound infection. Initial burn wound care involves:[4]

- Cleaning and debridement
- Burn wound assessment
- Ensuring adequate oxygenation of tissues
- Dressing of the burn wound:
  - Open or exposure method
  - Occlusive or semi-occlusive method

Cleaning and Debridement

The area is thoroughly washed with an antiseptic solution and normal saline to remove all the debris. All the loose nonviable tissues are removed with minimum trauma. Management of blisters remains controversial. Theoretically, the fluid in an intact blister is sterile. However, it is rich in proteins that cause it to set into a gelatinous form, which is an ideal culture medium for bacterial growth if the fluid happens to get contaminated. This fluid retards the local immunity by impairing the normal function of inflammatory cells and also retards the fibrinolytic process, thus delaying wound healing.[5] While very small blisters (<5 cm) may be allowed to be kept intact, the larger blisters (>5 cm) run the risk of rupture and are preferably deroofed at the time of initial dressing. Another way to manage blisters is to aspirate them with a needle to allow the blister membrane to stick to the wound. Some authors consider the blister skin as dead and necrotic tissue and prefer to deroof all blisters **(Figs. 8A and B)**.

Burn Wound Assessment

After a thorough cleaning, a proper appraisal of the depth of burns is done and it should be properly charted in the "burn chart" for future reference **(Fig. 9)**. This chart contains detailed observations of the wound. Any surgical procedure performed can also be noted in the chart. Any change in burn wound depth can also be charted in the same form at a later date to follow the progress of the burn wound.

Ensuring Adequate Oxygenation of Tissues

A continuous supply of oxygen is essential for all phases of wound healing. Following burns, the blood supply to the burn wound is reduced because of edema and impaired circulation leading to poor oxygenation of tissues. This reduced tissue oxygenation not only impairs wound healing but also favors bacterial invasion of the wound. The result is that the wound heals poorly and with excessive scarring. To counter this, some burn centers have used hyperbaric oxygen to assist wound healing. However, it has not been used widely.[6,7] Simpler measures can also be taken to ensure adequate oxygenation of burn wounds.

- All encircling bracelets, rings, and other jewelry on the burn victim are removed because they can act as tourniquets once edema sets in, causing distal ischemia.
- Constricting dressings and casts should be avoided, and the burned extremities should be elevated.
- Early escharotomies/fasciotomies should be done to avoid compromising circulation in case of circumferential full-thickness/electrical burns respectively **(Figs. 10A and B)**.

Dressing of the Burn Wound

After cleansing, the wounds are dabbed dry with sterile gauze and then the appropriate method of further wound management is selected, i.e., exposure method (open method) or closed method (occlusive method) of dressing. In most patients, neither of these methods used alone is ideal for local care, and frequently both methods are used in different areas of the body in the same patient for best results.

Open or Exposure Method

The open method of burn treatment has been used since eternity but was reintroduced by Wallace in 1948.[8] It is especially useful for burns of face and perineum, which cannot be adequately dressed. Extensive nonsalvageable burns >90% of total body surface area (TBSA) may also be managed by this method decreasing the requirement for manpower, material, and cost. This technique consists

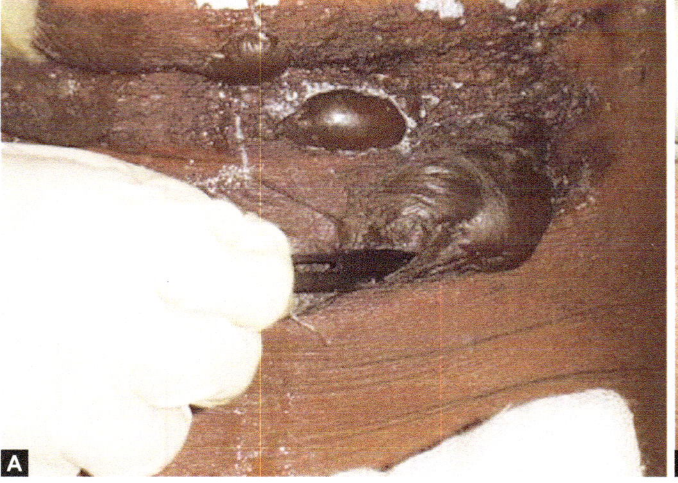

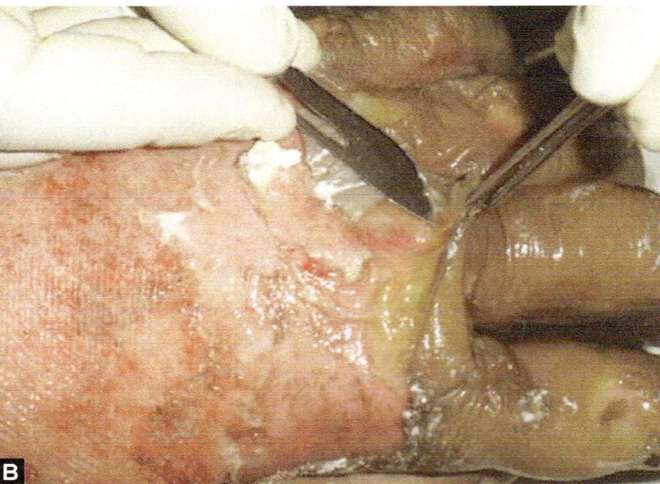

FIGS. 8A AND B: (A) Blister being incised; (B) Deroofing of blister being done surgically—underlying coagulum seen.

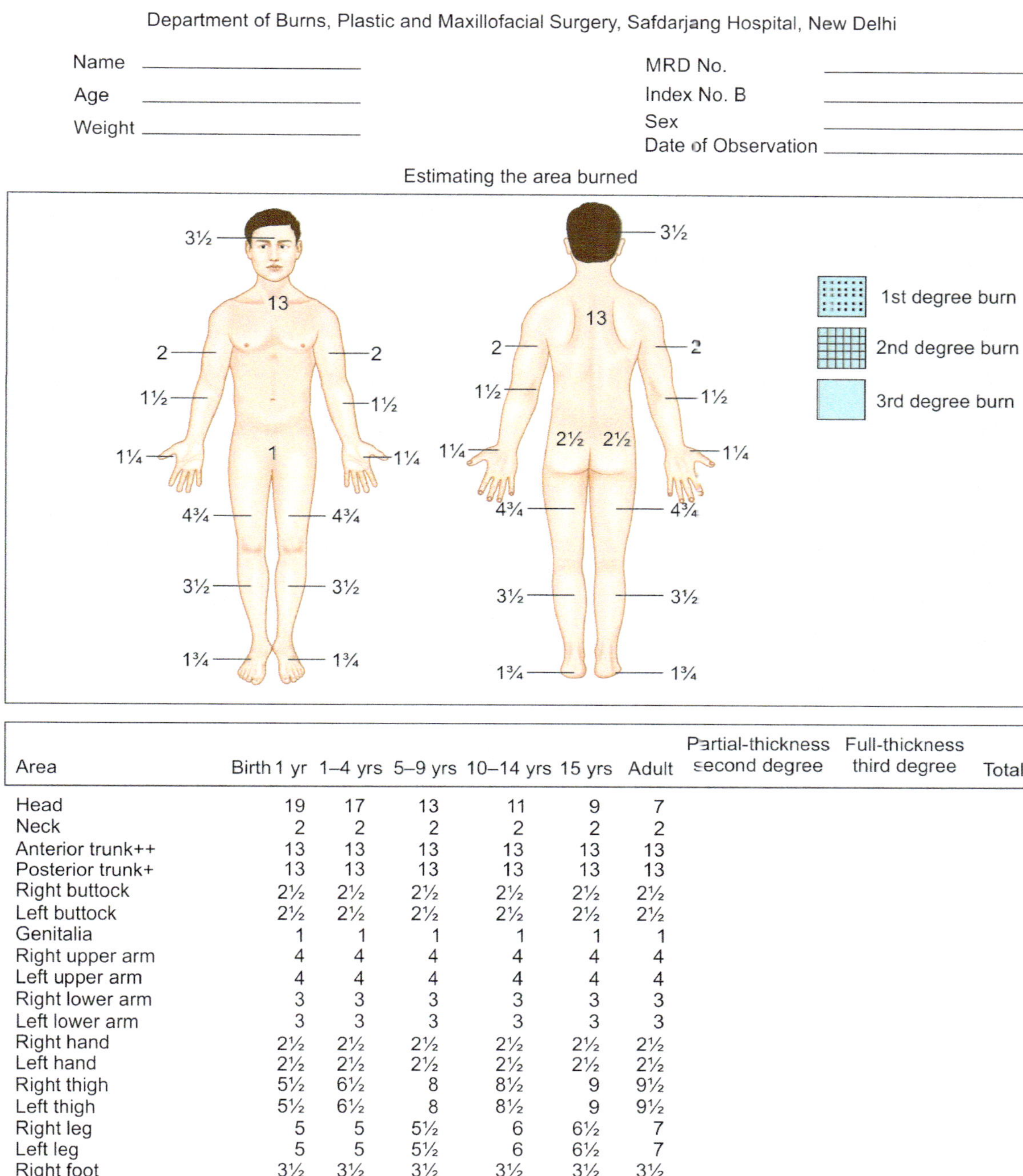

Department of Burns, Plastic and Maxillofacial Surgery, Safdarjang Hospital, New Delhi

Name ____________ MRD No. ____________

Age ____________ Index No. B ____________

Weight ____________ Sex ____________

Date of Observation ____________

Estimating the area burned

Area	Birth 1 yr	1–4 yrs	5–9 yrs	10–14 yrs	15 yrs	Adult	Partial-thickness second degree	Full-thickness third degree	Total
Head	19	17	13	11	9	7			
Neck	2	2	2	2	2	2			
Anterior trunk++	13	13	13	13	13	13			
Posterior trunk+	13	13	13	13	13	13			
Right buttock	2½	2½	2½	2½	2½	2½			
Left buttock	2½	2½	2½	2½	2½	2½			
Genitalia	1	1	1	1	1	1			
Right upper arm	4	4	4	4	4	4			
Left upper arm	4	4	4	4	4	4			
Right lower arm	3	3	3	3	3	3			
Left lower arm	3	3	3	3	3	3			
Right hand	2½	2½	2½	2½	2½	2½			
Left hand	2½	2½	2½	2½	2½	2½			
Right thigh	5½	6½	8	8½	9	9½			
Left thigh	5½	6½	8	8½	9	9½			
Right leg	5	5	5½	6	6½	7			
Left leg	5	5	5½	6	6½	7			
Right foot	3½	3½	3½	3½	3½	3½			
Left foot	3½	3½	3½	3½	3½	3½			
Total									

FIG. 9: Burn chart used in the author's unit—depth of burns in different areas can be charted.

of placing the patient on a clean, dry, sterile sheet under a cradle after cleaning and debriding the wounds. The wounds are left exposed to air without any topical agents or any covering agents. The exudate from the wounds dries up and along with the layers of destroyed skin forms a scab or an eschar. The latter acts as a "dressing" protecting the underlying tissues from bacterial colonization **(Fig. 11A)**. Although the dry cool air inhibits bacterial growth, pathogenic organisms can grow from the deep surface of the crust. Under these circumstances, the activity of the organisms is usually low, and the body is able to fight them and hence, healing can take place. The drying process, however, may retard the spread of epithelium which is faster under moist conditions. For deeper wounds, open treatment may be less satisfactory as the dry eschar takes a long time to separate. The patient

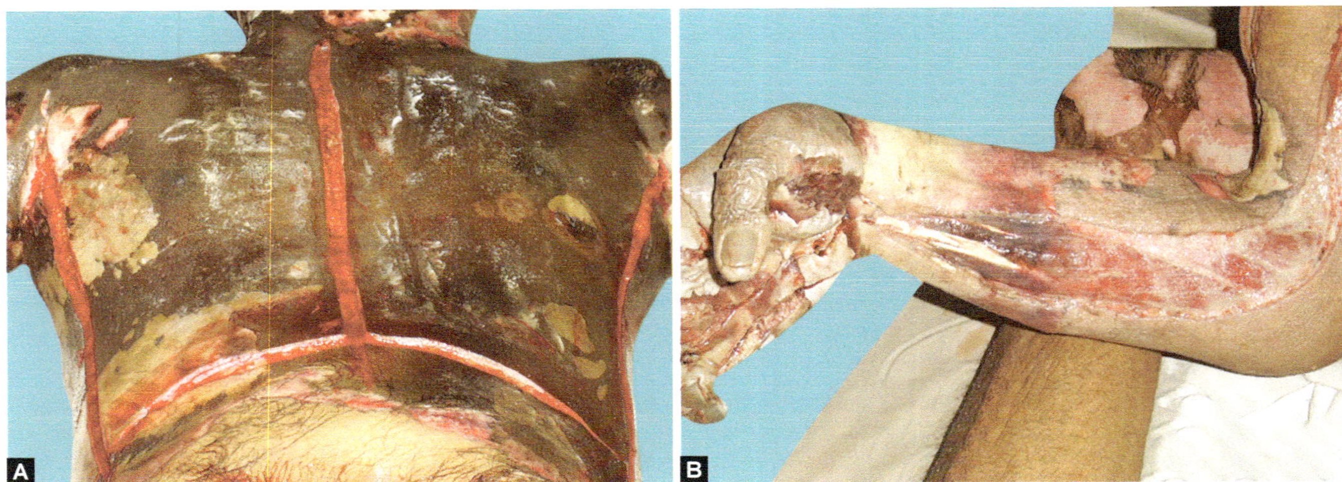

FIGS. 10A AND B: (A) Escharotomy incisions for full-thickness circumferential burn; (B) Fasciotomy incision over arm in electrical contact burn.

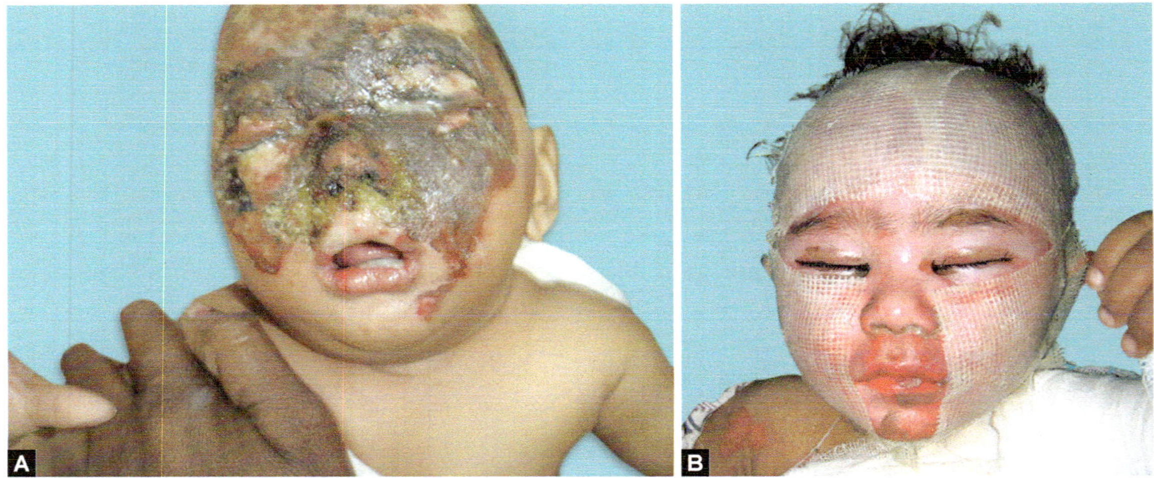

FIGS. 11A AND B: (A) Facial wounds treated by exposure technique–exudates from the wound dry up and form a scab, which acts as an external dressing to protect underlying tissues from infection; (B) Exposure technique but with the application of antibiotic-impregnated paraffin gauze—this transports exudates to the surface of the gauze so that the scab does not adhere to the wound surface and gauze can be removed easily without causing pain or bleeding from the wound surface.

and his/her attendants also may find the exposed wounds unsightly and uncomfortable. This method is not very suitable for wounds over joints as the scabs over a joint surface may crack repeatedly and bleed. In case of hands, exposure method allows full range of movements at all joints which avoids deformities of the hand.

A modification of the open technique is to apply a thin layer of antibiotic ointment over the wounds after cleansing and drying them daily, especially on the face. Sometimes an antimicrobial impregnated gauze is used on exposed wounds and this gauze acts as a wick to transport the exudates to the gauze surface where it dries up forming a scab. The advantage with this technique is that the scab does not adhere to the wound and the gauze can be removed easily without the risk of bleeding from the wound or else damage to the newly formed epithelium **(Fig. 11B)**.

If the burned area is of superficial partial thickness, the whole scab/gauze begins to separate after a week or so and this is trimmed gently and repeatedly with scissors and it finally comes out in 15–21 days to leave a well-healed skin surface. If the scab does not separate by 3 weeks, the burn is treated as a deep partial-thickness burn, and the management is changed to the technique of occlusive dressings, which hastens the separation of eschar. For patients treated by exposure method, appropriate maintenance of the environmental temperature in the range of 28–32°C and humidity at about 40% is important as leaving the wounds exposed increases the evaporative losses as well as body heat loss.

The advantages of open method are:
- Wound examination is easier
- Earlier detection of wound infection
- Early physiotherapy
- Easier control of hyperpyrexia
- Wound environment is not conducive to bacterial colonization.

The disadvantages of open method are:
- Delay in eschar separation
- Evaporative losses increase
- Chances of hypothermia
- Not possible where isolation is not available

Occlusive Dressing or Closed Technique

This method is most useful for patients with circumferential burns of extremities and torso **(Fig. 12)**. Occlusive dressings are avoided in burns of face, neck, and perineal region.

The advantages of occlusive dressings are:
- Reduces evaporative losses
- Provides a mechanical barrier to prevent bacteria from contaminating the wounds
- Absorbs exudates from the wound surface
- Maintains a moist environment which encourages epithelialization
- Patient is more comfortable

Dressing technique: The technique of dressing a burn wound determines the final outcome of burn wound treatment program. All burn dressings should be done with proper aseptic precautions to prevent wound contamination. All doctors and nursing staff should be properly gowned and gloved. Majority of the dressings can be performed without general anesthesia. Usually, sedation with opioid analgesics (e.g., morphine) is adequate.

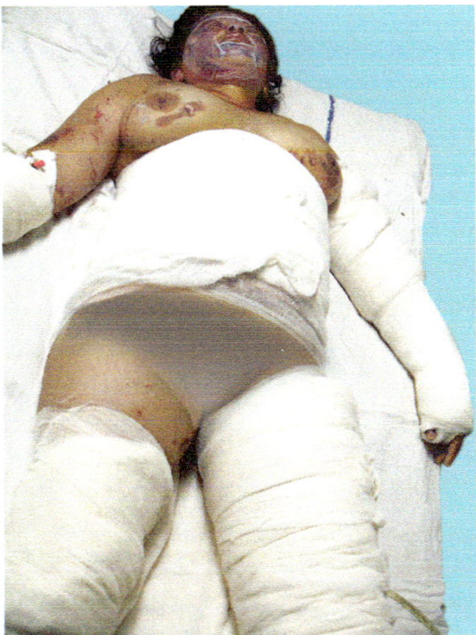

FIG. 12: Closed dressing technique.

A satisfactory burn dressing is one that can absorb all the fluid exuded from the burn wound and distribute evenly so that there is no collection of the exudate on the wound surface. The material that fulfills these requirements is the Gamgee pad, which consists of cotton wool sandwiched between two layers of absorbent gauze. These are easy to prepare and can be made in assorted sizes suitable for small as well as extensive areas. These are prepared, sterilized, and kept ready to use so that they are available at all times.

The innermost layer of occlusive dressing consists of a layer of an antimicrobial agent over which a wide mesh gauze impregnated with paraffin or petroleum jelly is applied. This tulle grass is nonadherent so that pain and trauma to the regenerating neoepithelium can be minimized at the time of change of dressing. After the nonadherent gauze and antimicrobial agent are applied, multiple layers of gauze and Gamgee pads, depending on the expected amount of exudate, are applied and kept in place with a gentle compression bandage. This dressing prevents edema formation, splints the wound, and facilitates absorption of discharge. However, it should not be constricting in any way. This outer layer of the dressing should be porous to allow evaporation of water and prevent inner layers from becoming soggy as that encourages microbial growth **(Figs. 13A to D)**.

The frequency of dressing change depends upon the depth of burns and the degree of infection in the burn wound. In case of partial-thickness burns, when there are no signs of infection, the first dressing can be left intact for 3–5 days. In case of full-thickness burns, the dressing should be changed every 3 days. Earlier change of dressing is indicated if there is soakage in dressing or any sign of infection of burn wound which includes local pain, unexplained fever, foul smell from dressing, and increased purulent discharge from wound. The topical agent being used on wound should also be changed if discharge increases. There are various antimicrobial agents and dressing materials used for burn dressings that are discussed later in this chapter.

TOPICAL ANTIMICROBIAL THERAPY

A variety of local medicaments have been used on burn wounds since eternity, which ranged from tinctures (600 BC), vinegar-soaked dressing (430 BC), greasy dressing

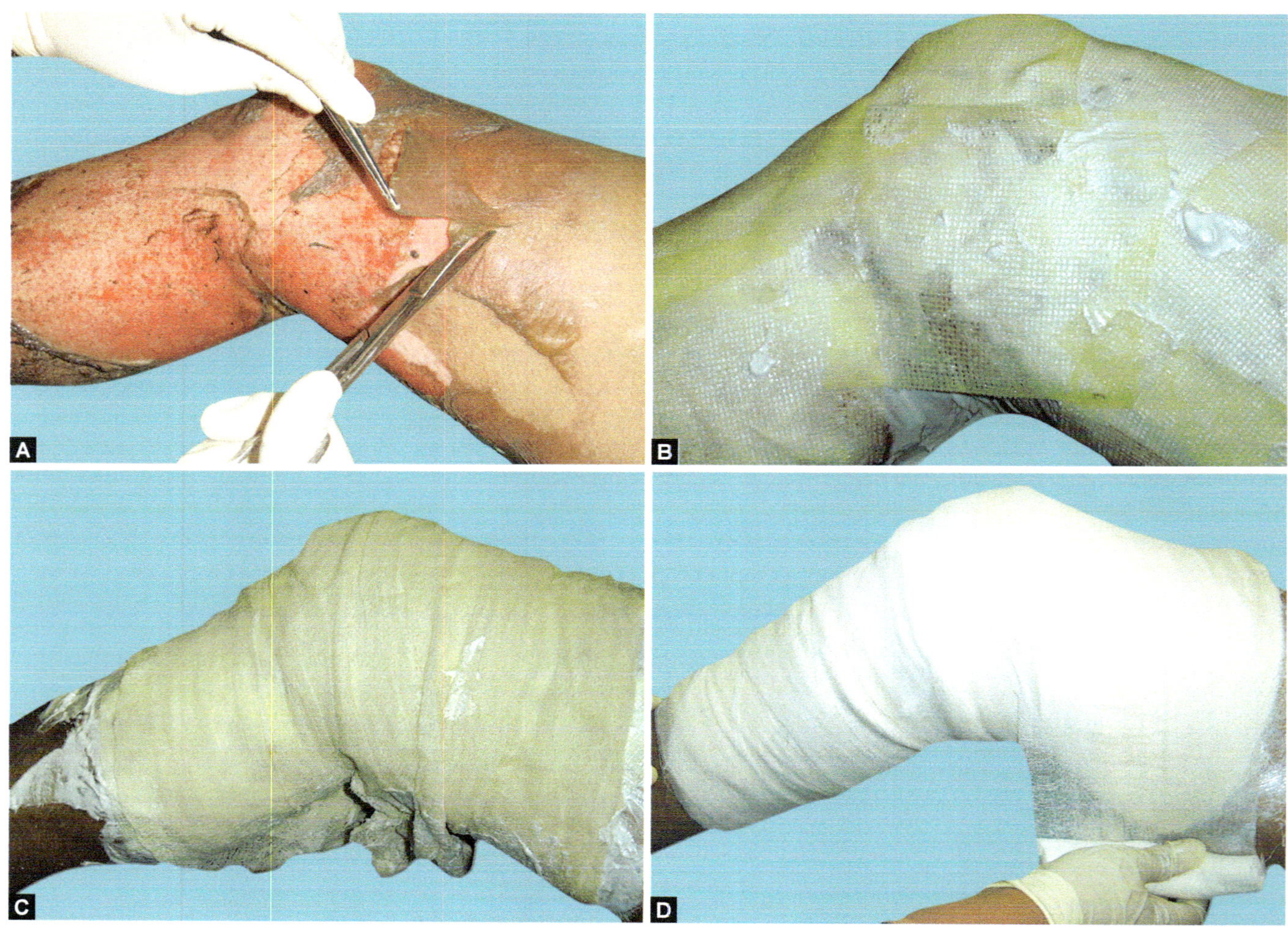

FIGS. 13A TO D: (A) Removal of loose dead skin; (B) Application of silver sulfadiazine over paraffin gauze; (C) Application of gauze and Gamgee; (D) A light compressive bandage over the limb.

(1596), tannic acid by Edward Clark Davidson (1894–1933) to Gentian violet by Aldridge in 1933 to Petroleum gauze by Harvey Allen in 1942. All these methods, however, fell into disrepute because of local and systemic toxicity or ineffectiveness of these substances. This initiated research for finding newer topical agents that are more effective and have fewer side effects.

History of Topical Antimicrobial Agents

The topical therapy of burn wounds dates back to the beginning of civilization. Throughout history, a number of famous philosophers, physicians, and scientists have contributed to the knowledge of burn wound management, including such notables as Hippocrates, Celsus, Pliny the Elder, Galen, Aristotle, Rhases, Clowes, Paré, Hildanus, Marjolin, Dupuytren, and Syme. A variety of substances have been advocated as effective topical burn treatments including some plants, gums, milk (goat milk and milk from "a women who has given birth to a son"), tea leaves, roasted angle worms, oak bark extract, honey, cork, bear fat, bran, ashes, vinegar, wine, fat from "very old wild hogs", calcium chloride soaks, moss "from the skull of a person hung", red sandalwood, cold water, saline baths, lemon strips soaked in oily dressings, soot, spider webs, linseed oil mixed with lime water, picric acid, medicated paraffin, carbolic acid, cod liver oil, and "portions of a genuine mummy". At the beginning of the 20th century, it was believed that the systemic derangements seen in burn patients resulted from a release of "toxins" from the burn wound, and thus the goal of topical therapy was to bind or leach toxins before they can be absorbed.[9] A secondary goal was to dry out the burn wound or to create a hard coagulum to minimize exudate, drainage, or fluid loss. A number of "escharotics", including 5% or 10% silver nitrate solution, gentian violet,[10,11] "triple" dyes, trinitrophenol, and tannic acid were employed, either alone or in combination. Over the years, the goals of topical burn treatment have changed. There was a drastic change in the treatment of burn wounds with dressings along with an antiseptic agent in 1868 following discovery of the concept of antiseptics by Lister. Carbolic acid, mercurial compounds, and aniline dyes were used as an inner layer of burn dressing. Unfortunately, they were unselective in their action and damaged normal tissues along with bacteria colonizing the wound surface. Hence, their use was discontinued. In the mid-twentieth century, phenol-containing dressings were highly recommended. Davidson at the Henry Ford Hospital first described the use of tannic acid spray in 1925 and believed that this modality reduced pain and produced a cleaner wound bed.[10,12] In 1935, Bettman added 10% silver nitrate to a 2.5% tannic acid solution, which allowed wound tanning to occur in seconds. Reports of liver necrosis in patients treated with tannic acid began to appear in the 1930s, although liver necrosis was often ascribed to the burn injury itself. Additionally, pus tended to accumulate under the coagulum formed by tannic acid application. McClure (1944), also from Henry Ford Hospital, reported that tannic acid was a hepatotoxin and the use of this agent was discontinued.

Work by Aldrich, Teplitz, Lindberg, and others established that septicemia in burn patients, a major cause of mortality, frequently originated in the burn wound.[11] Attention then turned to the application of various topical antimicrobials to the burnt surface and the development of mafenide (Sulfamylon®), silver nitrate, silver sulfadiazine (SSD), and others revolutionized burn care.

In early part of World War II, Marfanil which was later called Mafenide was used by the German army and was found to reduce the incidence of gas gangrene. Subsequently, it was used by the United States (US) Army for traumatic wounds as it was found to be effective against clostridial and enteric organisms. Its efficacy in controlling burn wound sepsis was discovered by Moncrief in 1964. Although it was found to be very effective against *Pseudomonas,* especially in the treatment of established infections, it was relatively inactive against gram-positive organisms, especially streptococci which was the main cause of burn wound infection at that time. In 1965, Moyer and colleagues showed excellent prophylactic use of 0.5% silver nitrate against *Pseudomonas*. However, it had no role in established infections and also caused dyselectrolytemia and the patient was uncomfortable because of the black staining and continuous wet feeling. So, its use fell into disrepute. In 1968, a new antimicrobial, namely SSD, was discovered by Fox for use in burns. Even half a century later, no serious side effects have been reported despite its widespread use. Many other antibiotics and antiseptics have been used singly and in various combinations for burn dressing, namely, gentamicin, neomycin, bacitracin, polymyxin, framycetin, nitrofurazone, and chlorhexidine, etc. Many of these have proved useful under certain circumstances. However, they have all failed to prevent serious systemic infections in extensive burns, especially *Pseudomonas* infection, which is now the most common organism responsible for burn wound sepsis worldwide.

Basis for Topical Therapy

Immediately following burns, the surface of the burnt skin is sterile, and the only organisms present are deep in the skin appendages and these are not very pathogenic. Some of these organisms come to the surface following burn but a sterile dressing and use of an antimicrobial agent can kill these organisms. In the case of closed dressings, presence of exudates in the dressings, warmth, and lack of light under the dressing are ideal conditions for the proliferation of organisms after they gain entry to the skin surface through exogenous or endogenous routes, resulting in infection. This can be avoided by using a broad-spectrum antimicrobial agent which has action against both gram-positive and gram-negative organisms. The topical agents used for burn wound dressing should have a dual purpose—first to control any organisms on the surface of the burn wound and secondly to prevent entry of new organisms from the exterior.

By the end of the first week postburn, the deeper surface of eschar especially around the hair follicles shows active proliferation of organisms, which can penetrate deeper into tissues and adjacent viable tissue as well, if not controlled. This can again be checked by the application of topical antimicrobial agents that have a good eschar penetration. The deeply burned areas are avascular, which not only provide a favorable environment for bacterial proliferation but also prevent penetration of systemically administered antibiotics into the burn wound surface. This is better tackled by topical antimicrobial agents and obviates the need for systemic antibiotics. It is very important to understand that topical therapy does not sterilize the burn wound. It only controls the bacterial proliferation and confines it within the limits of the burn wound. Topical agents are also no substitute for meticulous wound care which includes proper debridement of devitalized tissues and deroofing of sub escharotic abscesses. On the other hand, proper and judicious use of topical agents can prevent the conversion of superficial burns into deeper wounds and decrease the incidence of systemic sepsis.

Criteria for a Good Antimicrobial Agent

Criteria for a good antimicrobial agent are as follows:

- It should have a broad spectrum of activity against organisms that are most commonly isolated from the burn wound, for example, *Pseudomonas aeruginosa, Staphylococcus aureus, Klebsiella,* and *Enterococci,* etc.
- It should penetrate the eschar but not have a significant systemic absorption.
- There should be minimal emergence of resistance amongst organisms against the agent.
- It should cause minimal or no discomfort to the patient.
- It should be economical and easily available.
- It should have minimal side effects.
- Application should be simple and easy.

Topical Agents

The topical antimicrobial agents, most frequently used for burn wound dressings, are discussed below.

Silver Sulfadiazine[13-15]

Silver sulfadiazine is a white crystalline, highly insoluble compound synthesized by Fox in 1968 by reacting silver nitrate with sodium sulfadiazine. It is the most frequently used topical agent in the form of a water soluble cream base at 1% concentration, which provides the same amount of elemental silver as 0.5% silver nitrate solution (30 mEq/L). At this concentration, the amount of agent at the surface is more than that necessary in vitro to inhibit the growth of sensitive organisms.

Mode of action: The mechanism of action is due to both silver ion and sulfadiazine moiety, which are released at the wound surface by gradual dissociation. Sulfadiazine is a competitive inhibitor of para-aminobenzoic acid (PABA) which is a metabolic precursor. The ionic silver acts by impairing DNA replication, denaturing of proteins and enzymes, and increasing the permeability of the cell walls. It is primarily bacteriostatic and is active in vitro against a wide range of organisms which include *Staphylococcus aureus, Escherichia coli, Proteus, Enterobacteriaceae,* and Herpes virus. Clinical trials have shown reasonable prophylactic effect against gram-negative bacteria. It delays wound colonization by gram-negative bacteria in extensive burns.

In spite of the dissociation of the compound, there is no absorption of the silver from the wound. On the other hand, sulfadiazine levels of 1.5–4 mg/100 mL have been reported in the blood. There is also some grayish silver discoloration of the wound because of minimal precipitation of silver chloride or silver sulfide following oxidation of silver by exposure to sunlight.

Technique of application: It is applied as 1% cream to the burn wound in a thickness of approximately 0.5–1 cm either twice a day in case of exposed treatment or once a day in closed method. The substance has to be washed off between applications in order to debride the wound properly.

Advantages: It is an odorless cream, easy to apply, and causes minimal to no pain on application. It does not stain the skin or linen, unlike silver nitrate. It has an intermediate penetration capacity into the eschar. Bacterial resistance to SSD, even after prolonged therapy, has not been reported.

Disadvantages: Crystalluria has been occasionally reported. Methemoglobinemia is a well-known side effect of sulfonamide, although seen very rarely. Transient leucopenia can occur in patients treated with SSD after 2–3 days of starting treatment. This resolves spontaneously within a few days despite continued use of the agent. A macular rash is seen in <5% patients and is a cutaneous sensitivity reaction to SSD. A thin proteinaceous gel called "Pseudoeschar" forms on the wound surface after topical application of SSD. This can confuse an inexperienced observer during assessment of the depth of burn. With prolonged use of topical SSD, there is a risk of sulfadiazine-resistant gram-negative bacilli, especially Enterobacteriaceae group, developing plasmid-mediated resistance. Inhibition of epithelial regeneration with the use of 1% SSD has been demonstrated experimentally.

Silver Nitrate Solution (0.5%)[9]

Silver nitrate has been used for the treatment of burn wounds for over a century but fell into disrepute because of its side effects. Silver nitrate was used as a caustic and escharotic agent for burn care in the early 20th century in the form of a 10% solution, but was largely abandoned by the time of World War II as it was found to be toxic at such high concentrations. It was reintroduced by Moyer in 1965 as 0.5% solution and later popularized by Monafo as a topical agent for burn wound treatment. At this concentration, it is not toxic to the epithelium and has bacteriostatic action. For many years, 0.5% silver nitrate has also been used as a topical agent for patients with toxic epidermal necrolysis (TEN).

Mode of action: The free silver ion released is effective against the common microbial flora seen in the burn wound especially gram-negative bacteria. It is mainly bacteriostatic. There is no known resistance seen to this agent and if properly used, it is very effective as a prophylactic agent. There is minimal absorption of silver through the open wounds into systemic circulation because its salts are insoluble. Instead, there is precipitation of its salts, i.e., silver chloride and silver sulfide which cause the characteristic black discoloration of the burn wounds.

Mode of application: The technique of application of silver nitrate solution is as described by Monafo and Moyer. After cleaning and debriding the loose tissues in the wound, it is covered with 8–10 layers thick gauze dressing, which is then soaked with warm 0.5% silver nitrate solution. The dressing has to be wetted every 2 hours to ensure that the concentration does not become caustic (>2–3%). The advantage of this bulky wet dressing is that it minimizes evaporative loss.

Advantages: Application of silver nitrate is painless. No patient hypersensitivity has been reported to it. No resistant organisms have been isolated after its use. Its use helps in rapid debridement of the eschar because of twice daily change of the bulky gauze dressing. Its continuous use decreases evaporative water loss, which further helps in decreasing metabolic rate and improves the nutritional status of the patient.

Disadvantages:

- 0.5% silver nitrate has been found to be ineffective in established burn wound infections and its ability to penetrate the eschar is poor.
- It stains all the linen and floor brown or black. Thus, its use necessitates use of disposable linens and stain-resistant floor and wall coverings, which can increase the cost of treatment.
- There are severe electrolyte derangements noticed with its use. Use of distilled water as a vehicle for application of silver nitrate leads to a markedly hypotonic solution and it causes absorption of large volumes of distilled water into the tissues and eventually into the bloodstream. There is leaching of sodium by reverse mechanism, which results in hyponatremia, which can lead to convulsions, if severe. This can be prevented by administering large quantities of sodium chloride orally or intravenously. The precipitation of silver as silver chloride and silver sulfide salt results in hypochloremia, which can also be corrected by infusing saline. Hypokalemia and hypocalcemia can result from leaching of potassium and calcium. Ideally, 40–120 mEq of potassium and 4–8 g calcium along with vitamin supplements are necessary either orally or intravenously. It is recommended to replace about 350 mEq of sodium per square meter of wound surface in order to maintain adequate serum levels. The electrolyte imbalance with the use of silver nitrate is noticed mainly in infants and children and in patients with larger burns particularly >20% TBSA, unless the replacement therapy is maintained. In extremes of age, dyselectrolytemia can occur within 6–8 hours of its use and therefore, less frequent saturation of wound dressings is recommended in these age groups.
- The black discoloration of the burn wound surface interferes with clinical assessment of the wound.
- Some of the gram-negative bacteria especially *Enterobacter cloacae* metabolize nitrate ion to nitrite, which when absorbed through the wound results in methemoglobinemia. Though it is a rare complication, it has to be suspected if there is cyanosis or slate gray discoloration of skin without any pulmonary injury and arterial blood is brown in color even though PaO_2 is normal. Diagnosis can be confirmed by estimating methemoglobin levels in the blood. Management of this condition includes withdrawal of silver nitrate dressing and intravenous administration of reducing agents like methylene blue or ascorbic acid.

Mafenide (11.1%)[16-19]

Mafenide is a methylated sulfonamide, which was introduced for clinical use as a topical agent for burn wounds in 1964 by Moncrief. It is presently used as a cream with 11.1% concentration of the drug in a water-miscible base.

Mechanism of action: It is active against most gram-positive organisms and a wide spectrum of gram-negative organisms including *Pseudomonas*. It is particularly effective against Clostridial species. It has minimal antifungal action. Its mechanism of action is not known but it is primarily bactericidal only in higher concentrations. It actively penetrates the burn wound and minimal amount is left on wound surface after 3 hours. After 10 hours, the tissue level is below the concentration required to inhibit bacterial growth. Therefore, to maintain therapeutic levels of the agent in the wound, it has to be reapplied after 12 hours.

Mode of application: The cream is applied to the wound with a gloved hand in a thickness of 3–5 mm with or without a covering dressing. As the patient is free to move about in bed, the joint activity is maintained. Usually, twice-a-day application suffices as a means for controlling burn wound sepsis, but reapplication may be required in some areas. During reapplication, the remaining cream on the wound surface has to be wiped off with wet gauze.

Advantages: Mafenide is the most useful topical antibacterial agent for control of established or incipient burn wound sepsis where the bacterial invasion has started or extensive colonization is present. This is mainly because it has the best eschar penetration ability.

An overall reduction in mortality of 50% was noticed with the use of mafenide in a number of studies.

Disadvantages: Application of mafenide is associated with significant pain which is probably because of its high osmolarity and hygroscopic effect of the sulfonamide suspension. The painful sensation persists for several minutes, thereby earning its nickname of "white lightning". Alternatively, the application of mafenide cream can be limited to no more than 20% of the body surface area (BSA) at any one time. The sites of mafenide applications can then be rotated every 2 hours until the entire burn has been treated. It is also advisable to alternate mafenide and silver sulfadiazine creams on badly contaminated wounds as a form of "pulse therapy". 5% of the patients develop maculopapular rash, which is characteristic of sulfa sensitivity. It can be easily controlled by oral antihistamines. Experiments have shown that its use also leads to inhibition of epithelial regeneration. The most significant complication of the use of topical mafenide is compensated metabolic acidosis, which results from its carbonic anhydrase inhibiting effect that decreases the reabsorption of bicarbonate from the renal tubule. The acidic breakdown product of mafenide adds to the acid load. In addition, the bicarbonate is converted to carbon dioxide in the lung and excreted during hyperventilation, which is a compensatory mechanism. This is usually seen in patients with >40% TBSA burns being treated with mafenide. If the patient is only hyperventilating, it may not be a big problem. However, if the patient shows signs of respiratory distress in the form of use of accessory muscles, the drug has to be immediately removed from the burn wound surface and some other topical antimicrobial agent has to be applied. Additionally, ventilatory support and metabolic support in the form of sodium bicarbonate as per the laboratory test reports are also to be provided in these circumstances. Patients treated with mafenide also exhibit inappropriate polyuria, which results from significant reduction in evaporative water loss from the burn wound (because of 95% water content of the cream base) as well as the osmotic load on the kidney due to the breakdown product of mafenide. Hemolytic anemia is a rare complication seen with the use of mafenide.

Despite its disadvantages, mafenide is still one of the best topical agents for the control of established burn wound infection. Its use should be reserved for a short duration of time and withdrawn before significant side effects become evident.

Gentamicin[11,20,21]

Gentamicin is an aminoglycoside used as a 0.1% ointment or cream in burn wound dressing. It is a relatively safe broad-spectrum antibiotic.

Mode of action: It is primarily bactericidal. It is not effective against viruses or fungi. It is effective against both gram-positive and gram-negative organisms, particularly *Pseudomonas aeruginosa*. It acts by inducing defective protein synthesis. Indiscriminate use of gentamicin for serious systemic infections has shown development of resistant strains.

Technique of application: It is applied as 0.1% ointment or cream as a thin layer to the wound surface twice a day without dressing or with a light dressing. The application is painless and absorption rate from wound is low. Therefore, the incidence of ototoxicity and nephrotoxicity with topical application is negligible.

It has good eschar penetration, but its absorption decreases as the water content of the eschar decreases. Later, as the eschar separates and granulation tissue appears, the rate of absorption of drug again increases. The absorption of the drug is faster if applied as a cream base than from the ointment base. Therefore, if an occlusive dressing is used, it should be applied as ointment rather than as cream.

Advantages: Its application is easy and painless. It actively penetrates the eschar. There is a low incidence of toxicity when used topically and has a good antipseudomonal action.

Disadvantages: If used indiscriminately, there are high chances of developing resistant strains, especially of *Pseudomonas*. There are chances of ototoxicity and nephrotoxicity with prolonged use.

Although gentamicin gives good results as a topical agent on the burn wound, its use should be reserved exclusively for systemic use.

Bacitracin

Despite the lack of efficacy against common gram-negative burn pathogens, bacitracin remains popular in burn care, particularly on partial-thickness face burns. Whether this beneficial effect is due to the antibiotic itself or simply to the bland petroleum base remains controversial.

Less Commonly Used Topical Agents

Chlorhexidine gluconate: It has been used in moderate burn injuries either as such or in combination with 0.5% silver nitrate as a prophylactic agent. Its absorption and toxicity are not documented fully and hence, it is not used routinely.

Povidone iodine (Betadine®): It has been used as a water-miscible base (10%) for burn wound dressing. Though it is effective against gram-negative, gram-positive organisms, fungi, viruses, and protozoa, it has little effect on *Staphylococcus* strains. Its use is restricted because of certain disadvantages like its painful application. If used in large quantities in extensive burns, there can be absorption of large quantities of iodine leading to high iodine levels in the blood.

Soframycin, Polymyxin B: These have been used only for dressing of small burn wounds and are not indicated for extensive burns because of systemic toxicity resulting from absorption of these drugs from the extensive wounds.

Newer Dressing Materials

Collagen **(Figs. 14A to C)**: It is a biomaterial that has been shown to provide a moist wound healing environment. The dressing may be in the form of sheets, pads, or gels containing animal-source collagen. Collagen sheet dressings are thin, porous, and flexible, and thus can be applied easily to the wound. Many such dressing materials are available in the market such as Skin Temp,® Diacoll-S,™ Puracol,® and Revitalize-M.™ These are especially useful in superficial dermal burns and can also be used to treat facial burn wounds with exposure method.[22,23]

Hydrofiber dressings **(Figs. 15A to E)**: This consists of nonwoven carboxymethylcellulose fibers that convert into a gel when it comes in contact with wound fluid. This aids in creating an optimal environment for wound healing by locking in the moisture. The dressing material contours well to the wound bed, thus minimizing any dead space. Aquacel® is a hydrofiber dressing material, and benefits of silver are also available in another version of this dressing material. Aquacel Ag® incorporates 1.2% silver, which is released in a controlled manner into the wound.[24]

Polyurethane foam dressing **(Figs. 16A to C)**: This is a nonadhesive dressing material that absorbs the exudates and retains moisture to optimize wound healing. It conforms closely to the wound bed owing to its foam structure. Biatain Ag® is one such dressing that also incorporates a patented silver complex that is

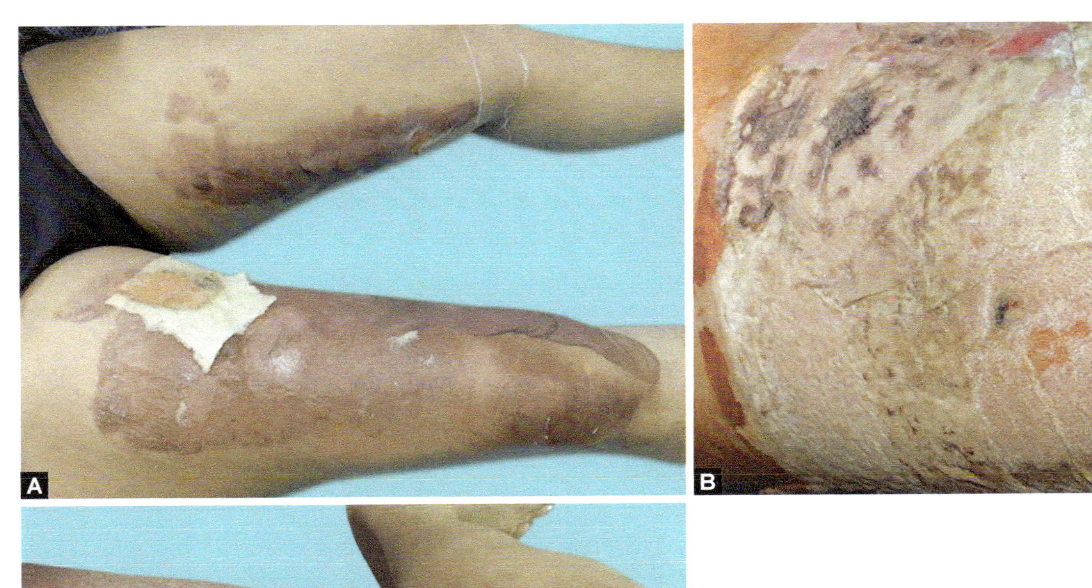
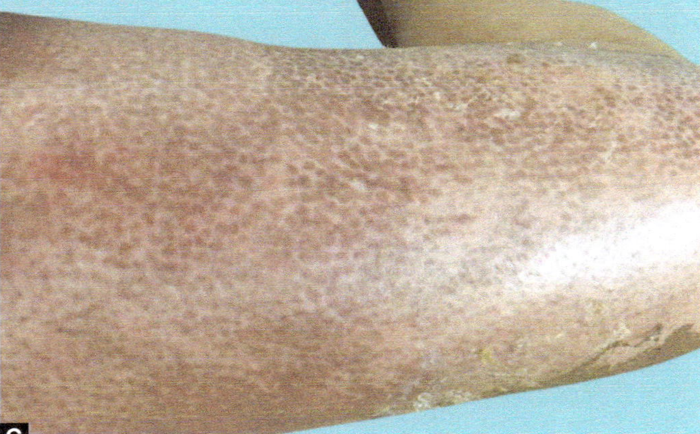

FIGS. 14A TO C: (A) Superficial dermal burns; (B) Dressing with collagen sheet—skin Temp® (C) Healed scar.

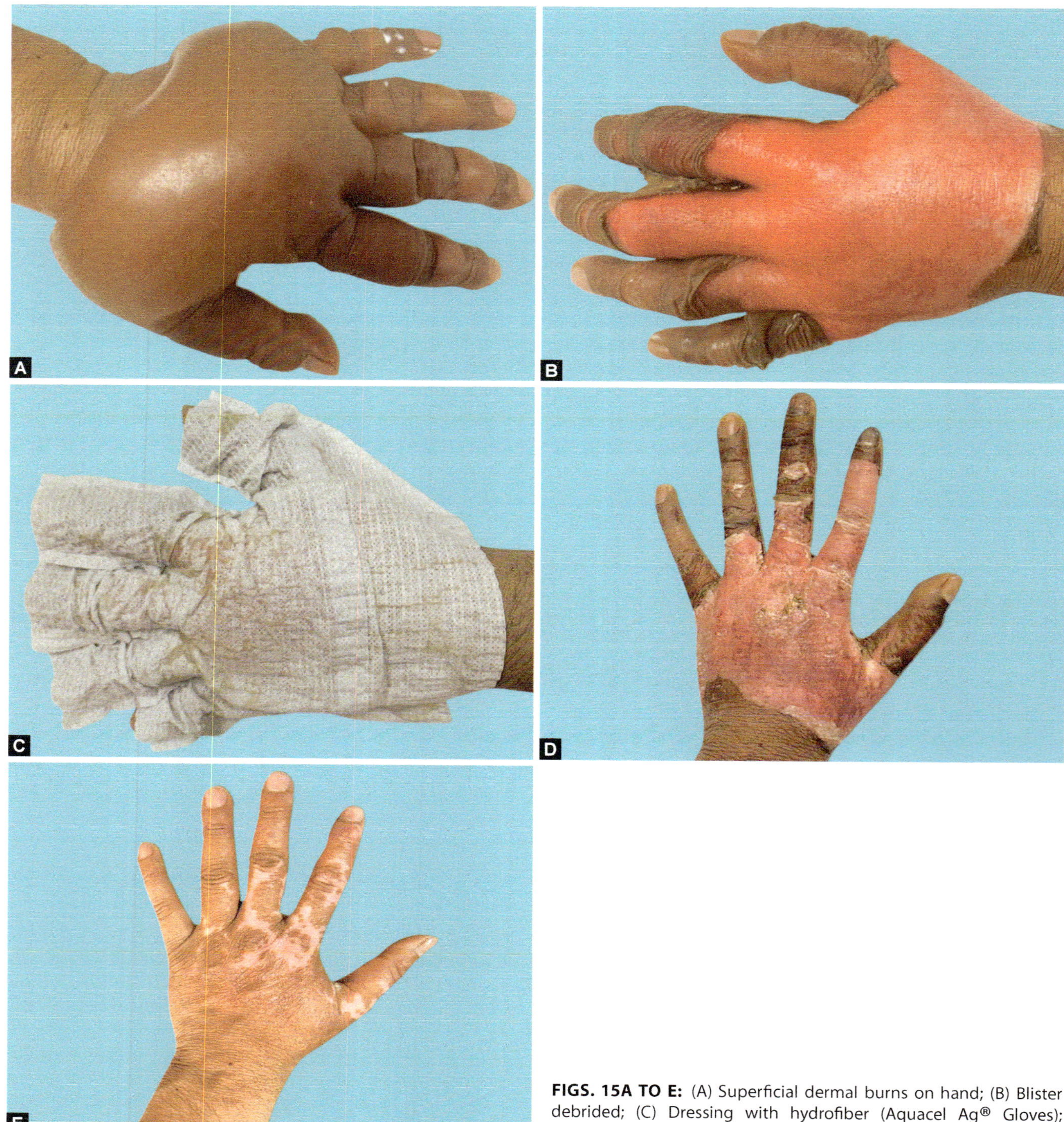

FIGS. 15A TO E: (A) Superficial dermal burns on hand; (B) Blister debrided; (C) Dressing with hydrofiber (Aquacel Ag® Gloves); (D) Healed area after 1 week; (E) Scar after 6 months.

released slowly into the wound for a sustained action. Mepilex Ag® is also a foam dressing that has a soft silicone wound contact layer.[25]

Nanocrystalline silver **(Figs. 17A to E)**: In the traditional silver containing antimicrobial agents, such as silver nitrate and SSD, most of the silver carries a strong positive electrical charge which makes it highly soluble, but it also reacts readily with substances such as chloride from the salt in the wound forming silver chloride which is ineffective. Most of these compounds allow an initial release of silver ions and then are rapidly inactivated. Therefore, it is necessary to apply these agents frequently.

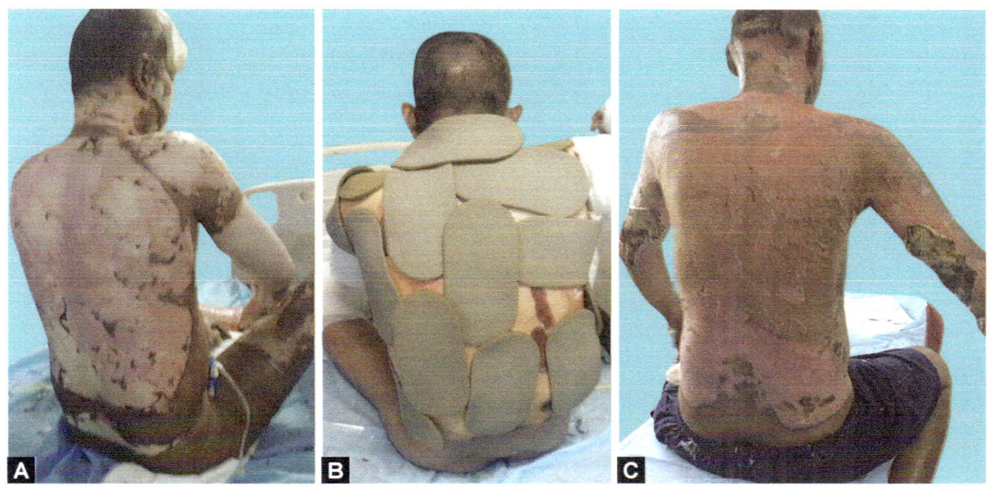

FIGS. 16A TO C: (A) Deep dermal burns of back; (B) Dressing with Mepilex Ag© foam dressing; (C) Healed area after 2 weeks.

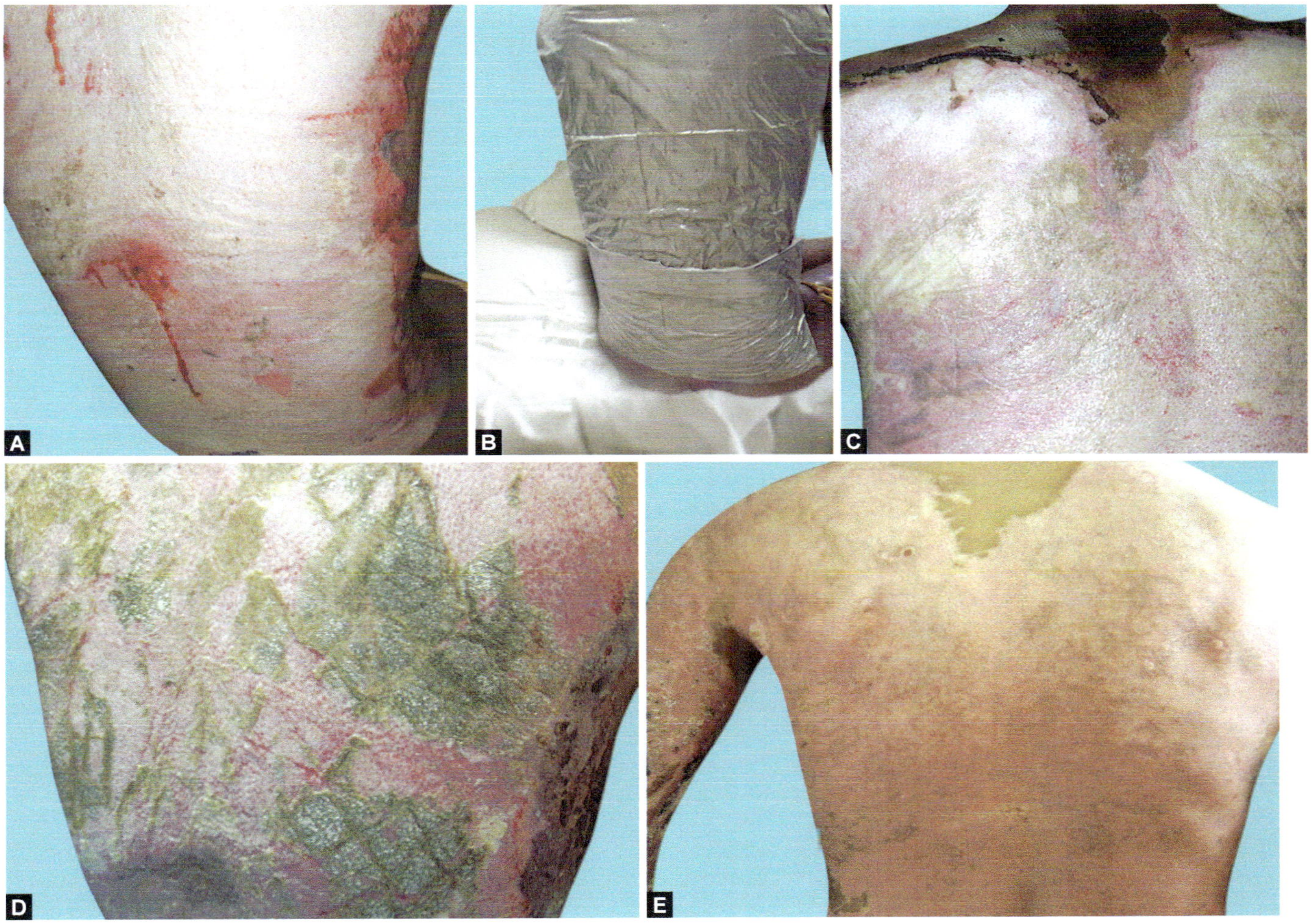

FIGS. 17A TO E: (A) Superficial to deep dermal burns of the back; (B) Nanocrystalline silver dressing (ACTICOAT)® applied to the burns on the back; (C) Wound in healing phase after first dressing with ACTICOAT®; (D) Wound almost healed after three dressings with ACTICOAT, i.e., after 12 days, showing gray staining because of metallic silver; (E) Same patient after 1 month with well-settled scars.

The newer nanocrystalline dressings such as Acticoat™ provide sustained bactericidal action due to the presence of Ag^0 form of silver, which is far less deactivated. Ag^0 is the uncharged form of metallic silver. Free silver cations have a potent antimicrobial effect, which destroys micro-organisms immediately by blocking cellular respiration and disrupting the function of bacterial cell membranes. They act by binding to tissue proteins, causing structural changes in the bacterial cell membranes, which in turn cause cell death. Silver cations also denature the bacterial deoxyribonucleic acid (DNA) and ribonucleic acid (RNA), thus inhibiting cell replication.

Nanocrystalline dressings are layered dressing constructs of a silver mesh containing silver nanocrystals applied to either side of a rayon/polyester core. They are manufactured by passing electric current through a chamber containing Argon gas that acts as an anode and silver as a cathode. The silver atoms knocked out are deposited on the substrate as nanocrystals measuring around 15 nanometers across, containing 30–50 atoms resulting in a metastable, high energy form of silver, by a process called physical vapor deposition. The smaller the particles of silver, the greater the wound surface area that will be in contact with silver, thus increasing bioactivity and silver solubility. These dressings release as much as 30 times less silver than other topical products but the silver released is more effective as it is not bound by halide and is released over a longer period of time.

In vitro and animal studies have shown that the nanocrystalline dressings are effective against a broad spectrum of microorganisms including the most common strains of bacteria, multiresistant organisms, and fungal spores. They have been shown to reduce the number of viable bacteria to very low levels within 30 minutes of application. These can be left in place for a longer period of time reducing wound manipulation and causing less trauma to the new epithelial growth. Apart from the antibacterial effects, these also decrease the level of matrix metalloproteinases (MMP) in patients with chronic wounds. Human studies show that nanocrystalline dressings are cost-effective, reduce burn wound infection, have decreased pain levels during dressing changes, and reduce bioburden. Additionally, they have no in vivo evidence suggestive of toxicity against keratinocytes and fibroblasts.

Nanocrystalline dressings are thus an effective way to manage burn wounds. They are effective at reducing inflammatory process, promote wound healing, and are less toxic than other forms of silver dressings.[26-28]

Summary

The use of topical antimicrobial agents in burn wound care can prevent or minimize burn wound infections and sepsis. It is important to understand that any one single topical agent cannot be used in all patients in all circumstances. All agents are effective if used in the right circumstances, and at the same time, indiscriminate use of any one single agent can be harmful in the long run. It is, therefore, imperative to use the topical antimicrobial agents judiciously, selecting the right agent for the right patient at the right time. Thus, the main aim of topical therapy is to control burn wound sepsis and improve the condition of the deep wounds so that they can be closed as early as possible by skin grafting/flap cover.

ROLE OF ESCHAROTOMY/FASCIOTOMY

In full-thickness circumferential burns of limbs, neck, and chest, the tight dry eschar with underlying edema may produce a tourniquet effect resulting in ischemic injury. This has to be diagnosed early in order to avoid vascular compromise to distal extremities and respiratory impairment. The following clinical signs and symptoms are indicative of ischemia: Cyanosis of distal unburned skin, delayed capillary filling in nails of fingers or toes, and paresthesias or deep tissue pain. This can be confirmed by a reduced flow on a color Doppler. An early escharotomy is warranted in such cases to prevent ischemic changes from setting in. An incision made through the full thickness of the eschar releases the constricting effect **(Figs. 18A and B)** and decompresses the underlying structures, thus improving the distal blood supply.[29,30]

Technique: The procedure is done bedside using a sterile technique. Anesthesia is not required as the eschar is dead tissue, and hence painless. Sites for incisions for escharotomy are given in **Figures 18A and B**; care should be taken to avoid injury to major peripheral nerves. The

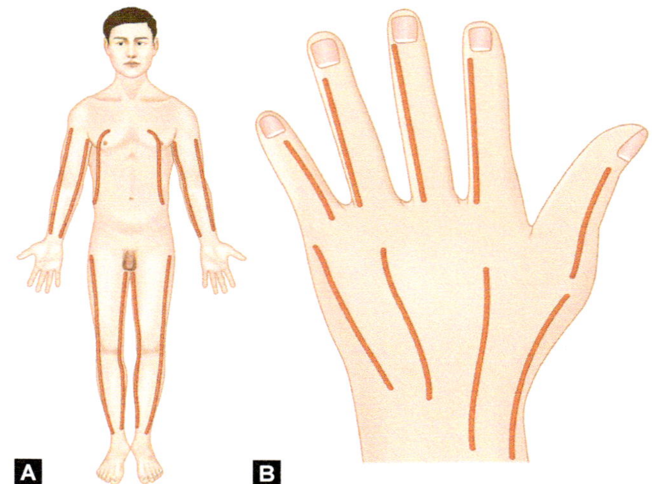

FIGS. 18A AND B: (A) Escharotomy incision lines; (B) Escharotomy incisions for hand.

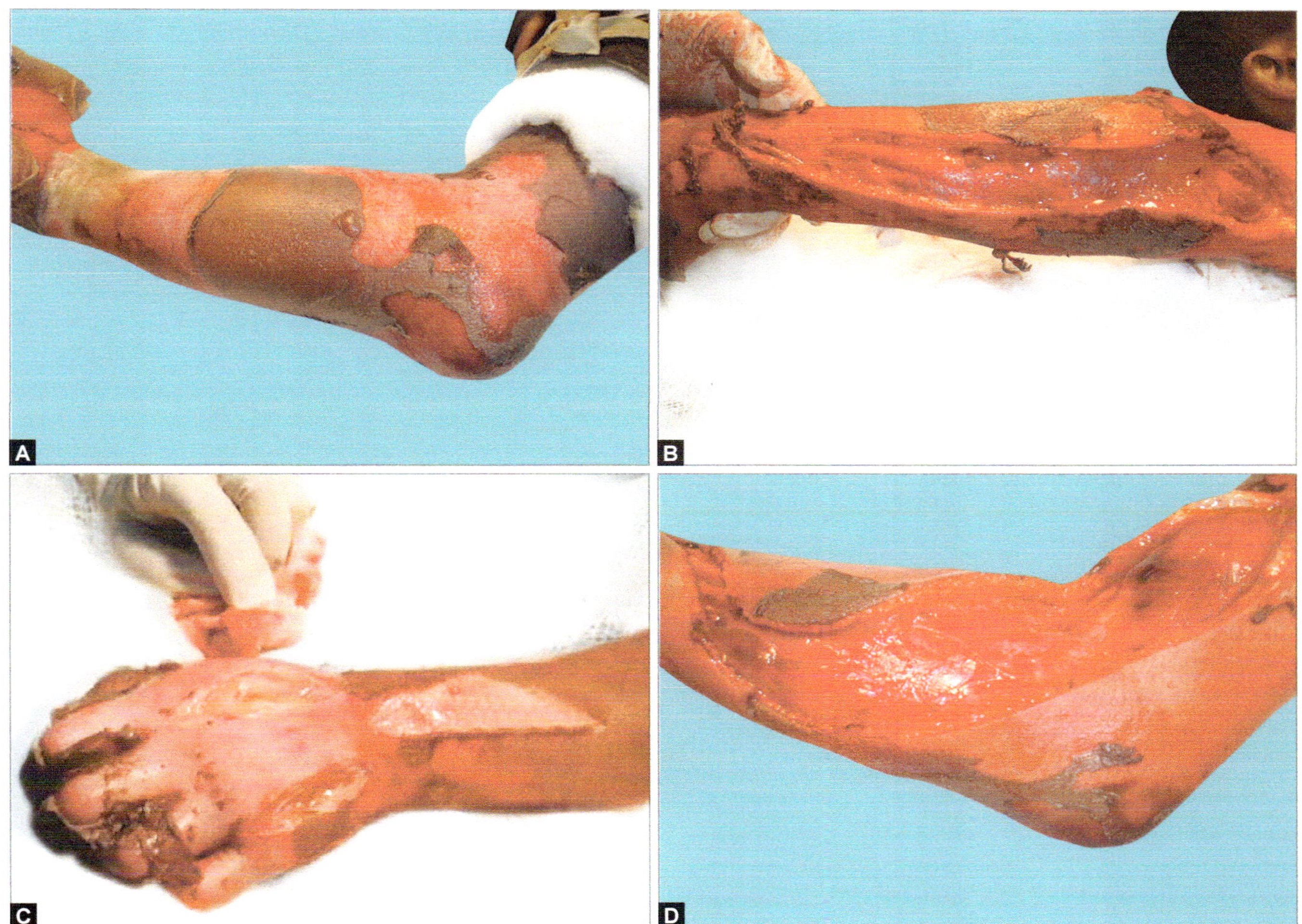

FIGS. 19 A TO D: (A) Electrical contact burn in the arm causing gross edema of limb and distal circulation compromised due to compartment syndrome, demanding urgent fasciotomy; (B) Incisions given till deep fascia, releasing the compartment pressure; (C) Fasciotomy incisions over the dorsum of the hand; (D) Following fasciotomy, the underlying muscles bulge out and bleeding on the surface is seen.

incision has to be first given across the mid-lateral line involving joints and throughout the length and thickness of the eschar. If perfusion does not improve, mid-medial incision is given to increase the decompression. Blood loss is usually minimal because the incision goes through the avascular eschar only.

In high-voltage electrical injury where the muscles are also involved, there can be edema under the deep fascia which raises the compartment pressure. A fasciotomy is required in such cases to decompress the compartment **(Figs. 19A to D)** and is done as soon as the patient is adequately resuscitated. Local anesthesia may be required for giving incisions in the unburnt skin. The carpal tunnel has to be opened in the hand to release the pressure on the nerves **(Figs. 20A and B)**. Fasciotomy incisions are given from proximal to distal direction, so that the pressure is released gradually and immediate profuse bleeding does not occur interfering with the incisions. If there is significant bleeding during fasciotomy, it can be controlled by pressure dressing for a brief duration or by using electrocautery. Since the incisions expose the underlying healthy tissues to a risk of infection by bacteria colonizing the burn wound, it is important to give cover by topical antimicrobial agent during dressing (refer to Chapter 21 for details).

FURTHER MANAGEMENT OF THE BURN WOUND

After the initial resuscitative measures and acute burn wound management, the patient comes out of the shock phase and the general condition stabilizes. Now, all the attention is paid toward the burn wound as that would then be the greatest threat to the survival of the patient. Apart from supportive care, proper wound management helps in the spontaneous healing of the partial-thickness burn wounds and successful resurfacing of the full-

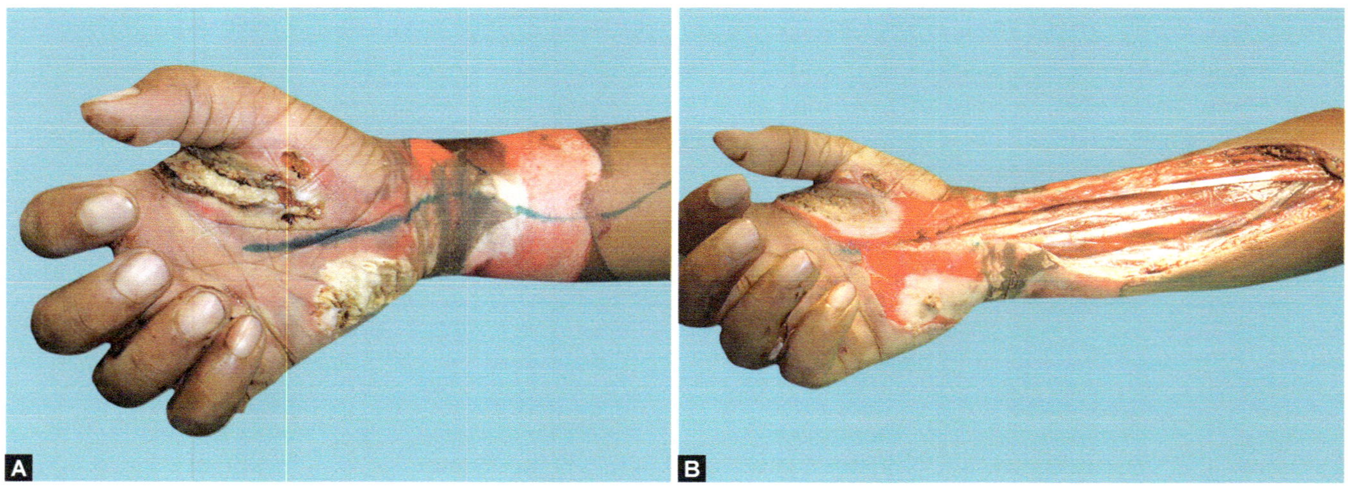

FIGS. 20A AND B: (A) Incision for opening carpal tunnel to decompress nerves; (B) Incision extended into forearm—circulation to hand restored and hand saved by timely intervention.

thickness wounds. Further wound care varies according to the depth of the burn wound. Burn wounds can either be managed with early surgical intervention or conservatively with regular dressings and delayed grafting, if needed.

Early Excision and Grafting

This is indicated for full-thickness or deep dermal burns, where the wounds either cannot heal on their own or where they heal with severe hypertrophic scarring or development of contracture. These surgical techniques are used in different patients or different areas in the same patient. The main aim of treatment is to close the burn wound as soon as possible, usually within 3–5 days of the burn injury. The excisional surgical procedures are described in the Chapter 15 in further detail.

Conservative Management

Conservative treatment involves regular dressings with conventional or newer dressing materials, allowing wounds to heal spontaneously or else reveal granulating wounds, which can be split skin grafted. The main aim of dressing is to:

- Decrease evaporative losses and pain
- Prevent and control colonization of wounds by bacteria
- Isolate the burn wound from the other sources of contamination
- Maintain an environment that promotes epithelialization of the partial-thickness wounds and prevents damage to neoepithelium

Conservative management is indicated for superficial dermal burns, which have the potential to heal own their own. The aim of this local treatment is to prevent their conversion into deeper burns by avoiding infection and providing optimal conditions for healing.

It is also indicated in deep dermal and full-thickness burns where immediate excision and grafting are not possible. This is usually seen in developing countries where early excision and grafting are not routinely done because of paucity of technical support, manpower, postoperative monitoring, and overload of burn patients. In these situations, a majority of the patients are managed by conservative treatment. In deep dermal wounds, the aim is to prevent infection and conversion to full-thickness wounds. Dressings are continued till the wounds heal. In full-thickness wounds, dressings are continued till a graftable bed is achieved. An eschar usually develops in full-thickness burns, and if it is still adherent at 21 days, late surgical excision of eschar can be considered as an option **(Figs. 21A to D)**. Another option is *grid escharotomy* **(Fig. 22)**. In this, incisions are given in a grid fashion so as to allow the introduction of surface bacteria underneath the adherent eschar and the subsequent pus formation allows the eschar to be lifted off the surface. Once the eschar is loosened, it is debrided mechanically, and the remaining nonviable tissue is best removed by repeated dressings with eusol. This is a wet-to-dry type of dressing, which involves direct application of eusol-soaked gauze followed by dry gauze and bandage. Eusol (Edinburgh University solution) is a good desloughing agent and contains the following: [31]

- Calcium hypochlorite, 1 part by weight
- Boric acid, 1 part by weight
- Water, 80 parts by weight

If a patient complains of pain, it can be diluted with normal saline to half or quarter strength. Gauze well

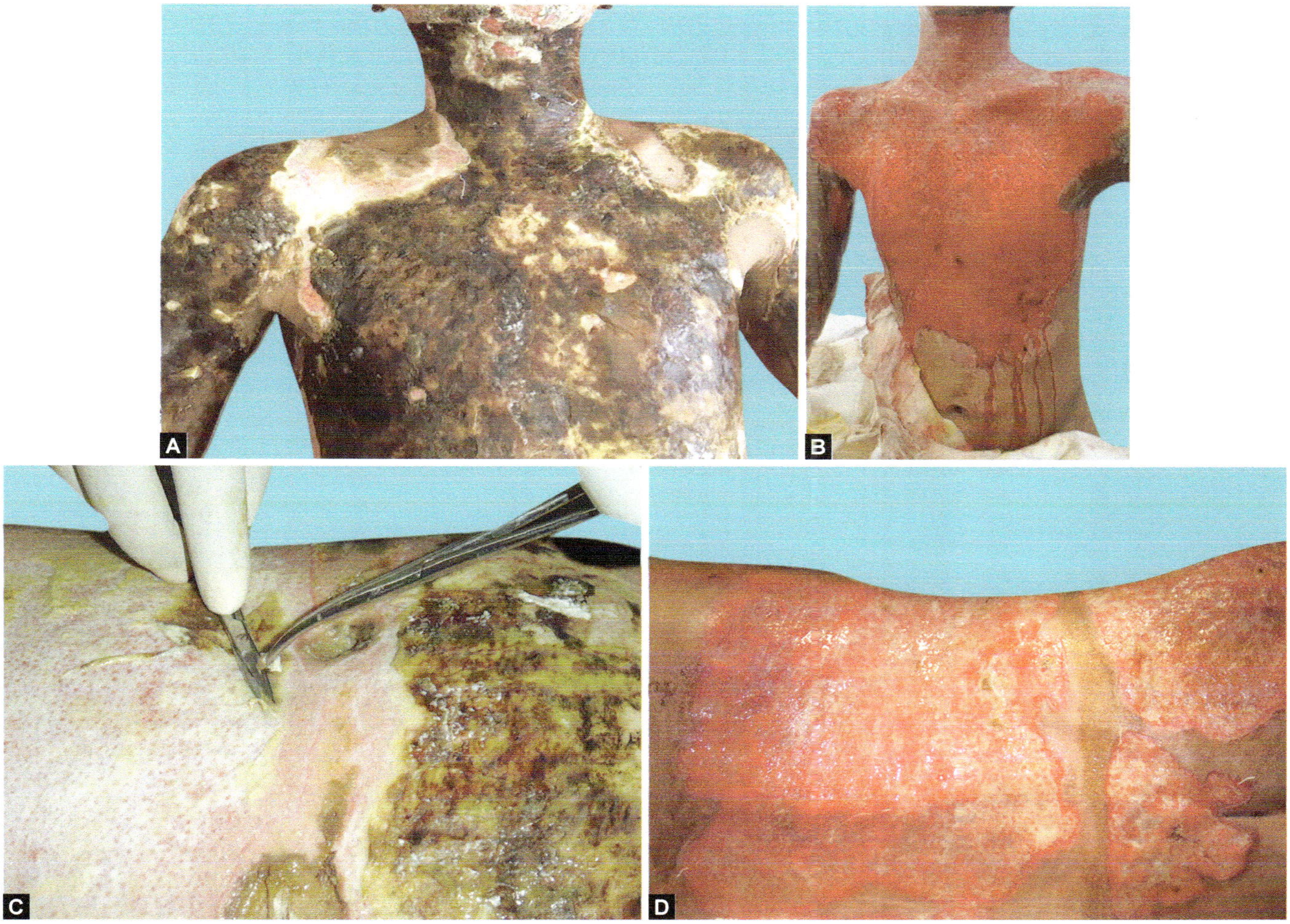

FIGS. 21A TO D: (A and B) Traditional wound management—eschar separation by autolysis; (C and D) Granulating burn wound following separation of eschar.

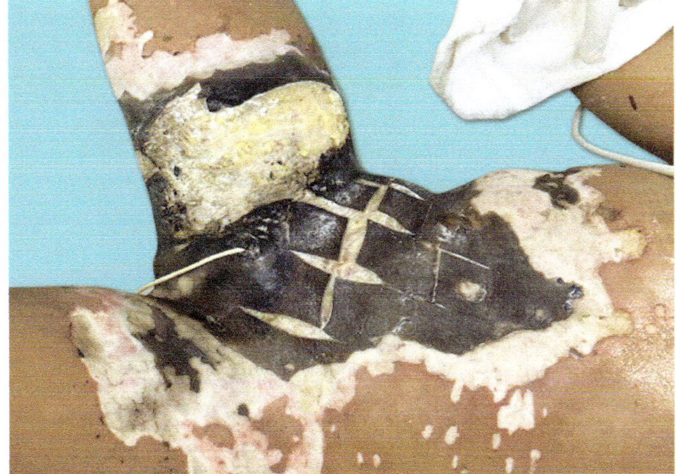

FIG. 22: Grid escharotomy—allows introduction of surface bacteria under eschar leading to suppuration and separation of eschar.

soaked in eusol and lightly squeezed out is directly applied to the wound without any paraffin gauze or any other nonadherent layer and covered further by Gamgee pads and bandage. Since this is an adherent dressing, it has to be soaked well with normal saline on removal during dressing change to avoid pain. Ideally, eusol dressings should not be allowed to dry for greater efficacy. It is advised to repeat the dressing 3–4 times a day as the action of hypochlorite is transient. As this is not feasible, the dressing is changed on a daily basis. Although the action of eusol has not been studied by any clinical trial, it has been used by surgeons for decades and found to be very effective.

Role of Debridement

Debridement is the removal of necrotic tissue, foreign material, and biofilm from an acute or chronic wound, and is the cornerstone of burn wound management that accelerates the healing process. The most direct form of debridement is surgical debridement and it is also the most efficient method. Other methods of debridement are mechanical debridement, autolytic, biological, and enzymatic debridement.

Enzymatic debridement is the application of exogenously derived proteolytic enzymes to a wound to accelerate a controlled degradation and removal of necrotic tissue. It is easy to apply and negates all the disadvantages of surgical debridement. There have been many agents that have been tried. Christopher Columbus used pineapple juice to promote healing of burn wounds. Since then enzymes derived from microorganisms such as *Clostridium histolyticum* like collagenase, varidase, papain (from papaya), and bromelain (BRM) (from pineapple) have been used. The use of enzymatic debridement seems to be very effective to treat patients with burns of indeterminate depth for enzyme's ability to selectively act on necrotic eschar without adverse effects on viable skin.[32-34]

NexoBrid® (NXB, MediWound Ltd., Yavne, Israel), another enzymatic debriding agent, contains a concentrate of proteolytic enzymes enriched in BRM. It has been proven to effectively and selectively remove burn eschar in a single 4-hour application, reducing the need for surgical eschar removal. BRM is extracted from the stem of the pineapple plant (*Ananas comosus*). It is available in the form of gel, which is spread on the surface of the necrotic area which is then covered with an occlusive bandage to protect the lesion. BRM acts on fibrin, denatured collagen, and elastin, removing selectively the necrotic tissue and preserving the dermis on the wound that is still viable and able to stimulate its spontaneous re-epithelialization.[35]

However, the results of enzymatic debridement are highly variable and further surgical debridement might still be needed. Furthermore, repeated applications may result in local infection and promote sepsis.[36] Therefore, the decision has to be individualized to the wound and also depends on the surgeon's experience with such debriding agents.

Hydrosurgery

The Versajet hydrosurgery system (Smith & Nephew, London, UK) is a specialized powered surgical and debridement tool which makes use of an innovative technology that can excise targeted tissue and preserve viable tissue, based on the Venturi effect.

The system is made up of five separate components. The pedal operated by the foot activates the power console and sterile saline flows through low-pressure tubing to the power console where it becomes pressurized. The pressurized saline is then forced through a small jet nozzle at the end of the hand-piece. A high-velocity stream of sterile saline jets across the operating window and targeted tissue can be excised. Additionally, a vacuum is created at this point (the "Venturi effect") and all debris and contaminants produced by the procedure are sucked into an evacuation tube, and deposited in a separate waste container. There are a number of power levels on the unit, the lowest will function mainly as a vacuum, but by increasing power, harder and tougher tissue can be removed. The hand-piece provides control to hold targeted tissue during irrigation. As the hand piece is single-use only, the incidence of cross-infection is minimized.

This treatment is well tolerated by the patient and drastically reduces the bacterial load and has several other advantages over standard surgical scalpel debridement such as it can be done in the ward, like a usual dressing; it is less aggressive and more selective, allowing a superior sparing on healthy tissue; prevents the diffusion of microbial contamination deeper into the wound; induces only minor bleeding; and is less painful. It can create a smoother, less irregular ulcer surface ready to receive a skin graft or other suitable dressings.

The high cost of the disposable handpiece represents a disadvantage of Versajet, but from a pharma-economical point of view, it shortens the hospitalization and the healing time, promoting a quicker debridement, thus allowing a total saving in wound management.[37]

Hydrotherapy

Hydrotherapy involves washing the burn wound or giving a bath to the entire patient prior to dressing change. This can be given in the form of a shower or immersion-in-saline bath (Arzo bathtub) or Hubbard tank **(Figs. 23A and B)**. The advantages of hydrotherapy are:

- It improves general hygiene and decreases the number of bacteria.
- Patient has a feeling of well-being.
- Dressings can be removed easily, and wounds can be cleaned painlessly.
- Active exercises can be performed during hydrotherapy, which prevents stiffness of joints.

Ambulatory patients are managed by using shower bath whereas nonambulatory patients or those with extensive burns are best managed in a saline bath or Hubbard tank. Minor debridements can also be carried out during this procedure. The main disadvantage of using bathtubs or tanks is the risk of cross contamination amongst the patients. Additionally, this is a cumbersome procedure involving a team of doctors, nurses, and therapists.

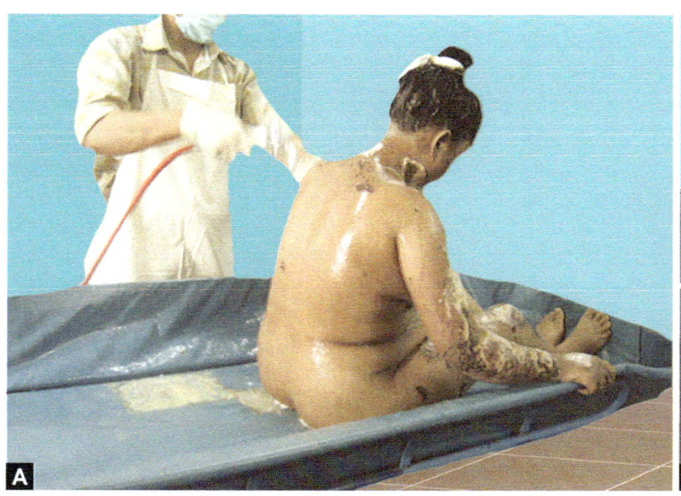
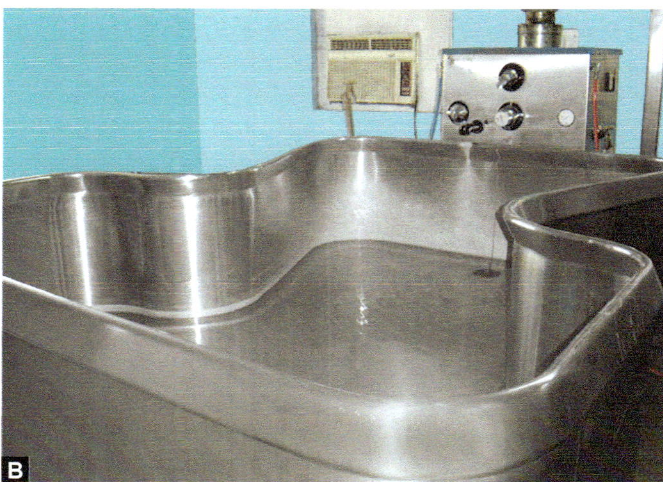

FIGS. 23 A AND B: (A) Shower bath on a shower trolley; (B) Saline bathtub used in the author's unit.

SKIN GRAFTING OF THE BURN WOUND

Skin grafting is done to achieve the final goal of wound closure. The grafts used are split skin grafts taken from unburnt areas of the body.

History

The history of skin grafts dates back to 1869 when Reverdin published his method of skin grafting. He took 1-2 mm diameter skin pieces from a donor area of the patient and transferred them to the granulation tissue of the skin defect.[38-40] This method was soon introduced throughout Europe despite French surgeons objecting that this method of producing new wounds encourages the risk of erysipelas. Reverdin believed in principle that the advancing edge of epithelialization makes the wound heal faster. This was also the basis for meshing of the graft. Pollock[41] at St. George's Hospital started performing skin grafting in Great Britain in 1870. Reverdin's discovery led to many more clinical experiments that explained the type of granulation tissue best suited for grafting and how the thickness of the skin graft affected the speed of epithelialization.

In 1870, Ash[42] concluded that thinner the graft, the quicker the spread of epithelium around it. With the discovery of the fact that complete coverage of wounds with grafts produced better scars, arose the need for larger grafts. In 1872, Ollier[43] a Frenchman, used grafts as big as 8 cm^2.

Gradually, surgeons performing eyelid surgery succeeded in covering a wound surface with full-thickness skin graft (FTG). In 1870, Lawson[44], a British surgeon applied this technique for upper eyelid reconstruction. In 1875, Wolfe[45] pioneered the FTG, which were then called "Wolfe grafts" or "Wolfe Krause" grafts after Krause gave his experiences with large size FTG in Germany in 1893.[46]

Till this time, no importance was given to the wound bed and apart from the patient's own skin, other humans as well as animals were used as donors, which led to a lot of disappointing results. The next important criteria for skin grafting were laid down by Thiersch, a German surgeon[47] who, on the basis of years of his experience, concluded that grafting should always be done from patient's own skin and grafts should be placed on fresh wound bed and if granulation tissue was present on wound bed, it should be excised to improve graft "take" and lastly, split skin grafts and not the FTG should be used to cover wound surface.

Thiersch procured grafts using a razor and they were thicker in the middle than at the edges. Therefore, for many years efforts were made to find new ways of improving harvesting techniques in order to get thin grafts of uniform thickness.

Skin grafts were applied only after granulation tissue had appeared, although graft application after excision in case of burns on eyelids on 6th postburn day was also reported.[48,49]

Methods of skin grafting fell into disrepute at the end of the 19th century because of the technique and the disappointing results. Interest in Reverdin's technique was reinvoked at the beginning of the 20th century with modifications. Davis referred to the modified version of Reverdin grafts as "Small deep grafts"[50] which were later renamed as "Pinch Grafts" by Gatch.[51] Douglas et al called them "Steele grafts" after Steele, one of the first British surgeons to apply the skin grafting techniques.

It was in 1929 that Blair and Brown described their successful technique of split skin grafting. They differentiated and elaborated on the advantages and disadvantages of thin, intermediate, and FTG. Split skin grafting for burn wounds with their technique became an accepted procedure from 1930 to 1950. The techniques were improved and more importance was given to the preoperative, peroperative, and postoperative care. In 1934, Humby formulated various criteria for graft cutting instruments and though his first device did not function too well, he introduced the "Humby" knife in 1936, which was a greatly simplified version.[52,53] The original Humby knife was a razor with a guard, which did not allow precise control over the thickness of the grafts. Further modifications were made to increase its reliability.

Another instrument that could be adjusted to procure grafts of a uniform width with varying thickness was the "dermatome". In 1924, Hagen developed a mechanical dermatome, which was driven with a flywheel. In 1939, Earl Padgett, a surgeon and Hood, a mechanical engineer, designed the Padgett-Hood dermatome in the USA[54] which could be set at a specific thickness. Brown, another surgeon, developed the "Brown dermatome" with the help of Barron, a mechanical engineer.[55] This had a rapidly vibrating knife driven by an electric motor.

Preparation of Wound for Grafting

Once granulation tissue appears, swab cultures are always taken to look for microbial growth and its sensitivity pattern to various antibiotics before taking up the patient for skin grafting. A healthy bed that is ready for grafting shows clean red granulations devoid of any necrotic areas and does not bleed readily on touch (**Figs. 24A to C**).

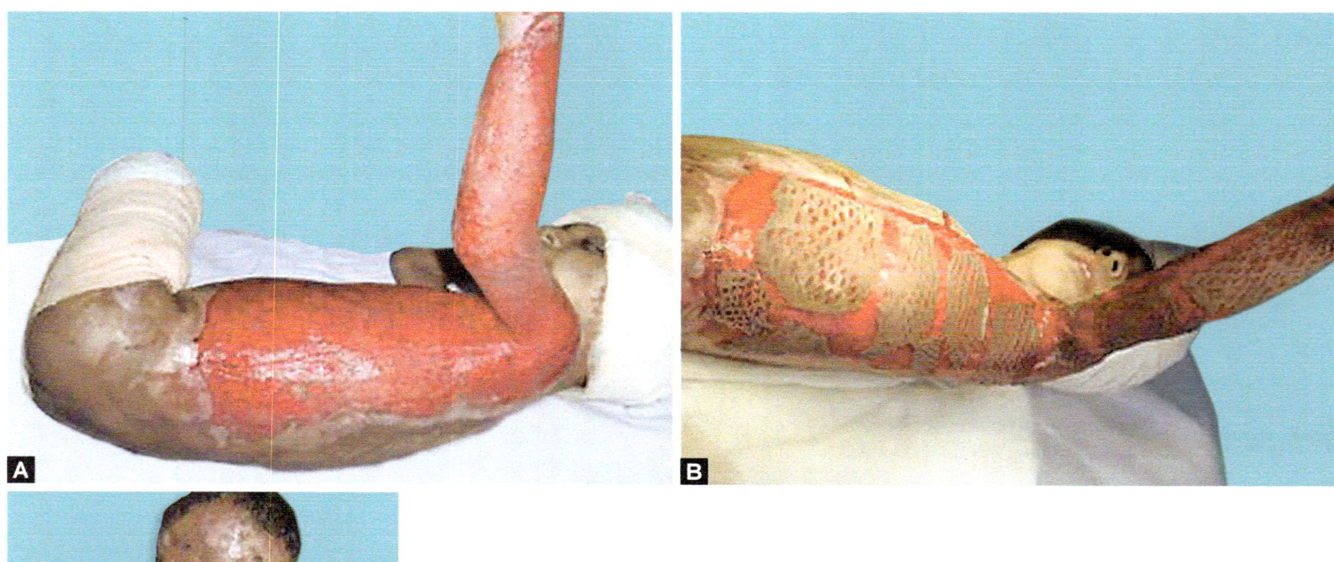

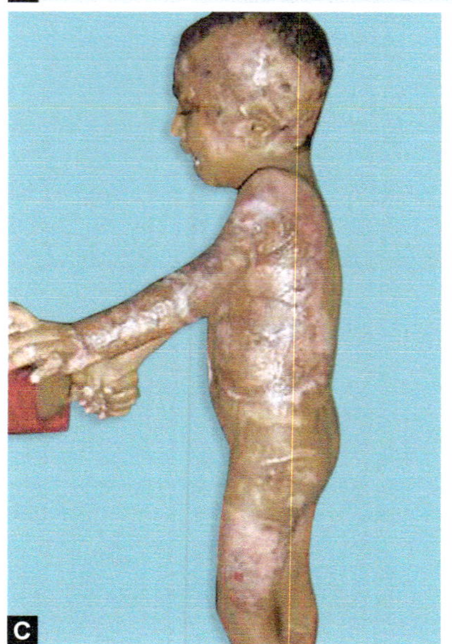

FIGS. 24A TO C: Healthy granulating wounds covered with split skin graft.

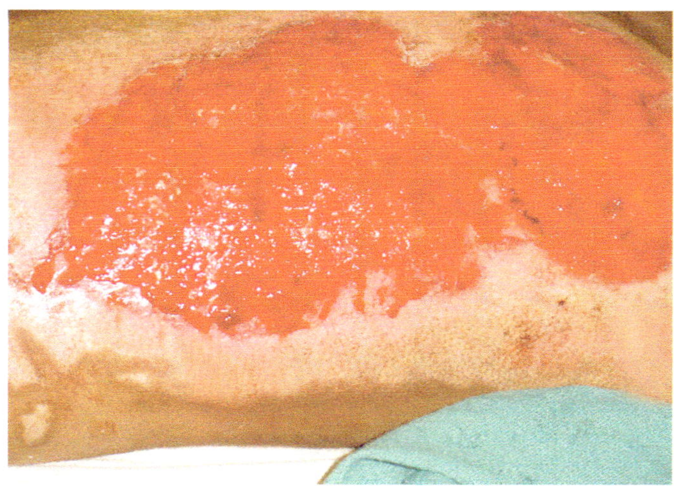

FIG. 25: Fragile granulation tissue bleeding profusely on touch—indicating streptococcal infection.

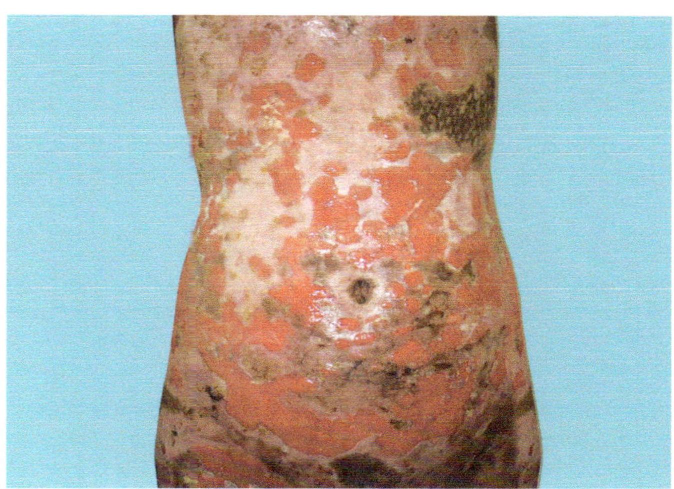

FIG. 27: Loss of skin grafts with methicillin-resistant *Staphylococcus aureus* (MRSA) infection.

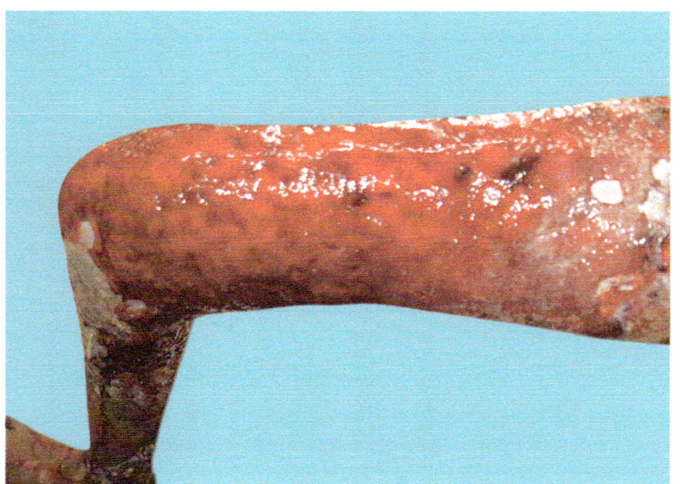

FIG. 26: Slimy dirty granulation tissue with copious discharge—indicating *Staphylococcus* infection.

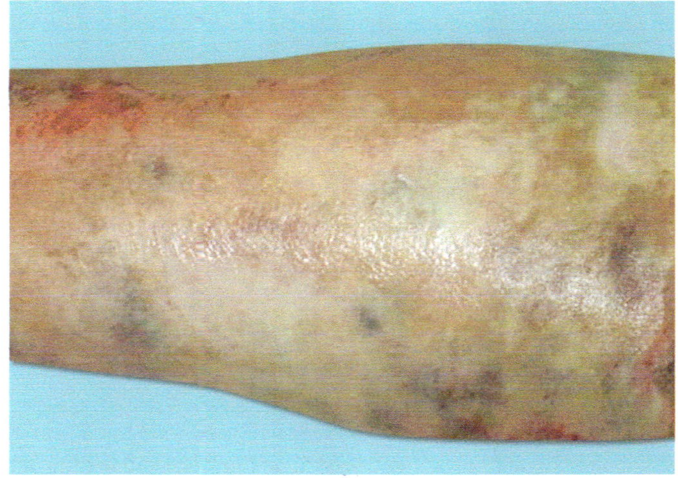

FIG. 28: Greenish discoloration of wound indicative of *Pseudomonas* infection.

If the wound looks angry red and granulation tissue is very fragile and bleeds readily on touch with unhealthy copious discharge, it is suggestive of beta-hemolytic *Streptococcus* infection **(Fig. 25)**.

This is an absolute contraindication for skin grafting of wound. *Streptococcus* is sensitive to large number of broad spectrum antibiotics which should be started immediately and continued till swab culture is negative. If the granulation tissue appears slimy, it is suggestive of *Staphylococcus* infection **(Fig. 26)**.

In these cases, systemic antibiotics, based on wound swab culture-sensitivity data are administered, and local dressings are done with antistaphylococcal agents like Fucidin or mupirocin. Presence of *Staphylococcus* infection in the wound bed results in loss of graft after initial "take" and gives an eaten-up appearance **(Fig. 27)**. Skin grafting is done only after *Staphylococcus aureus* is cleared

Bluish green pus discharge from the wound suggests *Pseudomonas* growth **(Fig. 28)**. In these cases, dressing with 1% acetic acid solution is very effective or else mafenide can be used. If there is edematous, hypertrophic granulation tissue, gentle compressive dressings using crepe bandages should be done to reduce edema. Local steroid cream is also effective. Sometimes the burn wounds are neglected, and they turn into chronic fibrosed wounds. These wounds cannot be prepared by dressing alone and require excision of the fibrotic bed till a healthy soft and supple vascular bed is reached before the application of split skin graft **(Figs. 29A to C)**.

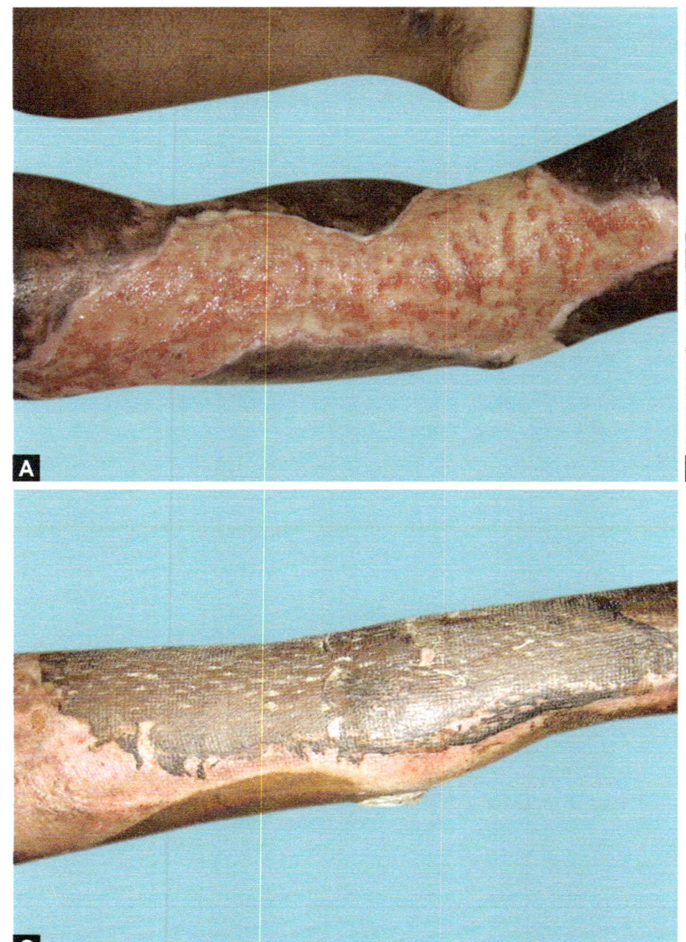

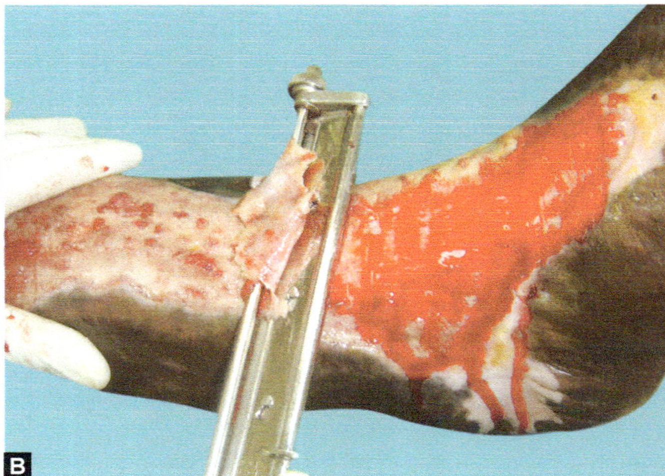

FIGS. 29A TO C: (A) Old neglected postburn raw area with fibrosed bed having slough and no granulation. This wound needs to be excised to remove the unhealthy tissue; (B) Excision of the same wound; (C) 10 days after application of skin graft, which is fully taken up on the healthy bed postexcision.

Types of Skin Grafts

There are different criteria for classifying skin grafts.

Based on the Anatomy

- *Split-thickness skin graft (SSG)*: It is most effective for postburn raw area coverage. It includes epidermis and part of dermis and undergoes significant primary contraction. Donor sites of SSG heal spontaneously by re-epithelialization from epithelial cells lining the hair follicles and sweat glands within 10–21 days. Skin graft can be reharvested from the donor site, once the wound epithelializes.
- *FTG:* These include epidermis with entire dermis. They require better vascular bed for survival as well as good vascularity from the margins. They undergo minimal primary contraction. Their sensory recovery is better than that of SSG. They are preferred for covering postburn contracture release. The donor areas for FTG cannot resurface spontaneously because of lack of epithelial elements and the defect needs to be closed primarily.

Based on Thickness

- Thin SSG that has a thickness of 0.006–0.012 inches
- Intermediate thickness graft that has a thickness of 0.012–0.018 inches
- Thick SSG that has a thickness of 0.018 to 0.030 inches

For treating burn patients with skin grafts, apart from age and sex, there are many more factors to be considered when deciding the thickness of the graft to be harvested. For most of the burn wounds, grafts should be thin because their "take" is better. However, because they undergo greater primary contraction, thicker grafts (intermediate thickness) are preferred for regions like face, especially eyelids and lips, so that they contract less postoperatively. In children and the elderly, usually thin grafts are harvested as the dermis is thin. If a donor site is to be reused more than once for procuring grafts as in patients with extensive burns, thin grafts should be harvested. This is because the donor sites may not heal due to loss of dermis if thick SSG are harvested repeatedly.

Based on Size and Technique

- *Pinch grafts*: These are "small deep grafts" that are not used at present because of the extremely ugly scarring of the donor site. The donor area chosen, therefore, is a hidden area usually the thigh or groin. The procedure involves lifting the skin with a needle and a 0.5 cm fragment is cut to obtain a graft which is thicker in the center and tapering toward the edges. The resulting wounds can even be closed primarily. The grafts are transferred to the wound at regular intervals, distance between them being about 5 mm. This method is now of historical importance only.
- *Stamp grafts*: These are SSG which, after harvesting, are cut as square or rectangular pieces of skin of different sizes. They are applied to the wound and held in place with occlusive dressings. The intervening areas between the stamps heal by epithelialization from the margins of the graft. As a result, these areas undergo hypertrophy and give unsightly scars. This method may be of use in cases of very extensive raw areas.
- *Sheet grafting* : It is the most widely used grafting at present as the grafts can now be easily harvested with the help of Watson skin grafting knife or dermatome. Large sheets about 10 cm wide or more can be procured easily, and they can cover large raw areas. This gives good aesthetic results especially on the face. These sheets can be meshed to increase their size to cover larger areas.
- *Meek grafting*: This was described in 1958 by an American surgeon, CP Meek. It involved the use of a "Meek-Wall" dermatome to obtain postage stamp autografts, which are expanded using double-pleated gauzes. This produced a regular distribution of autograft islands with a nine-fold expansion but required donor areas of suitable size and shape. It was discontinued for a while after the introduction of Mesh grafts in 1964, because of problems encountered with the old technique of Meek grafting. The Meek grafting technique was redesigned to overcome the imperfections of the original method. A special spray called "Meek adhesive" was developed and the prefolded gauzes were manufactured with expansion ratios of 1:3, 1:4, 1:6, and 1:9. This required very small donor areas and the graft islands were evenly placed in a regular pattern. The epithelialization and hospitalization time are reported to be shorter with this technique, compared to the mesh graft method. This method is preferred in extensive burns where the donor areas are very limited.[56,57]

Indications for Skin Grafting in Burns

Skin grafting is indicated in the following situations in burns:

- Following excisional surgery of burn wounds
- To cover postburn raw areas
- Following the release of postburn contractures
- Following excision of postburn scars like hypertrophic or hypopigmented scars, etc.

Essential Criteria for Skin Grafting

The essential criteria for skin grafting are as follows:

- Grafting of postburn raw areas should be done as soon as the granulation tissue is healthy. If delayed for long, the granulating areas become fibrotic and graft "take" is less than satisfactory.
- The granulation tissue should have a healthy red appearance, i.e., it should be a well-vascularized bed.
- The wound bed should be free from infection. The presence of beta-hemolytic *Streptococcus pyogenes* is an absolute contraindication for grafting as it does not allow the graft to "take" at all as it eats the fibrinogen which is responsible for graft adhesion to the bed. Presence of other bacteria like *Pseudomonas aeruginosa, E. coli, Klebsiella* is not a contraindication for grafting if present in <10^5 organisms/g of tissue. Although *Staphylococcus aureus* allows graft to "take" initially but it eats away the graft progressively to an unacceptable degree and it is not advisable to graft a wound until it has been eradicated.
- The general condition of the patient should be stable. Anemia should have been corrected by blood transfusion(s). Hemoglobin should be a minimum of 10 g%. The patient should be built up nutritionally (both enteral and parenteral).

Donor Areas

Skin grafts can be harvested from any area of the body. The most common sites whenever available are the lower limbs and upper limbs. The thigh is the most commonly used in the lower limbs, especially the anteromedial and anterolateral thighs. The back and buttocks are useful sites, if thighs are also burned. If the limbs and back is burnt, the chest, abdomen, or scalp can be used as donor areas. In these areas, adrenaline saline (1 in 200,000) can be injected subcutaneously to eliminate the depressions of the intercostal areas or the curvatures of the abdominal wall or bony prominences in order to form a flat base from which it becomes easier to harvest a good sheet of graft. Similarly, scalp is shaved and infiltrated with adrenaline saline solution before harvesting the graft. The advantage with scalp is that grafts can be harvested

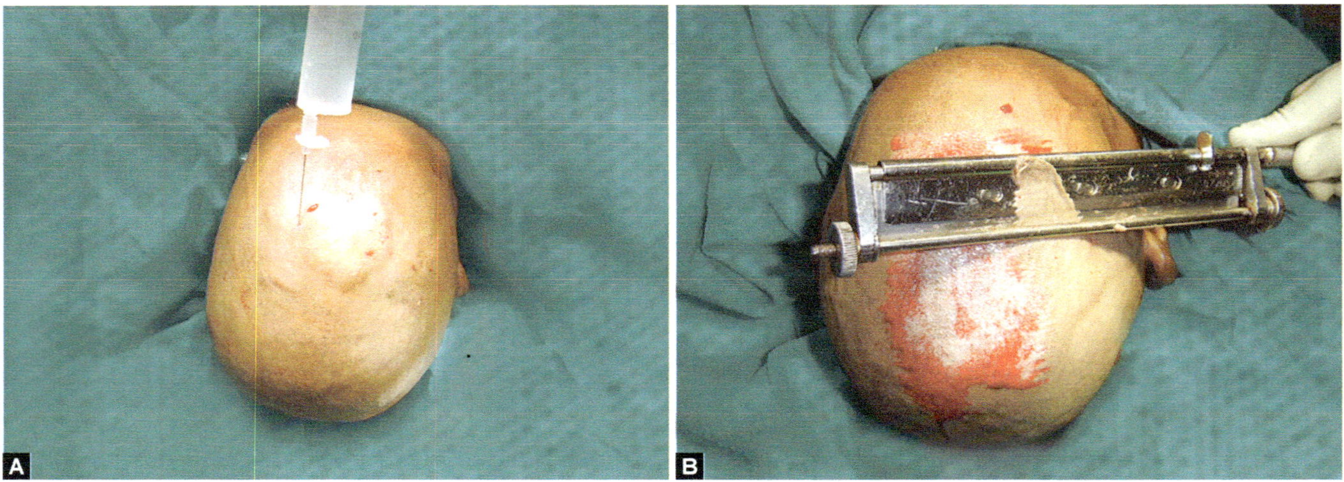

FIGS. 30A AND B: (A) Scalp as donor area—saline infiltration being done; (B) Graft being harvested from the scalp.

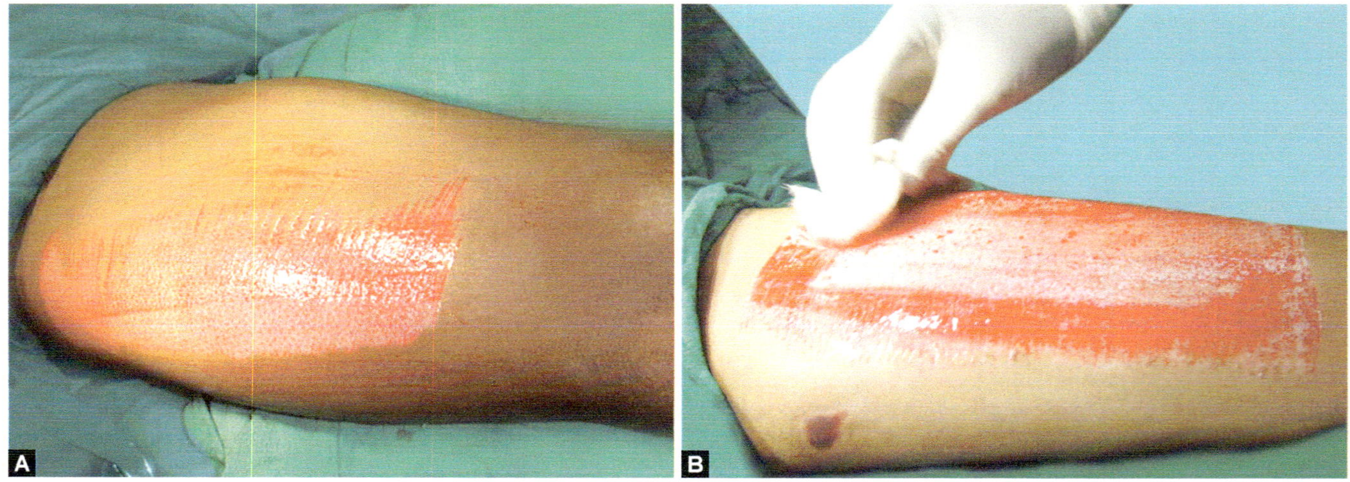

FIGS. 31A AND B: (A) Donor area of thin split-thickness skin graft (SSG)—bleeding points are small but numerous; (B) Donor area of thick SSG—bleeding points are larger but fewer.

repeatedly, every 10 days, as epithelialization is very fast from the epidermal lining of the large number of hair follicles **(Figs. 30A and B)**. While harvesting grafts from a hairy region, it is important to take thin grafts as thicker grafts contain undesirable hair follicles which lead to hair growth in the recipient area.

The donor areas of the split skin graft heal in 10–21 days. The donor areas are dressed by application of paraffin gauze, which may or may not be antibiotic-impregnated followed by gauze and then Gamgee pads and a compressive bandage. This bandage usually gets loosened up in 2 weeks and gauze falls off when opened in 3 weeks as majority of the superficial donor area re-epithelializes by 12 days. The other dressings that have been used for donor areas include collagen dressings, Biobrane®, and Opsite®. All these have been found to reduce pain, act as a barrier to bacteria, hasten healing, and reduce the bulk of dressing. However, they are very costly.

Blood Loss from Donor Areas

It is important to know about the blood loss while harvesting graft since majority of the burn patients have borderline hemoglobin levels. It is believed that older patients bleed less compared to younger patients who are well-nourished and have a good layer of subcutaneous fat. The back and buttocks bleed more than other areas of the body. Bleeding is more after harvesting thicker grafts than thinner grafts **(Figs. 31A and B)**. However, on average, while harvesting SSG, there is a loss of 23 mL blood from approximately 1% of the TBSA donor area.

This was studied by Robinson in 1949. However, it will vary according to the thickness of the graft taken.

Instruments for Grafting

There are various skin grafting knives available and they have been modified from time to time to improve the quality of graft which can be harvested with their help.[58] The earliest free-hand instrument to be used for grafting was the *Blair knife*, which required manual sharpening regularly. Then came the *Humby knife* which had a fixed blade but an adjustable roller guard, which adjusted the thickness of the graft harvested. The amount of pressure applied to the instrument on the surface of the skin also altered the thickness of the graft, i.e., the greater the pressure applied, the thicker the graft, and lesser the pressure, thinner the graft. There were various modifications to the Humby knife with a disposable blade, for example, *Braithwaite knife*, in which the roller guard moved longitudinally as well as rotated on its axis so that the graft tends to roll on to the rod and its edges were ragged. Then came another modification—*Bodenheim knife*, in which the roller guard moved only to and fro but did not rotate on its axis. The latest is the *Watson's modification* of Humby skin grafting knife **(Fig. 32A)** in which the guard is fixed and immobilized so that the edges of the graft are clean cut rather than ragged and the graft does not roll on to the rod as the knife proceeds forward. This is the most commonly used manual skin grafting knife at present. For procuring smaller sized grafts, "silver" knife has been used for many years **(Fig. 32B)**. The adjustment of the guard for varying the thickness of the graft in Watson's skin grafting knife is done by the screws present at both ends of the roller guard according to the calibrations present on proximal screw and then tightening the distal one. Another method for assessing the required gap between the blade and the guard is by holding the knife against the light so that the gap between roller guard and the disposable blade can be seen and the screws tightened. Increasing or decreasing the distance between guard and the blade produces thicker or thinner grafts, respectively. Even increasing the angle at which the knife is kept on the surface of skin and the pressure exerted varies the thickness of graft harvested.

The free-hand knives have been replaced by dermatomes **(Figs. 33A to D)**. *Padgett-Hood dermatome* was a mechanical drum dermatome in which the depth of cut could not be modified. After this, the *Brown dermatome* was introduced which was driven by an electric motor. The advantage of these motorized dermatomes was that they produced uniform long grafts with predetermined width and depth. The *air Zimmer dermatome* powered by compressed, water pumped nitrogen was introduced which has now been replaced by electric dermatome. Dermatomes may not be useful when the donor areas are narrow.

Technique of Harvesting Split Skin Graft (Figs. 34A to D)

Once the donor site has been selected, the graft can be harvested under general anesthesia, regional nerve blocks, or even local anesthesia. Infiltration of local anesthesia with adrenaline reduces the amount of blood loss from the donor area. The area is lubricated with Vaseline or paraffin and saline. An assistant gives traction to the skin from one end of the donor site while the operating

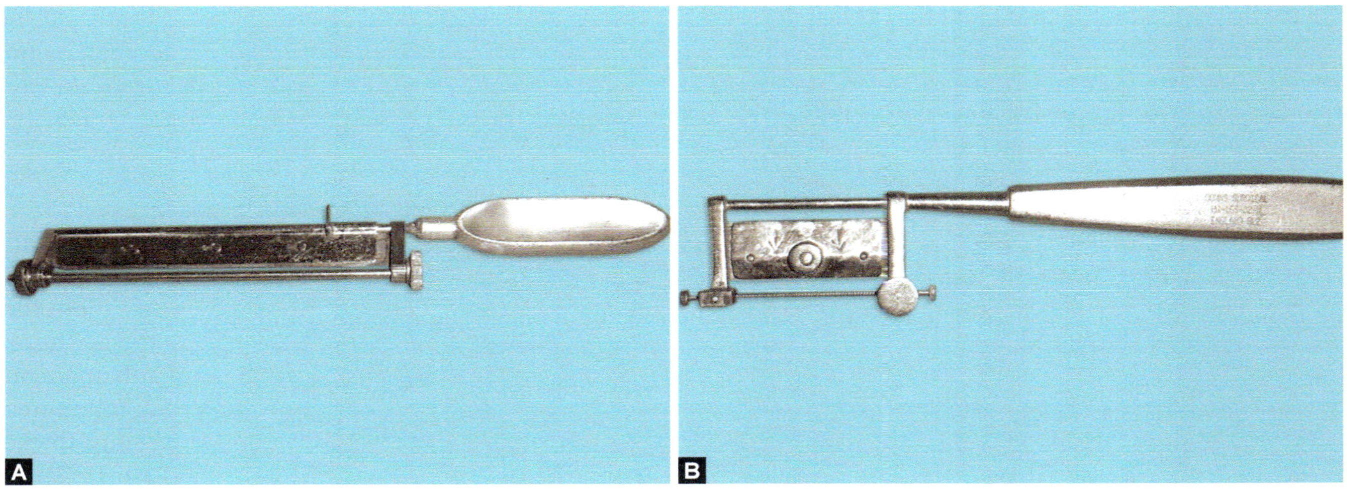

FIGS. 32A AND B: (A) Watson's modification of Humby's knife—most commonly used manual skin grafting knife; (B) Silver knife—used for harvesting small grafts.

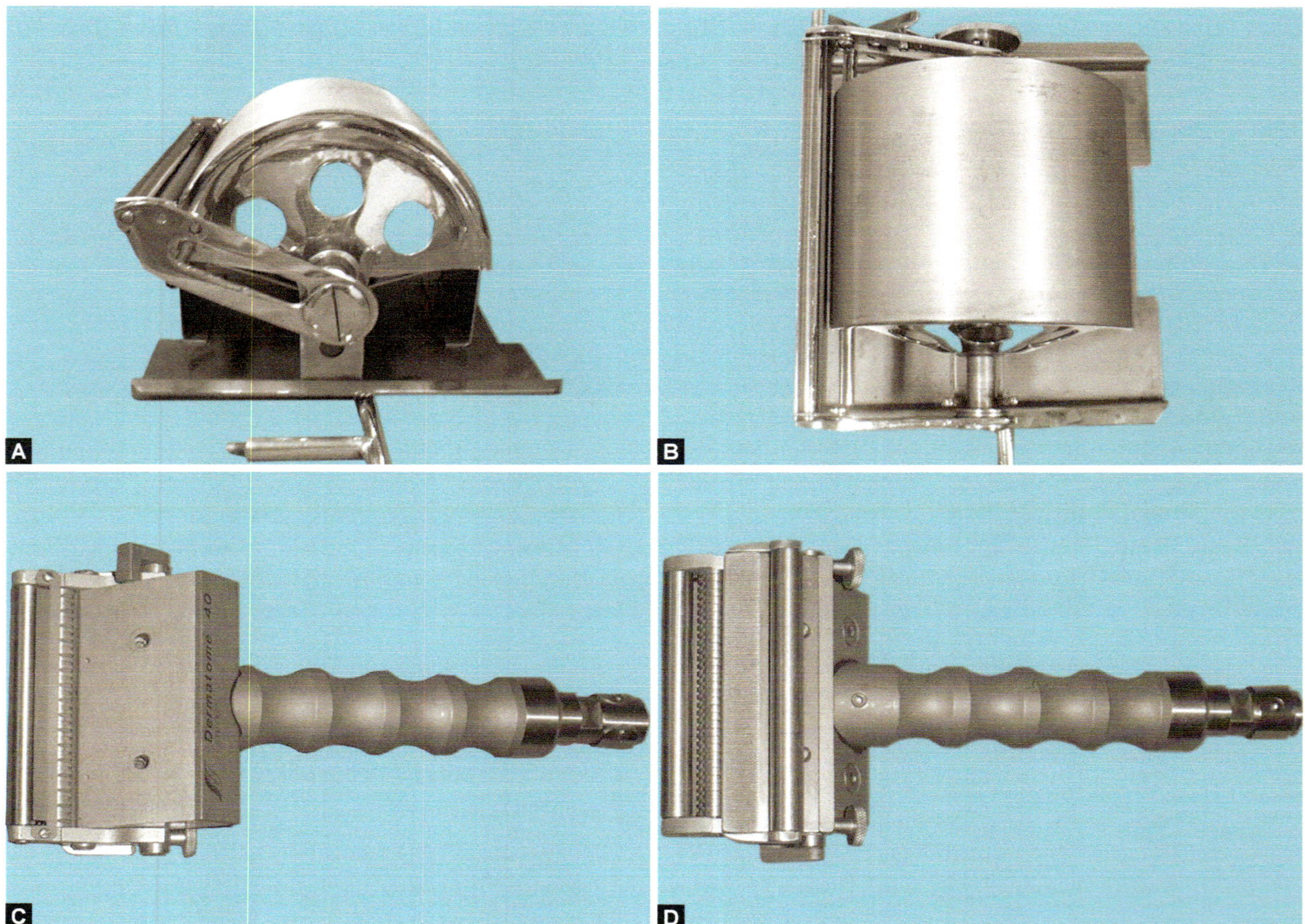

FIGS. 33A TO D: (A) Padgett's drum dermatome; (B) Same dermatome showing the surface of the drum on which the glue is applied when placed in contact with the skin; (C) Electric dermatome; (D) Electric dermatome—another view.

surgeon gives countertraction from the opposite side. Wooden/metallic graft (Gabbroo) boards are frequently used for applying the traction and counter traction. The knife is placed parallel to the surface of the skin and then moved "to and fro" with moderate pressure and gradually moved ahead with moderate speed till a long sheet is removed. The width of the graft harvested can be adjusted according to the area available. In the case of dermatome, it is kept on the skin surface at an angle of 30–45°, the throttle is pressed, and the dermatome is advanced flat to the skin with gentle downward pressure. Once the sheet of graft is harvested, the dermatome is angled upward and lifted off the donor site cutting the graft.

Meshing of Graft (Figs. 35 and 36)

Meshing of a skin graft is an old technique first described by Lanz of Amsterdam in 1907[59] when it was done manually. It was reintroduced by Tanner, Vandeput, and Olley (1964) with a new instrument.[60] They used a device that made slits in the graft at regular intervals producing a net-like structure when the graft is stretched. Tanner et al. were inspired by Dragstedt and Wilson (1937)[61] who used the same technique in FTG for drainage of fluid from the wound bed. They, in turn, were impressed with the "sieve" graft developed by Douglas (1930)[62] in which circular holes were cut in an FTG by leaving small islands of skin on the donor site for re-epithelialization.

The principle behind meshing a graft is to gain expansion by making incisions parallel to the longitudinal axis of the graft and the maximum advantage of meshing is gained when the long axis of the meshes parallel the stress lines of the area to be grafted. Earlier, incisions in grafts were made using a roller, which was rolled over a bed of small blades. Later, the graft was placed on a plastic carrier with slanting grooves and both the carrier and graft were drawn through a sort of mill with revolving blades. The technique has been steadily improved with

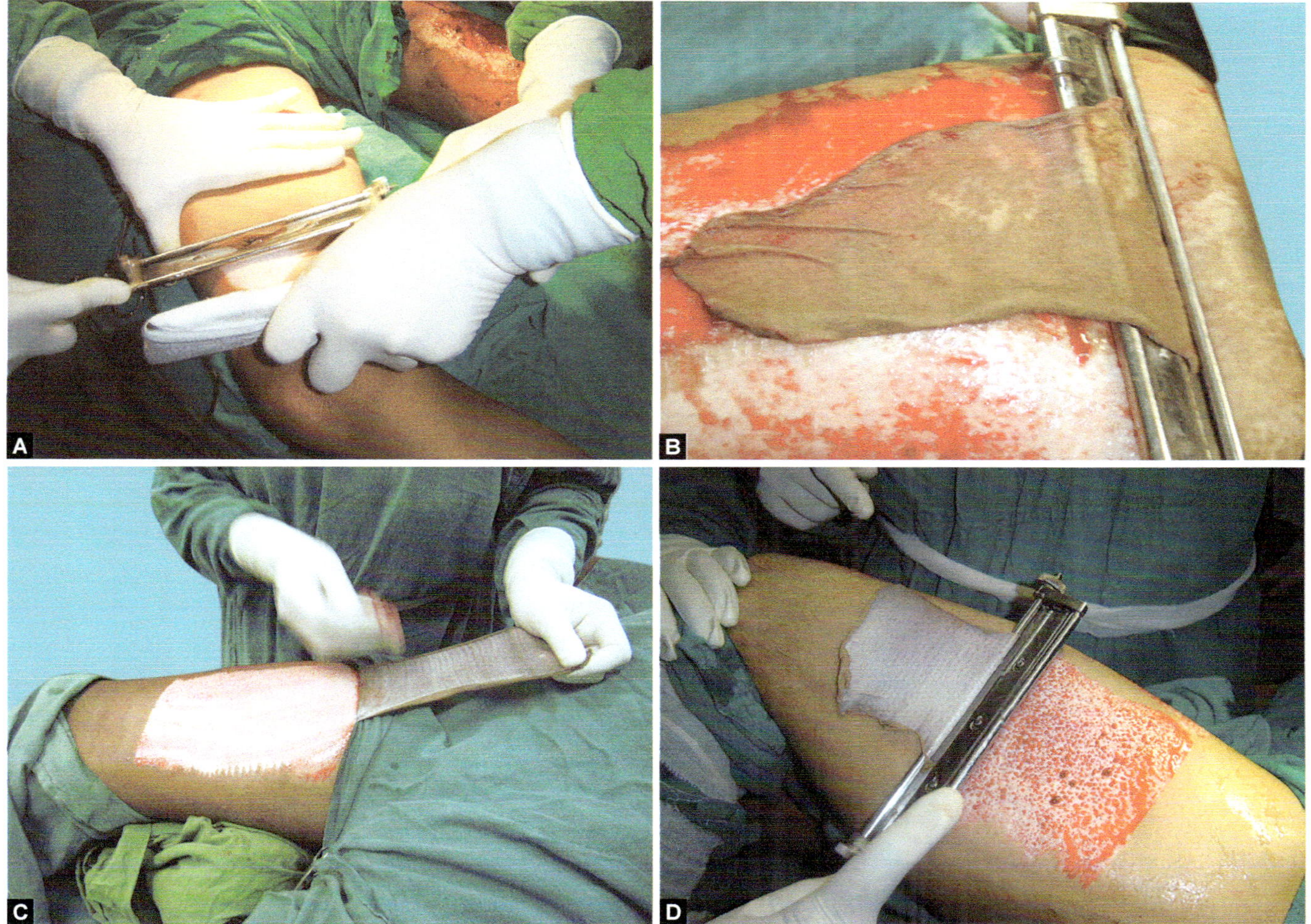

FIGS. 34A TO D: (A) Technique for harvesting skin graft with Watson's knife; (B) Thin split-thickness skin graft; (C) Intermediate-thickness skin graft; (D) Thick split-thickness skin graft.

modifications added to the older meshing instruments like Padgett's mesher. The latest is Zimmer's mesher in which the carrier with the graft can be pulled through the mesher with the help of a handle or lever. By adjusting the lengths of the cuts, the resulting size of the graft can be changed, and expansion of 1.5–9 times the original size can be gained. Minimal expansion should be used depending on the availability of the skin graft in relation to the size of the raw areas. In order to get good expansion by meshing, the grafts should not be too thin otherwise they tend to get torn.

The advantages of meshing are as follows:

- It expands the graft.
- Discharge can escape through the gaps in the graft and consequently, the accumulated discharge does not lift the graft off the wound surface.
- The meshing gives a larger edge for the production of new epithelial cells than the stamp grafts or strip grafts.
- A meshed graft conforms better to the wound surface and can be placed on uneven or convoluted surfaces.

The disadvantages of meshing are:

- The checkered board pattern or cobblestone appearance can be displeasing, especially in aesthetically important areas like face.
- The secondary epithelium in the meshed area is not of the same quality as the grafted skin and this is visible for the rest of life.

Application of Graft

Before the application of the graft to the wound bed it has to be ensured that proper hemostasis is achieved, especially if the unhealthy granulation tissue on the wound bed has been excised with a scalpel. Hemostasis is achieved by using adrenaline saline soaked (1 in 200,000) gauze pieces with pressure dressing or by fibrin glue which is being used of late (Tissel®).[63,64] The

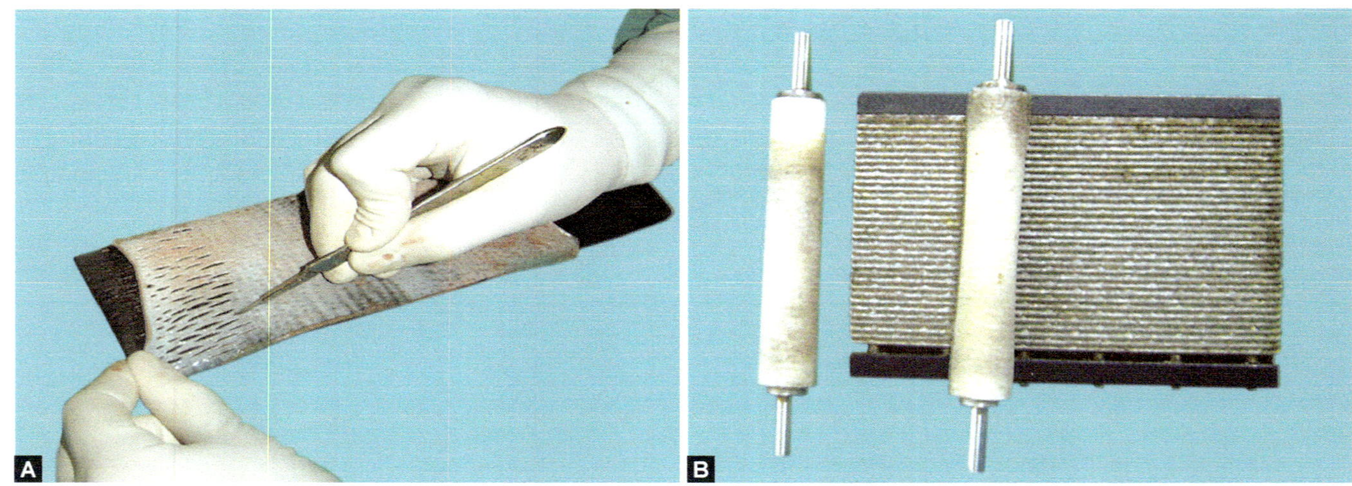

FIGS. 35A AND B: (A) Meshing of graft being done by hand; (B) Padgett's roller skin graft mesher.

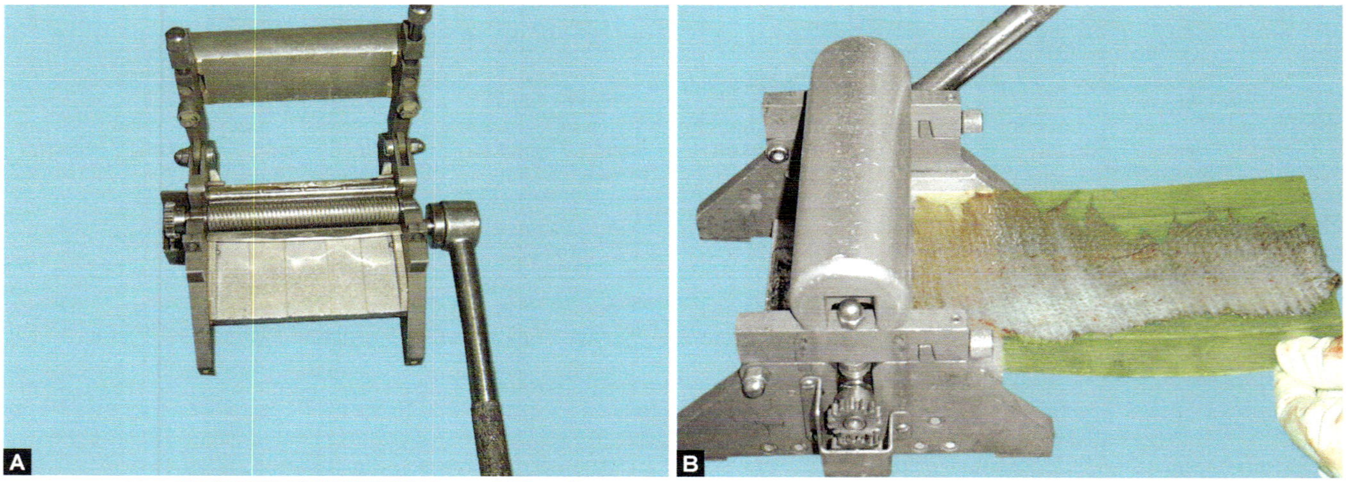

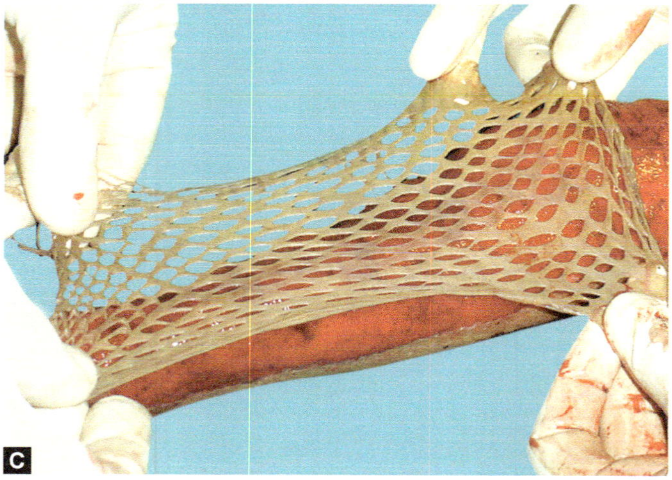

FIGS. 36A TO C: (A) Zimmer's skin graft mesher; (B) Graft being meshed by passing it through the mesher; (C) Meshed graft being applied on raw area.

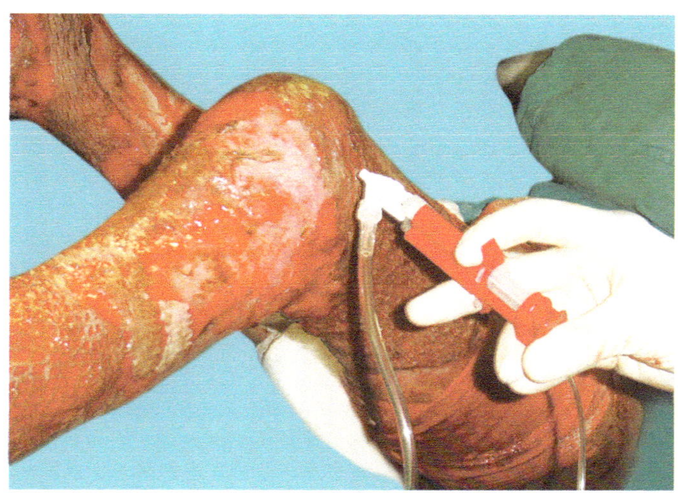

FIG. 37: Fibrin glue applied as a spray for anchoring graft to raw area.

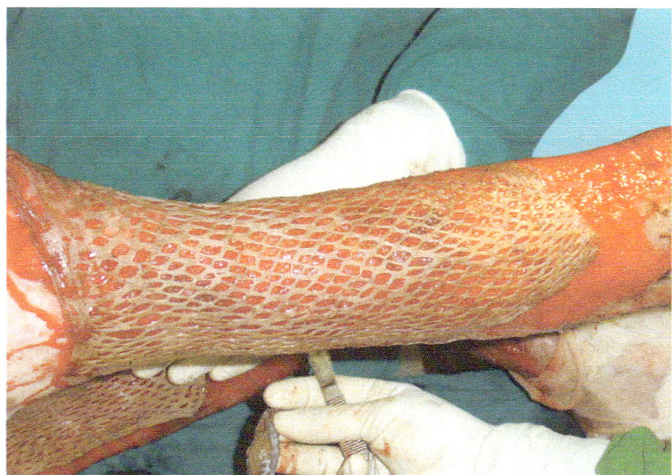

FIG. 38: Graft spread on the wound as a sheet, edges rolled out.

graft is then spread over the wound with the help of a graft spreader or with the back of forceps ensuring that the edges of the graft are properly spread out as these have a tendency to roll over. This can then be held in place with suture or surgical staples if areas are small or with fibrin glue **(Fig. 37)**. The graft can also be applied on the raw areas without using the above and covered with nonadherent gauze **(Fig. 38)**.

In the past, it was routine to do an occlusive dressing after any split skin grafting because it was considered that pressure over a graft was essential for its "take". However, with time and experience with different techniques, it has been clearly demonstrated that a graft can "take" satisfactorily over granulating areas as long as it is not mechanically displaced or lifted off from its bed by hematoma or pus formation and that occlusive dressings are not a must. Areas like the anterior chest, abdomen, and back of trunk where constant motion during respiration may displace the grafts by producing shearing between the dressing and the wound bed are better treated by exposure method after applying the graft. This is also true for the neck **(Figs. 39A to C)**.

If dressings are used as in the limbs, it is imperative to give an even gentle compression dressing with proper immobilization of the extremity **(Figs. 40A and B)**. The general principle is to immobilize a joint above and below the grafted area to minimize limb movements, and thus avoid shearing forces. In the case of mobile areas like the axilla or neck, stent dressing is advisable.

If the grafts are left without dressing, they should be inspected daily for initial 4–5 days to check for any displacement or any seroma or hematoma. However, if meshed graft is used it is advisable to apply a layer of paraffin gauze and a single layer of wet gauze till epithelialization of the interstices has occurred. Otherwise, the intervening raw areas tend to dry up and epithelial migration is inhibited. The same holds true for stamp grafts.

Skeletal traction can be applied on the extremities to elevate and immobilize the extremity following circumferential grafting of the limb by exposure technique. Suturing of graft edges is not favored in extensive raw areas as it can result in hematoma and at times microabscesses at each suture site resulting in graft loss. If adequate graft is available, it is preferred to overlap the adjacent graft edges slightly so as to avoid intervening raw areas. Although the intergraft raw areas heal by epithelial proliferation from the graft margins, it results in hypertrophic scarring which is aesthetically ugly and at times functionally poor.

Where homografts are available and donor area is limited, alternate strips of autograft and homograft are applied. In such cases as the homograft starts getting rejected after 14 days, the epithelialization from the margins has already covered quite a distance under the homograft. If homograft is not available and there are many small pieces of graft as in "postage stamp" grafts, they can all be spread on paraffin gauze with raw surface upward keeping a distance of 1 cm between two pieces. The paraffin gauze is then reversed and applied to the wound surface so that grafts adhere to the bed. "Postage stamp" autografts are also useful on multiple small areas of granulation. The Meek grafting is another method of obtaining extensive meshing to produce postage stamp grafts for coverage of extensive areas, as has been described earlier in this chapter **(Figs. 41 and 42)**.

Exposure technique is also preferred if the wound cultures show gram-negative organisms as these organisms are known to proliferate in the dark, moist, and warm condition provided by a dressing and will float

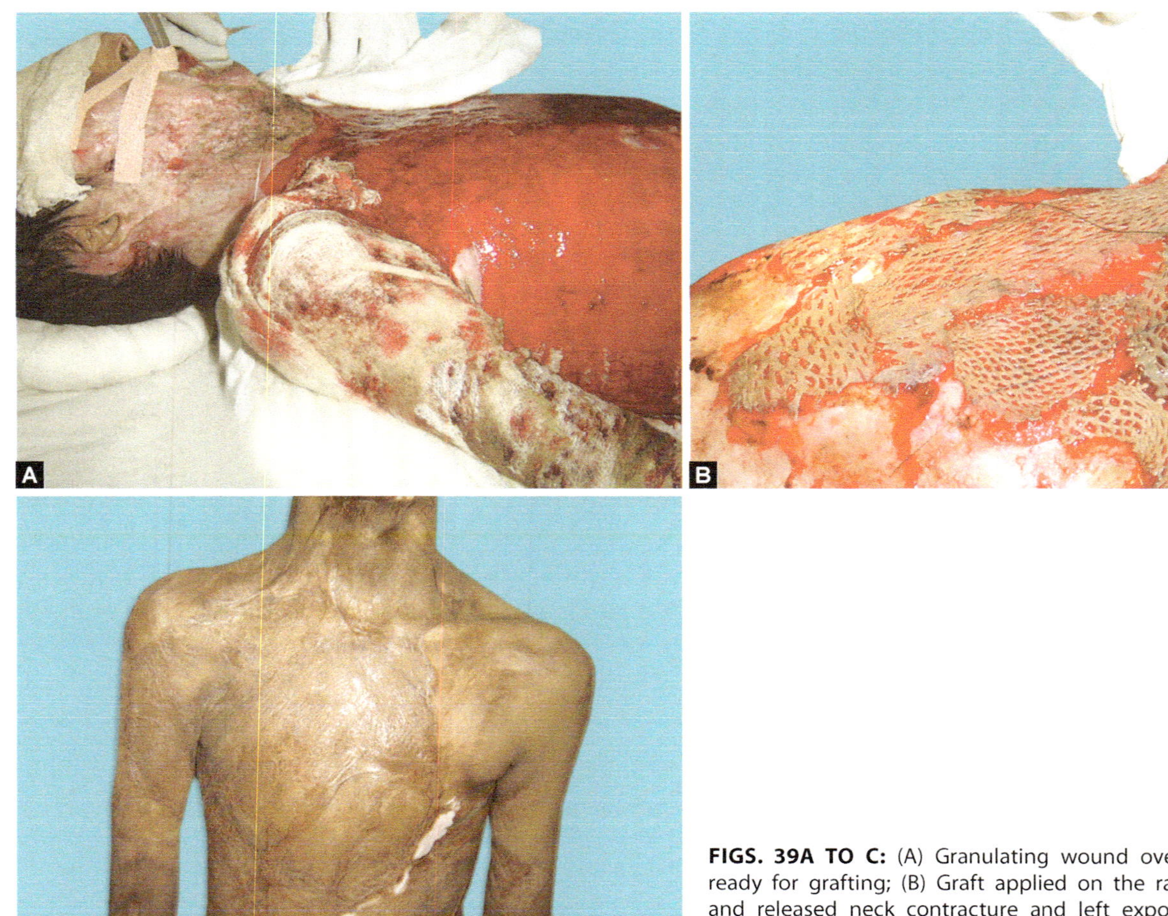

FIGS. 39A TO C: (A) Granulating wound over chest and neck, ready for grafting; (B) Graft applied on the raw area over chest and released neck contracture and left exposed; (C) 2 months postoperative picture of the same patient with completely healed areas with no hypertrophy.

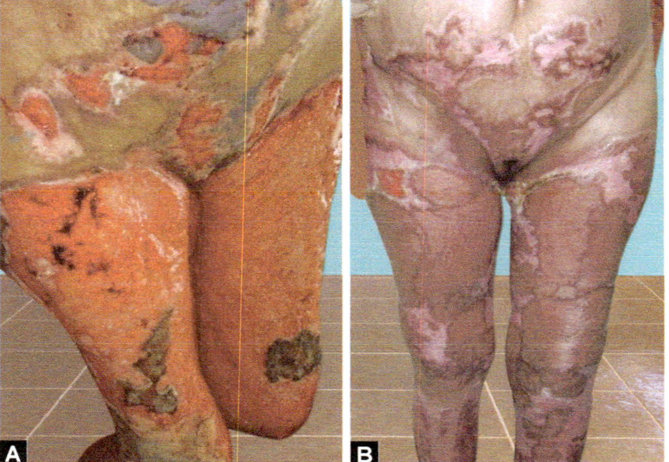

FIGS. 40A AND B: (A) Extensive granulating wounds over both lower limbs; (B) Wound closure with split-thickness skin autografts.

the grafts off the bed because of the volume of pus they produce. If these are kept exposed the activity of these organisms is decreased and chances of graft survival are better. After the fourth day, usually the time by which the grafts have adhered fairly well to the wound bed, closure method of treatment is started.

Delayed Application

At times in an anesthetized patient, it may be difficult to dress certain areas and there may be a risk of grafts getting displaced during recovery from anesthesia as is seen in neck, trunk, and face, and in heavy patients. In such cases, it is advisable to store the grafts and apply them to the wounds after a day when the patient is fully conscious and cooperative. The grafts can be applied bedside without any anesthesia. Delayed application of graft is preferred if slough or granulation has been excised and oozing from the raw area cannot be controlled.

Dressing Change

All postburn raw areas are potentially contaminated wounds. Therefore, it is of utmost importance to change the first dressing by 48–72 hours postgrafting. This should be done with full precautions to avoid moving the grafts. They are only dabbed with saline gauze to remove all the exudate and express out any seromas

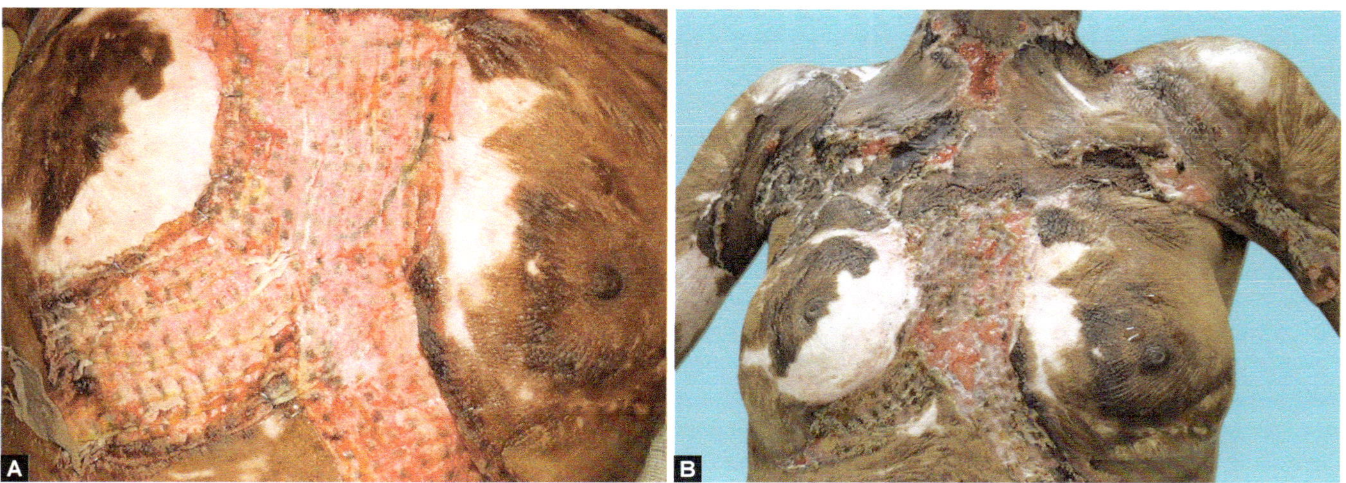

FIGS. 41A AND B: (A) Meek grafting technique used to resurface extensive defect created following release of contracture in a patient with multiple contractures and donor area deficit; (B) Healing areas with meek grafts.

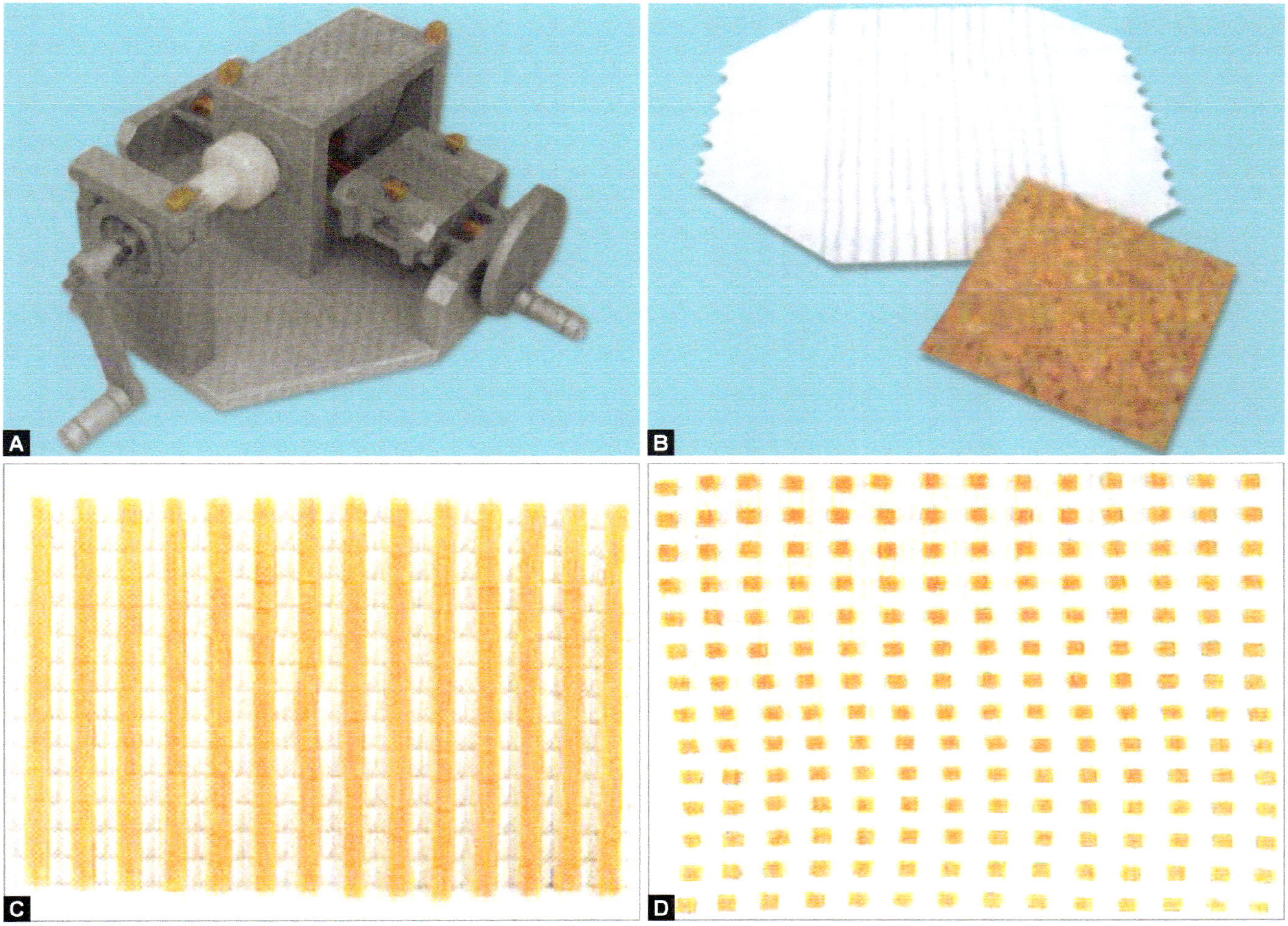

FIGS. 42A TO D: (A) Meek machine for "Meek grafting" with the cork plate and prefolded gauze; (B) The graft is spread on the cork plate and cut into small pieces by passing through the mesher. After the epidermal side of graft is sprayed with an adhesive, the graft is transferred to a prefolded gauze and the cork plate is removed. Expansion is achieved by unfolding the gauze; (C) First in one direction; (D) and then in the other direction.

Courtesy: Humeca Engineering group, Netherlands.

through the mesh or by giving a slit in the graft. A new dressing of the same type is reapplied. If delayed beyond 72 hours, in the author's experience, bacterial autolysis of graft or the purulent collection under the graft can lead to the loss of significant areas of graft and prolong the healing process.

The second dressing change can then be done at 5 days postgrafting and dried-up graft overlapping the normal skin can then be debrided and exposed dressing can be changed to a closed dressing, which will be less bulky. Thereafter, the dressing can be changed as often as required till the areas heal completely. Sutures or staples, if applied, can be removed on the third dressing. Once the grafts have taken up, movements of joint can be allowed during dressing change to avoid stiffening of the joints. Proper physiotherapy with full range of movements should be resumed only after all dressings are removed and healing is complete.

At times for one reason or the other, there can be small areas of graft failure. If they are more than 1 cm wide, patch grafting in a second stage may be required. However, if they are less than 1 cm wide, trials at repeated grafting may fail. In these circumstances, the areas should be cleaned thoroughly and dressed with topical antibiotic over mesh gauze along with a topical steroid preparation. The use of topical steroids allows the hypertrophic granulations to settle and the epithelium from the surrounding graft grows and spreads over the remaining raw areas.

Graft Survival

Graft survival has been studied in detail during the past century. By definition, skin graft is a piece of skin that is transferred from one place on the body to another after severing its blood supply, lymphatic system, and nerve supply. So, it is essentially skin transplantation and it derives its blood supply and innervations from the recipient area.

Serum Imbibition

Immediately after a skin graft is applied to the wound bed, the process of vascularization of the graft starts. Initially, the graft depends on the serous exudates or plasma which leaks out from the recipient venules, arterioles, and capillaries and fills up the space between the graft and host bed. This plasma is absorbed by the graft and is the source of its nourishment. This process was called "phase of serum imbibition" by Converse, Uhlschmid, and Ballantyne[65] and originally called "Plasmatic circulation" of graft by Alubscher and Goldman. Once the graft is lifted off the donor area, its vessels go into spasm squeezing out old blood and serum. When it is applied on the host bed, the cut ends of these vessels and the porous dermis start absorbing the serum collected between the graft and host bed passively. This makes the graft edematous and its weight also increases with the accumulation of waste products due to anaerobic metabolism till 48 hours until revascularization starts. In this phase, there is a growth of endothelial cells from the host into the graft as well.

Graft Revascularization

There have been various theories regarding how the graft gets revascularized. The earliest was the theory of "Abouchment" given by Beat[66] in which he noted microscopic anastomosis between host bed and graft. This was supported by Thiersch who termed the process of anastomosis between cut ends of host vessels and vessels of the graft as "inosculation" in an FTG. 25 years later, many researchers proposed that the original vasculature in the skin graft degenerates and endothelial cells and capillary buds from the host invade the graft by 9 hours and form a vascular network, and flow through the graft is established by the 4th postoperative day. These were confirmed by various histochemical, injection, and histologic studies. Another theory proposed by Henry[67] stated that though the original vasculature of the graft degenerates, the acellular basal lamina persists and acts as a conduit for endothelialization to start from the host capillary buds into the skin graft. This is also seen within 48 hours.

Thus, all the theories are by and large proposing the same explanation for the graft revascularization. To summarize, the vascular connections establish within 24 hours after grafting allowing inflammatory cells to invade the graft. By 4th postoperative day, blood inflow through the graft from the host bed is established. The graft now appears pink and blanches on pressure. This flow continues to increase till venous outflow from the graft back to the host bed is also started and by 1 month after grafting, the vascularization phase is completed.

The revascularization process is similar in both SSG and FTG. However, SSG survive longer without revascularization than an FTG because they contain fewer cellular elements to be nourished. The serum imbibition has to take place through a shorter distance through the dermis which is thinner. In an FTG, on the other hand, the full-thickness of the dermis acts as a barrier to the serum diffusion and hence, it depends more on the supply through the edges of the host bed with which it is in contact. Thus, in all granulating raw areas or areas with poor vascularity, a thin SSG survives better than a thicker graft and should be used.

Once the process of revascularization is understood, it is easier to understand why a hematoma or seroma under a graft inhibits its "take". Though they allow initial serum imbibition, they prevent the vascular ingrowth from the host bed into the graft which eventually dies out. Thus, it is important to evacuate any hematoma or collection under the graft before 72 hours by inspecting it on the first dressing which is advisable by the 3rd day. After evacuating the hematoma, the undersurface of the graft in that area where it is lifted off the bed, also needs to be scraped or rubbed with a gauze so that the tenuous lining of the proliferating epithelium which forms on the undersurface of the graft over the hematoma is removed. Otherwise, it can inhibit the graft's "take" once it is kept back on the host bed.

Graft Maturation

After the graft is vascularized, it matures over a period of time. An immature graft is soft, pink in color, blanches on pressure, may be thick, and shows scaling. The process of maturation takes about 6–12 months. During this phase of maturation, both the wound and the graft appear to undergo contraction. This process of graft contraction is actually a manifestation of the wound bed contraction mediated by the myofibroblasts. The myofibroblasts are differentiated fibroblasts with features resembling the smooth muscle cells, hence they contract the bed. This, in turn, causes the graft to contract to the dimensions of the underlying bed. This process is called "Secondary Contraction" of a skin graft.

Primary contraction of graft, on the other hand, is an inherent property of every skin graft and occurs immediately after the graft has been harvested. It is due to the recoil of the elastic fibers in the dermis. Therefore, primary contraction is more in an FTG as compared to a SSG because of a greater amount of dermis and elastic fibers.

An FTG has minimal secondary contraction compared to a SSG. The reason for this appears to be the full thickness of dermis in these grafts, which inhibits myofibroblasts differentiation. In a SSG, the lesser the amount of dermis, the lesser the inhibition of myofibroblasts differentiation, therefore the bed tends to contract more. Thus, after the application of SSG to postburn raw area, splintage and pressure are required for a long time postoperatively to avoid the secondary contraction. Besides greater secondary contraction in SSG, it tends to have lesser growth potential. This is important in the pediatric age group. In children with burns, treated with SSG, contracture formation is more as the graft does not grow with age and with respect to the rest of the body. An FTG on the other hand has a better ability to grow with age but is rarely used in pediatric burn wounds for reasons already stated.

In darker races, it has been observed that the graft is susceptible to hyperpigmentation. Thus, exposure to sun should be avoided for at least 1 year after grafting.

REINNERVATION OF GRAFT

The nerve fibers in the graft degenerate in 3 days after transfer to the recipient site. The new nerve fibers invade the graft from the periphery as well as the recipient bed at 40 days travelling along the empty Schwann sheaths or along the blood vessels. At 2–3 months, as these fibrils increase in number they reach the end organs in the graft, i.e., hair follicles, sweat glands, and sensory end organs, and gradually the sensation returns in the graft. Pain is the first sensation to return followed by touch, temperature, and tactile discrimination, although the sensation does not match that of the normal skin. In fact, in the first year of postgrafting, the graft may be hypersensitive. The sensations are better in FTG as compared to a SSG skin graft.

Sweat glands present in the dermis of the skin graft start functioning only after the reinnervation of the graft is established. Therefore, there is no sweating in the graft for 2–3 months postgrafting. Till such time, the graft remains dry and scaly and needs to be protected by moisturizing creams. Once the sweat glands are reinnervated, their behavior is similar to that of the recipient bed and not the donor site.

Hair growth is rarely seen in thin SSG because of damage to the majority of the hair follicles. But in a thick SSG and FTG, hair growth resumes and resembles that of the donor area. This is significant when FTG from the scalp is used for eyebrow reconstruction following burns.

Complications of Skin Grafting

The complications of skin grafting are as follows:

- The main complication of skin grafting is the failure of graft to "take". The various causes of graft failure are:
    - *Infection:* It is the most common reason for graft failure, especially with beta-hemolytic *Streptococcus*.
    - *Hematoma:* Hematoma under the graft prevents the graft from getting vascularized. Therefore, proper hemostasis in the bed prior to the application of graft should be ensured.
    - *Ineffective immobilization:* Failure to immobilize the grafted area is another important cause for the failure of graft "take". Therefore, it is important to avoid shearing between the graft and the wound bed.
    - *Poorly vascularized bed:* It is not able to sustain a graft and leads to graft failure.

- Blister formation and breakdown in graft occur in the extremities especially weight-bearing lower limbs in which the increased hydrostatic pressure causes venous congestion in graft. This is also seen as a purple discoloration of the graft.

Postoperative Care of Skin Graft

The grafted area can be left exposed if there is no loss by 10 days. By 14 days, patient can be allowed to have a bath. By 3 weeks, the graft is usually strong enough to withstand reasonable wear and tear.

In lower limbs, hanging of feet over the side of the bed can be allowed for short intervals of time at 10 days postoperatively. Weight bearing in grafted lower limbs can be started only after 2 weeks and gradually by 3 weeks walking can be resumed but only with the protection of a pressure garment or crepe bandage.

Repeated scaling in the graft is seen because of the absence/diminished number of sweat and sebaceous glands in the graft. Hence, they require lubrication for the rest of their life. Continuous pressure using pressure garments has to be applied over grafted areas to prevent inter-graft hypertrophy. In lower limbs, the pressure support is essential for 3–6 months. Apart from preventing hypertrophy in grafts, they also prevent venous congestion and breakdown in the graft. They have to be worn throughout the day and night, especially during ambulation.

SUMMARY

Burn wound healing is an important determinant of patient recovery and thus, wound management is an integral component in the care of a burn patient. Depth determination is of utmost importance as it determines the further course of management. Although early excision and grafting have become the treatment of choice for deep dermal and full-thickness burns, conservative management still maintains an important role in their management at many burn centers. Newer dressing materials are being developed to overcome the challenges of slow wound healing, pain, infection, and scarring of burn wounds. Skin grafting is the mainstay of treatment of deeper burn wounds. Development of skin substitutes that are cost-effective and can reduce the need for autologous skin are the future of local burn wound care.

REFERENCES

1. Johnson RM, Richard R. Partial-thickness burns: Identification and management. Adv Skin Wound Care. 2003;16(4):178-87.
2. Tiwari VK. Burn wound: How it differs from other wounds? Indian J Plast Surg. 2012;45(2):364-73.
3. Kowalske KJ. Burn wound care. Phys Med Rehabil Clin N Am. 2011;22(2):213-27.
4. Saffle R, Schnebly WA. Burn wound care. In: Richard RL, Staley MJ (Eds). Burn Care and Rehabilitation Principle and Practice. Philadelphia: FA Davis Company; 1994. pp. 119-67.
5. Rockwell WB, Ehrlich HP. Fibrinolysis inhibition in human burn blister fluid. J Burn Care Rehabil. 1990;11(1):1-6.
6. Cianci P, Lueders HW, Lee H, Shapiro RL, Sexton J, Williams C, et al. Adjunctive hyperbaric oxygen reduces the need for surgery in 40-80% burns. J Hyperbar Med. 1988;3:97-101.
7. Wiseman DH, Grossman AR. Hyperbaric oxygen in treatment of burns. Crit Care Clin. 1985;1(1):129-45.
8. Wallace AB. Treatment of burns; a return to basic principles. Br J Plast Surg. 1949;1:232-44.
9. Moyer CA, Brentano L, Gravens DL, Margraf HW, Monafo WW Jr. Treatment of large human burns with 0.5% Silver nitrate solution. Arch Surg. 1965;90:812-67.
10. Monafo WW, Fredman B. Topical therapy for burns. Surg Clin North Am. 1987;67(1):133-45.
11. MacMillan BG, Hill EO, Alteimer WA. Use of topical silver nitrate, Mafenide and Gentamicin in the burn patient: A comparative study. Arch Surg. 1967;95(3):472-81.
12. Harrison HN, Blackmore WP, Bales HW, Reeder W. The absorption of C-14 labelled Sulphamylon acetate through burned skin. I. Experimental methods and initial observations. J Trauma. 1972;12(11):986-93.
13. Fox CL Jr, Monafo WW Jr, Ayvazian VH, Skinner AM, Modak S, Stanford J, et al. Topical chemotherapy for burns using Cerium salts and silver sulphadiazine. Surg Gynaecol Obstet. 1977; 144(5):668-72.
14. Bridges K, Lowbury EJ. Drug resistance in relation to the use of silver sulphadiazine cream in a burn unit. J Clin Pathol. 1977; 30(2):160-4.
15. Moncreif JA, Lindberg RB, Switzer WE, Pruitt BA Jr. Use of topical antibacterial therapy in the treatment of the burn wound. Arch Surg. 1966;92(4):558-65.
16. Afshari A, Nguyen L, Kahn SA, Summitt B. 2.5% Mafenide Acetate: A Cost-effective Alternative to the 5% Solution for Burn Wounds. J Burn Care Res. 2017;38(1):e42-7.
17. Shuck JM, Thorne LW, Cooper CG. Mafenide acetate solution dressings: An adjunct in burn wound care. J Trauma. 1975;15(7):595-9.
18. Pruitt BA Jr. Diagnosis and treatment of infection in the burn patient: Presidential address. Arch Surg. 1986;121:13-22.
19. Lindberg RB, Moncrief JA, Switzer WE, Order SE, Mills W Jr. The successful control of burn wound sepsis. J Trauma. 1965;5(5): 601-16.
20. Stone HH, Kolb LD, Petit J, Smith RB. The systemic absorption of antibiotic from the burned wound surface. Am Surg. 1968; 34(9):639-43.
21. Moncrief JA. Management of burns. Monogr Surg Sci. 1966; 3:175.

22. Singh O, Gupta SS, Soni M, Moses S, Shukla S, Mathur RK. Collagen dressing versus conventional dressings in burn and chronic wounds: A retrospective study. J Cutan Aesthet Surg. 2011;4(1):12-6.
23. Singh A, Bhatnagar A. Management of Superficial Partial Thickness Burn with Collagen Sheet Dressing Compared with Paraffin Gauze and Silver Sulfadiazine. Ann Burns Fire Disasters. 2020;33(3):233-8.
24. Barnea Y, Weiss J, Gur E. A review of the applications of the hydrofiber dressing with silver (Aquacel Ag®) in wound care. Ther Clin Risk Manag. 2010;6:21-7
25. Chaganti P, Gordon I, Chao JH, Zehtabchi S. A systematic review of foam dressings for partial thickness burns. Am J Emerg Med. 2019;37(6):1184-90.
26. Fong J, Wood F. Nanocrystalline silver dressings in wound management: A review. Int J Nanomedicine. 2006;1(4):441-9.
27. Nadworny PL, Wang J, Tredget EE, Burrell RE. Anti-inflammatory activity of nanocrystalline silver-derived solutions in porcine contact dermatitis. J Inflamm (Lond.). 2010;7:13.
28. Moreira SS, Camargo MC, Caetano R, Alves MR, Itria A, Pereira TV, et al. Efficacy and costs of nanocrystalline silver dressings versus 1% silver sulfadiazine dressings to treat burns in adults in the outpatient setting: A randomized clinical trial. Burns. 2022;48(3):568-76.
29. de Barros MEPM, Coltro PS, Hetem CMC, Vilalva KH, Farina JA Jr. Revisiting Escharotomy in Patients with Burns in Extremities. J Burn Care Res. 2017;38(4):e691-8.
30. Orgill DP, Piccolo N. Escharotomy and Decompressive Therapies in Burns. J Burn Care Res. 2009;30(5):759-68.
31. Leaper DJ. Eusol. BMJ. 1992;304(6832):930-1.
32. Grünherz L, Michienzi R, Schaller C, Rittirsch D, Uyulmaz S, Kim BS, et al. Enzymatic debridement for circumferential deep burns: The role of surgical escharotomy. Burns. 2023;49(2):304-9.
33. Fischer S, Haug V, Diehm Y, Rhodius P, Cordts T, Schmidt VJ, et al. Feasibility and safety of enzymatic debridement for the prevention of operative escharotomy in circumferential deep burns of the distal upper extremity. Surgery. 2019;165(6):1100-5.
34. Hirche C, Kreken Almeland S, Dheansa B, Fuchs P, Governa M, et al. Eschar removal by bromelain based enzymatic debridement (Nexobrid®) in burns: European consensus guidelines update. Burns. 2020;46(4):782-96.
35. Rosenberg L, Krieger Y, Silberstein E, Arnon O, Sinelnikov IA, Bogdanov-Berezovsky A, et al. Selectivity of a bromelain based enzymatic debridement agent: A porcine study. Burns. 2012;38(7):1035-40.
36. Krizek TJ, Robson MC, Groskin MG. Experimental burn wound sepsis—evaluation of enzymatic debridement. J Surg Res. 1974;17(4):219-27.
37. Mosti G, Iabichella ML, Picerni P, Magliaro A, Mattaliano V. The debridement of hard to heal leg ulcers by means of a new device based on Fluidjet technology. Int Wound J. 2005;2(4):307-4.
38. Reverdin JL. Greffe epidermique. Bulletin de la Société Impériale de Chirurgie de Paris. 1869;101:511-5.
39. Reverdin JL, Sur La. Greffe epidermique. Comptes Rendus Hebdomadaires des Séances de lAcadémie des sciences (Paris). 1871;73:1280-2.
40. Reverdin JL. Greffe epidermique. Comptes Rendus des Séances de la société de Biologic Et de ses Filiales (Paris). 1871;23:147.
41. Pollock GD. Skin grafting and skin transplantation. BMJ. 1870; 2:565.
42. Ash V. The rationale of skin grafting (letter to editor). Lancet-2. 1870;913.
43. Ollier LXEL. Greffes cutanees ou autoplastiques. Bulletin de l' Académie Nationale de Médicine (Paris). 1872;1:243-50.
44. Lawson G. On the successful transplantation of portions of skin for the closure large granulating defects. Medical Times and Gazette. 1870;2:631.
45. Wolfe JR. A new method of performing plastic operations. BMJ. 1875;2:360-1.
46. Krause F. Uber die transplantation grosser ungestielter Hautlappen. Verhandlungen der Deustschen gesellschaft fur Chirurgie 1893;22:46-51.
47. Thiersch C. Ueber Hautverpflantzung. Verhandlungen der Deutschen Gesellschaft fur Chirurgie 1886;15:17-19.
48. Raehlmann E. Therapeutische Erfahrungen uber Lidkanten-operation sowie uber Haut und Schleihauttransplantation am Auge. Deutsche Medizinische Wochenscrift 1891;17:4-9.
49. Davis JS. The use of deep small grafts. JAMA. 1914;63:985-9.
50. Gatch WD. Report of a case of extensive Thiersch skin graft. Bull Johns Hopkins Hosp. 1911;22:84-5.
51. Douglas SR, Colebrook L, Fleming A. On skin grafting: a plea for its more extensive application. Lancet-2. 1917;5-12.
52. Humby G. Apparatus for skin graft cutting. BMJ. 1934;1:1078.
53. Humby G. Modified graft cutting razor. BMJ. 1936;2:1086.
54. Padgett EC. Skin grafting from a personal and experimental viewpoint. Springfield: Charles C Thomas; 1942.
55. Brown JB, Mc Dowell F. Skin grafting of burns. Philadelphia: JB Lippincott; 1943.
56. Meek CP. Successful microderma grafting using the meek-wall microdermatome. Am J Surg. 1958;96(4):557-8.
57. Lari AR, Gang RK. Expansion technique for skin grafts (Meek technique) in the treatment of severely burned patients. Burns. 2001;27(1):61-6.
58. Ameer F, Singh AK, Kumar S. Evolution of instruments for harvest of the skin grafts. Indian J Plast Surg. 2013;46(1):28-35.
59. Lanz O. Over transplantatie Nederlands Tijdschrift voor Geneeskunde. 1907;51:1335-7.
60. Tanner JC, Vandeput J, Olley JF. The mesh skin graft. Plast Reconst Surg. 1964;34:287-92.
61. Dragstedt LR, Wilson H. A modified sieve graft: A full-thickness skin graft for covering large defects. Surg Gynaecol Obstet. 1937;65:104-6.
62. Douglas B. The sieve grafts—a stable transplant for covering large skin defects. Surg Gynaecol Obstet. 1930;50:1018-23.
63. Jabs AD Jr, Wider T, Debellis J, Hugo N. The effect of fibrin glue on skin grafts in infected sites. Plast Reconst Surg. 1992;89(2):268-71.
64. Currie LJ, Sharpe JR, Martin R. The use of fibrin glue in skin graft and tissue engineered skin replacements: A review. Plast Reconstr Surg. 2001;108(6):1713-26.
65. Converse JM, Uhlschmid GK, Ballantyne DL Jr. Plasmatic circulation in skin grafts. The phase of serum imbibition. Plast Recons Surg. 1969;43(5):495-9.
66. Mathes SJ. Plastic Surgery, Volume 1: General Principles, 2nd edition. United States: Saunders; 2006. pp. 293-316.
67. Henry L, Marshall DC, Friedman EA, Goldstein DP, Dammin GJ. A histologic study of human skin autograft. Am J Pathol. 1961;39(3):317-32.

CHAPTER 15

Surgical Excision of Burn Wound and Skin Grafting

Pramod Kumar

INTRODUCTION AND HISTORY

Ever since fire has been known to human beings, not only it has been an undoubted boon but also a bane to some extent. The treatment of oldest (59,000–48,000 BC) known historic burn wounds with herbs and roots has been recorded in cave paintings of Neanderthal man. Later in 1500 BC, Egyptian Smith papyrus used salve of resin and honey for treating burn wounds.[1] Sushruta, the famous surgeon of ancient India (800–600 BC) and regarded all over the world as father of plastic surgery, in his book Sushruta Samhita[2] (Section 1: *Sutrasthana*, Chapter 12: *Agnikarma Vidhi Adhyaya*) has described the procedure of branding by fire (*Agnikarma vidhi*), burns (*Dagdha*)—types and treatment, suffocation due to smoke (*Dhumopahata lakshana*), and sun burn (*Atapadi dagdhana*).[2]

Although Jackson (1954) is regarded as the pioneer of early burn wound excision and grafting, Janzekovic[1] (1970) showed that early return to work (about 1 week post burn) is possible after tangential excision and split-skin grafting by days 3–5. In 1970, a brief article in Journal of Trauma by a Yugoslavian plastic surgeon, Zora Janzekovic, went unnoticed. In 1974, Monafo advocated excision and grafting for larger burns. In 1974, Burke used fascial excision for large burns with a huge increase in survival and decrease in hospital length of stay.[1] Later, Janzekovic gained considerably more attention when she reviewed her experience again as the Evans lecturer for the American Burn Association in 1975.[3] Until her observations were published, nearly all excision and grafting procedures were limited to full-thickness burns, and skin and subcutaneous tissues were removed beneath the burn to the level of the investing fascia. Due to disappointing results with excessive graft loss following infection from an adjacent nonexcised area, she along with many others abandoned early operation. Dr Janzekovic knew that deep donor site could be overgrafted with the thinner autograft, thereby hastening the healing and improving the appearance. Realizing that graft would survive on viable dermis, she applied this technique to dermal burns by progressive shaving off of thin layers of burnt dermis until she reached a bed that appeared viable and she immediately autografted it successfully. Between the years 1961 and 1974, Dr Janzekovic treated 2,615 of 4,370 burned patients with this form of early tangential (or sequential) excision and sheet autografting. Most of the burns were small [<20% total body surface area (TBSA)] but the hospital stay, pain, and need for reconstructive surgery reduced considerably and led to her opinion "Aesthetic disability" reduced considerably.[4] Though Tanner (1964) developed meshed skin grafting technique, Alexander (1981) showed advantages of using widely meshed autograft and its coverage with cadaveric graft. Development of artificial skin, Integra™ (bi-layered skin substitute made from collagen with plastic cover) by Burke (1981) and development of tissue-cultured grown skin by Bell made a substantial improvement in the management of larger burns using excisional surgery.[1]

Davies in 1990 reported that in India, 22% of burn patients died in the first 48 hours due to inappropriate or inadequate fluid therapy, 36% by day 7 postburn due to circulatory or respiratory complications, and virtually all the deaths during weeks 2, 3, and 4 after burns were due to overwhelming sepsis.[5] Incidence of contractures and hypertrophic scar is more if skin grafting is not done early and wounds are allowed to granulate. Baxter[6] documented the possibility of minimizing wound infection by topical use of 1% silver-sulfadiazine. Barret and Handerson[7] in their study concluded that burn wound excision significantly reduces bacterial colonization. Patients who underwent topical treatment and delayed burn wound excision exhibited greater bacterial colonization and increased rates of infection. Burke et al.[8] noted that the time required for closure of the open burn wounds using primary excision and skin grafting was reduced to 1½ time compared to topical therapy alone.

Modern advances and better understanding of burns treatment, especially in burns resuscitation, infection control, and nutrition along with early excisional surgery and skin grafting, have led to significantly reduced overall morbidity and to some extent burn wound sepsis and mortality.[4] Uninfluenced by the survival statistics, excisional surgery has become the treatment of choice for all deep dermal and full-thickness burns due to reduced cost of treatment, better functional result, early rehabilitation with return to work, and a reduction in long-term morbidity.

TYPES OF BURN WOUND EXCISION

The burn wound excision may be broadly classified into the following:

- *Primary excision*: This is followed by skin grafting in the same session.
    - *Immediate excision*: In case of small burns, where the wound is obviously deep and patient is physiologically fit for anesthesia and surgery, it may be taken for surgery between 0 and 2 days, Immediate excision and skin graft are ideal for appropriate small burn cases.[9]
    - *Early excision*: It is done within 2–10 days following burn (ISBI Practice Guidelines of Burn Care[10]). The delay of 48 hours helps to stabilize (resuscitation and correction of physiological derangements) the patient prior to surgery.
    - *Delayed excision*: Timing of delayed excision is not clearly defined, but usually delayed excision is done between 10 and 21 days. Delay in excision may lead to increased chances of complications due to infection and graft loss.

  Primary excision is further subclassified into tangential, sequential, and fascial excision, depending upon the technique used. However, many authors prefer to subclassify as tangential excision and en bloc excision.
- *Secondary excision*: This is basically a procedure for preparing the wound bed for grafting by removing the eschar and delayed skin grafting. It is synonymous with surgical toilet or debridement. This was practiced earlier for partial- and full-thickness burns in which the nonviable eschar is excised with a skin grafting knife till minimal bleeding bed is encountered. This bed is, then, covered with a biological dressing and reassessed after 48–72 hours to look for the remaining dead tissue which is again excised and dressed till healthy granulation tissue appears. This is secondarily grafted. This procedure is somewhere between primary excision and secondary grafting following conservative management of burn wounds as it takes 7–10 days for the healthy granulation tissue to appear following excision of dead tissue. It is suitable for cases where primary excision cannot be done due to medical reasons or associated injuries.

Types of Primary Excision

- *Tangential excision*: It is used typically for deep dermal burns. In this technique, the wound is excised with Watson's skin grafting knife/dermatome till healthy viable dermis is reached over which split-skin graft is applied immediately. In sequential excision, burnt/necrotic tissue is sequentially excised until viable tissue is encountered which can be either viable deep dermis or viable fat or fascia. This area is also immediately skin grafted. This technique is most effective for mixed deep dermal and full-thickness burns in which sequential excision helps in saving viable dermis or fat which would otherwise be sacrificed if the entire necrotic area were to be removed in one slice with Watson's skin grafting knife/dermatome or in en bloc excision of burnt tissue with a surgical blade leading to cosmetic problems.
- *Suprafascial full-thickness excision*: It is indicated for full-thickness burn wounds. In this, full thickness of burned skin with subcutaneous tissues is excised with a surgical knife till the deep fascia. This can be immediately grafted because fascia is a healthy bed for graft "take".
- *Subfascial/fascial excision* It involves excising till deep to the deep fascia, thus reaching the muscles. In these cases, the chances of graft "take" are poorer compared to suprafascial excision.

En bloc excision: In very deep burns, all burnt tissues including skin, fascia, fat, muscle, etc., are excised using knife in one block, and the deep viable tissues may be covered by skin graft, flap, or other suitable available methods depending on bed created. En bloc tissue excision is the terminology that can be used to replace terminologies like suprafascial and subfascial excision.

ANATOMICAL AND PHYSIOLOGICAL BASIS FOR EXCISION

The principle and type of excision can be explained by the anatomy of skin and depth of burn. For excisional purposes, the depth of burns is broadly classified into partial-thickness and full-thickness burns. The partial-thickness burns are those which involve the epidermis and upper part of dermis and they can heal without intervention. Full-thickness burns are those which involve the entire epidermis and dermis, and these do not heal on their own and require surgical intervention. In between these two are deep dermal burns which involve the epidermis and two-thirds of dermis, and these heal in a long time with severe hypertrophic scarring and contracture formation. So, in these cases if tangential excision is done it would not only improve morbidity but even mortality is reduced dramatically. The deep dermis is still viable; therefore, it needs to be covered with split-skin graft following excision.

INDICATIONS

Early excision is especially appropriate for flame and dry heat injuries, whereas a more conservative approach is needed for scald injuries which are often associated with less severe second-degree burns that are likely to heal well without excessive scarring. The results of a prospective randomized study in a pediatric population showed that scalded patients should be observed for approximately 14 days, after which the need for operative intervention can be reassessed.[11-15]

Dermal preservation during early tangential excision of thin slices sequentially plays a vital role to obtain superior healing and better scar outcome.[16]

Size of burn: It is a general agreement that small full-thickness, indeterminable, and deep dermal burns can be excised safely and grafted with good result (short hospital stay, reduced morbidity, reduced burn wound pain and sepsis, reduced nursing care turnover in critical care area, and reduced scar-related problems). Larger burns due to paucity of skin donor area may require homograft, synthetic skin substitutes, or cultured epithelial autograft. In massive burns (>60% TBSA) the problem of inadequate donor area can be tackled by using widely expanded (meshed 1:4 or 1:6) autologous split-thickness graft that can be overlaid with unexpanded (with hand meshed) homologous (cadaver) split-skin graft.[12,13,17,18] Bilayer skin substitutes have also been used to cover such wounds temporarily prior to covering them with autograft.[19]

Burns of 30–40% BSA may be excised and covered with autograft in two sessions at 10–14-day interval. The excision of 15–20% BSA in one session is safe in healthy individuals, although some surgeons set the limit even up to 40%.[11] In life-threatening burns, one should aim at covering larger areas (i.e., area easy to excise and easy to graft, e.g., trunk) rather than getting better functional result (i.e., excision of hand burn and finger burn that requires more time to cover less area).[20]

Timing of excision relative to changes in the wound itself is crucial to minimize risks: Primary excision in small burns can be done at the earliest as resuscitation and physiological correction may not be required in these cases for safe anesthesia and surgery, and chances of infection are significantly reduced. Tangential excision in larger burns is usually done between 3rd and 5th day following burns. The rationale for not doing it earlier is to give adequate time for resuscitation, especially in extensive burns, and to avoid unnecessary excision of deeper tissues where perfusion is restored after resuscitation is completed. After 5 days, there is a significant bacterial colonization of the wound which may inhibit graft "take". After 7 days, there is softening of the surface of wound which makes excision technically difficult (5% povidone iodine solution-soaked gauze dressing on the day prior to excision makes tissue stiff and excision becomes relatively easier). Early primary excision can be done up to 10 days and delayed primary excision may be done after 10 days up to 3 weeks.

Colonization of the wound develops during the first week, and manipulation of the colonized or infected wound runs an increasing risk of bacteremia. The reduced rates of wound infection and sepsis in the past three decades have been the result of many factors, of which early excision has been advocated as one of the major factors. Barret and Handerson[7] have shown that burn wound excision significantly reduces bacterial colonization. Patients undergoing topical treatment and delayed burn wound excision exhibit greater bacterial colonization and increased rates of infection. They have also advised acute burn wound excision for all full-thickness burns. Early excision of >30% TBSA burns in adults has not been universally accepted.[17] Desai et al.[21] have advocated that near-total excision of large burn within the first 24 hours reduces blood requirement and morbidity without adversely altering hemodynamic stability and increasing mortality risks. They have shown that blood loss in large burn injuries (>30% TBSA) was significantly decreased when surgical excision was performed within the first 24 hours after injury compared to those performed between the 2nd and 16th day after injury. Reduced blood loss was noticed in the second 24 hours after injury; however, this was not significant compared to blood loss between postburn day 2 and 16. Blood loss in burns treated conservatively with grafting on granulation tissue was also less when compared to blood loss from excision during post burn day 2 through 16. Hence, the size of the planned excision must be determined based on a clear understanding of increasing the risks of blood loss and bacteremia.

Early excision and grafting are not justifiable in conditions like charred hand where paratenon is affected and flap surgery is indicated. Excision and grafting should be avoided in the presence of inhalation injury.

Criteria for Early Excision

The diagnosis of deep burn must be established (only areas that do not blanch on applying pressure by fingertips are excised), patient should have enough donor area for autograft or bilayer skin substitute[19] homograft should be available for temporary cover, and patient's condition should permit major operation. Inhalation injury is often considered as contraindication for early excision and grafting.

GENERAL PRINCIPLES FOR BURN WOUND EXCISION AND GRAFTING

- The patient must be hemodynamically stable before considering excision.
- The potential for significant blood loss must be recognized and adequate amount of blood and its components, if indicated, must be available before starting excision. Significant blood loss in a major burn should be replaced with blood products.
- Pulmonary problems require a plan of management in the operating room. In the postoperative period, mechanical ventilation may be required.
- Hypothermia must be prevented during surgery. All the areas should not be exposed at a time. Operating room temperature should be maintained between 28 and 32°C and fluid warmer should be used. The patient's body temperature should be monitored.
- The stress induced by anesthesia and surgery must be limited to that which the patient can safely tolerate. Each operative period should be limited to 2–3 hours.

As suggested by various authors,[4,22,23] the following points should be considered when deciding to proceed with operation:

- Experienced surgeon is required for early excision. Inadequate excision can lead to loss of graft placed over it and thus increasing the raw area created.
- Small burns that eventually heal and offer little threat to life if allowed to heal over several weeks: In this group, patient selection should be such that if excised, operative mortality remains nonexistent.
- Small burns that can be managed and taken care of by the patient till healing at minimal cost without missing work may be treated conservatively.
- Small deep burns can be treated on an outpatient basis initially and then excised electively and grafted on the day surgery is scheduled.
- Loss of income due to hand and feet burns can be significantly minimized by early excision and skin grafting.
- Life-threatening-associated problems including trauma must be well controlled so that operation can be done with low morbidity and essentially no mortality. Herndon et al.[23] have shown that the presence of preadmission shock and inhalation injury were early determinants of mortality with secondary renal, pulmonary, or cardiovascular collapse being the later predictors of mortality.
- Large superficial burns with scattered small deep components are best treated conservatively until the shallow areas are healed.
- *To avoid problems of excessive wound-related pain and slough,* excision and grafting may be one of the options. Thomson et al.,[22] based on their study of the effect of early excision on major thermal injury, have indicated that results with early excision and grafting of major burn wounds (>50%) may prove to be equal to or better than those achieved with conservative methods of topical antimicrobial, delayed eschar separation, and grafting.
- *Burns over sole and palm*: Though early excision and grafting were recommended as the preferred form of treatment in patients with deep second-degree and third-degree flame burns of dorsal hand,[24] it is generally agreed that tangential excision and spilt-skin graft are not advised on palm and sole as there is a high possibility of damage to the digital nerves and vessels. Singh and Prasanna[25] in a study of five children with burns of feet have found that the tangential excision and split-skin grafting for acute burns of feet help in avoiding pain associated with repeated dressing, reducing the need for reconstructive procedures and hospital stay. It also allows preserving sensate unburned skin and normal growth of the foot.
- *Burns over scalp*: Tangential excision of the scalp is not practiced widely. Dickson et al.[26] in their study concluded that it is preferable to manage scalp burns conservatively and grafting as a secondary procedure. The earlier reports of tangential excision of scalp and grafting showing that it promotes faster healing thus reducing chances of hypertrophic scar and preserving hair growth have not been confirmed by the study of Dickson et al.[26] Furthermore, in their study, the major disadvantages of this technique had been recurrent blistering, breakdown, and infection. True milia cyst formation was not encountered in their study.
- *Burns of face*: Wound debridement and grafting is indicated for face burns that do not heal within 3 weeks and that the procedure yields results that permit the burn victims to return to society and minimizes the time off work or out of school.[27]

INVESTIGATIONS

- *Hematological*: Hemoglobin, total and differential leukocyte count, platelet counts, preoperative coagulation profile [prothrombin time (PT)/partial thromboplastin time (PTT)/international normalized ratio (INR)]
- Routine urine examination (sugar, protein, and microscopic examination)
- *Bacterial culture*: Wound swab, and if indicated blood culture
- Serum electrolytes
- Serum protein level (albumin globulin), immunoglobulin level (IgG, IgM)
- Renal function tests
- Myoglobin in urine (if urine is smoky or tea-like coloration), investigation for rhabdomyolysis: Creatine kinase (CK), aldolase, lactate dehydrogenase (LDH), serum glutamic-pyruvic transaminase (SGPT), and other enzymes
- *In electric burns*: ECG, CK [also known as phosphocreatine kinase or creatine phosphokinase (CPK)], and CK-MB.
- Arterial blood gas analysis, X-ray of chest, bronchoscopy (if indicated)
- Investigations to rule out other organ dysfunction (if indicated)
- Investigations for comorbid conditions (diabetes, hypertension, etc.) and preexisting illnesses (e.g., sickle cell disease)
- Blood group

TANGENTIAL EXCISION

Tangential excision **(Figs. 1 to 5)** is indicated for deep dermal wounds. In tangential excision, burnt dermis is excised sequentially with Watson's knife/hand-held dermatome or power-driven dermatome. Since excision is done tangent to the wound and often multiple thin slices of the tissue are excised till viable bleeding tissue is reached, the method of excision is called tangential excision.

Anesthesia during excision and grafting: During excision, the following anesthesia-related problems are encountered:

- *Setting up of intravenous (IV) line*: Due to burn wounds, it is difficult to get IV line at usual sites and to fix it by adhesive tape. Very often, a jugular line is started during anesthesia. Central line is started as the last option. Protecting the line during surgery and changing the patient's position under anesthesia may be difficult.

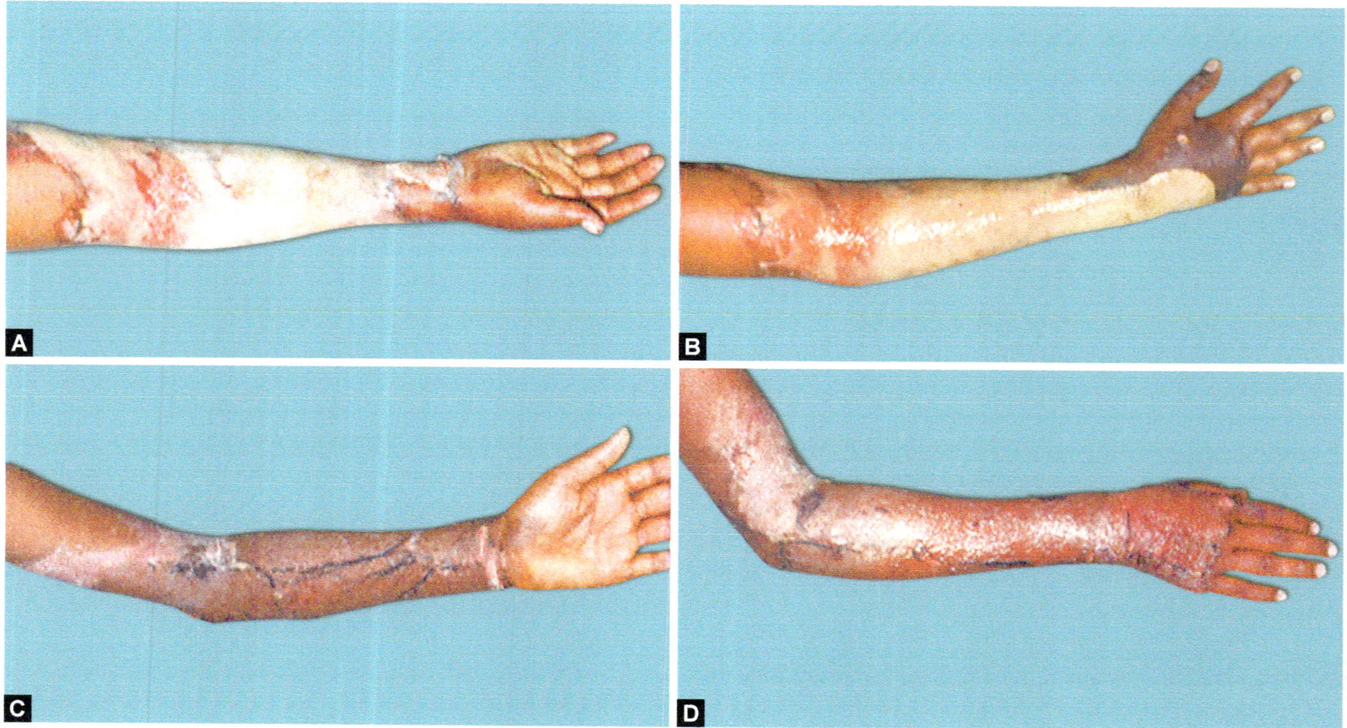

FIGS. 1A TO D: (A) Preoperative view: Deep dermal burn of right upper extremity—extensor aspect; (B) Preoperative view: Deep dermal burn of right upper extremity—flexor aspect; (C) Postoperative view of the same patient following tangential excision and grafting of deep dermal burn of right upper extremity—extensor aspect; (D) Postoperative view—flexor aspect.

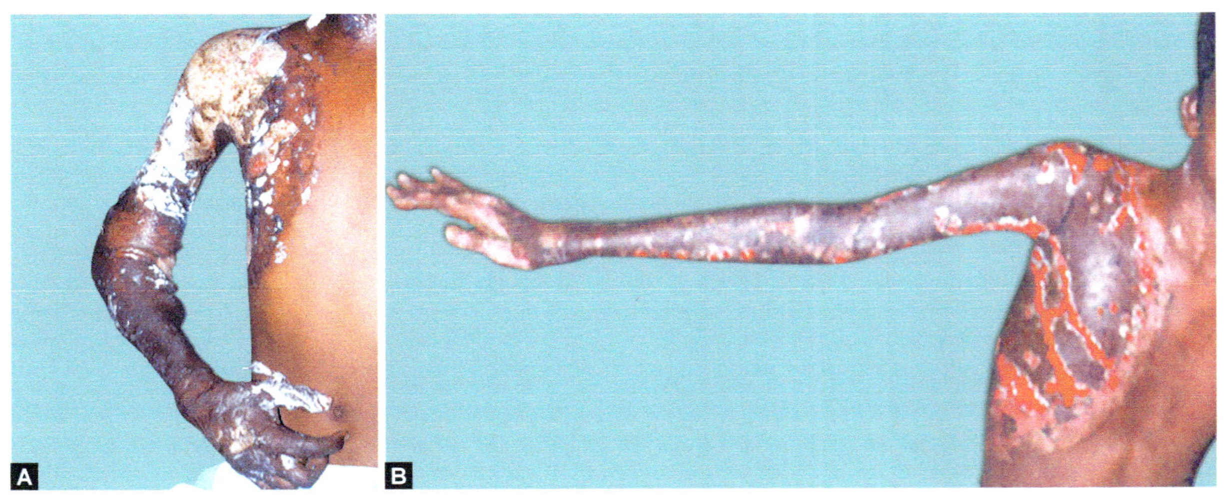

FIGS. 2A AND B: (A) Deep second-degree burn of right upper extremity; (B) Result after tangential excision and split-skin grafting.

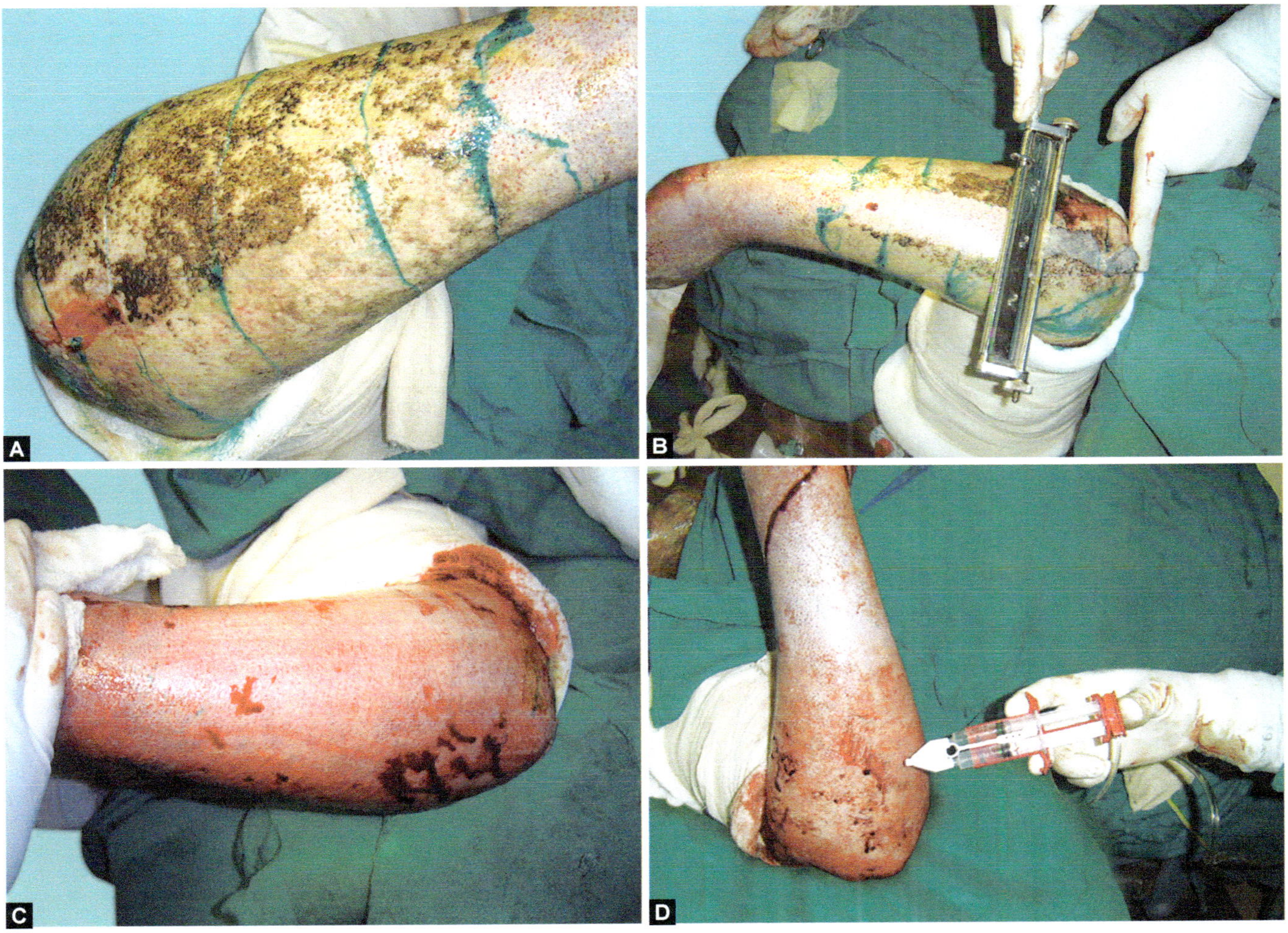

FIGS. 3A TO F: *Continued*

Continued

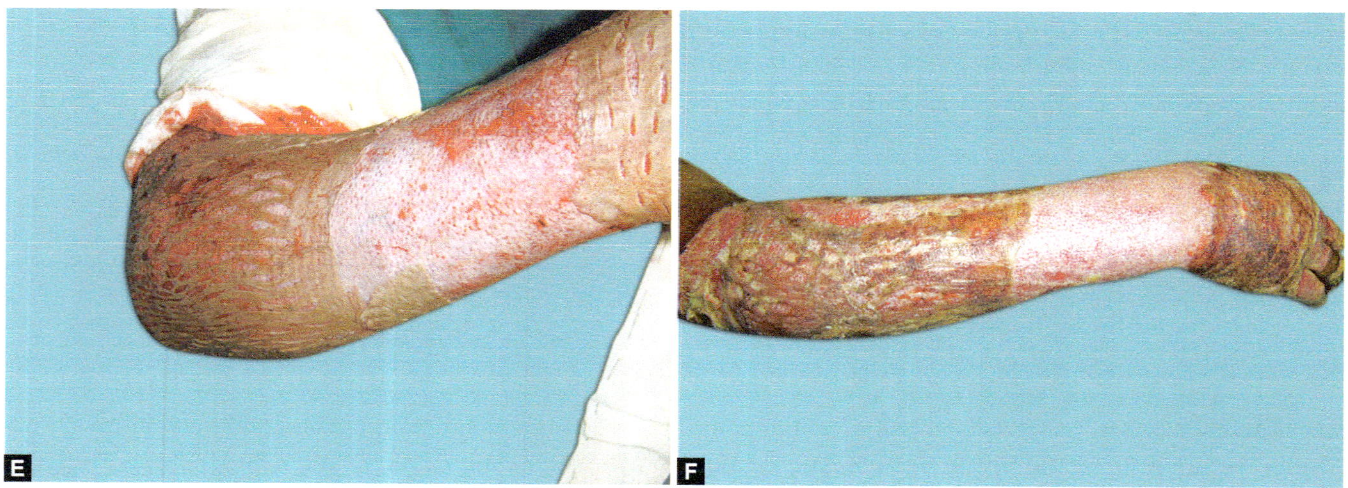

FIGS. 3A TO F: (A) Areas of deep dermal burns mapped in forearm prior to excision; (B) Watson's knife used to excise dead skin layers only in the mapped-out areas; (C) Healthy reticular dermis layer reached; (D) Fibrin sealant applied locally for hemostasis; (E) Split-skin graft applied after bleeding is controlled; (F) Second postoperative dressing after 8 days showing graft fully taken up and area healed.

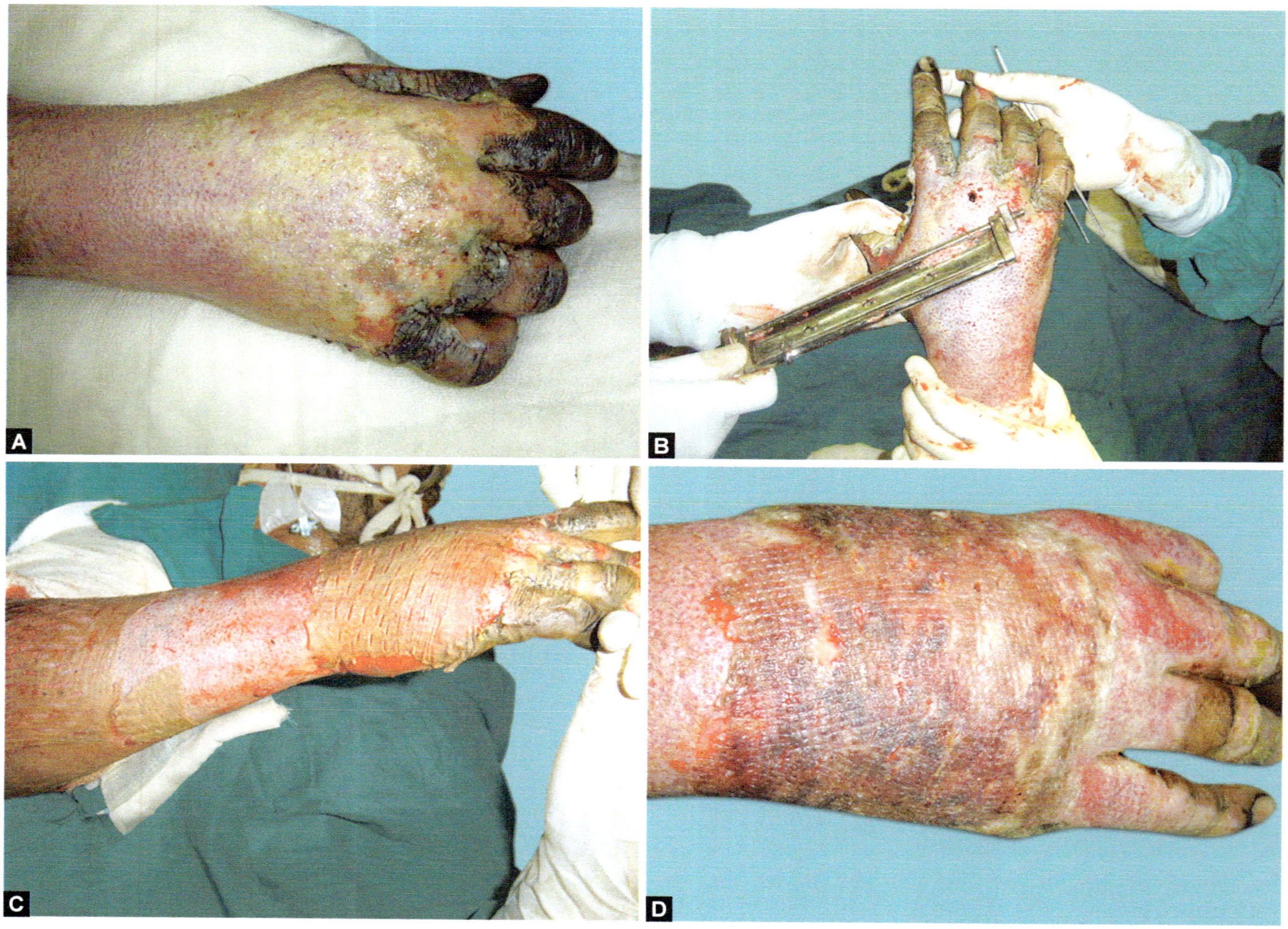

FIGS. 4A TO D: (A) Deep dermal burns of dorsum of hand; (B) Tangential excision being done with Watson's knife; (C) Graft applied after excision on dorsum of hand; (D) Postoperative picture showing complete take of graft on healthy bed.

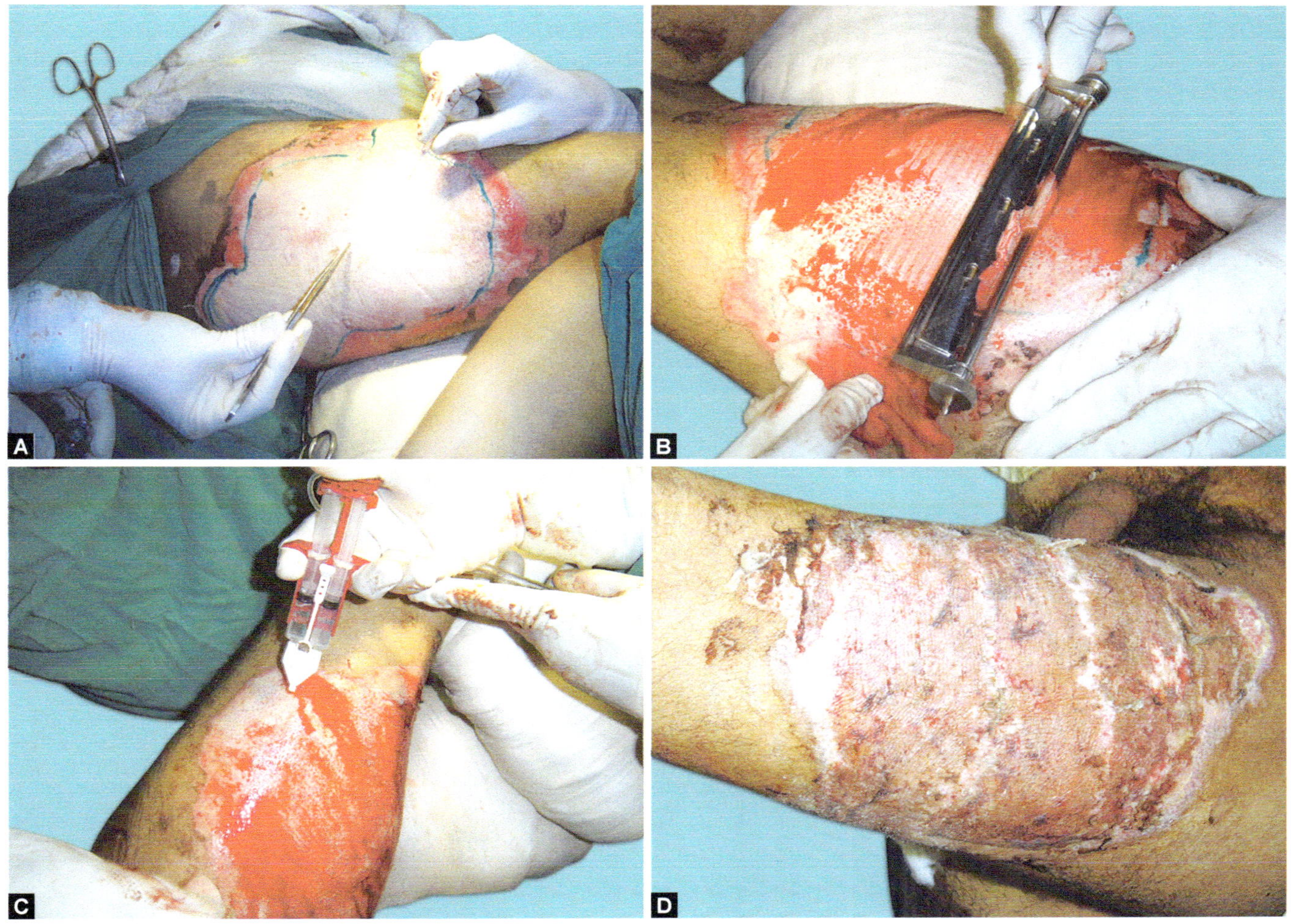

FIGS. 5A TO D: (A) Deep dermal burn over thigh—area marked; (B) Dead layer tangentially excised; (C) Hemostasis being achieved with fibrin sealant; (D) 2 weeks postoperative picture showing completely healed area.

- *Patient monitoring*: Continuous monitoring of ECG, pulse, and blood pressure may be difficult in burn patients as compared to other patients. This may be due to the pattern of burn, extensive nature of the burn, and unusual position of the patient on the operation table. By using a precordial stethoscope or use of esophageal stethoscope, one can continuously monitor heartbeat. Continuous monitoring of blood pressure may be done by starting an arterial line as the last option. It may be difficult to place standard ECG electrodes. Therefore, ECG leads are placed at a position that is convenient to both the anesthesiologist and the burn surgeon. Many a times, the site of the sphygmomanometer cuff and finger probe for monitoring oxygen saturation has to be changed from one place to another to enable the surgeon to complete the operation.
- *Difficult intubation*: Intubation may be difficult due to upper airway edema. Once intubated, fixation by adhesive tape may not be possible in facial burns. In this situation, the endotracheal tube is tied around the neck with a bandage and the bandage is fixed on the tube at an appropriate site with an adhesive tape.
- *Muscle relaxant*: In acute burns (like immobilized patients or those patients who had repeated sepsis), the use of suxamethonium (succinylcholine) is known to be potentially dangerous due to exaggerated hyperkalemia.
- Sudden blood loss from multiple sites during excision may produce serious problems during anesthesia. Excision may have to be stopped for sometime if deemed necessary by an anesthesiologist. Large quantities of fluid may need to be transfused in a short duration. In appropriate cases, it is better to start blood replacement from beginning of the operation.
- *Hypothermia*: Uncovered burnt areas, excised areas, and donor areas result in quick loss of heat. Keeping the areas that have been operated covered (by sterile plastic sheet which is a bad conductor of heat as well as it allows excised areas to be visible, if transparent, for any alarming bleeding), using fluid warmer for fluids

being transfused, monitoring patients' temperature, controlling operating room temperature, using warm saline mops, and limiting the duration of surgery reduce the problem of hypothermia.

- *Hypovolemia*: Sudden loss of large volumes during surgery may cause oliguria, anuria, and finally renal failure. Urinary output measurement at the beginning of surgery, hourly during the surgery, and in postoperative period helps in minimizing the problems.
- *Postoperative ventilatory support*: Maintenance of oxygen saturation may be difficult due to inadequate chest wall movement or chest complications making it necessary to ventilate these patients in the postoperative period.

Technique of Tangential Excision

First of all, the area of deep dermal burn to be excised is mapped and marked **(Figs. 3A, 4A, and 5A)**. The area that blanches and refills on release of pressure quickly is superficial and heals on conservative treatment. Usually, deep dermal areas are stained by betadine used during part preparation. For tangential excision with Watson's skin grafting knife, the knife is set to take thin split-skin graft. Saline is used to keep the area wet and help in easy movement of knife. Slices of burned tissue are excised till viable tissue with brisk bleeding is encountered **(Figs. 3B and C, 4B, and 5B)**. Viable dermis appears shiny white in color with multiple bleeding points. Small deeper (third-degree) burnt areas in the deep dermal burn wound may be excised till viable bright yellow fat is exposed and nonviable brown fat is completely excised. "Take" of skin graft over the fat is relatively poorer as compared to that on viable dermis. If fat is exposed in larger areas, it is better to cover with limited access dressing (LAD)[28] with/without dermal matrix[29] like MatriDerm®, which accelerates revascularization or use of bilayer skin substitute like Integra® or BTM® (biodegradable temporizing matrix) for 7–10 days prior to skin grafting which markedly improves the graft take **(Figs. 6A to E)**. To avoid sudden loss of a large volume of blood, one smaller area is excised and perfect hemostasis is achieved before starting excision over another area. Topical application of adrenaline

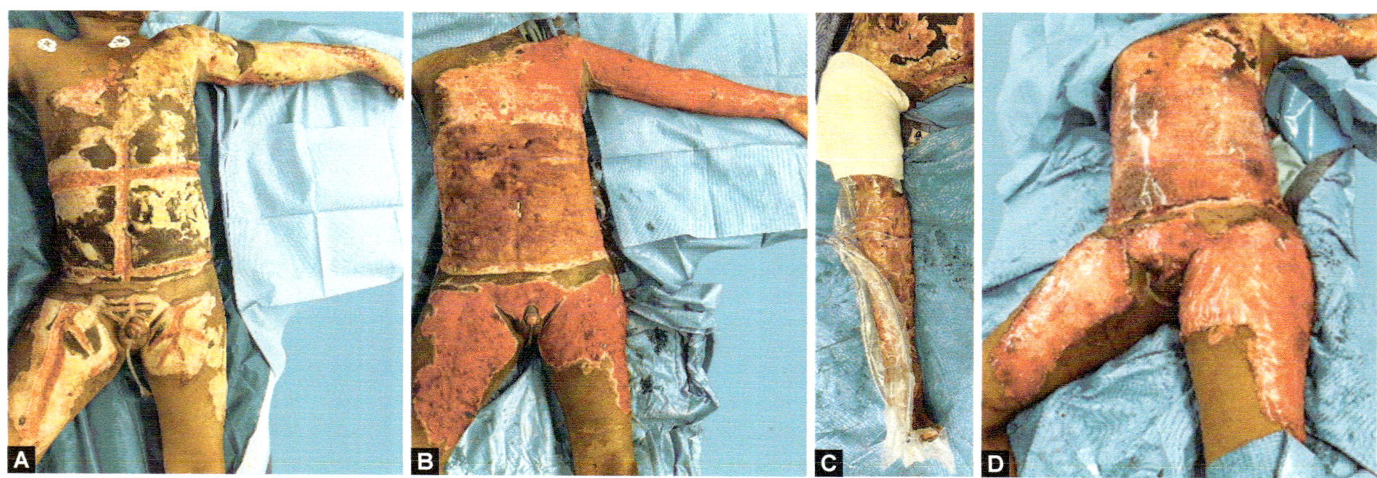

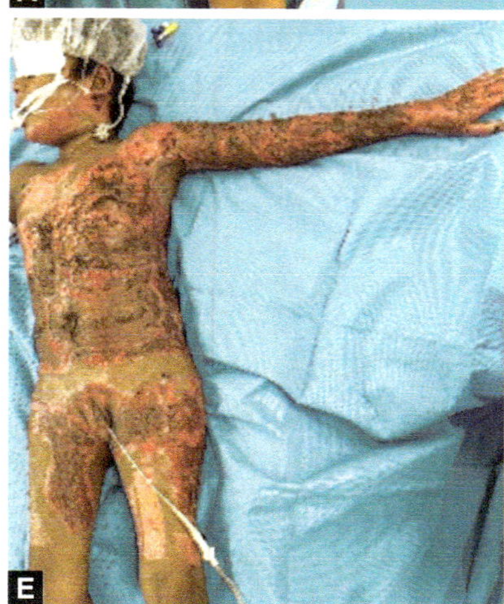

FIGS. 6A TO E: (A) TBSA 40% deep burn involving face, trunk, left upper limb, and both lower limbs in a 12-year-old boy. Escharotomy was done on the second postburn day. (B) Abdomen and thigh wound was excised early on fifth day and bilayered skin substitute was used to cover the wound. (C) Left upper limb wound was excised and prepared under limited access dressing. Other areas were prepared by povidone iodine-solution soaked gauze. (D) Thigh wound was grafted first after silastic epidermis of bilayered skin substitute was removed. (E) In multiple sittings, the whole body was covered by 1:6 meshed graft.

solution for 5–10 minutes and then use of slow water jet over excised area to localize bleeding points for bipolar cauterization are commonly used to achieve hemostasis. Exposed viable dermis and other tissues are covered immediately by adrenaline solution-soaked gauze/sponges to avoid its desiccation followed by cover with split-thickness skin graft **(Figs. 3E and F, 4C, and 5C)**.

Smaller areas of burn surrounded by unburnt skin are difficult to excise by a Watson's knife. Hence, smaller knives like Silver or Goulian-type Weck knife are used. The author uses pinch technique, in which the skin adjacent to the wound is pinched to lift burnt area from the unburnt area as a skin fold and the excision is performed by Watson's skin grafting knife.

For harvesting graft from uneven areas like chest wall, scalp, and areas with loose skin in emaciated patients, it is advisable to inject saline in subcutaneous tissues.

Blood Loss during Excision

Operative blood loss during excision can be calculated by the following formulae:

- By measurement of pre- and postoperative hematocrit value:

  Blood loss in mL =

  $$\frac{(\text{Preoperative RBCV}) + (\text{T} \times \text{RBCV}) - (\text{Postoperative RBCV})}{\text{Postoperative hematocrit} \times 0.01}$$

  where,

  RBCV = Red blood cell volume

  Preoperative RBCV (mL) = Body weight (kg) × 80 (mL/kg) × [preoperative hematocrit (%) + 0.01]

  Postoperative RBCV (mL) = Body weight (kg) × 80 (mL/kg) × [postoperative hematocrit (%) + 0.01]

  T × RBCV = Total mL of whole blood administered during surgery × 0.03

  Desai et al.[18] have shown that:

  - Average amount of blood loss for >30% TBSA burns when excised in the first 24 hours after injury was 0.41 ± 0.06 mL/cm^2.
  - Average amount of blood loss for >30% TBSA burns when excised between 2 and 16 days after injury was 0.75 ± 0.04 mL/cm^2.
  - Average amount of blood loss for >30% TBSA burns when excised > 16 days after injury was 0.49 ± 0.07 mL/cm^2.

- *By measurement of pre- and postoperative hemoglobin values*: This formula implies that decrease in hemoglobin is due to intraoperative blood loss along with hemodilution because of large volume of intraoperative crystalloid transfusion.

  Blood loss in mL =

  EBV × [(preoperative Hb – postoperative Hb)/average Hb] + Tx

  where,

  EBV = Estimated blood volume (70 mL/kg of body weight)

  Preoperative Hb = Preoperative hemoglobin in g/L

  Postoperative Hb = Hemoglobin in g/L at 24 hours postoperatively

  Average Hb = Mean of preoperative and postoperative hemoglobin in g/L

  Tx = Total intraoperative and 24-hour postoperative transfusion volume received in mL

  Using this formula, Cartotto et al.[30] calculated the blood loss (mean ± SD) to be 211 ± 166 mL/% TBSA excised. Blood loss can be minimized by limb elevation; application of topical epinephrine with or without thrombin to excised wounds and/or donor sites; the subcutaneous infiltration of vasoconstrictors such as epinephrine, phenylephrine, or vasopressin at donor and/or excision sites; the administration of systemic vasopressin; controlled intraoperative hypotension; electrocautery, performing excision with laser; staged excision and grafting; and use of limb tourniquets.[30] Topical hemostatic agents (recombinant thrombin or fibrinogen),[31] like Tissel® or ReliSeal®, are now available for use over such excised areas for control of bleeding **(Figs. 3D and 5D)**. However, there is no uniform, complete, and consistent approach to reduce intraoperative blood loss. From time to time, concerns have also been raised over assessing viability of recipient bed when tourniquet is used or subeschar epinephrine is used to reduce blood loss. This is because such methods interfere with bleeding from the viable tissues left after excision.

To reduce blood loss from donor area and burnt areas (to be excised) where tourniquet application is not possible, epinephrine solution 1:5,00,000 may be infiltrated subcutaneously until they become firm (i.e., tumescent). After harvesting graft, epinephrine saline solution (1:2,00,000) soaked gauze may be used topically.

To reduce blood loss during excision from the burnt areas over extremities, tourniquet is inflated 100 mm Hg above systolic pressure. After excision is complete, topical epinephrine solution may be used for 10 minutes before release of the tourniquet. After release of the tourniquet, the limb is again wrapped in epinephrine solution-soaked gauze for another 5 minutes.

For assessment of viability of the tissues after excision under tourniquet and epinephrine solution, the appearance of the tissues left is observed: The dermis must be pearly white, with no hemorrhagic staining; minor vessels on the wound surface must be patent; the fat must be pale yellow, firm, and moist (dry or golden-brown fat is unhealthy); and the excised wound rapidly becomes hyperemic, even under tourniquet control. In particular, shortly after what appears to be adequate excision, the white dermis and pale-yellow fat appear to develop hemorrhagic staining. Although this usually represents reperfusion, it can easily be confused with the staining that characterizes thermally injured tissue. Thus, there may be a tendency to unnecessarily re-excise the area. Hence, the level of excision is most easily determined with the initial passes of the debriding blade and should not be altered thereafter unless there is convincing evidence of inadequate excision (e.g., tissue fails to reperfuse, remains dry or contains thrombosed vessels on the wound surface).[30]

The order of excision: In cases of extensive burns, the first aim of excision should be toward coverage of the area (large and easily excisable areas, e.g., trunk) rather than toward functional recovery (excision of small and difficult-to-excise areas like hand).

Advantages

As compared to en bloc excision, tangential excision produces less contour problems and better cosmetic result. This technique results in better texture of grafted skin and greater sensitivity.

Complications

The immediate complication is failure of graft "take" which may be due to inadequate excision, infection, hematoma, and lack of proper immobilization. In authors' experience, take of 1:1.5 meshed graft is relatively better.

Problems

- Cyst formation, probably as a result of blockade of the ducts of adnexal glands
- Overhanging skin graft margin
- Pinhead dark spots from inspissated secretions which disappears after meticulous cleaning
- Epithelial bridging showing hair follicle at the undersurface of the epithelium[16]

Limitations: Paucity of graft donor area in extensive burn is taken care by use of allograft, homograft, or synthetic skin temporarily till cultured autokeratinocytes are available. Intermingled xeno/homograft and autograft may be used in the absence of keratinocyte culture facilities.[32] Use of negative-pressure dressing using LAD to prevent infection and possible use of leech effect in extensive areas may improve the result.[28]

EN BLOC EXCISION

En bloc excision **(Figs. 7 and 8)** is indicated for third-degree burns and involves removing the burnt skin and all underlying burnt tissues (that may include fat, deep fascia, and burnt muscle) en bloc till healthy bleeding tissue. This can be done with scalpel, electric cautery, or laser scalpel.[20] When excision is done up to the level of deep fascia (sometimes including muscle fascia), it is called fascial excision **(Figs. 7A and B)**.

In fascial excision, skin, subcutaneous tissue, and deep fascia are incised by knife and scissors. Traction is applied over the tissue to be excised and lifted from the plane deep to the deep fascia and burnt tissue is excised en block. If muscle is involved, it is debrided thoroughly. During en bloc excision **(Figs. 8A to D)**, fewer and larger vessels are

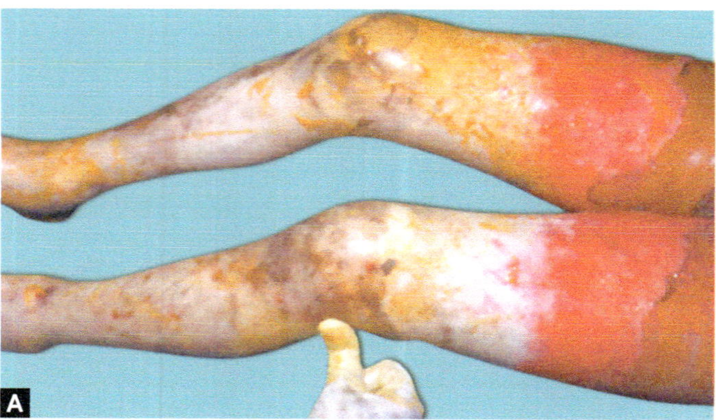

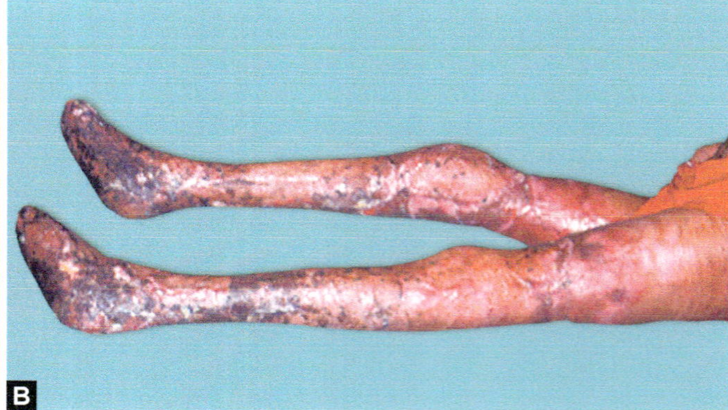

FIGS. 7A AND B: (A) Third-degree burn of both lower extremities; (B) Result after fascial excision and split-skin grafting.

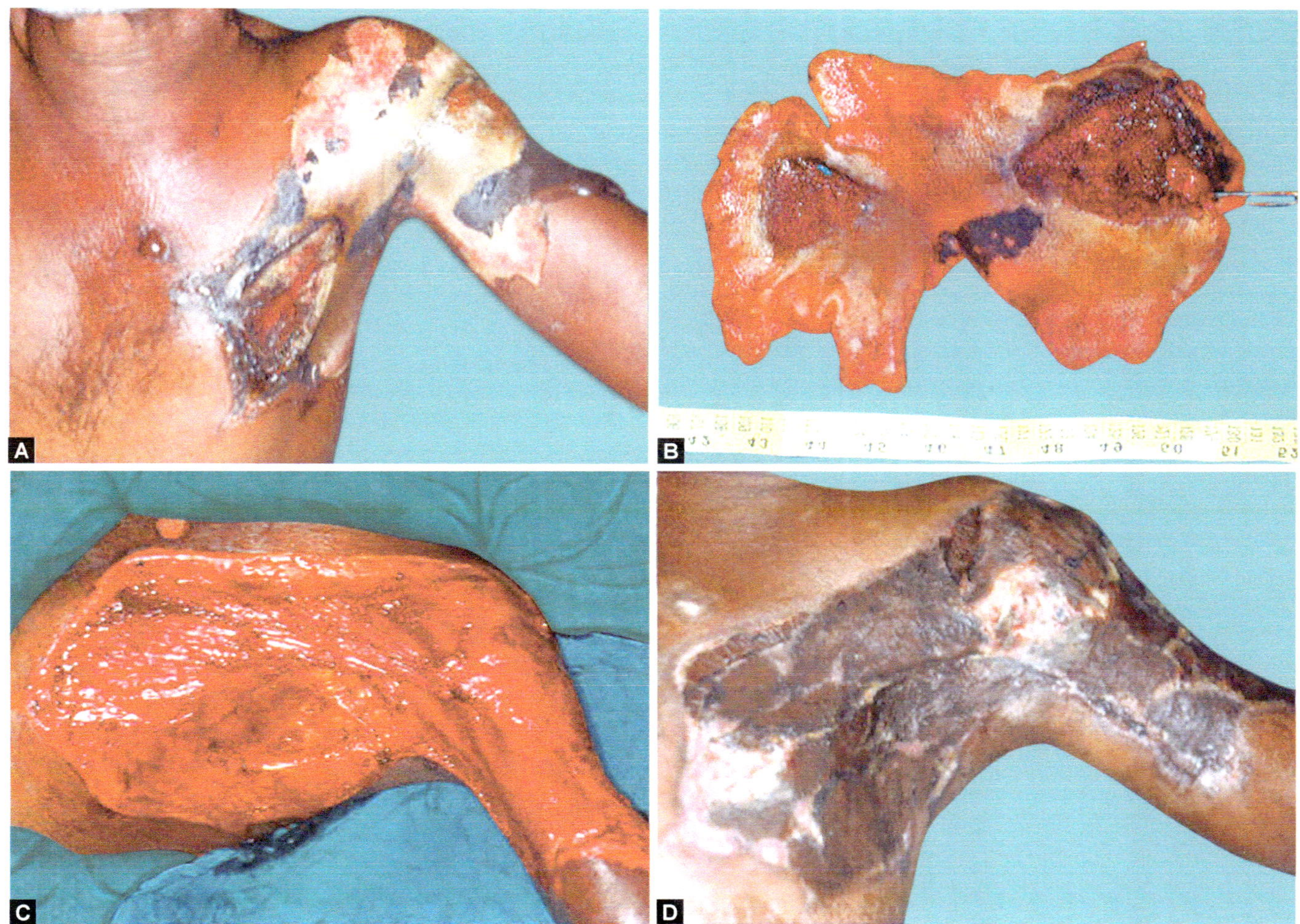

FIGS. 8A TO D: (A) Third-degree burn of chest and right upper extremity; (B) Excised tissue; (C) Viable tissue following en bloc excision; (D) Result after en bloc excision of burnt tissue including superficial muscle.

encountered. To reduce blood loss, these vessels should be divided after ligating or cautery application. To ensure good graft "take", perfect hemostasis is achieved before covering the area with skin graft.

Advantages

Blood vessels are easily identified at the level of deep fascia and hence tackled easily to reduce blood loss. Graft "take" is usually better than that on fat exposed after excision of burn involving full thickness of dermis.

Problems

- Excision of subcutaneous tissues alters body contours (aesthetically poor result) and results in poor texture of grafted skin and poor sensitivity. Hence, whenever possible, fat should be preserved over face, hands, dorsum of foot, and areas around the joints. In females, one should attempt to preserve as much mammary parenchyma as possible.
- While excising over tendoachilles and tendons over dorsum of hand and foot, the importance of staying in correct plane cannot be overemphasized in order to avoid exposure of bare tendons. If tendons or other vital structures are exposed, dermal substitutes like MatriDerm® or BTM® may be used undercover of LAD to promote vascularization.

Whatever technique is used, there is no substitute for experience of the surgeon and good facilities in a center where routine excisional surgery is performed.[4]

Immunological benefits of wound excision and closure: Wound excision and closure causes decrease of proinflammatory mediators, decreased endotoxemia, and restoration of contact hypersensitivity. It has been shown that burn injury inhibits cytotoxic T lymphocyte (CTL) function (which is involved in antigen recognition, processing, and elimination) in a size-dependent manner, and total wound excision significantly improves both CTL function and survival after injury. Therefore, it has been suggested that early excision may help to restore host immunocompetence and may decrease the infectious complications of thermal injury.[33]

Wound debridement: In cases where early burn excision and split-skin grafting are not done due to medical or other reason(s), excision of dead tissue, i.e., wound debridement (escharectomy, slough excision) is done, if needed, repeatedly at 48–72 hours intervals followed by repeated dressings till healthy granulation tissue (fit for split-skin grafting) appears. The author has used LAD extensively as well as dermal substitutes over excised or debrided areas to prepare the wound for grafting **(Figs. 6A to E)**.[28]

POSTOPERATIVE MANAGEMENT

In the immediate postoperative period, hemoglobin, packed cell volume (PCV), and serum electrolytes level is checked to assess blood loss and appropriate action is taken as per report. Hourly vital signs and urine output are measured and IV fluid is administered as per requirement. Antibiotics, as per culture and sensitivity report, analgesic and supportive treatment are instituted. Depending on gut function, oral feeding is started after 6 hours or later.

Depending on wound condition, dressing is done on day 3–5 and then on alternate days. Donor area heals in 10–14 days. Physiotherapy is started after 7 days. Any splint, if required, is delivered at the time of discharge or during follow-up visits.

SUMMARY

- Early wound excision and skin grafting are an established method of treatment for deep dermal, indeterminable depth, and deep burns.
- Technique-wise, excisional surgery is classified as tangential or en bloc excision. Based on the time of excision, it may be classified as immediate (within 24 hours), early (within 2–10 days), or delayed (from 10 to 21 days) excision.
- Excisional surgery has led to reduced overall morbidity significantly and to some extent burn wound sepsis and mortality. It has also led to reduced cost of treatment, reduced wound-related pain, better functional result, early rehabilitation, and reduced long-term morbidity with reduced time away from work.
- As compared to en bloc excision, tangential excision produces less contour problems and better cosmetic result. This technique results in better texture of grafted skin and greater sensitivity.
- Experience of the surgeon and facilities available at the center where excision is done is important. Less than 20% TBSA excision is safe. If treated with excision and grafting 20–40% TBSA burn patients appear to have fewer infectious wound complications and a shorter hospital stay.
- A significant increase in blood loss should be expected with wound excisions after 5–6 days as infection and inflammation of the viable tissue below eschar might increase its vascularity. Clotting abnormalities at this stage can also be a major problem.
- Chances of sepsis increase if excision is delayed by >5 days.
- By early excision and grafting, full functional recovery may be achieved within 2 weeks, whereas in the conventional method, desloughing alone requires 3 weeks and the shortest possible time for full healing is therefore about 5 weeks.
- Scarring (hypertrophy, contractures) is less if wound is closed early and there is reduction in the need for reconstructive procedures.

REFERENCES

1. Cinat ME, Smith MM. Acute burn management. In: Sood R, Achauer BM (Eds), Burns Surgery Reconstruction and Rehabilitation. Philadelphia: Elsevier Inc; 2006. pp. 50-76.
2. Murthy KRS (Translator in English language). Illustrates Sushruta Samhita (Text, English Translation, Notes, Appendices and Index), 2nd edition. Varanasi: Choukhansha Orientalia; 2004. pp. 70-7.
3. Janzekovic Z. The burn wound from the surgical point of view. J Trauma. 1975;15:42-61.
4. Heimbach DM. Early burn excision and grafting. Surg Clin North Am. 1987;67:93-107.
5. Davies JWL. The problems of burns in India. Burns 1990;(Suppl 1): S4-24.
6. Baxter CR. Topical use of 1% silver sulphadiazine. In: Polk HC Jr, Stone HH (Eds), Contemporary Burn Management. Boston: Little Brown & Co.; 1971. p. 217.
7. Barret JP, Handerson DN. Effect of burn wound excision on bacterial colonization and invasion. Plast Reconstr Surg. 2003;111:744-9.
8. Burke JR, Bondoc CC, Quinby WC. Primary burn excision and immediate grafting. A method of shortening illness. J Trauma. 1974;14:389.
9. Phelan HA, Jschke MG, Collins KA. Treatment of deep burns. [online] Available from https://www.uptodate.com/contents/treatment-of-deep-burns. [Last accessed May, 2024].
10. ISBI Practice Guidelines Committee. ISBI Practice Guidelines for Burn Care. Burns. 2016;42:953-1021.
11. Desai MH, Rutan RL, Herndon DN. Conservative treatment of scald burns is superior to early excision. J Burn Care Rehab. 1991;12:482-4.
12. Nguyen TT, Giplin DA, Meyer NA, Herndon DN. Current treatment of severely burned patients. Ann Surg. 1996;223:14-25.

13. Prassanna M, Singh K, Kumar P. Early tangential excision and skin grafting as a routine method of burn wound management: an experience from a developing country. Burns. 1994;20:446-50.
14. Kumar P, Chirayil PT, Chittoria R. Then and now: Burns in Manipal (letter). Burns. 2000;26:66-7.
15. Kumar P, Chirayil PT, Chittoria R. Ten year's epidemiological study of pediatric burn in Manipal, India. Burns. 2000;26:261-4.
16. Edmondson SJ, Ali Jumabhoy I, Murray A. Time to start putting down the knife: A systematic review of burns excision tools of randomised and non-randomised trials. Burns. 2018;44(7): 1721-37.
17. Herndon DN, Barrow RE, Rutan RL, Rutan TC, Desai MH, et al. A Comparison of conservative versus early excision: Therapies in severely burned patients. Ann Surg. 1989;209:547-53.
18. Alexander JW, McMillan BF, Law E, Kittur DS. Treatment of Burn with widely meshed skin autograft and meshed skin allograft overlay. J Trauma. 1981;21:433-8.
19. Kumar P. Classification of skin substitutes. Burns. 2008;34:148.
20. Klasen HJ. Early excision and grafting. In: Settle JAD (Ed), Principles and Practice of Burns Management. New York: Churchill Livingstone; 1996. pp. 275-87.
21. Desai MH, Herndon DN, Broemeling L, Barrow RE, Nichols RJ Jr, Rutan RL. Early burn wound excision significantly reduces blood loss. Ann Surg. 1990;211:753-62.
22. Thomson P, Herndon DN, Abston S. Effect of early excision on patients with major thermal injury. J Trauma. 1987;27:205-7.
23. Herndon DN, Gore D, Cole M, Desai MH, Linares H, Abston S, et al. Determinants of Mortality in pediatric burns with greater than 70% full-thickness total body surface area thermal injury treated by early total excision and grafting. J Trauma. 1987;27:208-12.
24. Shin HS, Lee JW, Jang YC. Clinical Experiences in management of the extensive flame burns dorsal hand by early excision and graft. J Korean Soc Plast Reconstr Surg. 2000;27:234-9.
25. Singh K, Prasanna M. Tangential excision and skin grafting for ash burns of the foot in children: a preliminary report. J. Trauma. 1995;39:560-2.
26. Dickson WA, Sharpe DT, Roberts A. Tangential excision of scalp burns: experience from the Bradford fire disaster. Burns. 1988;14:151-5.
27. Cole JK, Engrav LH, Heimbach DM, Gibran NS, Costa BA, Nakamura DY, et al. Early excision and grafting of face and neck burns in patients over 20 years. Plast Reconstr Surg. 2002;109:1266-73.
28. Kumar P. Exploiting potency of negative pressure in wound dressing using limited access dressing and suction-assisted dressing. Indian J Plast Surg. 2012;45(2):302-15
29. Ryssel H, Germann G, Kloeters O, Gazyakan E, Radu CA. Dermal substitution with Matriderm® in burns on the dorsum of the hand. Burns. 2010;36:1248-53.
30. Cartotto R, Musgrave MA, Beveridge M, Fish J, Gomez M. Minimizing blood loss in burn surgery. J Trauma. 2000;49:1034-9.
31. Browning JA, Cindass R. Burn Debridement, Grafting, and Reconstruction. [Updated 2023 Jan 22]. In: StatPearls [Internet]. Treasure Island (FL): StatPearls Publishing; 2023 Jan. [online] Available from https://www.ncbi.nlm.nih.gov/books/NBK551717/[Last accessed May, 2024].
32. Chih-chun Y, Tsi-siang S. Resurfacing acute extensive deep wound. In: Jackson IT, Sommerland BC (Eds). Recent Advances in plastic surgery. Edinburgh: Churchill Living Stone; 1985. pp. 155-67.
33. Hultman CS, Cairns BN, Deserres S, Frelinger JA, Meyer AA. Early, complete burn wound excision restores cytotoxic T lymphocyte function. Surgery. 1995;118;421-30.

CHAPTER

16

Anesthesia for the Thermally Injured

PK Verma, Bhavya Krishna

INTRODUCTION

The first written documentation describing the treatment of thermally injured dates back to almost four millennia.[1] However, it is only in the last 60 years that any significant improvements in morbidity and survival have occurred. The three factors that determine mortality are presence of inhalational injury, >40% total body surface area (TBSA) burns and age >60 years.[2] Currently, most deaths occur several weeks after injury and are due to multiple organ failure, often in association with sepsis. Improved survival rates are due to effective resuscitation, modern critical care, early burn wound excision, infection control, and ability to counteract the hypermetabolic response.[2]

Anesthetic management of the patient with burns can be complex due to physiological as well as anatomical difficulties following a burn comprising >20% TBSA. The patient with severe burns poses added challenges of airway management, fluid resuscitation, and vascular access besides the hemodynamic changes due to direct trauma to the skin and soft-tissue structures. An integrated approach is necessary for the anesthetic management of a patient with severe burns, emphasizing the interprofessional team in evaluation and treatment and involvement of a skilled and knowledgeable anesthesiologist.

PATHOPHYSIOLOGY

It is important to understand the early pathophysiological changes that occur with thermal injury as successful ongoing management relies on the response to resuscitation. Thermal injury produces many of the changes that are seen in any major trauma but are more profound and longer lasting.

Cardiovascular Changes

After a burn injury, especially > 20% TBSA burn, there is a loss of capillary integrity, in both normal and burned tissues, resulting in a loss of plasma volume into the interstitial space and the burn wound. During this resuscitation phase, lasting 72 hours, aggressive fluid replacement is essential to maintain the perfusion of the vital organs. In addition, adequate intravenous (IV) analgesia is administered not only for the comfort of the patient but also because the pain alters the vital signs that are so useful to monitor resuscitation.

The fluid shifts in the early postburn period decrease the cardiac output independent of the status of intravascular volume. Reduced cardiac contractility results from circulating humoral factors, reduced responsiveness, and decreased coronary blood flow. The magnitude of cardiac impairment is more in the older patients. Systemic vascular resistance also increases, coincident with the decrease in cardiac output.

After successful resuscitation in the first 24–48 hours after a burn, the myriad of inflammatory mediators and cytokines released change the cardiovascular response into the classical systemic inflammatory response syndrome (SIRS). This syndrome is manifested by an increased cardiac output and reduced systemic vascular resistance and reflects a marked increase in the metabolic rate. The consequences of this are important. These SIRS manifestations are identical to those seen in sepsis and care must be taken to avoid antibiotic use in the absence of other evidence of systemic infection. In addition, this syndrome is the prime cause of hypermetabolism seen in a severely burned patient.

Respiratory System Changes

In burns, airway obstruction can be due to direct inhalational injury or edema due to the burns. Risk factors for upper airway obstruction are burns to head and face, inhalational injury, associated trauma, and burns inside mouth.[3] Upper airway injuries result from inhalation of superheated air or steam and toxic compounds found in smoke. Brief exposure of the epiglottis or larynx to either dry air at 300°C or steam at 100°C leads to massive edema and rapid airway obstruction. In children, this may result in macroglossia, epiglottitis, and laryngotracheal bronchitis. Even patients with a mild upper airway injury are at risk for development of progressive airway obstruction as tissue edema develops. The clinical signs **(Box 1)** that should alert the clinician to the possibility of upper airway involvement are facial burns, singed nasal vibrissae, bronchorrhea, and sooty sputum **(Fig. 1)**. If severe, patient may appear dyspneic, use accessory muscles of respiration, and sit upright. Hoarseness and dysphagia are common. Flow-volume curves and nasopharyngoscopy may aid the initial diagnosis of upper airway burns and are particularly useful in assessing trends in airway impairment. The American Burn Life Support (ABLS) indications for early intubation include: Signs of airway obstruction (hoarseness, stridor, accessory respiratory muscle use, and sternal retraction), TBSA burns > 40–50%, extensive and deep facial burns, burns inside mouth, significant edema or risk for edema, difficulty in swallowing, signs of respiratory compromise (inability to clear secretions, respiratory fatigue, poor oxygenation or ventilation), decreased levels of consciousness where airway protective reflexes are impaired, and anticipated patient transfer of large burn with airway issue without qualified personnel to intubate enroute[4] (ABLS) **(Fig. 2)**. In fact, any delay may make a subsequent attempt at intubation physically impossible due to loss of identifiable landmarks as a result of severe edema of all the structures above the larynx. It may be wise to avoid performing a tracheostomy on these patients as this procedure is associated with a high mortality **(Fig. 3)**.[5]

BOX 1 Clues to inhalational injury.

- Exposure in a closed space
- Loss of consciousness
- Nasal, oral, or facial burns
- Singed nasal vibrissae
- Carbonaceous sputum
- Hoarseness or stridor
- Upper airway changes on bronchoscopy
- Flow–volume curves
- Chest radiograph showing pulmonary edema
- Carboxyhemoglobin levels > 10%

Note: Hypermetabolic state manifests clinically as a persistent tachycardia (despite adequate resuscitation), hyperpnea, and marked muscle wasting.

The oropharynx and upper airway are efficient heat exchangers. Therefore, thermal burns to the lower airway are rare unless steam or chemicals have been inhaled. The clinical signs described for upper airway injury are also applicable to lower airway injuries. In addition, the patient may give a history of being confined in a smoke-filled, closed space and may exhibit raised levels of carboxyhemoglobin. The airway remains reactive for months after the incident. If the thorax is burned, chest wall compliance may be decreased by edema, by the formation of an inelastic circumferential eschar and possibly by the application of tight bandages. Lung compliance and

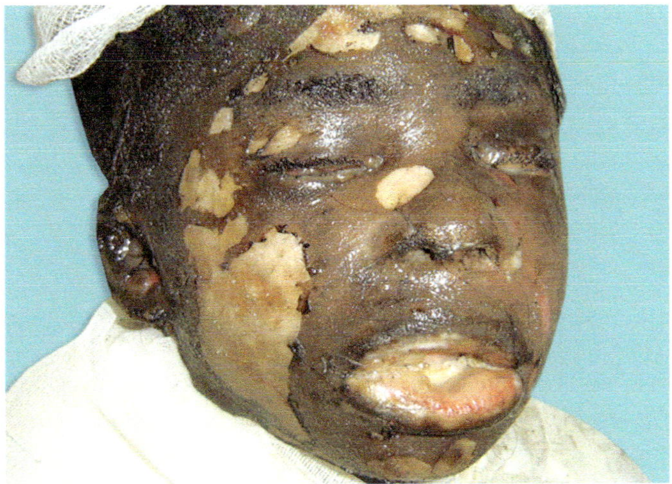

FIG. 1: Patient with face burns along with inhalation injury.

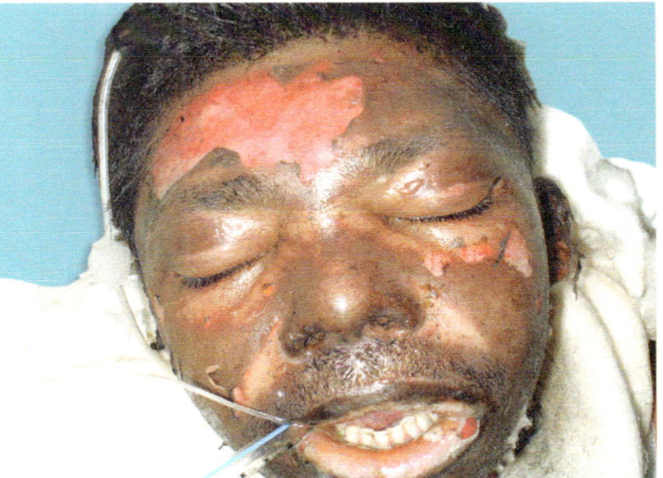

FIG. 2: Patient with inhalation injury requiring intubation for mechanical ventilation.

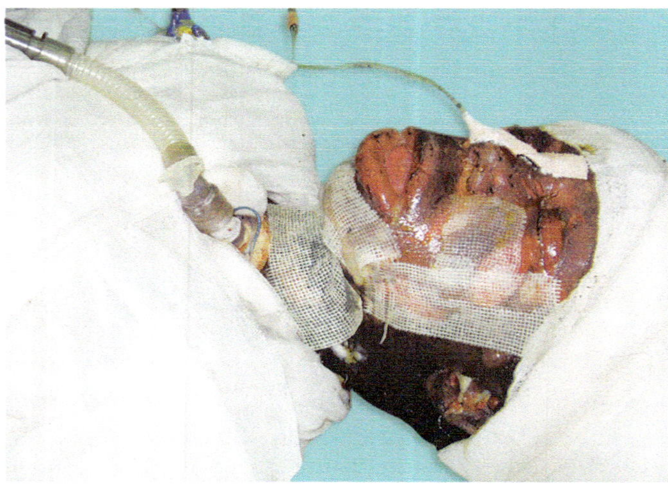

FIG. 3: Patient with severe inhalation injury requiring tracheostomy for ventilation.

functional residual capacity (FRC) may also be reduced. Minute ventilation and the alveolar/arterial gradient for oxygen increase, mainly because of edema and reduced cardiac output. Hypoxia coupled with increased work of breathing may exhaust the patient. These considerations reinforce the necessity for early tracheal intubation, high concentrations of oxygen, and controlled ventilation.

Metabolic Changes

The burn injury results in a massive catecholamine output. The outcome is a hypermetabolic state characterized by protein catabolism, urea genesis, lipolysis, and gluconeogenesis. In patients with burns of >50% of the TBSA, the basal metabolic rate may be doubled.

The loss of skin and the increased metabolic rate impair the thermoregulation of the patient who responds by increasing his core temperature to 38.5°C. This persistent pyrexia may mask the early signs of sepsis which is the most common cause of death once the patient has reached a burns unit. A high index of clinical suspicion, supported by hematological and bacteriological surveillance, is essential and aggressive antibiotic therapy and wound debridement must be initiated early.

Ambient temperature has an important effect on the metabolic rate in burn patients. A study of patients with a mean burn size of 44% TBSA showed that patients at thermoneutral ambient temperature (28–32°C) had metabolic rates 1.5 times those of unburned controls. However, when ambient temperature was decreased to 22–28°C, the metabolic rate increased in proportion to burn size. Thus, ambient temperature less than thermoneutral range should be avoided, whether in the burn unit or in the operating room, to minimize further increase in metabolic rate.

The increase in metabolic rate has implications for nutritional support in the postburn period. Early feeding decreases muscle catabolism and may reduce bacterial translocation through the intestinal mucosa. Adequate pain control, alleviation of anxiety, a thermoneutral environment, and an aggressive treatment of infection are all important steps in limiting catecholamine secretions and thus, hypermetabolism which diverts calories from the healing tissues.

Immunologic Changes

Sepsis and multiple-organ failure are a major cause of death among burned patients. Large areas of dead tissues are easily colonized with bacteria as a result of impaired white blood cell function and reduced levels of fibronectin and gamma globulins.

ANESTHETIC MANAGEMENT

Convalescence from a thermal injury can be divided into three phases. The anesthetic requirements during the three phases are different and will be discussed separately. First is the resuscitation phase, which starts at the time the patient sustains the burn. This phase deals with maintenance of the airway, acute fluid replacement, and cardiovascular stabilization and analgesia **(Box 2)**. All anesthesiologists must be familiar with the acute resuscitation of victims of major burns. Hemodynamic stability and adequate urine output should be established within 72 hours after injury and the resuscitation phase is now complete. This is followed by the hypermetabolic stabilization phase (when skin grafts are used to cover the defects). This phase may last up to 90 days or more. Finally, the third phase, i.e., the reconstructive phase deals with the restoration of form and function of damaged tissues and the release of contractures.

Resuscitation Phase

The role of an anesthesiologist in the acute resuscitation of a severely burnt patient varies from institution to institution.

The special skills of the anesthesiologist in airway management, fluid management, and percutaneous, IV,

BOX 2 **Problems encountered by the anesthesiologist in the resuscitation phase.**

- Airway management
- Cardiovascular stabilization
- Fluid replacement
- Analgesia
- Life-saving surgical interventions

and arterial catheterization may be required. The detailed discussion of the management during this phase is beyond the scope of this chapter and has been discussed elsewhere.

Anesthesia during resuscitation phase should be provided only for life-saving procedures. Common surgical problems which may require anesthesia are usually injuries associated with burns, for example, amputation of nonviable limb, exploratory laparotomy, or thoracotomy for penetrating injuries, etc. All else should be postponed till the patient has been resuscitated and stabilized. In the presence of injuries like fractures, abdominal, or thoracic trauma which are commonly associated with blood loss, blood replacement may be required in addition to resuscitation fluids. Ketamine may be the safest agent for anesthesia during this period and may be used in combination with a nondepolarizing neuromuscular blocking agent (NMBA) if relaxation is required. Suxamethonium may be used to facilitate intubation from the time of injury to 48 hours after injury but should be carefully avoided thereafter till up to 1 year since the burn.[6] Increased oxygen demand, tachycardia, and decreased compliance may make mechanical ventilation (MV) mandatory both, preoperatively and postoperatively. Adequate analgesia must be provided in the perioperative period and great care must be taken to ensure continued adequate resuscitation during anesthesia.

Hypermetabolic Stabilization Phase

Some of the commonly performed operations during this phase include primary excision and skin grafting, dressings, and debridement.

The pathophysiological state of the patient presenting for surgery and anesthesia varies depending on the percentage of TBSA burnt, location of burns, age of the patient, time elapsed since initial injury, and adequacy of the treatment received in the resuscitation phase **(Box 3)**. Blood loss due to increased wound vascularity, hypothermia, and plasma potassium levels are the predominant considerations during surgery on the burn patients in this phase.

BOX 3 **Factors modifying the pathophysiological state of the patient.**

- % TBSA burnt
- Location of burns
- Age of the patient
- Time elapsed since initial injury
- Adequacy of the treatment received in the resuscitation phase

(TBSA: total body surface area)

Preoperative Assessment and Preparation (Box 4)

Successful anesthesia for excision and grafting of a burn patient requires planning. Because burn patients often undergo many operative procedures, it is important for the anesthesiologist to establish good rapport with the patient and explain all movements and procedures in advance, especially if they may be painful.

A brief history should be obtained, either from the patient or from the progress notes. The cause of the

BOX 4 **Considerations in preoperative evaluation/ during preoperative visit of the burned patient.**

- Reassure the patient; establish rapport; and explain the procedure in advance
- Obtain history of the patient
  - Ascertain the cause of burn (chemical, electrical, inhalational, etc.)
  - Review any past history of relevance
- Perform physical examination
  - Record the extent of burn and other injuries
  - Assess current IV access and whether the current site needs a change
  - Assess the airway and predict if a difficult intubation is likely
  - Assess for adequacy of resuscitation (mental status, skin color, capillary refill, hematocrit, oxygen saturation, and urine output) and correct any deficiency.
  - Evaluate cardiovascular system (ECG, BP, CVP, pulmonary artery catheterization, if indicated)
  - Ascertain the respiratory status (X-ray chest and ABG)
  - Look for evidence of any coagulation abnormality (Hb/ hematocrit, electrolytes, and coagulation profile)
  - Any evidence of acute renal failure (blood urea, serum creatinine, serum electrolytes, urine output, and urine osmolality)
- Interact with the burn surgeon (nature and extent of excision, amount of blood loss, and operative time)
- Arrange for the estimated blood loss
- Premedication:
  - Provide adequate analgesia
  - Brief period of fasting
- Take a decision about the monitoring and care to be provided during transport
- Consider antithrombotic prophylaxis
- Record any additional point(s) of relevance

(ABG: arterial blood gas; CVP: central venous pressure)

burn should be ascertained. Electrical burns may cause myocardial damage. Chemical burns are associated with a high incidence of renal or hepatic damage. Exposure to toxic fumes or concurrent inhalational injury may interfere with respiratory function. Past medical history, allergies, recent medications, previous surgery, and previous anesthetics should be reviewed.

Physical examination may be limited by dressings, dyskinesia, or pain. The extent of the burn and other injuries should be ascertained from the recorded notes. The respiratory and cardiovascular system should be examined as in any other assessment. The sites of possible venous access should be evaluated as these may be limited and difficult to find. A vein finder is often useful in these scenarios.[7] The assessment of the airway and predicting, if a difficult airway is likely, is important in these patients at this stage. Finally, adequacy of resuscitation is confirmed. Simple parameters like assessment of mental status, skin color, capillary refill, hematocrit values, oxygen saturation, and urine output should be employed fully. Noninvasive blood pressure measurement and electrocardiographic (ECG) monitoring should be a routine, but unusual sites may be required for the cuff and electrodes. Placement of a sterile cuff over burned areas is acceptable or an unsterile cuff may be placed over a thin occlusive dressing. Invasive arterial and central venous pressure monitoring may be helpful, particularly for patients with extensive burns or an inhalational injury. However, these carry significant risk of infection.

Of all the parameters available, urine output is probably the most useful. If resuscitation is adequate, the urine output should be at least 0.5 mL/kg body weight/hour and the osmolarity of the urine in the range of 600–1,000 mOsm/L. In the presence of myoglobinuria, mannitol may be given to promote diuresis. In these patients, the urine output is no longer a reliable guide to the adequacy of resuscitation. If resuscitation is inadequate, this is the time to take corrective measures.

Respiratory status of the patient should be assessed carefully during the preoperative assessment and strategy to deal with the findings planned accordingly. A patient with burns around the airway (e.g., singed nasal hair) should be intubated as early as possible. Direct inhalational/thermal injury and fluid resuscitation may make delayed intubation more difficult secondary to upper airway edema, as discussed earlier. Physiologic derangements due to injury to lower airways may include pulmonary edema and acute respiratory distress syndrome (ARDS). Additionally, burn patients can be severely hypermetabolic with corresponding increased carbon dioxide production. These patients may have high-peak inspiratory pressures (PIPs) and high-minute ventilation requirements. High level of positive end-expiratory pressure (PEEP) may be helpful in these patients. Other possible effects of severe burns include: decreased lung and chest wall compliance, decreased FRC, increased alveolar-arterial oxygen gradient, increased carboxy hemoglobinuria, and increased methemoglobinuria. Chest radiograph and arterial blood gases (ABG) should be asked for to evaluate the progress of the patient's condition.

Cyanide can be part of inhalational injury related with burns and its poisoning causes clinical spectrum ranging from headache, dizziness, tachycardia, and tachypnea to lethargy, seizures, and respiratory failure. The treatment consists of amyl nitrate inhalation until IV access is secured, then a combination of IV sodium nitrite and sodium thiosulfate along with 100% oxygen therapy. IV hydroxocobalamin plus 100% oxygen therapy can also be instituted. Hydroxocobalamin is usually the recommended treatment option in burn patients, because it is safer in patients with inhalational injuries. During the initial smoke inhalation injury, the patient is also exposed to other chemical products of combustion, such as ammonia, nitrogen dioxide, and sulfur dioxide which are airway irritants causing bronchospasm, edema, and mucous membrane ulceration predisposing the patient to the development of recurrent infections and pneumonia.[8]

Septicemia and chest infections are generally associated with respiratory failure and are indications for controlled MV.

The variations of urea and electrolytes in blood should be corrected preoperatively. An element of renal failure associated with inadequate resuscitation may be present. The blood sugar is usually elevated and may cause an osmotic diuresis with a concomitant loss of electrolytes. Coagulopathies may result directly from the burn injury, especially in the 2nd week of postburn, as well as from rapid replacement of blood loss during operative procedure and should be monitored closely. Coagulation profile, hemogram, hematocrit, and electrolyte reports should be analyzed to monitor the condition of the patient. The hematocrit, if all else is normal, indicates the level of hydration.

Preoperative anemia is, in part, dilutional in the early days, but levels below 8 g/dL should be corrected before surgery. The attention to anticipated amount of blood loss should be given at this visit. Postoperative oozing into dressings can be considerable and this loss should also be taken into account when ordering blood to maintain the hemoglobin concentration above 10 g/dL. It is important (during this preoperative visit) for the surgeon and anesthesiologist to decide collectively, about the nature and extent of the excision, the amount of blood loss anticipated and the anticipated operative time in view of the patient's condition. The endpoints for surgical excision in large burns are: (i) Operative time of 2–3 hours; (ii) core temperature of 35°C; or (iii) blood loss of 10 units of packed red blood cells. The violation of any of these parameters invites coagulopathy and increasing problems with hemostasis and vital signs stability.

Burns patients are hypermetabolic and are usually underfed in terms of their higher caloric requirement. Repeated fasting for multiple surgeries also hampers their nutritional requirements, hence, preoperative fasting guidelines have been modified in burns. Achieving adequate caloric intake in patients with major burns is difficult and nutritional support is frequently supplemented with nasogastric tube feedings. Thus, minimizing the fasting period before operation is beneficial. It is advisable not to discontinue enteral feeding before operation in patients who are already intubated with cuffed endotracheal tubes and some guidelines recommend intraoperative feeding in intubated patients; in nonintubated patients, feeding should be stopped 2 hours prior to surgery.[6] This improves preoperative nutrition without apparently increasing the risk of aspiration.

Premedication is required to provide adequate analgesia and anxiolysis since burns patients are in pain and often anxious. If a patient does not have a secure airway in place, it is important not to oversedate and risk losing the airway, especially if the patient appears to be a potentially difficult intubation. Patients who present for excision and debridement are often already intubated and sedated. It is important to continue this sedation in the perioperative period.[8] An antisialagogue such as glycopyrrolate may also be included in the premedication.

The effect of the premedicant analgesic should be noted because these patients may be unduly sensitive or apparently resistant to analgesics. Ketamine continues to have a role in premedication for children via the oral or rectal routes.

Antithrombotic prophylaxis should be considered, balancing the hypercoagulable state of the major burn with the risk of disseminated intravascular coagulation (DIC) and the potential for deep vein thrombosis in any nonambulatory patient against the risk of hematoma formation under skin grafts or skin substitute.

Preoperative visit is also the time to plan the ways to transport the patient (depending on the condition) from ward to the operating room. The patient may be brought to the operating room on the ward bed as any movement to and from a transport trolley causes unnecessary pain. For patients with severe ARDS, transportation may pose formidable challenges with regard to ventilation. Cardiopulmonary monitoring must be continued during transport; the ventilation system used in transport must be capable of delivering high minute volumes, PEEP, and inspiratory pressures. These requirements may not be satisfied by standard bag-valve systems and may require a high-quality transport monitor.

The following conditions may be considered as contraindications for surgery:[c]

- Inadequate resuscitation
- Abnormal electrolytes
- Respiratory or metabolic acidosis
- Abnormal clotting studies
- Incipient septicemia
- Unexplained rapid temperature changes
- Changed consciousness level
- Instability in respiratory or cardiovascular parameters

Intraoperative Period

While there is no single technique that may be regarded as ideal, a number of general principles apply while giving anesthesia to burn patients **(Box 5)**. Skin-grafting or free-tissue transfer must not be jeopardized by poor perfusion during or after anesthesia. The use of hypotensive techniques, smooth balanced anesthesia, and excellent analgesia with good fluid/blood replacement contribute to a successful outcome.

Regional techniques are rarely feasible, given the multiple surgical sites for harvesting and skin grafting. Laryngeal mask airways (LMAs), in general, are not recommended for major burns, given the potential for significant fluid resuscitation and subsequent airway edema, as well as the frequent repositioning of patient intraoperatively. LMAs, however, are invaluable for shorter procedures, avoiding repetitive laryngeal instrumentation and for their ability to maintain the difficult airway while deepening the anesthetic or as an aid to intubation with or without the fiberoptic bronchoscope **(Fig. 4)**.[11]

Induction of Anesthesia

The patient should be brought to the induction room on the ward bed (if facilities exist), as any movement to and from a transport trolley causes unnecessary pain. Induction of anesthesia can be performed on the bed and the patient transferred to the operating table once profound analgesia has been obtained. Noninvasive monitoring should be placed in site prior to induction of anesthesia **(Fig. 5)**. A second anesthesiologist is helpful to assist in induction. A surgeon should be available in the induction room. He may be called upon to perform a cut-down on a vein if percutaneous venous access is not possible. Securing venous access is a prerequisite to burn excision and grafting procedures. This may be established the night before surgery to ensure adequate hydration. For most cases, a minimum of two large-bore peripheral IV lines or one peripheral and one

BOX 5 Anesthetic consideration for excision and grafting of major burns.[10]

- *Premedication*:
  - Provide adequate analgesia
  - Brief period of fasting
- *Vascular access*:
  - Establish large-bore IV access
  - Consider invasive monitoring
- *Induction*:
  - Volume resuscitated: Propofol/Thiopentone
  - Volume depleted: Ketamine
- *Securing the airway*:
  - Consider alternatives to direct laryngoscopy
  - Consider awake intubation
- *Ventilation*:
  - Ventilation requirement, due to:
    - Hypermetabolism
    - Parenteral alimentation
  - Smoke inhalation/circumferential burns/ARDS may necessitate ICU-type ventilator
- *Fluid and blood*:
  - Blood loss can be extensive
  - Check coagulation profile
  - N-saline/Ringer lactate @ 8–10 mL/kg/hour
  - Keep urine output 0.5–1 mL/kg/hour
  - Continue parenteral nutrition
- *Temperature regulation*:
  - Warm all fluids and keep operation theater warm
  - Humidify gases
  - Warming blanket/reflective head cover
- *Selection of anesthetic agent*:
  - Include opioids with all techniques
  - Catecholamine (endogenous and exogenous) levels are increased: Choose/use compatible inhalational agents
- *Muscle relaxants*:
  - Avoid succinylcholine.
  - Resistance to NMBAs (nondepolarizing muscle relaxant)
- *Recovery/postoperative state*:
  - Opioid requirements are large
  - Keep the patient warm
  - Check coagulation profile
  - Continue cardiopulmonary monitoring
  - Oxygen administration
  - Consider initiating enteral nutrition as early as possible

(ARDS: acute respiratory distress syndrome; NMBAs: nondepolarizing neuromuscular blocking agent)

central line should be used. Ultrasound-guided venous access can be obtained. These may be inserted under local anesthesia with xylocaine and used for induction. Insertion of large-bore cannulae can be performed under

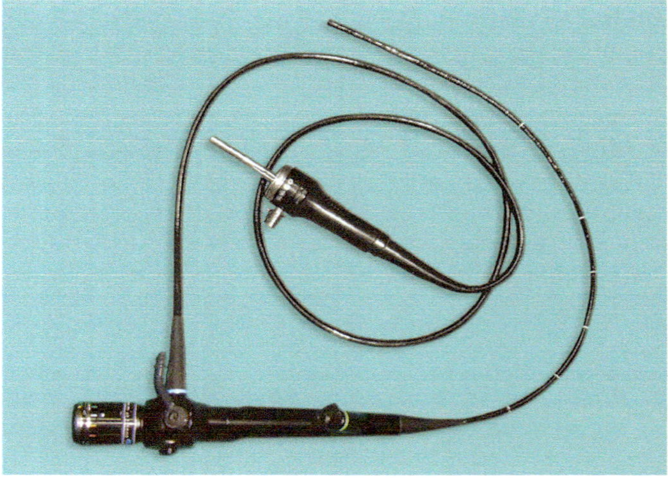

FIG. 4: Fiberoptic bronchoscope set.

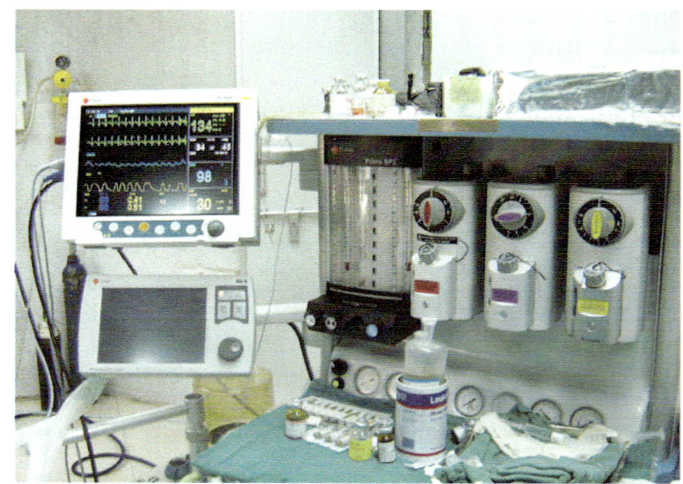

FIG. 5: Anesthesia workstation with attached noninvasive monitors.

general anesthesia. The positioning of both IV access and monitoring should be discussed with the surgeon with respect to the operative site.

Preoxygenation is advisable because of the high-metabolic rate, tachycardia, and increased oxygen needs. If the trachea is assessed as being easy to intubate and patient is adequately volume-resuscitated, fentanyl at 3–5 mg/kg body weight may be given by slow IV injection.

Ketamine has been considered the induction agent of choice in burns with a dose of 2 mg/kg since it has analgesic effects, has sympathetic stimulant properties, and maintains airway reflexes. Other agents like propofol (1–2 mg/kg) may be used.[6] This technique allows for rapid recovery and minimizes postoperative cognitive disturbances. Alternatively, thiopentone (3–5 mg/kg) may also be used. Xylocaine (1–1.5 mg/kg) may be given prior to intubation to depress the cardiac response to intubation and enhance the potency of fentanyl. If the patient is intravascularly volume-depleted, ketamine (1–3 mg/kg) is recommended. Patients with extensive burns (>30% TBSA) develop a decreased sensitivity to NMBAs; therefore, 1.5 times the usual intubating dose of NMBAs is recommended: Vecuronium (1.5 mg/kg), or rocuronium (1.5 mg/kg). If rapid sequence induction is indicated, high-dose rocuronium (2 mg/kg) can be used. Sugammadex, if available, is useful in difficult airway cases where rocuronium is used for early reversal.[12] Succinylcholine is contraindicated during this phase (i.e., when injury is >48 hours old) because of potentially lethal efflux of potassium ions from muscle. This abnormal response probably occurs because the entire muscle membrane, rather than just the myoneural junction becomes a receptor.

In case, a difficult intubation is anticipated, alternative plans should be sought for. Most injuries leading to difficult intubation will have burns around the face and neck which are likely to be infected. If a tracheostomy is performed, it may lead to septicemia, mediastinitis or chest infection, ultimately causing the demise of the patient. Facial burns, with a raw area on the face, may make placing a face mask difficult on the face. A sterile Gamgee pad, with a hole in the area of nose and oral aperture, may be used to cover the raw area and the face mask can be kept on the pad. The other methods of intubation which can be considered include inhalational induction followed by awake fiberoptic intubation **(Figs. 6A to C)**, cricothyroidotomy with jet ventilation, cricothyroid puncture, and retrograde cannulation or percutaneous tracheostomy. The LMA has proved its worth and is an acceptable alternative method to try for shorter procedures **(Fig. 7)**. Securing the endotracheal tube (ETT) can be difficult in the presence of facial burns **(Fig. 8)**. Alternatives to taping the ETT include suturing the tube to the lip or using a circumferential tie around the patient's head.[13]

Maintenance of Anesthesia

Controlled ventilation, facilitated with muscle relaxants, is the method of choice for all but the shortest procedures, i.e., dressing changes. This technique reduces oxygen consumption and makes it possible to increase the minute

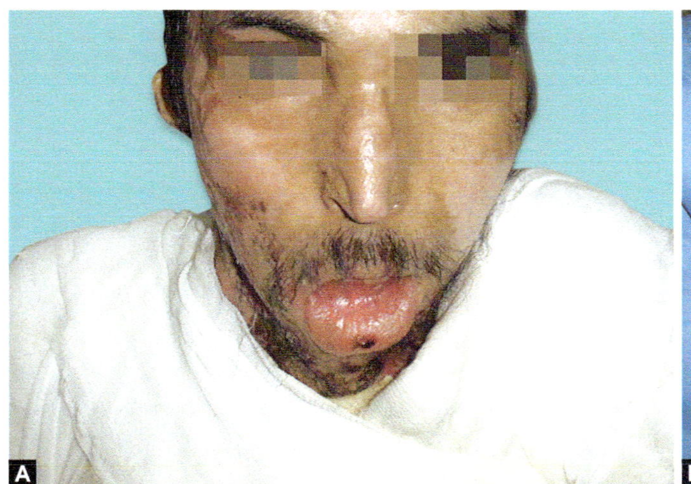

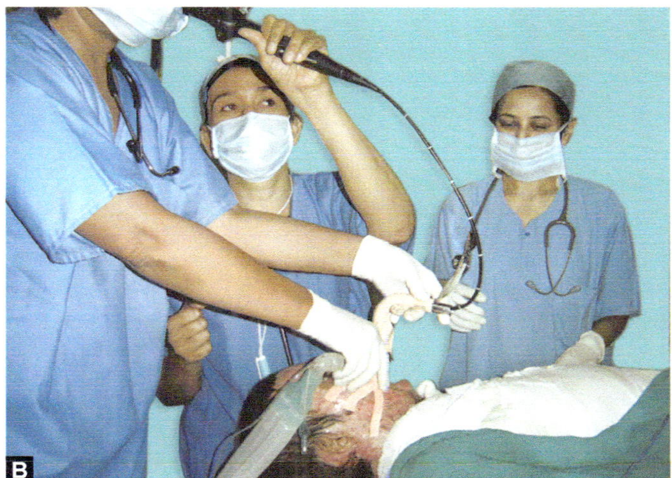

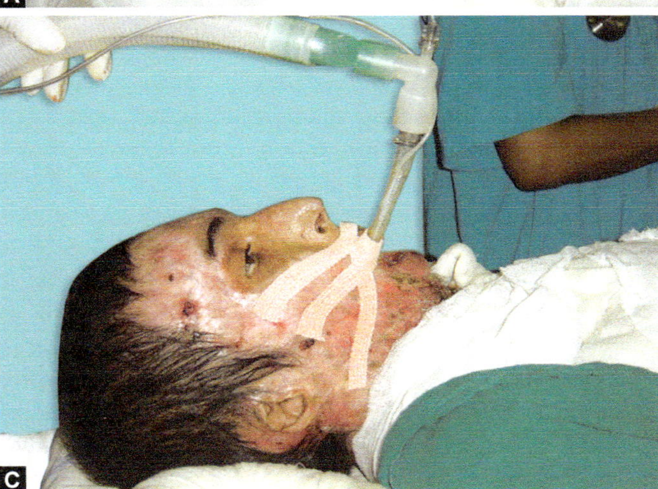

FIGS. 6A TO C: (A) A patient with chronic postburn raw area with contracture of neck with difficult airway. (B) Fiberoptic bronchoscopy through intubating laryngeal mask airway (LMA) being tried for the same patient through oral route because of pinched nostrils. (C) Same patient successfully intubated orally.

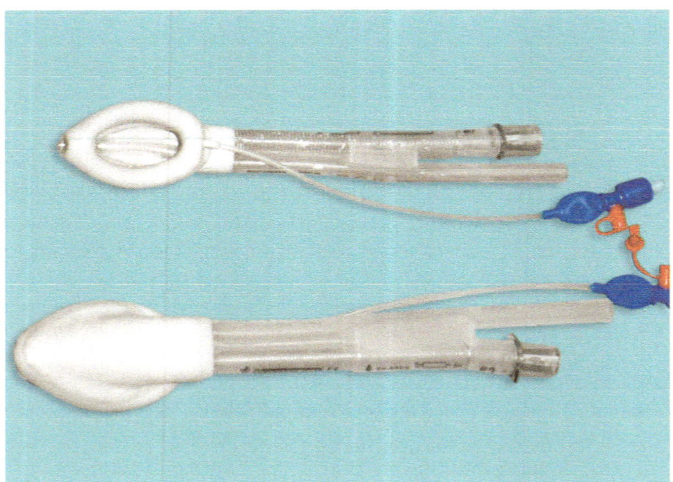

FIG. 7: Laryngeal mask airway (LMA).

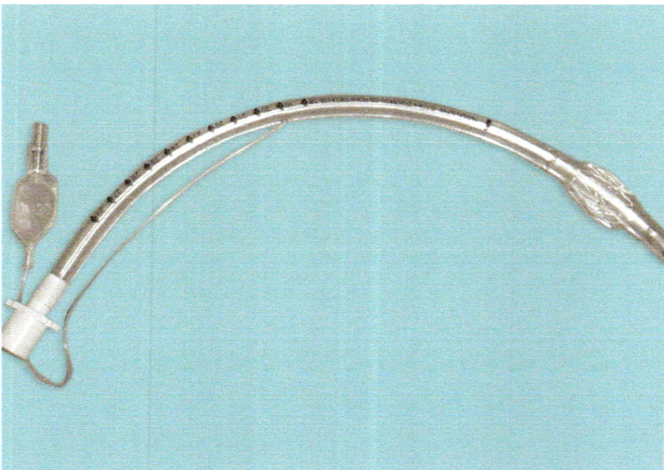

FIG. 8: Endotracheal tube.

volume to ensure that normal carbon dioxide levels are maintained in these highly catabolic patients. Care should be taken to assess a patient's ventilatory requirements preoperatively and lung protective ventilation should be continued throughout the intraoperative period. Patients who have also suffered an inhalation injury may have increased requirements for oxygen and PEEP. For these patients, it is particularly important to avoid alveolar derecruitment with the loss of PEEP during transfer to a transport or theater ventilator. As the hypermetabolic response suffered by patients with burns leads to increased oxygen consumption and carbon dioxide production, higher than expected oxygen concentrations and minute volumes may be required.[14] Physiologic derangements of the respiratory system (poor gaseous exchange and a low compliance) and a hypermetabolic state may require high inspiratory pressures, PEEP, and other ventilatory adjuncts to maintain oxygenation. Depending on equipment availability, an ICU ventilator may be necessary. The effect of positive pressure ventilation, PEEP, and hypovolemia may summate to have a deleterious effect on the cardiac output and renal function and must be avoided by ensuring adequate intravascular volume and, if required, by the use of inotropic agents.

Inhalational agents may be used to provide balanced anesthesia. Intraoperatively, burn surgeons commonly use epinephrine-soaked sponges to decrease blood loss. Systemic absorption of epinephrine causes tachycardia and increases the probability of dysrhythmias; therefore, it is better to avoid halothane or desflurane. Isoflurane and sevoflurane are acceptable. The prolonged or repeated use of nitrous oxide may decrease erythropoiesis by inhibition of vitamin B12. This can be overcome by hydroxocobalamin injections.

Circumferential burns may require the patient to be moved during the procedure. An armored tracheal tube and a lightweight coaxial breathing system, such as the Bain system may be preferred. The cornea should be protected with eye ointment and pressure points should be padded. Facial burns may make eye closure difficult, and a temporary tarsorrhaphy may be required after prior discussion with the patient.

Adequate analgesia should be given during the intraoperative period and should continue in the postoperative state. It is humane to complete the dressing and place the patient on the ward bed before terminating anesthesia. Inadequate postoperative analgesia may make the patient restless; this, in turn, may provoke bleeding under the skin grafts (and their subsequent loss) or alternatively, displacement of the grafts. If large volume resuscitation has occurred intraoperatively, there is a possibility of clinically significant airway edema; use caution before extubating a patent airway.

Monitoring

Monitoring methods which are taken for granted in nonburn patients may be difficult in the burned patients. The blood pressure cuff may be applied to a lower limb when both upper limbs are to be operated upon. The blood pressure cuff may be rotated from one extremity to another to accommodate the surgery or an arterial catheter may be inserted. Surface electrodes may not adhere even after tincture of benzoin has been applied, in which case percutaneous needle electrode may be required. Transesophageal electrodes may be the method of choice even though they are expensive. The pulse rate can usually be measured manually, by the arterial waveform or by ECG tracing. The pulse oximeter is a useful monitor which indicates hemoglobin saturation as well as the pulse rate.

A suitable pulse for the sensor may be difficult to find. Alternative sites include the earlobe and nasal septum. It is important to remember that pulse oximetry cannot be relied upon to detect carbon monoxide (CO) poisoning as it continues to overestimate the oxygen saturation.[15]

An esophageal stethoscope can be used to monitor both heart and breath sounds. Capillary refilling can be easily observed and the patient's color is noted. These clinical observations may be all that is available in certain patients and conditions. Because of increased metabolic rate and carbon dioxide production, increased alveolar ventilation may be required. ABG analysis must, therefore, be assessed early and frequently throughout the anesthetic procedure. Constant monitoring of expired carbon dioxide is very helpful during intraoperative management. However, one must be cognizant of the possibility of significant differences between arterial and expired carbon dioxide values as a result of shunting and dead space ventilation in patients with severe pulmonary injury.

All patients with major burns have a urinary Foley catheter in place. Adequate fluid replacement ensures a good urine output but a decreased output is a late sign of inadequate replacement.

Temperature control is a major problem and heat loss can be enormous. Both core and peripheral temperatures must be monitored. Heat loss is minimized by warming all fluid, especially those used to prepare skin for surgery. The thermoneutral temperature for these patients is between 31°C and 33°C. This can be extremely uncomfortable for the working staff. Burn operation theaters (OT's) can be uncomfortable for staff. Raising the ambient temperature aims to compensate for the loss of temperature regulation by the skin and the hypermetabolic response with severe burns that results in a core temperature elevation to approximately 38–38.5°C, thought to be due to a hypothalamic set point mechanism.[16] Ambient temperature target is 28–33°C.[14]

Areas not being operated upon must be covered; overhead heaters and heating blankets should be used, especially on children; and simply covering the head may make a noticeable difference. A falling peripheral temperature may be due to an inadequate plasma volume if the core temperature is remaining static.

The most important feature of the intraoperative course is monitoring and replacing patient's blood loss. The expected blood loss may be 100–200 mL/% BSA excised or 3.4% of total blood volume for each % of TBSA excised and grafted. Therefore, one must be familiar with the surgical approach to burn excision. During a tangential excision, a patient might lose three to five times more blood than during excision down to fascia. Bleeding risks are increased in patients with infected burn tissue, deeper thickness burns and by prolonged operative time. Intraoperative tourniquet use on burned extremities reduces overall blood loss and also decreases the rate of loss, making intraoperative hypovolemia less likely. Some centers use postoperative compression dressing after excision and grafting to reduce blood loss. Epinephrine solution (1 in 200,000 in normal saline) injected subcutaneously in both donor and excision sites are also used to reduce blood loss during excision and grafting procedures. Although high levels of catecholamines in the blood have been measured with this technique, complications such as dysrhythmias are uncommon. After burn injury, cardiovascular responses to catecholamines are attenuated because of a reduced affinity of the β-adrenergic receptors for ligands and decreased second messenger production. Blood loss is also quite dependent on the expertise of the surgical team. Hypotensive anesthesia has also been advocated as a means to decrease blood loss. Exact estimation of the blood loss is difficult because of bleeding into dressings, sponges and packs, and on to the floor. Other indicators of circulating blood volume, such as urine output, central venous pressure, arterial pressure, and shape of the arterial waveform, whenever possible, must be closely monitored. Blood loss should be replaced adequately. For patients without contraindications to hemodilution (e.g., coronary artery disease and anemia), it is often better to delay packed red blood cells transfusion until major blood loss is complete. If sudden decrease in blood pressure occurs during very rapid transfusion of blood (>150 mL/min), using calcium to counteract the chelating effect of citrate is considered. However, one should be cautious to avoid over transfusion especially in a small child or in an elderly. The use of near-patient coagulation studies such as thromboelastography may be superior to standard laboratory-based tests in detecting coagulation abnormalities and may be of value to direct blood product use intraoperatively.[17]

Total parenteral nutrition should be continued throughout the procedure in order to avoid large changes in blood sugar levels which may occur when parenteral nutrition is constantly interrupted by surgical procedures. Difficulties are encountered due to the effects of stress response on the uptake and hormonal control of fluids. Intermittent hourly monitoring of blood sugar under anesthesia can help to prevent excessive hyper- or hypoglycemia. In children, the rate of infusion of glucose solutions must be adjusted to maintain a normal blood glucose level throughout the operative and recovery periods.

Postoperative Care

Excellent analgesia during the operation is imperative and relative overdose must not be reversed with antagonists.

It is better to support ventilation for a few hours than to reverse analgesia and subject the patient to the subsequent pain or discomfort that ensues. If the patient wakes up complaining of pain, an opioid should be titrated intravenously to obtain the required effect.

Normal cardiopulmonary monitoring should be continued during transportation and in the postoperative period. Blood replacement, if required, should continue in the postoperative period. Clotting studies indicate whether fresh frozen plasma (FFP) or platelet concentrate needs to be administered. Fluid replacement should be done to ensure a urine output of at least 0.5 mL/kg/hour.

Rewarming the patient is another priority in the recovery phase. This decreases shivering and, thus, oxygen consumption; it also reverses the anticoagulant effect of hypothermia. Tramadol is sometimes beneficial to treat immediate postoperative shivering.

Oxygen administration is always indicated in the recovery period and should be guided by ABG analysis and saturation.

As with other critically ill patients, the enteral route of nutrition is preferred. Postpyloric feeding may be required if gastric stasis is impairing calorie delivery as it may also help to reduce the risk of aspiration, especially in patients requiring multiple interventions under general anesthesia. Parenteral nutrition is rarely required, but when used, caution should be exercised because of the associated risks including infection, overfeeding, and erratic blood glucose control.[14]

Reconstructive Phase

By the time, patient reaches this phase, skin coverage has been complete, and all the burn wounds have healed. Caloric requirements are supplied in excess of those needed and the anabolism has begun. The pulse rate, respiration, and thermoregulation have stabilized. The anesthesia required is usually remarkably straightforward unless the face, neck or airway is compromised in any way.

Reconstruction of shape and function involve release of contractures and skin grafting, use of flaps, tissue expanders, etc. The major anesthetic problems during this phase are airway management, placement of IV catheters, and psychological disorder, including posttraumatic stress disorder or depression. These patients may return to the OT for many years, so the problems tend to recur. It is important for the members of the burn team to support them psychologically and plan the surgery well ahead. Adequate reassurance and premedication are essential.

Contractures may limit mouth opening and neck movements in the patient undergoing reconstructive surgery **(Figs. 9 and 10)**. Visual assessment and examination of the patient may aid in the diagnosis of a difficult airway. If the epiglottis and posterior larynx can be seen in a seated patient with neck extended, mouth wide open and tongue fully protruded, one may predict that the trachea can be successfully intubated. Neck mobility can be evaluated by asking the patient (in the sitting position) to place the chin on the chest and look downward and then bring the head and neck all the way to look upward toward the ceiling behind the head. Restricted neck mobility can make the intubation difficult. Another useful predictor is the "3-3-2" rule. The first "3" in the rule refers to the ability to place three fingers in the patient's mouth. This examines the adequacy of mouth opening. The second "3" refers to the space from the mentum to the hyoid bone. Three fingers placed side by side should fit into this space. This indicates adequate mandibular dimensions to permit access to the airway. The "2" in the rule requires that two fingers be placed between the thyroid notch and the floor of the mouth (i.e., the hyoid bone). This indicates that the larynx is sufficiently low within the neck to permit access by the oral route.

Contracture release on the neck may require special skills from the anesthesiologist as the airway may be particularly difficult to intubate. At times, the surgeon may be required to release them under local anesthesia, facilitating the intubation **(Fig. 9)**. Awake fiberoptic intubation is the best solution for intubating such difficult airways **(Figs. 10A to E)**. An entire armamentarium of video laryngoscopes is also now available for use in difficult airways.

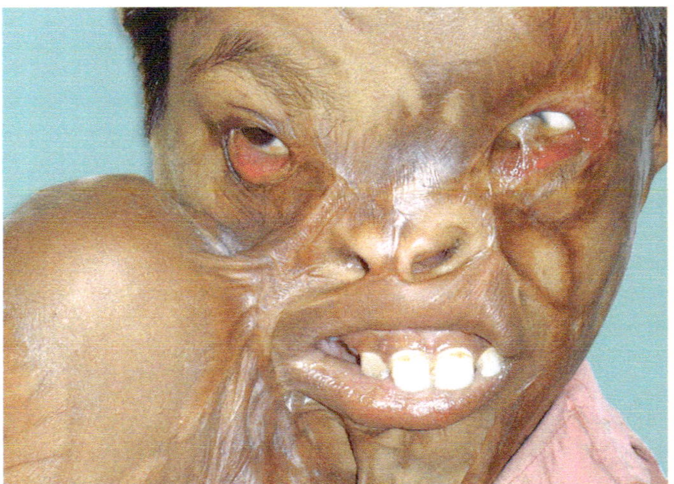

FIG. 9: A 7-year-old child with severe anterolateral contracture of neck and face distorting the facial structures and airway structures completely. Difficult mask ventilation and intubation both because of restricted mouth opening and inability to extend neck due to contracture.

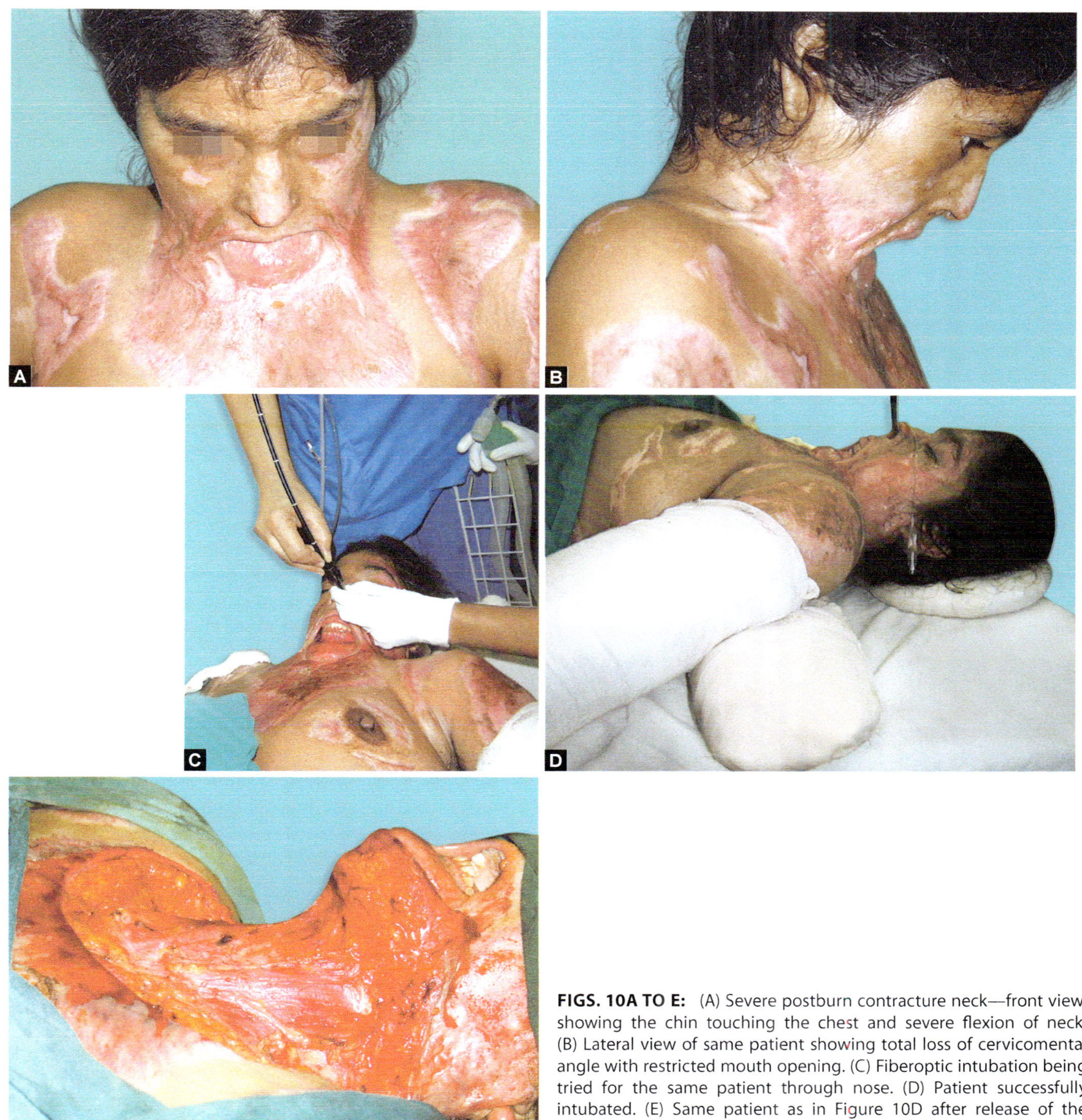

FIGS. 10A TO E: (A) Severe postburn contracture neck—front view, showing the chin touching the chest and severe flexion of neck. (B) Lateral view of same patient showing total loss of cervicomental angle with restricted mouth opening. (C) Fiberoptic intubation being tried for the same patient through nose. (D) Patient successfully intubated. (E) Same patient as in Figure 10D after release of the contracture showing restoration of the cervicomental angle. Neck can now be extended for easy intubation for future surgeries.

Many times, tissue expanders are placed under normal skin adjacent to the scarred area. The bag is slowly inflated with saline solution over a period of weeks until the skin has been expanded to the desired size **(Fig. 11)**. At times, the inflated expander may cause problems for the unwary anesthesiologist. An expander in the occipital area may cause difficulties with the extension of the neck in preparation for intubation. Similarly, an expander in the neck has the potential to cause tracheal deviation or compression. Provided that the problem is recognized, the surgeon can be asked to deflate the expander immediately before the induction of anesthesia. Other methods of

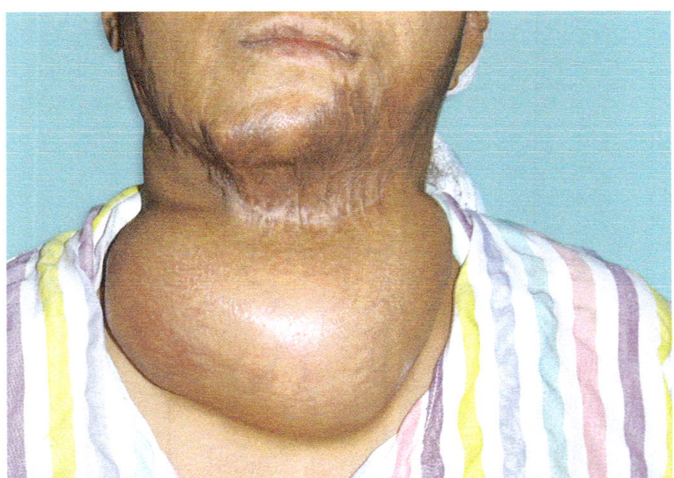

FIG. 11: Patient with scar on lower face with tissue expander in neck—can create problems during intubation.

intubation, as mentioned earlier, should be kept in mind and strategy is planned accordingly. The LMA during this phase is safe, has proved its worth, and is an acceptable alternative method to try, whenever indicated.

Suxamethonium is contraindicated during this phase. NMBAs can be safely used. In order to lessen blood loss and operate in a bloodless field, it is common to use dilute solutions of adrenaline. The anesthetic agents selected must be compatible with the surgical use of adrenaline.

Sometimes, skin grafting or local pedicle flaps may be inappropriate or unavailable respectively for reconstructive surgery and the surgeon decides to use a "free" flap. These operations require intricate microvascular surgery and may be lengthy. Blood loss is slow but persistent. It is vitally important that the patient's circulation be maintained in an optimum condition to ensure that blood flows freely throughout the newly anastomosed blood vessels. A degree of hemodilution is desirable, but the circulatory blood volume must be meticulously maintained and vasoconstriction avoided.[18] The anesthetist can make useful contribution to survival of the flap. The patient must be kept warm throughout the procedure. Cardiovascular status should be carefully monitored. All blood loss should be replaced, but crystalloid or colloid rather than blood should be used initially to achieve an optimum hemoglobin concentration of 10 g/dL. A hematocrit of 30–35% will provide adequate oxygen transport, while minimizing viscosity. Tissue perfusion can be further improved by the administration of dextran 40 and vasodilators, which act directly on the smooth muscles of the blood vessels in both the flap and surrounding tissues.[19]

After surgery, it is essential to provide adequate analgesia, because pain causes vasoconstriction and impairs flap perfusion. In addition, surgeon may request intraoperative anticoagulation in the form of heparin.

For the operations during this phase, feeding postoperatively is usually not a problem although a smooth awakening is important. Coughing, restlessness, and shivering are to be avoided, as bleeding may occur under graft/flap or graft may be dislodged by movement. The goal should be a sedated but arousable patient.

LOCAL AND REGIONAL ANESTHESIA

Infiltration of donor sites with local anesthetic agents with a vasoconstrictor reduces both the blood loss and the pain produced by these wounds. If the donor site is small, topical application of EMLA cream is highly effective if anesthesia is not indicated.

The burn wound is classified as an infected area. Thus, peripheral nerve blocks and regional techniques are relatively contraindicated as the risk of introducing infection is high. If the burn is small and the area limited such as a hand burn, a brachial block may be contemplated.

In major burns, regional anesthesia is not considered very effective as it has several limitations like (1) Limited noninfected/nonburned area available for needle insertion; (2) vasodilation with central neuraxial blockade (CNB) may accentuate hypotension in already volume depleted burns patients; (3) loss of normal skin barrier may increase chance of infections especially with CNB.[6] Probably, the greatest limitation to the use of regional technique is the extent of the surgical field. Most patients with major burns have multiple operative sites along with the need to harvest skin graft/flaps from areas too extensive to be easily blocked by a regional technique.

During the reconstructive phase when these patients are no longer considered as potentially infected cases, local and regional techniques may be used. The sympathetic blockade produces to improve blood flow to flaps by dilating vessels and facilitating tissue transfer.

ANESTHESIA AND ANALGESIA FOR BURN DRESSINGS

The frequency with which dressings are changed depends on the condition of wound and type of dressing material used. A severely burned patient requires many dressing changes during his/her recovery. The procedure is frequently painful and if the pain is not relieved adequately, the patient may become psychologically disturbed whenever a dressing change is due. It is also stressful for the nurses and doctors who must inflict pain to the patient. At the same time, excessive sedation following anesthesia is neither necessary nor desirable as oral nutrition gets compromised. Prior to general anesthesia, a period of fasting is necessary, which makes the administration of an adequate calorie intake extremely difficult. It has also been said that the need for fasting makes the routine use of general anesthesia impractical.[20] It is better to have an organized anesthesia service as a part of burn management team, for the regular dressing of these patients. The benefits of such organized service certainly outweigh the disadvantage.

Opioids alone, in general, are often insufficient as pain is severe and response varies from patient to patient. Hence, individual titration to effect and frequent reassurance is important. In addition, most burned patients rapidly develop tolerance to opioids.

Ketamine is a popular choice with a maximum of 4 hours of fasting before the dressing change. Ketamine is administrated in subanesthetic doses of 0.5 to 1 mg/kg body weight, together with midazolam (0.5 mg/kg body weight). At these doses, the patient is not deeply unconscious and may even talk and is pain free. Recovery is usually complete in 20–30 minutes. If necessary, the initial dose of ketamine can be supplemented with 20 mg boluses at approximately 10 minutes intervals. The duration of sedation and a number of disturbing psychological sequelae, however, at times, limits its use. IV propofol and fentanyl in combination can also be used for dressing changes of shorter duration. The other alternatives include remifentanil infusion and general anesthesia. General anesthesia is reserved for major burns, for the very young child or for intricate dressings, e.g., to the hand, which take a considerable time.

Psychological care/rehabilitation: A multidisciplinary team of physiotherapists, psychologists, nurses, councilors, and occupational therapists are vital to aid rehabilitation and reduce long-term impairment.[21]

SPECIAL CONSIDERATIONS

Electric Burns

The burn from electrical current results from the conversion of high-voltage electrical energy to thermal energy. Determinates of damage include the area of contact, the duration of current flow and the varying resistance of the body.

Electrical burns can be associated with gangrene of limbs and other injuries that may not be immediately obvious. The extent of injury is also unpredictable. The surface injury is often small, but the extent of underlying tissue damage and necrosis is massive. Victims often have concurrent injuries such as fractures of vertebrae or long bones, ruptured organs, myocardial injury, or numerous contusions. These patients may be admitted in coma with seizures. Muscles immediately surrounding the bone are usually more affected than superficial muscles because bones tend to provide maximum resistance to the current flow and in the process produce maximum heat which causes damage to the deeper muscles. Early fasciotomy is needed to preserve the blood flow to extremities. It necessitates general anesthesia during the first day of injury at the time when fluid shifts, hyperkalemia, and myoglobinuria are maximal. Massive myonecrosis and hemolysis may result in hyperkalemia as well as myoglobinuria and hemoglobinuria. In the presence of hemoglobinuria or myoglobinuria, an increased urine flow of at least 2 mL/kg bodyweight/hour should be ensured by the administration of increased fluids and mannitol. Alkalization of urine prevents the precipitation of these proteins in the renal tubules. Follow-up of patients with electrical injuries often reveals unpredictable sequelae, which may manifest months to years later; these injuries may occur in organs or areas that do not appear abnormal during the acute course of illness. These late complications frequently include neurologic dysfunction, ocular damage, damage to the gastrointestinal tract, changes in the ECG, and delayed hemorrhage from large vessels. Electrical burns, most often, require much more fluid administration than is suggested by the extent of surface burn because of extensive damage of deeper tissues. Therefore, use of standardized fluid algorithm is not appropriate in these cases.

Pediatric Burns

Thermal injury in children is a common occurrence, accounting for up to 40% of burn patients and majority of these are minor scalds. Children are not just small adults, especially when burnt. There are many differences to be considered.[22]

Throughout childhood, the body surface area-to-weight ratio is increased, tending toward the adult ratio the older the child gets. This results in more severe physiological responses to the burn injury. The rise in temperature may cause febrile convulsions and it may be necessary to actively cool the child. The resuscitation formulae must be adjusted to the needs of the child. Drug dosage, fluid requirements, and nutritional needs are more accurately assessed if based on the surface area rather than the weight.

The inability to communicate well in the younger child presents the anesthesiologist with a frightened, often crying child at the preoperative visit. It is important to attempt to gain the child's confidence at this time. Preoperative sedation is desirable for children to reduce the stress of fasting, transport to the operating room, and induction of anesthesia. Sedation, amnesia, and sufficient drying of secretions are provided with a premedicant dose of trimeprazine supported, if necessary, by a further dose of IV morphine at the time of induction.

As IV access may be difficult, an inhalation induction can be performed and a cannula placed into a vein when the child is asleep. The use of EMLA cream helps allay the fears associated with blood-sampling and IV cannulation. Heat loss is greater in the child because of the greater surface area to weight ratio, thin skin, and higher cardiac output. Every effort must be made to maintain normal temperatures during surgery. Smaller children can be operated upon under infrared heaters. Intraoperative monitoring may prove difficult as previously mentioned, but the size of the patient adds to these difficulties. Fluid replacement, blood loss, and drugs need special care as these are affected by the basal temperature, the cardiac output, the size of the burn, the size of the child and the nutritional status. The nutritional requirements are high and preoperative starvation should be kept to an absolute minimum. Hypoglycemia is common in very small children and must be guarded against by constant monitoring and an adequate dextrose infusion.

Ketamine has been used in children as the occurrence of postoperative problems associated with hallucinations is reported to be low. This may be due to inadequacy of communication skills in the child. Other techniques which include titrated doses of various drugs like propofol, morphine, etc. as indicated are preferred that ensure minimal starvation, swift recovery, and early feeding.

Blood loss, when over 10% of the estimated blood volume, should be replaced, as erythropoiesis is impaired and there is an increased need of good oxygen transport so that satisfactory healing occurs.

Pain relief should be measured objectively. Smiling faces instead of the visual analog scale may prove successful. Children of school-going age can be taught to use a patient controlled analgesic device.[23] Oral analgesics should be instituted as early as possible. Many novel ways of administering analgesia have been tried, all with some success. These include fentanyl lollipops, fentanyl skin patches, and intranasal fentanyl.

SUMMARY

The anesthetic management of burn patients must include an understanding of the altered physiology and pharmacology associated with burns. Proper psychological support for the family and patient can be greatly facilitated by a thoughtful and considerate anesthesia care. The anesthesiologist is often the friend of such patients if he/she provides periods free of pain, including the time of transport from intensive care unit to the OT. It is important to remember that a normal personality resides in that devastatingly injured body and we must remain sympathetic and supporting at all times and under all circumstances.

REFERENCES

1. Bryan CP. Chapter 12: Minor Surgery. In: Bryan CP (Ed). The Papyrus Ebers. New York: Appleton; 1931.
2. Barash PG, Cullen BF, Stoelting RK, Cahalan MK, Stock MC, Ortega R. Clinical anesthesia, 7th edition, Print + e-book with multimedia. Philadelphia, PA: Lippincott Williams and Wilkins; 2013.
3. American College of Surgeons. Advanced trauma life support: Student Course Manual, 10th edition. United States: American College of Surgeons; 2018.
4. American Burn Association. (2018). American Burns Life Support Guidelines. [online] Available from https://ameriburn.org/wp-content/uploads/2019/08/2018-abls-providermanual.pdf [Last accessed May, 2024].
5. Eckhauser FF, Billote J, Burke JF, Quinby WC. Tracheostomy complicating massive burn injury: a plea for conservation. Am J Surg. 1974;126:418-23.
6. Black RG, Kinsella J. Anaesthetic management for burns patients. BJA CEPD Rev. 2001;1(6):177-80.
7. Nizamoglu M, Tan A, Gerrish H, Barnes D, Dziewulski P. Infrared technology to improve efficacy of venous access in burns population. Eur J Plast Surg. 2016;39:37-40.
8. Lovich-Sapola JA. Anesthesia for burns. In: Smith CE (Ed). Trauma Anesthesia. United Kingdom: Cambridge University Press; 2015. pp. 666-88.
9. Judkins KC, Lord WD. Thermal injury: Anesthesia. analgesia and intensive care. In: Healing TEJ, Knight PR (Eds). Wylie and Churchill Davidson's A Practice of anesthesia, 7th edition. London: Arnold Press; 2003. pp. 1105-33.
10. MacLennan N, Heimbach DM, Cullen BF. Anesthesia for major thermal injury. Anaesthesiology. 1998;89:749-70.
11. Frei FJ, Ummen Hofer W. Difficult intubation in paediatrics. Paediatr Anaesth. 1996;6:251-63.
12. Ezri T, Boaz M, Sherman A, Armaly M, Berlovitz Y. Sugammadex: An Update. J Crit Care Med (Targu Mures). 2016;2(1):16-21.
13. Jensen NF, Kealey GP. Securing on endotracheal tube in the presence of facial burns or instability. (Letter) Anaesth Anal. 1992;75:641-2.
14. McGovern C, Puxty K, Paton L. Major burns: part 2. Anaesthesia, intensive care and pain management. BJA Educ [Internet]. 2022;22(4):138-45.
15. Dorsch JA, Dorsch SE. Understanding Anesthesia Equipment, 5th edition. Baltimore, MD: Wolters Kluwer Health; 2014.

16. Stapelberg F. Challenges in anaesthesia and pain management for burn injuries. Anaesth Intensive Care [Internet]. 2020;48(2):101-13.
17. Marsden NJ, Van M, Dean S, Azzopardi EA, Hemington-Gorse S, Evans PA, et al. Measuring coagulation in burns: an evidence-based systematic review. Scars Burn Heal. 2017;3:205951311772820.
18. Sutcliffe AJ. Burn patients. In: Grande CM (Ed). Textbook of trauma anesthesia and Critical Care. St Louis: Mosby; 1993. pp. 594-605.
19. Aps C, Cox RG, Mayou BJ, Sengupta P. The role of anaesthetic management in enhancing peripheral blood flow in patients undergoing free flap transfer. Ann R Coll Surg Engl. 1985;67(3):177-9.
20. Rylah LTA, Harper N. Anesthesia for the thermally injured. In: Kaufman L, Ginusburg R (Eds). Anesthesia Review 12. London: Churchill Livingstone; 1995. pp. 215-32.
21. Bishop S, Maguire S. Anaesthesia and intensive care for major burns. Continuing Education in Anaesthesia, Critical Care and Pain. Br J Anaesth. 2012;12(3):118-22.
22. Cote CJ, Lerman J, Anderson B. A Practice of Anesthesia for Infants and Children Book, 6th edition. Amsterdam, Netherlands: Elsevier; 2019.
23. Cote CJ. Burn debridement. In: Stehling L (Ed). Common Problems in Pediatric Anesthesia, 2nd edition. St. Louis: Mosby yearbook; 1992. pp. 207-18.

CHAPTER

17

Biological Dressings and Skin Substitutes in Burns

PK Bilwani, Suvashis Dash

INTRODUCTION

A early coverage of the wound is the main goal of burn wound management. In partial thickness burns, reepithelization leads to wound closure. In such burns, the antimicrobial creams and nonstick moist dressings promote reepithelization, prevent infection and damage to the regenerating neoepithelium until complete epithelialization from the remaining epidermal appendages takes place. In full thickness burns, the wound is closed by applying autografts over the raw areas after the dead skin is removed surgically by excision or gradually by suppuration. Biological dressings and skin replacements when applied to the burn wounds lessen pain, limit fluid and protein loss from exudation and evaporation, and reduce the risk of infection from contamination. However, in cases of severe burns, the critical threshold at which the donor area runs out is between 30 and 40%. Therefore, until autografts are available, the wounds must be temporarily covered with a biological covering or skin substitute. As per calculations, a 70 kg medium built person will require 150 cm^2 graft per 1% burned area of skin to cover the wound.

There are various types of biological dressings and skin substitutes.[1-3] Skin substitutes are a heterogeneous group of wound coverage materials that aid in wound closure and replace the functions of the skin, either temporarily or permanently, depending on the product characteristics.[4] An ideal skin substitute should be inexpensive, readily available, nonantigenic, sterile, durable, flexible, and permeable enough but should not allow excessive water loss. At the same time, it should provide an effective barrier to microbes. Unfortunately, such a material does not exist. The available skin substitutes can be subdivided into two types, namely temporary and permanent. There are different proposed classifications, where individual skin substitutes are classified with all the attributes.[5,6] The authors classify them as given in **Flowchart 1**.

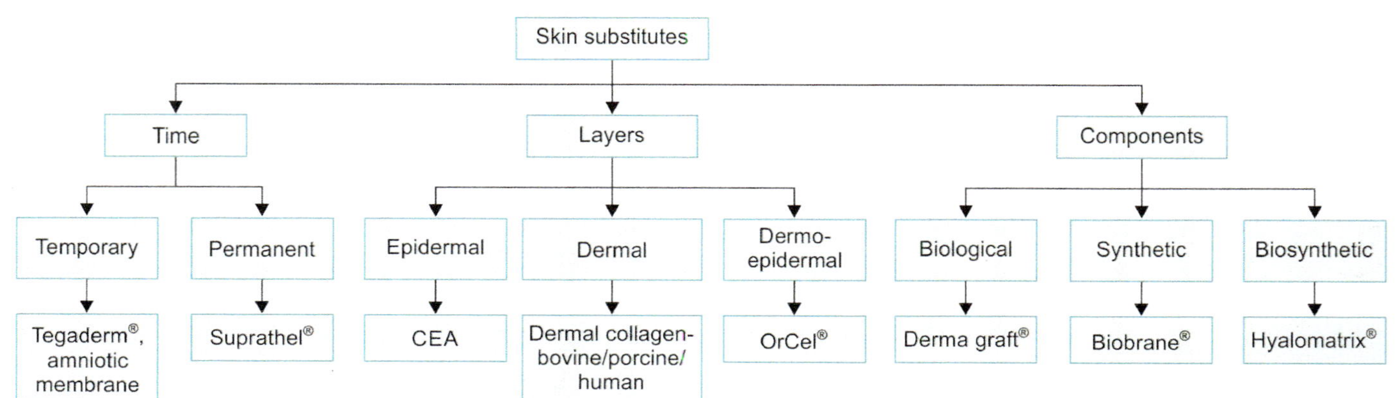

FLOWCHART 1: Different classes of skin substitutes and dressing materials.
(CEA: cultured epithelial autograft)

TEMPORARY SKIN SUBSTITUTES

Temporary skin substitutes are materials which are used temporarily to cover the burned area. These can be of different materials, such as biological or synthetic. Amniotic membrane, collagen, and allograft are examples of biological temporary skin substitutes, whereas Biobrane®, Transcyte®, Omniderm®, Apligraf®, etc., are examples of synthetic temporary skin substitutes.

Biological Temporary Skin Substitutes

Amniotic Membrane

Amniotic membrane facilitates re-epithelialization of partial-thickness burn wounds. Both human and bovine amnion has been used as a dressing material.[7] Amniotic membrane can be used in two forms: (1) Combined amnion and chorion as a whole for deep burns and (2) only amnion for superficial burns.[8] The application of an amniotic membrane to a partial-thickness skin damage helps in re-epithelialization.[9,10] Amnion from both humans and bovine has been utilized as a dressing material. Amnion can cover enormous areas and is easily accessible and affordable. Even though it does not get vascularized, it offers a fantastic temporary covering for a few days and improves reepithelization in donor areas for split skin grafts or clean second-degree burns. In full-thickness wounds, it also promotes epithelial ingrowth from the wound borders. Additionally, it promotes angiogenesis that makes the wound bed's capillary density higher. Amnion can be sterilized, dried, and kept at room temperature for up to 9 months after being treated with 0.25% sodium hypochlorite and 200,000 units of penicillin. However, as it's use can increase the chance of spreading infections such as acquired immunodeficiency syndrome (AIDS), etc., appropriate investigations need to be carried out on donor beforehand. The placenta is obtained preferably from cesarean deliveries. When handling the placenta, all aseptic and antiseptic procedures are used. Using a sterile gauze swab, the placental membrane is separated from the blood clots. After that, it is cleaned with sterile saline and applied to the burn wounds. Whether the membrane's chorionic or amniotic side meets the wound is irrelevant. Because it does not get vascularized, the body does not reject it, allowing for its repeated use.[8]

Amnion can be kept in sterile bottles with a 0.25% sodium hypochlorite solution for a period of 2–3 days. It lessens discomfort during dressing changes, lessens leaking, and safeguards regenerating tissues underneath. It is usually advocated in developing countries where other products are expensive hence out of reach. Amniotic membrane can be impregnated with antibiotics, but the membrane must be changed/replaced every 2–3 days. Nowadays, decellularized human amniotic membranes are used for wound coverage as they are durable, easy to store, and have antibacterial properties by zinc oxide nanoparticles **(Figs. 1A to C)**.[9]

Collagen

Collagen is a fibrous protein of vertebrates and forms the chief constituent of the fibrils of connective tissue. It can be isolated and purified in large quantities from tissues of animals. It constitutes 25–30% of body protein. Collagen is hydrophilic and very suitable for cell adhesion. It has very low antigenicity and like amnion, it does not get vascularized and therefore adheres to the wounds poorly. It is commercially manufactured and is readily available as preserved wet as well as dried sheets **(Figs. 2A to C)**.[10,11]

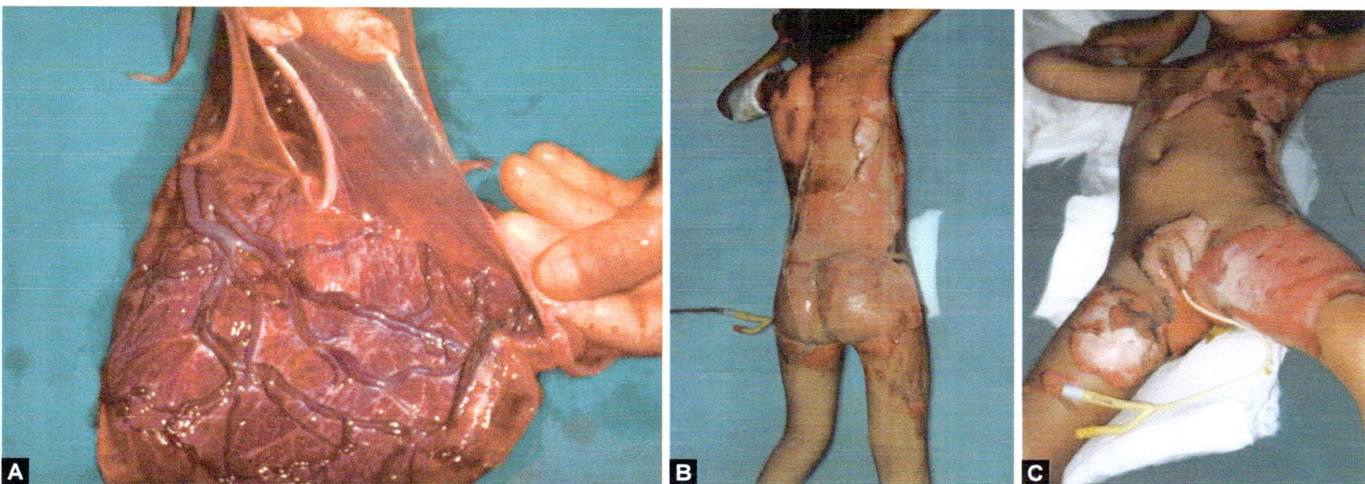

FIGS. 1A TO C: (A) Harvest of the amniotic membrane from placenta; (B) amniotic membrane is used for dressing of pediatric burns wound; and (C) appearance of wound after 1 week with starting of epithelialization of the wound from periphery.

The method of application is the same as for amniotic membrane. The wet collagen sheet is rinsed in normal saline and spread over cleaned wounds. Thereafter, it is left exposed to get dry and stick firmly to the wound. In case of dry collagen sheets, the surface of the wound is made wet with saline before application of the collagen sheet and then covered with a dressing of gauze and Gamgee. In second-degree superficial dermal burns, epithelization occurs under the collagen sheet. It is also helpful for skin graft donor sites for improved healing **(Figs. 2D and E)**. When healing is complete, the dried collagen automatically falls off. Thus, it provides good biological temporary cover in superficial and deep partial-thickness burns. It also reduces pain and evaporative losses and forms a barrier for microorganisms, thus minimizing the chances of wound infection.[10,11]

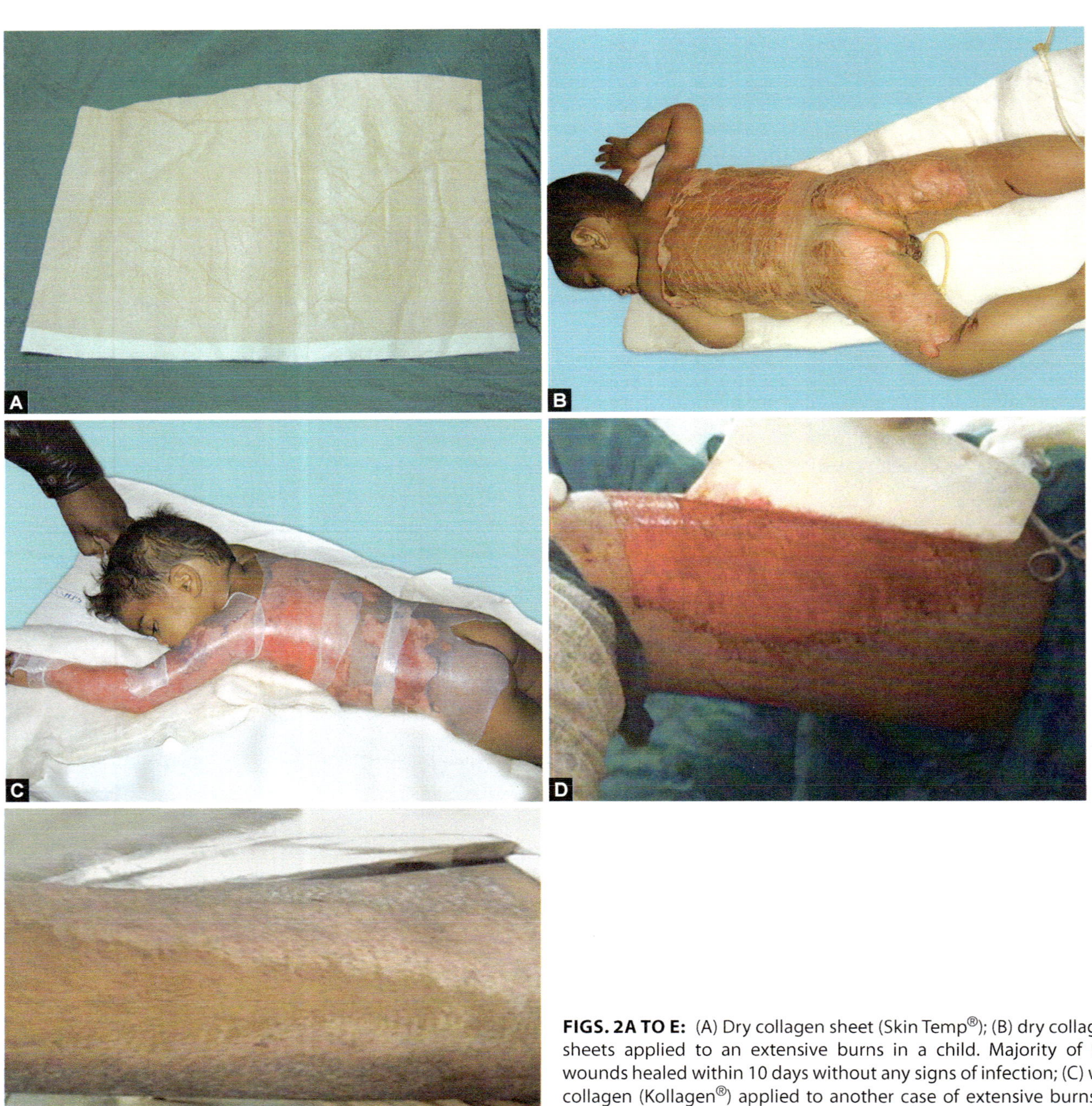

FIGS. 2A TO E: (A) Dry collagen sheet (Skin Temp®); (B) dry collagen sheets applied to an extensive burns in a child. Majority of the wounds healed within 10 days without any signs of infection; (C) wet collagen (Kollagen®) applied to another case of extensive burns in a child. The wounds are sealed from the environment and heal fast; (D) skin graft donor site dressed with dry collagen (Skin Temp®); and (E) appearance of the donor site at 10 days—healed without any complications.

Homograft (Allograft) (Figs. 3 and 4)

Homografts (live or cadaveric) are used in burn patients with the following objectives:

- *Temporary wound coverage*: They are used as a temporary dressing and provide some pain relief and promotes re-epithelialization.
- *Reduces risk of complications*: They help protect the wound from infection, fluid loss, and provide a moist environment for healing.
- *Wound bed preparation*: When the wound bed is contaminated, surgeons sometimes use allografts for the wound bed preparation before autografting[12,13] **(Figs. 3 and 4)**.

Furthermore, the homografts can be classified as follows: (1) *Viable*: Fresh (freshly harvested from donor or refrigerated) or cryopreserved and (2) *Nonviable*: Lyophilized (glycerol) or irradiated (gamma irradiation). Freshly harvested homografts are superior in terms of "take" and resistance to infection.[14]

Homografts are usually stored in skin banks. However, due to the nonavailability of skin banks in all burn units and lack of public education about skin donations, the surgeons of developing countries procure homograft from live donors, preferably near relatives as a life saving technique especially in children. Nevertheless, the use of homografts from live donors is not a routine in India. Nonavailability of artificial skin mandates salvage of major burns by homograft.[13]

Homografts are mostly required in patients where adequate donor area is not available for auto graft harvest. Multistage early excision (3rd–7th day) followed by coverage with homografts gives a chance of survival in these groups of patients with major burns. In children with 30–60% burns, homografting saves lives. However, it is not always possible to do early excision due to obvious reasons and these patients are treated expectantly with close monitoring till all second-degree burns have healed and the third-degree burns start granulating. Thereafter, the important areas are covered with whatever autografts are available and the rest are covered with homografts. Once these grafts settle (10–12 days), the patient's general condition improves fast. The homografts get vascularized or "take" exactly like an autograft. They survive for 3–10 weeks before getting rejected by the body's immune system. They should be removed from the wound before the signs of rejection appear as the rejection reaction can deteriorate the condition of the wounds. For the coverage of resultant raw areas, autografts can be easily reharvested. It is usually suggested not to do meshing in stored homografts as the epithelium does not spread in the meshed areas. However, in our experience, meshing (1:2) helps in increased "take" of the grafts and graft expansion. The major drawbacks for homografts are availability and availability and concerns regarding disease transmission.[12,14]

Heterograft (Xenografts)

Due to the difficulty in obtaining homografts, surgeons have used skin from sources such as pigs, cattle, fish, and dogs. However, because the xenografts do not develop blood vessels, they have weak tissue adhesion and are not very successful at stopping bacterial growth. They do reduce pain and stop evaporative losses. Regarding the sources of the xenografts, the patient's religion or other beliefs presents an obstacle.[15,16]

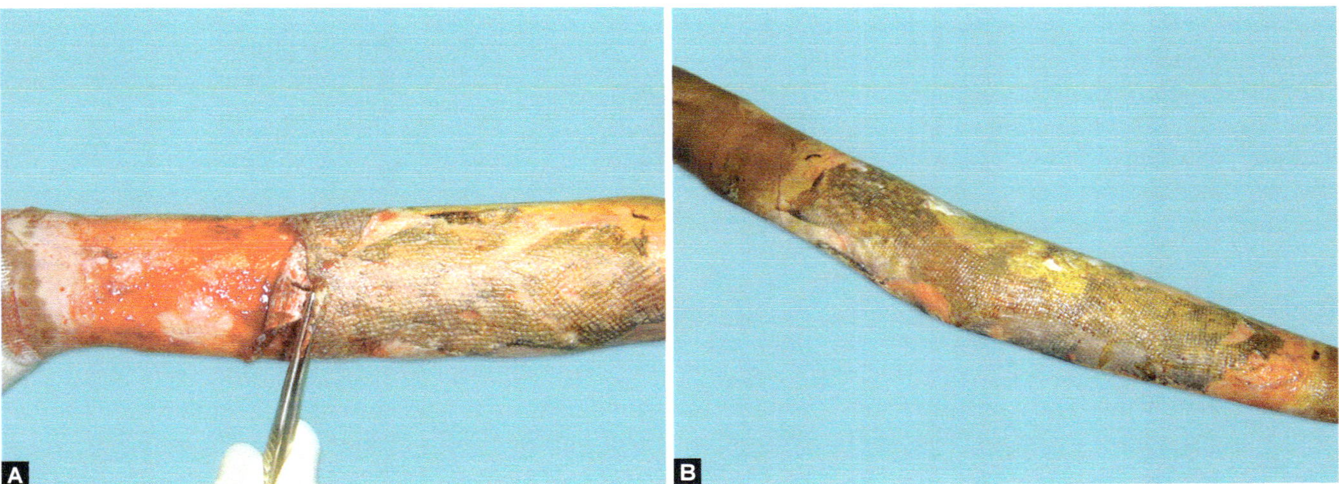

FIGS. 3A AND B: (A) Homograft from related donor applied to a patient with extensive burns—on removal of the homograft, it shows healthy, granulating wounds. (B) After removal of homograft, autograft was applied and fully "taken" up.

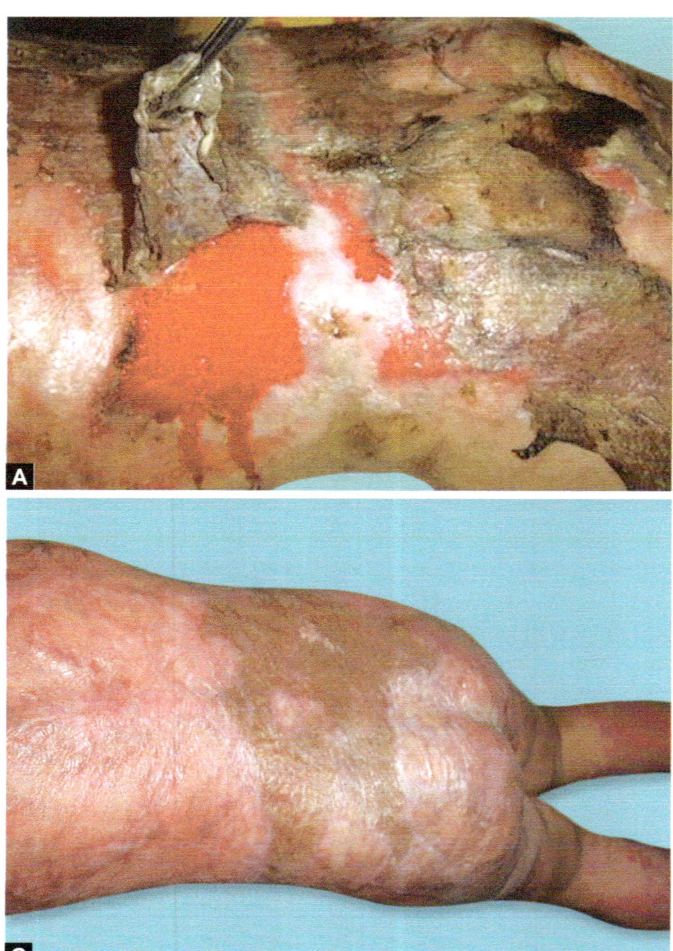

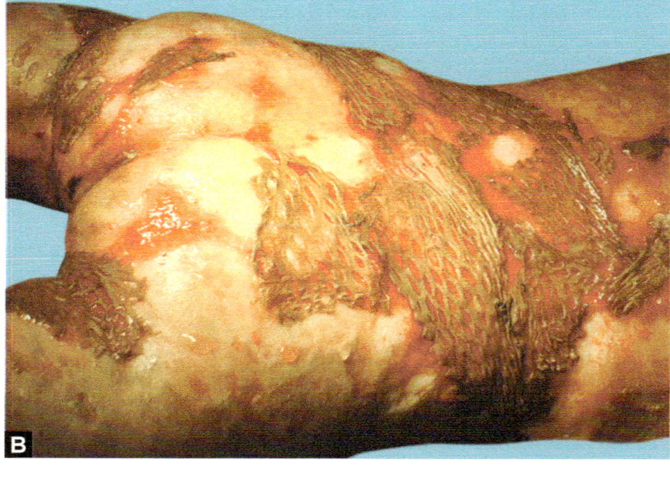

FIGS. 4A TO C: (A) Homograft from mother applied in a 4-year-old with extensive burns—being removed in multiple sittings for autograft application; (B) autograft applied on healthy raw areas; and (C) completely healed areas after 1 month.

Synthetic Temporary Skin Substitutes[17,18]

The synthetic skin substitutes (synthetic dressing materials), though available "off-the-shelf," lack property of adhesion and hence, submembrane suppuration is common. The various synthetic skin substitutes consist of films such as polyurethane (Opsite® and Biobrane®); foams such as polyurethane foam (looms); gels such as Amiderm®, DuoDERM®, and Kaltostat®; and sprays such as polyhydroxyethylmethacrylate.

Biobrane (Winthrop Pharmaceuticals, Santa Ana, CA)

Biobrane® is a two-layered, temporary, synthetic skin substitute. The outer layer is composed of ultrathin layer of silicon rubber which is semipermeable and permits the exit of water vapors but prevents entry of bacteria from the exterior. The inner layer is tightly woven nylon fabric. Both layers have porcine collagen peptides covalently bonded, which allow the sheet to adhere to the wound by integration of tissues without causing inflammation. The collagen is slowly replaced with host tissue. Biobrane **(Fig. 5)** is translucent, allowing observation of wound healing through it. It is elastic and confirms to irregular surfaces. When donor sites for autografts become available, the silicon sheet is removed and autografts are applied. It should preferably be removed in about 2 weeks to prevent fibroblast ingrowth into the mesh.[18,19]

Transcyte® (Dermagraft-TC®)

Transcyte® is a temporary, synthetic covering composed of a semipermeable silicone membrane along with newborn human dermal fibroblasts cultured on a porcine collagen-coated nylon mesh.[20] These neonatal fibroblasts are cultured and proliferated for 4–6 weeks on an inner layer of nylon mesh that is embedded with an outer silicone layer.[21] This dermal template contains human matrix proteins and multiple growth factors.[22] Evidence shows this skin substitute to be as effective as allograft and effective for temporary coverage after burns wound excision.[23] It has the following advantages, including easy availability, hassle-free storage, and can help in visual

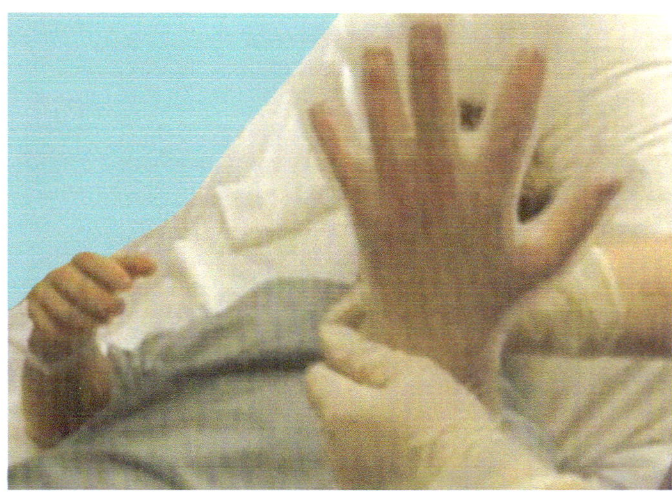

FIG. 5: Biobrane applied over hand burn.
Courtesy: Smith and Nephew Ltd.

monitoring of the wound bed as it is transparent.[24] It is indicated for use as a temporary covering for excised burns prior to autografting or burns that do not require autografting (partial thickness burns). This material is applied to the burn and will peel away as the burn heals or it must be removed or excised prior to grafting full-thickness wounds. It has been recommended for use as a temporary covering for burns after surgical debridement and before autografting or in partial-thickness burns.

Omniderm (Omikron Scientific Ltd, Rehovat, Israel)

Omniderm® is a temporary synthetic skin cover which is thin, transparent, flexible membrane of polyurethane. It is hydrophilic, absorbs water, and is elastic in nature. It is permeable to liquid and can be used as an interface for skin grafting (as a layer between graft and the dressing). It allows water vapor to evaporate and allows antibiotics to permeate inside.[17,18]

Apligraf (Graftskin) (Organogenesis Inc., Canton, MA)

Apligraf® manufactured skin analog is composed of two layers, namely the epidermal layer made of human foreskin-derived neonatal keratinocytes and the dermal layer made of neonatal fibroblasts seeded in bovine type 1 collagen lattice. This has been shown to improve the cosmetic results when applied over widely meshed grafts.[17,18]

Opsite/Cling Film/Via Film

Opsite is a synthetic adhesive vapor-permeable dressing made up of modified polyvinyl chloride. Although it is permeable to water vapor, it is impermeable to bacteria. The permeability to water is low; at times, can lead to collection under this dressing. Pain relief, lack of bulky dressings, and early healing are the advantages.[17,18]

Polylactic Acid Polymers Sheet

Suprathel® is a synthetic caprolactone dressing made of polylactic acid, trimethylene carbonate, and e-caprolactone made by PolyMedics Innovations GmbH in Dockendorf, Germany. In superficial burns and in the split-skin donor sites, suprathel is indicated. It is an absorbable, one-time application membrane. It's microporous surface, adapts to the surface of the wound, and adheres upon contact. The polylactic acid copolymer being synthetic in origin, is nonimmunogenic. It is applied to the wound site and left there until re-epithelialization is complete.[25]

Once it is applied to a healthy, clean wound bed, the membrane turns translucent; there is no need to change the suprathel® membrane; only the outer dressing needs to be changed and it separates with epithelialization with no need for surgical removal. In a study with a 3-month follow-up assessment, it exhibits less hypertrophic scarring.[26] Suprathel® also significantly decreases patient discomfort, resulting in fewer dressings changes and significant pain reduction.

PERMANENT SKIN SUBSTITUTES

Epidermal Replacement—Biological

Cultured Epithelial Autograft

Split-thickness skin grafts (STSG) are the "gold standard" for burn wound closure and continue to be the cornerstone of care to provide long-term wound coverage and promote healing. However, in certain extensively burned individuals, donor sites are limited. In such cases, use of cultured human keratinocytes has made it possible to cover the burn wounds quickly and easily by rapidly growing large areas of cultured epithelium from a small skin biopsy in laboratory setup.[27,28]

Cultured epithelial autograft (CEA) is expensive to use and very sensitive to infection. It requires meticulous wound care and more time and effort than procedures with conventional autografts.[28] However, the use of CEAs for the treatment of extensive third-degree burn wounds is definitely a life-saving procedure. It allows coverage of very extensive lesions, where conventional methods would falter and should probably be used only in cases where traditional treatment has a poor chance of success [65–70% total body surface area (TBSA) full-thickness burns].[27,28] CEAs can now be made available sooner by taking advantage of the rapid expansion possible via the Rheinwald and Green culture system, followed by seeding the keratinocytes to a membrane, and thus eliminating the need to prepare post confluent sheets.[29] Recently, the addition of fibroblasts to the cultured graft will definitely result in superior wound repair in terms of functional and aesthetic results and will provide permanent closure. At present, an emerging consensus indicates that temporary closure with allograft, following early excision, provides the best CEA take.[27,28] The best and most practical option would be the two-step Cuono technique in which the wound is covered first by a living fresh or cryopreserved allogenic skin graft (not glycerol preserved allograft) that would allow incorporation of dermal elements into the wound bed. The allogenic graft is subsequently dermabraded after a period of 3–4 weeks and covered with CEA sheets.[22,23] Undoubtedly, this requires an autologous keratinocyte culture facility in addition to a skin bank capable of providing cryopreserved allografts both of which can be practically available only in large referral and research centers. Despite its cost and sensitivity to infection, CEA remains a crucial intervention for extensive burn injuries.[30-32]

Dermal Replacement—Synthetic

Integra® (Integra Life Sciences Corporation, NJ) (Figs. 6A to H)

Integra® is a synthetic, bilaminate product designed to provide permanent skin cover, with outer epidermal substitute made up of silicone (polysiloxane polymer) layers, which controls moisture loss from the wound bed. The deeper dermal analog is made up of bovine tendon collagen arranged in a three-dimensional porous matrix and cross-linked with glycosaminoglycan (chondroitin-6-sulfate, derived from shark cartilage). With its use, the dermal layer is infiltrated by fibroblasts. This is followed by capillary invasion which vascularizes and leads to deposition of collagen by fibroblasts and the dermal matrix gradually biointegrates with the wound. The silicone layer separates out in 2–4 weeks' time when a thin-split skin graft coverage shall be required to cover the neodermis.[33]

Integra® has been used since 1981 (Burke et al.) and subsequent trials have concluded that hypertrophic scarring was less, late contractures were rare, and artificial skin-grafted areas demonstrated growth with the growth of the child.[33]

The Integra have four distinct phases of dermal regeneration—imbibition, fibroblast migration, neovascularization, and remodeling and maturation. The first phase imbibition occurs within minutes and the fibrin in the wound exudate enters the matrix. The matrix swelling occurs in this period. At the end of 1st week, the fibroblasts migrate into the matrix. The myofibroblasts migrate and start collagen production within the matrix by end of 3rd week. At 4th week, the host collagen replaces the matrix collagen and the neodermis is fully vascularized. Initially, the neodermis is thicker than host dermis, but during the maturation, the neodermis becomes thin and pliable.[34] The use of Integra has slowly grown and has now become an important consideration in both acute and chronic burns management.

Dermagraft® (Advanced Tissue Sciences, La Jolla, California)

This synthetic bioabsorbable dermal matrix is made by seeding neonatal fibroblasts on to a polyglactin mesh by Cooper method.[35] It can be used as a temporary or

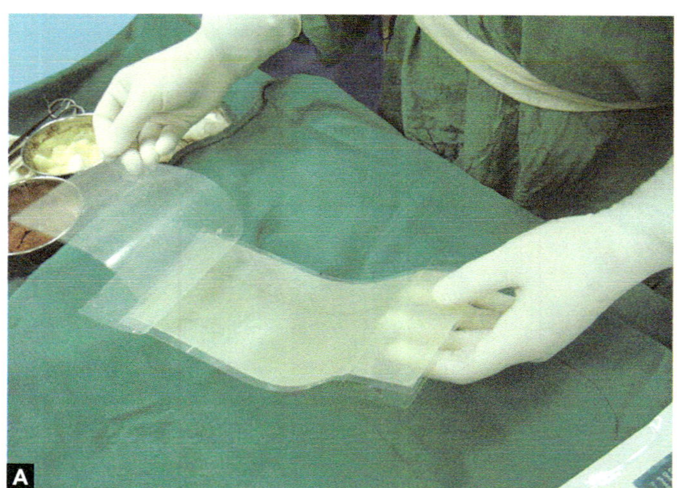

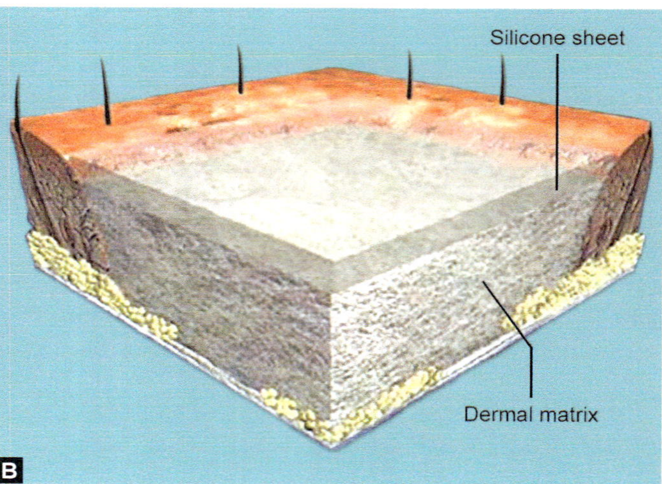

FIGS. 6A TO H: *Continued*

Continued

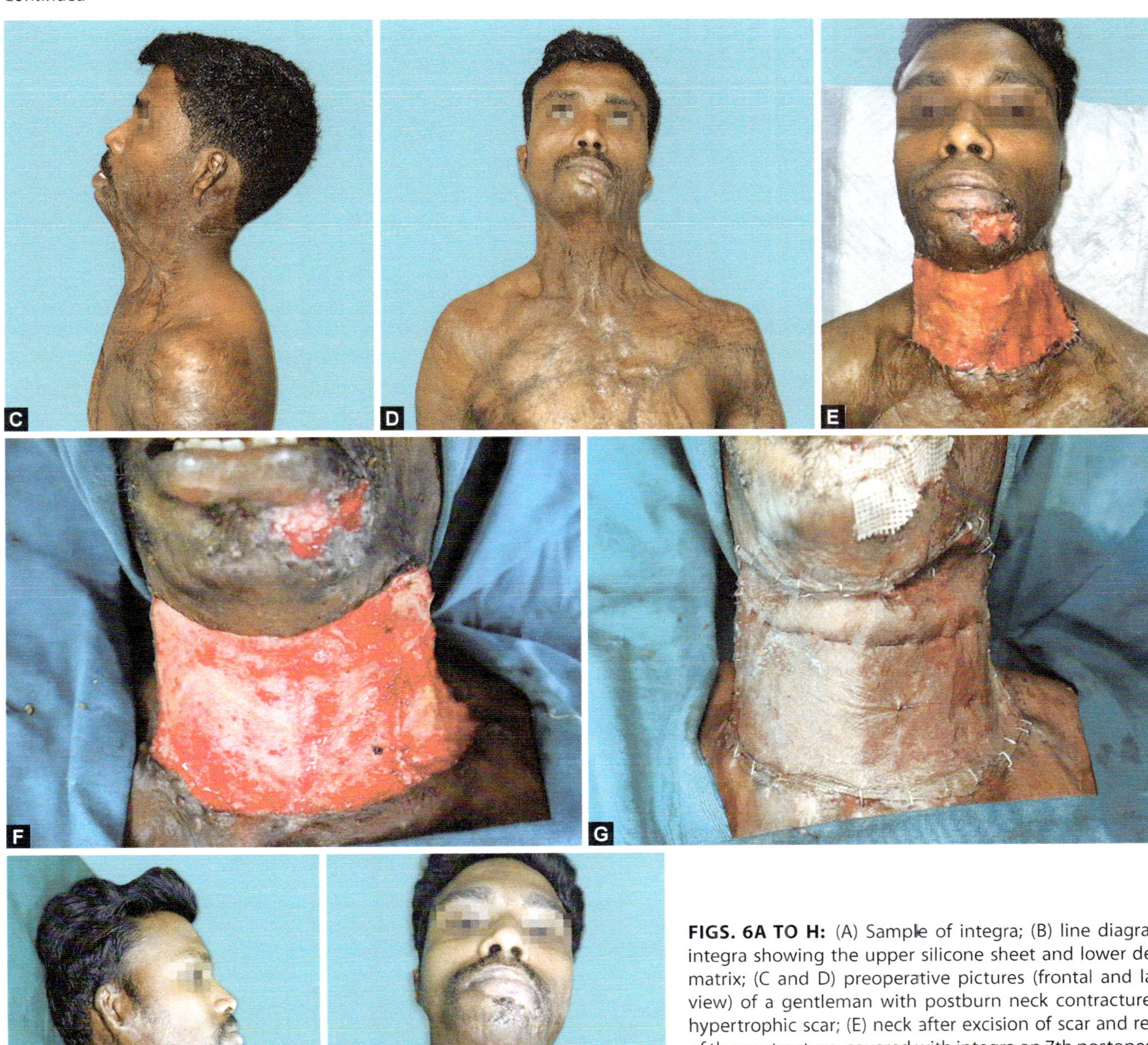

FIGS. 6A TO H: (A) Sample of integra; (B) line diagram of integra showing the upper silicone sheet and lower dermal matrix; (C and D) preoperative pictures (frontal and lateral view) of a gentleman with postburn neck contracture and hypertrophic scar; (E) neck after excision of scar and release of the contracture, covered with integra on 7th postoperative day (first stage); (F) good integration of the integra and ready for skin grafting on 3rd postoperative week; (G) after integration of dermal regeneration template—the silicone layer is removed and covered with split-thickness skin graft; and (H) postoperative result showing 100% take of graft with good cosmesis (frontal view); and lateral view showing improved neck contour.

Courtesy: Contributed by Dr Sujata Sarabahi, VMMC and Safdarjung Hospital.

permanent burn wound covering. It is usually used on excised burn wounds with a split-skin autograft. This material should be used over wounds with adequate blood supply. Gradually over a month, the mesh gets absorbed. The graft uptake on the matrix is slightly less than autograft alone but shows more resistance to bacterial contamination. Regarding wound infection, wound exudate, wound healing time, wound closure, and graft take, this dermal substitute seems to perform as well as allograft. It has a much greater level of patient satisfaction and is easier to remove than an allograft.[23,24,36,37] No adverse reactions to Dermagraft® have been reported and there is no evidence of rejection, early degeneration, or detachment from the site.[24,36,37]

Dermal Replacement—Biological

Alloderm

Alloderm is decellularized allograft dermis. It is prepared by a special biochemical process to make the human dermis acellular. It is used as a dermal transplant in deep, second-degree and third-degree burns. Donors are screened for human immunodeficiency virus types 1 and 2 (HIV 1 and 2), hepatitis B (HBV), hepatitis C (HCV), human T-cell leukemia/lymphoma virus 1 (HTLV-1), and syphilis serologically. Then the material is freeze dried and stored. After wound excision, the dermal matrix is grafted on to the fresh wound and covered with split-skin graft. There are fewer incidences of inflammation and infection.[20-22]

Matriderm® (Figs. 7A to E)

Matriderm® is a dermal regeneration substitute composed of bovine collagen (types I, III, and V) and elastin, decellularized with gamma rays.[38] It can be either used in single stage or two stages; for single-stage use, thinner 1 mm Matriderm® templates are used. While the thicker 2 mm and 3 mm Matriderm® templates are used in two-step procedures. Compared to the commonly used dermal templates, Matriderm® has the advantage of being used in single-stage procedure.[38] The elastin component of the matrix increases the stability and flexibility of the regenerated tissue while acting as a support structure for the ingrowth of cells and blood vessels. Moreover, elastin-based dermal replacements may lessen wound contraction and enhance the functionality and look of scars.[39] The elastin in the Matriderm helps in early integration and neovascularization, hence, split-skin grafts can be applied in single-step surgery. Matriderm is indicated for coverage of full-thickness or deep dermal burns and postburn reconstruction. Due to its inherent nature, it is useful for coverage of hands or joints with good functional outcome.[40,41] It is has shown to be effective in wound coverage in a single-step process in critically ill patients with good graft take. It is especially useful in the pediatric population to enhance scar quality.[40,42]

Hyalomatrix®/Hyalograft 3D®

This is a biodegradable bilayer and its matrix is made of esterified hyaluronic acid having an outer silicone layer. The wound bed gradually receives hyaluronic acid from the matrix, followed by cellular migration and ingrowth of new capillaries. With colonization by fibroblasts and extracellular matrix (ECM) components, this matrix integrates.[43] Like other templates, the silicone membrane in this product also acts as a temporary barrier.[44] Hyalomatrix helps in wound healing by either spontaneous re-epithelialization or provide a suitable dermal layer for autologous skin grafting. It is indicated in deep burns and burn reconstruction. A variant of this product is Hyalograft 3D®. This contains autologous fibroblasts that help in rapid healing of wounds.[44]

Biodegradable Temporizing Matrix® (Figs. 8A to G)

It is synthetic polyurethane dermal matrix called the NovoSorb®. Biodegradable Temporising Matrix (BTM) is used to rebuild difficult wounds, such as deep dermal and full-thickness burns, necrotizing fasciitis, and free-flap donor sites. This template has 2 mm-thick biodegradable polyurethane open-cell foam covered by a nonbiodegradable layer. BTM is applied in a two-stage procedure. After the debridement of the wound, the wound is cleaned and BTM is fixed to the wound bed and in the second stage (after 2–3 weeks), the overlying nondegradable membrane is removed and a split-skin graft is applied over the granulating surface. BTM has been successfully used to reconstruct deep dermal and full-thickness burns.[45,46]

COMPOSITE EPIDERMAL AND DERMAL REPLACEMENT

Composite (Dermal–Epidermal) Cultured Grafts

Although cultured epidermal sheets have been successful in some cases, they have the following disadvantages: (1) Epidermal sheets lack dermis and therefore do not vascularize adequately on full-thickness wound beds and hence, do not adhere satisfactorily. (2) Epidermal sheets lead to extensive scar formation. (3) In normal skin, presence of rete ridges at dermal epidermal junctions (DEJ) provides resistance against shearing forces. However, following application of cultured epidermal sheets in full-thickness wounds, the epithelium is unstable due to the lack of rete ridges and may get detached easily.

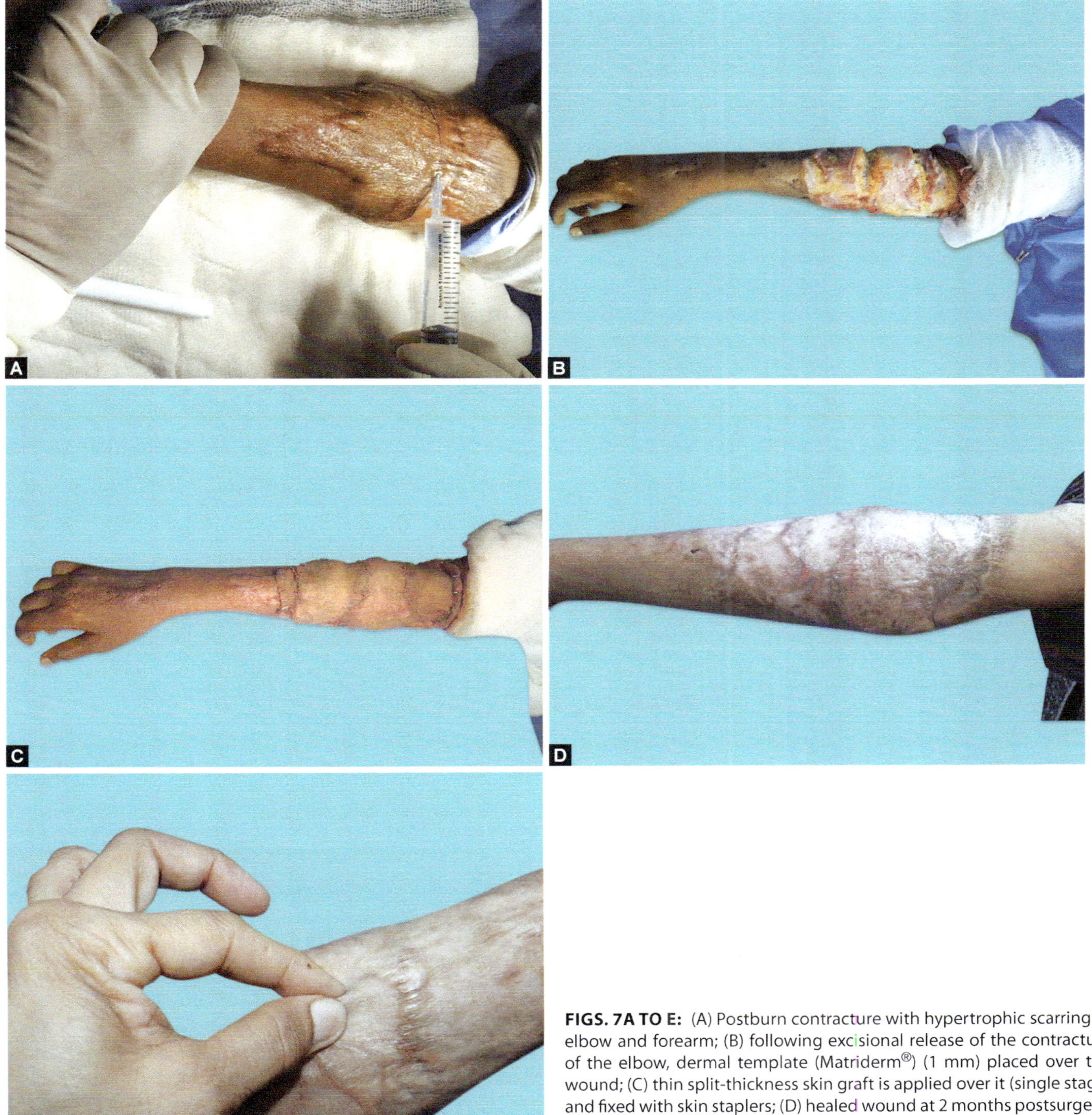

FIGS. 7A TO E: (A) Postburn contracture with hypertrophic scarring of elbow and forearm; (B) following excisional release of the contracture of the elbow, dermal template (Matriderm®) (1 mm) placed over the wound; (C) thin split-thickness skin graft is applied over it (single stage) and fixed with skin staplers; (D) healed wound at 2 months postsurgery; and (E) healed area is soft and supple appreciated by pinch test.
Courtesy: Contributed by Dr Sujata Sarabahi, VMMC and Safdarjung Hospital.

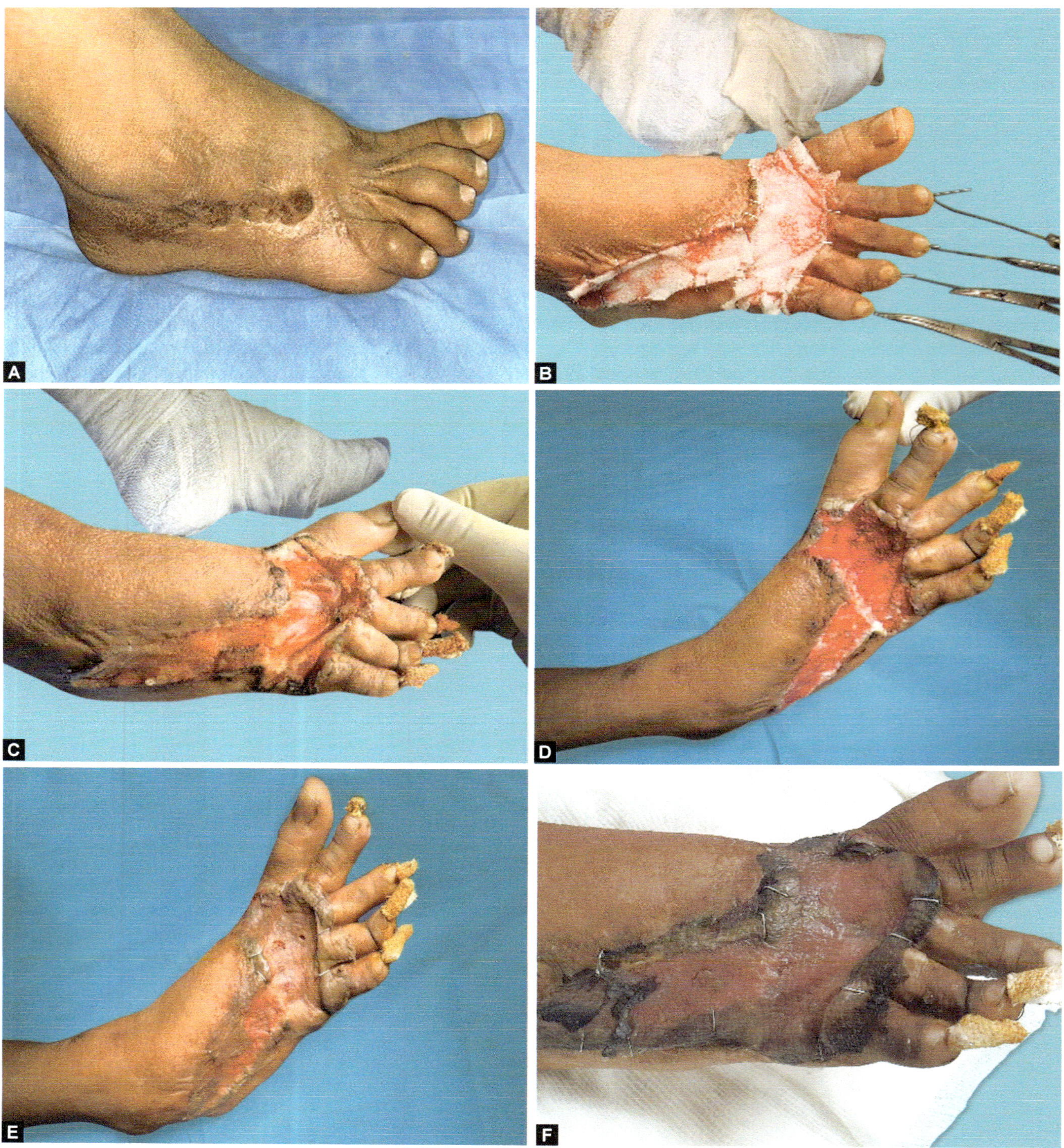

FIGS. 8A TO G: *Continued*

Continued

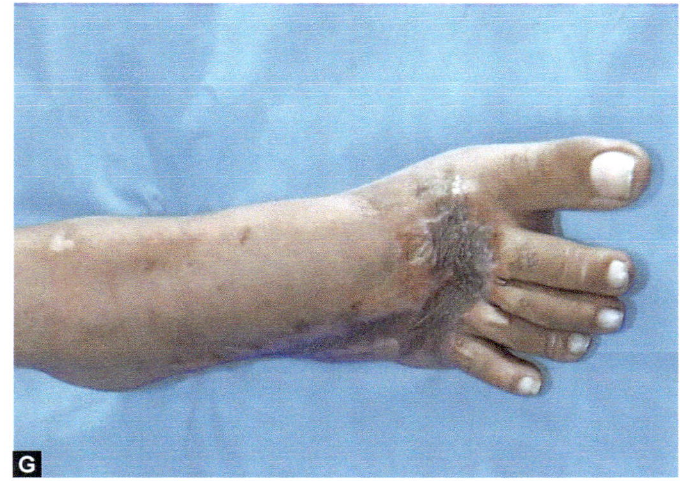

FIGS. 8A TO G: (A) Postburn contracture of dorsum of foot. (B) Following incisional release of the contracture of the foot, BTM® dermal template is applied over the wound (first stage) and fixed with skin staplers and dressed. (C) At the end of 3rd week postsurgery, the BTM® is integrated with wound. The nonabsorbable glossy layer (sealing membrane) of BTM is appreciated. (D) After removal of the nonabsorbable glossy layer (sealing membrane) of BTM, the appearance of wound on 3rd week. (E) A split-thickness skin graft was applied over the wound. (F) Appearance of the wound on end of 1st week with full take of the graft. (G) Appearance of the scar after 1 month of surgery with improved range of movement of the toes.

The above-mentioned disadvantages with the use of cultured epidermal sheets clearly indicate that dermal component is essential for satisfactory wound healing. Hence, for optimal wound healing, dermal-epidermal grafts have been developed by growing epithelium on a dermal substrate. The dermal substrate is derived from either collagen gel fibroblast or allograft dermis.

SUMMARY

Dermal substitutes are advanced alternatives for treating burn wounds. These engineered biomaterials mimic the skin's structure and function, providing a temporary scaffold for cell regeneration. They protect the wound, promote cell migration, and stimulate tissue formation. Dermal substitutes offer advantages over traditional methods by reducing scarring and eliminating the need for additional donor sites. They are particularly beneficial for patients with limited healing potential. Challenges include optimizing cell integration, vascularization, and long-term durability. Overall, dermal substitutes show promise in burn wound treatment, enhancing healing, and minimizing donor graft requirements. Continued research is needed to improve their efficacy and clinical application.

REFERENCES

1. Alsbjorn BF. Biologic wound coverings in burn treatment. World J Surg. 1992;16:43.
2. Brown AS, Barot LR. Biological dressing and skin substitute's. Clin Plast Surg. 1996;13(1):69-74.
3. Norton L, Chvapil M. Comparison of newer synthetic and biologic wound dressings. J Trauma. 1981;21:463.
4. Halim AS, Khoo TL, Mohd Yussof SJ. Biologic and synthetic skin substitutes: An overview. Indian J Plast Surg. 2010; 43(Suppl):S23-8.
5. Quinby WC, Hoover HC, Scheflan M, Walters PT, Slavin SA, Bondoc CC. Clinical trials of amniotic membranes in burn wound care. Plast Reconstr Surg. 1982;70:711.
6. Sawhney CP. Amniotic membrane as a biological dressing in the management of burns. Burns. 1989;15:339.
7. Sangwan VS, Burman S, Tejwani S, Mahesh SP, Murthy R. Amniotic membrane transplantation: a review of current indications in the management of ophthalmic disorders. Indian J Ophthalmol. 2007;55(4):251-60.
8. Robson MC, KrizekTJ, Koss N, Samburg JL. Amniotic membrane as a temporary wound dressing. Surg Gynacol Obstet. 1973;136: 904-6.
9. Ramasamy P, Krishnakumar R, Rekha R, Vaseeharan B, Saraswathi K, Raj M, et al. Bio-Fabrication of Human Amniotic Membrane Zinc Oxide Nanoparticles and the Wet/Dry HAM Dressing Membrane for Wound Healing. Front Bioeng Biotechnol. 2021;9:695710.
10. Chhatre MG, Mani MM. Biological Dressings and skin substitutes. In: Ramakrishnan M, Hanumadas M (Eds). Handbook of Burns Management. New Delhi: Jaypee Brothers Medical Publishers (P) Ltd.; 1991. pp. 135-9.
11. Yang JY. Clinical application of collagen sheet as a burn wound dressing. YCWM. 1990;16:457.
12. Bilwani PK. Skin Donation an overview of 26 years experience. Indian J Burns. 2005;13:18.
13. Bilwani PK, Sheth H. Use of Lyofoam as a dressing for split skin graft donor sites. Indian J Plast Surg. 1988;21:38-40.
14. Gupta S, Mohapatra DP, Chittoria RK, Subbarayan E, Reddy SK, Chavan V, et al. Human Skin Allograft: Is it a Viable Option in Management of Burn Patients? J Cutan Aesthet Surg. 2019;12(2):132-5.
15. Chiu T, Burd A. "Xenograft" dressing in the treatment of burns. Clin Dermatol. 2005;23(4):419-23.

16. Luze H, Nischwitz SP, Smolle C, Zrim R, Kamolz LP. The Use of Acellular Fish Skin Grafts in Burn Wound Management-A Systematic Review. Medicina (Kaunas). 2022;58(7):912.
17. Chester DL, Papini RPG. Skin and skin substitutes in burn management. J Trauma. 2004;6:87-99.
18. Bar-Meir E, Mendes D, Winkler E. Skin substitutes. Isr Med Assoc J. 2006;8(3):188-91.
19. Fan C, Pek CH, Por YC, Lim GJS. Biobrane dressing for paediatric burns in Singapore: a retrospective review. Singapore Med J. 2018;59(7):360-5.
20. Pham C, Greenwood J, Cleland H, Woodruff P, Maddern G. Bioengineered skin substitutes for the management of burns: A systematic review. Burns. 2007;33:946-57.
21. Bello YM, Falabella AF, Eaglstein WH. Tissue-engineered skin. Current status in wound healing. Am J Clin Dermatol. 2001;2(5):305-13.
22. Hansbrough J. Status of cultured skin replacement. Wounds. 1995;7(4):130-6.
23. Purdue GF, Hunt JL, Still JM Jr, Law EJ, Herndon DN, Goldfarb IW, et al. A multicenter clinical trial of a biosynthetic skin replacement, Dermagraft-TC, compared with cryopreserved human cadaver skin for temporary coverage of excised burn wounds. J Burn Care Rehabil. 1997;18:52-7.
24. Ruszczak Z. Effect of collagen matrices on dermal wound healing. Adv Drug Deliv Rev. 2003;55:1595-611.
25. Hundeshagen G, Collins VN, Wurzer P, Sherman W, Voigt CD, Cambiaso-Daniel J, et al. A Prospective, Randomized, Controlled Trial Comparing the Outpatient Treatment of Pediatric and Adult Partial-thickness Burns with Suprathel or Mepilex Ag. J Burn Care Res. 2018;39:261-7.
26. Schwarze H, Küntscher M, Uhlig C, Hierlemann H, Prantl L, Ottomann C, et al. Suprathel, a new skin substitute, in the management of partial-thickness burn wounds: Results of a clinical study. Ann Plast Surg. 2008;60:181-5.
27. Atiyeh BS, Costagliola M. Cultured epithelial autograft (CEA) in burn treatment: three decades later. Burns. 2007;33(4):405-13.
28. Atiyeh Bishara S, Gunn William S, Hayek Shady N. New technologies for burn wound closure and healing—review of the literature. Burns. 2005;31:944-56.
29. Guilbaud J. Problems created by the use of cultured epithelia. Ann Medit Burns Club. 1993;4:176-8.
30. Wright KA, Nadire KB, Busto P, Tublo R, McPherson JM, Wentworth BM. Alternative delivery of keratinocytes using a polyurethane membrane and the implications for its use in the treatment of full thickness burn injury. Burns. 1998;24:7-17.
31. Chester DL, Balderson DS, Papini RPG. A review of keratinocyte delivery to the wound bed. J Burn Care Rehabil. 2004;25:266-75.
32. Cuono CB, Langdon R, Birchall N, Barttelbort S, McGuire J. Composite autologous-allogeneic skin replacement: development and clinical application. Plast Reconstr Surg. 1987;80:626-37.
33. Yannas IV, Burke JF. Design of an artificial skin. I. Basic design principles. J Biomed Mater Res. 1980;14(1):65-81.
34. Moiemen NS, Vlachou E, Staiano JJ, Thawy Y, Frame JD. Reconstructive surgery with Integra dermal regeneration template: histologic study, clinical evaluation, and current practice. Plast Reconstr Surg. 2006;117(7 Suppl):160S-74S.
35. Cooper M, Hansbrough J, Spielvogel R, Cohen R, Bartel RL, Naughton G. In vivo optimization of a living dermal substitute employing cultured human fibroblasts on a biodegradable polyglycolic acid or polyglactin mesh. Biomaterials. 1991;12:243-8.
36. Van Der Veen VC, van der Wal MBA, van Leuwen MCE, Ulrich MMW, Middelkoop E. Biological background of dermal substitutes. Burns. 2010;36:305-21.
37. Hansbrough JF, Mozingo DW, Kealey GP, Davis M, Gidner A, Gentzkow GD. Clinical trials of a biosynthetic temporary skin replacement, Dermagraft Transitional Covering, compared with cryopreserved human cadaver skin for temporary coverage of excised burn wounds. J Burn Care Rehabil. 1997;18:43-51.
38. Shores JT, Gabriel A, Gupta S. Skin substitutes and alternatives: a review. Adv Skin Wound Care. 2007;20:493-508.
39. Bloemen MCT, van Leeuwen MCE, van Vucht NE, van Zuijlen PP, Middelkoop E. Dermal substitution in acute burns and reconstructive surgery: a 12-year follow-up. Plast Reconstr Surg. 2010;125:1450-9.
40. Rnjak J, Wise SG, Mithieux SM, Weiss AS. Severe burn injuries and the role of elastin in the design of dermal substitutes. Tissue Eng. 2011;17(2):81-93.
41. Haslik W, Kamolz LP, Manna F, Hladik M, Rath T, Frey M. Management of full-thickness skin defects in the hand and wrist region: First long-term experiences with the dermal matrix Matriderm. J Plast Reconstr Aesthet Surg. 2010;63:360-4.
42. Kolokythas P, Aust MC, Vogt PM, Paulsen F. Aktuelle Ubersicht zum Dermisersatz mit Kollagen-Elastin-Matrix Matriderm bei Brandverletzungen [Dermal subsitute with the collagen-elastin matrix Matriderm in burn injuries: a comprehensive review]. Handchir Mikrochir Plast Chir. 2008;40(6):367-71. [German].
43. Gravante G, Delogu D, Giordan N, Morano G, Montone A, Esposito G. The use of hyalomatrix PA in the treatment of deep partial-thickness burns. J Burn Care Res. 2007;28:269-74.
44. Myers SR, Partha VN, Soranzo C, Price RD, Navsaria HA. Hyalomatrix: A temporary epidermal barrier, hyaluronan delivery, and neodermis induction system for keratinocyte stem cell therapy. Tissue Eng. 2007;13:2733-41.
45. Lim P, Li H, Ng S. Novosorb® Biodegradable Temporising Matrix (BTM) and its Applications. Surg Technol Int. 2023;42:sti42/1608.
46. Li H, Lim P, Stanley E, Lee G, Lin S, Neoh D, et al. Experience with NovoSorb® Biodegradable Temporising Matrix in reconstruction of complex wounds. ANZ J Surg. 2021;91(9):1744-50.

CHAPTER

18 Skin Banking

Amrita More, Sujata Sarabahi, Deepak Nanda

INTRODUCTION

Skin is the largest organ of the body. It is the body's first line of defense against external physical, chemical, and microbial insults and has thermoregulatory properties that are essential to maintaining homeostasis. Ideally, any wound that is incapable of spontaneous healing should be resurfaced with autologous skin grafts at the earliest. However, if the wounds are extensive, donor sites may not be adequate to provide sufficient skin for coverage. In extremes of age and sick patients with associated comorbidities, harvest of large volumes of grafts can be detrimental. With longer life expectancy and increase in incidence of chronic illnesses and comorbidities, the prevalence of nonhealing wounds has increased.

All these conditions have created a market for various biologic dressings made of human, animal, and synthetic components that can be used to resurface wounds and have greatly enhanced our ability to effectively manage complex wounds. With today's technology, it is now possible to biologically engineer autologous tissues. Burns are a major problem of the developing world and affect the middle- and lower-income strata more commonly. Cost and availability are prohibitive for use of the above modalities in most scenarios. Skin is the best biologic dressing. Homografts have been used for many decades for resurfacing of wounds. When timely applied on a prepared wound bed, it temporarily takes up thus protecting the body from infection and reducing pain by covering the raw nerve ends. This helps in stabilizing the patient, reducing the wounds, and buys us time till the conditions are suitable for autologous grafting.

Skin can be obtained from living donors or cadavers and amputated parts. It is best when it is freshly sourced, but that is not always possible. Skin banks provide a facility to procure, process, and store human skin that can be retrieved when needed. With the establishment of skin banks in association with major burn centers, the morbidity of extensive burns has reduced dramatically.

HISTORY OF SKIN BANKING

The clinical use of skin graft was first described in 1869 by Reverdin.[1] In 1871, George Pollock demonstrated the use of his own skin along with the patient's skin (both autograft and homograft) in a pediatric burn patient.[2] Cadaveric skin graft was first used by Girdner in 1881.[3] The viability of skin graft begins to decline as soon as it is lifted off the donor site. In the 1940s, Webster and Matthew independently reported successful storage of skin grafts at 4–7°C for 3 weeks.[4,5] Cryopreservation or storage at subzero temperatures was found to further prolong graft viability in various experiments by Baxter in 1948 and Billingham and Medawar in 1952.[6,7]

With the World War II and the Vietnam War, long strides were made in reconstructive surgeries and there was an increasing demand for allogenic skin, bone, and other tissues. Storage and processing methods were also undergoing rapid development at this time. The first skin bank was established by the United States Navy in 1949 at Maryland. By the 1960s, many tissue banks were established in the United States and across Europe.[8,9] In Asia, Burma Tissue Bank was established at Rangoon in 1981 and Bangkok Biomaterial Centre in Thailand was established in 1984.[10]

Tissue banking in India started by eye banking at Regional Institute of Ophthalmology at Chennai in the year 1945. The first skin bank in India was established in the year 1978 at Bai Jerbai Wadia Hospital in Mumbai by Dr Manoj Keswani, but the project was not successful due to financial constraints and lack of awareness. Tata Memorial Hospital (TMH) Tissue Bank was started in 1988 in Mumbai with the help of International Atomic Energy Agency (IAEA) and recognized with the Health Services, Maharashtra state. It stored lyophilized tissues sterilized by 25 kGy gamma radiation like amnion, dura mater, bone, and skin from live donors and cadavers. TMH tissue bank initiated another tissue bank at the Defence Laboratory at Jodhpur which also used gamma radiation for sterilization.[11] In 2000, Dr Madhuri Gore established a skin bank at Lokmanya Tilak Municipal Medical College and Sion Hospital, Mumbai. From 2000 to 2006, skin grafts were cryopreserved at –70°C with 15% glycerol but after that a high-concentration glycerol preservation method developed by the Euro Skin Bank was used.[12] In the year 2009, RCBN Skin Bank was established in National Burns Centre at Airoli, Mumbai, by Dr Sunil Keswani, with financial and technical support from Rotary International and Euro Skin Bank, respectively. It has run a continuous public awareness campaign with the help of several nongovernment organizations to raise cadaver donations and was the first successful skin bank model in India. They further helped to establish several other skin banks across the country. Today, there are 23 registered skin banks in India as of now **(Table 1)**.

TYPES OF SKIN BANKING

The main factor that influences the clinical behavior of the allograft is the viability of the cells in the graft rather than the technique of processing and storage.[13] Allografts stored by refrigeration have viable cells, but viability reduces rapidly with time. Cryopreservation maintains cell viability and the shelf life is longer than refrigeration, but it varies with the method of processing and storage. Glycerol-preserved allografts are nonviable but have the advantage of storage at 2–5°C. Freeze drying or lyophilization and high concentration solute preservation kill all the viable cells, but the mechanical structure is well preserved and can be stored at room temperature indefinitely. Both cryopreserved and glycerol preserved skin allografts are used as temporary biological dressing. The main difference is their biological activity and mechanism of rejection. Viable grafts incite an immunologic response. Nonviable allograft has no immunogenic potential but provides a scaffold for regeneration. It is generally believed that viable allografts are better in terms of neovascularization, granulation tissue formation, and wound healing rate, especially in chronic nonhealing wounds. However, some

TABLE 1: Skin banks in India.

State	Skin Bank
Maharashtra	• LT Medical College and Hospital Skin Bank, Sion, Mumbai (2000) • RCBN Skin Bank, Navi Mumbai (2009) • Rotary Surya Hospital Skin Bank, Pune (2011) • Rotary Ochri Skin Bank, Nagpur (2015) • Rotary Vedant Skin Collection Centre, Nasik (2016) • Masina Hospital, Byculla, Mumbai (2017) • Rotary Sushrut Hospital Skin Bank, Sangli (2018)
Tamil Nadu	• Ganga Hospital Skin Bank, Coimbatore (2014) • Skin Bank, Right Hospital (2014) • Skin Bank, Kilpauk Medical College (2014) • Skin Bank, Stanley Medical College (2016)
Karnataka	• Rotary Ashirvad Bangalore Medical College and Research Institute Skin Bank, Victoria Hospital, Bangalore (2016) • KLES Skin Bank, Belgaum (2018) • Rotary Kasturba Hospital, Manipal Skin Bank (2020)
Gujarat	Civil Hospital, Ahmedabad (2024)
Delhi	• Safdarjung Hospital (2023) • All India Institute of Medical Sciences (2023)
Odisha	Sum Hospital Skin Bank, Bhubaneshwar (2015)
Madhya Pradesh	Choithram Hospital Skin Bank, Indore (2011)
Telangana	Osmania General Hospital, Hyderabad (2021)
Rajasthan	Sawai Man Singh Hospital Skin Bank, Jaipur (2022)
Chhattisgarh	Jawaharlal Nehru Hospital and Research Centre Skin Bank, Bhilai (2022)

TABLE 2: Differences between viable and nonviable skin allograft.

Type of allografts	Viable	Nonviable
Method of processing and storage	• Simple refrigeration (4°C) • Deep freezing • Cryopreservation	• Freeze drying or lyophilization • High-concentration solute preservation, e.g., glycerolization • Glutaraldehyde preservation • Irradiation
Viability	Cells are viable	Cells are not viable
Shelf life	• *Refrigeration*: Autografts for 2 weeks and cadaver allografts for 7–8 days • *Freezer (–20°C)*: 60 days • *Ultra-low-temperature freezer (–80°C)*: 1 year • *Liquid nitrogen (–196°C)*: 5 years	• *Freeze drying*: Indefinitely • *Glycerol preservation*: 3–5 years
Immunologic properties	High antigenicity, can cause immunologic hypersensitivity in the next sitting	Low antigenicity, does not cause immunological hypersensitivity
Graft rejection	9 to 10 days	13 to 14 days
Transplantation performance	Performance is good on gross and microscopic evaluation but less than fresh graft	Performance is good on gross evaluation but less than fresh and cryopreserved allograft
Mechanism of graft rejection	Immunologic basis	Nonimmunologic; depends on the rate of wound healing
Graft appearance during rejection	Edema with petechial hemorrhages followed by epithelial necrosis	Graft hardens but remains adherent to bed and slowly separates from the periphery to the center

authors argue that this may not be due to the viability of cells and there are insufficient standardized studies to prove one's superiority over the other **(Table 2)**.[14]

Guidelines for Skin Bank

Tissue banks follow certain guidelines and are regulated by the respective national legislations. The US Navy Tissue Bank was the first to lay down standards for donor screening, tissue recovery, and processing that are relevant even today. At the time, tissue banks were mostly unrecognized and unregulated units, developing and working independently. In the early 1990s, the Centers for Disease Control and Prevention (CDC) reported a human immunodeficiency virus (HIV) infection after transplantation of an imported bone allograft in the United States. After this, donor screening and record keeping became mandatory and in 2005, federal laws pertaining to tissue banking and transplantation were passed. US Food and Drug Authority (FDA) has regulatory authority over tissue banks in the United States. The American Association of Tissue Banking (AATB), established in 1975, publishes extensive guidelines and technical manuals in tissue banking, keeping abreast of the latest FDA, CDC, and American Burns Association (ABA) recommendations. These have been incorporated in the guidelines of many tissue banks around the world. AATB offers accreditation to tissue banks in the world over that run as per their recommended guidelines.

The European Association of Tissue Banks (EATB) was established in 1991, and it laid down the EATB standards of tissue banking and banking of skin substitutes in 1998. In 2004, European Union directives outlining good manufacturing practices (GMPs) were adopted by 27 European Union members to align tissue banking standards across Europe. GMP guidelines are for monitoring and maintenance of strict environmental parameters to check particulate and microbial contamination, equipment calibration, and aseptic processing of tissues in tissue banks. In addition to these, there is national legislation and guidelines by national associations and organizations such as the British Association of Tissue Banks in the United Kingdom.

In Australia, tissue banks need to be licensed by the Therapeutic Goods Administration (Therapeutic Goods Act 1989) and comply with the Australian code of GMP for human blood, blood components, human tissue, and human cellular therapy products.

In the 1990s, national guidelines or legislations for tissue banking in Asia, Middle East, and Africa were nonexistent and accreditation by AATB was an expensive and exhaustive process, not entirely suitable for developing countries at nascent stages of tissue banking. In 2003, the IAEA established the International Standards for Tissue Banks and Guide for Legal and Regulatory Authority based on the American and European guidelines, and these were adopted by 30 countries. The Latin American

Tissue Banking Association also has given guidelines that few central and South American countries follow. The Asia Pacific Association of Surgical Tissue Banking (APASTB), established in 1988, developed the standards for safety and ethics in tissue banking in the Pacific rim region. The Japanese Society of Tissue Transplantation also published documents on guidelines and standard operating procedures in tissue banking. The Asia Pacific Burns Association (ABPA) has developed the Asia Pacific Skin Banking Guidelines and launched it at the 12th Asia Pacific Burns Congress at Singapore in August 2019.[14]

Tissue banking is allowed in India only for therapeutic purposes and not for research. In India, the Transplantation of Human Organ Act of 1994 dealt with legalities of organ transplantation and prevention of its commercialization with the main emphasis on thoracic and abdominal organs like liver, kidneys, lung, etc. As most tissues that are banked did not come under the definition of organ as stated in this act and the rules related to organ transplantation could not be practically applied to tissue banking, skin banking remained largely outside its purview. In 2011, this act was amended to include tissue transplantation and it is now known as Transplantation of Human Organ and Tissues Act. In 2014, the Ministry of Family Health and Welfare implemented the "Transplantation of Human Organs and Tissue Rules." With this amendment, tissue transplantation has been recognized as a specific entity, registration of tissue banks has become mandatory, and unauthorized tissue donation and commercial use of tissue are punishable.[15] National Organ and Tissue Transplant Organization (NOTTO) is a national-level organization set up under Directorate General of Health Services, Ministry of Health and Family Welfare, Government of India located at 4th and 5th floors of Institute of Pathology (ICMR) Building in Safdarjung Hospital, New Delhi. It is the nodal networking agency for Delhi for procurement, allocation, and distribution of organs and tissues in Delhi and an apex center for all-India activities of coordination and networking for procurement and distribution of organs and tissues and maintaining a transplant registry in the country. Each state has a State Organ and Tissue Transplantation Organization (SOTTO) which comes under one of five Regional Organ and Tissue Transplantation Organization (ROTTO) for North, South, East, West, and North-East regions.

In order to maintain quality control, ISO 9000 standards were adopted by AATB in 1996 and then later by other tissue banks. Further, ISO 9001 and ISO 19011 guidelines in 2015 and 2018, respectively, have helped organizations to have standardized traceable quality management and auditing systems. The World Health Organization has also given out key safety requirements for human organ and tissue transplantation, especially on ethical concerns and non-commercialization of tissue banking.

INFRASTRUCTURE AND PERSONNEL

The skin bank should be run as per the national laws and regulations. The three main aspects are the infrastructure, laboratory equipment, and personnel. The infrastructure should consist of adequate space to carry out the processing and storage of skin grafts safely. The laboratory needs to be a contamination-controlled area with high-efficiency particulate air filter with positive pressure, constant thermo-hygrometric parameters, and monitoring for particle/microbial contamination. As per GMP, the aseptic processing of allograft should be undertaken in a grade A room or a grade A area in a grade B background zone. This can be achieved by using a laminar airflow cabinet **(Table 3)**.

A biosafety cabinet provides a sterile workstation with laminar flow and UV radiation. All handling of the graft takes place inside this. A shaking incubator is used to incubate the grafts or for cell culture. It provides steady temperatures and frequent orbital agitation that promotes cell aeration and equal distribution of nutrients

TABLE 3: Classification of clean rooms (goods manufacturing practices guidelines).

Grade	Maximum permitted number of particles ≥ 0.5μ/m³ At rest μm/m³	Maximum permitted number of particles ≥ 0.5μ/m³ At operations	ISO class At rest/at operations
A	3,250	3,250	Level 5/level 5
B	3,520	352,000	Level 5/level 7
C	352,000	3,520,000	Level 7/level 8
D	3,520,000	Not defined	Level 8/not defined

Notes: Grade A requires a laminar airflow; sinks and drains are prohibited in grades A and B; grades C and D are for less critical operations like assembly and cleaning of instruments/equipment prior to sterilization. ISO (International Standards Organization) class is based on the count of particulate matter in the air, class 1 being the cleanest and class 9 being the dirtiest among clean rooms.

Source: GMP Facility: Understanding grade A, grade B, grade C & D.[online] Available from https://www.mecart-cleanrooms.com/learning-center/gmp-facility-understanding-grade-a-grade-b-grade-c-and-d/. [Last accessed May, 2024].

in cell cultures. There is usually a changing room where the laboratory worker can change into sterile gear prior to entering the processing area. Apart from this, basic equipment required for sterilization of laboratory equipment and storage containers like the hot air oven and autoclave machine is needed. A cold room or walk-in freezer is needed if grafts are stored in large quantities.

The personnel consist of a manager, a team for skin graft harvest, and technical staff for graft processing and quality control personnel. The harvest team may be doctors or other medical or nonmedical professionals trained in skin graft harvest. The technical staff is either trained laboratory workers or nursing staff.

DONOR SCREENING

Donor criteria exist to ensure good quality of allograft and minimize risk of disease transmission. Once a donor is available, the tissue bank coordinator is notified. The coordinator verifies relevant data like age, gender, cause of death, time of death, and refrigeration.

- Preliminary screening is performed by a review of medical records, and the treating physician is also contacted if any additional information is needed.
- A donor risk assessment interview is conducted with the patient's next of kin to rule out high-risk behavior and recent travel history.
- In case of multiorgan donors, the serological reports are usually available. If the serological reports available are not within 7 days prior to death of the patient, a blood sample can be obtained via femoral or cardiac puncture at the time of skin harvest. Serological testing is done for HIV, hepatitis C virus (HCV), hepatitis B surface antigen (HBsAg), and venereal disease research laboratory (VDRL).
- Testing for human T lymphotrophic virus, cytomegalovirus, ABO, and Rh blood typing is optional.
- A thorough physical examination of the body is conducted to examine the skin condition, especially at the donor sites. The body is examined for skin lesions, recent IV puncture wounds, recent tattoos, piercings, and any evidence suggestive of high-risk behavior for IV drug abuse, HIV, and other sexually transmitted diseases. These are documented as per a standard protocol.

Once a donor is found meeting the selection criteria, the procurement team needs to reach the site where the body is kept. This may be the hospital or the patient's home. Skin donations are acceptable within 18 hours postmortem time if refrigerated (12 hours if the body is not refrigerated). However, most centers in India accept donation within 6 hours. Adult donors between the age of 18 and 60 years are preferred so that adequate quantity and good-quality skin can be procured per harvest.

The absolute contraindications are history of malignancies (except primary brain tumors), sepsis, drowning, tuberculosis, and slow viral disease. The relative contraindications are history of diabetes mellitus, long-term IV drug abuse, long-term corticosteroid use, at-risk behavior for HIV, or any other transmissible diseases. Patients having afflictions of the skin like autoimmune dermatoses, postinfective skin damage, systemic collagenosis, nephrogenic fibrosing dermopathy, porphyria, burns, or trauma at the site of skin procurement are not suitable donors.[16,17]

ALLOGRAFT PROCUREMENT AND TRANSPORT

Written informed consent is obtained from the next of kin. Usually, skin is harvested from the limbs and trunks only, but other areas can also be used depending on the consent and after prior information to the relatives taking into consideration religious and cultural sentiments during the last rites. Donor sites are shaved and prepared. Parts are painted with povidone iodine, isopropanol, or chlorhexidine as per manufacturer guidelines and the donor sites draped with sterile sheets. Skin grafts are harvested taking all aseptic and antiseptic measures similar to surgical operations being carried out in live patients. A sterile field should be established which is cleaned and draped. The technical team should don cap, masks, OT gown, shoe cover, and sterile gloves. The surgical instruments required should be sterile, and date and mode of sterilization should be documented for each batch of harvest. Strips of split-thickness skin grafts are harvested of thickness varying between 0.25 and 0.35 mm. An electric dermatome is preferred over manual grafting handles and blades to ensure even thickness and dimensions of grafts. Use of dermatomes also has a faster learning curve. The donor site is then dressed with absorbent dressing and wrapped in a plastic sheet to avoid leakage of bodily fluids from the donor sites during transport of the body.

The transport medium and temperature during transit varies depending on the type of processing, time taken for transit and the skin bank protocol. As per Euro Skin Bank (Netherlands) protocol the graft is processed by glycerolization and transported in glycerol 98% and NaCl 0.9% (50/50 v/v) with 1 g of streptomycin sulphate and 1,000,000 IU of sodium penicillin G, mean time from harvest to next stage in processing being 4.2 hours (range 1 to 12 hours).[17] Skin Bank at University Hospital of Siena, Italy use Ringer lactate or Roswell Park Memorial Institute (RPMI) 1,640 supplemented with 320 mg/L gentamicin,

500 mg/L vancomycin, and 600 mg/L lincomycin (per 100 mL of transport medium, respectively).[14] Burn Wound Centre, Queen Astrid Military Hospital, Brussels, Belgium use 800 mL custom-made medium for culturing epithelial cells, consisting of Dulbecco's Modified Eagle Medium (DMEM)/Ham's F12 nutrient mix and 10.6 g/L sodium bicarbonate 3:1, supplemented with 200 mL of custom-made Cambridge antibiotic solution, consisting of gentamycin sulfate 4 g/L, primaxin 0.2 g/L, polymyxin B 0.2 g/L, vancomycin 0.05 g/L, and nystatin 2,500,000 U/L in medium 199 with 25 mM HEPES) in refrigerated tanks at +4°C and kept for minimum 24 hours (maximum 72 h) at 2–8°C before further processing.[18] At the Hannover Skin Bank, Germany, each skin graft is rolled in a gauze, placed in a separate sterile absorbent bag, tightly sealed, placed in a transport box (Transmed, Regensburg, Germany) and transferred at room temperature within 30 minutes for immediate processing.[19]

STERILISATION OF SKIN ALLOGRAFT

One of the main concerns in allograft use is contamination. Even the presence of one microorganism in the graft is defined as contamination. Contamination rate is the proportion of graft samples that are positive for contaminants at different stages of graft processing. Bioburden refers to the quantitative measure of contaminants per gram of the sample. Disinfection is the process or intervention to reduce the bioburden in the graft after harvest.

Most common organisms found in the grafts as derived from cultures taken just after harvest are *Staphylococcus* and *Propionibacterium* species. Other commonly found contaminants are *Acinetobacteria*, *Streptococcus epidermidis*, *Micrococcus*, *Candida albicans*, *Bacillus* species, and *Escherichia coli*. The contamination rate at the time of harvest can vary from 10 to 95% and can be minimized by taking strict aseptic precautions while harvest and transport and ensuring the transport media is sterile. When banking viable allografts, all traces of the antimicrobial prepping solutions should be removed completely as it can be cytotoxic.

The method of sterilization varies depending on viability of allograft and the regional protocol. Nonviable allograft can be sterilized with chemical methods like peracetic acid, ethylene dioxide, or irradiation as cell damage is not a concern. Gamma radiation generated from Cobalt-60 or electron beam accelerator is effective for most microbes, although some viruses need a higher dose and duration of exposure. The standard dose is 25 kGy but various skin banks use a radiation dose ranging from 15 to 35 kGy. However, these methods can cause ultrastructural changes and the dose and exposure time are selected accordingly.

Glycerol and cryopreservation are as such inhibitory to microbial growth. In addition, a combination of antibiotics and antifungals in the transport media and/or initial incubation media have shown to reduce the contamination and discard rate significantly. However, there is no consensus on the combination, its dose, or the media used. The usual combinations are Penicillin + Streptomycin + Amphotericin B. Use of kanamycin, gentamicin, vancomycin, lincomycin and nystatin is also documented.[20-22] Almost all antibiotics are effective at normothermic temperature (37°C) but when incubating at lower temperatures, only antibiotics effective at these temperatures should be used. The exposure time should be longer when using cooler temperatures.

Graft samples are sent for culture after processing prior to the final storage. Random sampling of stored grafts is also carried out frequently. If found to be contaminated at any stage, the media is changed with glycerol or antibiotics and incubated for 3 months and then recultured. If found to be contaminated again, this process is repeated two more times and if the sample still comes out to be positive, it is discarded.

PROCESSING AND STORAGE OF SKIN ALLOGRAFT

Refrigeration

The viable cells in the skin graft utilize nutrients and oxygen from its environment and release salts and toxic metabolites. As graft metabolism continues and toxins accumulate, the cells begin to die. When stored at 4°C, cell metabolism is slowed and cell viability can be prolonged up to 3 weeks.

Grafts are folded dermal side on itself and stored in saline-soaked or paraffin gauze as sheets or rolls, in a sterile container and refrigerated at 2–5°C. This is done in most burn units with leftover autografts in a surgery or when wound bed is not prepared and grafts are required within a short period of time.

Isotonic solutions like normal saline or Hartman's solution provide few electrolytes and dilute the ions and toxic metabolites, but grafts stored in these solutions are usually edematous and have low cell viability. 10–33% human serum nourishes the graft as well as buffers the toxins.[23] Several culture media have also been experimented with such as University of Wisconsin (UW) solution, histidine-tryptophan-ketoglutarate (HTK) solution, Roswell Park Memorial Institute-1640 (RPMI) solution, etc. Among these agents, RPMI solution shows better quality and highest percentage of viable cells over time but none have significantly prolonged storage time.[24-26]

Deep Freezing

Tissues are directly frozen by the refrigeration or liquid nitrogen vapor at ultra-low temperatures of –70 to –100°C. Deep freezers maintain a temperature of –80°C and the newer deep freezers can even maintain a temperature of –150°C. During this process, ice crystals form inside the cells which cause mechanical damage and it also changes intracellular hyperosmolality which affects cell viability. Cryoprotective agents help in reducing the cell damage during the process. In controlled cooling, the viability of keratinocytes and fibroblasts is maintained but the immunogenicity is reduced. This method is simple and allografts can be stored for 1–5 years.

Cryopreservation

Cryopreservation is a technique of preservation at subzero temperatures for prolonged periods of time, taking care of the cell viability. It can be done by two methods: Slow cooling and vitrification.

Slow Cooling

Each cell type has an "optimal cooling rate." As a tissue has different types of cells and it is not possible to maintain different cooling rates for various cells in the same tissue, here comes the role of cryoprotectants.

Glycerol and dimethylsulfoxide are the most common cryoprotectants used in practice. They act by entering the cell and preventing shrinkage of cells and by providing a medium for buffering of salts and toxins. The rate of entry of cryoprotectants into the cell is temperature dependent and at higher temperatures they can be toxic. Thus, it is also necessary to regulate the duration and temperature at which the cells are exposed to these cryoprotectants. Apart from this, the basal media in which the cryoprotectant is mixed is another variable. Basal media acts like a solvent for various salts that are produced during cell metabolism, and it buffers them. Buffering capacity of most media reduces with drop in temperature and for the purpose of cryopreservation, zwitterionic buffers are preferred.

Another type of cryoprotectants is membrane-impermeable cryoprotective agents which remain in the extracellular space and provide higher dimensional cryoprotection. Examples are polyvinyl pyrrolidone, hydroxyethyl starch, 2-methyl 2,4-pentanediol, and other sugars and polymers. Sericin is a protein derived from silkworm cocoons that has been used for cryopreservation of hepatocytes, human adipose-derived stem cells, and other progenitor cells. Proteins isolated from fishes have also shown potential as an antifreeze agent.

A cooling rate of –1°C per minute is safe for most cells with the use of cryoprotectants, and this is achieved by a controlled cooling apparatus. Leukocytes and macrophages are more susceptible to die with faster cooling as compared to keratinocytes. This property has been taken advantage of by a cooling rate of –30°C/min which preserves the keratinocytes as well as makes the allograft less immunogenic. This concept is called the "cooling rate-dependent immunogenicity".

Once the skin is cooled to –80°C, the graft can be cryopreserved in liquid nitrogen at –130°C at which no more cell death can occur. Each batch of allograft is aseptically packed in rolls and placed in a tube or as sheets in metallic laminated pouches and placed in the cryoprotectant agent and sealed in sterile double plastic bags that are then placed in the liquid nitrogen with several other such packets. As there is a higher risk of cross contamination in liquid nitrogen if a single packet is perforated, the vapor phase of liquid nitrogen is preferred.

When needed for use, it is transported in liquid nitrogen (–130°C) or in dry ice (–79°C) sealed containers to the location. Then it is put in a 37°C water bath until just thawed after which the inner pack is removed aseptically and the contents of the inner pack are emptied in a sterile kidney tray, where the cryoprotectant is washed off. As use of saline can be hypo-osmolar for the graft containing intracellular hyperosmolar molecules of cryoprotectant, sucrose is added to the saline solution used initially to make it more hyperosmolar and gradually diluted. As soon as the thawing process is complete, it should be applied to the bed immediately.[14]

Vitrification

The liquid state of water in the cells is directly converted to solid or glass state without crystallization. This is done by employing high concentration of cryoprotective agents and very high cooling rate using liquid nitrogen. A careful balance needs to be maintained between the cooling rate, warming rate, sample volume, and sample viscosity. Handling is difficult, and the risk of contamination is high. This method has been found to be very effective at preserving oocytes, sperm, and embryos and is now also finding application in preserving more complex tissues like blood vessels, articular cartilage, and heart valves. Research is going on to find an ideal vitrification protocol to produce sufficient allograft of acceptable viability. This process can also be used to produce other skin substitutes.[27]

Glycerol Preservation

Until 1984, the Dutch National Skin Bank used the cryopreservation method of skin banking. Glycerol, which was routinely used as a cryoprotective agent, was found to have antibacterial and antiviral properties. In 1984, they devised the glycerol preservation technique. This method was simple and cost effective and did not require complex equipment. This method shows good preservation of cell viability and ultrastructure, especially the elastic-skeleton structure in comparison to other methods.[28,29] With encouraging clinical outcome and growing demand, this method has become commonly used at many skin banks all over the world, including India.

This method includes three aseptic phases:

1. Cadaver skin graft is harvested under aseptic precautions and placed in a solution of equal quantities of 98% glycerol and 0.9 % saline in sterile tubes. This is transported to the skin bank at room temperature. This time period from placing the graft in the glycerol solution to the next stage in processing is called "first glycerolization", and this can range from 1 to 12 hours (mean 4.2 hours).
2. Once in the skin bank, the grafts are sorted and good-sized and even-thickness grafts are meshed and placed in sterile tubes containing 70% glycerol solution and placed in a shaking incubator at 33°C for 3 hours. This is the "second glycerolization" and ranges from 4 to 18 hours.
3. Then they are again removed and placed in 85% glycerol solution and incubated in a shaking incubator for a further 3 hours at 33°C. After this, the graft is removed, trimmed, sizes recorded and placed in sterile tubes, labeled, and stored in 85% glycerol in the refrigerator at 2–5°C, ready for use.

When needed, the preserved allograft is retrieved, rinsed with lukewarm saline for 10 minutes to remove the glycerol, and applied to the graft bed.[17]

Lyophilization

Lyophilization involves first freezing the tissue and then applying vacuum so that the frozen water in the tissue sublimes to its gaseous state and the tissue is completely dehydrated to less than 5% water content. It is then stored at room temperature in sterile packets. The tissue is nonviable, but the tissue architecture remains well preserved and can be used even after years. De-epidermized dermis (DED) is commonly preserved by this method. When needed, it is immersed in a saline bath at 37°C for 30 to 60 minutes.[30-32]

Gamma Radiation

Infection in the recipient due to contaminated grafts is a serious complication and disinfection of the graft is a crucial step. This is a process of sterilization of nonviable tissue grafts by gamma rays from radionuclide isotopes of Cobalt-60 and Cesium-137. The reference dose of 25 kGy is advised by the IAEA, though some tissue banks prefer a lower dose to protect the biomechanical properties of the tissue. A dose above 25 kGy can cause collagen denaturation in the graft. The reduction of bioburden in the graft depends on the dose and it is practical to reduce the initial bioburden by disinfecting the graft prior to irradiation. The tissue is processed by freezing and a radioprotective agent is added and then irradiated. After this, it can be stored at room temperature and used for up to 1 year.

It is quite popular for musculoskeletal grafts but for skin grafts, some architectural changes have been reported and it stiffens the graft to an extent.[33] A study by Rooney et al. reports no physical and histological alterations or cytotoxicity in grafts processed by 20% glycerol and irradiated with 25 kGy gamma radiation.[34] There are several case reports of successful use of these skin grafts in difficult wounds, but there are no comparative studies with grafts preserved by other methods.[35,36]

QUALITY CONTROL

Quality management systems exist to ensure that the grafts in skin banks are of good quality, contamination free, and safe for use. It includes proper organizational structure with trained personnel who have delineated responsibilities, written standard procedures and processes, and the necessary resources. Proper record keeping of each step in the procurement, processing, storage, and handling of the grafts is also equally important so that in case of an issue, all the data can be traced to identify the source of the problem. Periodic self-assessments and internal and external peer-audits or third party audits are recommended. Several guidelines and regulations in tissue banking deal with this aspect in great detail.

Microbiological surveillance: A skin sample from the graft is cultured in aerobic and anaerobic media. As certain bacteria like the *Mycobacterium* species are slow growing, grafts incubated up to 2 weeks can identify additional contaminants or a polymerase chain reaction (PCR) test can be done. Yeasts and fungi are tested by culture on Sabouraud agar medium for 3 weeks. Skin sampling is performed at the time of procurement, after rinsing with antibiotics and incubation period and after processing prior to storage. If even a single colony-forming unit is identified, specific cultures and biochemical tests are performed to identify the exact species followed by antibiograms. If contaminated by few nonpathogenic bacteria, then the graft is reglycerolized, antibiotics are applied as per antibiogram and then tested again. This time if the graft is negative for bacteria, it is used. Skin grafts contaminated with *Staphylococcus aureus, Streptococcus pneumoniae*, gram-negative bacilli, enterococci, *Clostridium*, and spore-forming organisms are discarded. Periodic microbiological analysis of laboratory surfaces, processing media, and glove print of the personnel are also performed.

Viability assessment: Viable grafts are believed to perform better clinically as compared to nonviable grafts although there is no level I evidence to prove that one is superior to the other. In stored viable skin grafts, it is important to assess cell viability prior to application.[14,37,38] Histopathological examination of random graft samples is performed to assess the graft quality. Cell viability can be assessed by colony-forming efficiency, dye exclusion method, or various metabolic assays. It depends on the freezing protocol, temperature at which it is stored, time since storage, and also the initial tissue viability before processing. Frozen or deep frozen grafts lose up to 50% cell viability in the first 2 weeks and then more gradually over months. In cryopreserved skin at 1 year, cell viability varies from 50 to 70% and it is higher in cryopreserved tissue as compared to frozen. There are also changes in tissue architecture in frozen skin over time that do not occur in the cryopreserved graft. So, although these tissues remain viable over years, there is no clearly defined period up to which it can be used clinically.

Transplantation performance: The most important test is how the graft performs when placed on a live body. Although not routinely done, this employs placing the graft on a live rat or mice and then assessing the graft adherence by gross and histological examination.

DISTRIBUTION AND APPLICATION OF SKIN BANK PRODUCTS

In addition to skin allografts, other skin bioproducts can be derived from skin such as DED, homologous keratinocyte culture, autologous keratinocyte culture, autologous fibroblast culture, autologous endothelial cell culture, and autologous stem cells. The main indication for use of skin allografts is burns. Apart from burns, skin bank products also have a role in reconstruction of other surgical wounds and nonhealing ulcers. Since the regulations on animal testing have become very stringent, cadaver allograft provides an alternative for in vitro testing of the effects of various toxins, pharmacological drugs, and therapeutic agents on skin biology (**Box 1**).[39]

Extensive burns have limited donor sites for autografts, and early wound coverage with a skin graft offers several advantages like reduction in pain, desiccation, hypermetabolism, and infection and promotes healing and early mobilization. Cryopreserved allograft and glycerol-preserved allografts are the most commonly available. Although the former is viable graft and the latter is nonviable, there has not been found much difference between the two in terms of graft take, rejection, and overall clinical outcome. For partial-thickness wounds, it acts like a dressing and promotes healing. In deep partial thickness and full thickness, it is used as a temporary dressing or a dermal template.

BOX 1 **Indications for use of skin allograft.**

Clinical indications

- Nonhealing ulcers
  - Venous and arterial ulcers
  - Pressure ulcers
  - Diabetic foot ulcers
  - Pyoderma gangrenosum
  - Post-traumatic lesions
- Surgical wounds
  - Moh surgery
  - Reconstructive surgery
  - Wound cover in critical areas
  - Aesthetic surgery
- Other nondermatological indications
- Bullous diseases
  - Congenital epidermolysis bullosa
  - Lyell's syndrome

Experimental indications

- In vitro toxicology
- In vitro investigations in skin biology

Source: Reproduced from Fimiani M, Pianigiani E, Di Simplicio FC, Sbano P, Cuccia A, Pompella G, et al. Other uses of homologous skin grafts and skin bank bioproducts. Clin Dermatol. 2005;23(4):396-402.

Conventional technique: In deep burns, when autograft is not immediately available, burn wounds are excised within 7 days of injury and covered with allografts. The graft adheres to wound bed initially and when the allograft is rejected it appears necrosed or separated from the wound bed, the allografts are then removed and covered with autografts. This usually occurs around 2 weeks later. It helps in preparing the wound bed for autografting. Since it acts like a scaffold for some dermal regeneration, the final graft quality is superior as compared to direct autografting.

Sandwich technique: This is indicated in burns wounds where the amount of autograft available is less than needed. The autograft is meshed 1:3 and used to cover a larger area, and this in turn is covered with an allograft that is meshed 1:1. While the autograft takes, the interstitial raw areas are protected by the overlying allograft. As the allograft is slowly rejected, complete epithelialization occurs. In this, glycerol-preserved allograft is preferred as it is less antigenic and causes a lesser immune response. Although this allows faster healing and reduced number of procedures, there is a risk of maceration and infection if the allograft is rejected before epithelialization takes place.

Allograft template and delayed keratinocyte application: Cultured epidermal autografts (CEAs) were first used for burn wounds in 1981, but they did not take well on full-thickness wounds. The more popular method is the two-staged method in which allograft is first applied as a dermal template for dermal regeneration followed by delayed application of autologous or homologous keratinocyte culture. This method is associated with lesser infection and improved take of the keratinocytes.

De-epidermized dermis: Derived from cadaveric skin, this acts as a biological scaffold for dermal regeneration. This can be used as a composite skin substitute along with a thin autograft or homologous or autologous keratinocyte cultures on full-thickness wounds. As compared to skin graft alone, use of DED on full-thickness wounds is associated with lesser contractures and good aesthetic outcome. As both the dermal and epidermal components require vascularization, there is a risk of loss of graft if the dermal component does not take and gets infected. It is used in the treatment of small burns or wounds in critical areas such as palms, soles, neck, and peri-articular areas, with or without ultra-thin autograft and has shown reduced scarring and good color match. AlloDerm® (Lifecell Corporation, Branchburg, New Jersey) has been used to correct defects of the anterior and medial cranial fossa, as dural replacement during craniotomy, diaphragm prostheses in cases of congenital agenesis, endoscopic surgical reconstruction of perforations of the nasal septum and tympanoplasty.[39]

Keratinocyte culture: Skin is digested with enzymes and then can be grown in cultures of specific cells like keratinocyte, melanocyte, and fibroblasts based on the cell culture media used. The first successful in vitro human keratinocyte culture was done by Rheinwald and Green in 1975. This was achieved in a xenobiotic medium and since then, a number of xenobiotic-free media have been developed so as to minimize the risk of human transmission of animal diseases.

Homologous keratinocyte culture: It is known to encourage epithelial regeneration and stimulate angiogenesis in wounds. A skin biopsy is obtained from the patient and then processed. Keratinocytes have been used as a noncultured epidermal suspension in a spray form, often along with a widely meshed graft or else the keratinocyte culture is prepared in a bioengineering laboratory and transplanted on the wound as single-cell suspension or CEA. The processing takes about 3 weeks and the cost involved is prohibitive for its regular clinical use. This along with keratinocyte–melanocyte co-culture are used in treatment of vitiligo.

Autologous keratinocyte and fibroblast cultures: Dermal fibroblasts play a key role in wound healing by producing various growth factors and extracellular matrix proteins. Allogenic de-epidermized acellular dermis seeded with autologous keratinocytes, fibroblasts, and endothelial cells cultured from individual patient biopsies has been used in composite grafts. The process takes about 6 weeks and is not suitable for acute burns. The use of allogenic cultured keratinocytes and fibroblasts in a bilayered construct containing murine collagen called StrataGraft® (Stratatech Corporation, Madison, Wisconsin) has recently been approved by the FDA for use in deep dermal burns.

Autologous endothelial cell, autologous stem cell culture: Transplantation of autologous endothelial progenitor cell cultures has been used in vascular diseases like ischemic stroke. In preclinical animal model studies, use of mesenchymal stem cells, adipose-derived stem cells, embryonic pluripotent stem cells, and mesenchymal stem cells, have been found to promote wound healing by stimulating angiogenesis and collagen deposition. It can potentially halt the zone of stasis in acute burn wounds and regenerate skin appendages and reduce scarring.[40-43]

SUMMARY

We have come a long way in the treatment of burns, but skin graft remains the gold standard for coverage of burn wounds. In today's times, access to skin bank facilities is essential for a burn center. A skin bank is not only a source of allografts but can also produce various skin bioproducts and bioengineered skin substitutes in bulk. Efforts to universally standardize tissue banks can one day hopefully allow collaboration between tissue banks all over the world for clinical as well as research purposes.

REFERENCES

1. Reverdin JL. Greffeepidermique, experiencefaitedans le service de M le docteurGuyon, a l'hopitalnecker. Bull Imp Soc Chir Paris. 1869;10:511-5.
2. Pollock GD. Cases of skin grafting and skin transplantation. Trans Clin Soc Lond. 1871;4:37-54.
3. Girdner JH. Skin-grafting with grafts taken from the dead subject. Med Record NY. 1881;20:119-20.
4. Webster JP. Refrigerated skin grafts. Ann Surg. 1944;120(4): 431-9.
5. Matthews DN. Storage of skin for autogenous grafts. Lancet. 1945;2:775-8.
6. Baxter H, Entin MA. Experimental and clinical studies of reduced temperatures in injury and repair in man. III. Direct effect of cooling and freezing on various elements of the human skin. Plast Reconstr Surg. 1948;3:303-34.
7. Billingham RE, Medawar PB. The freezing, drying, and storage of mammalian skin. J Exp Biol. 1952;19:454-68.
8. Barker CF, Markmann JF. Historical overview of transplantation. Cold Spring Harb Perspect Med. 2013;3(4):a014977.
9. McCauley RL. The skin bank. In: Herndon DN (Ed), Total Burn Care, 1st edition. Philadelphia, PA: Saunders; 1996. pp. 159-63.
10. Nather A, Zheng S. Evolution of allograft transplantation: A comprehensive guide for tissue banks 2010:3–19. [online] Available from http://www.worldscibooks.com/etextbook/7539/7539_chap01.pdf [Last accessed May, 2024].
11. Gajiwala AL. Setting up a tissue bank in India: The Tata Memorial Hospital Experience. Cell Tissue Bank. 2003;4:193-201.
12. Gore MA, De AS. Deceased donor skin allograft banking: response and utilization. Indian J Plastic Surg. 2010;43(S01):S114-20.
13. Kearney JN. Guidelines on processing and clinical use of skin allografts. Clin Dermatol. 2005;23(4):357-64.
14. Tognetti L, Pianigiani E, Ierardi F, et al. Current insights into skin banking: storage, preservation and clinical importance of skin allografts. J Biorepository Sci Appl Med. 2017:41-56.
15. Gajiwala AL. Regulatory aspects of tissue donation, banking and transplantation in India. Cell Tissue Bank. 2018;19(2):241-8.
16. Heck E. Banking of skin. Essentials of Tissue Banking. New York: Springer; 2010. pp. 81-92.
17. De Backere AC. Euro Skin Bank: large scale skin-banking in Europe based on glycerol-preservation of donor skin. Burns. 1994;20:S4-9.
18. Verbeken G, Verween G, Vos DD, Pascual B, Corte PD, Richters C, et al. Glycerol treatment as recovery procedure for cryopreserved human skin allografts positive for bacteria and fungi. Cell Tissue Bank. 2012;13(1):1-7.
19. Schlottmann F, Strauβ S, Ziesing S, Reineke C, Ipaktchi R, Weyand B, et al. Organization of Hannover Skin Bank: Sterile culture and procurement protocols for viable cryopreserved allogeneic skin grafts of living donors. International Wound Journal. 2024;21(1):e14374.
20. Pirnay JP, Verween G, Pascual B, Verbeken G, De Corte P, Rose T, et al. Evaluation of a microbiological screening and acceptance procedure for cryopreserved skin allografts based on 14 day cultures. Cell Tissue Bank. 2012;13:287-95.
21. Pianigiani E, Ierardi F, Cuciti C, Brignali S, Oggioni M, Fimiani M. Processing efficacy in relation to microbial contamination of skin allografts from 723 donors. Burns. 2010;36(3):347-51.
22. Neely AN, Plessinger RT, Stamper B, Kagan RJ. Can contamination of a patient's allograft be traced back to the allograft donor?. J Burn Care Res. 2008;29(1):73-6.
23. Marrangoni AG. An experimental study on refrigerated skin grafts stored in ten per cent homologous serum. Plastic Reconstruct Surg. 1950;6(6):425-34.
24. Cram AE, Domayer MA. Short-term preservation of human autografts. J Trauma. 1983;23(10):872-3.
25. Başaran Ö, Özdemir H, Kut A, Şahin Fİ, Deniz M, Sakallıoğlu EA, et al. Effects of different preservation solutions on skin graft epidermal cell viability and graft performance in a rat model. Burns. 2006;32(4):423-9.
26. Boekema BK, Boekestijn B, Breederveld RS. Evaluation of saline, RPMI and DMEM/F12 for storage of split-thickness skin grafts. Burns. 2015;41(4):848-52.
27. Jaiswal AN, Vagga A. Cryopreservation: A Review Article. Cureus. 2022;14(11):e31564.
28. Biagini G, Poppi V, Cocchia D, Ruboli G, Damiani R, Laschi R. Skin Storage in Liquid Nitrogen: An Ultrastructural Investigation. J Cutan Pathol. 1979;6(1):5-17.
29. Eldh J, Bartholdson L, Mobacken H. Histological and histo-chemical studies on effects of some storage solutions on human split thickness skin grafts. Scand J Plastic Reconstruct Surg. 1974;8(3):202-6.
30. Castagnoli C, Alotto D, Cambieri I, et al. Evaluation of donor skin viability: fresh and cryopreserved skin using tetrazolium salt assay. Burns. 2003;29(8):759-67.
31. Ferrando PM, Balmativola B, Cambieri I, Scalzo MS, Bergallo M, Annaratone L, et al. Glycerolized reticular dermis as a new human acellular dermal matrix: an exploratory study. PLoS One. 2016;11(2):e0149124.
32. Schiozer WA, Gemperli R, Mühlbauer W, Mendonça Munhoz A, Castro Ferreira M. An outcome analysis and long-term viability of cryopreserved cultured epidermal allografts. Assessment of the conservation of transplantable human skin allografts. Acta Cir Bras. 2013;28(12):824-32.
33. Singh R, Singh D, Singh A. Radiation sterilization of tissue allografts: A review. World J Radiol. 2016;8(4):355.
34. Rooney P, Eagle M, Hogg P, Lomas R, Kearney J. Sterilisation of skin allograft with gamma irradiation. Burns. 2008;34(5):664-73.
35. Rosales MA, Bruntz M, Armstrong DG. Gamma-irradiated human skin allograft: a potential treatment modality for lower extremity ulcers. Int Wound J. 2004;1(3):201-6.
36. Agarwal P, Jain A, Sharma D. Assessment of biological response of lyophilized cadaveric skin allograft in post burn raw area and nonhealing ulcers. Indian J Burns. 2016;24(1):13-7.
37. Brubaker SA. Establishing a quality system. Essentials of Tissue Banking. New York: Springer; 2010. pp. 191-215.
38. American Association of Tissue Banks. Standards for tissue banking. Processing, preservation, quarantine, and storage. Virginia: American Association of Tissue Banks; 2012. pp. 53-66.
39. Fimiani M, Pianigiani E, Di Simplicio FC, Sbano P, Cuccia A, Pompella G, et al. Other uses of homologous skin grafts and skin bank bioproducts. Clin Dermatol. 2005;23(4):396-402.
40. Wang C, Zhang F, Lineaweaver WC. Clinical Applications of Allograft Skin in Burn Care. Ann Plast Surg. 2020;84(3S):S158-60.
41. Chua AW, Khoo YC, Tan BK, Tan KC, Foo CL, Chong SJ. Skin tissue engineering advances in severe burns: review and therapeutic applications. Burns Trauma. 2016;4:s41038-016.
42. Francis E, Kearney L, Clover J. The effects of stem cells on burn wounds: a review. Int J Burns Trauma. 2019;9(1):1-12.
43. Li Z, Maitz P. Cell therapy for severe burn wound healing. Burns Trauma. 2018;6:13.

CHAPTER

19

Keratinocyte Culture and Cell Therapy

RP Narayan, Mula Rohit Babu

INTRODUCTION

Skin is the primary target organ in thermal burn with loss of its structural and functional integrity. Restoration and regeneration of damaged skin is primary goal of burn wound management. Coverage of full thickness burn wounds with autologous split skin graft is well established and time-tested procedure. The skin autograft provides epidermis and dermis for mechanical stability and is the gold standard for burn wound management. However, availability of split skin graft in adequate quantity in extensive burns is a major problem. Continuous efforts are being made to address this problem in the last five decades or so. The skin replacement technologies introduced have positively impacted burn care. Efforts have been focused on finding temporary and ideal permanent replacements to native human skin. A large variety of skin substitutes and dressings are used to solve the problem. However, when available, the replacement material of choice is the patient's own (autologous) skin to treat acute burns. Autologous split-thickness skin graft is therefore closest to being an ideal skin substitute. One of the major problems in extensive burns is the relative lack of available autograft and the limitations of homograft are also well known. This brings to attention the importance of skin culture and how it can help us overcome the above problems.

Attempts to culture keratinocyte in laboratory were successful about five decades ago and it heralded a new era in burn wound management. Advances in cell biology and biotissue engineering have made it possible to regenerate a variety of tissues from stem cells. Cell therapy for wound closure is a process of delivery of autologous/homologous cellular component in wounds for repair and regeneration of damaged tissue to restore normal physiological function of skin.[1] In this chapter, we will review in brief how the cells from different sources/origin, processed in laboratory, can help to achieve wound closure in the shortest possible time **(Flowchart 1)**.

KERATINOCYTES (CULTURED EPITHELIAL AUTOGRAFT OR CEA)

Keratinocytes are specialized epithelial cells of epidermis which are regularly replaced by keratinocyte stem cell in the basal layer of epidermis. Melanocytes, Langerhans' and Merkel cells are other cells of epidermis.[2] Keratinocytes were the first cells which were cultured and used clinically for burn wound closure and are described in detail for better understanding of the entire cellular processing mechanism.

History of Keratinocyte Culture

Healing of partial thickness burn wounds (epithelialization) occurs from basal epithelial cells (keratinocytes) of epidermis and skin appendages (hair follicles and sweat glands). Attempts of growing autologous keratinocytes in laboratory for coverage of burn wounds have been in practice for several decades. Keratinocytes have been known to be difficult cells to grow because of their limited proliferation, early differentiation, and frequent contamination with fibroblasts. Cultured epidermis for human use in burns was first proposed by Pickerill in 1951[3] and in 1956. Basset, Evans, and Earle[4] also proposed that epidermal cell culture in massive quantities could provide a solution for wound closure in burns. Since then, efforts have been made to develop techniques for growing the transplantable epidermis (Karaseck, 1968)[5] in vitro. The importance of fibroblasts in epidermal

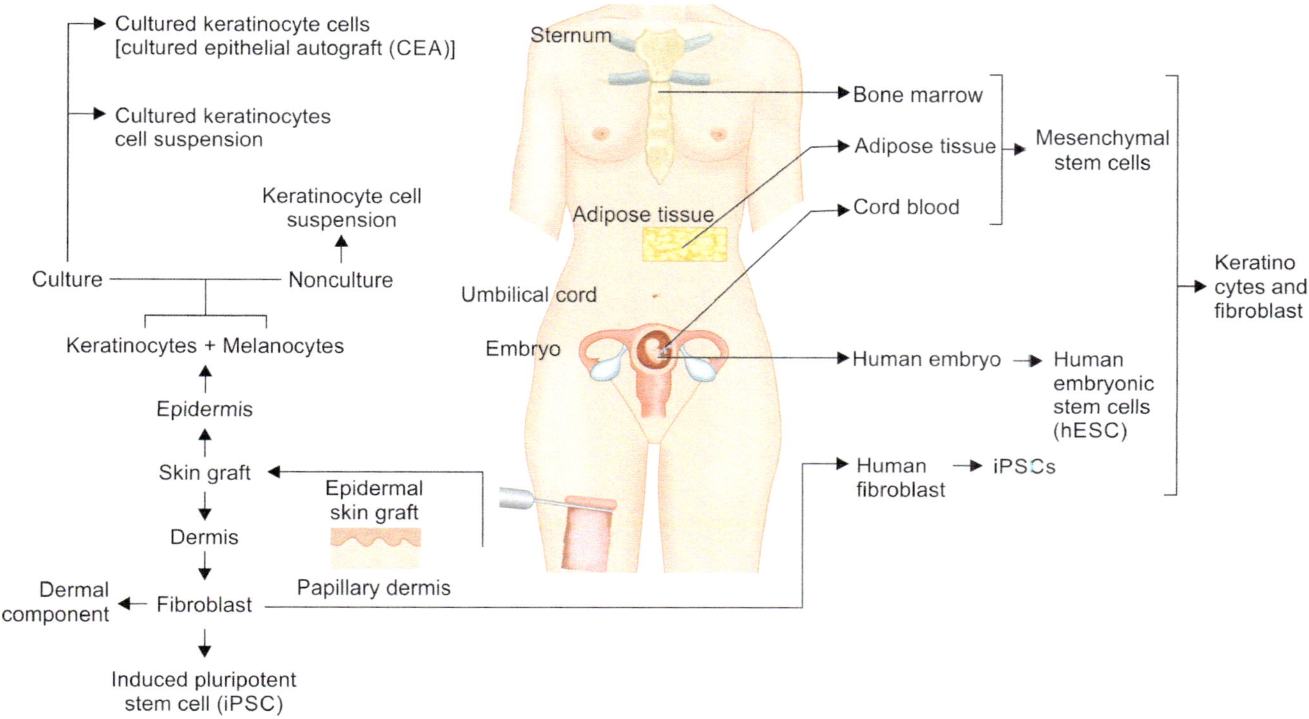

FLOWCHART 1: Source of cells for wound cover.

growth and differentiation has also been demonstrated. Later on, works by Green and associates (Rheinwald and Green, 1975[6] and Green et al., 1979[7]) demonstrated the techniques for serial cultivation and differentiation of keratinocytes and proposed logistical estimates for human application. The first clinical experience with cultured autologous epithelium was reported by O'Connor et al.[8] in 1981 and later by many other teams from all over the world (Gallico, 1985;[9] Cuono, 1986;[10] and DeLuca, 1992[11]). The biggest advantage of this technique is the enormous expansion potential of a small skin biopsy into a live-cultured epithelium ready for grafting large burn area in 3 weeks (Paddle-Ledinek et al., 1997[12]). Besides this, cultured epithelium has a wider application spectrum as in the treatment for skin ulcers (Hefton et al., 1986),[13] vitiligo patches (Plott et al. and Lontz et al., 1994),[14,15] and other skin defects (Green, 1991; Hafemann et al., 1994).[16,17] Human epidermal keratinocytes have been shown to grow from small biopsy samples of a patient by use of co-culture methods. They proliferate and form thin and multilayered epidermal sheets that have been used to resurface severely burned tissues. After transplantation, these epidermal sheets or CEAs form an organized epidermis and re-establish epidermal coverage, with formation of a new connective tissue or a neodermis beneath the new epidermis.

Autologous Keratinocyte Culture

It is a highly technical and skilled procedure requiring a sophisticated tissue culture laboratory. Briefly, it has the following components.

Patient Selection

Patients with extensive burns, generally taken as > 50% total body surface area (TBSA) burnt with majority being third-degree, in whom the raw areas exceed the available donor sites, are the ones suitable for this procedure. Patients having cutaneous tuberculosis, acquired immunodeficiency syndrome (AIDS) or hepatitis B are not suitable candidates for culture. Age is no contraindication. However, an elderly with a major medical problem is a definite contraindication as they compromise the prognosis. Inhalational injury is also not a contraindication.

Biopsy

There should be a minimum delay between the burn injury and the plating of keratinocytes. Preferably, it should be < 48 hours following burns. If it is delayed beyond 48 hours, there is usually a bacterial contamination of the skin requiring antibiotic treatment of the biopsy in vitro before processing. A split thickness skin biopsy of about 1–5 cm^2 is harvested with all aseptic and antiseptic precautions from a suitable unburnt site of the patient as soon as the patient is admitted to a burn center. The removed skin piece is transferred to tissue culture medium with antibiotics.

Keratinocyte Isolation

The harvested skin is thoroughly washed off the medium and subjected to differential trypsinization. The separated epidermal component is centrifuged and cell suspension is obtained.

Technique of Culture

The basic procedure for culture described by Green et al. (1979)[7,16] is followed at majority of centres. It is now a routine to culture keratinocytes on feeder layers to obtain sufficient cultured epithelium sheets. This feeder layer usually consists of fibroblasts which are either locally irradiated or pretreated with mitomycin. Usually, murine fibroblast line and normal human fibroblast are used as they allow similar growth rate of keratinocytes.

The isolated keratinocytes are seeded on to plastic Petri dishes/culture flasks containing mitomycin C treated mouse fibroblast 3T3 cells. The 3T3 cells are attenuated by treating with mitomycin C and frozen in liquid nitrogen and when required they are thawed, counted, and plated. The keratinocytes are grown in 3:1 mixture of Dulbecco's modified Eagle's medium supplemented (DMEM) with Hams F12 medium, 0.4 mg/mL of hydrocortisone, insulin, 5 mg/mL of transferrin, 8×10^{-4} mmol/L adenine, 2×10^{-2} mmol/L tri-iodothyronine, 10^{-10} mmol/L cholera toxin, antibiotics and 10% fetal calf serum. The cultures are incubated at 37°C in humidified atmosphere with 5% CO_2. After 3 days in culture, 10 ng/mL of human epidermal growth factor (EGF) is added to the medium. EGF acts when the differentiation and stratification begin in the center of the colonies and it promotes the migration of keratinocytes to the periphery. Cholera toxin and cyclic—AMP activators also increase the cellular growth rate. Once a good primary culture is established the keratinocytes are passaged "*n*" number of times depending upon the required graft area.

The keratinocytes adhere to the extracellular matrix synthesized by the irradiated/treated fibroblasts and produce three types of clones: (1) holoclones, (2) meroclones, and (3) paraclones. The basal cells are considered as stem cells and grow as holoclones and have the maximum growth potential allowing 5-6 subcultures. Suprabasal cells produce paraclones and have the lowest growth potential. During the cell culture, the holoclones progressively become meroclones and paraclones. As a result, only second and third passages are used for grafting. Each colony of the cultured cells expands by the peripheral cells dividing and moving outward. After 8–10 days when cultures are nearly confluent, all the cultures are seeded/reseeded with attenuated 3T3 cells.

Attempts have been made to avoid use of xenogeneic culture media for keratinocyte multiplication. Human fibroblast can replace murine fibroblast.[18] Replacement of fetal bovine serum is still under process[19] and may take some time for adoption.[20] The cultures are maintained by the same conditions until confluence and differentiation into multicellular epithelium is obtained **(Figs. 1 and 2)**. The epithelium is enzymatically detached from the culture

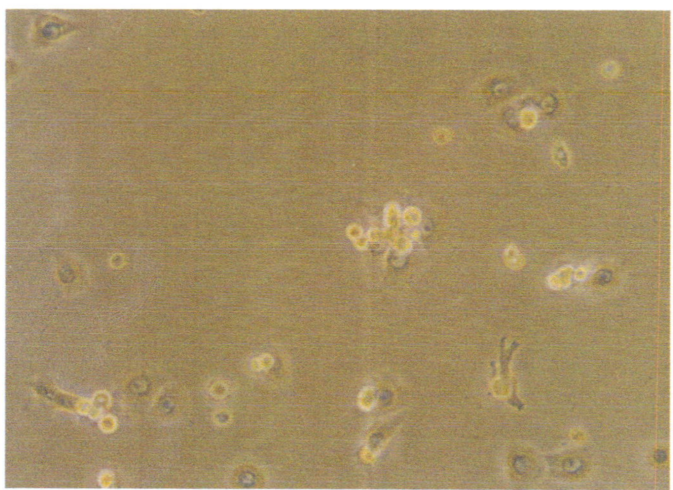

FIG. 1: Cell suspension of keratinocyte.

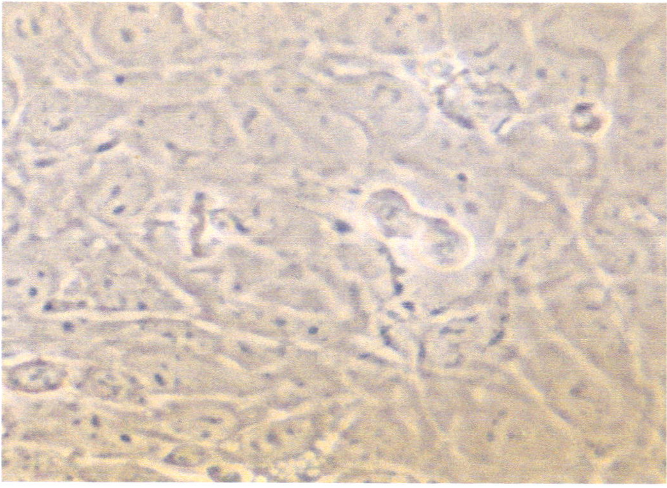

FIG. 2: Confluent keratinocyte on culture.

flask or dish by Dispase and rinsed in PBS. The epidermis is taken on to vaseline gauze of smaller mesh size by preserving the orientation of the graft in such a way that the basal cells are applied on to the wound bed **(Figs. 3 to 5)**. CEAs usually take about 2–3 weeks' time. The detached epithelium is assessed for cell viability (Green et al., 1979).[7]

During this intervening period when the keratinocytes are being cultured, the patient's wounds are serially debrided to remove all the dead tissues after the patient's general condition stabilizes, usually after the 3rd day post burn. The excision is done every 2–3 days and can vary from tangential to fascial depending on the depth of burns. The excised areas are covered with a variety of dermal skin substitutes available commercially or by cadaveric homograft.

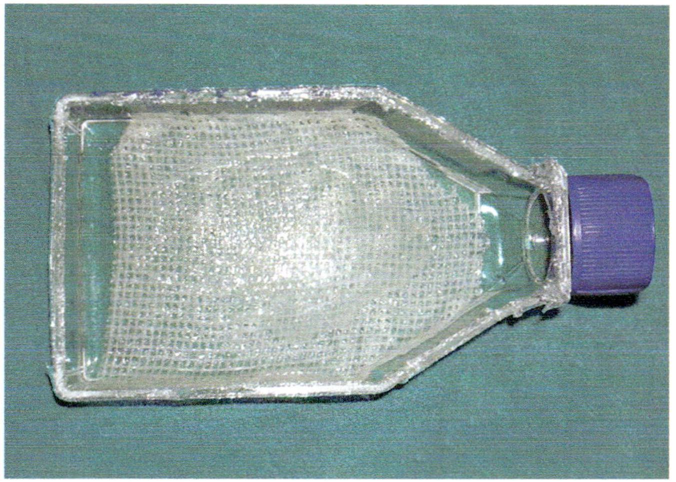

FIG. 3: Sheet of cultured keratinocytes on paraffin gauze before transfer.

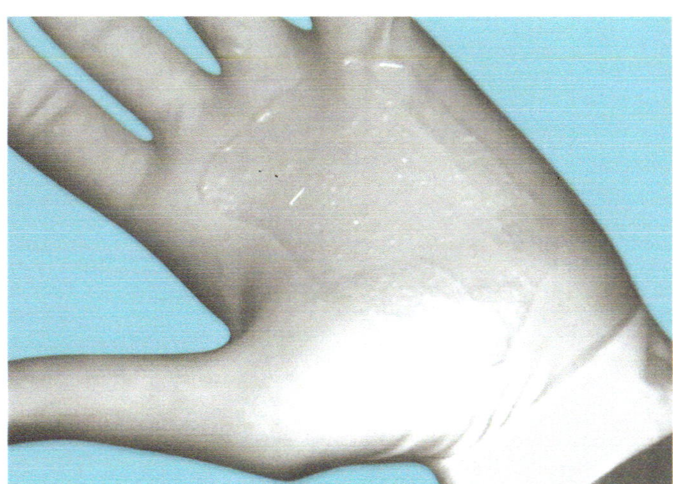

FIG. 4: Cultured keratinocyte sheet spread out on hand.

The cultured graft material is transported in aseptic conditions in petri dishes containing DMEM under 5% CO_2 to the operation theater, where the patient is prepared for transplantation under aseptic condition.

There are reports on use of dermal equivalents with different compositions along with keratinocytes.[21-24] Even though they do increase the possibility of graft "take", the high cost of these materials precludes their use for extensively burned patients who would require a large skin resurfacing in a short period of time. There have also been a lot of studies on using acellular fibrin gels as a biological support medium for keratinocyte cultures.[25] It has been observed that the keratinocytes cultured on fibrin gels are easier to handle and can be easily detached when prepared without using any enzymes so that the continuity of the layer of cells is preserved as use of enzymes reduces the adhesion potential of the cells.[26] Also, this method reduces the culture time to 15 days for producing sheet grafts.

Grafting Procedure and Postgrafting Care

The grafting is carried out as soon as the cultured graft material arrives in the operation theatre (OT). The graft material with carrier gauze is applied on to the wound bed after debridement without friction, air bubbles, and hematoma formation underneath the graft **(Figs. 6 to 8)**. The carrier gauze is covered with saline-soaked gauze followed by thick and dry gauze dressing. The first dressing change is done after 5 days and every 2 days thereafter. The carrier gauze is removed between day 6 and 8. The rest of the management is same as that routinely followed for skin grafting. Limitation of CEAs for full thickness loss is the failure of this approach to reconstitute dermal layer. Epidermal replacement also

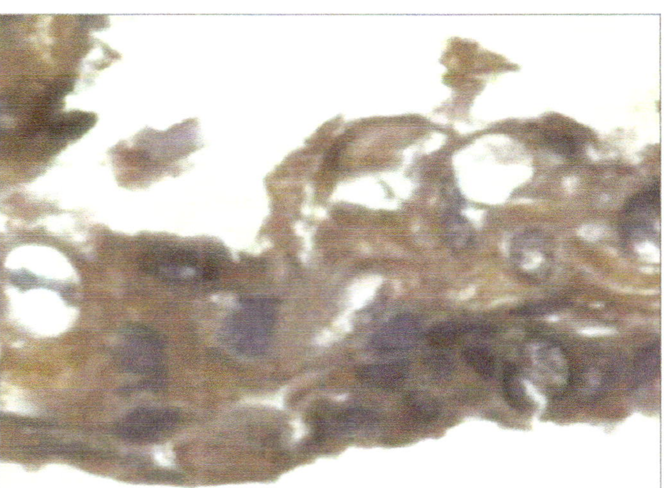

FIG. 5: Multilayer-cultured keratinocyte under high-power of magnification.

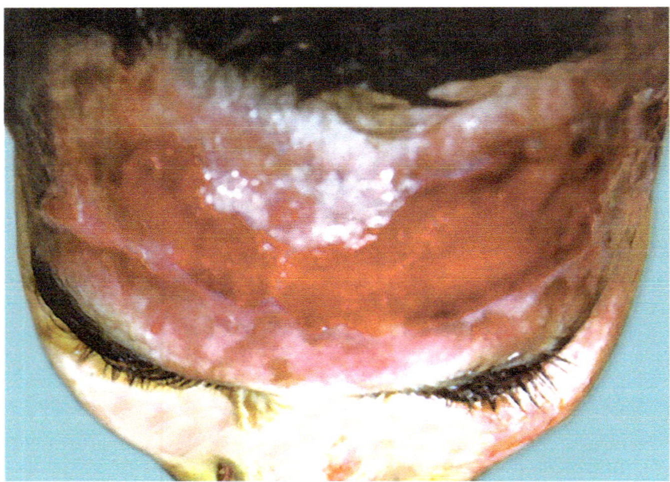

FIG. 6: Burn wound on forehead—preoperative.

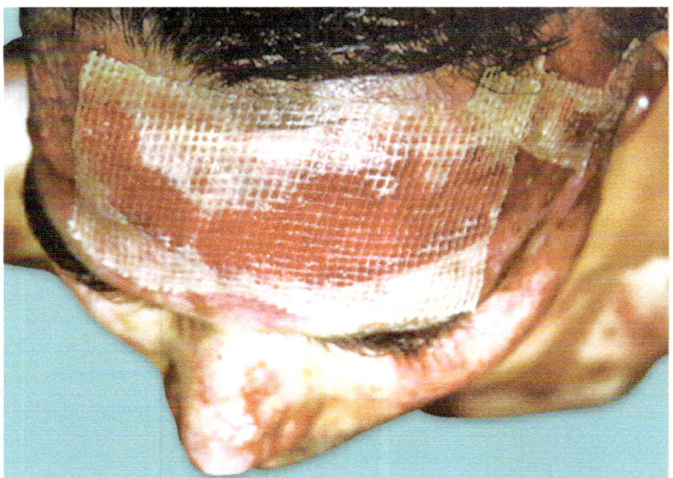

FIG. 7: Burn wound on forehead covered with cultured keratinocyte sheet.

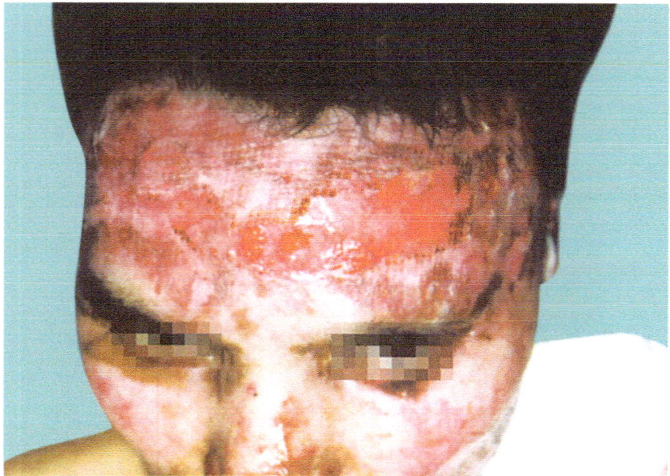

FIG. 8: Healed burn wound on forehead covered with cultured keratinocyte sheet after 2 weeks of application.

ignores the fundamental importance of the dermis in providing the skin with its integrity and durability. Clinical problems of poor durability, scarring and wound contraction are often encountered. Graft "take" can be improved by placing cultured keratinocytes autografts on a pregrafted cadaver dermis.

Disadvantages

Many of the drawbacks associated with cultured keratinocyte autografts can be attributed to the absence of dermal element. The keratinocyte culture contains no dermal matrix tissue and is placed on debrided full thickness burns that lack any dermal elements. Since it is the dermis which provides the elastic quality to the skin, healed wounds that lack dermis are thin and stiff. Cultured keratinocyte grafts placed directly on the muscles or subcutaneous tissues form the basement membrane very gradually. The basement membrane serves as an important attachment function and cultured epidermis lacks a well-formed basement membrane. It blisters and shears off easily. Graft fragility results in "delayed losses". However, even a partial "take" of epidermal cultured grafts can lead to complete wound healing by gradually progressing epithelialization from the islets. In the long term, it has been observed that these grafted areas tend to contract in the same manner as an autograft, though at the same time, the inflammatory reactions are weak and hypertrophic scarring rarely develops in these areas. The above drawbacks have limited their clinical applications and emphasize the need to develop keratinocyte culture methods on surfaces that mimic the human dermis or dermal equivalent.

Epidermal Allograft Culture

Several centers have used cultured keratinocyte allograft to treat burn wounds with varying success. The cultured epidermal allograft can be available at all times and are much less expensive to produce. However, they undergo rejection similar to cadaveric homograft. These cells work best as temporary coverage where a supply of autologous keratinocytes is available to replace the allograft after rejection. The concept is that it will prevent the desiccation of underlying wounds and there is release of unknown growth stimulating substances by the cells as they die which will stimulate native wound healing.

CULTURED KERATINOCYTE SUSPENSION

Cultured keratinocyte sheets usually take 3–4 weeks' time to reach transplantation stage in laboratory and are thereafter transplanted on burn wound. This time can be reduced to 5–7 days, if instead of sheets, subconfluent keratinocytes grown on polymer material are used for wound resurfacing.[27-30] Initial process of separation of keratinocyte and culture is same as described above. Cells are removed from culture flask just before single layer sheet is formed. The subconfluent keratinocytes can also be transferred to dermal substitute. The suspension can also be used with wide meshed auto- or allograft and can also be directly sprayed on wound. Large surface area of wound can be covered by the cell suspension/spray. Application of cultured keratinocyte on wound surface helps in reformation of organized epidermal structure.[31].

NONCULTURED KERATINOCYTE SUSPENSION

Culturing of keratinocyte requires cell culture laboratory facility and special transportation facility from laboratory to the hospital. Now it is possible to make the keratinocyte suspension at the site without the need of specialized laboratory. Epidermis from small piece of skin is separated from dermis by enzymes and cell suspension of keratinocyte, melanocyte, and Langerhans cell is made with in short time for immediate application.[32] The suspension can be sprayed on the wound directly, or sprayed on wide meshed skin autograft. For rapid epithelialization, the cell suspension can be used in 1:80–100 expansion ratio.[33] Due to presence of melanocytes in suspension, the problem of skin hypopigmentation is also reduced and it can also be used for treatment of vitiligo depigmentation.[34-36] Devices to make keratinocyte suspension are now commercially available.

DERMAL SUBSTITUTE

Dermis is deeper layer of skin. Epidermis is securely connected with dermis by basement membrane. Fibroblasts are main cells which produce extracellular matrix like collagen, elastin fibers, proteoglycans, and aminoglycans. Unlike epidermis, dermis does not regenerate. It heals by fibrosis and scar formation. CEA sheets lack the mechanical strength which normal skin requires in day-to-day activity. Due to lack of dermal component, breakdown of epithelial sheets is very common. Dermal substitute containing biodegradable polymer scaffolding provides the much-needed support to CEA. Integra® and Matriderm® are few commercial products available. Different cell line can be seeded into them and applied to wound to simulate the natural skin appearance and function.

MESENCHYMAL STEM CELLS

Mesenchymal stem cells (MSCs) are obtained from autogenous or allogenic sources such as umbilical cord, cord blood cells, bone marrow, adipose tissue, and dermis.[37-39] These are pluripotent cells and can be modified into different cells lines like keratinocytes and sweat glands.[40,41] These cells are also capable of producing antifibrotic factors which can modulate hypertrophic scarring.[42] MSCs produce large variety of biofactors which are very helpful in wound healing[40,41,43-45] and tissue regeneration. These cells have shown great potential in vivo and large clinical trials are needed for their widespread use.

INDUCED PLURIPOTENT STEM CELLS

Human embryonic stem cells (hESCs) are obtained from human embryos and are known for their immense capability to differentiate into large variety of transplantable cell lines. These cells can be induced to differentiate into keratinocyte and multilayered epidermis[18,46-49] and fibroblast[50] in vitro. There are ethical issues involved in the sourcing of these cells from human embryos and their alternative has been found. Dermal fibroblast cells harvested from human adult can be induced, by using complex retroviral system in laboratory, to become pluripotent cells capable of producing different cell lines. Cells generated from this modulation are very similar to the human embryonic stem cells.[51]

SUMMARY

Regeneration and repair of damaged tissue by cell therapy is a new concept of wound healing. Future of cell therapy is very promising. When Rheinwald and Green described the cultivation of strains of human epidermal keratinocytes with the formation of colonies of these cells from one single cell, there were claims by scientists that it had revolutionized the burn care since it provided quick and easy cover of burn wounds following excision. Though it was thought that autologous keratinocyte culture was a boon for coverage of an extensively burnt patient, but it is not universally accepted because of many of the imperfections associated with it, which are mainly unstable wound coverage, high cost, time consuming and sophisticated technology. The absence of dermal component produces frequent disruptions of overlying epithelium. Therefore, efforts to find suitable dermal component to be used along with epidermal cells started and limitations of this technology were overcome by further research, improving acceptability of the dermal substitutes manifold.

With rapid development in cell bioengineering, it is expected that in near future there will be no shortage of biocellular wound cover material for clinical application. The survival rate of extensive burn patient will improve considerably by use of laboratory produced wound cover products. At the same time the concept of tissue engineering using "stem cells" is being explored but the full potential of stem cells has not yet been fully exploited. If successful, it would have a dramatic impact on burn wound care and it may even take over the skin culture in near future. It is possible that the use of autologous split skin graft for wound cover may be consigned to the history books in the distant future.

REFERENCES

1. Li Z, Maitz P. Cell therapy for severe burn wound healing. Burns Trauma. 2018;6:13.
2. Horst BT, Chouhan G, Moiemen NS, Grover LM. Advances in keratinocyte delivery in burn wound care. Advan Drug Deliv Rev. 2018;123:13.
3. Pickeril HP. On the possibility of establishing skin banks. Br J Plast Surg. 1951;4:157-65.
4. Basset C, Evans V, Earle W. Characteristics and potentials of long term culture of human skin. Plast Reconstr Surg. 1956;17:421-9.
5. Karaseck MA. Growth and differentiation of transplanted epithelial cell cultures. J Invest Dermatol. 1968;51:247-52.
6. Rheinwald JG, Green H. Serial cultivation of human epidermal Keratinocytes: The formation of keratinizing colonies from single cells. Cell. 1975;6:331-44.
7. Green H, Kehinde O, Thomas J. Growth of cultured human epidermal cells into multiple epithelial suitable for grafting. Proc Natl Acad Sci USA. 1979;76:5665-8.
8. O'Connor NE, Mulliken JB, Banks-Schlegel SB, Kehinde O, Green H. Grafting of burns with cultured epithelium prepared from autologus epidermal cells. Lancet. 1981;1:75-8.
9. Gallico GG 3rd, O'Connor NE, Compton CC, Kehinde O, Green H. Permanent coverage of large burn wounds with autologus cultured human epithelium. N Engl J Med. 1985;311:448-51.
10. Cuono C, Langdon R, Mc Guire J. Use of cultured epidermal autografts and dermal allografts as skin replacement after burn injury. Lancet. 1986;1:1123-4.
11. De Luca M, Bondanza S, Cancedda R, Tamisani AM, Di Noto C, Muller L, et al. Permanent coverage of full thickness burns with autologus cultured epidermis and re-epithelialization of partial thickness lesions induced by allogenic cultured epidermis: A multicentre study in the treatment of children. Burns. 1992;88:S16-9.
12. Paddle-Ledinek JE, Cruickshank DG, Masterton JP. Skin replacement by cultured Keratinocytes grafts: An Australian experience. Burns. 1997;86:204-11.
13. Hefton JM, Caldevell D, Bizoes DG, Balin AK, Carter DM. Grafting skin ulcers with cultured autologous epidermal cells. J Am Acad Dermatol. 1986;14:399-405.
14. Plott RT, Brysk MM, Newton RC, Raimer SS, Rajaraman S. A surgical treatment for vitilgo: Autologus cultured epithelial grafts. J Dermatol Surg Oncol. 1989;15:1161-6.
15. Lontz W, Olsson MJ, Moellmann G, Lerner AB. Pigment cell transplantation for treatment of vitiligo: A Progress report. J Am Acad Dermatol. 1994;30:591-7.
16. Green H. Cultured cells for treatment of diseased. Sci. Amer. 1991;11:64-70.
17. Hefemann B, Heltich R, Ennslen S, Kowol B, Zuhlke A, Ebert R, et al. Treatment of skin defects using suspensions of in vitro cultured keratinocytes. Burns. 1994;20:168-72.
18. Kidwai FK, Liu H, Toh WS, Fu X, Jokhun DS, Movahednia MM, et al. Differentiation of human embryonic stem cells into clinically amenable keratinocytes in an autogenic environment. J Investig Dermatol. 2013;133:618-28.
19. Jubin K, Martin Y, Lawrence-Watt DJ, Sharpe JR. A fully autologous co-culture system utilising non-irradiated autologous fibroblasts to support the expansion of human keratinocytes for clinical use. Cytotechnology. 2011;63:655-62.
20. Lamb R, Ambler CA. Keratinocytes Propagated in Serum-Free, Feeder-Free Culture Conditions Fail to Form Stratified Epidermis in a Reconstituted Skin Model. PLoS One. 2013;8:e52494.
21. Kamolz LP, Luegmair M, Wick N, Eisenbock B, Burjak S, Koller R, et al. The Vietnamese culture method: cultured human epithelium obtained on a dermal matrix based on fibroblast containing fibrin glue gels. Burns. 2005;31:25-9.
22. Maruguchi T, Maruguchi Y, Suzuki S, Matsuda K, Toda K, Isshiki N. A new skin equivalent: keratinocytes proliferated and differentiated on collagen sponge containing fibroblast. Plast Recons Surg. 1994;93:537-44.
23. Boyce S, Hansbrough J. Biologic attachment, grow and differentiation of cultured human epidermal keratinocytes on a graftable collagen and chondroitin-6-sulphats substrate. Surgery. 1988;103:421-31.
24. Saintigny G, Bonnard M, Damour O, Collombel C. Reconstruction of epidermis on a chitosan cross linked collagen–GAG lattice: effect of fibroblast. Acta Dermatol Venerol. 1993;73:175-80.
25. Kaiser HW, Stark GB, Kopp J, Balcerkiewicz A, Spilker G, Kreysel HW. Cultured autologous keratinocytes in fibrin glue suspension, exclusively and combined with STS–allograft (preliminary clinical and histological report of a new technique). Burns. 1994;20:23-9.
26. Currie LJ, Sharpe JR, Martin R. The use of fibrin glue in skin grafts and tissue engineered skin replacements: a review. Plast Reconstr Surg. 2001;108:1713-26.
27. Tay AG, Phan TT, See P, Teik LS, Song C. Cultured subconfluent keratinocytes on wound polymer dressings in the treatment of burns and chronic wounds. Wounds. 2000;12:123-9.
28. Chua AW, Ma DR, Song IC, Phan TT, Lee ST, Song C. In vitro evaluation of fibrin mat and Tegaderm wound dressing for the delivery of keratinocytes—implications of their use to treat burns. Burns. 2008;34:175-80.
29. Burt AM, Clarke JA. Transfer of autologous keratinocytes grown on a polymer reduces time taken from biopsy to graft. Ann Burns Fire Disast. 1997;10.

30. Myers SR, Partha VN, Soranzo C, Price RD, Navsaria HA. Hyalomatrix: a temporary epidermal barrier, hyaluronan delivery, and neodermis induction system for keratinocyte stem cell therapy. Tissue Eng. 2007;13:2733-41.
31. Fei X, Seah CS, Lee ST. Human keratinocyte cell culture for the burns patients—a preliminary report. Ann Acad Med Singap. 1991;20:493-7.
32. Gerlach JC, Johnen C, Ottomann C, Bräutigam K, Plettig J, Belfekroun C, et al. Method for Autologous Single Skin Cell Isolation for Regenerative Cell Spray Transplantation with Non-Cultured Cells. Int J Artif Organs. 2011;34(3):271-9.
33. Esteban-Vives R, Young MT, Zhu T, Beiriger J, Pekor C, Ziembicki J, et al. Calculations for reproducible autologous skin cell-spray grafting. Burns. 2016;42:1756-65.
34. Paul M. Autologous non-cultured basal cell-enriched epidermal cell suspension transplantation in vitiligo: Indian experience. J Cutan Aesthet Surg. 2011;4:23-8.
35. Stoner ML, Wood FM. The treatment of hypopigmented lesions with cultured epithelial autograft. J Burn Care Rehabil. 2000;21:50-4, 114.
36. van Geel N, Ongenae K, De Mil M, Haeghen YV, Vervaet C, Naeyaert JM. Double-blind placebo-controlled study of autologous transplanted epidermal cell suspensions for repigmenting vitiligo. Arch Dermatol. 2004;140:1203-8.
37. Ding D, Shyu W, Lin S. Mesenchymal stem cells. Cell Transpl. 2011;20:5-14.
38. Liao Y, Itoh M, Yang A, Zhu H, Roberts S, Highet AM, et al. Human cord blood-derived unrestricted somatic stem cells promote wound healing and have therapeutic potential for patients with recessive dystrophic epidermolysis bullosa. Cell Transplant. 2014;23:303-17.
39. Duscher D, Barrera J, Wong VW, Maan ZN, Whittam AJ, Januszyk M, et al. Stem cells in wound healing: the future of regenerative medicine? Gerontology. 2016;62:216-25.
40. Pittenger MF, Mackay AM, Beck SC, Jaiswal RK, Douglas R, Mosca JD, et al. Multilineage potential of adult human mesenchymal stem cells. Science. 1999;284:143-7.
41. Sasaki M, Abe R, Fujita Y, Ando S, Inokuma D, Shimizu H. Mesenchymal stem cells are recruited into wounded skin and contribute to wound repair by transdifferentiation into multiple skin cell type. J Immunol. 2008;180:2581-7.
42. Foubert P, Zafra D, Liu M, Fajoria R, Gutierrez D, Tenenhaus M, et al. Autologous adipose-derived regenerative cell therapy modulates development of hypertrophic scarring in a red Duroc porcine model. Stem Cell Res Ther. 2017;8:261.
43. Ren G, Zhang L, Zhao X, Xu G, Zhang Y, Roberts AI, et al. Mesenchymal stem cell-mediated immunosuppression occurs via concerted action of chemokines and nitric oxide. Cell Stem Cell. 2008;2:141-50.
44. Le Blanc K, Frassoni F, Ball L, Locatelli F, Roelofs H, Lewis I, et al. Mesenchymal stem cells for treatment of steroid-resistant, severe, acute graft-versus-host disease: a phase II study. Lancet. 2008;371:1579-86.
45. Kwon HM, Hur SM, Park KY, Kim CK, Kim YM, Kim HS, et al. Multiple paracrine factors secreted by mesenchymal stem cells contribute to angiogenesis. Vasc Pharmacol. 2014;63: 19-28.
46. Guenou H, Nissan X, Larcher F, Feteira J, Lemaitre G, Saidani M, et al. Human embryonic stem-cell derivatives for full reconstruction of the pluristratified epidermis: a preclinical study. Lancet. 2009;374:1745-53.
47. Ji L, Allen-Hoffmann BL, de Pablo JJ, Palecek SP. Generation and differentiation of human embryonic stem cell-derived keratinocyte precursors. Tissue Eng. 2006;12:665-79.
48. Green H, Easley K, Iuchi S. Marker succession during the development of keratinocytes from cultured human embryonic stem cells. Proc Natl Acad Sci USA. 2003;100:15625-30.
49. Bilousova G, Chen J, Roop DR. Differentiation of mouse induced pluripotent stem cells into a multipotent keratinocyte lineage. J Invest Dermatol. 2011;131:857-64.
50. Shamis Y, Hewitt KJ, Carlson MW, Margvelashvilli M, Dong S, Kuo CK, et al. Fibroblasts derived from human embryonic stem cells direct development and repair of 3D human skin equivalents. Stem Cell Res Ther. 2011;2:10.
51. Itoh M, Umegaki-Arao N, Guo Z, Liu L, Higgins CA, Christiano AM. Generation of 3D skin equivalents fully reconstituted from human induced pluripotent stem cells(iPSCs). PLoS One. 2013;8:e77673.

CHAPTER

20

Burn Wound Infection

VK Tiwari, Sujata Sarabahi, Anoop S

INTRODUCTION

The management of patients with extensive burns has improved drastically over the years, greatly improving their survival rate. Yet microbial infections and resultant complications are the most important factors in burns mortality. Extensively burnt patients are immunocompromised and far more susceptible to infection than normal individuals despite the use of systemic and topical antimicrobials. Burn wounds at the onset are considered sterile. The amount of heat sufficient to cause damage to skin kills the microorganisms in and around the burnt area as well. Colonization by patient's normal skin flora, i.e., *Staphylococcus aureus* and *Streptococcus pyogenes* occurs within 48 hours following a burn injury as these organisms are located deep within the sweat glands and hair follicles surviving the thermal insult. Subsequent contamination of wound either by endogenous (gut flora) or by exogenous sources occurs shortly thereafter, usually within 5–7 days.[1-3] Blisters and eschar represent superficial and deep burn respectively and are part of dead and devitalized tissue and they are potential sites for colonization and bacterial invasion. The pattern of bacterial and fungal colonization is related in part to the topical or systemic antibiotic(s) used for prophylaxis and treatment of infection and varies with the area burnt. For example, burns of lower limbs are more frequently contaminated with enteric flora.

ETIOPATHOGENESIS OF BURN WOUND INFECTION

Simple colonization of the burned surface does not necessarily indicate infection but it can be dangerous as it can be followed by rapid proliferation of bacteria which eventually invade healthy tissues. Burn wound colonization may be diagnosed when bacteria are present at low concentrations [$<10^5$ colony-forming units (CFU)] on the wound's surface. No surrounding erythema or cellulitis is evident, but deterioration of the wound surface can be observed. Infection is defined as the presence of high concentrations ($>10^5$ organisms/g of tissue) of bacteria in the burn wound and scab. However, no evidence exists that the infection is invasive. The presence of cellulitis is the foundation of the clinical diagnosis. Burn wound cellulitis can be observed when the area of erythema extends beyond what would be expected for the injury alone.[4] With tissue invasion, local arteritis and thrombosis occur producing characteristic satellite lesions around the burn wound. Septic emboli eventually also enter the bloodstream producing abscesses in the liver, kidney, and brain. The blood-borne bacterial dissemination can be documented through positive blood cultures although this is true for gram-positive bacteria only. The absence of bacteria in blood cultures with clinical signs of sepsis indicates gram-negative toxemia. This is due to exotoxins liberated from the primary site of infection rather than the circulating bacteria per se.[5]

Older literature emphasized on *Streptococcus* and *Staphylococcus* as the most commonly isolated organisms in the burn wound. However, the frequency of these infections was gradually exceeded by gram-negative infections including those due to *Pseudomonas*, *Escherichia coli*, *Klebsiella*, *Enterobacter*, *Citrobacter*, *Proteus*, and *Bacteroides*.[6] With increasing use of topical and systemic antimicrobial agents over the past five decades, the fungal infection of burn wounds is becoming a growing problem and even viral infections have also gained significance. *Staphylococcus aureus*, especially MRSA (methicillin-resistant *Staphylococcus aureus*), is again emerging as the most common cause of burn wound infection (BWI) in many centers at present.[7-10]

Pseudomonas aeruginosa has been reported to be the second most frequent agent followed by *Acinetobacter*, *Klebsiella*, etc. One of the most dangerous aspects of post-burn infection by *Pseudomonas* and *Acinetobacter* species is the multidrug resistance (MDR) of these organisms which is fast becoming a therapeutic problem. Even the bacteremia caused by gram-negative organisms is associated with a high mortality in burn patients.[11,12]

According to a recent study, *Staphylococcus aureus* accounted for the largest proportion, followed by *Staphylococcus epidermidis*, *Enterococcus faecalis*, and *Staphylococcus haemolyticus* among the gram-positive organisms. *Klebsiella pneumoniae* and *Acinetobacter baumannii* ranked first among the gram-negative bacteria, followed by *Pseudomonas aeruginosa*.[13]

Acinetobacter species is gaining concern in burn infections because of increased resistance to anti-microbials. The increased incidence can be attributed to carriage on human skin, particularly in tropical climate, longer hospitalization, and presence of intra-vascular lines for longer duration. Studies show resistance to majority of antibiotics including piperacillin tazobactam, ciprofloxacin, amikacin, gentamicin, etc. Although carbapenems are active against *Acinetobacter* strains, emergence of enzymatic and membrane-based mechanism of resistance hinders the clinical utility of this class of antimicrobials.[14]

The incidence of invasive infection depends on the type of organisms present in the eschar.[15,16] *Pseudomonas* produces enzymes and other metabolic products and has flagella which enhance their potential for invasion and rapid spread. On the other hand, gram-positive organisms form different sized microabscesses in the eschar and subcutaneous tissues but rarely invade more deeply. *Candida* species also rarely invades deeper tissues. On the other hand, filamentous fungi like *Aspergillus* are more aggressive invaders of the subcutaneous tissues.

The most distinct pathologic response in burn wound is demonstrated in *Pseudomonas* infection which evolves from intraeschar colonization to subeschar invasion. The diagnosis may be suspected when areas of hemorrhagic discoloration are seen in and around the burn wound though the actual infective focus may be hidden by the thick eschar. On histopathology of necrotic hemorrhagic tissues, it can be seen invaded by scores of bacilli. The reason for these lesions is attributed to vasculitis and effects of bacterial endotoxins. Typical colonization of bacilli seen in the walls of the blood vessels in case of *Pseudomonas* infection is far in excess of what is seen in infection with *Proteus* and other gram-negative bacteria.

A superficial wound infection caused by *P. aeruginosa* typically will have a characteristic yellow/green color and a malodorous fruity smell. This may become an invasive infection or ecthyma gangrenosum, causing blue-purplish "punched-out" lesions in the skin. This picture indicates local thrombosis of vessels and requires urgent debridement to remove the newly necrotic tissues.[4]

MICROORGANISMS AND THEIR SOURCES IN BURN WOUND CONTAMINATION

Microorganisms can contaminate a burn wound from either endogenous or exogenous sources.

- *Endogenous*—Bacterial source is patient's own body.
    - Patient's normal skin flora—*Streptococcus* and *Pseudomonas*
    - Upper respiratory tract—*Staphylococcus*
    - Fecal flora—*E. coli* and other enteric bacteria
- *Exogenous* can be from:
    - *Community-acquired infection*: This is caused by *Streptococcus* and other less virulent bacteria that are sensitive to first line of antibiotics.
    - *Hospital-acquired (nosocomial) infection*: Existing bacterial flora of ICU/Ward contaminates the burn wound. *Staphylococcus* (MRSA), *Pseudomonas*, *Acinetobacter*, and *Klebsiella* are the common organisms which are usually resistant to the first line of antibiotics. The nosocomial transmission of microorganisms to the burn wound occurs by transfer from the hands of healthcare personnel or through immersion hydrotherapy[17,18] or through contaminated surfaces such as patient's mattresses, blankets, etc.

The various routes for invasion of pathogens into the wound are as follows:

- *Burn wound*: The burn wound with its exudates and necrotic tissue makes an excellent nutrient medium which favors growth of microorganisms. Patients suffering from electrical burns with massive muscle necrosis, which produces an anaerobic environment, tend to get infected with *Clostridium tetani* and *Clostridium perfringens* and may manifest the disease frankly. With regular use of tetanus immunization in the pediatric age group and following trauma, the incidence of tetanus has now reduced greatly.
- *Pulmonary*: Infection of the lower respiratory tract is an important cause of death from sepsis in burns. This is common in patients with inhalational injury, especially those requiring endotracheal intubation or tracheostomy and patients who do not receive proper chest physiotherapy.
- *Indwelling cannulae*: Intravenous cannulations and venesections, if not carried out with proper aseptic and antiseptic precautions or if performed through

the burnt skin or if kept for a prolonged period of time, may lead to suppurative thrombophlebitis and multiple abscesses along the length of the vein. This is an important cause for sepsis as well as sudden thromboembolic deaths in burn patients.

- *Urinary tract*: Prolonged catheterization, which very often is unnecessary, can lead to urinary tract infection. However, prolonged catheterization may be imperative in children and female patients to prevent soilage of dressings on thighs and perineum.
- *Gastrointestinal tract*: Translocation of bacteria through the gut is a very frequent occurrence in burn patients who have not been resuscitated well and are hypovolemic for a long time after sustaining burns. This is due to the sustained splanchnic vasoconstriction leading to gut mucosal erosions and migration of bacteria and their toxins through the gut wall into the peritoneum. This is an important cause for sepsis in burn patients.
- *Miscellaneous*: Escharotomy incisions, burned areas which involve cartilage, e.g., the burns of pinna, are particularly susceptible to infection. Suppurative chondritis, endocarditis, and arthritis also form a focus of infection in a burn patient which can, in rare cases, lead to sepsis.

TYPES OF ORGANISMS IN BURN WOUND CONTAMINATION

From 1960 till date, *Pseudomonas aeruginosa* has remained the most common organism isolated from the burn wound. Prevalence of this organism is around 60% in most of the burn units. Average distribution of different microorganisms is given in **Table 1**.

TABLE 1: The various types of microorganisms isolated from burn wound, their incidence, and sensitivity in the authors' unit.

Type of organisms	Name	% incidence	Source	Antibiotic susceptibility	Remarks
Gram +ve cocci	*Staphylococcus* MSSA	1–2	Community acquired	Amoxicillin and cephalexin	• Present in burn wound of patients • Treated at other hospital for 5–7 days before coming to burns unit
	Staphylococcus MRSA	10–12	Nosocomial	Vancomycin and teicoplanin	Cause of fulminant sepsis in extensive burns
	Streptococcus haemolyticus	0.5–1	Endogenous	Crystalline penicillin	100% graft failure if present in burn wound
	Streptococcus faecalis	0.5–1	Endogenous	Crystalline penicillin	In immunocompromised extensive burns patient, can cause fulminant sepsis
Gram –ve bacilli	*Pseudomonas aeruginosa*	65–70	Nosocomial	• Beta-lactamase producing • Sensitive to cefoperazone + sulbactam and piperacillin + tazobactam ESBL sensitive to carbapenems (second generation)	Rapidly develops multidrug resistance by efflux pump mechanism
	Klebsiella	10–12	Nosocomial	Gr. 2 beta-lactamase and extended-spectrum beta-lactamase producing, sensitive to cefoperazone + sulbactam, piperacillin + tazobactam, amino glycosides and carbapenems (second generation)	More likely to cause fulminant lung infection
	Proteus	2–5	Nosocomial	Gr. 2 beta-lactamase producing, sensitive to amino glycosides, cefoperazone + sulbactam, piperacillin + tazobactam, carbapenems	Usually respond to proper timely intervention
	Acinetobacter	2–5	Nosocomial	ESBL producing, sensitive to carbapenems (also known as gram –ve bacilli equal to MRSA)	Fulminant pulmonary complication
Fungal infection	*Candida* species	50–60	Endogenous	Azoles, caspofungin	Mainly in patients on prolonged antibiotic combinations, TPN, diabetics

(ESBL: extended-spectrum β-lactamase; MRSA: methicillin-resistant *Staphylococcus aureus*; MSSA: methicillin-sensitive *Staphylococcus aureus*; TPN: total parenteral nutrition)

TERMINOLOGY USED IN BURN WOUND INFECTION

There are many terms used while defining different stages in BWI. They are as follows.

Colonization

Surface culture from burn wound shows presence of pathogenic organism and count is $<10^5$ organisms/g of surface tissue. This is also termed as supraeschar colonization. This supraeschar colonization through dead hair follicles may invade eschar tissue usually termed as noninvasive wound infection.

Noninvasive Wound Infection

Infection is limited to eschar and subeschar tissues. Bacterial count in eschar may be $>10^5$/g of tissue. Subeschar infection helps in early eschar separation. In extensive burns and low-resistance individuals, this subeschar colonization may lead to invasion of healthy tissues and BWI.

Burn Wound Infection

Invasion of normal nonburned tissues by microorganisms is known as BWI. Quantitative bacterial count is $>10^5$/g of tissue.

Bacteremia

Presence of viable bacteria in blood is known as bacteremia.

Septicemia

Systemic illness caused by the spread of microbes or their toxins via the bloodstream is known as septicemia.

Systemic Inflammatory Response Syndrome

If two of the following four signs are present, the patient is labeled as having systemic inflammatory response syndrome (SIRS).

1. Oral temperature is >38°C or is <36°C
2. Respiratory rate of >20 breaths/min or arterial partial pressure of carbon dioxide ($PaCO_2$) < 32 Torr
3. Heart rate > 90 beats/min
4. Total leukocytes count > 12,000/mm^3 or < 4,000/mm^3 or over 10% immature forms or bands

In the pediatric population, the definition is modified to a mandatory requirement of abnormal leukocyte count or temperature to establish the diagnosis, as abnormal heart rate and respiratory rates are more common in children.[19]

Sepsis

Systemic inflammatory response syndrome with proven microbial etiology in any patient is termed as sepsis.

Sepsis Syndrome

Sepsis and one more sign of organ dysfunction such as hypertension, metabolic acidosis, alteration of mental status, oliguria, acute respiratory distress syndrome (ARDS), or platelets count < 0.1 million/mm^3.

Multiple Organ Dysfunction Syndrome

It is dysfunction of more than one organ requiring intervention to maintain homeostasis like ventilatory support for ARDS and dialysis for renal failure, etc.

The microbial status of burn wound can be further classified according to the depth of involvement into:

Stage I is the stage of colonization:
- *Superficial colonization*: Organisms are present only on the superficial surface.
- *Microbial penetration*: Microorganisms invade the eschar.
- *Subeschar proliferation*: Microorganisms proliferate in subeschar space.

Stage II is the stage of invasion of viable tissue:
- *Microinvasion*: Microscopic foci of organism in viable tissue below burn wound
- *Generalized invasion*: Diffuse penetration into viable subcutaneous tissue
- *Microvascular invasion*: Organisms invade into burned blood vessels and lymphatics

IMMUNE PROFILE OF EXTENSIVELY BURNT PATIENT[20-26]

The natural resistance of human body to infection in any kind of wound is primarily a function of the innate immune system. Following burns, the innate immune system responds by stimulating localized and systemic inflammatory reaction. But in extensive burns, patients are usually immunocompromised due to:
- Alteration in the function of neutrophils, lymphocytes, and macrophages
- Alteration in immunoglobulin kinetics

This results in depression of both cellular and humoral immunity. As a result, the burn victim gets predisposed to infectious complications. The host response to thermal injury is mediated to some extent by arachidonic acid and cytokinin cascade and the combined effect of this cascade being release of various endotoxins, such as prostaglandin E_2 (PGE), thromboxane $A_2\alpha_2$-vasoconstrictor, and TNF (tumor necrosis factor). The alteration in the immune system has a combined effect of increasing the burn patient's exposure to pathogens and decreasing the natural defenses responsible for counteracting them. Because of impaired function of the neutrophils, natural killer cells, and macrophages, the body's immune system is unable to eradicate the pathogens to which the wounds are exposed. Thus, burn patients are more susceptible to wound infections, sepsis, and multiorgan failure. Even the reduction in levels of circulating immunoglobulins such as IgG and IgM has been associated with high BWI rate and mortality. Briefly, there is a marked diminution of serum IgG concentration, total and all subclasses. The maximum fall occurs at 2–3 days after injury when the mean concentrations of IgG, IgA, IgM, IgD, and IgE have been shown to be 30, 44, 49, 35, and 22% respectively of the level found in healthy controls. Their concentration returns to normal level after 19, 9, 7, 30, and 11 days, respectively.

CLINICAL FEATURES

Early diagnosis of burn wound infection can be made on the basis of local wound and systemic changes **(Figs. 1 to 3)**.

Local Signs of Burn Wound Infection

- Black or dark brown focal areas of discoloration
- Increasing eschars
- Increase in the depth of burn injury
- Increasing inflammation and edema in normal skin adjacent to burn margin
- Increased bleeding from granulation tissue during dressing
- Rashes or papule in skin surrounding burn wound and/or distant part of body

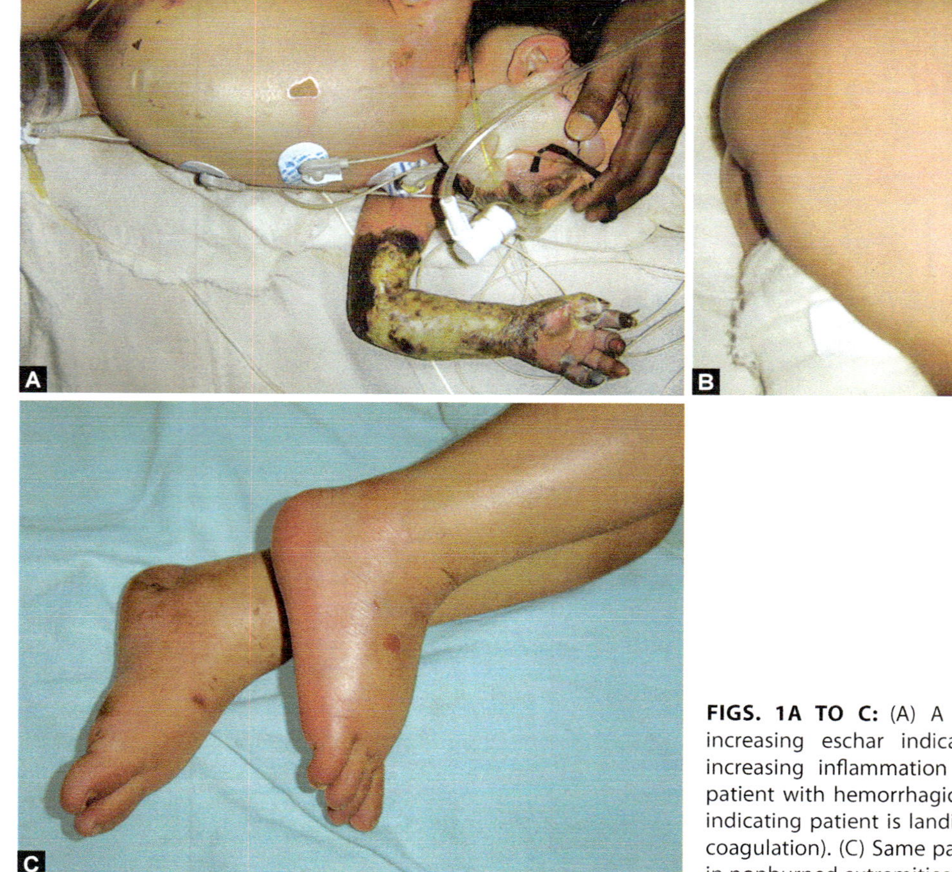

FIGS. 1A TO C: (A) A 2-year-old child with 20% burns with increasing eschar indicating increasing depth of burns with increasing inflammation and edema in normal skin. (B) Same patient with hemorrhagic patches with edema of uninvolved skin indicating patient is landing up in DIC (disseminated intravascular coagulation). (C) Same patient with rashes, papules, and erythema in nonburned extremities indicating invasive gram-negative sepsis.

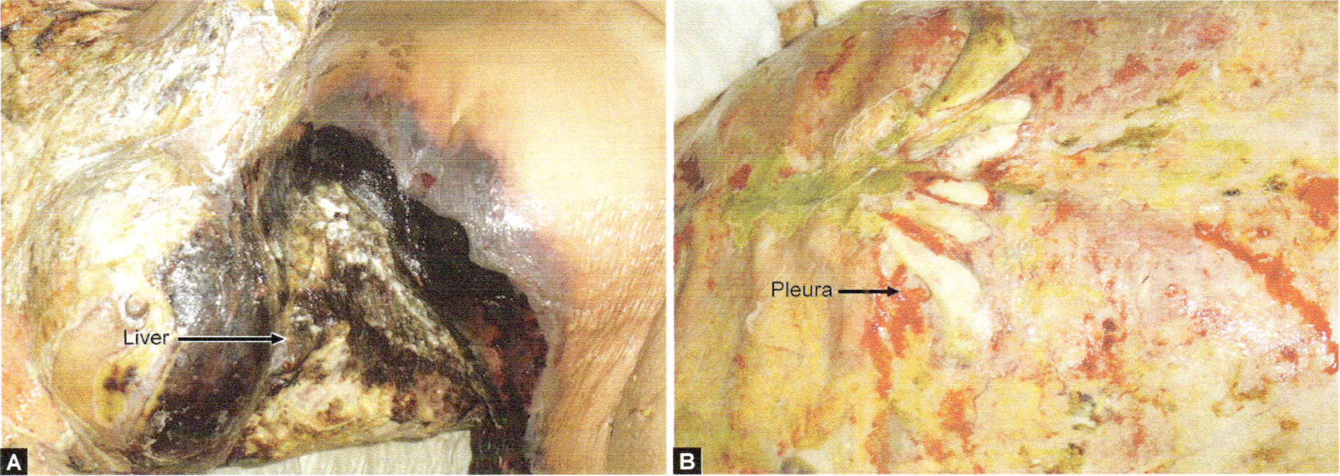

FIGS. 2A AND B: (A) Synergistic gangrene of abdominal wall following uncontrolled burn wound infection. The chest wall and abdominal muscles are totally necrosed which is likely to expose the underlying structures. (B) Neglected patient showing deepening of burn wound up to ribcage with exposed pleura.

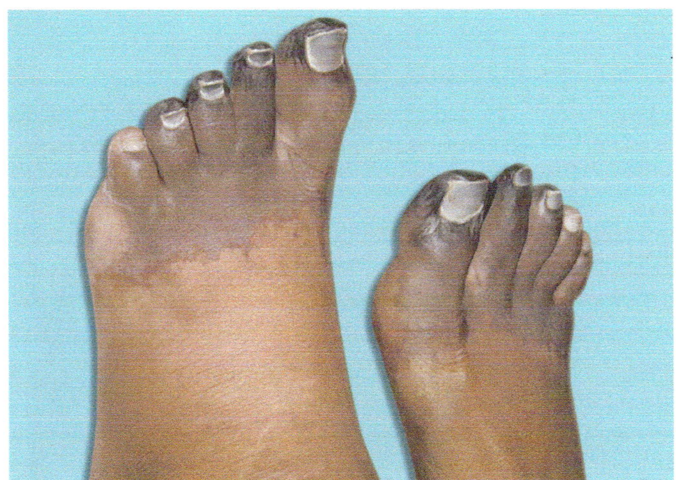

FIG. 3: Patient in gram-positive sepsis throwing septic emboli causing bilateral gangrenous changes in distal foot.

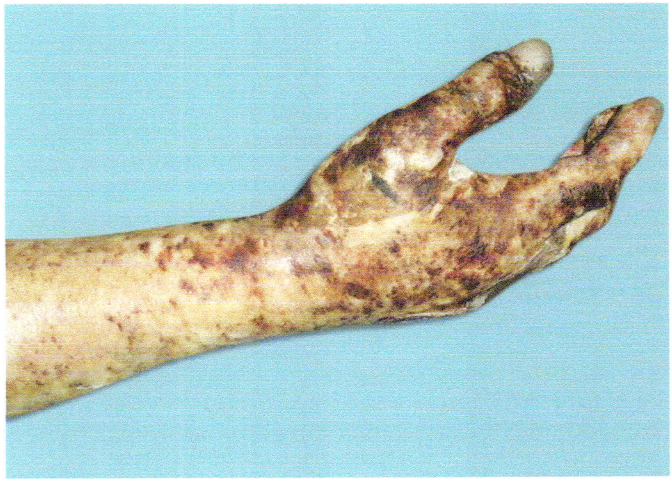

FIG. 4: Superficial burns converting to deep burns indicating burn wound infection—black areas of discoloration, thickening eschar.

Systemic Signs of Burn Wound Infection

- *Signs of gram-negative septicemia*: Rapid onset of symptoms within 8–12 hours characterized by hyperthermia (100–103°F), tachycardia, and tachypnea. Patient is well perfused with bounding pulse. Systolic blood pressure is initially normal or raised (high-output shock). Pulse pressure is usually varied as vasodilatation may reduce diastolic pressure to a considerably low limit. Later on, if sepsis remains untreated, systolic pressure also drops (low-output shock). Mental clouding and diarrhea are sometimes presenting symptoms of BWI leading to sepsis. Multiorgan failure in late stage may involve any system causing renal failure, paralytic ileus, and ARDS. Jaundice and disseminated intravascular coagulation (DIC) are very late manifestations and usually have very poor prognosis. Decrease in platelet counts is another diagnostic sign of beginning of sepsis.
- *Signs of gram-positive septicemia*: Symptoms are gradual and usually start with hyperpyrexia (temperature >105°F) and leukocytosis. Hypotension, paralytic ileus, and oliguria are common with initial gram-positive septicemia.

The most reliable clinical sign of an invasive BWI is the conversion of an area of partial thickness injury to full-thickness necrosis **(Fig. 4)**. Any change in wound appearance mandates immediate biopsy of the area for

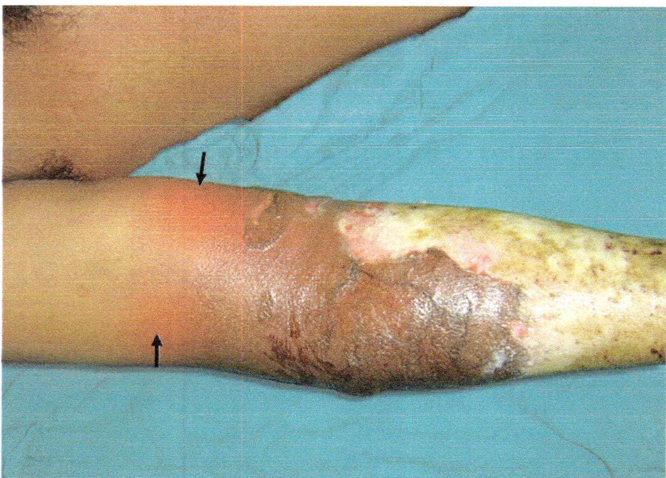

FIG. 5: Streptococcal burn wound infection with extending erythema into surrounding normal skin from burn wound margin.

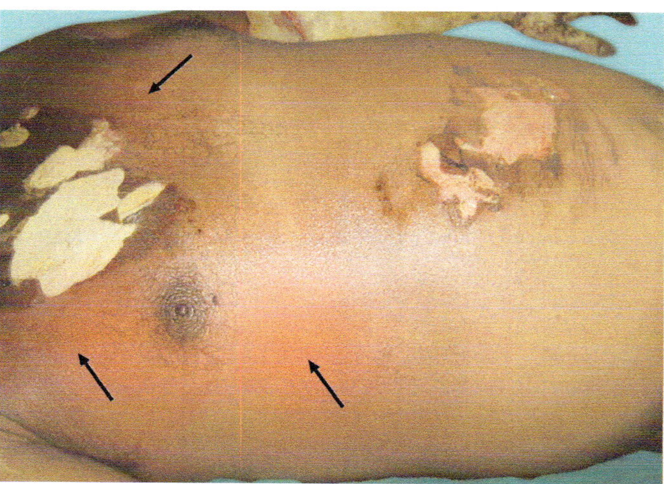

FIG. 6: Another patient with streptococcal erythema involving unburnt skin of chest and abdomen.

histopathology and culture sensitivity as wound biopsy is the only reliable way of differentiating microbial colonization from invasive infection. Beta-hemolytic streptococcal infection may be manifested by an increase in erythema at the margins of the burn wound, like in cellulitis, with inflamed and edematous burn wound **(Figs. 5 and 6)**.

Colonization of burn wound by *Pseudomonas* is evidenced by bluish-green discoloration of the wound which is due to pyocyanin or there can be erythematous, violaceous, or necrotic escharified nodular lesions in the unburned skin, called as ecthyma gangrenosum **(Figs. 7A to C)**. When there is a foul-smelling odor with purulent discharge, *Proteus* organism should be suspected.

Following excision of a burn wound, if the surface is left exposed, the wound surface undergoes desiccation which creates a neo-eschar. This should not be mistaken for infection-related necrosis. Therefore, excised areas should always be covered immediately either by autograft or homograft.

FUNGAL INFECTION IN BURNS

Although fungal growths were noticed in burn wounds prior to the use of topical antimicrobial therapy, with their extensive use for burn dressings, the incidence of fungal colonization in burn wounds has increased. In fact after the introduction of mafenide for burn dressing, there was a fourfold increase in the incidence of fungal BWI.[27] This trend continued with incidence of bacterial infections decreasing over the years till such a period when fungi represented the most common BWI.[28] The fungi most frequently isolated include *Candida*, *Mucor*, *Rhizopus*, *Aspergillus*, and *Alternaria* species.

The fungi can be grouped into three categories:

1. *Aspergillus*-like morphology
2. Mucor-like morphology (zygomycosis/mucormycosis)
3. Yeast-like morphology (*Candida*)

Candida albicans has been reported as the most frequent pathogenic species causing nosocomial fungal infection in burn patients with an incidence of 3%,[7] with mortality ranging from 38 to 50%.[29,30] The incidence of candidiasis increases as the duration of stay in the hospital increases. It has been reported from the authors' unit that the incidence of candidiasis is 5% in less than 7 days post-burn patients and it increases to 58% in more than 7 days post burn.[31] This is attributed to long-term use of systemic antibiotics, central lines, use of total parenteral nutrition, immunosuppression, and ventilatory support.

Although *Candida* plays a major role in fungal BWIs, there is an increasing prevalence of non-*Candida albicans* species, such as *Candida tropicalis*, *Candida parapsilosis*, *Candida krusei*, and *Candida glabrata* is being seen. They are associated with higher mortality rates and a decreased susceptibility to the widely used fluconazole and other antifungal agents.

The earliest gross findings of fungal infection are hemorrhagic area(s) of discoloration in burn wound. Some of the fungi especially *Mucor* and *Aspergillus* have a preference for vascular invasion and, therefore, produce widespread ischemic necrosis of soft tissues which may be so severe as to produce gangrene of an entire limb. Necrosis and saponification of subeschar fat beneath the burn wound are also characteristic of fungal infection and these are seen as a cheesy yellow appearance of subeschar

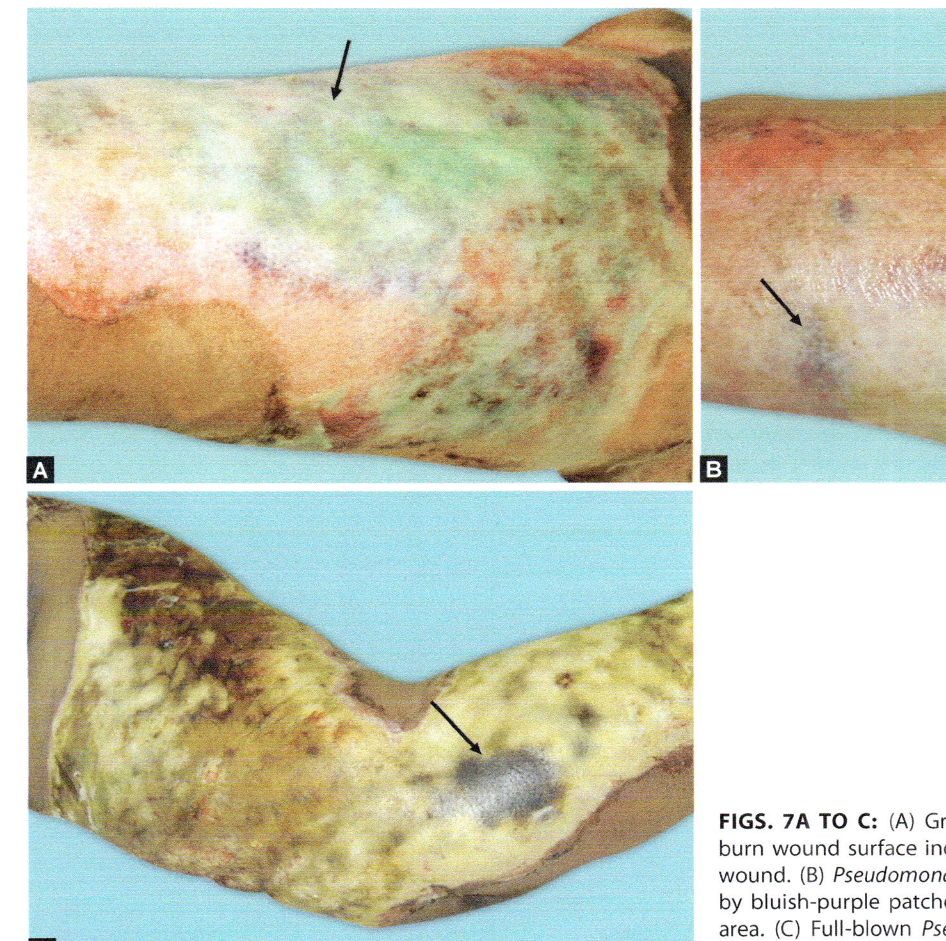

FIGS. 7A TO C: (A) Greenish discoloration of the dressing and burn wound surface indicating *Pseudomonas* colonization of the wound. (B) *Pseudomonas* invasion of the same wound indicated by bluish-purple patches appearing in the depth of the burned area. (C) Full-blown *Pseudomonas* invasive sepsis—hemorrhagic patches with thickening eschars, increasing soakage from wound.

tissues when the burn wound is debrided **(Figs. 8 and 9)**. Histopathologic examination of wound biopsy is required for differentiating fungal infection from the other bacterial infection.

The fungal involvement of burn wound is classified into fungal wound colonization (FWC) and fungal wound infection (FWI).

Fungal wound colonization is defined as presence of fungus in the burn eschar without penetration to the level of viable tissues. Fungal wound infection is defined as invasion into viable tissue deep to the eschar.

Fungal infections in burn wounds typically manifest during or after the second week post-thermal injury, particularly in patients who have undergone multiple antimicrobial treatments.

A significant number of fungal infections often go undetected due to a lack of clinical awareness, compounded by their presentation similar to bacterial infections and the limited availability of mycology laboratories. Timely diagnosis and treatment of these mycoses can be crucial for saving lives, especially considering the otherwise high mortality rates. It is essential to identify the specific fungal species for appropriate topical and systemic antifungal therapy.

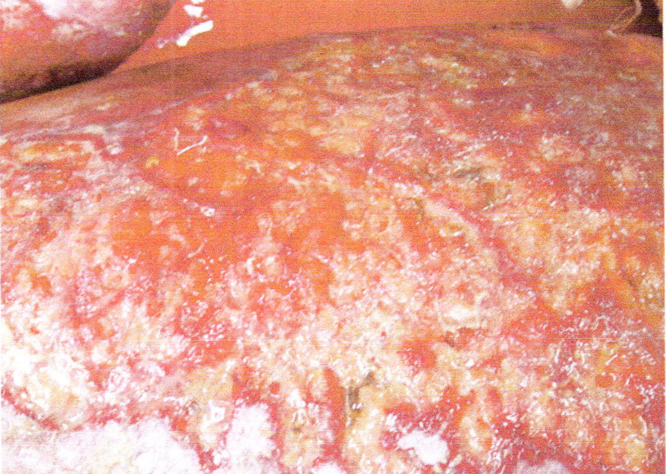

FIG. 8: Close-up view of invasive fungal sepsis due to *Aspergillus* infection.

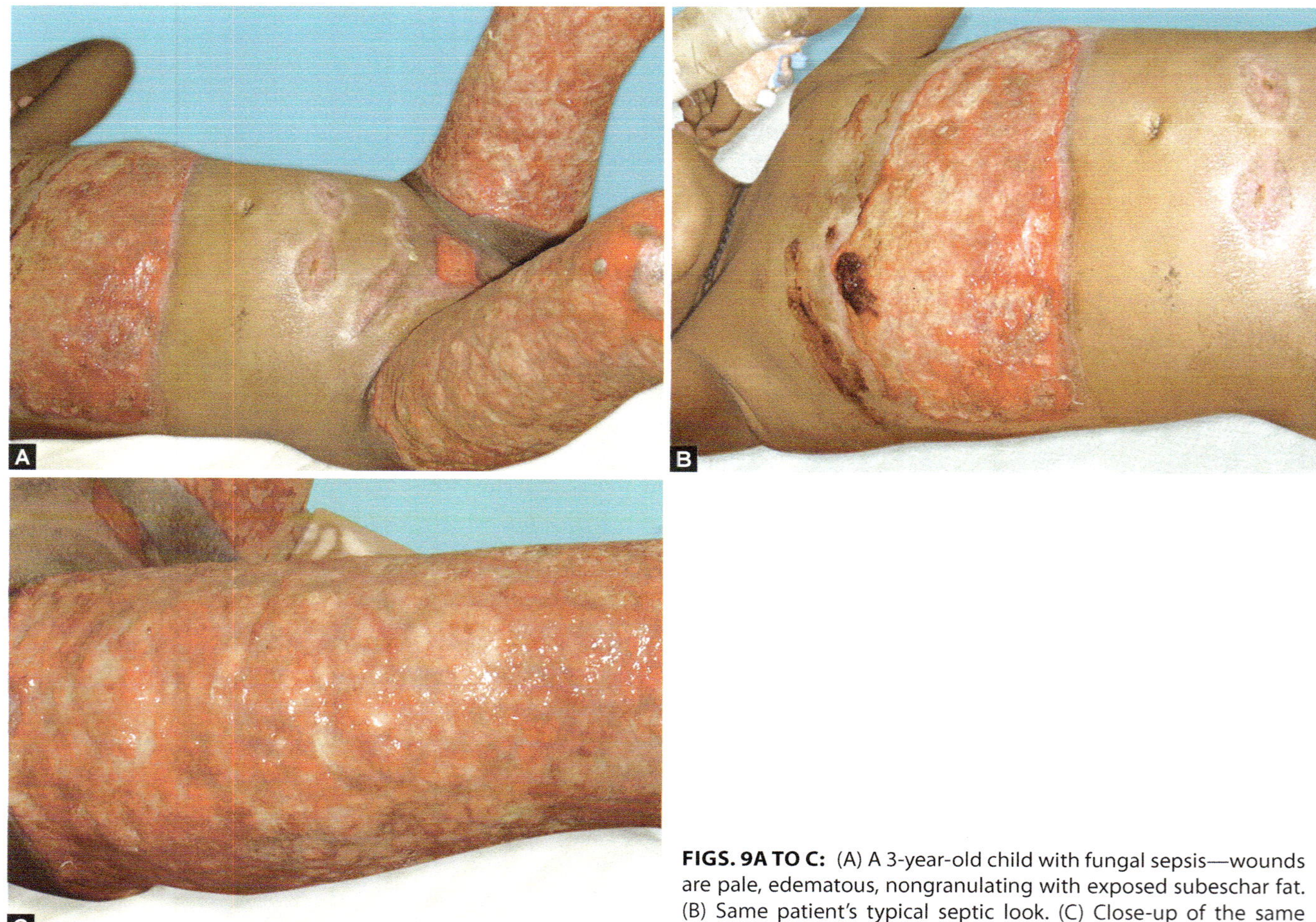

FIGS. 9A TO C: (A) A 3-year-old child with fungal sepsis—wounds are pale, edematous, nongranulating with exposed subeschar fat. (B) Same patient's typical septic look. (C) Close-up of the same invasive fungal wound.

Deep-tissue biopsies are evaluated by standard mycological procedures using direct microscopy, culture and histopathological examination. Patients with FWC should be treated by aggressive surgical debridement. In cases of FWI, surgical debridement is complemented by the administration of an intravenous antifungal medication, commonly either amphotericin B or caspofungin. Subsequent to this, the treatment strategy involves de-escalating to voriconazole, itraconazole, or fluconazole, depending on the specific fungal species or susceptibility to antifungal agents, when the culture and sensitivity reports are available. As the duration of the wound's existence prolongs, the susceptibility to fungal infection increases. Hence, expediting wound closure, administering topical and systemic antifungal treatment based on antifungal susceptibility can enhance the prognosis for severely burned victims.[32]

Prolonged and frequent utilization of fluconazole has resulted in the emergence of drug-resistant strains of *Candida albicans*. Recently published guidelines strongly advocate for caspofungin as the primary choice, followed by fluconazole, especially for patients who are deemed unlikely to harbor a fluconazole-resistant *Candida* species. Voriconazole is approved to be the first choice in non-*Candida* infections, followed by liposomal amphotericin B. Caspofungin can be considered in combination with voriconazole against invasive aspergillosis and *Fusarium* in severe or refractory cases. Due to the reported rise in resistance to these antifungal agents, the development of newer drugs becomes crucial in the fight against fungal BWI.

VIRAL INFECTION IN BURNS

Viral infection in burn patients has not received much attention in the past but BWI by herpes-varicella viruses and *Cytomegalovirus* has been reported.[33] The reason given for this is the lowered immune status of

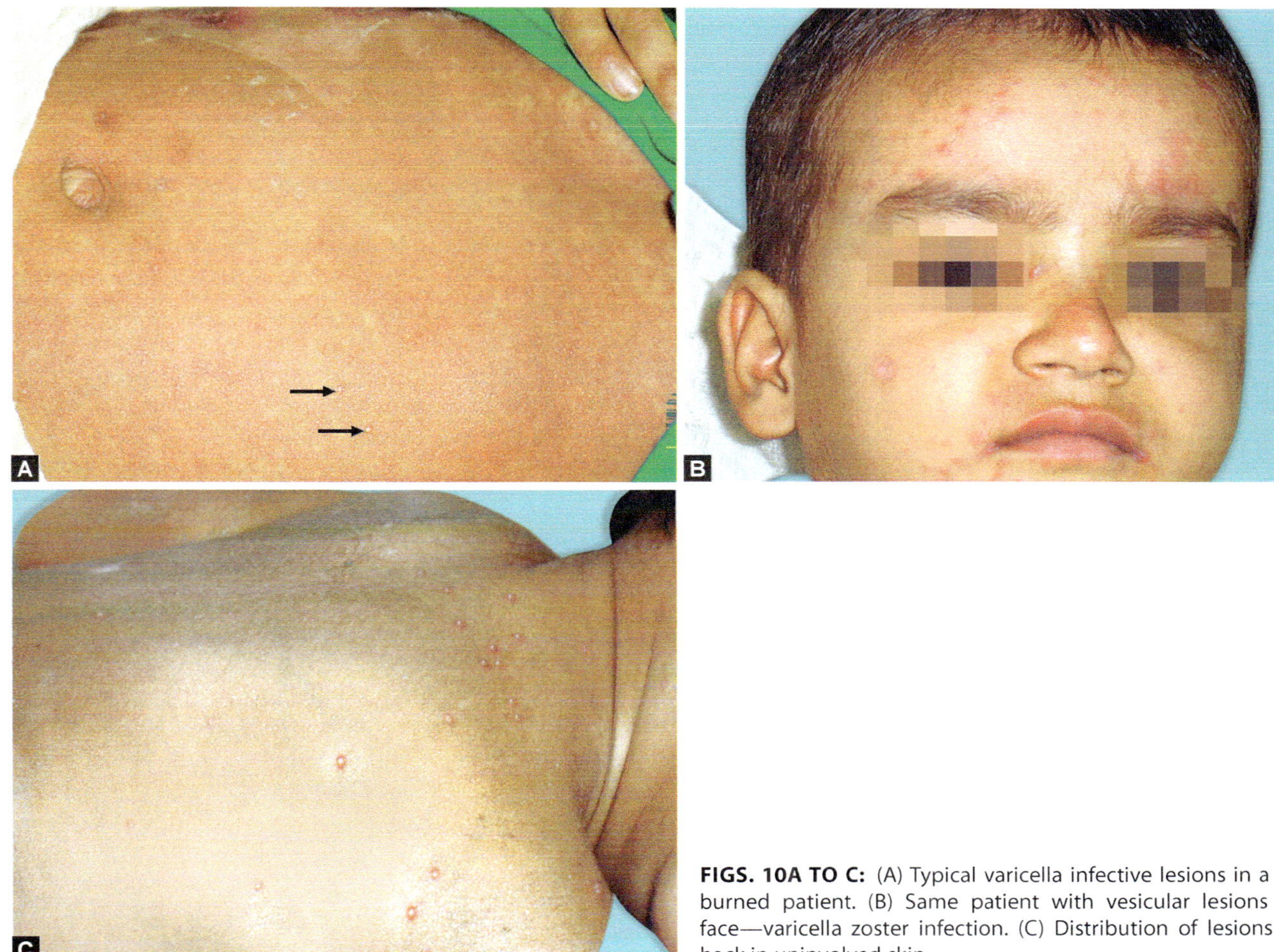

FIGS. 10A TO C: (A) Typical varicella infective lesions in a healing burned patient. (B) Same patient with vesicular lesions on the face—varicella zoster infection. (C) Distribution of lesions on the back in uninvolved skin.

the patient which allows the latent viruses to manifest themselves. The lesions usually occur in the area of healing second-degree burns and present as vesicles and superficial erosions with secondary bacterial infection. Extensive cutaneous herpetic infection or varicella zoster (chickenpox) infection may develop in some burn patients and the systemic dissemination to liver, adrenals, respiratory, and gastrointestinal system along with secondary bacterial infection of cutaneous lesions may be fatal **(Figs. 10A to C)**. Only a biopsy of an early lesion will manifest signs of infection by herpes-varicella group because rapid colonization by *Staphylococcus* and *Pseudomonas* later can obscure the viral nature of the lesions. Usually shave biopsy of entire vesicle provides adequate tissue for diagnosis. Diagnosis can also be established by measuring neutralizing or complement fixing antibodies in acute and convalescent phase sera because viruses cannot be isolated from older lesions.

MANAGEMENT OF BURN WOUND INFECTION

There are three levels of management of BWI:

1. Prevention of burn wound contamination from exogenous source (primary line of management)
2. Prevention of BWI and septicemia in wounds which are already contaminated by microorganisms from exogenous or endogenous sources (*secondary line of management*)
3. Early diagnosis and treatment of infected burn wound (*tertiary line of management*)

Primary Line of Management (Aseptic Techniques)

The saying, "An ounce of prevention is better than tons of cure", holds true when dealing with BWI. The principles are same as what we follow and practice in any surgical discipline for wound care management, comprising of aseptic and antiseptic techniques.

- Primary line of management for burn wound starts as soon as the patient enters the casualty or even earlier at the site of accident. Wounds are essentially sterile at the time of burns. Prevention of wound contamination is, therefore, of utmost importance. The public should be taught to cover the burn wounds with cleanest sheet available. In the casualty, the first dressing should not be done in hospital's main casualty, unless the hospital has a separate burns casualty manned by proper trained staff. If extensive burns are being received in hospitals main casualty, they should be wrapped in sterile sheet with sterile rubber Mackintosh sheet placed underneath the victim and transported to burns unit for dressing. Practice of applying coloring agents such as Gentian violet and Mercurochrome creates problems in burn assessment; hence, it should be discouraged.
- *Dressing stations*: The dressing stations are an important site for transmission of infection from healthcare workers to the wound as well as from one patient to another. During dressing of any extensive burn, there is heavy contamination of the air inside the room. There should be a gap of at least 30 minutes between two dressings. The ideal burn dressing room should have total exchange of sterile air between two dressings. Room air can be decontaminated within minutes by the use of laminar airflow system with bacterial filters and fixed air asepticizers. HEPA filter (high-efficiency particulate air filter) fitted laminar airflow rooms, providing sterile environment, are the ideal dressing station and patient care cubicles. Plenum ventilated dressing stations are now replaced by fixed air asepticizers to get round the clock sterile environment.
- *Dressing technique*: "No Touch Technique" is a must in treating the burn wound. Burn dressing is a highly skilled job and should be carried out by the person well trained in that. Three teams are responsible for change of one dressing only, which includes doctors, nurses, and dressers. First team, which involves a nurse and dresser, is for dressing removal only and is usually known as "dirty" or "unsterile" nurse. Second team is the main dressing team who does the sterile dressing work. Third team is responsible for floor work, known as "floor nurse". Once the dressing of one patient is completed, the entire team changes for next dressing. Minimum of two to three such teams should be there in a "heavy" burns unit, where 8–10 extensive dressings are being done daily. In minimal touch technique, instruments are mainly used for doing dressings, burns wounds are touched by sterile gloved hands only. Priority of dressing should be for clean, less extensive and pediatric dressings first, extensive and "dirty" dressings to be done later. All workers in the dressing room should follow strict operation theater norms.
- Invasive procedure such as urethral catheterization and venesections or CVP (central venous pressure) cannula insertion is often found to be major source of septicemia. Ideally, peripheral cannulae should be changed every 3 days. Prolonged use of catheters and long lines requires proper maintenance for avoiding major source of infection, especially infective deep vein thrombosis which often is the triggering point of burn septicemia.
- *Prevention of infection in burn ICU*: Extensive burns patient requires isolation as well as maximum nursing care and monitoring in a burn ICU. Barrier nursing, patient isolation, and environmental sterilization are few methods to prevent cross infection. All healthcare personnel should be appropriately gowned and gloved at each entry into the patient's room. Simple hand wash during ward rounds, before and after seeing the burn patient, is the easiest way to prevent cross contamination. Bacillocid® spray, 30 minutes before receiving a new patient is equally effective and less toxic than fumigation. All equipment in each patient's room should be regularly cleaned with appropriate disinfectants.
- Culture of environment of burn ward, burn ICU, and all other burn stations by exposing culture disk for 15 minutes and culture from beds, monitors, and other equipment are done every 3 weeks. If found positive, their remedial process is very important aspect of burn wound prevention. Formalin fumigation and carbolization of bed and equipment have largely been replaced by modern environment-friendly safe procedures like Bacillocid® spray of walls and equipment. Ultraviolet light can be installed to reduce bacterial count in vacant areas (without patient). Usually a combination of the following procedures is used to minimize environment and fomite contamination.

Procedures that predispose the patient to cross-contamination, such as use of hydrotherapy tanks, are better avoided or kept to a minimum. Cohort nursing care is another component of environmental control in a burn unit. Nurses and other health workers are assigned to work as a team for one specific patient or a group of patients and the movement between patients is strictly limited. Convalescing patients are kept separate from the acute patients since they form a reservoir of more antibiotic-resistant organisms which are acquired during their hospital stay. Thus, after the ICU, there is a step-

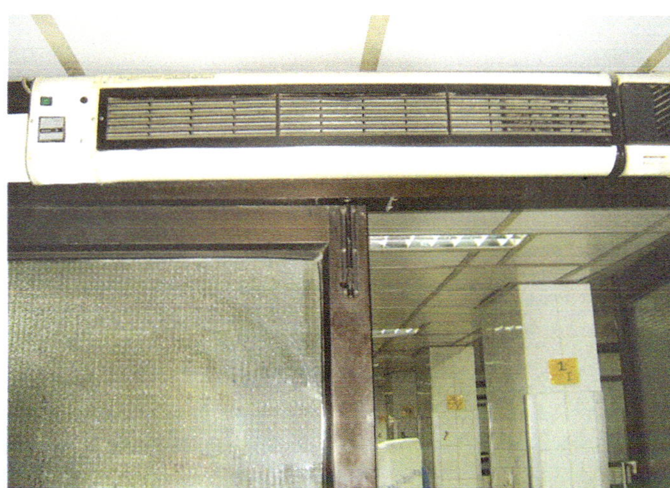

FIG. 11: Fixed air asepticizer at the entrance of burns ICU and wards to reduce bacterial count.

down ICU where the patient is shifted after he/she is fully resuscitated and stabilized and thereafter, there should be a chronic ward where patients are prepared for skin grafting of the raw areas.

- *Physical*:
  - Laminar air flow system with HEPA filters (high-efficiency particulate air filters)
  - Fixed or mobile air asepticizer **(Fig. 11)**
  - Ultraviolet (UV) light exposures
- *Chemical*:
  - Formalin fumigation, carbolization, and Bacillocid spray®

Secondary Line of Burn Wound Management (Antiseptic Methods)

- Prophylactic antibiotics
- Local chemotherapeutic agents
- Biological dressings
- Early wound closure
- Immunotherapy

Prophylactic Antibiotics

Role of prophylactic antibiotics in burns is debatable. Extensively burned patients are usually immunocompromised and may require prophylactic antibiotics. A diabetic burn patient and the one coming late to a burn center from far-flung areas with open wounds have fair chances of wound contamination and invasion.

Recommendations for management of burn patients do not provide clear guidance on whether prophylactic antibiotics should be administered or not. A Cochrane systematic review concluded that the antibiotic prophylaxis does not demonstrate reduction in BWI, invasive infections, or mortality associated with infection.[34] The findings from the review suggested a reduction in the incidence of pneumonia. International Society for Burn Injury (ISBI) practice guidelines 2016 also state that prophylactic systemic antibiotics do not reduce sepsis and should be avoided. A retrospective study conducted in our department suggests not to routinely use antibiotic prophylaxis in burns patients, but there seems to be benefit in certain subgroups like patients with inhalational burns and burn patients with pneumonia.[35]

Local Chemotherapeutic Agents

1% silver sulfadiazine (SSD) cream for extensive burns usually takes care of surface contaminants or endogenous contamination from hair follicles with painless acceptable eschar penetration and minimal toxicity. Therefore, it is the ideal topical antimicrobial cream for extensive burns.

Silver sulfadiazine cream, however, is relatively short-acting, requires reapplication at least daily, and ideally needs to be applied twice daily.[36]

Silver-impregnated dressings have tried to overcome these limitations by releasing additional silver from the material thus maintaining a steady supply of silver on the wound surface. For clinical use, various silver commercially available-impregnated dressings are available, for e.g., ActiCoat®, Aquacel-Ag®, UrgoTul Ag®, etc. These silver-impregnated dressings are covered with a four-layer moistened gauze followed by four layers of dry gauze and pads whose purpose is to absorb the surplus amount of fluid. The dressing is held in place with a bandage. It is changed 3 to 7 days after application depending on the exudate. Silver-impregnated dressings significantly reduce the frequency of burn dressings which reduces the pain for patient and workload for the burn management team.[37]

Biological Dressings

Collagen dressings and other biological dressings seal the wound from external environment and thereby reduce the chances of wound contamination.

Early Wound Closure

Excision of deep dermal and full-thickness burns with immediate skin grafting reduces the morbidity. Elimination of the necrotic tissues and raw areas, in turn, reduces the chances of infection and septicemia.

Immunoprophylaxis

Apart from active and passive tetanus prophylaxis, many other vaccines are available for gram-negative and gram-positive bacteria. Their efficacy is not established. However, there is a definite role of immunoglobulins in prevention and management of BWI and septicemia. The availability of refined preparations of immunoglobulins and widespread increase in prevalence of multidrug-resistant bacteria have brought immunoglobulins to the forefront during the last decade. The role of intravenous gamma globulins in burn patients has been studied extensively in the past.[22,23] Recently, the use of IgM-enriched immunoglobulins to enhance the humoral response has emerged as a valuable tool in the management of burn patients with infection. Experimental in vitro and animal studies on IgM-enriched immunoglobulins have demonstrated that elevated titer of antiendotoxin antibodies correlates significantly with decreased mortality due to gram-negative sepsis. Besides neutralizing antigen, IgM-enriched immunoglobulin also activates compliment factor like opsonins. To enhance immune response against bacteria, IgM immunoglobulin has been shown to have a synergistic action with beta-lactam antibiotics as well as a beneficial immunomodulating effect.[24,25]

Tertiary Line of Management of Burn Wound Infection

Early Diagnosis and Treatment (Figs. 12A to N)

Early diagnosis of BWI and septicemia and specific treatment for the same is the key for decreasing mortality in extensive burns. Going by the definition of SIRS, almost all extensive burn patients are in SIRS. They have to be regularly observed for signs of septic syndrome. Patients with diabetes or other immunocompromised conditions are more likely to land in septic complications. Following local signs and symptoms, if present, are the starting point for invasive infection:

- Unexplained pain or discomfort in burn wound
- Excessive soakage
- Unexplained fever
- Inflamed burn wound margins. In facial burns, especially if ears are involved, increased cephaloconchal angle is the first sign of inflammation.

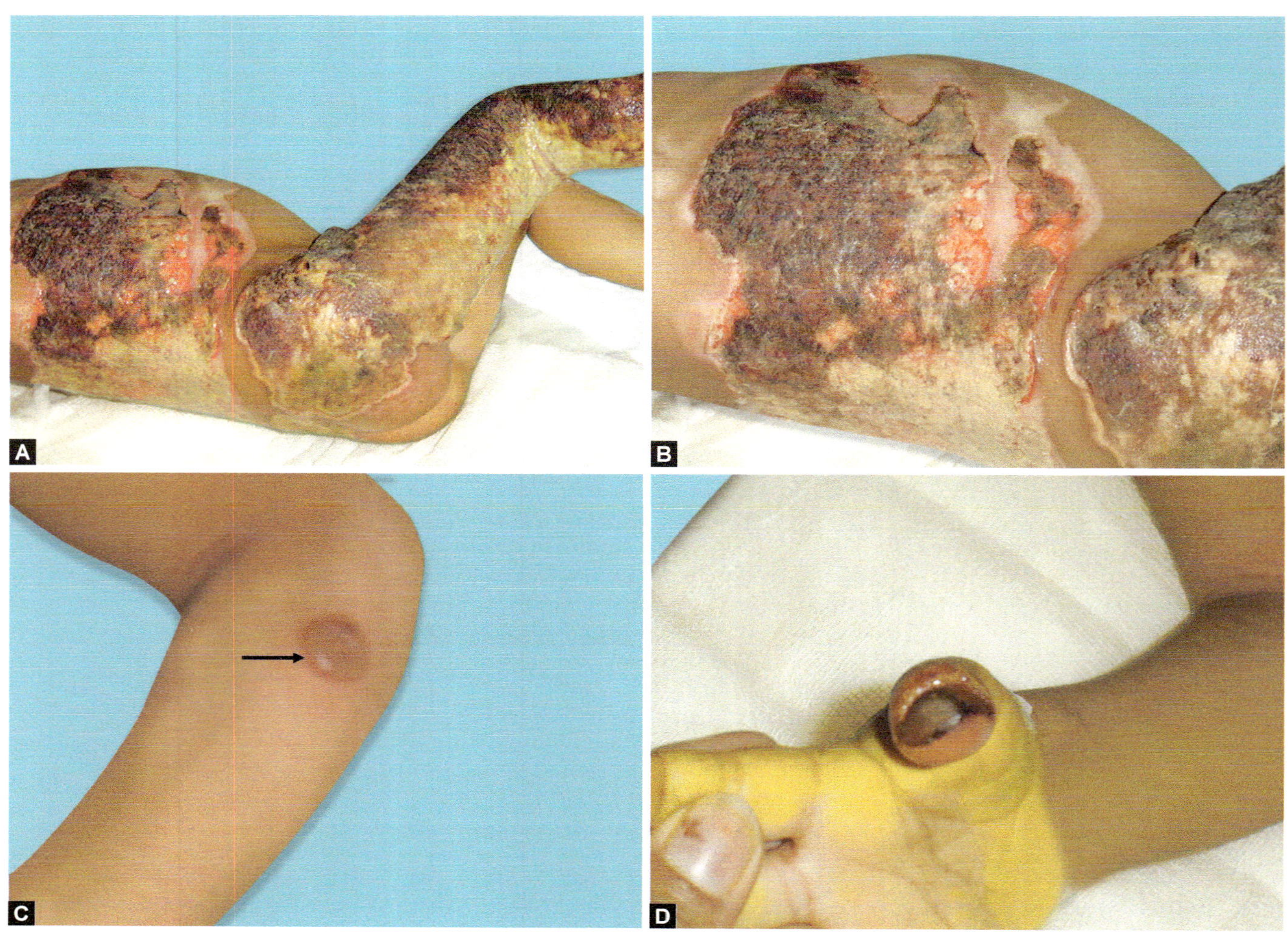

FIGS. 12A TO N: *Continued*

Continued

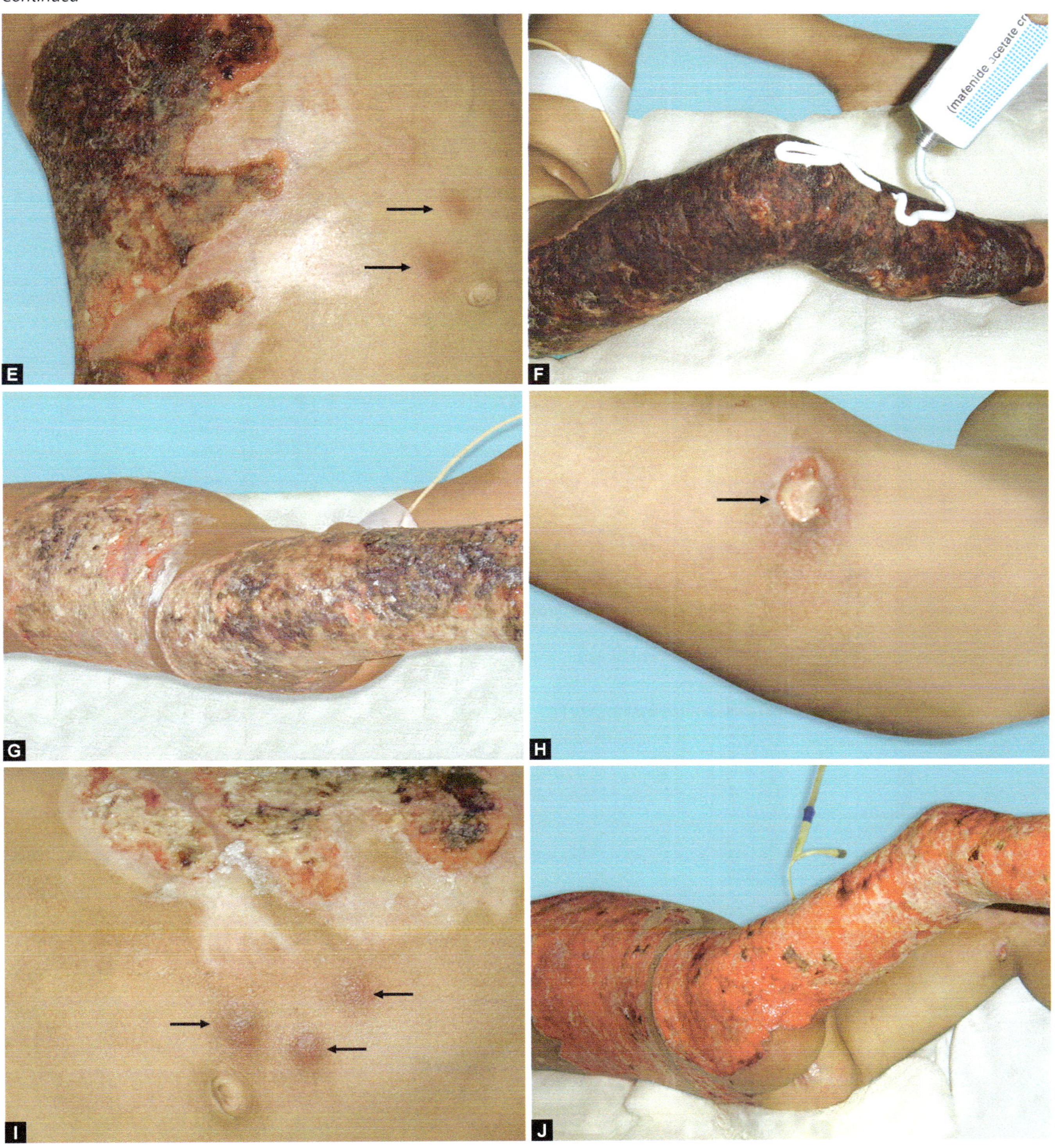

Continued

Continued

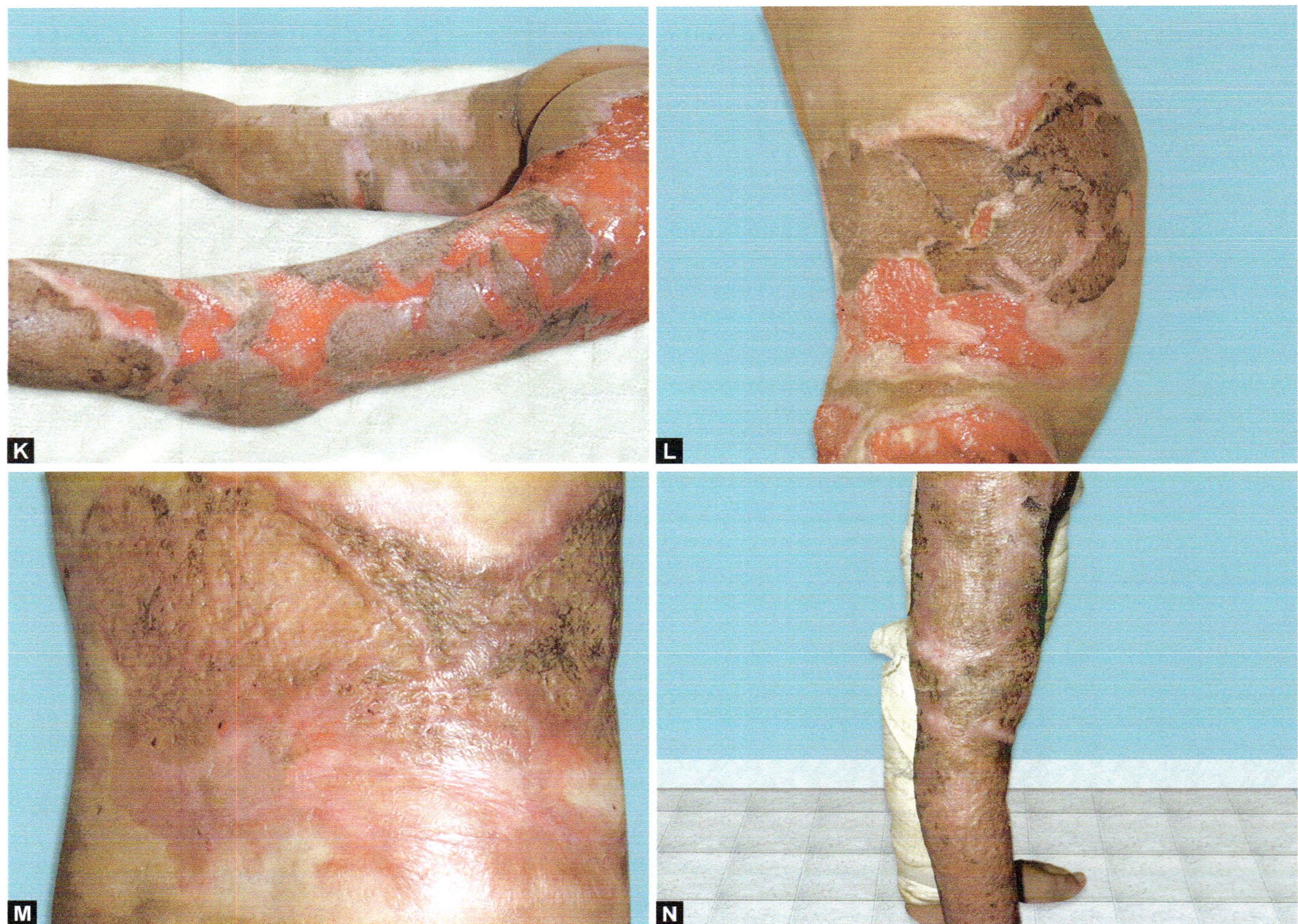

FIGS. 12A TO N: (A) Patient with invasive gram-negative burn wound sepsis—hemorrhagic discoloration of entire eschar. (B) Close-up view of same wounds. (C) Typical nodular satellite lesions in uninvolved skin—ecthyma gangrenosum. (D) Infective gangrenous changes in thumb indicating septic embolization. (E) Nodulo-papular lesions in adjacent unburned skin over the abdomen and chest with edema of the skin with distension abdomen. (F) Patient managed with change of local antimicrobial from SSD to mafenide and third line of systemic antibiotic—carbapenems with aminoglycoside. (G) Improving wounds—eschar penetrated by mafenide to reach subeschar tissue, tissue edema reduced and general condition improved. (H) Ecthyma gangrenosum reduced. (I) Satellite nodules drying up. (J) Healthy granulating wound after 10 days of change in treatment. (K) Same wounds grafted in stages on lower limbs—full graft uptake. (L) Successfully grafted back of same patient. (M) 1 month postoperative picture of the back of same patient. (N) Legs of the same patient.

(SSD: silver sulfadiazine)

- Gastrointestinal symptoms in the form of loose motions and or abdominal distension
- Abnormal behavior, intermittent irrelevant talks, and oliguria despite adequate perfusion are sometimes the presenting features of sepsis.

Investigations

Investigations along with these preliminary signs and symptoms help in diagnosing the specific organism invading the burn wound.

- *Leukocyte count and platelet count*: Importance of total leukocyte count in relation to infection is well documented. Leukocytosis in early sepsis and leukopenia in late sepsis are often diagnostic. Persistently decreasing platelet count is often the first sign of impending septic syndrome in extensive burns.
- Invasive BWI usually starts after the 5th post-burn day in extensive burns. Initial surface culture report, if available, is the best guide for the type of organism and its antibiotic sensitivity.
- Blood culture is usually noninformative as 75% cases are in gram-negative septicemia in which only the toxins are present in blood. In gram-positive septicemia, blood culture report is usually more informative.

- *Wound biopsies*: Quantitative wound analysis is helpful in some cases not responding to treatment as bacterial counts >10^5 organisms/g of tissue demand for a multipronged approach for burn sepsis. Serial biopsies are essential to follow the progress of infection. Any change from stage Ia to stage Ic (as mentioned earlier) demands immediate change in wound care management. If stage II is diagnosed, excision of the eschar and underlying infected tissues should be carried out as soon as possible. If gram-negative invasion is present, the topical antimicrobial agent being used is changed to mafenide cream should be used till excision is performed. Wound biopsy is also indicated for fungal infection, usually superimposed, once bacterial infection is being successfully treated with higher antibiotics.

Treatment

Depending on extent of body surface area burnt, the type of infecting organism, and the general condition of the host, the treatment should be planned against the infecting microorganism using:

- Local and systemic antimicrobial agents
- Increasing the host resistance to infection by using immunoglobulin
- Enteral and parenteral nutrition including albumin and blood transfusions
- Controlling concomitant diseases like diabetes, hypertension, etc.

Local wound dressings: Early BWI requires change of antimicrobial agent to the one which is effective against the suspected organism(s). Unfortunately, very few agents are available for use in extensive burns with good eschar penetration. If 1% SSD cream is being used and subsequently *Pseudomonas* infection is suspected, changeover to 11.1% mafenide cream is advised **(Figs. 13A to C)**. This should be applied twice a day. If MRSA (methicillin-resistant *Staphylococcus aureus*) is the causative agent, silver ion is more effective and a thick

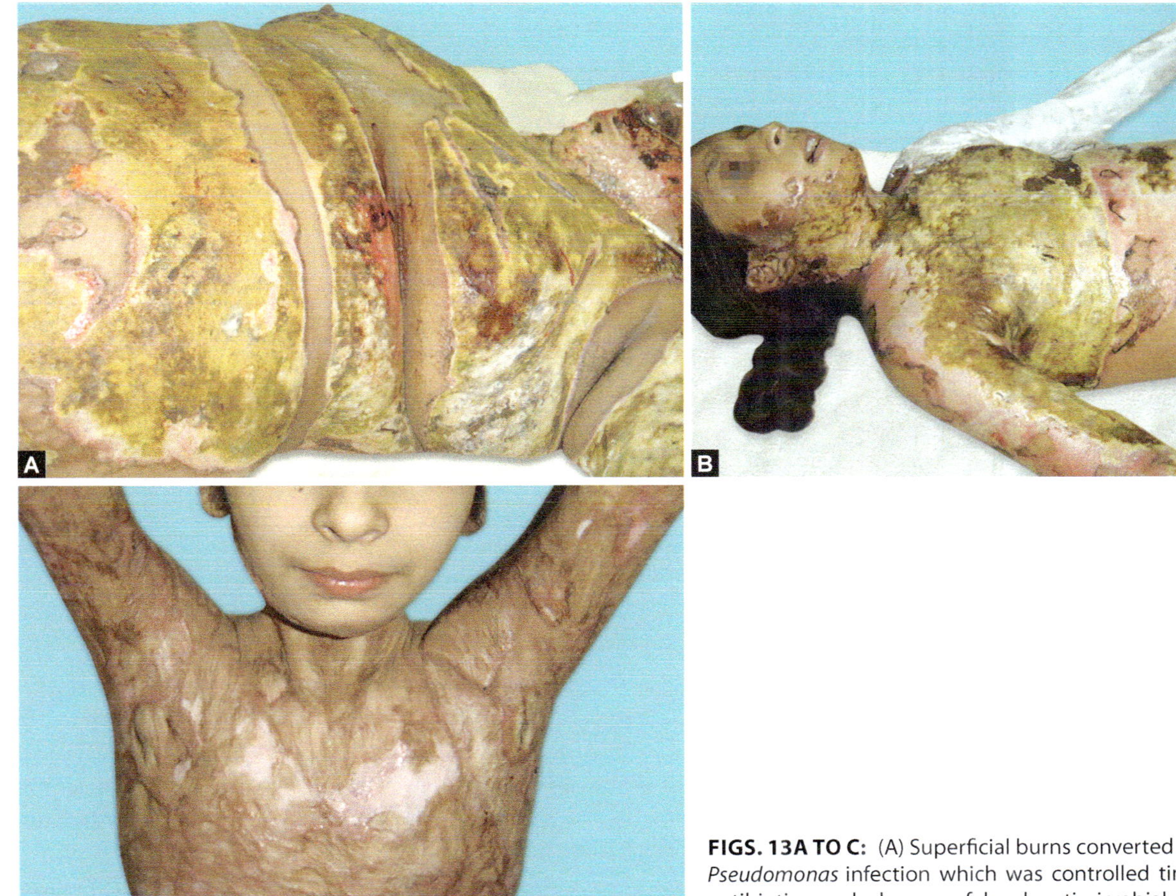

FIGS. 13A TO C: (A) Superficial burns converted to deep burns by *Pseudomonas* infection which was controlled timely by systemic antibiotics and change of local antimicrobial agent. (B) Same patient with wounds showing improvement. (C) Finally grafted wounds of same patient—2 months postoperative picture.

coating of SSD is to be applied and dressing needs to be changed every 8 hours.

Nanocrystalline silver dressings (e.g., Acticoat) slowly release silver, which is toxic to microorganisms. Although silver dressings are toxic to bacteria, there is some in vitro evidence that they inhibit keratinocytes and fibroblasts in wound bed, which can potentially prolong healing time.[38-40]

Systemic antibiotics: In stage IIc, hematogenous and lymphatic dissemination demands systemic antibiotic therapy. Ideally systemic antibiotics should have been started much earlier so as to prevent progression to this stage which may ultimately lead to multiorgan failure.

Appropriate systemic antibiotics should be started depending on the culture sensitivity report. If, however, the report is not available, empirical antibiotic therapy has to be started as per the ward antibiogram. Every burn unit should formulate its own antibiotic policy according to which the treatment can be started. In the authors' unit, it is a standard practice to use cefoperazone + sulbactam or piperacillin + tazobactam and amikacin for beta-lactamase producing *Pseudomonas* and *Klebsiella* and *vancomycin* for MRSA. Extended-spectrum beta-lactamases (ESBLs) (metalloenzyme) producing *Pseudomonas* and *Klebsiella* require second-generation carbapenems, i.e., imipenem + cilastatin or meropenem along with aminoglycosides.

It is important to diagnose the type of fungal infection accurately because no antifungal provides optimal coverage for all fungi. Because of this varying spectrum of activity of each antifungal agent, it is important to identify the infecting fungi accurately, often down to the species level. Intravenous amphotericin B still has the broadest antifungal spectrum especially against *Candida* and *Aspergillus* species. The older azole agents, fluconazole and itraconazole, cover most *Candida* species but have limited action against molds. The newer broad-spectrum azole, voriconazole, has improved mold coverage as well as *Fusarium* and *P. boydii* but no action against *Zygomycetes*. The newer agents such as caspofungin, micafungin, and echinocandin have good action against *Candida* and *Aspergillus* but do not cover *Zygomycetes*, molds, and *Cryptococcus*.

Antimicrobial resistance: Alexander Fleming, who discovered Penicillin, had announced the risk of the inevitable phenomenon of antibiotic resistance which turned out to be accurate. The inappropriate use of antibiotics hastens up the development and spread of bacteria resistant to them.

The worldwide emergence of antimicrobial resistance among the majority of human bacterial and fungal burn wound pathogens makes the therapeutic options limited for effective treatment of BWI.[41,42] MRSA and methicillin-resistant coagulase-negative *Staphylococcus*, vancomycin-resistant enterococci, and multiple resistant gram-negative bacteria which have several types of beta-lactamases including ESBL, amp-C beta-lactamases, and metallo-beta-lactamases are emerging as serious pathogens in hospitalized burn patients.[43]

Bacteria are able to inactivate antibiotics through numerous molecular mechanisms:[44]

- Production of inactivating enzymes
- Changes and alterations in the antibiotic target
- Reduced cellular permeability
- *Increased outflow*: Antibiotics taken up into bacteria cell are removed by energy-driven drug efflux systems.

The risk factors for acquisition of antibiotic-resistant organisms include treatment with antibiotics prior to the development of infection, prolonged hospital stay, previous hospitalization, invasive procedures, and advancing age.

In 2015, the WHO decided to adopt the Global Action Plan on Antimicrobial Resistance, based on five strict objectives:[45]

1. To improve awareness and understanding of antimicrobial resistance
2. To strengthen knowledge and the amount of data
3. To reduce the incidence of infections through effective hygienic measures
4. To optimize the use of antimicrobial drugs in human and animal health
5. To increase investment in new drugs, diagnostic tools, vaccines, and other interventions

Even fungi especially *Candida* species have become an important opportunistic pathogen due to widespread inappropriate use of broad-spectrum topical and systemic antibacterial agents in burn patients and are now showing increasing degree of drug resistance.[46,47]

The antibiotic utilization should be rotated or changed on a regular basis as per the changing antibiotic resistance and sensitivity patterns.

Strict infection control practices and appropriate empirical antimicrobial therapy are essential for reducing incidence of infection by these resistant organisms.

The use of subeschar clysis[48] with a broad-spectrum antipseudomonal agent has also been recommended with number 20 spinal needle (half of the dose mixed in 1,000 cc saline) to fight the infection locally. This can be repeated just before excision to reduce intraoperative dissemination of viable bacteria and toxins.

Newer antibiotics: Polymyxins are class of antibiotics approved for management of systemic infections caused by susceptible strains of multidrug-resistant organisms such as *Pseudomonas aeruginosa*. Polymyxin B and polymyxin E (colistin) are the two drugs within this antibiotic class used primarily in clinical practice. They are useful in treating infections of the urinary tract, meninges, and bloodstream by susceptible strains of *Pseudomonas aeruginosa*, *Enterobacteriaceae*, and *Acinetobacter baumannii*. They act by destabilizing the phospholipids and lipopolysaccharides (LPS) present on the outer membrane of gram-negative bacteria.

Most of the approved compounds target carbapenem-resistant *Enterobacteriaceae* and other pathogens (of high and medium priority) included in the WHO's list. Both omadacycline and eravacycline are derivatives of tetracyclines. A promising new combination of β-lactam antibiotic and β-lactamase inhibitor, presenting activities against *Klebsiella pneumoniae* carbapenemase (KPC), has been approved. This is the combination meropenem and vaborbactam (a β-lactamase inhibitor).

Against MRSA, the most recently approved antibiotics include dalbavancin, tedizolid, oritavancin, and delafloxacin.

Plazomicin is a new aminoglycoside derived from the modification of sisomicin (a specific antibiotic against gram-negative infections). Plazomicin, blocks most of the aminoglycoside-modifying enzymes (AMEs) specifically in *Enterobacteriaceae* species.

Burn Unit Antibiogram

All burn units should routinely determine the specific pattern of burn wound microbial colonization and the changes in the microbial flora with time and the susceptibility profiles of the organisms. This information can be obtained by periodic sampling of burn wounds and other anatomic sites and with a proper liaison between the treating clinician and the microbiologist, antibiogram data can be analyzed periodically. This can then help in selecting and administering appropriate empirical systemic antibiotic, at the slightest sign of sepsis, even before the microbiological culture and sensitivity report is available. This saves precious time required to control invasive infection.

Surgical Treatment of Infected Burn Wound

The excision of infected wound should be done under general anesthesia, with a scalpel and all the tissues above deep fascia should be excised. In case there is involvement of fascia or subfascial tissues, they also need to be excised. If it is definite that all the infected tissues have been excised, the resulting wounds should be split skin grafted or covered with skin substitute or biological dressing. However, if there is any doubt regarding the depth of excision, the wounds should be dressed with gauze soaked in 5% mafenide or 0.5% silver nitrate solution. The wounds should be reexamined 24–48 hours later for further excision.

Fungal infection **(*Figs. 14A to E*)**: *Candida*-infected burn wounds do not require surgical excision as they rarely invade healthy tissue. For these cases, dressing with topical antifungal agent such as clotrimazole cream is usually effective. If infection is not controlled with the above treatment and involves more tissues locally, excision may be necessary. Invasion of the wound is usually seen in filamentous fungi as previously stated, the most aggressive being *Phycomycetes* followed by *Aspergillus* species and merits a complete excision of the infected wound followed by twice daily application of topical clotrimazole cream. Extensive involvement or systemic invasion requires systemic amphotericin B or other antifungal agents as per sensitivity pattern. In some of these cases, if muscles are also involved, an amputation of the limbs may be necessary.

Viral infection:[33] If a patient has unexplained hypotension or other signs of systemic sepsis with no other source and rapidly spreading cutaneous herpetic lesions, the possibility of systemic herpes simplex virus should be entertained and acyclovir therapy should be instituted.

BURN WOUND IMPETIGO

It is characterized by multiple small superficial abscesses, the causative organism being *Staphylococcus*. If not controlled in time, it can cause extensive destruction of grafted areas or even healed partial thickness burns and donor areas **(Figs. 15A and B)**. Treatment for this condition involves deroofing of all abscesses and application of topical antibacterial ointments like Mupirocin (T-bact®, Bactroban®) or Fusidic acid (Fucidin®) twice a day. Vancomycin is required if there is a disproportionate systemic response to this infection.

SUPPURATIVE THROMBOPHLEBITIS (FIGS. 16 AND 17)

Very often, thrombophlebitis is the cause for septicemia in burn patients as these patients require intravenous (IV) fluids and frequent parenteral hyperalimentation fluids for a long time with an impairment of host defenses due to burn injury. The incidence of catheter-associated infections has been found to be inversely proportional to the distance of the line insertion site from the burn wound. Catheter infections in burn patients usually arise from the adherence and migration of burn wound flora

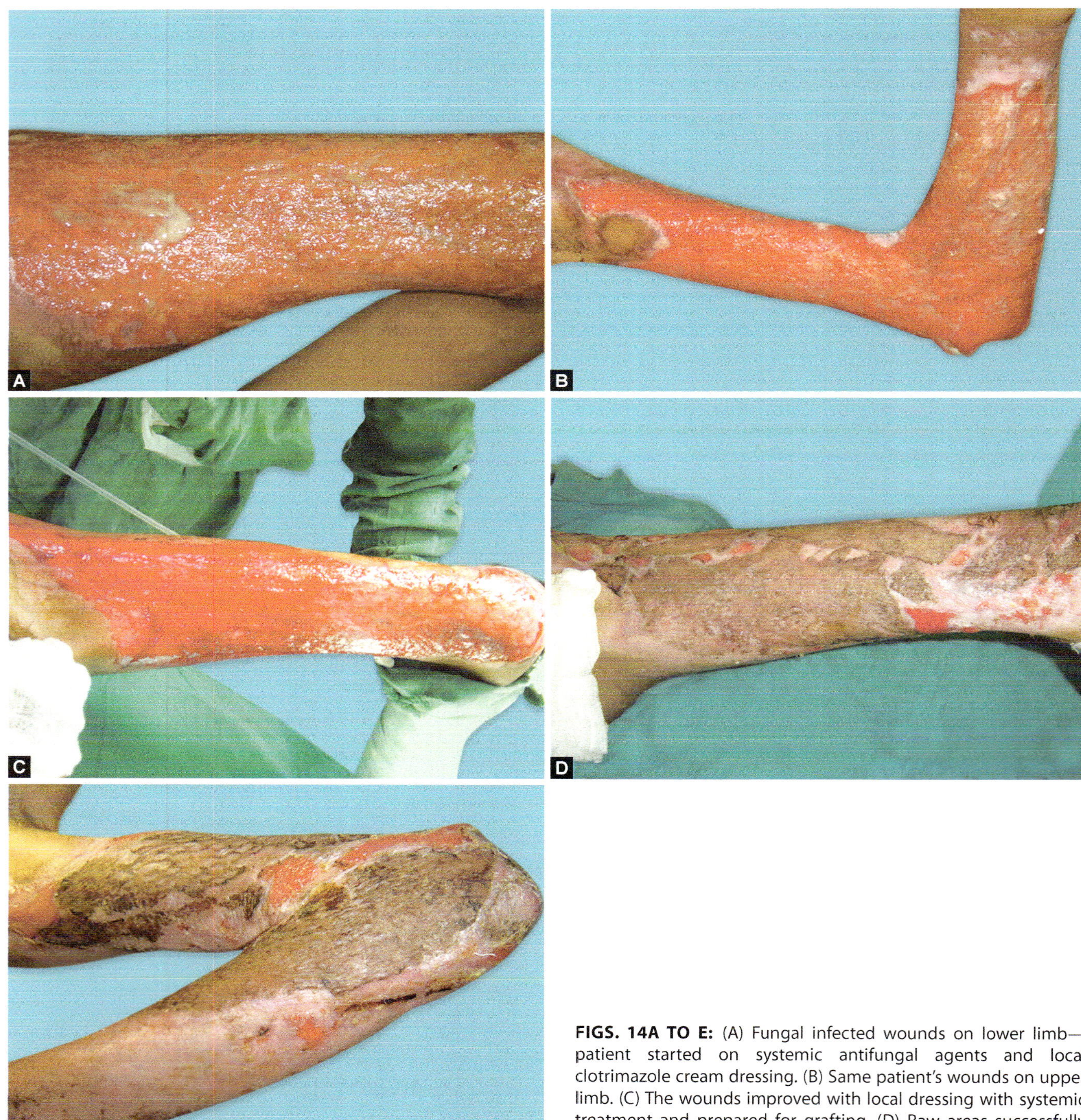

FIGS. 14A TO E: (A) Fungal infected wounds on lower limb—patient started on systemic antifungal agents and local clotrimazole cream dressing. (B) Same patient's wounds on upper limb. (C) The wounds improved with local dressing with systemic treatment and prepared for grafting. (D) Raw areas successfully grafted on lower limb—2 weeks postoperative picture. (E) Same patient's upper limb healed with skin graft in 2 weeks.

microorganisms along the catheter surface to the tip.[7,49] Though peripheral and central venous catheters should ideally be inserted through normal skin, this may not be possible in case of extensive burns. At times, it may be necessary to cut down into a vein through the burn wound itself if other veins have been exhausted in a patient with extensive burns. All veins, which have been cannulated, have to be examined. Usually there is a red streak seen along the length of infected vein with tenderness indicating thrombophlebitis. If the vein is incised and there is a brisk flow of blood from proximal segment, this condition can be excluded as the cause for sepsis. But,

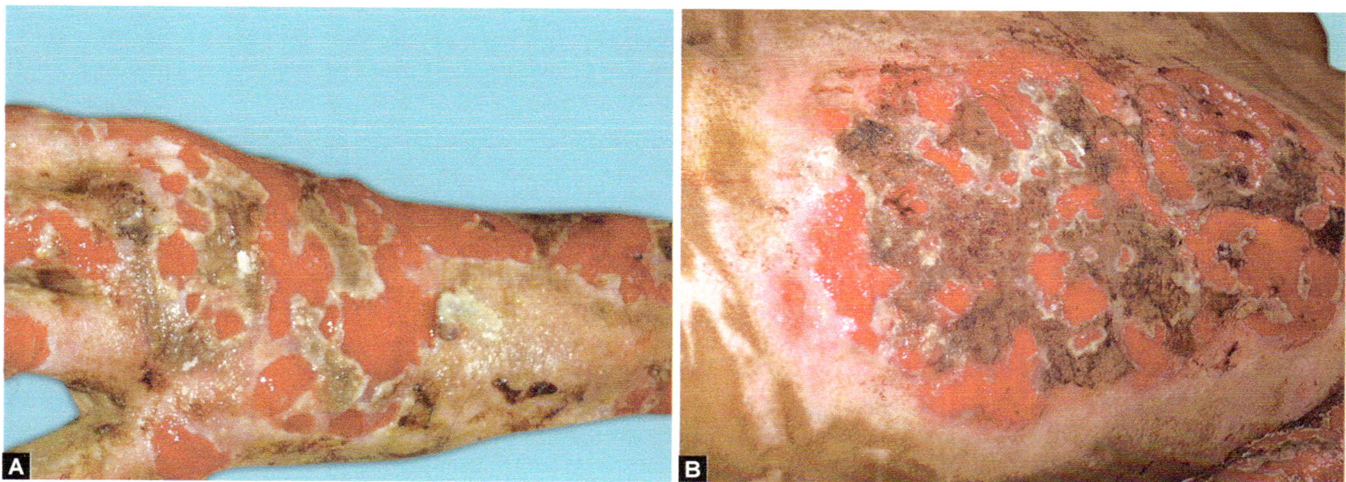

FIGS. 15A AND B: (A) Staphylococcal infection postgrafting—typical eaten up appearance of graft applied on hands and arm. (B) Same patients grafted chest showing graft eaten up by *Staphylococcus*—required change of local antimicrobial agent to mupirocin and systemic antibiotics with antistaphylococcal action.

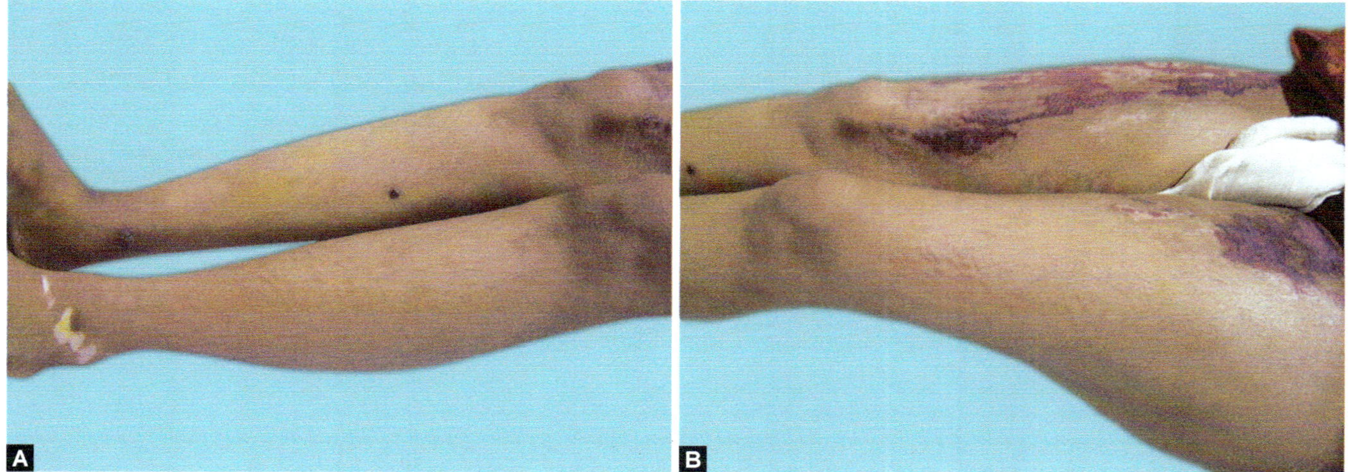

FIGS. 16A AND B: (A) Deep vein thrombosis in a patient on prolonged central venous line in left lower limb showing gross edema of lower limb and color Doppler showed thrombus extending in popliteal V, femoral vein till external iliac V. (B) Grossly edematous left thigh of same patient.

if there is pus in the vein, culture of the pus should be taken and the entire involved vein till the point where it is grossly normal should be excised completely. Systemic antibiotics are also essential at the same time. To avoid this complication, the IV site should be changed every 3 days.

TETANUS IN BURNS

Despite the widespread immunization with tetanus toxoid in childhood, which is till date the most effective vaccine, tetanus is still a problem in many underdeveloped and developing countries. Since tetanus prophylaxis is an integral part of management of all patients with burns, the incidence of tetanus in patients admitted with thermal burns is very rare. In the author's unit, tetanus is noticed mostly in electric burn patients and patients who are referred late without receiving proper tetanus prophylaxis.

In addition to tetanus, gas gangrene and mixed clostridial infections are also seen in burn patients especially with full-thickness burns or electric burns with extensive muscle necrosis which is a suitable environment for anaerobic organisms.

Tetanus Prophylaxis

For burn patients who have history of receiving 3 doses of basic immunization series, 0.5 mL of tetanus toxoid (TT)

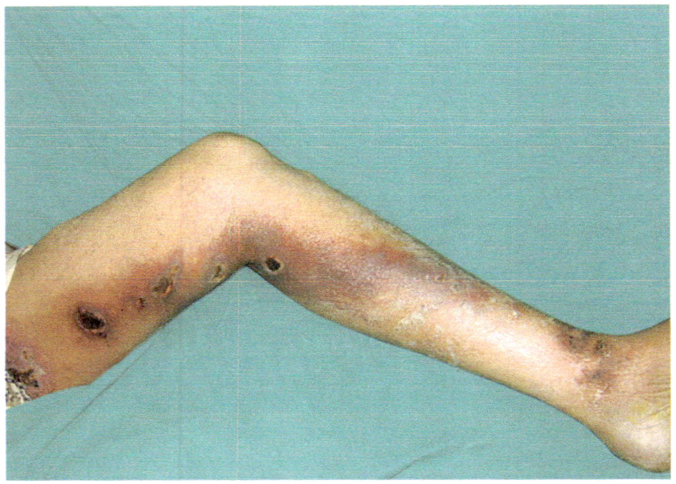

FIG. 17: Septic thrombophlebitis all along the length of the great saphenous vein with abscesses presenting superficially at multiple sites with overlying skin necrosis—required drainage of pus with excision of the entire length of vein.

given IM at initial treatment of burn is usually adequate prophylaxis. In case, interval from last booster dose is more than 5 years or if there is a delay from time of burning to treatment, 500 units of human tetanus globulin should be given IM in addition to tetanus toxoid with a different syringe at a different site. Patients who have not received basic immunization as per schedule should receive initial 0.5 mL tetanus toxoid at time of burns followed by 2 injections of 0.5 mL TT at 4 weeks interval and then at 6 months to 1 year after the last injection. In addition, 500 units of human tetanus immunoglobulin should be also given IM.

Treatment of Tetanus in Burns

There are three stages of tetanus—first stage is the "focus of infection" stage, wherein there is deposition of Clostridial tetani in the burn wound. This infection is well localized as the organism does not have strong invasive powers. During this stage, only local wound care is sufficient, failing which the second stage sets in. This is the stage where the organism releases highly diffusible neurotoxin into the body fluids. Treatment during this stage is by neutralization of the toxin with tetanus antitoxin which may be present in the body from active immunization or should be administered passively. If this stage is not controlled in time, the third stage or neurological stage sets in wherein the toxin fixes to the neuromotor cells in the central nervous system. At this stage, the antitoxin has no effect on the tetanus neurotoxin. The neurological or clinical tetanus is diagnosed based on clinical signs and symptoms and can be mild, severe, or fulminating depending upon the amount of toxin combined with the nervous system cells. Tetanus typically begins with increase in tone of various muscle groups especially spasm of masseter muscle leading to difficulty in opening mouth or clenching of teeth with a fixed smile called "risus sardonicus". The patient is irritable and complains of inability to swallow, i.e., dysphagia. As the disease progresses, there will be stiffness of neck, back, and abdominal muscles. Violent contractions of muscles or tetanic spasms produce opisthotonus, abdominal rigidity, and extension of extremities and these can be initiated with the slightest stimulus. These can even lead to difficulty in respiration which may manifest with hypoxia, cyanosis, and even sudden death.

Treatment of established tetanus involves the following steps:
- Neutralization of circulating toxin by administering 3,000 units (1,500–10,000 U) of human tetanus immunoglobulin once only at different sites deep intramuscular.
- Removal of source of toxin, by excision of presumed site of entry, which is the burn wound, is possible only in small burns. Excision of major burns for treating tetanus is not recommended.
- Sedation to control tetanic spasms in the form of diazepam is useful though toxic doses should be avoided.
- *Maintenance of respiration*: All patients with tetanus should undergo tracheostomy and ventilator should be kept ready, if needed.
- *Supporting care*: Fluid electrolyte balance, renal function, ventilation, nutrition, and prophylaxis for pulmonary and urinary tract infections have to be looked into as well.

SUMMARY

Infection remain a leading cause of mortality among burn victims despite improved survival rates even in extensive burns, due to their compromised immune systems. The chapter details the different stages of infection, from superficial colonization to invasive infection, with systemic infections leading to septicemia and end organ damage. Key pathogens include gram-positive bacteria, gram-negative bacteria, and fungi. Multidrug resistant organisms, especially *Pseudomonas* and *Acinetobacter* species, present significant treatment challenges.

Management strategies for burn wound infections are categorized into three levels: primary, secondary, and tertiary. Primary management focuses on preventing wound contamination through aseptic techniques starting from the accident site. Secondary management involves preventing infection and septicemia in already contaminated wounds, while tertiary management emphasizes early diagnosis and treatment of established infections. The use of systemic and topical antimicrobials, along with proper wound care protocols, plays a crucial role in these management strategies.

The chapter underscores the importance of early intervention and rigorous infection control measures to mitigate the risk of infections in burn patients. Ongoing research and adaptation of treatment protocols are needed to address the challenges posed by multidrug resistant organisms and emerging pathogens.

REFERENCES

1. LeVoyer T, WG Cioffi Jr, Pruitt L, Shipper R, Mc Manus WF, Mason AD Jr, et al. Alterations in intestinal permeability after thermal injury. Arch Surg. 1992;127:26-9.
2. Manson WL, Klasen HJ, Saver EW, Olieman A. Selective intestinal decontamination for prevention of wound colonization in severely burned patients: a retrospective analysis. Burns. 1992;18:98-102.
3. Ryan CM, Bailey SH, Carter EA, Schoenfeld DA, Tompkins RG. Additive effects of thermal injury and infection on gut permeability. Arch Surg. 1994;129:325-8.
4. Norbury W, Herndon DN, Tanksley J, Jeschke MG, Finnerty CC. Infection in Burns. Surg Infect (Larchmt). 2016;17(2):250-5.
5. Teplitz C. Pathology of burns and the fundamentals of burn wound sepsis. In: Artz CP, Moncreif JA, Pruitt BA (Eds). Burns: A team approach. Philadelphia. WB Saunders; 1979. p. 69.
6. Mac Millan BG. Local care and infection in burns. J Trauma. 1965;5:292-306.
7. Santucci SG, Gobara S, Santos CR, Fontana CA, Levin AS. Infections in a burn intensive care unit: Experience of 7 years. J Hosp Infect. 2003;53:6-13.
8. Taylor GD, Kibsey P, Kirkland T, Burroughs E, Tredget E. Predominance of staphylococcal organisms in infection occurring in a burns ICU. Burns. 1992;18:332-5.
9. Gang RK, Sanyal SC, Bang RL, Mokaddas E, Lari AR. Staphylococcus septicemia in burns. Burns. 2000;26:359-66.
10. Wisplinghoff H, Perbix W, Seifert H. Risk factors for nosocomial bloodstream infection due to *Acinetobacter baumanni*: a case control study of adult burns patients. Clin Infect Dis. 1999;28: 59-66.
11. Mason AD Jr, McManus AT, Pruitt BA Jr. Association of burn mortality and bacteremia. Arch Surg. 1986;121:1027-32.
12. Lachiewicz AM, Hauck CG, Weber DJ, Cairns BA, van Duin D. Bacterial Infections after Burn Injuries: Impact of Multidrug Resistance. Clin Infect Dis. 2017;65(12):2130-6.
13. Zhou S, Xiao S, Wang X, Wang X, Han L. Risk Factors and Pathogens of Wound Infection in Burn Inpatients from East China. Antibiotics. 2023;12(9):1432.
14. Meshram P, Wanjare V. Acinetobacter in Burn Wound Infection: Emerging problem in Central India. Int J Health Sci Res. 2017;7(4):127-31.
15. Pruitt BA Jr. Infections of burns and other wounds caused by Pseudomonas aeruginosa. In: Doggett RG (Ed). Pseudomonas aeruginosa. New York: Academic; 1979. pp. 339-66.
16. Pruitt BA Jr, Mc Manus AT. The changing epidemiology of infections in burn patients. World J Surg. 1992;16:57-67.
17. Cardany CR, Rodeheaver GT, Horowitz JH, Kenney JG, Edlich RF. Influence of hydrotherapy and antiseptic agents on burn wound bacterial contamination. J Burn Care Rehabil. 1985;6:230-2.
18. Mayhall CG. The epidemiology of burn wound infections: then and now. Clin Infec Dis. 2003:37:543-50.
19. Chakraborty RK, Burns B. (2023). Systemic Inflammatory Response Syndrome. [online] Available from https://www.ncbi.nlm.nih.gov/books/NBK547659/. [Last accessed May, 2024]
20. Arturson G, Hogman CF, Johansson SGO, Killander J. Changes in immunoglobulin level in severely burned patients. Lancet. 1969;1:546-8.
21. Munster AM, Hoacland HC, Pruitt BA Jr. The effect of thermal injury on serum immunoglobulin. Ann Surg. 1971;172:965-9.
22. Dominioni L, Dionigi R, Zanello M, Chiaranda M, Dionigi R, Acquarolo A, et al. Effect of high dose IgG on survival of surgical patients with sepsis score of 20 or greater. Arch Surg. 1991;126:236-40.
23. Rodriguez A, Rello J, Neira J, Maskin B, Ceraso D, Vasta L, et al. Effect of high dose of I/V immunoglobulin and antibiotics on survival for severe sepsis undergoing surgery. Shock. 2005;23(4):298-304.
24. Stephen W, Dichtelmuller H, Schedel I. Properties and efficacy of a human Ig M preparation for Intravenous administration. Arzneim Forsch/Drug Res. 1985;35(1):933-6.
25. Balikcioglu S, Schedel I, Berger D. Rationale of anti-endotoxin therapy of sepsis and septic shock with polyclonal immunoglobulin. Third International Congress on the immunomechanics and therapeutic approaches; 2-5 March; 1995; vol 20. Munich edited by: Eugeu Fairst, Artheu EB, Lambert T.
26. Bergquist M, Hästbacka J, Glaumann C, Freden F, Huss F, Lipcsey M. The time-course of the inflammatory response to major burn injury and its relation to organ failure and outcome. Burns. 2019;45:354-63.
27. Nash G, Foley FD, Goodwin MN, Bruck HM, Greenwald KA, Pruitt Jr BA. Fungal burn wound infection. JAMA. 1971;215: 1664-6.
28. Becker WK, Cioffi WG, McManus AT, Kim SH, McManus WF, Mason AD, et al. Fungal burn wound infection. A 10-year experience. Arch Surg. 1991;126:44-8.
29. Robert F, Lebreton F, Bougnoux ME, Pangam A, Wasserman D, Schlotterer M, et al. Use of random amplified polymorphic DNA as a typing method for albicans in epidemiological surveillance of a burn unit. J Clin Microbio . 1995;33:2366-71.
30. Mac Millan BG. The control of burn wound sepsis. Intensive Care Med. 1981;7:63-9.
31. Gupta N, Haque A, Latiff AA, Narayan RP, Mukhopadhyay G, Prasad R. Epidemiology and molecular typing of Candida isolates from burn patients. Mycopathologia. 2004;158:397-405.
32. Capoor MR, Sarabahi S, Tiwari VK, Narayanan RP. Fungal infections in burns: Diagnosis and management. Indian J Plast Surg. 2010;43(Suppl):S37-42.

33. Foley FD, Greenwald KA, Nash G, Pruitt BA Jr. Herpes virus infection in burned patients. N Eng J Med. 1970;282:652.
34. Barajas-Nava LA, Lopez Alcalde J, Roque i Figuls M, Sola I, Bonfill Cosp X. Antibiotic prophylaxis for preventing burn wound infection. Cochrane Database Syst Rev. 2013;(6):CD008738.
35. Muthukumar V, Arumugam PK, Bamal R. Role of systemic antibiotic prophylaxis in acute burns: A retrospective analysis from a tertiary care center. Burns J Int Soc Burn Inj. 2020;46: 1060-5.
36. MacGregor L. International Consensus "Appropriate Use Of Silver Dressings In Wounds". An expert working group consensus. London: Wounds International; 2012.
37. Jain A, Husain J, Singh A. Evaluation of Nano-Crystalline Silver Dressings in Superficial Partial Thickness Burns. J Clin of Diagn Res. 2019;13(11):PC05-8.
38. Khansa I, Schoenbrunner AR, Kraft CT, Janis JE. Silver in Wound Care-Friend or Foe?: A Comprehensive Review. Plast Reconstr Surg Glob Open. 2019;7(8):e2390.
39. Poon VK, Burd A. In vitro cytotoxicity of silver: Implication for clinical wound care. Burns. 2004;30(2):140-7.
40. Widgerow AD. Nanocrystalline silver, gelatinases and the clinical implications. Burns. 2010;36(7):965-74.
41. Clark NM, Patterson J, Lynch JP. Antimicrobial resistance among gram negative organism in the ICU. Curr Opin Crit Care. 2003;9:413-23.
42. Heggars JP, McCoy L, Reisner B, Smith M, Edgar P, Ramirez RJ. Alternate microbial therapy for vancomycin resistant enterococci burn wound infections. J Burn Care Rehabilit. 1998;19:399-403.
43. Embil JM, McLeod JA, Al- Barrak AM, Thompson GM, Aoki FY, Witwicki EJ, et al. An outbreak of MRSA on a burn unit: potential role of contaminated hydrotherapy equipment. Burns. 2001;27:681-8.
44. Alekshun MN, Levy SB. Molecular mechanisms of antibacterial multidrug resistance. Cell. 2007;128:1037-50.
45. World Health Organization. (2015). World Health Assembly Global Action Plan on Antimicrobial Resistance. [online] Available from https://iris.who.int/bitstream/handle/10665/193736/9789241509763_eng.pdf?sequence=1. [Last accessed May, 2024]
46. Baddley JW, Moser SA. Emerging fungal resistance. Clin Lab Med. 2004;24:721-35,vii.
47. Mousa HA, al-Bader SM. Yeast infection in burns. Mycoses. 2001;44:147-9.
48. Mac Manus WG, Mason AD Jr. Subeschar antibiotic infusion in the treatment of burn wound infection. J Trauma. 1980;20:1021.
49. Ramose GE, Bolgiani AN, Patino O, Prezzavento GE, Guastavino P, Durlach R, et al. Catheter infection risk related to the distance between insertion site and burned area. J Burn Care Rehabil. 2002;23:266-71.

SECTION

4

Burns of Special Types

CHAPTER

21

Electrical Burns

SP Bajaj, Aakanksha Goel, Arun Goel

"Like fire, electricity is a good servant but a bad master."

INTRODUCTION

Electricity is known to mankind since times immemorial. It is one of the most powerful forces on earth. Thales of Miletus in 6th century BC wrote that rubbing fur on amber would cause attraction between two substances. This was probably what we understand today as static electricity. The word "electricity" is derived from Latin "electricus", meaning amber-like. Luigi Galvani (1781) demonstrated that electricity was the medium by which nerve cells pass signals. The first report of a fatality from electricity in scientific literature was in 1879 from France where a stage carpenter was killed following a contact with an alternating current of 250 volts generated by a Siemens dynamo. In the USA, Samuel Smith was the first person to die from electrocution from a generator in 1881. Since then, mortality and morbidity from electricity has shown a steady increase all over the world consequent to its widespread use.

Very few developments have had such a great impact on mankind as electricity and its generation by a number of modes. Two hundred years ago, Michael Faraday invented the electric motor. Over the last more than one and a half century, electricity has changed the way we live, work, communicate and enjoy in a modern society. It has become a thing of absolute necessity rather than a luxury to mankind. In urban areas, apart from acting as source of light for illumination, every household has a number of gadgets which need electricity for their running. In modern times, our life is unimaginable without electricity. So much so that a nation cannot consider itself as developed unless every citizen in the remotest place gets this facility. It has greatly influenced the medical field as well by providing us with newer diagnostic and interventional techniques. Electricity has been used as electroconvulsive therapy for mental illnesses and for rhythm disorders of heart using defibrillators. It has also been used for pain relief using transcutaneous electrical nerve stimulator (TENS) and, unfortunately, as a method of torture and committing suicide. The speed with which government is making efforts to make it available to the remotest person in the country has not kept pace with making the public aware of how to use it safely and prevent oneself from its harmful effects. Probably, this is the reason, caution is not exercised by the lay person as well as electricians. Ever since electricity was first put into commercial use, in mid-18th century, electrical injuries have occurred. It is probably the most dangerous commodity which we use every day and in every moment of our lives. The term "electrical burn" is not clearly defined in literature and along with "electrical injury" is often loosely employed in referring to the same injury, i.e., an injury caused by electricity, both fatal and nonfatal.[1] So is the case in this chapter also.

EPIDEMIOLOGY[2-5]

In all major burn centers, electrical burns constitute the second most common cause of burn, thermal burns being the first. In various studies, they account for 4–8% of burn admissions but far higher percentages have also been reported. Li et al. reported 14.7% from China.[6] They are seen more commonly in rainy season because of greater chances of leakage of electric current. Most studies report more than half the cases to be work-related and majority of such cases are high-voltage injuries (up to four times).

Thus, majority of the victims are young male electricians and construction workers, <40 years of age, who are most likely to come in direct or indirect contact with "live"-wires as they are more commonly employed in these high-risk jobs (occupational hazard). These accidents result mainly from not using personal protection equipment and unsafe machine operations. Most of these cases eventually end up in litigation for negligence, product liability or worker compensation and are, thus, labeled medicolegal. At home, there may be faulty electrical appliances, exposed electrical sockets, broken extension cords, etc. Another mode of sustaining this injury is when a person tries to "steal electricity" by hooking street electricity supply. Kite-flying is a popular sport in children and young adults in India in rainy season with the attendant risk of electrical injury due to kite or its string getting caught in high-tension wires. In India, people frequently travel on the roof top of trains, especially during festive seasons when there is a great rush to visit their native places for celebrations. Some individuals may train-surf to avoid the cost of a ticket or as a recreational activity, while undertaking acts of "bravado". There is very rapid electrification of railways in our country by the government and unsuspecting commuters get electrical injuries by the overhead high-tension lines. One fact which is not known to public is that the very high voltage required to run the trains does not require a person to actually touch the "live" wire as in domestic settings to get contact electrical burn injuries. Electrical current can arc (jump) 2.5 cm from a power source or line for every 10,000 volts being carried. Thus, a person does not actually have to physically touch the source to sustain injury. These victims have additional injuries due to fall from height as well. High-tension wires going across the highways may fall on the vehicles due to heavy rain and wind speed. A high-tension "live" wire fallen in a field flooded with rainwater may also be a cause of electrical injury to an unsuspecting farmer. Toddlers and children, because of their inquisitive nature, tend to "chew" naked household electric wires causing full thickness perioral burns. They are also prone to domestic voltage electric burns by putting their fingers or metallic objects into electric sockets. Defective household appliances or their wrong use are a common cause in domestic injuries. Electricity is one of the most common causes of starting of fires due to short circuit in defective electrical equipment or substandard quality of cables and poor workmanship in wiring and other installations, etc. Consequently, it leads to not only flame burns in homes and workplaces but also loss of property.

Lightning is another cause for accidental extremely high-voltage electrical injury, quite often resulting in instant death of several persons standing together (see later).

PATHOPHYSIOLOGY

With the widespread use of electricity and injuries from it, all burn surgeons must know some fundamentals about physics of electricity apart from its pathophysiological effects on humans as well as their management in detail for an optimal outcome. Classical work of Kouwenhoven[7,8] provided the basic understanding about the effects of electricity on the human body. He also confirmed that the main mechanism of immediate death from electricity was by induction of ventricular fibrillation. As opposed to surface damage seen in purely thermal burns, an electrical injury produces tissue destruction in depth. The current enters the body at the first point of contact with source of electricity, traverses the body through the path of least resistance and exits the body at the point of grounding. These points have traditionally been called "entry" and "exit" points **(Figs. 1A and B)**. These points bear the brunt of high temperatures (leading to thermal burns) while the passage of electrical current through the body causes devastating damage to any of the tissues coming in its path. The spectrum of electrical injuries ranges from insignificant-sized burns on the skin to a threat to limb and life.

Electron, proton, and charge: Movement of electric charge is known as "electric current". Charge on electron and proton is same. Electron is negatively charged while proton is positively charged. This concept of negative and positive charge was given by Benjamin Franklin. Symbol "Q" is used to express the amount of charge and is expressed in Coulombs. Each electron or proton has a charge of 1.602×10^{-19} coulombs.

The effects of electricity on the human body are determined by a number of factors, viz., (1) Voltage, (2) Resistance of the body, (3) Type of current, (4) Amperage, (5) Duration of current, (6) Pathway of current, (7) Surface area of contact, and (8) Victim's individual susceptibility to electrical current.[9-11] Their serial numbers do not indicate order of their importance. Due to the large number of variables influencing the effect of current on the body, the exact pathophysiology of the electrical injury is not well understood yet. There can be a great number of permutations and combinations of these factors giving rise to a myriad form of injuries in any one patient. Each patient presents unique problems depending on the parameters of these factors with voltage and duration of contact being the principal determinants.

- *Voltage of current*: Electricity is a flow of electrons from atom to atom. In all conductors, they move in a random fashion until driving forces (electromotive forces) are applied to them. Voltage is the force that causes the electrons to flow and is expressed in "volts".

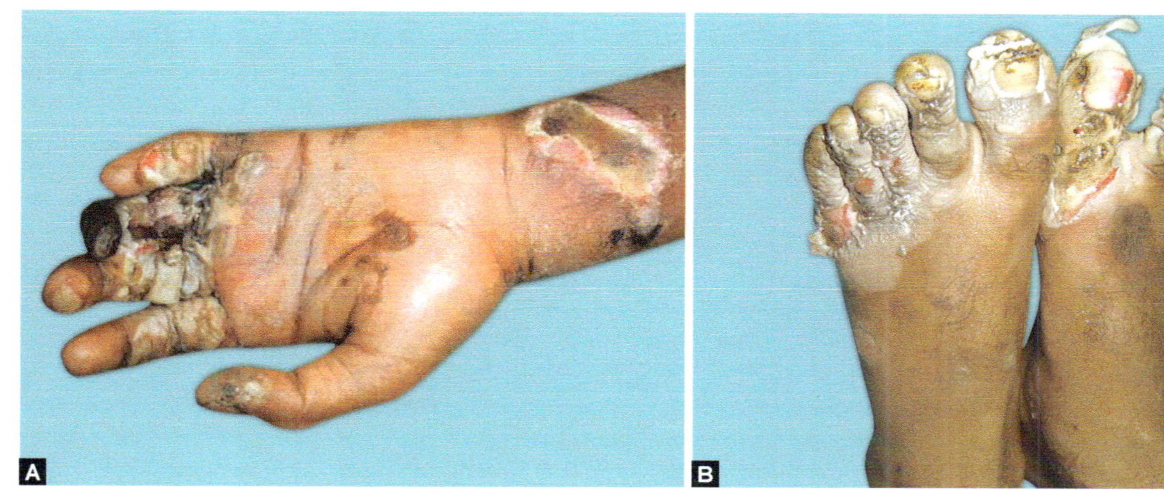

FIGS. 1A AND B: (A) Entry wounds in fingers due to contact with high voltage current and arc injury at wrist causing full thickness burn at wrist and (B) Exit wound in feet.

A large voltage exerts a large force which makes electrons to move more current in a short period. Thus, high voltages are used in all transmission cables. This also reduces the electricity losses due to leakage and heating. However, greater the voltage, lesser is the safety to human body. The thermal damage sustained by a victim of electrical contact burn is directly proportional to voltage. After any accident, it is only the voltage that is known to the victim or attendants. For this reason, electrical injuries have been arbitrarily grouped into low voltage (<1,000 volts) or high voltage (>1,000 volts). Although the former is classified as low voltage, the current capacity is large and is capable of causing substantial injury and permanent disability **(Figs. 2 to 4 and Table 1)**.

Apart from transmission cables, high voltages are also used to move electric trains and metro. In India, it is 25,000 volts. In the United Kingdom and some European countries, it is 11,000 volts. In Indian subcontinent, Europe, Australia, China, and most of Africa, domestic voltage is 210–220 volts with 50 cycles (Hertz, Hz) per second (A 50 Hz source will have 50 positive half cycles that alternate with 50 negative half cycles per second). Household current in American subcontinent is supplied at 110–120 volts with 60 Hz. Electric current of 110 volts is safer than 220 volts. Unfortunately, it is not possible now to convert to 110 volts in India and elsewhere because that will necessitate discarding all the existing equipment and gadgets creating a nationwide chaotic situation. Almost all pediatric burns are low voltage having been sustained at home but high-tension injuries are also seen.

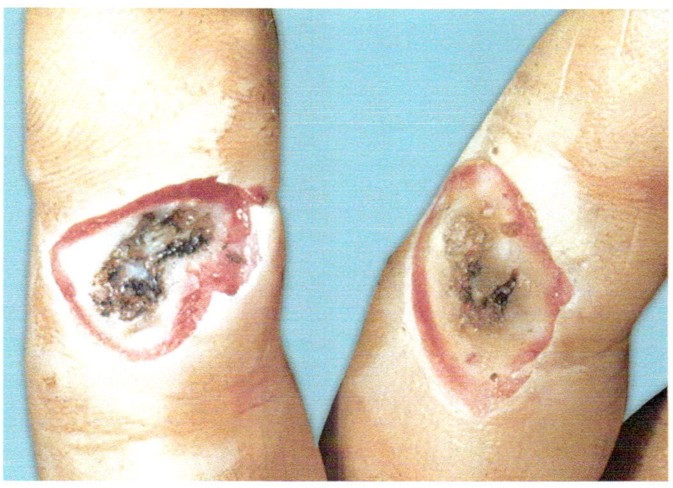

FIG. 2: Low voltage electrical burns of fingers treated by primary excision and grafting. No involvement of tendon and nerves.

A threshold of 24 volts has been described as safe. Lower voltages than this in any circuit have been found to have no lethal effects on the human body. Actually, it is the total current entering the human body which is of concern. This was best described by Hodgkin in 1974 as mentioned by Wu.[12] According to him, 1 mA of current leads to just tingling or perception which becomes painful when increased to 5 mA. At 60 mA, it leads to cardiac fibrillation, burns at 5,000 mA, and respiratory arrest at 10,000 mA. A person with high-voltage injury develops respiratory arrest because of spasm of respiratory muscles (asphyxial death) and is more likely to be revived as compared to a low-voltage injury where the heart goes into fibrillation and is less likely to be revived.

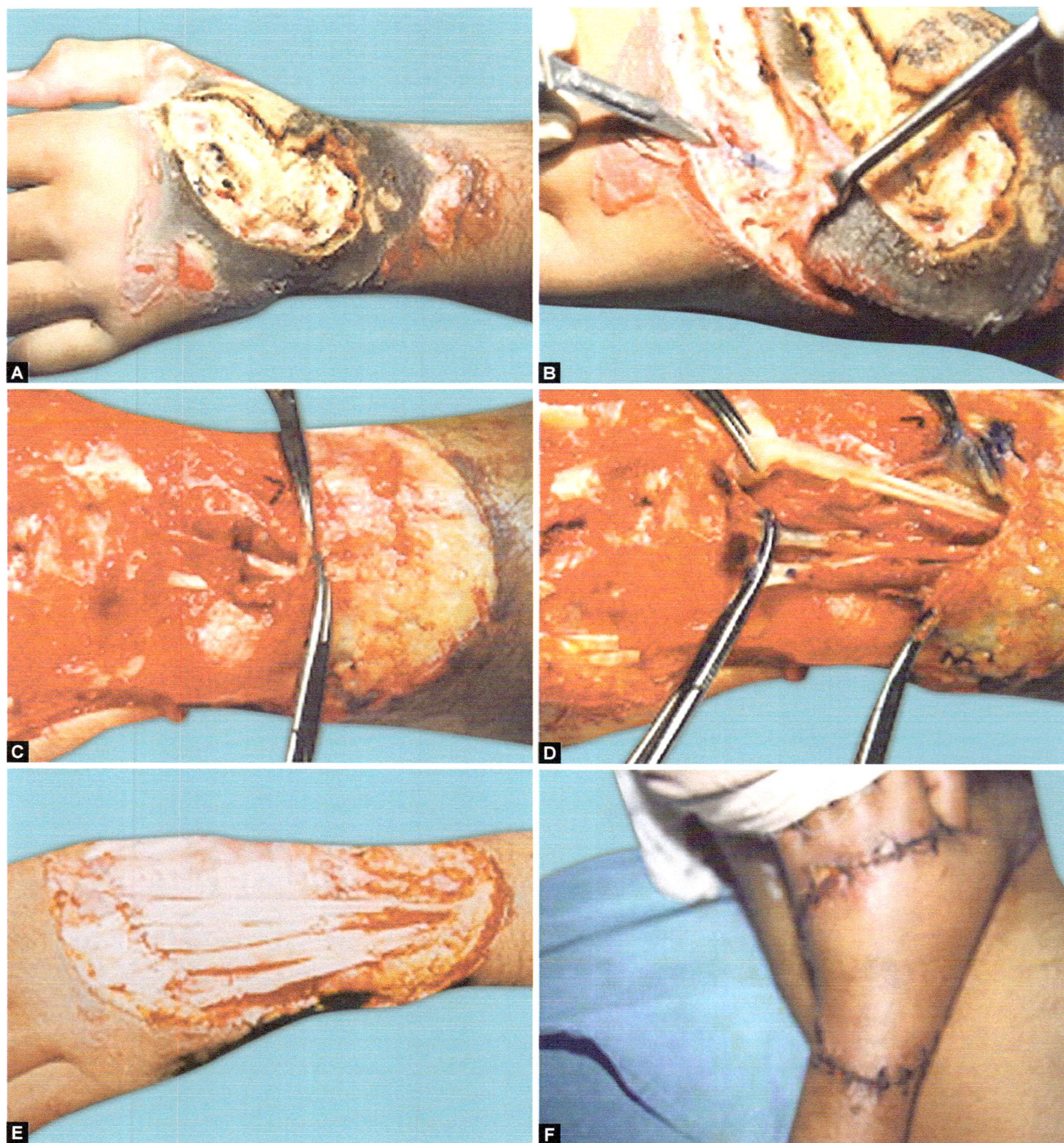

FIGS. 3A TO F: Low voltage electrical injury involving extensor surface of the hand. Showing different levels of involvement with in-between normal tissue while deeper necrosis of tendon or thrombosis of veins. Total reconstruction by providing tendon and cover. Cover by pedicle groin flap.

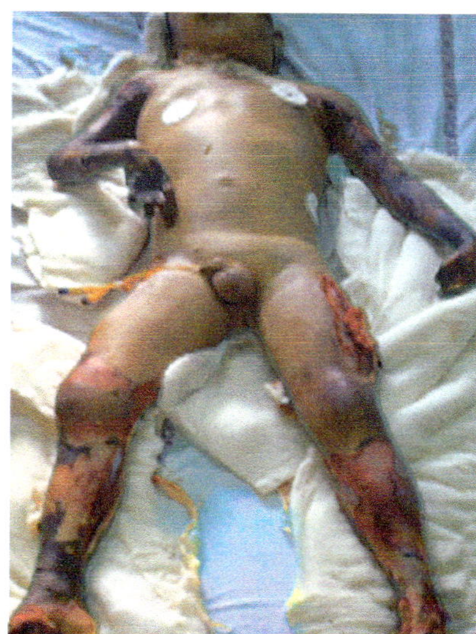

FIG. 4: High voltage electrical injury involving all four limbs, scalp, and back. Patient died from severity of injury.

- *Resistance of the body*: If it were not for the inability of electricity to pass through every substance easily, it would have been of no use to mankind and rather would have been a cause of morbidity and mortality. Different substances offer different resistance (hindrance) to the flow of electric current. Substances which have low resistance are called good conductors while those with high resistance are called bad conductors. In a bad conductor, the electrons are fixed and have hardly any movement (e.g., dry wood, porcelain, glass and rubber, also called insulators) while in a good conductor, the electrons are loosely placed (e.g., water, copper, and silver). Substances which have no resistance are called super conductors. The unit of measurement of resistance, that is, how difficult it is for current to pass through a material, is called an ohm.

TABLE 1: Comparison between high-voltage and low-voltage electrical injuries.

	High voltage	Low voltage
Voltage	>1,000 volts; present in high-tension transmission lines and electric supply to trains and metro. Practically, all these burns are contact in parallel (as the current passes out from the body to the ground leading to more damage to the body tissues	<1,000 volts, present in domestic supply (220 volts); electrical injuries by electric iron, kettle, hair dryers, lawn mower, desert air coolers, bathtubs and other home appliances are most common causes of low-voltage deaths. In industries, where three-phase current is in use, voltage may be 440 volts
Current	Less than 240 amperes	Less than 1,000 amperes
Duration of current	Short	Prolonged
Type of current	DC (in industries) or AC (in transmission lines, train, metro, etc.)	Mostly AC (domestic supplies)
Person involved	Usually, electricians and construction workers	Usually, children and young adults in domestic setting; Oral cavity and hand burns
Major threat	Electrothermal injury	Ventricular fibrillation
Type of injury	Electric arc is the most common type of injury	Contact and flash
Usual cause of cardiac arrest	Ventricular fibrillation	Ventricular fibrillation
Usual cause of respiratory arrest	Tetanic contractions of respiratory muscles or mechanical trauma due to falls	Tetanic contractions of respiratory muscles
Tissue injury	Usually extensive areas of dead skin, fat and muscles. More extensive injuries are present in high-tension injury (proves that electrical injuries are a "grand masquerader").	Injuries usually small and limited to areas of contact (e.g., hands, feet, mouth, etc.); "What you see is what you get" describes low-tension injury
Amputation	Very high incidence	Far less
Surgical interventions	Very high number with major reconstructions required	Less; commonly skin grafting only
Fractures	Can cause fractures	Less common

Continued

Continued

	High voltage	Low voltage
Muscle contraction	DC: single; AC: tetanic	Tetanic
Burns	Commonly deep	Usually superficial
Rhabdomyolysis	Very common	Possible
Systemic effects	Systemic effects are very common and involve all systems	Usually no systemic effects, however, sometimes ECG changes are seen in the form of elevated ST segment/ T-wave depression
Blunt injury (cause)	Muscle contraction and fall	Fall (uncommon)
Mortality (acute)	Moderate (higher than low voltage)	Lower than high voltage

A human body becomes an integral part of the electrical circuit when it comes in contact with a source of electricity and presents a number of resistors to the current. The resistance offered by different body tissues to current is different. The resistance of tissues to passage of current is largely dependent on their water content because the latter is a good conductor. Thus, while bone offers the greatest resistance, the fluid in the blood vessels provides least resistance and the best pathway for transmission. The other body tissues in descending order of offering resistance in between bone and blood are fat, tendon, skin, muscle, nerves, and blood vessels. It is the skin which encounters the electric current first. The resistance offered by skin at the point of entry shows great variations. The skin of sole of the feet and palm of hands is thick and cornified and offers greater resistance than thinner skin of other areas because of low water content in the former. Dry skin offers more resistance (up to 1 million ohms/ cm^2) as compared to wet skin due to say, sweating (35,000 ohms/cm^2), thoroughly wet approximately 10,000 ohms/cm^2 and finally, of a person immersed, in say, a bathtub just 1,000 ohms/cm^2. Moist mucous membranes have negligible resistance (100 ohms/ cm^2). Resistance is also low in children and at extremes of age because of thinner epidermis. Dermis has lesser resistance as compared to epidermis as body fluids and blood are good conductors because of their salinity. Skin, nonetheless, represents an initial barrier to flow of current and an electric insulator to deeper tissues. Thus, it can be understood how comparatively lesser voltage may cause fatality in an individual in a bathtub whereas similar voltage may cause minimal damage on coming in contact with thick and dry skin of heel pad. From a practical point of view, an electrical injury will have more local effects (i.e., burns due to conversion of electrical into thermal energy) when skin provides higher resistance and more severe systemic effects when the skin has lower resistance.

Resistance offered by the skin generates enormous amount of heat leading to evaporation of water content of the skin and underneath tissue. The resistance changes with the flow of current. The initial slow rise represents a progressive decrease in skin resistance. This is followed by an abrupt and rapid climb in amperage, coinciding with complete breakdown of resistance offered by skin and an unimpeded flow of current in the internal body tissues. The current flows through the structure which provides least resistance to its flow. After carbonization of skin from the conversion of electrical energy into thermal energy, an appearance of a flash indicates the termination of current flow. No further tissue damage is now possible.

Thus, entry point of high-voltage electric current appears as charred or whitish yellow area with a leathery texture, with markedly depressed central zone surrounded by hyperemic border. Exit wounds which can be in lower limb or opposite hand can be multiple and appear ruptured tanned black and give an impression that the current exploded while exiting because of explosive release of heat due to high-voltage current coming out. Thus, these two places show maximum resistance and, hence, maximum local damage is seen at these two sites.

It has been found that the cross-sectional area (or circumference) of the region of the body involved is more important than resistance of individual tissues. A combination of comparatively smaller cross-sectional area with high internal resistance of an extremity leads to a considerable drop in voltage when the current passes through it. The resulting conversion of electrical energy into thermal energy is maximal at the site of contact in the skin and adjoining structures. Thus, chest and abdomen with greater cross-sectional area provide lesser resistance, the amount of heat generated is much less, it dissipates over a larger area and thermal damage to viscera is rare. A finger with lesser circumference provides greater resistance and more damage is seen. Specific regions or "choke points" in the upper limb (e.g., wrist and elbow) having decreased cross-sectional area (increased current density) and highly resistant bone and tendons result in increased heat production and greater tissue damage. Similarly, current flow in the larger vessels with bigger circumference provides less resistance while smaller vessels provide more resistance and, hence, are more likely to get thrombosed. Current density has further effects on the human body. With arteries having rapidly moving blood, current density at any given point and at any given time becomes less because of rapid flow of blood. The current density is more in veins because of slower flow of blood. Therefore, thrombosis and stoppage of blood flow is higher in veins and comparatively lesser in arteries.

In reality, in a clinical scenario, the internal tissues of the body act as a single resistor and not as a compendium of multiple resistors.

- *Type of current*: Electric current exists in two forms: (1) Alternating current (AC, invented by Nikola Tesla) and (2) Direct current (DC, invented by Thomas Edison). AC is usually generated with a cyclic reversal of the direction of electrons and thus creates a sign wave. In DC, the electrons always travel in one direction (unidirectional flow) from the entry point in contact with electrical source to the exit point, usually in contact with the ground. There were considerations about safety and cost of electricity supply in 19th and early 20th centuries. At present, AC has entirely superseded DC as it is considered to be a far more efficient way of generating and distributing electricity, and is cheaper and easy to transform into any desired voltage. Use of DC is restricted to the chemical and metallurgical industry. It is also used in the automobiles. All batteries deliver DC. Use of uninterruptible power supply (UPS) and defibrillators is based on DC.

  The type of current, AC or DC, has significantly different effects on the human body. It is believed that AC is three times more dangerous to life as compared to DC of same voltage.[13] Skin offers greater resistance to DC than to AC. The latter produces a tetanizing effect on skeletal muscles. With increasing AC, the magnitude of contraction of muscles keeps on increasing and hold of the victim on the contact point becomes so intense that he/she is unable to "let go" from the electrical source (known as "no let go" phenomenon). This phenomenon occurs because of simultaneous contraction of stronger forearm flexors and weaker extensors. Maximum current a person can hold and still release at one's will is called "let go" current. Such strong muscle contraction may lead to fractures and/or dislocation of joints. Threshold for "let go" effect in both sexes is different, probably because of different muscle strength. It is 16 mA in men and 11 mA in women with 60 Hz of AC. The earlier commonly used terms "entry" and "exit" wounds are "misnomers" with respect to AC injuries as the flow of current reverses and re-enters through the two contact points alternately. They may, however, represent the patient's body part which first came into contact with electrical source.

  Direct current does not produce muscle contraction as produced by the AC and a person is thrown away after a short muscle contraction. Low voltage DC is not as dangerous as an equivalent voltage of AC. AC of 60 Hz with as low voltage as 60 volts can be fatal. Conversely, a high voltage of DC is more likely to be fatal when compared to AC of same voltage.
- *Amperage*: Amperage of the current that flows through the human body on coming in contact with an electrical source is extremely important as it determines the resulting damage. When 6.24×10^{18} electrons pass through a given point in 1 second, it is called passing of 1 ampere of current. 1 ampere of current represents 1 coulomb of charge. 1 ampere is almost equivalent to current flowing through a 100-watt lit light bulb.

  There is a definite relationship between intensity of current (ampere), force of current flow (voltage), and resistance to flow. This relationship was described by Ohm and is called Ohm's law. Ohm's law states that:

  Amperage (Intensity, I) is equal to voltage (E) divided by resistance (R).

$$I = E/R$$

  It means current is directly proportional to voltage and inversely proportional to resistance. More the voltage, more the current. More the resistance, less is the flow of current. The minimum current a human can feel is thought to be about 1 milliampere (mA) (1 mA = 1/1,000 of an ampere).

  Death caused by an electric current is referred to as electrocution. This can be accidental, suicidal, or as a method of execution in which the condemned person is subjected to a heavy charge of electric current, usually lasting about 2 minutes. Thus, this term is inappropriately used when patients are alive and being transported and admitted to hospitals. This term is also not generally used for patients who die several days later due to complications of electrical burns. Electric shock is a sudden violent response by a person to flow of electric current through any part of the body.

  With greater resistance, greater numbers of electrons collide with each other and generate more heat. In a clinical scenario, since the resistance is not known, it is difficult to find the true intensity of the current. The heat generated at "entry" and "exit" points is directly proportional to the amperage and resistance. Heat generated in a current source due to flow of current is the indicator of power. Watt is the unit of electrical power. 1 ampere of current flow through 1 Ohm of resistance in 1 second is 1 Watt of energy generated. 1 Watt per second produces 0.24 calories of heat.

This was described by Joule and is explained mathematically by Joule's Law.

Power (P) = Voltage (E) × Current (I); further, E = I × R

Therefore, $P = I^2 \times R$

As seen in Joule effect,

$$\text{Heat } (^\circ\text{C}) = 0.24 \times \text{Amperage}^2 \times \text{Resistance} \times \text{Time}$$

- *Duration of current*: The duration of contact with electrical current is an important determinant of injury. Longer the duration of contact, greater are the chances of damage to the vital structures. However, high voltages of even brief duration can cause massive injury to superficial and deeper tissues. Thus, an electric shock caused by AC will cause greater injury than that due to DC of the same amperage because the latter causes a single muscle contraction that "throws" the victim away from the power source, in effect minimizing the injury. The tetanizing effect of AC, preventing the interruption of contact with the electrical circuit, increases the duration of contact. These differences have practical significance only at low voltages. At high voltages, both currents have a similar effect. Prolonged contact may also ignite clothing leading to flame burns as well. In lightning strikes, the duration of contact is in milliseconds and thus, serious burns are infrequently seen. One of the most important differences between lightning and high-voltage electrical injuries is the duration of exposure to the current.
- *Pathway of current*: The pathway of current in the human body is of extreme importance. In general, the current passes from the point of entry into the body toward a site which is grounded, that is, toward lower resistance, the air being a bad conductor. Despite having low conductivity, the physical dimensions of earth are so massive that it offers practically nil resistance to electric current. Obviously, when the vital organs come in the path of electrical current, it is likely to be more severe and lethal. A vertical pathway is the most dangerous because it involves the brain, conducting system of heart, respiratory muscles and in a pregnant woman, the fetus as well. The most common pathway is from one limb to another while it is rarely through the head. The susceptibility of the heart to passage of current is also affected by the different times of its contraction cycle (first part of the T wave is most vulnerable). A current passing from upper extremity to ipsilateral lower extremity may not involve heart. A horizontal pathway from hand to hand will spare the brain but can still be fatal due to involvement of the heart and/or respiratory muscles. A pathway through the lower part of the body may cause severe local damage but probably will not be lethal. It must be noted that electricity seeks all paths and not just the path of least resistance to reach lower potential. It is not always possible to predict the path it has taken from examination of skin burns and is at best a clinical guess. The unpredictable course and the variations in response by individual tissues differentiate the electrical from the most common thermal burn injuries.
- *Surface area of contact*: Smaller the area of contact, greater is the density of current. Thus, more energy is converted into heat and greater is the local tissue destruction. Conversely, if the contact area is very large, the current density may not be able to produce any local lesion at all. However, skin being a poor insulator, the current may be sufficient enough to kill an individual. The importance of size of area of contact can be seen in domestic voltage accidents wherein a toddler sucks/chews a "live" wire but sustains deep burns to lips only without any systemic effects. On the other hand, a person lying in a bathtub or swimming pool gets killed immediately without any local lesions if he/she touches an ungrounded "live" electrical wire.
- *Individual susceptibility*: The victim's susceptibility to electrical current also determines the clinical presentation and outcome.

TYPES OF ELECTRICAL BURNS

Apart from conventional division into low (<1,000 volts) and high (>1,000 volts) voltage, electrical burn injuries have also been classified as follows. While contact and arc burns are "true" electrical burns, flash, and flame burns are "false" as electricity is only the causative agent and there are no local or systemic effects of electricity.

- *Contact burns*: These are considered as true electrical injury **(Figs. 5 to 7)**. The body becomes a part of the circuit by direct contact with the source and injury by the passage of current through the body is manifested by "entry" and "exit" cutaneous wounds. They can be either low or high voltage. The electric path from entrance to exit usually takes the shortest distance between the two points. Multiple exit wounds in some patients attest to the possibility of several pathways

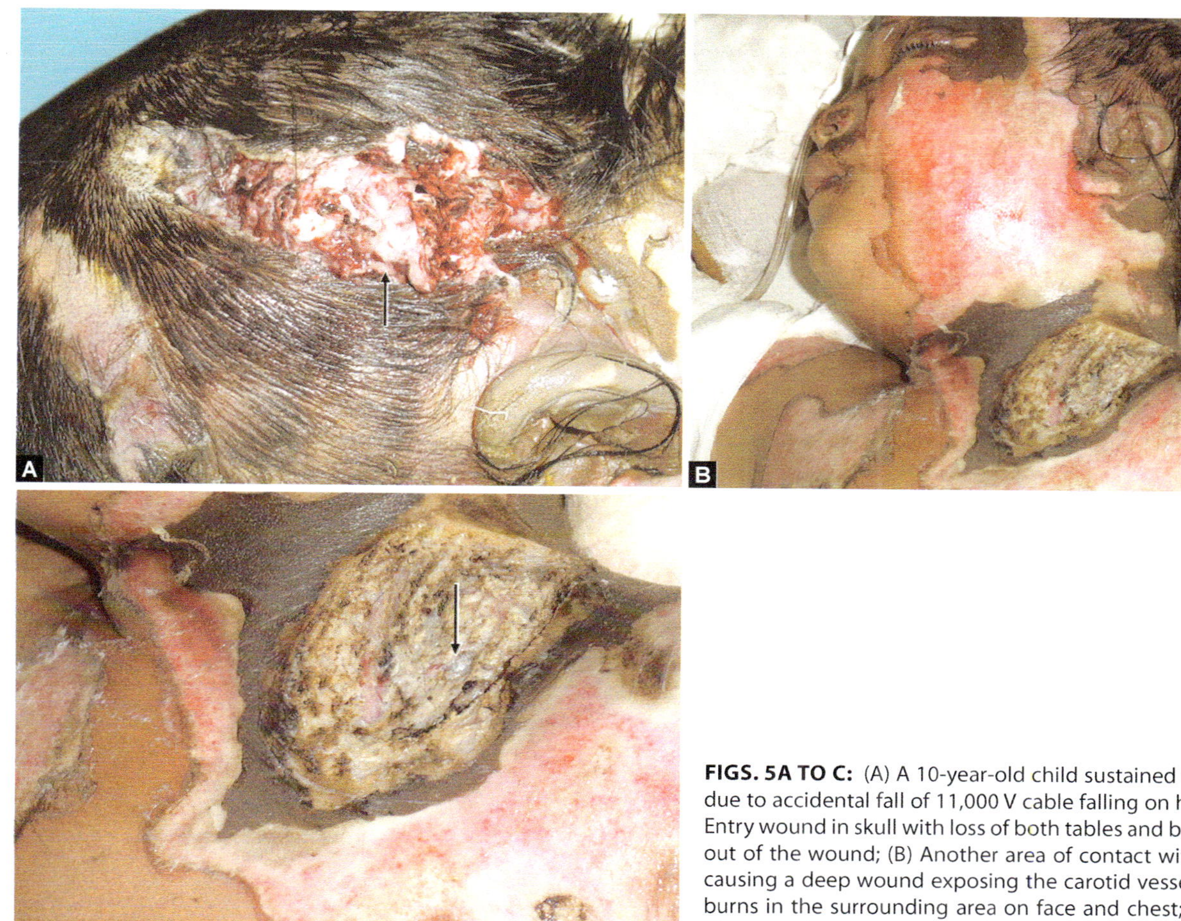

FIGS. 5A TO C: (A) A 10-year-old child sustained high tension injury due to accidental fall of 11,000 V cable falling on her while playing—Entry wound in skull with loss of both tables and brain matter coming out of the wound; (B) Another area of contact with wire in the neck causing a deep wound exposing the carotid vessels, with deep flash burns in the surrounding area on face and chest; and (C) Third area of contact in same patient below the axilla exposing pleura requiring chest tube drainage for pneumothorax.

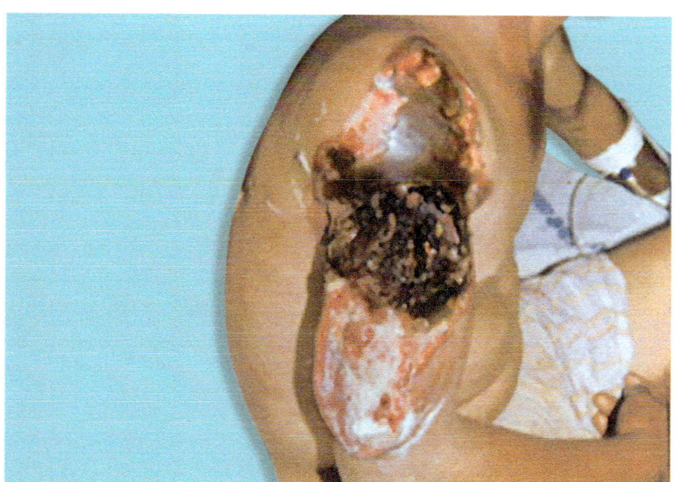

FIG. 6: Electric contact burns in series, no wound of exit or grounding. Maximum local damage by production of heat.

taken by the current. Burns caused by contact with a high-voltage alternating electric circuit conforms to two types: (1) burns from an electric current and (2) burns from an electric arc.

- *Arc burns*: Arc burns are highly destructive in nature. The permanent damage on the tissues is immediate and profound. It involves muscles, tendons, and bones and usually necessitates amputation of extremities. Often the lesion is bloodless, cold, and painless. An "arc" burn is produced by a current coursing external to the human body from the point of contact to the ground or above the surface to another part of the body. The electrical energy "jumps" from a high-resistance area to a low-resistance area. The arc has an intense and pale-violet light. It is made up of ionized gas or "plasma" which is a very good conductor of electricity. It is driven by high electromagnetic force (voltage) between the source and human body with air space in between. As a result, an arc can form a direct electrical connection and allow current to pass along its length without any mechanical contact or touching by the victim. As stated above, electrical current can arc (jump) 2.5 cm from a power source for every 10,000 volts. Once a high voltage arc has been established, it may extend for 10 feet before interruption of circuit occurs. Arc burns occur due to the high temperatures (4,000–20,000°C) which can even melt bone and volatilize metal. A high-voltage arc can also produce a considerable pressure wave blast in excess of 1,000 pounds/in^2 of pressure. Sometimes, the pressure wave throws the victim, usually an electrician, away from the arc-blast. While this may reduce further exposure to the thermal energy, serious physical injury, ruptured tympanic membrane, etc., may result. Although there is no true electrical current flow through the patient, it is difficult to determine this clinically in a patient. A common example of arcing is the flash that one sometimes sees when a domestic light switch is turned on or off. This is not dangerous because of the low voltage. Electric arc remains an important cause in high-voltage electrical injuries. Burns occur at the point where arc strikes the human body. These arc burns are mostly seen on the palmer surface of hand, flexor aspect of wrists, forearm, and flexor surface of the elbow joint **(Fig. 8)**. Usually, there is little or no systemic effect. Current takes the path of maximum conductivity. There is maximum damage to nerves which are burnt out at the site of the injury and where current passes, the veins get thrombosed. Tendons are charred and muscles show typical pale lusterless appearance with no contractility and become dead.

- *Flash burns*: Although the causative agent is electricity, flash burns are essentially surface thermal injuries, usually of the skin of exposed areas (unprotected by the clothing) of the body like face, forearm, and hands **(Figs. 9 to 11)**. In some cases, as compared to electrical arc burns injuries, the arc does not contact a person because of distance. In this situation, burns are caused by generation of intense heat due to electrical short circuit with random movement of electrons of the nearby electrical flash. It can be both, low and high voltage. They are similar to each other except that high-voltage flash burns are more extensive and deeper because of greater heat generated in high voltage. The current does not touch or enter the body at all. Hence, there are no systemic or local effects of electric current on the human body. The burn appears to be worse than actually it is, as the skin appears charred. The temperature in the spark may be as high as 4,000°C and it lasts for a fraction of a second. It is of great clinical importance to determine whether a high-voltage injury involved electric current flow through the body or not. In the latter case, management is as for thermal burns only.

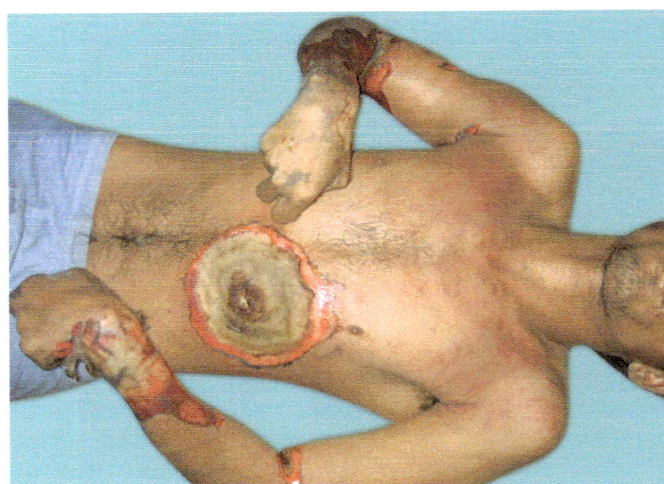

FIG. 7: Electrical contact burn in a young patient who was standing next to a wall and holding a pole with both his hands which accidentally touched a high-tension wire causing severe burn in both the hands—gangrene of both hands and exit wound in lower chest and abdomen which is less than the limb injury because of the larger circumference of the chest.

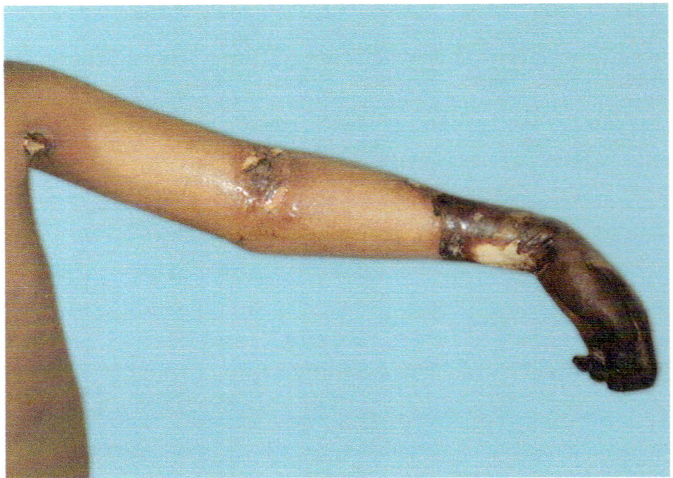

FIG. 8: Arcing of current or jumping of current from wrist to elbow to axilla with contact in the fingers.

- *Flame burns*: Faulty gadgets or electrical systems that are poorly designed or maintained or overloaded may overheat and generate arcs and sparks and start a fire. During short-circuiting, electrons randomly collide with each other producing electrical sparks. The intense heat and flash lasting for fraction of a second can ignite flammable and combustible materials and fire from these can produce deeper and extensive burns.

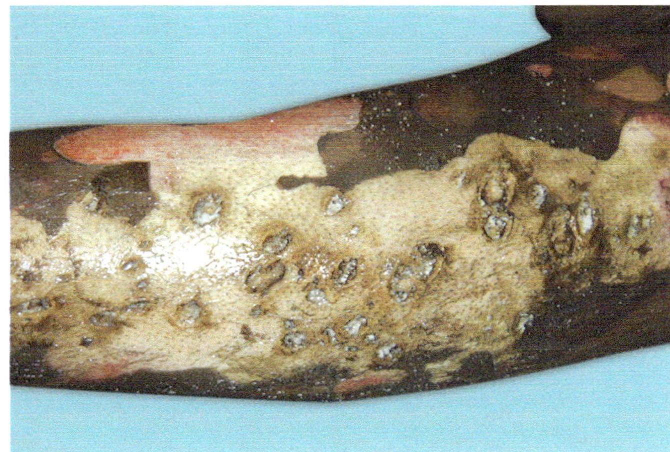

FIG. 9: Full thickness flash burns.

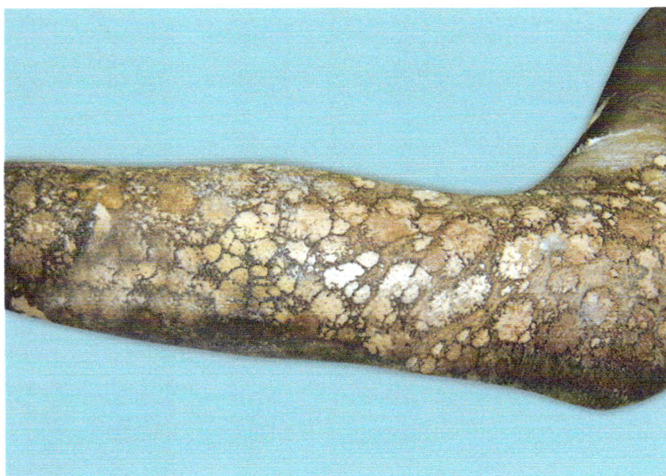

FIG. 10: Typical deep dermal injury in flash burns.

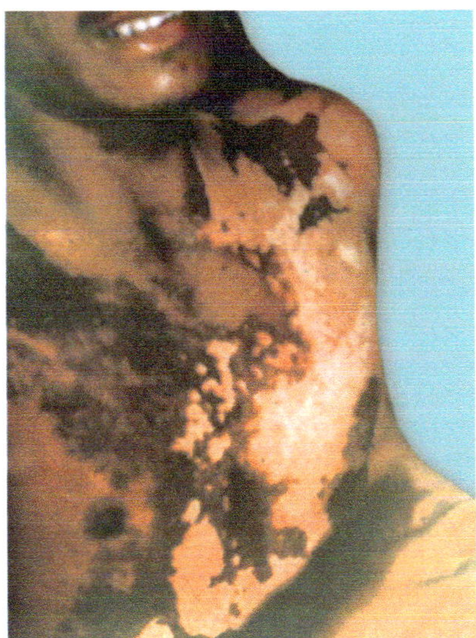

FIG. 11: Electrical flash burn.

- *Electric shock*: It is usually suffered by electricians who describe the feeling as balls of light (electrician's moons) when the current passes through the body followed by trembling, pallor, sweating, and feeling of apathy or euphoria. The patient may become unconscious because of cerebral edema and raised intracranial pressure. There may be temporary deafness or blindness with auditory hallucinations and stiffness or paralysis of limbs. These can last for a few minutes to hours. Altered sensorium may also be temporary. Many a times, there may be cardiac and respiratory arrest requiring cardiac massage and artificial respiration. An electric shock can kill without leaving burns.[14] Shock injuries are almost always associated with AC, while DC shock is rare. This is not only because AC use dominates home and workplace everywhere but also because excitation effects on nervous system are more with AC as compared to equivalent DC.
- *Lightning* is an extremely high voltage, high amperage, direct electrical current discharge of ultra-short duration natural phenomenon producing its own peculiar injury pattern (see later).

MECHANISMS OF INJURIES DUE TO ELECTRICITY

Effects of current on human body are well described. However, the mechanisms of action are not equally well understood. Electricity is said to cause injuries to human body by several mechanisms. Although the mechanisms are considered separately, in reality they can occur together in a victim.

- *Direct effect of electrical current on body tissues*: This can lead to ventricular fibrillation, asystole, or respiratory arrest (apnea).
- *Conversion of electrical energy into thermal energy resulting in burns*: Joule heating, the thermal energy generated by the electrical current, has long been attributed to be the primary cause of tissue damage inflicted when the body becomes part of a "live" circuit. There is transfer of energy with charged particles losing energy to the tissues in the form of heat. The temperatures may rise to supraphysiologic levels causing denaturation of macromolecules, which is usually irreversible. However, all clinical manifestations are not explained in this way. Different body tissues provide different resistance to the flow of current. Maximum resistance is provided by the deepest structure, i.e., bones and the most superficial structure, i.e., epidermis. They offer higher resistance and get heated up and coagulate. Tissues like nerves

and blood vessels offer lower resistance and transmit the current. However, the alternative view considers the human body to act like a volume conductor (with a resistance of 500–1,000 Ohms) with no effect of resistance of individual tissues. This view appears to be correct as it explains why there is far lesser incidence of damage occurring to abdomen and chest (with greater cross-sectional area) as compared to extremities at wrist or ankle level (with smaller cross-sectional area) (see above). However, deeper tissues, e.g., periosseous region in forearm, do retain more heat and present with more severe damage as compared to more superficial structures.

- *Electroporation*:[1,15-18] It is the process by which there is formation of aqueous pores in lipid bilayers of the cell membrane on exposure to a supraphysiologic electric field, allowing free passage of ions and fluid (membrane permeabilization). The pore formation likely allows calcium influx into the cytoplasm thereby triggering apoptosis and cell death. The cell membranes are disrupted directly resulting in cell death without generating heat. It is different from tissue damage by protein denaturation and coagulation due to heat in thermal burns.

    Studies have shown that electroporation is also a mechanism of electrical injury and can mediate skeletal muscle necrosis. This is significant because it directly addresses whether nonthermal mechanisms of cell damage can cause tissue necrosis. The cell does attempt to maintain its ionic gradients through great expenditure of energy. If the pores do not reseal, the cell eventually exhausts its energy reserves and dies. If the pores seal, the cell may eventually recover. However, the sealing process is considerably slower than the pore opening. Even if the pores close, secondary injury processes may be disruptive or even fatal to the cell. Unlike thermal heating, electroporation may not affect every cell in a specific region. In the human body, electricity encounters the greatest resistance when passing through any cellular membrane. For smaller cells, electricity may flow more readily around rather than through the cells. However, nerve and muscle cells are larger than other cells. Thus, electricity is more likely to pass through rather than around these cells. The larger the cell, the more likely it is to be injured by this mechanism.

    Due to electroporation and deep tissue heating, the damage caused is often nonuniform and difficult to interpret clinically. Electroporated muscle appears viable on gross inspection for hours and coupled with damage from tissue heating, initial diagnosis of the extent of the tissue undergoing necrosis remains problematic.

- *Secondary mechanical trauma*: High-voltage DC causes a single muscle contraction and throws the victim away from the source with likelihood of associated trauma. Lighting strikes are also DC and can cause mechanical injury by throwing away the victim or creating a blast effect. Arc injuries can also throw the victim away due to blast effect.

CLINICAL EFFECTS OF ELECTRICITY ON DIFFERENT BODY SYSTEMS[19-22]

Electric burn injuries not only have cutaneous involvement but can also have an involvement of cardiovascular, pulmonary, neurological, and renal systems. There is vascular damage and involvement of muscles of the extremities, involvement of abdominal wall and viscera, bone, and joint complications. Eyes are also affected. Clinical presentations range from a tingling sensation to a widespread tissue damage and even instantaneous death.

Cutaneous

After a high-voltage injury, seemingly minor skin burns may coexist with massive muscle necrosis as well as other internal organ injuries. The extent of damage seen on the skin is only the "tip of an iceberg". Often, the main symptom of an electrical injury is a skin burn only. Flash burns are usually superficial dermal. Burns are often most severe at the contact ("entry" and "exit") points and have typical features (see above). The former is usually in the hands or the head while the latter is often on the feet or hand. A specific type of burn, called the "kissing burn", occurs at the flexor creases (e.g., elbow and axilla) and is related to the current flowing through the opposing skin at the joint when the flexor muscles contract due to tetany.

Cardiovascular[23]

Both heart and lungs are well protected by comparatively avascular structures, namely, pericardium and pleura, respectively. Injury to the cardiovascular system is the most feared complication of both high- and low-voltage electric current because of the potential for instant cardiac arrest and death. The pathway of the electric current in the body is predictive of cardiac involvement. Thus, if the current enters through one upper extremity and leaves through the other or if it takes a vertical path from skull to chest to foot, involvement of heart is likely. The electrical injuries have a potential to change the normal cardiac electrical activity and this is seen as cardiac dysrhythmias being one of the most common complications. Cardiac arrest can occur both due to direct alteration of cardiac rhythm or to depression of respiration with consequent hypoxia. Cardiac arrest can be either complete standstill (asystole) or ineffective overactivity (ventricular fibrillation, VF). VF is the most common cause of death at the scene of accident and is more common with low-voltage AC, whereas asystole is more often associated with high-voltage AC or DC. Thus, domestic electrical injuries resulting in cardiac arrest are likely to be due to VF. The technique of cardiopulmonary resuscitation (CPR) and availability of defibrillators and their use should be taught to general public to save the life of these victims. An electrocardiogram (ECG) is done for all patients of electrical injury and cardiac monitoring should be done during transport and in the emergency room.[24] However, continued monitoring of only selected patients is required. Patients with history of documented cardiac arrest, cardiac dysrhythmia during transport or in the emergency room, an abnormal ECG upon arrival to emergency (other than sinus bradycardia or tachycardia) need ECG monitoring. Extensive total body surface area (TBSA) burns, elderly patients or those with preexisting cardiac pathology, etc., are other indications for monitoring. The abnormalities seen on an ECG are sinus tachycardia, nonspecific ST- and T-wave changes, atrial and ventricular ectopy, atrial fibrillation, first- and second-degree heart block, bundle branch block, and QT interval prolongation, etc. Multiple extrasystoles and atrial fibrillation may require administration of different cardiotropic drugs. Most of the cardiac effects recover spontaneously, long-term consequences being very rare. Late dysrhythmias are probably due to arrhythmogenic foci secondary to patchy myocardial necrosis. Direct myocardial injuries behave more like traumatic myocardial contusion rather than true myocardial infarction as they do not have consequences of atherosclerotic infarctions. Cardiac injury and rhythm disturbances can be due to anoxia secondary to respiratory arrest. Patients with no history of arrhythmia at the site of mishap, no syncope and no chest pain do not require further cardiac monitoring as they are unlikely to develop significant arrhythmias after 24–48 hours. Low-voltage (household) exposures in patients with no cardiac complaints and a normal initial ECG can even be safely discharged if no other indication for admission. Even victims of high-voltage injuries without initial ECG changes do not require cardiac monitoring. However, cardiac monitoring is still done by most clinicians in such patients for at least 24 hours.

Enzymatic assessment of cardiac damage may not be helpful because they may be elevated due to associated striated muscle damage and may not be cardiac muscle-specific. Changes in lactic acid dehydrogenase (LDH) levels may occur without ischemic changes in the heart as slight damage of cardiac muscle recovers spontaneously without any consequences. Creatine phosphokinase (CPK) and MB isoenzyme of creatine phosphokinase (CPK-MB) levels are also poor indicators of myocardial injury in the absence of ECG changes showing myocardial injury, especially in cases of significant skeletal muscle injury.

In patients with extensive necrosis over large blood vessels like in the neck and groin, there is always a danger of delayed hemorrhage (blow out) from them. This can be minimized by providing early vascularized muscle flap cover over these areas.

Pulmonary[25-27]

The most serious pulmonary complication from an electrical injury is respiratory arrest. It is usually due to underlying cardiac arrest. There is no specific injury to lungs or the airways directly due to electric current. There may be a direct injury to the respiratory control center leading to cessation of respiration. Tetanic contractions of the respiratory muscles may cause suffocation. The resistance of lung tissue is higher than that of other thoracic structures. This may be the reason for decreased incidence of direct pulmonary injury as more current flows through the surrounding structures with lower resistance. There may be loss of surfactant. Trauma from falls secondary to electrical exposure can cause pneumothorax or pulmonary contusion. Pleura may get damaged leading to effusion or collapse of lung necessitating intercostal drainage. Very rarely pulmonary edema, atelectasis, pneumonia, hemopneumothorax, pulmonary contusion, and laryngeal injuries may be seen. Finally, patients may develop pulmonary complications as part of ongoing treatment, e.g., acute respiratory dysfunction syndrome and ventilator-associated pneumonia, etc.

Extremities

The maximum impact of electrical injury is seen in the skeletal muscle and peripheral nerves. Involvement of upper extremity is more common as the victim is most likely to touch the "live" wire with his hands **(Figs. 12 to 16)**. The flexors being stronger than extensors, the hand becomes rigidly closed in a fist position when it touches AC. Lower extremity is more likely to be an exit point or else the patient might have stepped on a "live" wire. Linear flow of electrical current may cause muscle damage right up to axilla. Unfortunately, upper limb amputations are 2–3 times more common than the lower limb despite reconstructive procedures to salvage the limb. The damage may be to a particular group of muscles only or to all muscles and their neurovascular bundles.

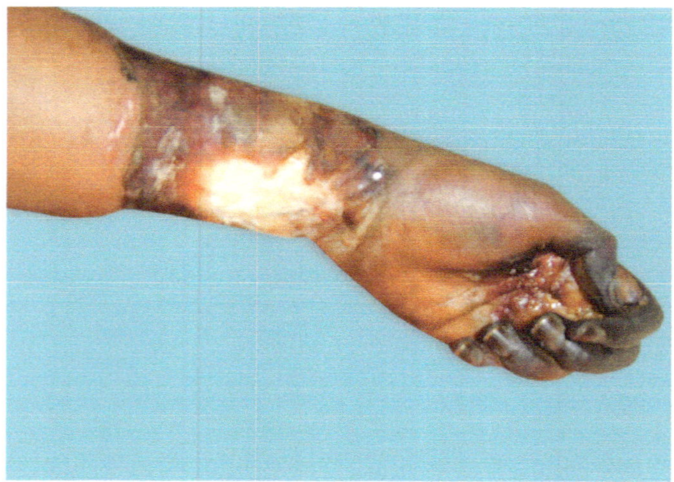

FIG. 12: High-voltage contact burn in palmar surface of hand with arcing causing full thickness circumferential burns in wrist and lower forearm causing compartment syndrome leading to ischemic damage to all fingers.

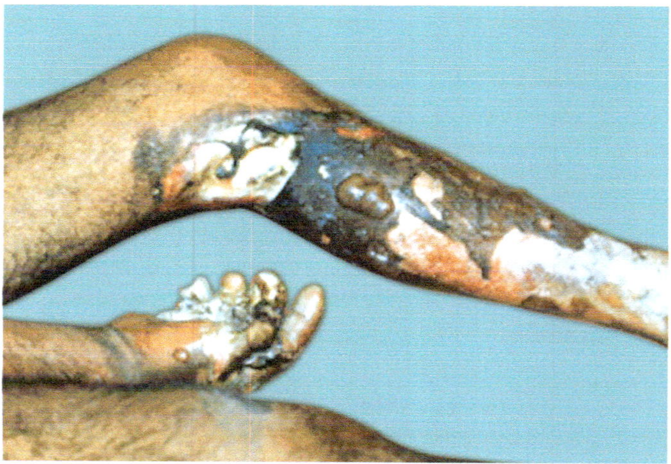

FIG. 13: Electrical contact burn on the right hand with full thickness burns on the left leg from clothes catching fire.

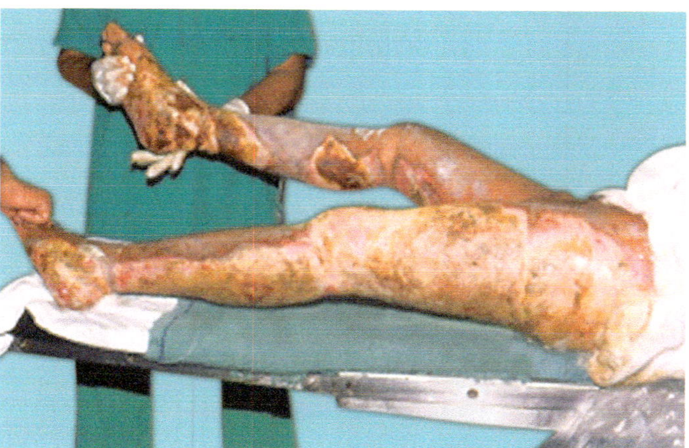

FIG. 14: Electrical contact burns of right lower limb showing patchy areas of normal skin with proximal and distal full thickness burns and flame burns of the lower extremity from clothes catching fire.

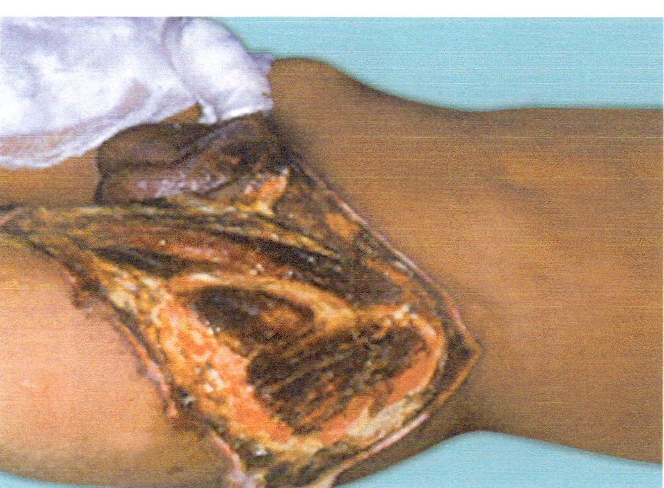

FIG. 15: High-tension electrical burn involving left groin. The patient was on a pole holding the pole by both the thighs.

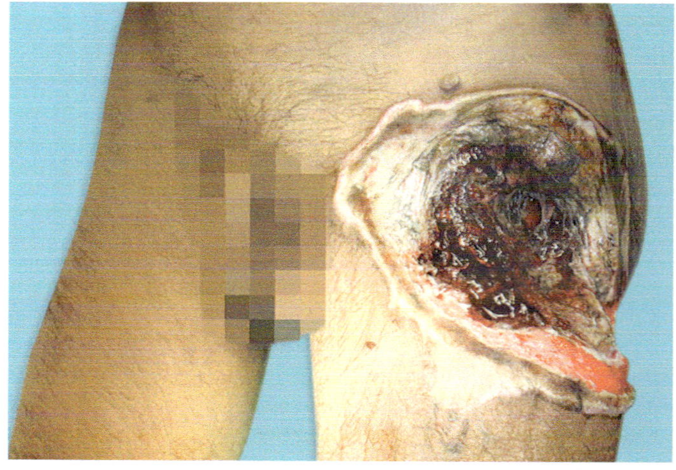

FIG. 16: Electrical contact burns on left thigh in an electrician sustained while working on an electrical pole with extensive muscle damage exposing hip joint.

It is not common to see deep muscle damage much beyond the point of entry with no superficial muscle damage. In the case of upper limbs where entry point of current is the finger, skin damage is seen at wrist, elbow, and at the axilla. This type of patchy skin damage is often described as "arcing of current" from finger to wrist and from wrist to elbow because of muscle contraction. It means these damages are indirect damage where current has flown from outside with air pocket in between, i.e., "jumping of current" across a flexed joint. As the current exits and re-enters the skin, a tremendous amount of heat is generated and the cutaneous injury in flexor creases can vary from minor erythema to explosive charring. However, in the author's (Dr SP Bajaj) opinion, after examining >60 cases of high-tension burns, this injury is because of flow of current through the blood vessels and at these points, i.e., at the wrist, elbow, and axilla, the blood vessels become superficial and these vessels give perforating vessels to the skin. Current transmitted through the blood vessels reach the superficial tissues in the skin and again resistance of skin leads to the heat production and full thickness skin damage occurs. Here, damage to the skin is based on changing direction and flow of current. However, distant damage is seen in muscles, arteries, and veins. More current flows through the muscle because of larger muscle mass and diameter with more water content. Blood vessels because of smaller diameter have more resistance. In arteries, because of rapid flow of blood, there is reduction in current density at any given point while in the veins because of slow flow of blood the current density is high. Therefore, chances of thrombosis of veins are higher which lead to increase in edema and rise in compartmental pressure leading to further damage to the muscles and compression of the arterial supply. The latter may also ultimately get thrombosed leading to death of the muscle. It appears that most of the damage in electrical burn is secondary to vascular damage.

All the extremities should be palpated and neurological, vascular, and motor examination done to look for acute compartment syndrome. It results from high-tissue fluid pressure in closed osseofascial compartments, e.g., in hand, forearm, and leg, and leads to reduced capillary perfusion below that required for tissue viability. Thus, increased compartment pressure is of great concern. Several explanations have been advocated for the mechanism of its development. However, it is the muscle ischemia and hypoxia that leads to edema, increased compartment pressures, and eventually ischemia of the distal limb necessitating fasciotomy. The diagnosis of compartment syndrome is made clinically. Adjunctive studies, such as measuring compartment pressures (>30 mm Hg) are unnecessary as these are not subtle injuries.

Fasciotomy: Muscle damage becomes irreversible after 6–8 hours of ischemia **(Figs. 17 and 18)**. A low threshold for fasciotomy is indicated because an early fasciotomy often limits further ischemic damage to distal tissues by removing the effects of vascular compression and thus, lowers the site of amputation and ensures least number

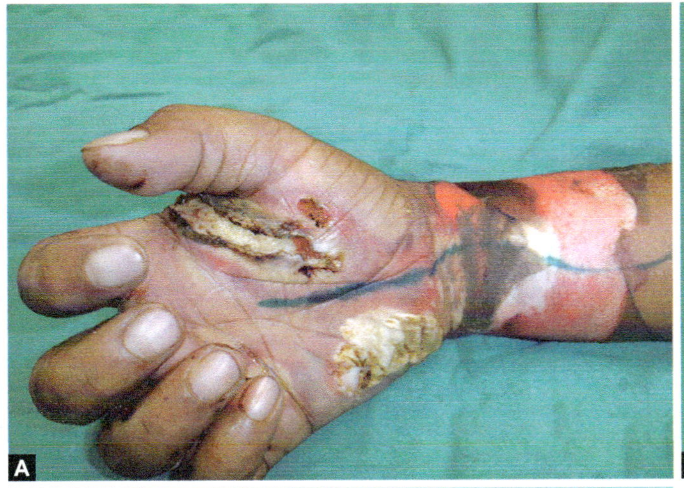

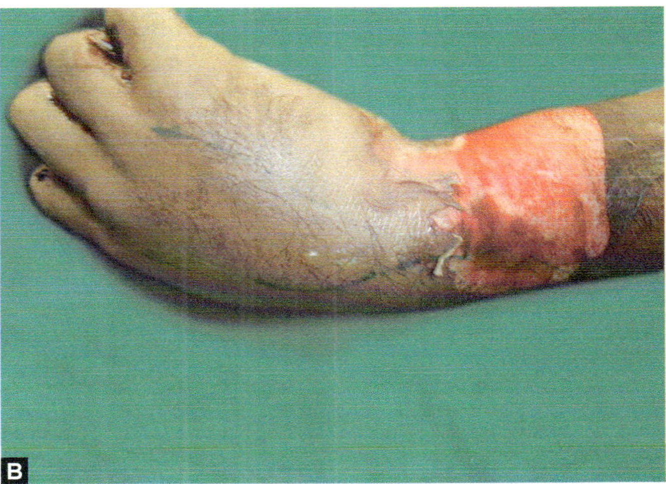

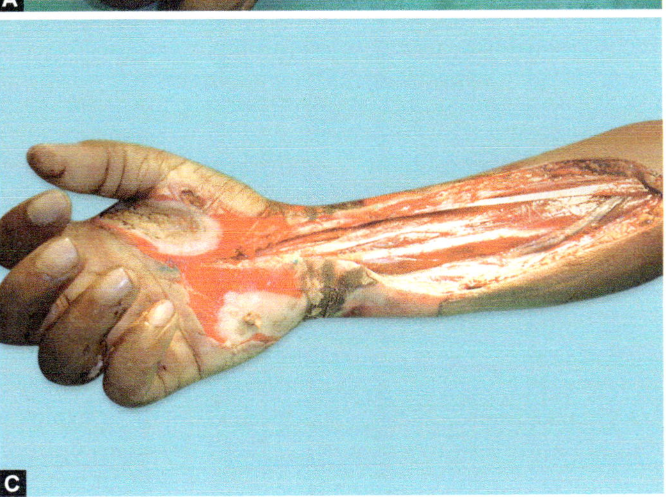

FIGS. 17A TO C: (A) Contact injury to hand and wrist causing proximal compartment syndrome in forearm and tight carpal tunnel; (B) Dorsum of same hand showing circumferential injury at wrist with edematous dorsum; and (C) Early fasciotomy done to release compartment syndrome and opened carpal tunnel showing thrombosed ulnar vessels.

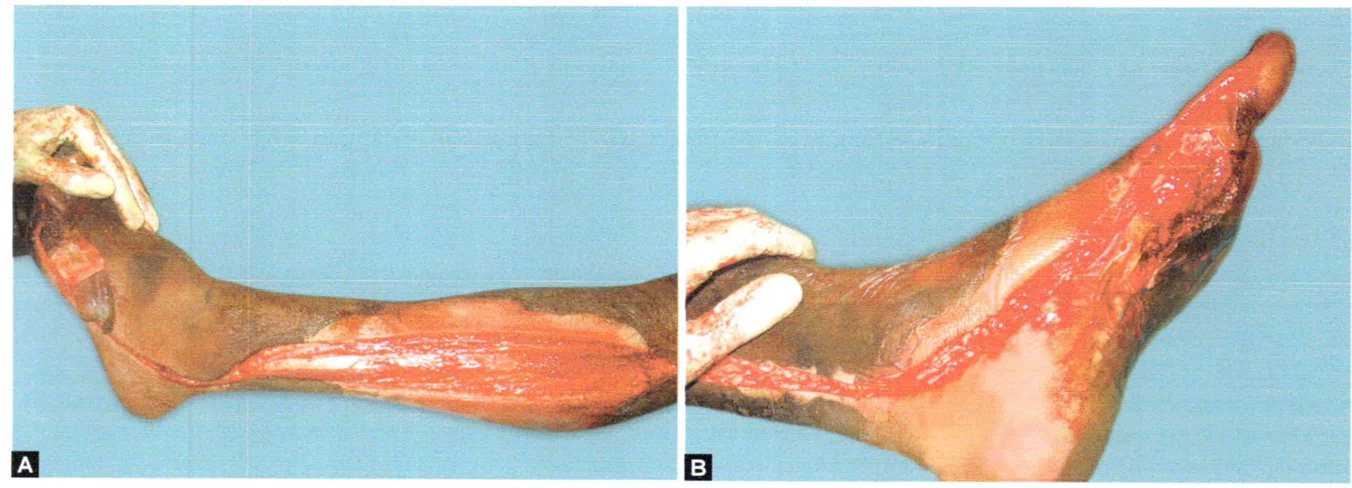

FIGS. 18A AND B: (A) Early fasciotomy in lower limb to release compartment syndrome and (B) Fasciotomy incision extending into foot.

of complications and better survival of body parts and life as well. The patient must be well resuscitated before fasciotomy so that the myoglobin released from the just perfused muscle are flushed out rapidly. The hallmark of compartment syndrome is pain with passive motion in the compartment containing the muscle groups responsible for that motion. Characteristically, the pain is unrelenting and may appear out of proportion to the visible injury. There may be paresthesia, hypoesthesia, or decreased motor function. Loss of pulses is a late sign of compartment syndrome. Fasciotomy also helps the surgeon in determining the extent of muscular necrosis earlier. For an adequate fasciotomy, all the four compartments in the forearm (superficial volar, deep volar, dorsal, and mobile wad of Henry) and 10 compartments in the hand (4 dorsal interossei, 3 palmar interossei, hypothenar, thenar, and adductor pollicis) must be released.[28] One incision on the volar aspect and another on the extensor aspect of the forearm are needed for release of all compartments. Occasionally, only a carpal tunnel release and possibly Guyon's canal release with a short proximal extension is required. Fasciotomy may even be required in the leg. The four compartments of leg which need fasciotomy are superficial and deep posterior compartments, lateral compartment, and anterior compartment. The four fasciotomy incisions can be made through two cutaneous incisions, one medial (a fingerbreadth behind medial border of tibia) and one lateral (over the fibula). Damage to underlying neurovascular structures must be prevented. Fasciotomy may involve considerable blood loss and, hence, best done under anesthesia in operation theater with facilities of diathermy, etc. Blood transfusion(s) may be required. The skin incision is made from distal to proximal and extended as required. The necrotic tissues of the affected limbs must be thoroughly debrided. The wound is covered with antimicrobial creams like silver sulfadiazine 1% or mafenide acetate 11.1%. Re-assessment at 24–48 hours later must be done during subsequent dressings of the wound and, if required, further debridement may be done. Fasciotomy wound closure generally requires skin grafting for wound coverage after the development of healthy granulation tissue. Skin substitutes can be applied till definitive closure with autografts. Early closure can often be facilitated with use of vacuum-assisted closure (VAC) therapy. It must be remembered that impaired circulation in the extremities after an electrical injury may be due to constrictive circumferential full thickness eschar and/or due to compartment syndrome due to subfascial edematous muscle. While the former requires escharotomy, the latter requires fasciotomy. Both may be present together in patients who have associated flame burns causing third-degree burns of skin. If escharotomy does not restore distal circulation, fasciotomy is done. This decision can usually be made by the bulging appearance of the muscles beneath the fascia. In case of doubt that the constricting fascia is responsible for the vascular compromise, a fasciotomy incision is definitely indicated.

Myoglobinuria and hemoglobinuria: Rhabdomyolysis[29-31] (literally, the dissolution of skeletal muscle) is characterized by leakage of muscle-cell contents, including electrolytes, myoglobin, and other sarcoplasmic proteins (e.g., creatine phosphokinase, lactate dehydrogenase, alanine, and aspartate aminotransferases) into the circulation. Myonecrosis can occur several days after the initial injury. Massive amounts of free hemoglobin from lysed red blood cells are also released. The products of breakdown of myoglobin and hemoglobin may lead to acute kidney injury which is a potential complication of severe rhabdomyolysis. The outcome of rhabdomyolysis is usually good provided that there is no renal failure. Thus, myoglobin and heme pigments and red blood cells in the urine must be looked for and cleared promptly. The presence of gross pigmenturia (variously described as dark tea or coca cola or mahogany-colored urine) in a patient with an electrical burn indicates significant muscle damage. Gross pigmenturia is diagnosed visually and confirmed positive on dipstick test for blood and negative on microscopy for red blood cells.[24] Once urine is grossly clear, it can be assumed that the pigments have been cleared. If the pigments are detected in the urine, aggressive treatment is started with volume loading to keep urine output at 1.5–2 mL/kg body weight/h (or 100 mL/h or 1.5–2 times the amount desired in thermal burns) till the urine is clear. Bolus dose of mannitol 25 g is given intravenously and repeated (12.5 g every 2–4 hours), if necessary. Mannitol, an osmolar diuretic, provokes (i) vasodilation of renal parenchyma, in effect improving renal perfusion and glomerular filtration; (ii) acts on the proximal convoluted tubules and contributes to the excretion of myoglobin, heme, and iron thereby minimizing the probability of myoglobin cast formation and its direct cytotoxic effects on epithelial cells; and (iii) decreases the oxidative stress in the tubular cells by its antioxidative action. Furosemide (a loop diuretic), although causes more intense diuresis, is not as effective as mannitol and also has the disadvantage of producing urine with low pH. Since metabolic acidosis is commonly seen in massive electrical burn patients, intravenous sodium bicarbonate ($NaHCO_3$, 50 mL of 7.5% solution as bolus or added to intravenous fluids) is administered. The aim is to have a urinary pH above 6.5 and a serum pH from 7.40–7.45. The alkaline pH of urine increases the solubility of myoglobin and limits the formation of myoglobin casts. It also impedes the degradation of myoglobin into heme and free iron which are nephrotoxic. The rationale behind mannitol and sodium bicarbonate therapy is to prevent precipitation of pigments in the renal tubules (acute kidney injury). In addition, $NaHCO_3$ also corrects hyperkalemia consequent to metabolic acidosis. Maintaining an adequate perfusion pressure and monitoring the acid-base balance are of vital importance.

The large necrotic muscle mass and dead tissue resulting from the passage of electrical current should be removed early. A massive release of intracellular contents into the blood, due to lysis of cells, may be at least partly responsible for systematic toxicity seen after the injury. This is well seen in the improvement in cardiac functions once an injured muscle or limb is removed. The policy of "wait and watch" for development of line of demarcation may lead to an increase in the secondary damage while early surgical interventions have no harm other than that the patient may require a second excisional surgery. In extensive cases, amputation remains the only option.[32]

Amputation as the first operative procedure is required only in obviously mummified and contracted limb. In general, necessary amputations can be done safely after 48–72 hours of injury once the patient has been thoroughly resuscitated. These early amputations should be preferably done under regional blocks as the myocardium remains sensitized to various drugs for 5–7 days following passage of electrical current through the heart. General anesthesia should be avoided. Commonly, the level of amputation may be higher than the cutaneous line of demarcation because the underlying muscle damage extends more proximal than the skin damage. In fact, for 6–8 cm proximal to the line of demarcation in the normal appearing skin, the underlying muscles may be dead. It is preferable not to close the amputation stump in the first operation as there may be a requirement for revision, more than once, to a higher level **(Fig. 19)**.

Injury to extremities can be both, by thermal and mechanical means. When voltage and current are sufficient to overcome the very high resistance of bone, large amounts of heat are generated in bone and periosteal tissues leading to osteonecrosis and periosteal burns. Electrical injuries are also very commonly associated with traumatic injuries due to falls from height. There can be associated fractures of skull, limbs, and spine with associated quadriplegia or paraplegia and dislocations (Secondary injuries). Mechanical injury can also be due to forceful muscular contraction as a result of electric current. Fractures can also occur in low-voltage exposures, although this is less common. Spinal trauma can occur due hyperextension following forceful muscular contraction.

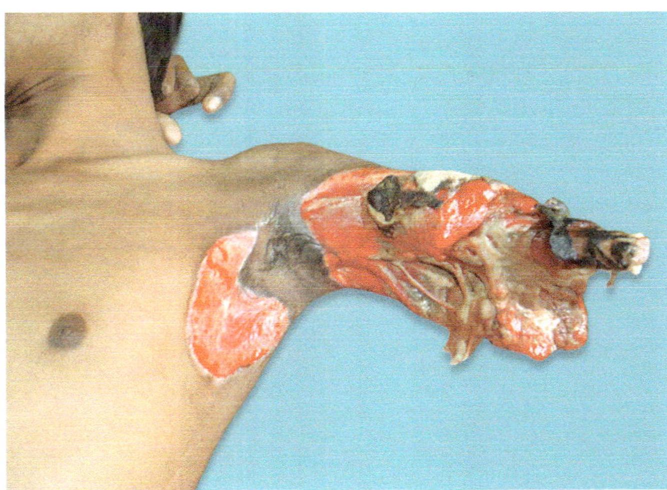

FIG. 19: Guillotine amputation done in midarm level showing residual dead muscles requiring revision of amputation.

Ligation of subclavian vessels may be required in case the entire length of upper limb is gangrenous and needs an amputation at shoulder level. This avoids blow out from axillary vessels at amputated site, if the damage extends till axilla or more proximal **(Figs. 20A to D)**.

Thermal injury versus crush syndrome controversy: There is a long-standing controversy as to whether electrical burns are thermal injury or crush injury in nature. "Electrical burn" is the term used to refer to an injury caused by exposure to supraphysiological electrical currents. By inclusion of "burn" in the term, reference is made to the long-held view that the mechanism of electrical injury is mediated by heat. The immediate damage to skeletal muscles of extremities is caused by heat and is usually patchy in distribution along the course of the current, often most severe near the bones. The theory of heat effect derives from the generation of heat as the current flows through a resistive path, with the amount of heat generated being proportional to the square of the current and the amount of resistance. This theory was initiated by Jaffe and his coworkers.[33,34] They concluded from their electrical experiments "it was the heat liberated in the obstructed vessel that was detrimental to the tissue of the vascular wall." Hunt et al. (1976), reporting on their experiments on animals, concluded that "an electrical burn is simply a thermal injury."[35] Many investigators adopted this theory to interpret the phenomena of electrical injuries. They believe that Joulean heat is generated during the passage of current and this heat destroys cells. However, some authors noted clinical differences between the electrical and the thermal burns.

Thus, Artz believed that electrical burns resemble a crush injury more closely than they do a thermal burn.[36,37] The damage below the skin where the current passes is usually far greater than the appearance of the overlying skin indicates. A crush injury affects the muscles and is

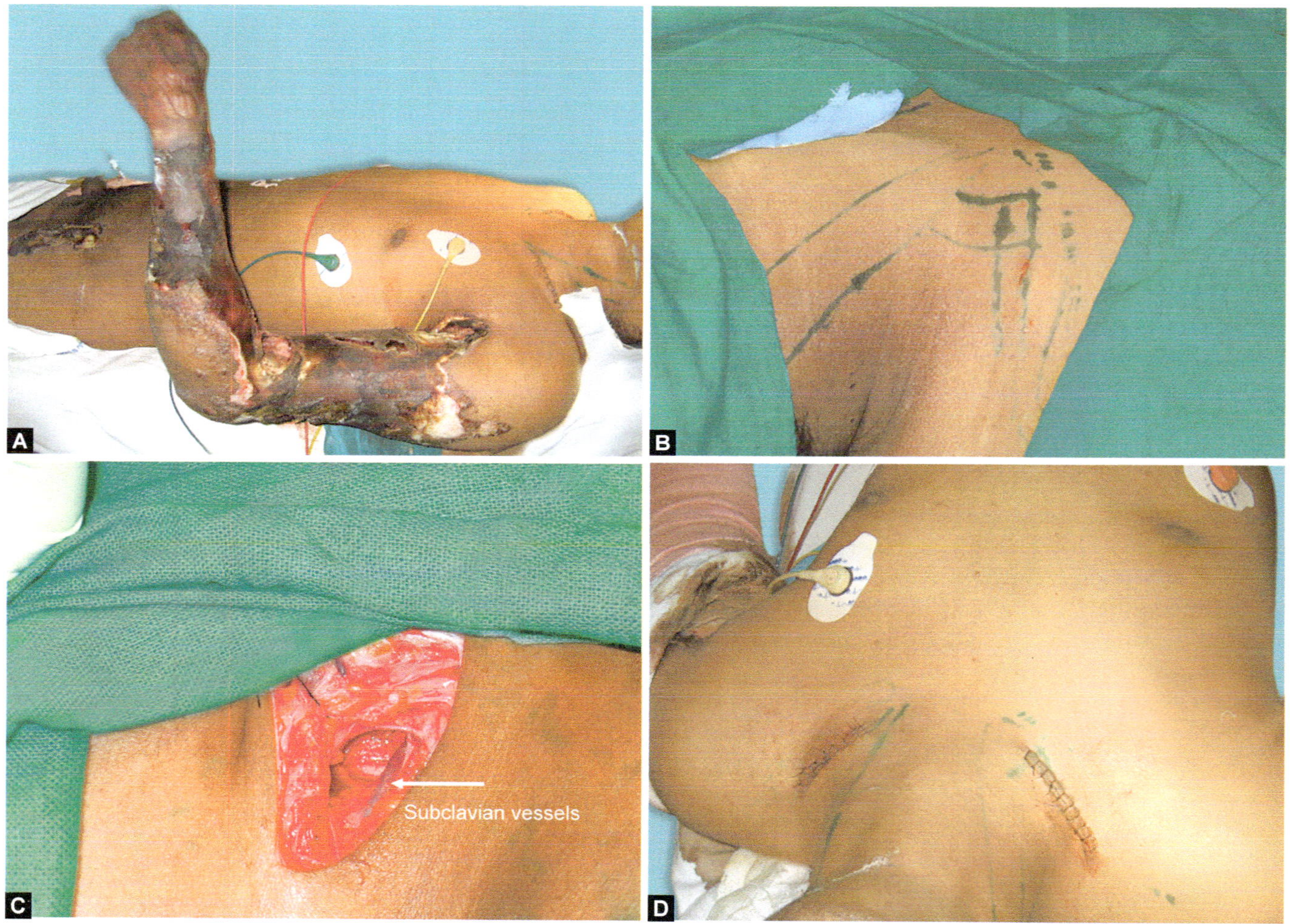

FIGS. 20A TO D: (A) Gangrene of entire length of upper limb because of high-voltage contact burns requiring amputation at the level of shoulders. Prior to amputation the subclavian vessel ligation was required so as to prevent their blowout postoperatively; (B) Marking for locating subclavian vessels; (C) Subclavian vessels exposed beneath the clavicle; and (D) Bilateral subclavian ligation achieved after which both the gangrenous limbs can be disarticulated safely at the shoulder.

followed by myoglobinuria. Likewise, an electrical injury that penetrates the deepest tissues causes destruction of muscles leading to myoglobinuria. Electrical injuries are associated with a far greater risk and incidence of acute renal failure (acute kidney injury) than are thermal burns. Sometimes, an electrical injury of an extremity resembles a burn and is treated as burn only to find development of clostridial infection in a few days because of the dead muscle. The clostridial bacteria invade the dead skin and the dead muscle leading to an overwhelming infection.[36,37]

Kidneys

The kidneys are of special importance in electrical injuries because of higher incidence of renal failure as compared to thermal burns. Renal damage is caused by a number of mechanisms as follows: (i) the high susceptibility of kidneys to anoxic/ischemic injury due to cardiopulmonary arrest, (ii) decrease in renal filtration pressure following hypovolemia secondary to systemic fluid losses that accompanies severe electrical injury, and/or (iii) direct electrothermal effect of high voltage electric current on the renal cortical tissues and vasculature affecting tubular ionic transport mechanisms. In addition, myoglobin and hemoglobin (hemochromogens) released into circulation may cause renal tubular damage leading to acute kidney injury. Myoglobin plays a dominant role in the pathogenesis of rhabdomyolysis-induced acute kidney injury. There is direct cytotoxic action of myoglobin on epithelial cells of the proximal convoluted tubules and myoglobin cast formation in the distal convoluted tubules. Greater incidence of myoglobinuria, hemoglobinuria, and hematuria in these patients is similar to that seen in "crush syndrome". Iatrogenic over resuscitation has also been blamed for renal failure. Acute renal failure, once developed, may need intervention by a nephrologist and renal replacement therapy (see chapter on "Management of Acute Renal Failure in Burns").

Neurological[19,38-40]

Many neurological complications have been described in electrical burn. Some are understandable while others are not fully understood. Electrical current can cause acute and delayed injury to the central and peripheral nervous systems. Acute central nervous system symptoms include altered mental status like confusion, impaired concentration, and disorientation. More severe cases may have loss of consciousness, depression of respiratory center, paralysis, and seizures. Injury or effects on peripheral nerves, median, ulnar, or radial and sometimes compound global brachial plexus injuries can also take place because of severe muscle contraction pulling the brachial plexus. Mostly, injuries to the nerves are confined to the local site where a nerve is directly damaged by the electrical current. In some cases, the nerve damage is secondary to increased intracompartmental pressure. The effects revert back to normal once the pressure is released. Where irreversible damage occurs, nerve grafting may be required. However, results of nerve grafting may not be good because of intense fibrosis and associated muscular damage in the region.

Patients who sustain electric burns with site of exit or entry being the scalp or skull are most likely to develop complications relating to the central nervous system. Spinal cord damage is the most common out of the permanent sequelae of electrical injury and occurs when the path of current is either from arm to arm or from arm to the leg. The paraplegia or quadriplegia may occur weeks to months after electrical injury. In these patients, motor symptoms are more pronounced than the sensory involvement. Mechanism of its development is not fully understood but appears to be due to slow development of cord ischemia. Damage to brain has also been described. The cause of this damage is not well understood. Often, a localized hemorrhagic infarct is seen in brain especially in the white matter areas such as thalamus and internal capsule **(Fig. 21)**. These are the areas where blood vessels are less protected and are more likely to have flow of current outside leading to damage. These cases develop extrapyramidal symptoms. The mechanisms which lead to delayed neurological presentations are not well understood. There may be peripheral neuropathies, nonfocal neurologic signs and symptoms, problems with gait and balance, seizures, personality changes, and even loss of memory.

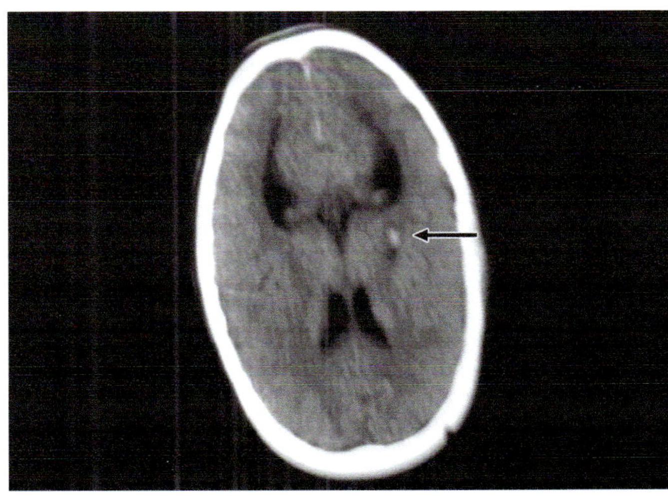

FIG. 21: CT scan showing hemorrhagic infarct in the area of internal capsule following electric contact burns.

Bone and Joint

Bone and joint injuries may be associated with electrical burns. These may be secondary to fall or because of strong muscle contractions. The heat generated from the passage of current through the bone can cause aseptic necrosis, burns to periosteum or complete destruction of bone matrix leading to autoamputation **(Figs. 22A and B)**. All victims of a high voltage electrical injury and/or fall must be treated as cases of spinal injury till proved otherwise. They should be managed with proper head and neck and spine immobilization during primary survey itself. Fall from heights can cause fractures of long bones and pelvis. Strong spasm of the back muscles causing vertebral fractures needs to be differentiated from fractures due to associated trauma. An orthopedic consultation is required for their management. Anterior and posterior shoulder dislocations from tetanic spasm of the rotator cuff muscles can occur during electric injuries. Besides these major sequelae, some patients may develop heterotopic bone formation, especially at the cut end of amputation stumps, bone cysts, periarticular ectopic calcification, especially around the elbow.

Scalp and Cranium

Scalp is third most common site involved in electrical burns after upper and lower limbs. In the presence of thick hair, these burns may be missed, if not looked for carefully. They are very important as late neurological sequalae are common and there can be medicolegal issues. All scalp burns are full thickness. Invariably, there is involvement of calvarium as well (outer table only or both tables). However, involvement of dura is the least common. These burns may have varying degrees of brain involvement **(Figs. 23 and 24)**.

When localized to scalp with no other life-threatening injuries and the patient is otherwise stable, they can be treated by primary excision of burned scalp and covering the defect with a split skin graft (over viable periosteum), or a local/free flap (e.g., latissimus dorsi flap with skin graft, anterolateral thigh flap, etc.), over bare bone. The flaps provide vascularity to the devitalized bone underneath and may allow it to regenerate (bone graft in situ). All obviously charred bone needs removal till bleeding areas. Even both tables of calvarium may need removal. Help of a neurosurgeon must be sought in such patients. Reconstruction is done with split calvarial bone or rib graft or a bone substitute covered with a flap.

In critically ill patients, who cannot be taken up for surgery early, these wounds are managed with dressings till spontaneous eschar separation occurs. Once the patient is fit for surgical intervention on scalp and the wound reveals healthy granulations, split skin grafting may be done. If dead and necrotic bone is revealed, it is chiseled out till bleeding bone and split skin graft may be applied immediately or when the granulations develop (usually 5 days). The wound, if small, can also be covered with local rotation flaps. For larger defects, distant free flaps may be needed, especially if both the tables have been removed. Transposition flaps are preferably avoided as they jeopardize the chances of tissue expansion which may need to be done later for final esthetic restoration of scalp. Drilling of holes into the outer table of calvarium, to permit growth of granulation tissue from the viable diploë to come onto surface and merge with each other to provide a split skin graftable bed, is no longer done. It leads to prolonged morbidity (a period of several months) apart from unstable areas and sinuses, discharging pieces of sequestrum off and on.

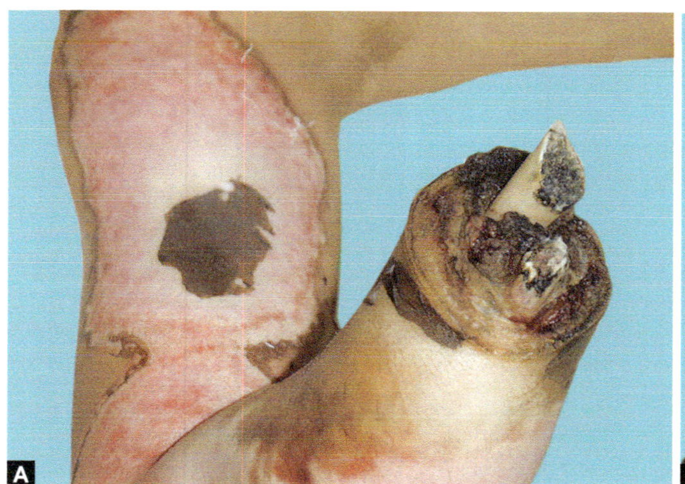

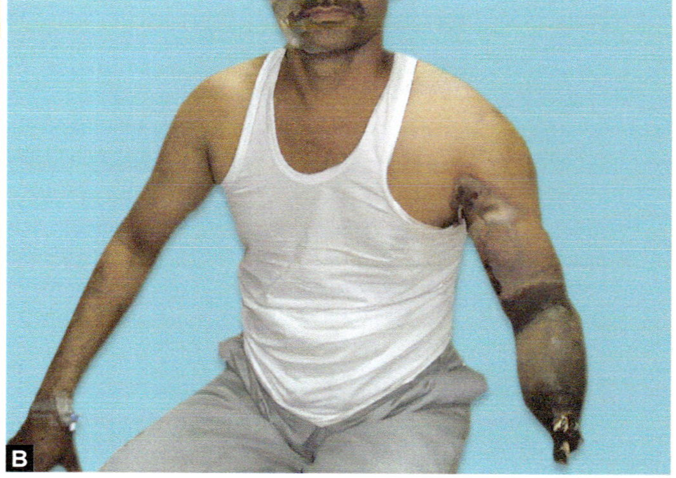

FIGS. 22A AND B: (A) High-voltage contact injury causing autoamputation at the level of forearm because of necrosis till bone and (B) Primary forearm autoamputation following high-voltage injury with visible proximal damage of elbow extending till axilla.

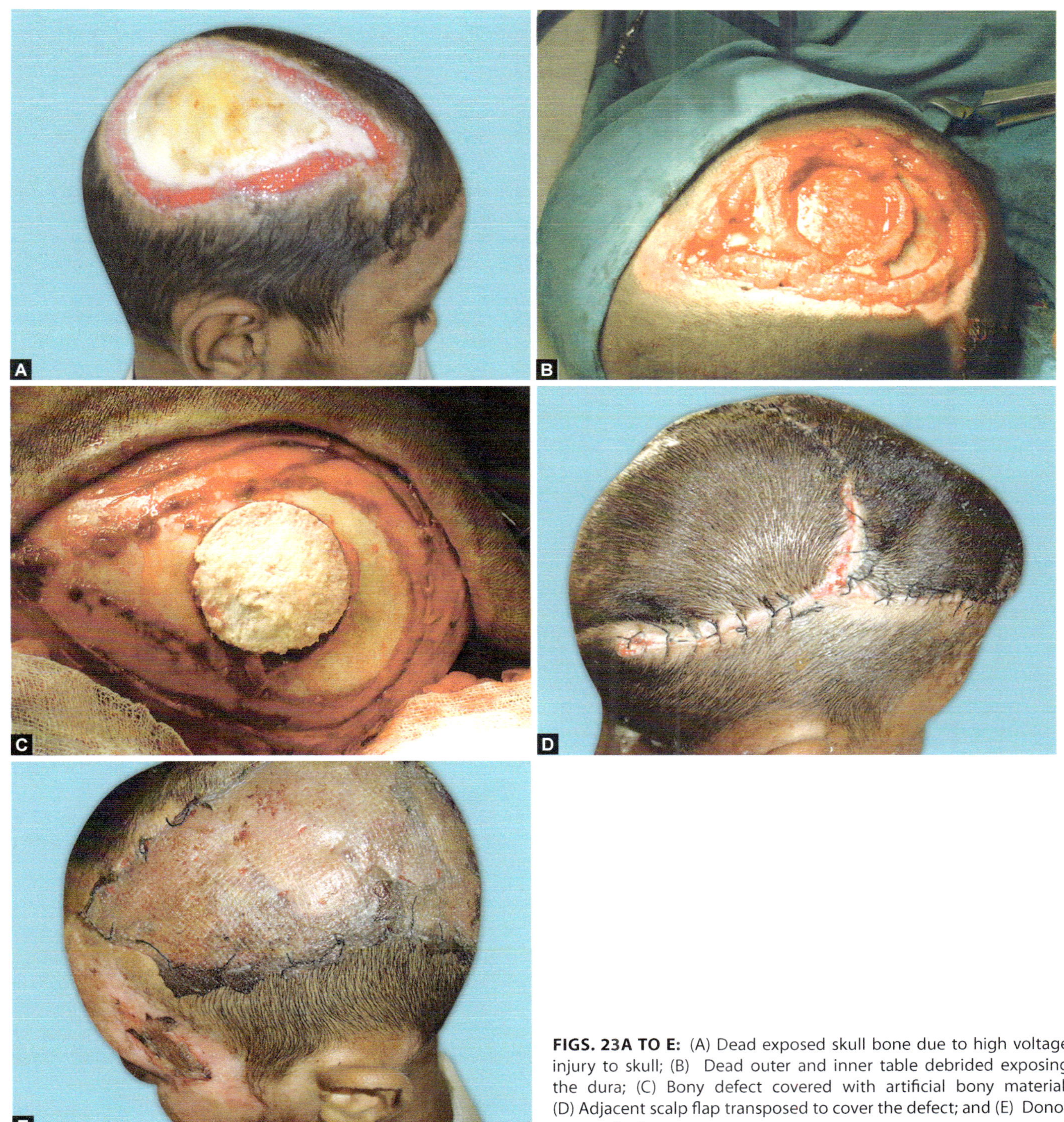

FIGS. 23A TO E: (A) Dead exposed skull bone due to high voltage injury to skull; (B) Dead outer and inner table debrided exposing the dura; (C) Bony defect covered with artificial bony material; (D) Adjacent scalp flap transposed to cover the defect; and (E) Donor area grafted.

Abdomen[41-43]

As stated above, due to its greater cross-sectional area and low resistance, which tends to dissipate the electrical energy, abdomen is rarely affected. Usually, intra-abdominal injury is prevented by a comparatively avascular peritoneum. However, when current enters through the abdomen, one gets direct injury to the intestines and colonic injuries are the most common. Electrical injuries can damage the abdominal viscera even without direct contact with the abdomen. Patients

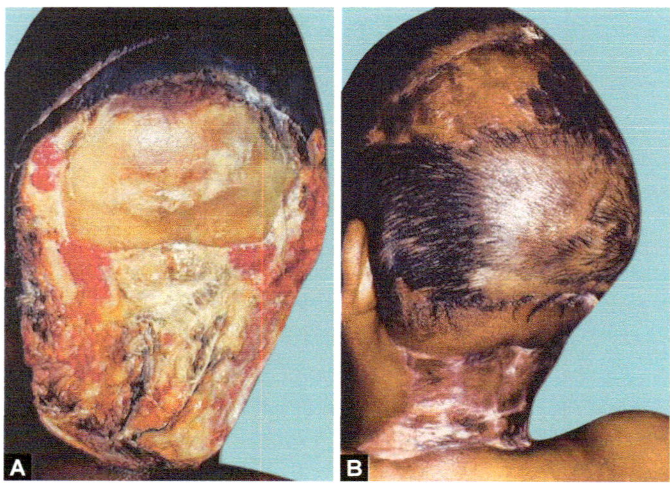

FIGS. 24A AND B: (A) Post electric burn exposed skull and neck tissues and (B) Transposition flap cover from adjacent scalp.

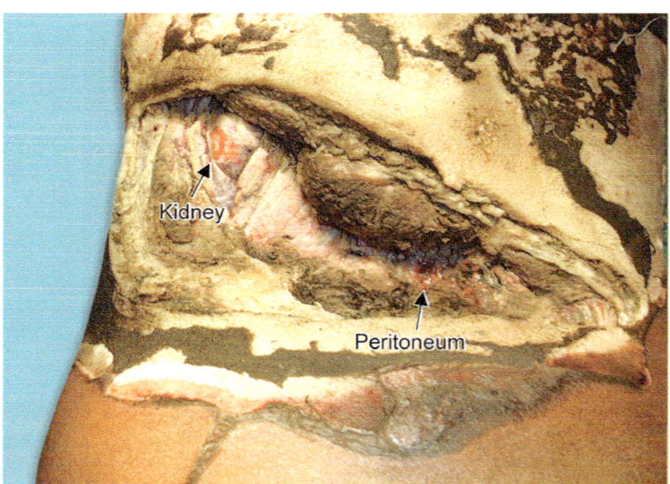

FIG. 26: Deep high voltage injury in trunk with extensive damage of all abdominal muscles exposing underlying viscera.

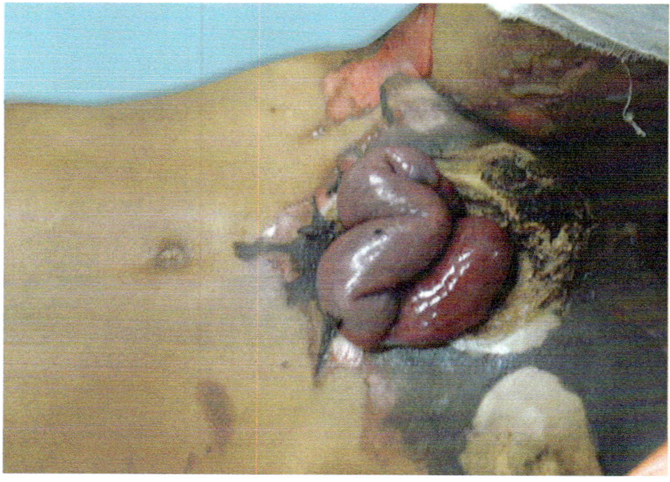

FIG. 25: A 14-year-old boy with electric contact burn over lower abdomen exposing the bowel with loss of external genitalia.

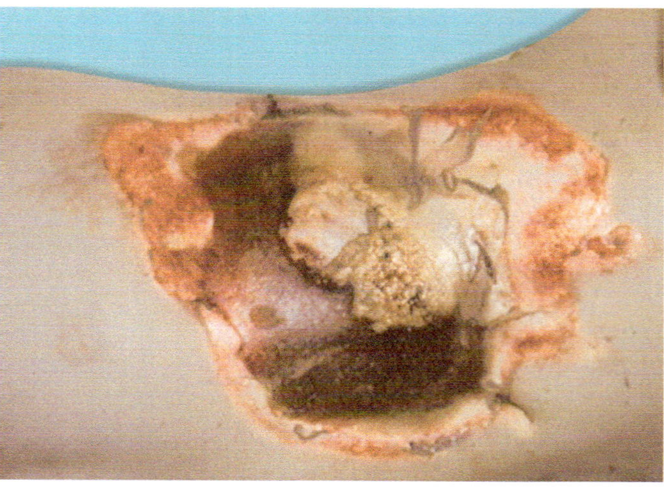

FIG. 27: High tension electrical burn of abdominal wall. Patient climbed on the roof top of electrified train.

with abdominal visceral damage, with an intact but burnt abdominal wall at the time of initial presentation, have a high mortality because clinical recognition is difficult in early stages. It may be difficult to know if the burn has involved full thickness of abdominal wall. These concealed injuries may present as "burst abdomen" after a few days.

In case of direct prolonged contact, local damage to the hollow viscous may be seen **(Figs. 25 to 28)**. There can be necrosis of intestines and perforations or even direct electrical damage to liver, pancreas, gallbladder, etc., which can be fatal. Curling's ulcers and gastrointestinal bleeding have also been reported.

Treatment consists of exploratory laparotomy and excision in case where there are signs of intra-abdominal injury which is confirmed by ultrasonography and CT scan. Injured hollow viscous are treated by colostomy or exteriorization of the colon or small bowel. Similarly, injuries to the urinary bladder and penis can also take place directly due to passage of current. It can lead to loss of male external genitalia. The abdominal wall defects can be reconstructed with different locoregional or free flaps, e.g., tensor fascia lata flap, free latissimus dorsi flap, etc. Penile reconstruction may require radial artery free forearm flap while silicone implants are used to restore testes.

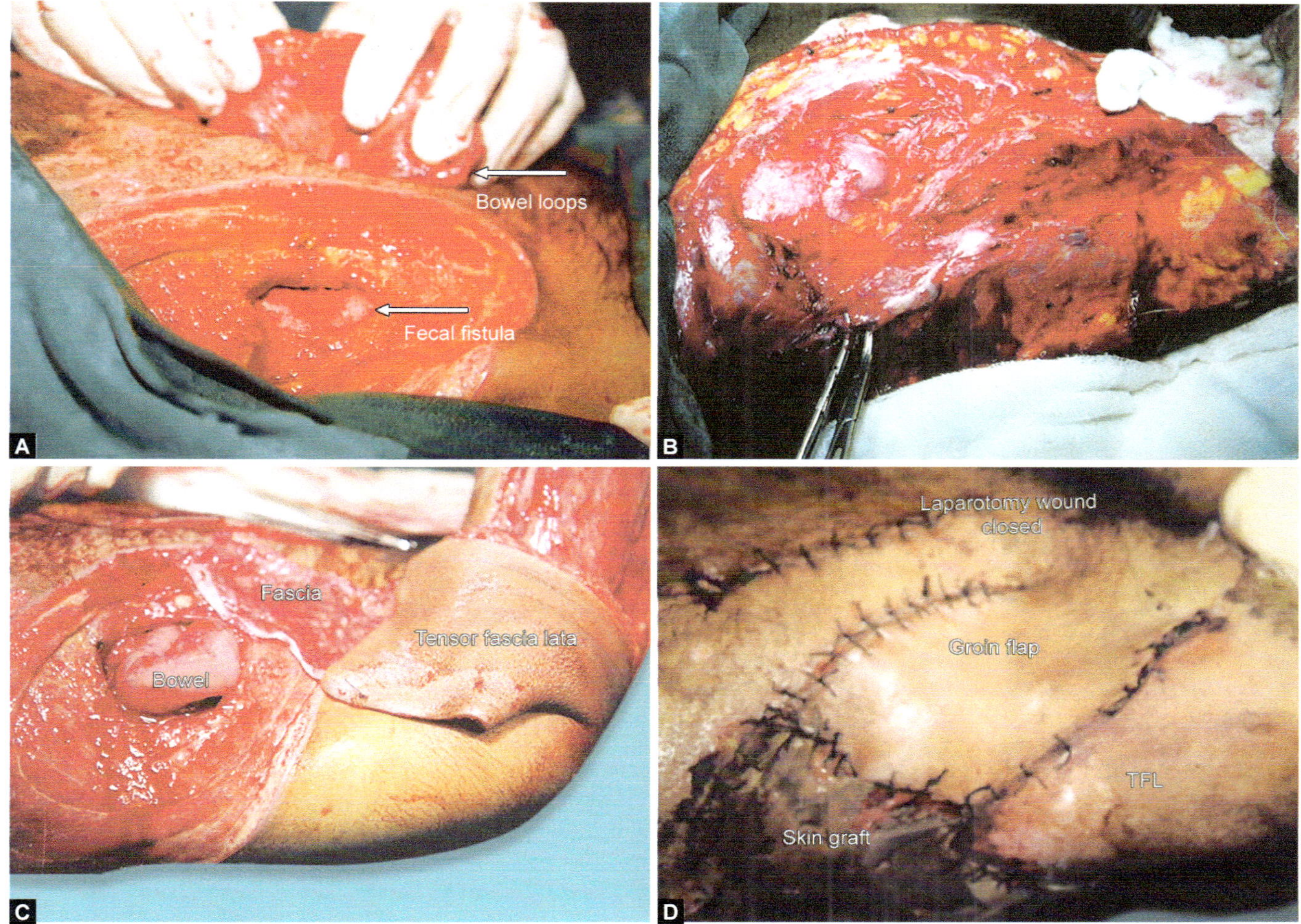

FIGS. 28A TO D: (A) Case of fecal fistula following electrical contact injury on abdomen. Patient taken up for laparotomy—bowel delivered from laparotomy wound; (B) Resection anastomosis of diseased bowel done; (C) Extended tensor fascia lata (TFL) flap raised to cover exposed bowel site but was insufficient; and (D) Laparotomy wound closed and defect covered by TFL and groin flap.

Electrical Burns and Pregnancy[44-46]

Ninety-five percent of electrical burns have been noted to occur in men. Therefore, involvement of women and that too a pregnant woman is very rare. The spectrum of effects of electricity ranges from transient unpleasant sensation to mother with no effect on fetus to instant maternal and fetal mortality. The hand-to-foot and vertical head-to-foot pathways of current appear to carry the worst prognosis for the fetus as they travel through the uterus, placenta, and amniotic fluid. It is not known whether the injuries are because of the effect of direct current on the fetus or else due to secondary effects of maternal burns. Uteroplacental vessels and amniotic fluid have low electrical resistance. Fetal skin has far lower resistance than the skin after birth. Amniotic fluid transmits current effectively and this can increase the risk of spontaneous abortions and fetal burns or death. Fetal exposure to an electric shock may cause a cardiac arrest which explains the cessation of fetal movements noted by mothers. The fetal injury may manifest immediately or postnatally. It is well known that nature always gives priority to the mother over her fetus and the latter is expelled out to save the mother. Thus, the pregnant women with electrical burn abort or expel their fetuses in natural way. In case pregnancy continues, placental abruption, oligoamnios, decreased fetal movements and asphyxia, fetal cardiac arrhythmias, growth retardation, and damage to central nervous system can occur.

Orofacial Burns[47]

These injuries are generally seen in infants and toddlers. An inquisitive child tries to explore the wire by taking it into the mouth and chewing it with the gum or newly erupting teeth. In majority of these cases both the wires,

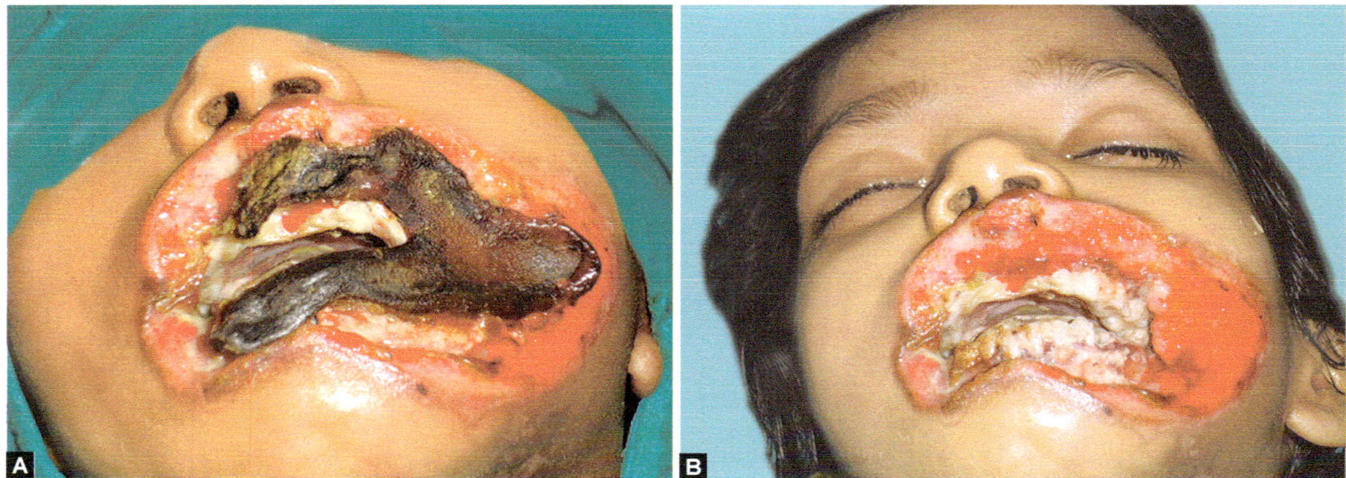

FIGS. 29A AND B: (A) An 8-year-old child with oral cavity burns due to accidental fall of high-tension wire over face, leading to necrosis of both upper and lower lips and left cheek and (B) Defect after removal of eschar exposing both alveoli and teeth requiring flap cover.

positive as well as negative, are taken into the child's mouth **(Figs. 29 and 30)**. Salty watery contents of the mouth allow the current to flow out through the same wire (contact burn in series). The child's mouth works like a resistance added in the flow of current. The current is converted into thermal energy leading to extensive local damage with eschar formation of the lips, commissure, mucous membranes of oral cavity and tongue, sometimes resulting in massive edema. Usually, it does not lead to any respiratory problem or any difficulty in swallowing. Excessive salivation and dribbling are seen. An occasional complication is a secondary hemorrhage from labial artery which occurs several days later when the eschar over the artery is dislodged by the child's tongue. The eschar is gradually replaced by granulation tissue which causes considerable deformity. There is another possibility of the current passing out from the body to the ground from child's wet diaper, feet, or buttocks (contact burn in parallel). This invariably leads to serious cardiac problem and may even prove fatal.

As these burns are confined to growing children, their management should take into consideration, growth, and further development. Electrical burns of mouth extend from angle of mouth to the upper and lower lip with injury to the gum, bone, and developing teeth. There are two views in the management of oral burns. One believes in early excision and primary cover. This provides sufficient vascularized tissue for the growth of bones and tooth buds. While trying to do the early excision, too much of tissues may get excised which otherwise would have recovered on their own. The other view is that as the mouth is a specialized structure, no reconstruction can be as perfect to take up all the normal functions. Hence, the consensus today is toward initial conservative management and early release of all tight contracting bands including tight oral commissure. Conservative management includes proper mouth care, topical antibacterial creams and providing splintage for 6–12 months. This provides a practically invisible scar but with a defect or deformity which is electively reconstructed later.

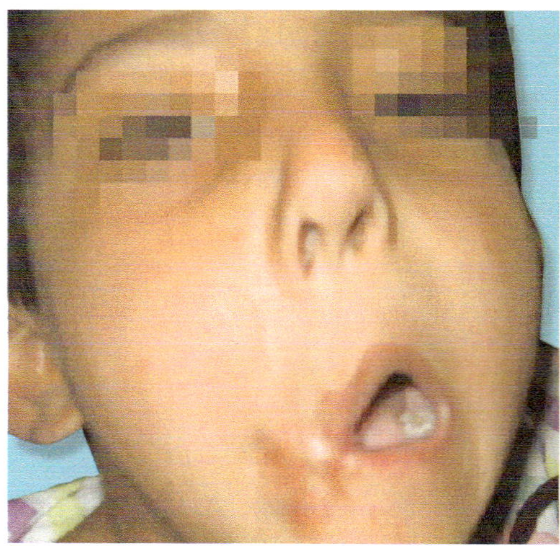

FIG. 30: Post electric burn deformity of mouth (microstomia).

Eye and its Adnexa[47,48]

Ocular complications following electrical burns are uncommon. While many of these appear immediately, the ones which impair vision (e.g., cataract) may develop slowly over a period of months to years.[49,50] The eyes may be involved in both, contact and flash electrical burns. Flash burns may lead to superficial and superficial dermal burns of the skin of eyelids and singeing of eyebrows and eyelashes. In contact burns, a number of changes have been described in conjunctiva, cornea, lens, iris, retina, and optic nerve. In high-tension electrical injuries, conjunctival hyperemia, swelling, and subconjunctival hemorrhages may occur. Corneal injuries include transient subepithelial/interstitial opacities, loss of corneal epithelial/endothelial cell layers, and loss of stromal keratocytes. In extensive injuries opacification, thinning, necrosis, and perforation can occur. Acute, mild, and transient or recurrent and severe iritis (uveitis), bullous keratopathy, and secondary glaucoma can occur.

The fact that an electrical injury can lead to development of cataract is known for 300 years **(Fig. 31)**. It is the most common ocular complication of electrical injuries with reported incidence of 5–20% of patients. The propensity for its development appears to depend partially on the magnitude of initial electrical injury with greater incidence being seen in patients with high voltage although it is not always necessary. It can occur following lightning injuries also. Both eyes are more commonly involved. It usually manifests with a latent period of 6–12 months after electrical injury but may develop earlier or later. The patient, whose all wounds might have healed, may present with complaints of gradual diminution of vision since injury. Thus, it mandates examination and documentation by the ophthalmologist in the acute stage of burns along with long-term careful follow-up as one may have to testify in the court of law later (for monetary compensation, etc.), about its causation as the burns were sustained long time back. They occur equally in patients who have obvious contact points on the face or head and in those who do not. Two-thirds do require surgical intervention.

Although the exact pathogenesis of the effect of electric current is unclear but it is believed to be due to coagulation of proteins of crystalline lens and the osmotic changes following damage to the subcapsular epithelium. Opacities form in the capsule and in the anterior subcapsular cortex. Posterior cortex may also be affected. Extensive epithelial damage is also considered to be the cause of the lenticular opacities. The lens in younger patients is more liable to be damaged than that of older patients.

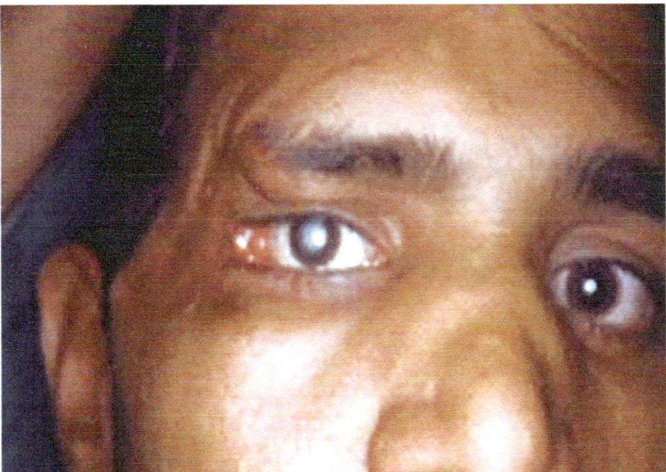

FIG. 31: Cataract development after electrical contact burn near zygoma.

Retinal and choroidal changes are seen rarely. There may be coagulative necrosis of vasculatures of these structures leading to intraretinal and subretinal hemorrhages. Retinal detachment, optic atrophy, and central retinal vein occlusion can occur.

The functional disabilities accompanying these lesions may be photophobia and blepharospasm while there may be transient to permanent bilateral visual loss. There may be concentric contraction of fields. An ophthalmologist's consultation must be taken early in all cases of electrical contact burns.

Gas Gangrene and Tetanus

Tetanus and gas gangrene due to clostridial infection have been reported following electric burns with massive amounts of necrotic muscle mass and other tissues. Over a period of last several decades, almost all the children in our country are regularly getting immunized against tetanus in infancy. A large segment of population also gets a dose, acting as a booster dose, whenever they sustain any injury. Unfortunately, many patients may not know of their immunization status. Despite the unparalleled effectiveness and safety of tetanus toxoid, the administration of human tetanus immunoglobulin (TIG) for passive protection for patients with suspicious symptoms or wounds grossly contaminated with soil is often highly desirable. 250 international units (IU), if 24 hours or less since injury or 500 IU, if >24 hours after injury, is given intramuscularly. In addition to tetanus, gas gangrene and mixed clostridial infections are also seen with extensive muscle necrosis which is a suitable environment for anaerobic organisms. Gas gangrene requires urgent management, i.e., amputation of the involved limb in order to save the patient's life along with medical management in the form of appropriate antibiotics (penicillin) and anti-gas gangrene serum. Topical therapy with mafenide cream also gives protection against clostridial infection.

PREVENTION AND FIRST AID

The tremendous load of morbidity and mortality consequent to electricity-related injuries can be reduced only by applying preventive strategies, both active and passive. The active measures include teaching about dangers of electricity and its safe use to children and general public via educational programs in schools, television and radio talks, etc. The passive measures include changes such as better design of electrical plugs, burying power lines, making high-voltage sources less accessible, etc., apart from the standardization of the quality of available electrical cables and other fittings and all electrical gadgets. All these can go a long way in decreasing the incidence of these injuries. The electrical and construction workers must abide by standard operating protocols for which the employers should have regular updates for their employees.

The first aid for any burn injury is provided by the lay person(s) available at the accident site and continues till the patient reaches a healthcare facility. Electrical mishaps pose the same threat to the rescuer(s) as they do to the victim. This is because if the victim is still in contact with the source of the current, as is more likely with AC, he/she becomes a conductor and may electrocute the rescuer. Similarly, in high voltage injuries, wet ground may conduct current to the rescuer(s). Hence, unless the source of the electrical current has been switched off or the victim has been moved away from the source of current using nonconductors like dry wooden or PVC table, chair, pole, etc., no attempt should be made to rescue the victim lest the rescuer becomes the next victim. Safety of the rescuer is of prime consideration. Although it is disheartening for anyone to see a person dying and not being able to help him, the loss of two lives is a worse consequence. Fortunately, contact with a victim of lightning injury does not pose any threat to the rescuer because the current duration is extremely short. Attention is now directed toward airway, breathing, and circulation of the patient and steps for basic life support have to be taken. For this, it is highly desirable that the general public should be conversant with the basic first-aid knowledge. The patient should then be shifted immediately to the closest hospital. Within few minutes of resuscitation, if possible, cardiac monitoring of the patient is done because most arrhythmias occur within the first few minutes to an hour after an electrical injury. Defibrillation at the scene of mishap or as soon as possible may save a patient's life. Spine should be immobilized prior to movement, if there is a fall.

MANAGEMENT

Medical Management

Electrical injury has been called as a "grand masquerader" of burn injuries because small surface wounds may be associated with devastating deeper injuries. That is why they should all be admitted. American Burn Guidelines state that all electrical burn patients need to be referred to burn centers. An extremely wide spectrum of injuries on the body of a victim ranging from a very minor, barely visible skin burn to severe damage requiring mutilating amputation(s) resulting in a crippled individual can be seen. The burnt areas are the most distracting injury in any patient. However, there may be one or more of other life-threatening injuries present as well. Thus, every patient with history of electrical injury must undergo primary survey followed by secondary survey as per advanced trauma life support (ATLS) guidelines. The Advanced Burn Life Support has also been developed by the American Burn Association along the same lines. Airway and cervical spine stabilization, breathing and ventilation must be assessed and taken care of appropriately. The consciousness of the patient is checked using Glasgow Coma Scale (GCS). The patient is completely undressed and a log roll is done to look for associated injuries. A warm environment for the patient must be maintained using warm intravenous fluids, blankets, and warmers.

The secondary survey is begun after the patient is stabilized in the primary survey. It begins with taking a brief history about the circumstances of the electrical injury. Was the current DC or AC? What was the voltage, low or high? The duration of contact? Whether the patient was thrown away or fell from height? Any history of loss of consciousness and whether any CPR was attempted at the scene? History of any other comorbid illness(es)/pregnancy/allergies, etc., if available, is recorded.

If the injury is due to electrical flash/flame burn, the management is same as for a thermal injury. However, in case of contact or arc burns, apart from all the requirements of managing a thermal injury, treatment also has to be focused on prevention of complications like compartment syndrome and acute renal failure due to rhabdomyolysis.

A complete head-to-toe evaluation of the patient is done to determine the percentage TBSA burnt in order to calculate fluid requirements. However, these patients require more fluid than that calculated as per Parkland or modified Brooke formulae for thermal burn patients. No burn formula can be used to estimate fluid therapy because all these formulae are based on TBSA. The volume of tissues destroyed in a patient of electrical injury is far greater than that destroyed in a thermal burn. These formulae do not take into account the injury to muscle and other deeper tissues. Additionally, there is a need for flushing out the pigments to save the victim from acute kidney injury. Fluid replacement is the single most important aspect of the initial resuscitation. Similar to thermal burns, electrical injuries also cause massive fluid shifts with extensive tissue damage and acidosis. Therefore, continuous monitoring of a patient's hemodynamic status is important. There is consensus that fluid formulae are starting points only. The rate of infusion needs meticulous titration. Hourly urine output monitoring and assessment of symptoms and signs of end-organ perfusion needs to be done to avoid over or under resuscitation. Fluid resuscitation should be commenced using two wide bore cannulas or venous cutdown. Choice of fluid remains Ringer lactate as for thermal burns. Colloids should be avoided in the first 24 hours. Urine output is the most important indicator of adequacy of perfusion and it must be maintained at 1.5–2 times the rate for thermal burns till urine is clear of pigments. An indwelling Foley urinary catheter is required for accurate volume measurements and, therefore, tissue perfusion. In addition, monitoring of color of urine is done by saving samples in small bottles/test tubes kept in a row **(Figs. 32A and B)**. In extensive injuries, bicarbonate and mannitol are administered (see above).

Once the urine is clear and adequate, the intravenous fluid can be titrated down to maintain an output of 1 mL/kg/h in adults and 0.5 mL/kg/h in children. In case the urine output is less or more than desired, the rate of infusion is increased or decreased. Central venous pressure (CVP) is another very important tool for monitoring fluid requirements in an electrical burn patient because while under-perfusion is definitely undesirable, even over-perfusion can also lead to abdominal hypertension, abdominal compartment syndrome, and acute kidney injury.

Along with assessment of extent of burn, simultaneously one must assess for depth of burn based on the clinical characteristics of the burn wound.

Management of pain relief, prophylactic therapy to prevent stress ulceration (Curling ulcer), nutrition, local wound infection, and systemic sepsis (and its complications) remain similar to any thermally burnt patient. Blood transfusion is rarely indicated during resuscitation of acutely burnt patient unless associated traumatic injury with significant blood loss is present. Later during the hospitalization, blood is transfused based on clinical assessment and laboratory parameters. It is generally not given to patients with Hb% of >10 gm% and should be administered as one unit at a time unless the patient is actively bleeding or undergoing operative intervention with blood loss. Next unit of blood is transfused after reassessment.

Investigations[51]

There are no clear guidelines regarding investigations which should be done following an electrical injury. Actually, there cannot be any because of the extremely vast spectrum of these injuries. Thus, to a large extent, it must be determined clinically on a case-to-case basis by the burn surgeon. The tests which may need to be done are:

- *Routine hematological studies*: (a) Complete blood count, viz., Hb%, hematocrit, total, and differential leukocyte count; (b) Renal function tests, viz., blood urea, serum creatinine, serum electrolytes (Na^+, K^+, and Cl^-); and (c) Blood sugar.
- *Arterial blood gas (ABG) analysis*: Acid-base imbalance has to be carefully monitored by doing ABG analysis since destruction of tissues due to electric current causes metabolic acidosis. It is also required in patients requiring ventilatory support or those with severe rhabdomyolysis who require alkalinization therapy.

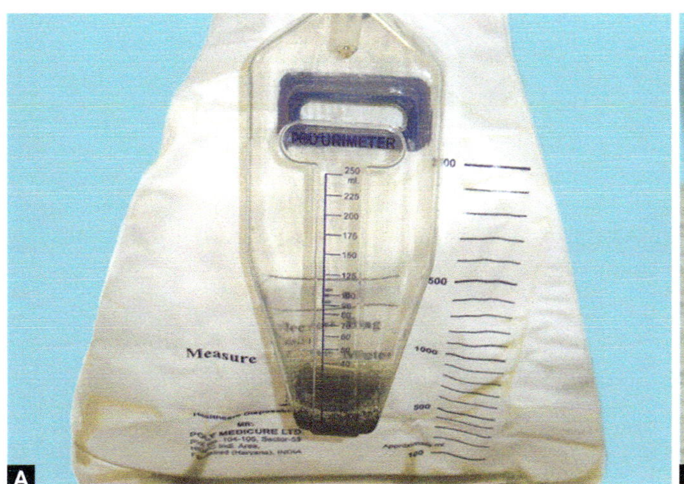

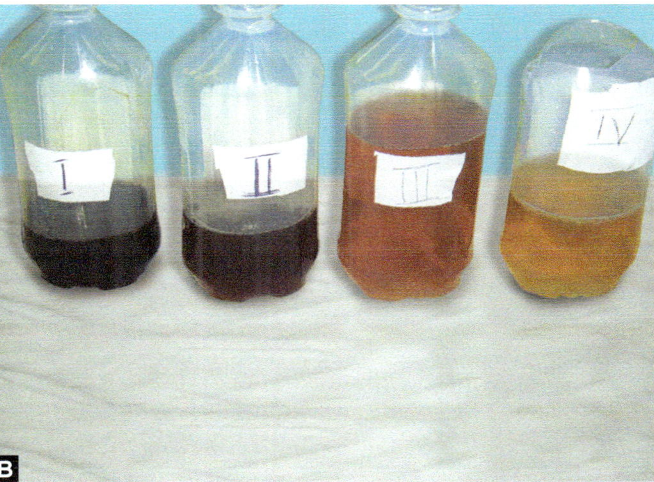

FIGS. 32A AND B: (A) Myoglobinuria indicated by reddish black urine requires vigorous resuscitation and (B) Gradual improvement in both color and quantity of urine with proper resuscitation, osmotic diuresis, and alkalinization of urine.

- *Enzyme studies:*[52] Creatine phosphokinase (CPK), an enzyme catalyzing the reversible phosphorylation of creatine by adenosine triphosphate (ATP), is found primarily in skeletal and cardiac muscles. The primary isoenzyme in the skeletal muscles is creatine phosphokinase-muscle unit (CPK-MM), while a significant amount of CPK-MB is contained in the cardiac muscles. Its levels are greatly elevated in patients who have massive myonecrosis, especially seen in high-voltage injuries. The serum CPK level peaks in the first 12–36 hours after sustaining an electrical injury but decreases steadily over the next several days. The half-life of CPK is 1.5 days. If the value of CPK-MB is elevated and the ratio of CPK-MB to total CPK (relative index) is >2.5–3, it is likely that the heart is damaged. A high CPK with a relative index below this value suggests that skeletal muscles are damaged. Assessing initial CPK levels can help in predicting the patients who can benefit from early fasciotomy to prevent subsequent amputations and the prevention of renal failure in the first few days after burn. Elevated levels also suggest prolonged hospital stay. There is a risk of amputation of limb when CPK enzyme is >4,000 U/L. Unfortunately, patients with elevated levels of these enzymes do have significant clinical findings for the clinician to take appropriate action, making these levels of academic importance only.
- *Urinalysis*: Specific gravity, pH, presence of RBCs, casts, myoglobin, and hemoglobin.
- Patients who require surgical intervention may need blood grouping and cross matching, prothrombin time, and activated partial thromboplastin time studies.
- *Imaging studies*: Choice of imaging studies is dictated by the history and presence of blunt trauma, altered mental status, cardiac or respiratory arrest, and the type of electrical exposure. One or more of the following may be required:
    - *Chest X-ray*: In patients with history of cardiac or respiratory arrest, shortness of breath, chest pain, hypoxia, CPR at the site of mishap or history of fall/blunt trauma.
    - *Computed tomography (CT) of head*: In cases with altered mental status, significant trauma, seizure, loss of consciousness, or focal neurologic deficits.
    - *Cervical spine imaging*: Patients with history of loss of consciousness or significant trauma must have their cervical spine immobilized and imaging studies done accordingly. An alert mental status without significant injuries may be clinically declared normal whereas others may require plain X-rays studies only. Patients with focal neurologic deficits or evidence of spinal cord injury should undergo full spinal imaging.
    - *CT scan/ultrasonography*: Depending on the amount of trauma sustained and the pathway of the current exposure, patients may require further imaging to evaluate for abdominal visceral injuries.
    - Radionuclide scanning with Xenon[133], Technetium-99m pyrophosphate (99m Tc Pyp), and Gadolinium-enhanced MRI have been shown to predict tissue damage. A 99m Tc Pyp muscle scan is safe, sensitive, noninvasive, and reliable diagnostic tool in defining the viability of muscles. Areas of muscle without uptake of isotopes are indicative of dead muscle. The test is extremely sensitive and many false positive results may be seen. However, these investigations add little to direct clinical evaluation.

    Other tests: ECG/cardiac monitoring. All patients should have an initial ECG and cardiac monitoring which should be continued in selected patients (see above).
- *Monitoring of physiological parameters*: Various physiological parameters including heart rate and blood pressure are useful in guiding resuscitation. Hourly assessment of peripheral circulation must be done with respect to skin color, edema, capillary refill, peripheral pulses, and skin sensation. CVP monitoring may be required in estimating fluid requirements and also in critically ill patients.

Surgical Management (Local Wound Therapy)[53,54]

The burn depth is greater in electrical burns as compared to thermal burns **(Figs. 33 to 36)**. Therefore, operative interventions are required in most of the electrical burn patients. Also, amputations and flap cover and complex

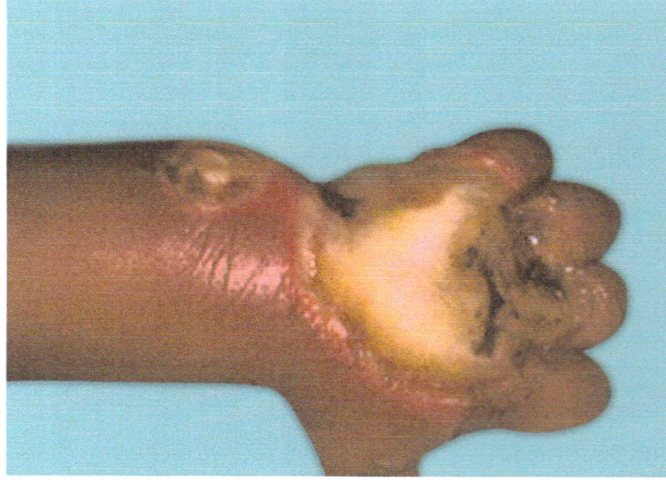

FIG. 33: Electrical burn in a child from domestic electric current 220–240 volts with involvement of extensor surface of hands and wrist.

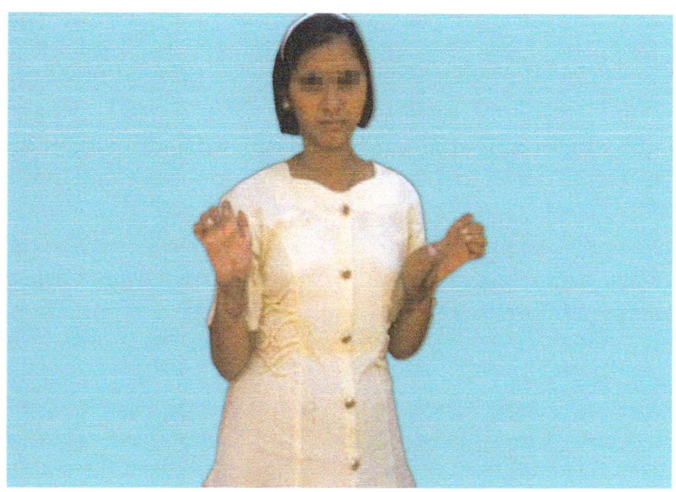

FIG. 34: High-tension electrical burn in female (electric arc). This young girl sustained arc burns while drying wet dupatta close to high-tension wires passing near the balcony. Her both hands were involved, involving both median and ulnar nerves. Thrombosis of both ulnar arteries. Damage to most of the flexor tendons. Both hands were saved by pedicled extended groin flaps.

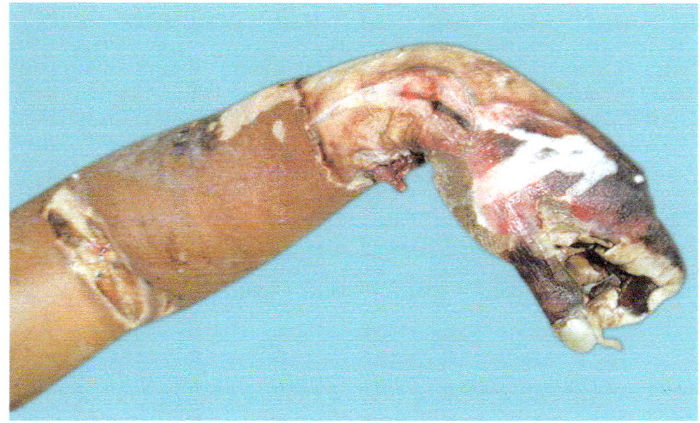

FIG. 35: High-voltage current causing primary gangrene of hand with arcing at elbow causing full thickness burns over elbow.

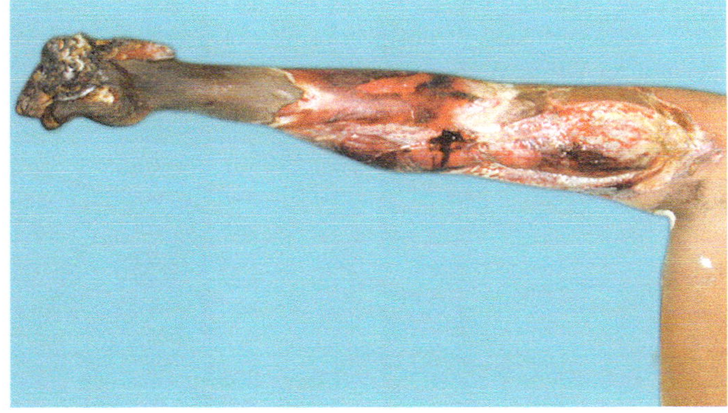

FIG. 36: High-tension injury showing extent of damage to deeper structures beyond the apparently damaged skin. Though the line of demarcation is till elbow, the muscles are seen necrosed much more proximally, thus requiring a higher level of amputation.

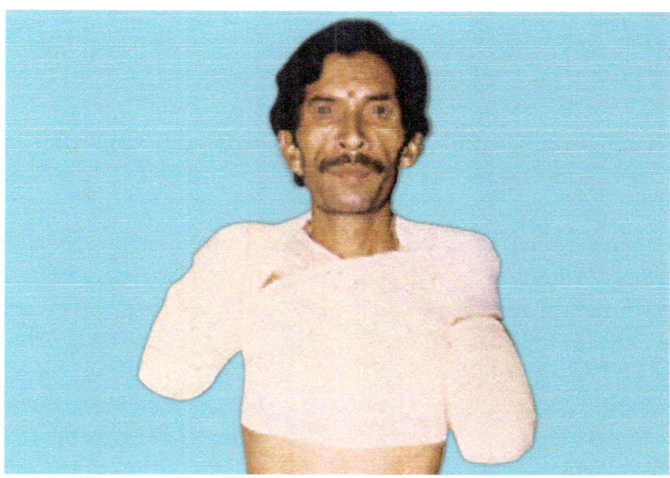

FIG. 37: A case of arm-to-arm transmission of high-voltage electricity leading to above elbow amputation of both the upper limbs.

reconstructions are more commonly required **(Fig. 37)**. Functional outcome after an electrical burn injury depends on the time lapsed before the start of appropriate surgical intervention on the wound and reconstructive procedure(s). Fasciotomies, escharotomies (see above) with early and adequate fluid resuscitation, and wound debridement are the key to salvage of compromised tissues and successful reconstructive procedures.

The controversy of progressive tissue necrosis:[5,53,55] A long-standing controversy about the electrical injuries is whether there is any progressive tissue necrosis or damage over a period of several days after sustaining an injury. This gains importance because an early wound closure is bound to result in a disaster with loss of precious flap and/or skin graft used to provide cover. Having problems of pus discharge from necrosed tissues under the flap or loss of graft is distressing both for the patient and the surgeon. Conversely, a delayed approach may be a cause of loss of precious tissues which are alive but may become dead in the absence of timely cover with consequent poor outcome. Progressive venous and arterial thrombosis may prevent the definitive diagnosis of the level of nonviable tissue for 2 weeks or so. As the injury is usually most severe in the small muscular branches which become thrombosed because of slower blood flow, complete damage is not initially evident. Jaffe et al. showed that vascular intima may be damaged without producing immediate thrombosis.[33,34] There is compression of tunica media, stretching of internal elastic membrane, and vasculitis following an electrical injury. It was proposed that such changes cause late vascular occlusion.[56]

Another alternative explanation for progressive tissue loss observed was provided by Robson et al.[57] They found increased production of various metabolites of arachidonic acid including prostaglandin F_{2a} and thromboxane

A_2. The increased amounts lead to local tissue ischemia (due to vasoconstriction and thrombosis), progressive ischemic necrosis, and further thromboxane production. They were also able to reverse the damage to some extent, in experimental animals, by pharmacological manipulation using thromboxane antagonists. This creates an illusion of "progressive tissue necrosis".

In a clinical setting, there is no doubt that burn surgeons have regularly experienced this progression in thousands of patients. As the surgeon debrides a wound up to live tissues and plans to cover the wound in next sitting, one finds that the previous assessment was "wrong" and more debridement is needed. This continues for several days and one is forced to conclude "progression". Hence, till the progression stops, wound closure and reconstruction cannot be done. However, experimental studies do not support and have convincingly shown that there is no progression of injury.[55]

Current opinion suggests that progressive tissue loss represents the surgeon's inability to accurately assess the extent of muscle necrosis with naked eye and is a significant consideration in the surgical intervention on the patient. If the superficial muscle is appearing live, there is no way a surgeon can know the status of deeper muscle where damage is actually up to several centimeters proximal to the skin demarcation line. As the debridement is done from a "top down" exposure, damage to deeper muscles is considered equal to superficial muscles and minimal incisions are made lest delicate neurovascular structures are injured. The phenomenon of electroporation also explains this damage which is not due to thermal conversion of electrical energy. The phenomenon of "progressive recognition"[55] may be largely explained by the occurrence of this nonthermally mediated tissue damage.

It is prudent to have a second look (or even third look) when there are doubts about the viability of the tissues. This prevents problems with both over and under debridement. Extensive debridement may also need blood transfusions. Frankly, necrotic and devitalized tissue should be removed in the first surgical intervention while indeterminate tissues are left for next intervention 48–72 hours later when definitive cover is provided. The disadvantage of this approach is one (or more) extra anesthesia and operation. Increased cost of treatment is another drawback. However, it saves the precious graft or flap which may be lost, if applied over necrotic bed. There is a gross limitation of local tissues being moved safely for reconstruction. Regional flaps or distant flaps (free or pedicled) may need to be done. These may be fasciocutaneous, myocutaneous, or muscle flaps with a split thickness skin graft. As the availability, versatility, and variability of microvascular free flaps have greatly increased in last two decades, the indications for their use in burn reconstruction have also expanded especially in electrical burns.[58] Out of the vast spectrum of reconstructive armamentarium of a plastic surgeon **(Figs. 38 to 45)**, one has to choose the best in a given scenario based on size of defect, available locoregional options, and availability of healthy vessels at recipient site for distant microvascular free flap. Free flap must be carefully planned and anastomotic site should be placed away from the site of injury.

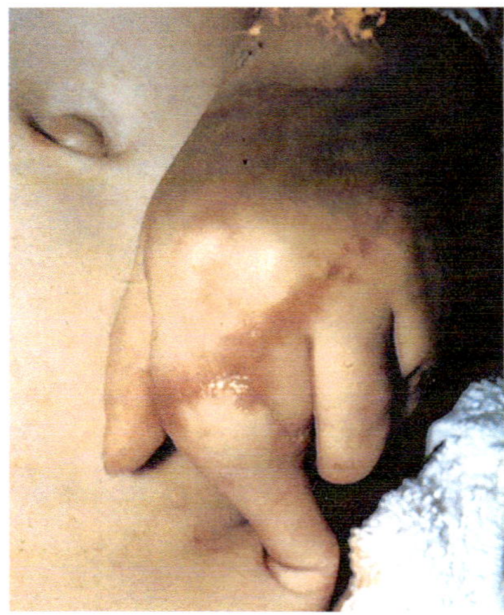

FIG. 38: A case of electrical socket injury involving index finger and dorsum of hand. Dorsum primarily excised and closed. Finger covered by pedicle groin flap.

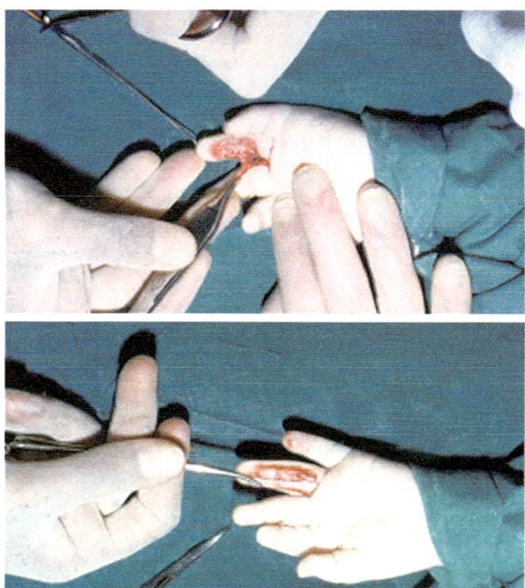

FIG. 39: Domestic electrical burn involving inner aspect of the ring finger. An electrical socket injury. Exposed tendon treated by cross finger flap cover.

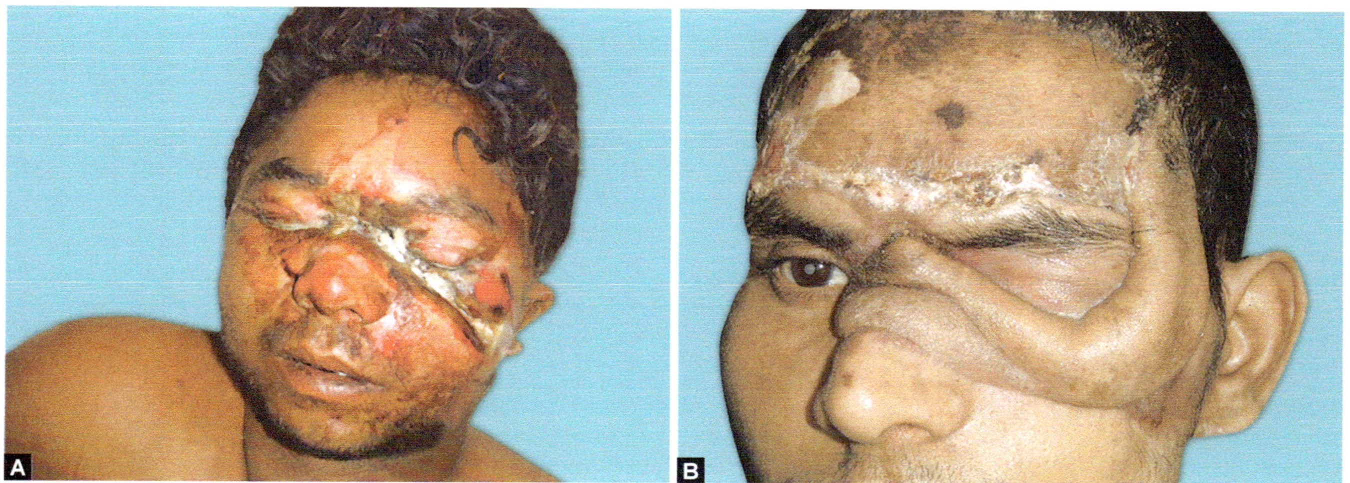

FIGS. 40A AND B: (A) Contact injury on face by wire falling accidentally causing deep injury on nose, left eye, and cheek with total loss of left eye and (B) Following debridement laterally based forehead flap cover given to cover the defect and cataract seen to have developed in the contralateral eye.

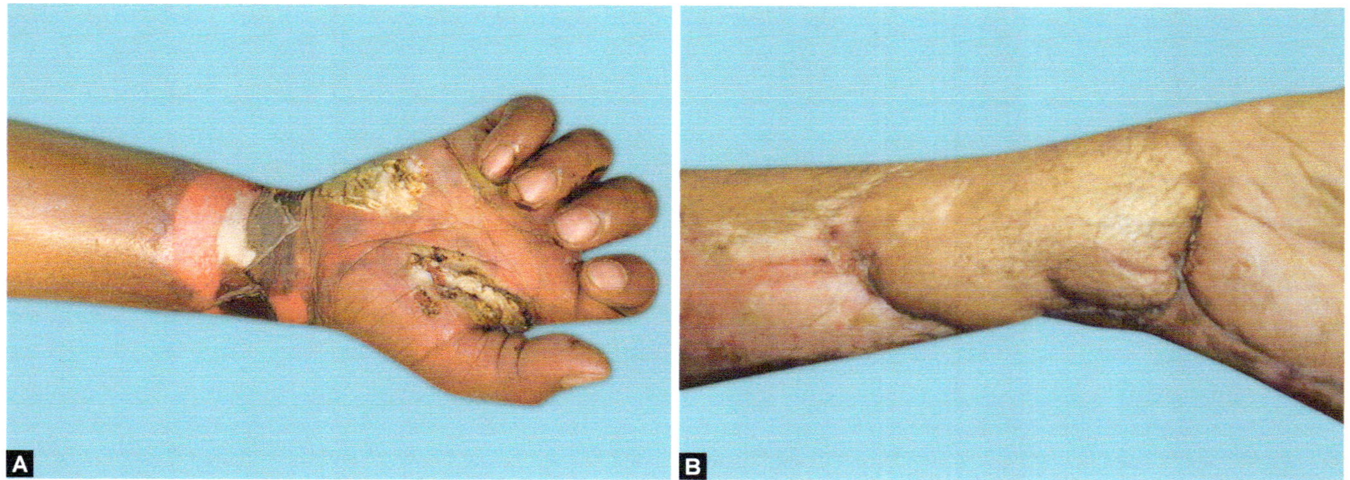

FIGS. 41A AND B: (A) Full thickness burns over wrist following contact with current in palm and (B) Wound debrided and exposed tendons and nerves covered by groin flap.

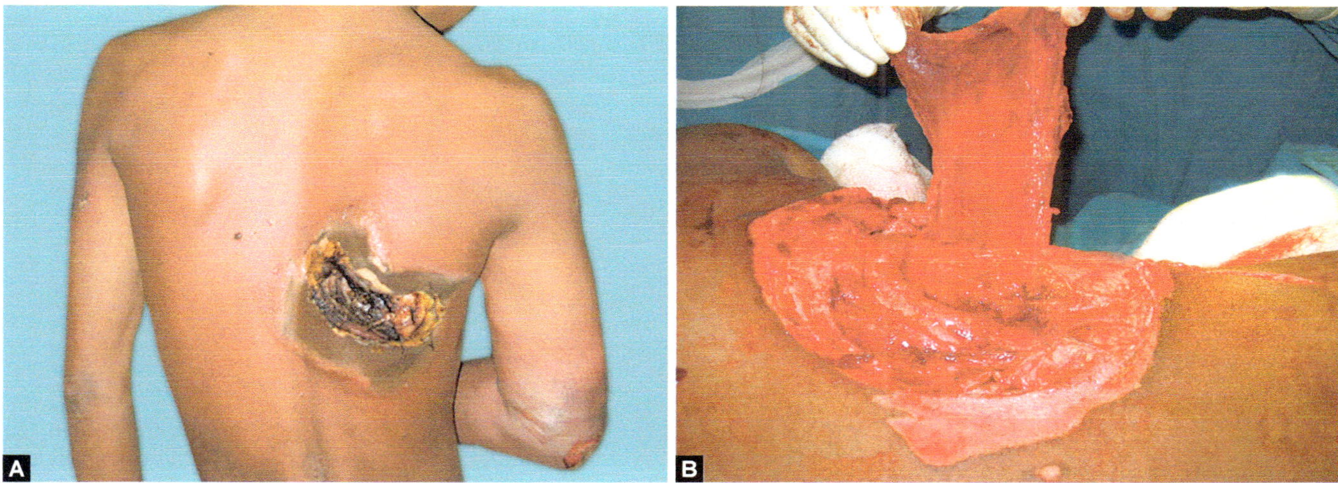

FIGS. 42A TO D: *Continued*

Continued

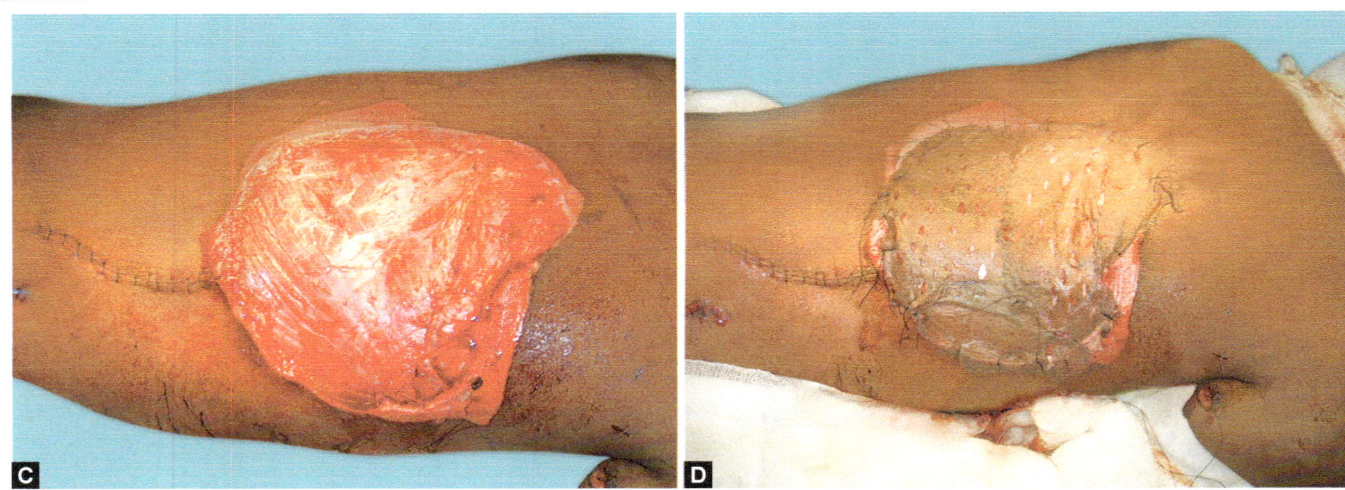

FIGS. 42A TO D: (A) High-voltage injury on the back of chest; (B) Wound debrided and exposed ribs with raised latissimus dorsi flap; (C) Latissimus dorsi flap covering the defect; and (D) Skin graft applied over muscle flap.

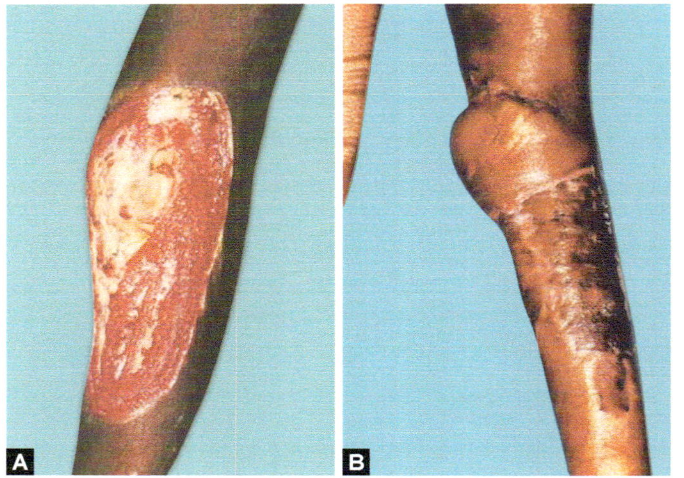

FIGS. 43A AND B: (A) Exposed knee joint following electric contact burns and (B) Covering knee joint by superiorly based fasciocutaneous flap.

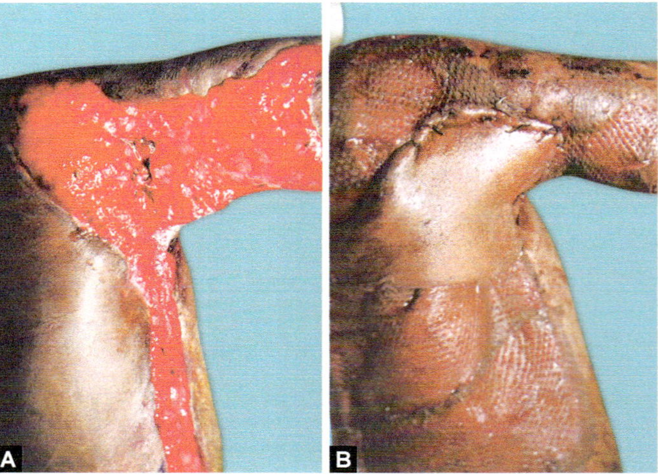

FIGS. 44A AND B: (A) Exposed axillary vessels following debridement of eschar from electric burns and (B) Cover over exposed vessels by latissimus dorsi musculocutaneous flap.

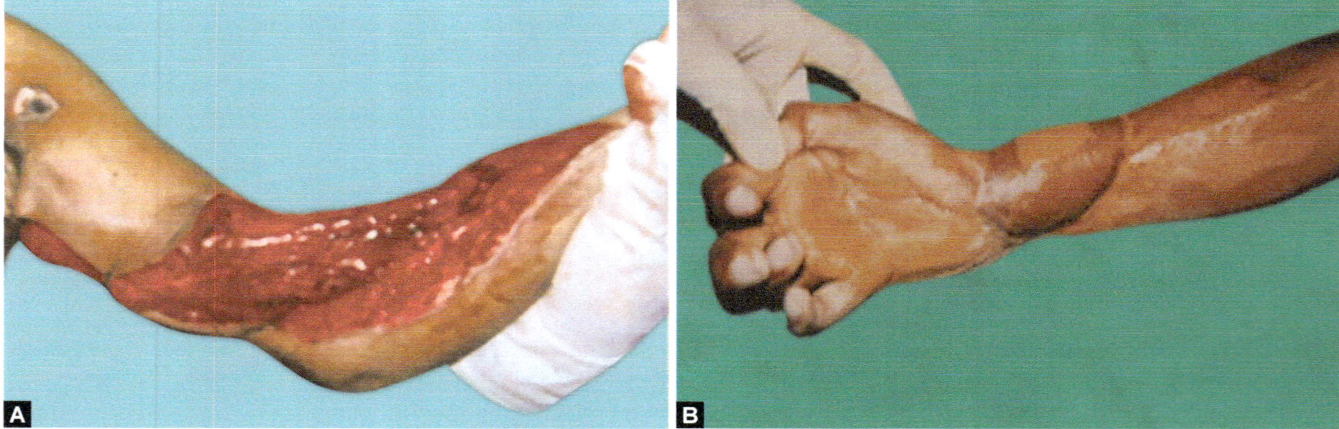

FIGS. 45A AND B: (A) Reconstruction to save the involved neurovascular bundle in elbow by providing muscle cover (latissimus dorsi muscle) and (B) Reconstruction of hand after electrical burn—functional gracilis muscle transfer for finger flexion with groin flap cover over exposed vessels and tendons in wrist.

In the author's opinion (Dr SP Bajaj) as there is far more damage to the venous system, an early excision and a pedicled flap cover helps in providing alternative venous channels which in turn prevents any further damage due to venous congestion.

Pedicled groin flap is a work horse flap for hand and wrist region. A random pattern flap from abdomen can also be planned. Cross finger flap and dorsal metacarpal artery flap are used for covering small defects over fingers. Surgical treatment of electrical injuries usually entails much more than just provides skin closure. Reconstructive procedures upon nerves, tendons, bones, and joints are quite commonly required to restore function.

Hand burns are seen in infants and toddlers due to putting the fingers into the electric sockets. However, with the development of better and safe childproof sockets, these electric burns in children have become much less. Electrical burns in children, because of soft pliability of skin, accumulate lots of fluids and are more likely to develop ischemic changes or median and ulnar nerve damage if burn involves wrist. An early surgery should always be considered in children and one must release the carpal and ulnar tunnel and also provide a flap cover. In fingers, a cross-finger flap, flag flap, or metacarpal artery flaps can be used to provide cover.

The areas of partial thickness burns (e.g., those following flash burns) require conservative management with dressings as for thermal burns while full thickness skin burns need split skin grafting done either after early excisional surgery or on granulating wounds after spontaneous eschar separation.

Many patients of electrical burns have complex or difficult wounds requiring not only the vast spectrum of armamentarium but also the ingenuity of a reconstructive plastic surgeon in their closure. Thus, (i) a wound with extensive loss of scalp along with both tables of calvarium and dura with exposed brain, (ii) chest wall wounds with extensive skin wound along with necrotic ribs and exposed lung, (iii) massive necrosis of abdominal wall with necrosed viscera, (iv) charred male external genitalia, etc., may need multiple operations over a period of months to years for the victim's return to useful life and "return to society".

REHABILITATION

Electrical burns are devastating injuries with both short- and long-term sequelae. They have greater severity, higher morbidity and mortality, need more complicated management including multiple surgical interventions, longer hospitalization period, and higher expenditures to patient or government exchequer in acute stage. They are also a heavy burden on families and society after the reconstructive surgery is over **(Fig. 46)**.

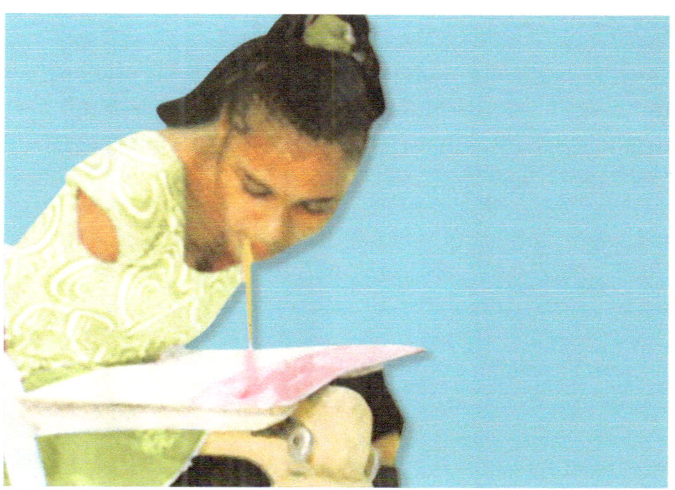

FIG. 46: A girl, who lost all her four limbs after 11,000-volt power line fell on her, paints with her mouth.

They are a major health problem for the developing as well as developed world. Most injuries are work-related. The quality of life (QoL) of these patients, especially amputees, is highly affected. It is not only very poor but job resumption is also almost impossible. They are unable to regain preinjury status and return to society. They may also become dependent on relatives and caregivers even for activities of daily living seriously affecting their psychology. Hence, serious efforts have to be made for prevention. Following healing of all wounds, rehabilitation of the patient with respect to both physio-occupational and psychological, especially if patient has undergone amputations, is extremely important in order for their successful "return to society". It is a matter of regret that the fear of losing financial compensation for the injury often keeps patients avoiding reconstructive surgery and remain out of work longer than is necessary. The long-term prognosis depends on the severity of the initial injury and the development and severity of delayed sequelae. Motivation of the patient is probably a very important factor in the functional prognosis of the patient. Prosthetic fitting and training must be an early consideration. In patients with bilateral upper limb amputations, the problems are manifold. Should it be impossible by any surgical technique to save even simple pinch or grasp in one or both hands, bilateral prostheses are required. All plastic reconstructive and orthopedic options need to be explored. Unfortunately, some form of attendant care may still be necessary throughout the rest of the patient's life in some of severely crippled patients.

LIGHTNING INJURIES[59-62]

The devastating power of lightning was viewed by mankind with awe and understandably, it was attributed to supernatural powers or divine presence. It was the sole cause of electrical injury since antiquity. The lightning strikes are usually freak accidents and one of most common causes of weather-related deaths. They strike the earth >100 times per second or 8 million times in a day. In India, a significant number of fatalities are caused by lightning every year. As per data from National Crime Records Bureau (NCRB), lightning accounted for 2,880 deaths, comprising 40% of all deaths caused by "forces of nature" in 2021.[63] Not all regions are uniformly affected with some areas being highly prone to it. Lightning frequency is highest in northeastern states and West Bengal, Sikkim, Jharkhand, Odisha, and Bihar. However, the number of lightning-related deaths is higher in central Indian states like Madhya Pradesh, Maharashtra, Chhattisgarh, and Odisha. Bihar is one of the most vulnerable states to lightning strikes with a significant number of deaths reported annually.

Lightning consists of transfer of electrical charge resulting from the sudden environmental discharge of static electricity sandwiched between an upper negatively charged region, such as thunderheads and a lower positively charged area on earth. When voltage between the two oppositely charged fields exceeds atmospheric resistance, discharge occurs. The most common types of lightning strikes are intracloud (the majority of discharges) and cloud-to-ground (some 20%) with ground-to-cloud and cloud-to-cloud lightning occurring only rarely.

There is a very rapid discharge of static electricity with voltages between 20 million and 1 billion volts. This can occur even in the absence of a thunderstorm. The current of a lightning strike rises to a peak in about 2 seconds, lasts for 1–2 milliseconds only and generate currents of 0.2 million amperes for 10s of milliseconds. The electrical energy gets converted to thermal energy with temperatures rising to 30,000°C and is accompanied by a shock wave of up to 20 atm that can contuse or perforate human organs. The clinical significance is that because the lightning discharge is actually completed within milliseconds, the victim can be immediately touched and CPR started without risk to rescuer. Apart from the duration of exposure to the current, lightning injuries differ from high-voltage electrical injuries in several other respects also. The voltage and current peaks reached by lightning are seldom attained in high-voltage injuries. However, lightning is a DC which is far less dangerous than AC which is more frequently associated with electrical injuries. Lightning causes ventricular standstill (asystole) as compared to fibrillation seen in AC because the former acts as a massive direct-current countershock, depolarizing the entire myocardium simultaneously.

With rapid intervention, many victims can be revived. The total amount of energy transferred is limited. Majority of the electrical energy flows over the victim's body (flashover effect) rather than through it. This is because lightning generally occurs in open spaces during rainy season and the highly conductive wet skin causes the energy to stay on the surface. This phenomenon is perhaps the reason which minimizes the corporal current flow so that the electrical injury to the tissues is less severe and mutilating than those with man-made high-voltage contact injuries. The injuries due to lightning can vary from minor burns to major burns from ignition of the victim's clothes or heating of the metallic objects on the victim's body like jewelry or coins, etc. The extremely short duration of lightning prevents struck objects from melting. The usual response of people during lightning strikes is to take shelter under a tree or a metallic roof and this tendency usually accounts for a greater number of casualties. When the lightning injuries occur inside a building, the current may travel through electrical wirings or through plumbing to cause electric shock to persons inside. There is always a possibility of further strikes and rescuers must be aware and take measures to protect themselves before moving the victim(s) to a safer place.

Lightning strikes result in multisystem dysfunction and survivors may experience prolonged disability following recovery from the initial insult. In lightning injury, burns are common and can be (a) arc burns, (b) flash burns to the surface, or (c) deeper burns. The cutaneous burns from lightning have been described variously as feathery, "fern-like," arborescent or a fine branching rash resembling bare tree branches. These "Lichtenberg" figures,[64] also known as keraunographic markings, are pathognomonic of lightning injury. There may be linear or punctate pattern also. These appear approximately 1 hour after a strike and disappear of their own within hours in survivors and thus, do not require much treatment. Their etiology is poorly understood. They are not burns and do not follow nerve or vessel pathways and are not associated with damage to the epidermis or underlying tissues. Their rapid resolution in survivors is more in keeping with temporary capillary dilatation rather than with interstitial hemorrhage or inflammation. Although victims of lightning show evidence of multisystem derangement, the most dramatic effects involve the cardiovascular and central nervous systems. Cardiopulmonary arrest is the most common cause of death in lightning victims and requires prompt resuscitation with cardiac massage and ventilation. If multiple persons are struck, attention must be directed first to those who are apparently dead because they may be in respiratory arrest and in urgent need of immediate

CPR. It must be remembered that CPR can be amazingly successful in lightning strike victims when done for a far longer time period than what seems reasonable in other situations. It has been postulated that lightning inhibits cellular metabolism by some unknown mechanism which delays the onset of degenerative processes. Autonomic dysfunction can cause pupils to become fixed and dilated or asymmetric.[65] This finding must not be used as a reason to stop CPR. Hence, the usually considered criteria of fixed dilated pupils and lack of spontaneous movements may not be applicable to diagnose death. Unconsciousness and other neurological complications can present in immediate period or delayed. There can be transient or permanent ischemic stroke or spinal cord injury or peripheral nerve symptoms.

Keraunoparalysis, also called Charcot's paralysis, is a common neurological complication immediately following lightning injury.[66] It consists of a transient weakness in one or more limbs (generally lower limbs) and is associated with vasomotor disorders from direct sympathetic stimulation reflected in arterial spasm or even complete loss of pulses, cold extremities and a pale or blue livid skin discoloration. Sensibility disturbances may give the victim a feeling of having no limbs. Generally, the paralysis, vasomotor disorders and sensibility disturbances disappear within an hour, rarely lasting for >24 hours.

Keraunoparalysis in both lower limbs occurs as a result of current flowing in opposite directions and is frequently seen in patients submitted to a high-step voltage. When a lightning bolt strikes the ground, the current is discharged into the mass of earth. As the current dissipates along the earth, a person standing in the direct vicinity where the lightning has struck is subjected to a potential difference between his feet when they are separated from each other. This potential drop causes the current to enter the body through one leg and exit through the other. The ground current decreases radially as distance from the strike point increases.

Damage to the central nervous system accounts for the second most debilitating group of injuries. These include immediate loss of consciousness, confusion, amnesia, even brief aphasia, weakness, intracranial injuries, paraplegia, quadriplegia, and cold pulseless extremities. There may be tympanic membrane rupture, temporary or permanent deafness, dilated or nonreactive pupils, transient blindness, retinal detachment, cataracts, etc. The rhabdomyolysis and myoglobinuria are uncommon. Many of injuries can be detected only by MRI examination. Electrocardiographic changes observed following lightning accidents are probably from primary electric injury or burns of the myocardium without coronary artery occlusion. Other organ systems injured by lightning include the gastrointestinal system, skin, and musculoskeletal system.

Ritenour et al. have described the following modes of injury by lightning:[67]

- *Direct strike*: Some victims, especially those standing in an open area or those carrying/wearing metallic objects, e.g., umbrellas, jewelry, watch, etc., experience a direct strike. These are usually fatal.
- *Contact injury*: It occurs when a person is touching a metallic object, e.g., a car or a metallic pole, which has been struck by lightning.
- *Side flash*: It involves current splashing from a nearby object or person onto the victim. Splashes occur when the direct pathway of current, e.g., through a tree, has a higher resistance than the air between the tree and the victim.
- *Ground (step) current*: Lightning strikes the ground in the vicinity of a person and passes underneath to enter into his/her body. These can be as serious as direct or side splash (see Keraunoparalysis above).
- *Blast injury*: A person is thrown violently from the lightning strike or the explosive force that occurs as surrounding air is superheated and rapidly cooled (sledgehammer blow). Lightning's blast effect or thunder may cause either primary or tertiary blast injury. Primary blast injury is often seen as rupture of tympanic membranes (in about two-thirds of patients) and internal organ contusion or perforation, whereas tertiary blast injury may present as blunt trauma when the victim falls or is thrown away.

The best treatment of lightning injuries is prevention.

SUMMARY

This chapter summarizes the current concepts in the management of patients with electrical injuries. Apart from understanding the pathophysiology of manifestations of these burns, both local and systemic, an early diagnosis of the extent of underlying tissue damage is equally important. An aggressive program of prompt and adequate resuscitation, timely fasciotomy, and early debridement including amputations and vascularized flap cover can decrease the incidence of renal failure, early toxemia and septicemia reducing the morbidity and mortality. The importance of progressive destruction of tissues in electric burns cannot be overlooked and necessitates repeated assessment and frequent debridements. Following healing of all wounds, rehabilitation of the patient, both physical/occupational and psychological, particularly if patient has undergone amputations, is very important in order to successfully rehabilitate the patient.

REFERENCES

1. Lee RC, Astumian RD. The physicochemical basis for thermal and non-thermal 'burn' injuries. Burns. 1996;22:509-19.
2. Pratap D, Sarabahi S, Tiwari VK, Annapareddy SNR. To Study the Incidence of Electrical Contact Burns and to Evaluate the Pattern of Injury in a Tertiary Burn Care Centre. Acad J Surg. 2019;2:40-4.
3. Ding H, Huang M, Li D, Lin Y, Qian W. Epidemiology of electrical burns: a 10-year retrospective analysis of 376 cases at a burn centre in South China. J Int Med Res. 2019.
4. Sokhal AK, Lodha KG, Kumari M, Paliwal R, Gothwal S. Clinical spectrum of electrical burns—A prospective study from the developing world. Burns. 2017;43:182-9.
5. Gandhi G, Parashar A, Sharma RK. Epidemiology of electrical burns and its impact on quality of life—the developing world scenario. World J Crit Care Med. 2022;11:58-69.
6. Li H, Tan J, Zhou J, Yuan Z, Zhang J, Peng Y, et al. Wound management and outcome of 595 electrical burns in a major burn center. J Surg Res. 2017;15:182-9.
7. Kouwenhoven WB. Effects of electricity on the human body. Elect Engin. 1949;68:199.
8. Kouwenhoven WB. The effects of electricity on the human body. Bull Johns Hopkins Hosp. 1964;115:425-46.
9. Fish RM, Geddes LA. Conduction of electrical current to and through the human body: a review. Eplasty. 2009;9:e44.
10. Koumbourlis AC. Electrical injuries. Crit Care Med. 2002;30: S424-30.
11. Edlich RF, Farinholt HM, Winters KL, Britt LD, Long WB 3rd. Modern concepts of treatment and prevention of electrical burns. J Long Term Eff Med Implants. 2005;15:511-32.
12. Wu YC. Electrical injuries—a literature review. Center for Consumer Product Technology. Report to: Consumer Product Safety Commission. Bethesda, Maryland: National Institute of Standards and Technology; 1979.
13. Jain S, Bandi V. Electrical and lightning injuries. Crit Care Clin. 1999;15:319-31.
14. Fish R. Electric shock, Part I: Physics and pathophysiology. J Emerg Med. 1993;11:309-12.
15. Lee RC, Kolodney MS. Electrical injury mechanisms: electrical breakdown of cell membranes. Plast Reconstr Surg. 1987;80: 672-9.
16. Lee RC. Injury by electrical forces: pathophysiology, manifestations, and therapy. Curr Probl Surg. 1997;34:677-764.
17. Lee RC, Zhang D, Hannig J. Biophysical injury mechanisms in electrical shock trauma. Annu Rev Biomed Eng. 2000;2:477-509.
18. Bryan BC, Andrews CJ, Hurley RA, Taber KH. Electrical Injury, Part I: Mechanisms. J Neuropsychiatry Clin Neurosci. 2009;21: iv,241-4.
19. Fish R. Electric shock, Part II: Nature and mechanisms of injury. J Emerg Med. 1993;11:457-62.
20. Fish RM. Electric injury, part I: treatment priorities, subtle diagnostic factors, and burns. J Emerg Med. 1999;17:977-83.
21. Fish RM. Electric injury, part II: Specific injuries. J Emerg Med. 2000;18:27-34.
22. Spies C, Trohman RG. Narrative review: Electrocution and life-threatening electrical injuries. Ann Intern Med. 2006;145:531-7. Erratum in: Ann Intern Med. 2006;145:936.
23. Waldmann V, Narayanan K, Combes N, Jost D, Jouven X, Marijon E. Electrical cardiac injuries: current concepts and management. Eur Heart J. 2018;39:1459-65.
24. Arnoldo BD, Purdue GF. The Diagnosis and Management of Electrical Injuries. Hand Clinics. 2009;25:469-79.
25. Schein RM, Kett DH, De Marchena EJ, Sprung CL. Pulmonary edema associated with electrical injury. Chest. 1990;97: 1248-50.
26. Masanès MJ, Gourbière E, Prudent J, Lioret N, Febvre M, Prévot S, et al. A high voltage electrical burn of lung parenchyma. Burns. 2000;26:659-63.
27. Chen CW, Lin YK, Yeh YS, Chen CW, Lin TY, Chang SH. Low-voltage Electricity-Associated Burn Damage of Lung Parenchyma: Case Report and Literature Review. J Emerg Med. 2021;60:e33-7.
28. Botte MJ, Gelberman RH. Acute compartment syndrome of the forearm. Hand Clin. 1998;14:391-403.
29. Bosch X, Poch E, Grau JM. Rhabdomyolysis and acute kidney injury. N Engl J Med. 2009;361:62-72. Erratum in: N Engl J Med. 2011;364:1982.
30. Somagutta MR, Pagad S, Sridharan S, Nanthakumaran S, Arnold AA, May V, et al. Role of Bicarbonates and Mannitol in Rhabdomyolysis: A Comprehensive Review. Cureus. 2020;12:e9742.
31. Culnan DM, Farner K, Bitz GH, Capek KD, Tu Y, Jimenez C, et al. Volume resuscitation in patients with high-voltage electrical injuries. Ann Plast Surg. 2018;80:S113-8.
32. Tarim A, Ezer A. Electrical burn is still a major risk factor for amputations. Burns. 2013;39:354-7.
33. Jaffe RH. Electropathology. Arch Path Lab Med. 1928;5:837-70.
34. Jaffe RH, Willis D, Bachem A. The effects of electric currents on arteries. Arch Pathol. 1929;7:244-52.
35. Hunt JL, Mason AD Jr, Masterson TS, Pruitt BA Jr. The pathophysiology of acute electric injuries. J Trauma. 1976;16: 335-40.
36. Artz CP. Electrical injury simulates crush injury. Surg Gynecol Obstet. 1967;125:1316-7.
37. Artz CP. Changing concepts of electrical injury. Am J Surg. 1974;128:600-2.
38. Bryan BC, Andrews CJ, Hurley RA, Taber KH. Electrical Injury, Part II: Consequences. J Neuropsych Clin Neurosci. 2009;21:iv.
39. Cherington M. Central nervous system complications of lightning and electrical injuries. Semin Neurol. 1995;15:233-40.
40. Andrews CJ, Reisner AD. Neurological and neuropsychological consequences of electrical and lightning shock: review and theories of causation. Neural Regen Res. 2017;12:677-86.
41. Bajaj SP, Pande S, Ahmad I, Arora S. Abdominoperineal electrical injury involving urogenital organs. Burns. 2000;26:664-8.
42. Sandhir RK, Tiwari IN, Goel A. Management of electrical injuries of the abdomen. Burns. 1992;18:253-5.
43. Srivastava R, Kumar R. Electrical burns of the abdomen. Indian J Plast Surg. 2013;46:587-90.
44. Sparić R, Malvasi A, Nejković L, Tinelli A. Electric shock in pregnancy: a review. J Matern Fetal Neonatal Med. 2016;29: 317-23.
45. Caballero-Carvajal JA, Manrique-Hernández EF, Becerra-Ar C, Alvarado-Socarras JL. Secondary maternal–fetal consequences to electrical injury: A literature review. Taiwanese J Obstet Gynecol. 2020;59:1-7.
46. Fish RM. Electric injury, part III: cardiac monitoring indications, the pregnant patient, and lightning. J Emerg Med. 2000;18: 181-7.

47. Thomas SS. Electrical burns of the mouth: still searching for an answer. Burns. 1996;22:137-40.
48. Al Rabiah SMH, Archer DB, Millar R, Collins AD, Shepherd WF. Electrical injury of the eye. Int Ophthalmol. 1987;11:31-40.
49. Boozalis GT, Purdue GF, Hunt JL, McCulley JP. Ocular changes from electrical burn injuries. A literature review and report of cases. J Burn Care Rehabil. 1991;12:458-62.
50. Kærgaard A, Nielsen KJ, Carstensen O, Biering K. Electrical injury and the long-term risk of cataract: A prospective matched cohort study. Acta Ophthalmologica. 2023;101:e88-94.
51. Sanford A, Gamelli RL. Lightning and thermal injuries. Handb Clin Neurol. 2014;120:981-6.
52. Singh S, Ahuja RB, Goel A. Utility of biochemical markers in the management of electrical burns. Germany: Lap lambert Academic Publishing GmbH & Co. KG; 2014.
53. García-Sánchez V, Gomez Morell P. Electric burns: high- and low-tension injuries. Burns. 1999;25:357-60.
54. Kidd M, Hultman CS, Van Aalst J, Calvert C, Peck MD, Cairns BA. The contemporary management of electrical injuries: resuscitation, reconstruction, rehabilitation. Ann Plast Surg. 2007;58:273-8.
55. Zelt RG, Daniel RK, Ballard PA, Brissette Y, Heroux P. High-voltage electrical injury: chronic wound evolution. Plast Reconstr Surg. 1988;82:1027-41.
56. Lees VC, Frame JD. Electrical burns. In: Settle JAD (Ed). Principles and practice of burns management. London: Churchill Livingstone; 1996. pp. 369-76.
57. Robson MC, Murphy RC, Heggers JP. A new explanation for the progressive tissue loss in electrical injuries. Plast Reconstr Surg. 1984;73:431-7.
58. Baumeister S, Köller M, Dragu A, Germann G, Sauerbier M. Principles of microvascular reconstruction in burn and electrical burn injuries. Burns. 2005;31:92-8.
59. Apfelberg DB, Masters FW, Robinson DW. Pathophysiology and treatment of lightning injuries. J Trauma. 1974;14:453-60.
60. Pfortmueller CA, Yikun Y, Haberkern M, Wuest E, Zimmermann H, Exadaktylos AK. Injuries, Sequelae, and Treatment of Lightning-Induced Injuries: 10 Years of Experience at a Swiss Trauma Center. Emerg Med Int. 2012;6:167698.
61. Craig SR. When lightning strikes. Pathophysiology and treatment of lightning injuries. Postgrad Med. 1986;79:109-12, 121-4.
62. Gatewood MO, Zane RD. Lightning injuries. Emerg Med Clin. 2004;22:369-403.
63. Yadava PK, Soni M, Verma S, Kumar H, Sharma A, Payra S. The major lightning regions and associated casualties over India. Nat Hazards. 2020.
64. Byard RW. Lichtenberg figures-morphological findings. Forensic Sci Med Pathol. 2023;19:269-72.
65. Jost WH, Schönrock LM, Cherington M. Autonomic nervous system dysfunction in lightning and electrical injuries. NeuroRehabilitation. 2005;20:19-23.
66. ten Duis HJ, Klasen HJ, Reenalda PE. Keraunoparalysis, a 'specific' lightning injury. Burns Incl Therm Inj. 1985;12:54-7.
67. Ritenour AE, Morton MJ, McManus JG, Barillo DJ, Cancio LC. Lightning injury: a review. Burns. 2008;34:585-94.

CHAPTER

22 Industrial and Chemical Burns

Mamta Sikroria, Mula Rohit Babu

INTRODUCTION

Industrial burns are similar to any other burns. The only major difference is labor and union problems, and one must be fully aware of the labor laws and compensation. Also, emphasis on safety measures is a must as the treatment of burns is a painful and prolonged process and also involves a lot of expenditure. Besides the loss to the company in terms of substantial manpower loss, the cost of treatment and subsequent compensation involved put a tremendous burden on the company. Any type of burn can occur depending on the type of industry the worker is employed with.

EPIDEMIOLOGY

The exact statistics of burns and the cost of treatment are not available in India. In America, a fatal injury occurs every 103 minutes and a disabling workplace injury occurs every 8 seconds. Workplace injuries cost Americans $125 billion in a year that is equivalent to nearly triple the combined profit reported by the top 5 Fortune 500 companies in the same year. Work-related burns account for 20–25%[1] of all serious burns. In India, approximately 1 million burns occur every year. The percentage of industrial burns is not exactly known in India. However, in a steel industry like ours, the work-related burns which need admission account for 10–15% of total burn admissions.[2]

Except for major disasters which occur once in a while, these burns are usually not very extensive and mortality is accordingly very low. Most of the work-related burns are seen in welders where flash burns and explosions are the most common injury-producing events. Another common form of injury is contact with hot metal (sometimes molten metal). These burns are very deep and cause severe morbidity but are rarely fatal.

Chemical burns again are quite frequently reported at workplace but they are rarely fatal. The greatest risk of phenol injury is associated with manufacturing of dyer, fertilizer, plastics, and explosives and in hospitals where it is used as a disinfectant. Workers involved with the glass etching process, petroleum refining, and air conditioner cleaning are exposed to the risk of hydrofluoric (HF) acid injury.

Anhydrous ammonia injury commonly occurs in agricultural workers. White phosphorus and mustard gas injuries mostly inflict on military personnel.[3] Risk of injury due to strong acids occurs in persons who are involved in the plating process and fertilizer manufactures. The greatest risk of strong alkali injury in the workplace is associated with soap manufacturing.

Flame burns are less common in factories; they usually occur in restaurant workers but are rarely serious enough to warrant hospital admissions.

Electrical current injuries are very common in line men working on high-tension wires. They usually present with very deep burns and even gangrene leading to multiple amputations. They are commonly associated with injuries like head injury or spinal injuries.

Electric flash burns are usually seen in workers who are checking transformers or electrical switch boards.

Employees of utility companies, electricians, construction workers (particularly those working with cranes), farm workers moving irrigation pipes, oil field workers, truck drivers, and individuals installing antennae are at a great risk of high-voltage electric injury.[4] Hot tar burn is common in workers involved in building and road construction. Cement burns (due to lime in it) though reported in Western literature are very rarely seen in India. Acid burns in the Indian subcontinent are usually homicidal and only a few cases are accidental. Accidents are usually domestic because of improper storage of chemicals used for cleaning toilets and drains. Work-related acid burns are seen very often in jewelers who use sulfuric acid for cleaning purpose. Phenol burns are commonly seen in hospitals where it is used for carbolization of wards and operation theaters.[1,5-8]

PATHOPHYSIOLOGY

Pathophysiology of thermal burns and electrical burns is discussed in detail in chapters dealing with them. Contact burns with hot metal are thermal burns, so pathophysiology remains the same. Here, we will only dwell upon the chemical burns. There are similarities between chemical and thermal burns, namely both involve protein denaturing and produce wounds which look superficially alike. On the other hand, important differences do occur. Thermal burns are typically produced by very short-term exposure to intense heat which is relatively quickly stopped.[5] Chemical injuries are more likely produced by longer exposure to chemicals and this exposure may still be continuing in an emergency room. In thermal injuries, there is a rapid coagulation of protein due to irreversible cross-linking reaction, whereas with chemical burn, the protein destruction is continued by other mechanisms. The most common mechanism is hydrolysis which is driven by pH disturbances. Thus, there is an additional problem of restoring tissue pH in order to stop cellular damage. These mechanisms may continue so long as traces of the offending agent are present, especially in the deeper layers. The degree of tissue damage as well as the level of systemic toxicity is determined by the chemical nature of the agent, its concentration, the duration of skin contact, and the mechanism of action. Chemical injuries are classified either by the mechanism of action on the skin or by the chemical class of the offending agent.

MECHANISM OF ACTION

With the exception of concentrated or fuming sulfuric acids, thermal injury rarely plays more than a minor role in chemical injury. The main mechanisms of action on living tissue can be placed into six categories. The cells may be damaged by:

1. Reduction
2. Oxidation
3. Corrosion
4. Protoplasmic poisons
5. Desiccation
6. Vesicant activity

Reduction: Protein denaturation is caused by the reduction of the amide linkages following exposure to reducing agents. Heat may also be a product of a chemical reaction, thereby causing a mixed picture. Reducing agents are rather rare and highly reactive chemicals, for example, alkyl mercuric compounds, diborane, lithium, aluminum hydride, and other metallic hydrides.

Oxidation: Some agents cause damage by inserting oxygen, sulfur, or halogen (most often chlorine) atoms to otherwise viable body proteins. In general, this destroys a protein's ability to function. Sometimes, the oxidation product can have very untoward effects as it becomes a competitor for active metabolic sites. Common examples are sodium hypochlorite, potassium permanganate, all peroxides, and chromic acid.

Corrosive agent: These substances severely denature proteins and erode skin. They behave differently as a class, but generally speaking, they cause a soft eschar that can develop into a superficial, indolent ulcer. The most frequent corrosive agents that are encountered are phenols. In a close second are the hydroxides of calcium, ammonium, potassium, and sodium.

Protoplasmic poisons: Certain poisons work by attaching to or inhibiting inorganic ions that are essential for regular, healthy cellular activity or by forming esters with proteins. Acetic and formic acids are representative of ester formers, but HF and oxalic acids are metabolic competitors or inhibitors.

Desiccants: They cause injury because they draw water out of tissues through the employment of hygroscopic substances. Since these reactions are typically exothermic, heat generation frequently makes the damage worse. The most well-known desiccant is sulfuric acid, fuming or concentrated.

Vesicants: These are characterized by their ability to produce cutaneous blisters and are potent chemical warfare agents. They include mustards, arsenicals, and halogenated oximes. Mustards are alkylating agents and the damage to DNA renders them toxic to proliferating cells. Following the death of the basal cells, proteases are released from lysosomes causing the epidermis to separate from the dermis. The result is a blister with the basement membrane on its dermal side.[9]

Chemical Classes

A noxious agent's chemical class is determined by the chemical reactions that it is likely to start. Effective wound management requires taking into account one of the most crucial properties of all harmful chemicals: Acidity/alkalinity or the capacity to alter pH. It should be mentioned that a chemical's reactivity is significantly influenced by its concentration. Concentrated solutions (>70% wt) release more heat during lavage or neutralization and are generally more viscous, reactive, and hygroscopic. The ease with which an acid surrenders its proton defines its strength; the avidity with which a base attaches its proton defines its strength. The pH scale, which is logarithmic and has a range of 1–14, is used to determine the strength of acids and bases. The pH of a strong base is 14, that of a strong acid is 1 and neutral pH is 7.

Numerous variables, such as the agent's pH, concentration, volume, duration of contact, and physical form, can affect how severe a chemical burn is. When solid alkaline pellets are consumed, the stomach is in contact with the substances for a longer period, which can lead to more serious burns. Furthermore, when diluted, concentrated versions of some acids and bases produce a lot of heat, which can cause thermal and caustic damage.[10]

Caustic dermal burns leave scars in their wake, and the severity of the scars varies according to the burn site. Ocular burns may cause the cornea to become opaque and result in total blindness **(Fig. 1)**. Gastric and esophageal burns may cause strictures to occur.

Acids

Acids release hydrogen ions and lower pH from a neutral 7 to as low as 0 because they are proton donors. Because they are reactive, hydrogen ions can protonate any carboxylic or amine site. A protein structure collapses as a result of this. Hydrogen ions eventually catalyze the breakdown of proteins into their component amino acids. Most acids cause coagulation necrosis by denaturing proteins, which results in the formation of a coagulum (such as eschar) that restricts the acid's ability to penetrate.

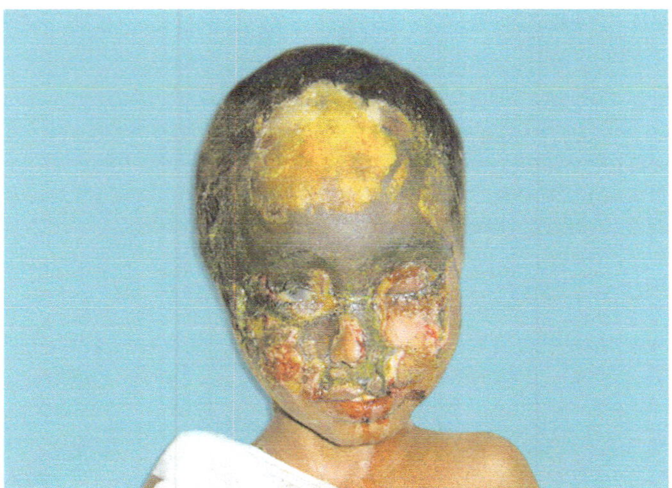

FIG. 1: Deep acid burns of the face and scalp in a 4-year-old child involving both eyes with complete loss of vision.

Mineral acids may also have additional effects, such as the creation of heat and desiccation in injuries caused by concentrated sulfuric acid, which results in a mixed injury. For example, phosphoric acid can also cause mixed damage by chelating calcium. Hydrofluoric acid differs from other acids in that it causes a necrosis known as liquefaction.

Bases

Proton acceptors are bases. The most common forms that can harm someone are mineral alkalis. Bases remove hydrogen ions from carboxylic and protonated amine groups. Bases catalyze protein hydrolysis, just like acids do, which results in the collapse of protein structure. As with the corrosives, bases can also result in mixed damage by generating salts and soaps, which can destroy tissue. Liquification necrosis is a more serious damage that is commonly caused by bases. Both protein denaturation and fat saponification are involved in this, which has little effect on tissue penetration. The most frequent substances that can harm someone are ammonia, lime, and the hydroxides of salt and potassium.

Numerous commercial and industrial goods have acids, bases, or other potentially harmful concentrations that can burn skin.

Some of the more common products are listed in the following text.

Acids

- Sulfuric acid is frequently used in the production of fertilizer, car battery fluid, drain cleaners, toilet bowl cleaners, and metal cleaners.
  Acid concentrations vary from 8% to nearly pure. The concentrated acid has a viscosity that is higher than that of water. When diluted, it produces a great deal of heat as well. Because of these qualities, sulfuric acid works well as a drain cleaner. Sulfuric acid concentrations are hygroscopic. Dehydration, heat injury, and chemical injury result in cutaneous injuries. It usually results in a brownish-black slough because it quickly converts glucose in the tissues into carbon **(Figs. 2 to 4)**.
- Common applications for nitric acid include electroplating, engraving, metal refining, and fertilizer production. Because of the xanthoprotein response, it results in the usual orange-yellow coloring of the skin.
- Common uses for hydrochloric acid include cleaning solutions for toilet bowls, metal, soldering fluxes, dye production, metal refining, plumbing, swimming pool cleaning, and laboratory supplies. The range of concentrations is 5–44%. Muriatic acid, another name for hydrochloric acid, causes the skin to turn yellow-brown **(Fig. 5)**.

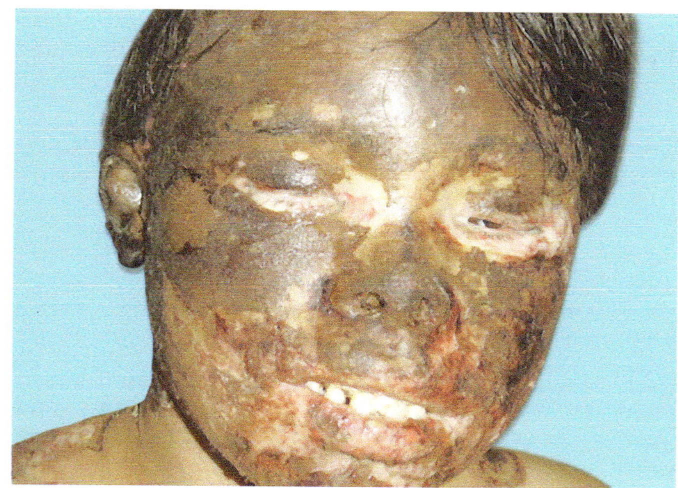

FIG. 2: Case of homicidal acid burns with superficial and deep dermal burns of the face due to sulfuric acid showing brownish discoloration of the skin and total loss of the right ear.

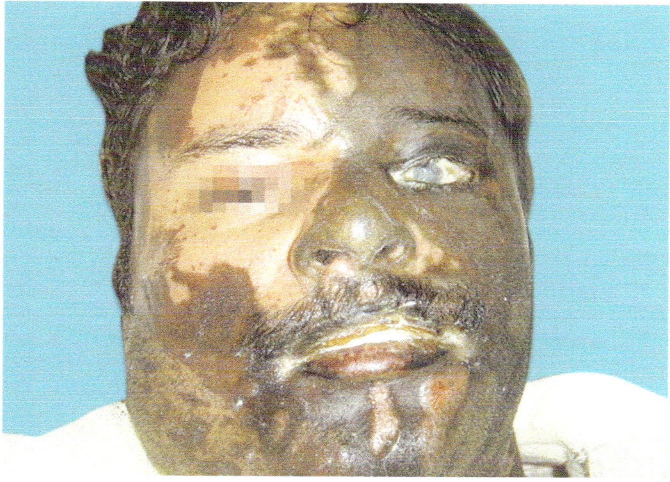

FIG. 3: Case of homicidal acid burns with brownish color eschar and involvement of the left eye.

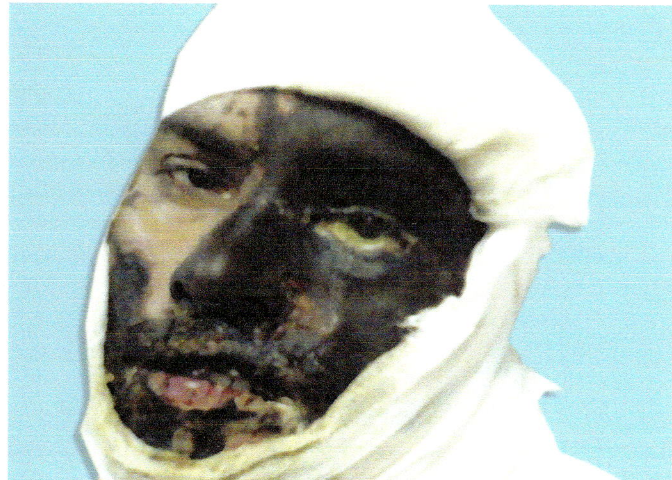

FIG. 4: Full-thickness burns due to concentrated sulfuric acid with discoloration of the sclera and black eschar on the face.

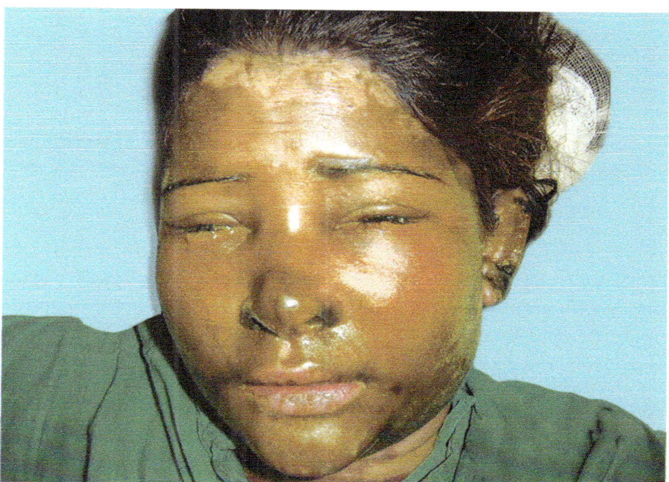

FIG. 5: Case of homicidal acid burns due to hydrochloric acid showing yellowish-brown discoloration of skin.

- Common uses for HF acid include tanning, semiconductors, glass etching, tyre and tile cleaning, rust removers, semiconductor production, and petroleum refining. Since it is a weak acid, it does not burn or hurt when it comes into touch when diluted.
- The production of fertilizer, detergents, disinfectants, rust-proofing, and metal cleansers frequently uses phosphoric acid.
- Acetic acid is frequently used in printing, hair wave neutralizers, colors, rayon, and hat making. It is diluted with vinegar.
- Formic acid is frequently used to make cellulose, glue, and tanning for airplanes.
- *Chloroacetic acids*: Phenoxyacetates, pigments, carboxymethylcellulose, and some medications are all made from monochloroacetic acid. Because it penetrates and stops the tricarboxylic acid cycle, which prevents cells from respiring, it has a high amount of systemic toxicity. It corrodes quite easily.
  - Chemicals are manufactured using dichloroacetic acid. It is not as strong as trichloroacetic acid and does not prevent cells from respiring.
  - Chemical industries and laboratories both employ trichloroacetic acid. It "fixes," or corrodes, tissues that come into contact with it. It does not stop cells from respiring.

Bases

- Oven and drain cleansers, Clinitest pills, and denture cleaners all include sodium and potassium hydroxide. They corrode quite easily. 45–50% of sodium hydroxide (NaOH) or potassium hydroxide (KOH) is present in Clinitest tablets. When diluted, solid or concentrated NaOH or KOH produces a lot of heat since they are

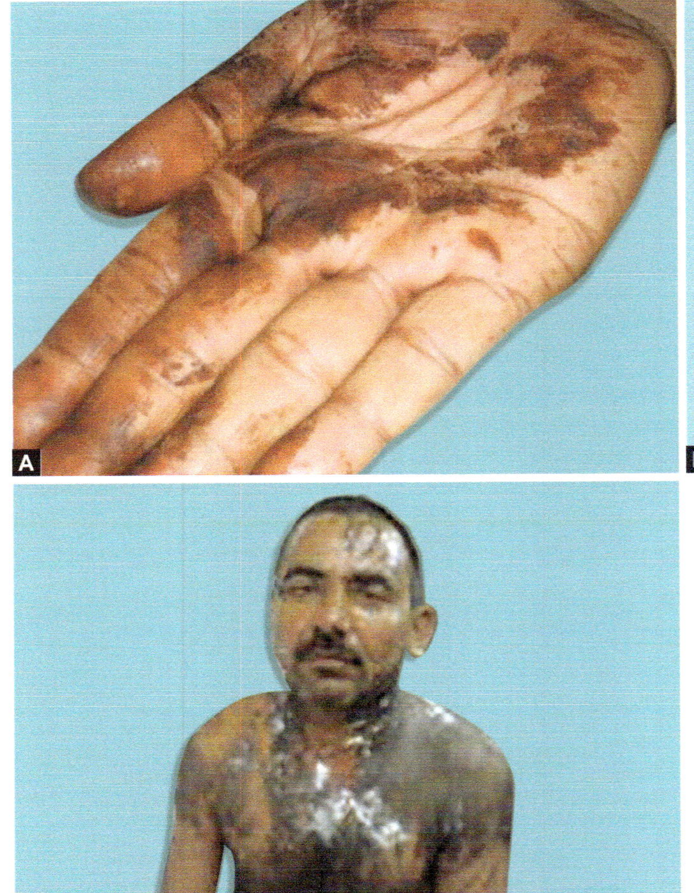

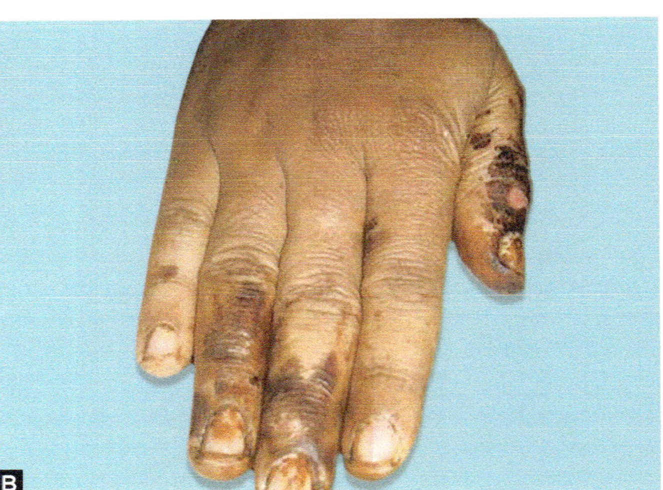

FIGS. 6A TO C: Case of homicidal acid burns due to hydrochloric acid showing yellowish-brown discoloration of the skin. (A) Accidental alkali burns of hand while using alkali in laboratory–palmar aspect; (B) Same patient's hand as in (A)—dorsal aspect; (C) Patient with alkali burns due to Drainex (NaOH).

denser than water. Burns are caused by both the alkalinity and the heat produced **(Figs. 6A to C)**.

- Another name for calcium hydroxide is slaked lime. It is utilized in cement, plaster, and mortar. Compared with calcium oxide, KOH, and NaOH, it is not as caustic.
- Common components of pool chlorinating solution and household bleach are calcium and sodium hypochlorite. Pool chlorinators are quite caustic because they have a pH of about 13.5 and contain NaOH as well. With a pH of about 11, household bleach is far less corrosive.
- The caustic component of cement is calcium oxide, sometimes referred to as lime. When diluted with water, it releases heat and can burn the skin thermally or caustically **(Fig. 7)**. In our country, lime is frequently used to get rid of warts and moles.
- Ammonia is used in cleaners and detergents. The dilute form is not very corrosive. Gaseous anhydrous ammonia is used in a number of industrial applications, particularly in fertilizer manufacturing. It is very hygroscopic (has a high affinity for water). It produces injury by desiccation and heat of dilution

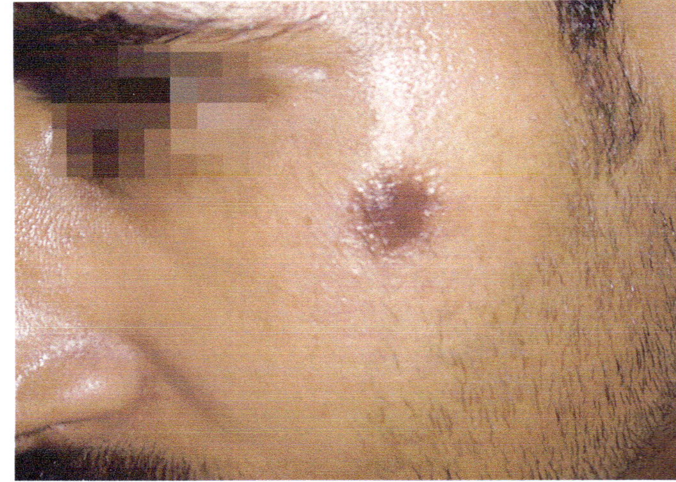

FIG. 7: Lime burn of the face (lime used for "treating" a mole).

in addition to causing a chemical burn. It can cause severe skin burns as well as pulmonary injury.

- A wide variety of cleaning products and detergents for the home frequently contain phosphates. Tribasic potassium phosphate, trisodium phosphate, and sodium tripolyphosphates are among the substances.
- Sodium silicate and sodium metasilicate are examples of silicates. In detergents, they take the place of phosphates. Dishwashing detergents are alkaline because they contain silicates and carbonates as their main builders. They have a little corrosive power.
- Detergents include sodium carbonate. It can be considered somewhat alkaline based on the amount present.
- Carbon dioxide is absorbed by lithium hydride in space technology applications. It interacts violently with water to produce lithium hydroxide and hydrogen. Both heat and alkaline burns may result from it.

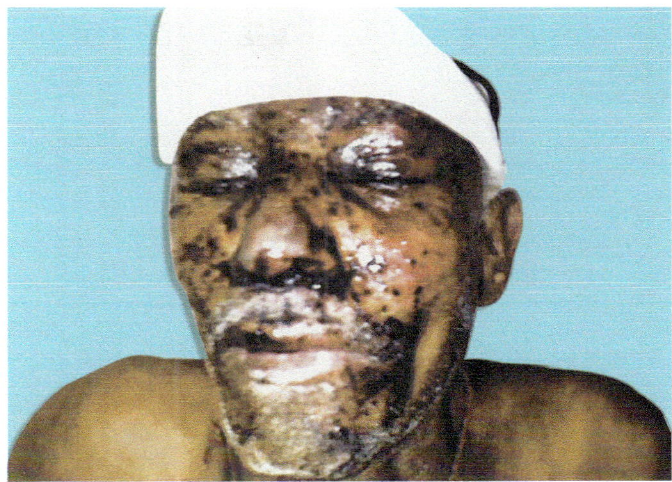

FIG. 8: Burns of the face due to blast from a mixture of sodium and potassium that the patient was grinding.

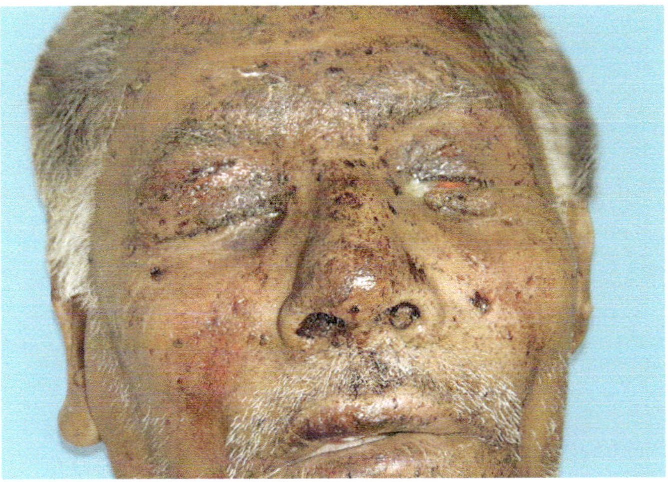

FIG. 9: Phosphorus burns on the face due to accidental bursting of a firecracker.

Organic Compounds

A wide range of organic compounds damage protein by direct chemical reactions and heat production. They may also act as solvents and disrupt the protein structure. Such agents include phenol and petroleum-based compounds.

- Phenol, sometimes referred to as carbolic acid, is a weak organic acid that is utilized in the production of disinfectants, medicines, resins, and polymers.
- Dihydroxybenzenes, or cresols, are employed as chemical intermediates, degreasing agents, and wood preservatives. These compounds can cause systemic toxicity through skin absorption and cause severe skin irritation.

Inorganic Agents

Apart from the mineral acid and alkalis referred to above, highly reactive elements damage skin by direct binding and salt formation as well as heat production. Sodium, phosphorus, lithium, and chlorine are excellent examples **(Figs. 8 and 9)**. Some salts, especially fluoride, can also cause damage.

Oxidants

- *Bleaches*: In the US, chlorates are the main compounds used as bleaches. Although household bleach has an alkaline pH of 11–12, it is sufficiently diluted to cause only minor skin irritation. Industrial-strength chlorates, which are more concentrated, can be more harmful to skin.
- *Peroxides*: Skin irritation is minor to nonexistent when using household-grade hydrogen peroxide (3%). 10% of concentrations have the potential to produce paresthesias and skin blanching. Blisters appear right away with concentrations of 35% or higher.
- *Chromates*: Common industrial chemicals such as potassium dichromate and chromic acid are used in tanning, waterproofing textiles, painting, printing, and as an oxidizing agent in chemical reactions. Chromates can cause severe burns on the skin, which can lead to systemic toxicity and even kidney failure.
- *Manganese*: Potassium permanganate is a potent oxidizer that is utilized as a sanitizer or disinfectant in diluted solutions. It causes very little skin irritation in diluted solutions. It can result in severe burns, ulcerations, and systemic toxicity when present in concentrated form or pure crystal form **(Figs. 10A and B)**.

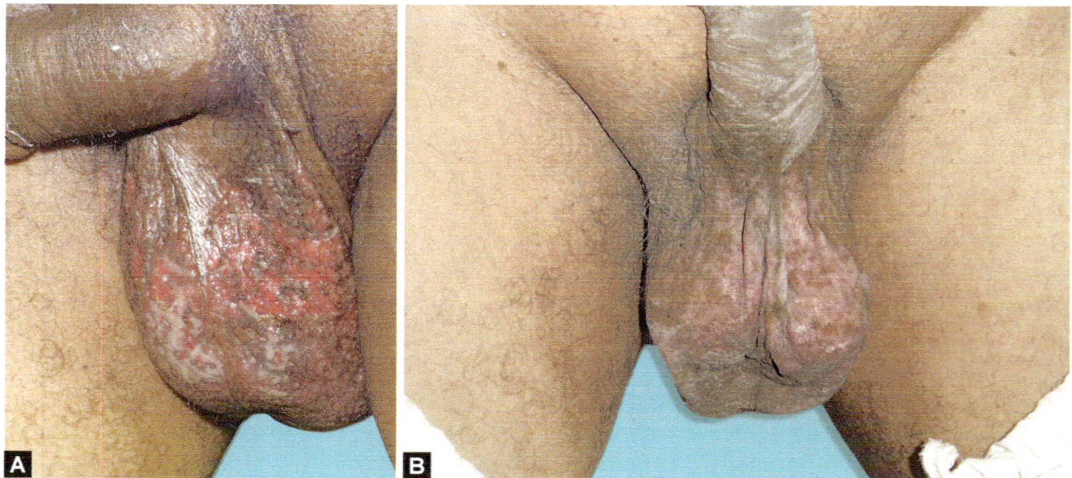

FIGS. 10A AND B: (A) Perineal burns due to potassium permanganate used for sitz bath; (B) Same patient after complete healing of wounds in 2 weeks.

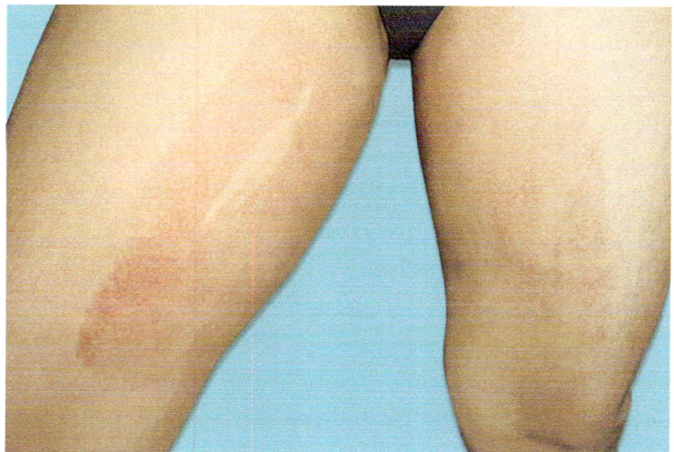

FIG. 11: Superficial burns caused by Savlon cleaning during dilatation and curettage operation in a female.

- Concentrated Savlon is another frequent corrosive that has been observed to produce burns **(Fig. 11)**.

MANAGEMENT

Management starts with on-site care and transfer to a specialized burn unit.

On-site Emergency Care of Burn Victims

Thermal burns brought on by contact with a hot surface, steam, flame, or liquid before medical assistance arrives:

- Use low-pressure water to end the fire
- First-aid assistance when necessary [cardiopulmonary resuscitation (CPR), etc.]
- Stop bleeding (bleeding does not occur from burns; if it does, there is another reason). Use pressure
- *Call for help*: Urgent medical aid call
- Use a blanket to keep the victim warm
- Stay with the victim till assistance comes.

Cool the tar with water to prevent burns. At the scene of the accident, never attempt to remove the tar.

Electric burn: It is caused by contact with electric current. Prior to the arrival of medical assistance:

- Before attempting rescue, if the victim is being held by the source, switch off the current or knock the victim away from the source using a nonconductive object (such as a wooden stick).
- Use low-pressure water to douse the flame of the clothing after the electrical contact is off.
- Perform CPR and first aid as necessary.[11]

Chemical burn: It is caused by contact with a hazardous chemical. Before medical help arrives:

- If the material is powdered, remove as much as possible using a brush before using water.[12]
- To remove the chemical right away, use a safety shower with low-pressure water.[13]
- When soaked in water, take off contaminated jewelry, clothing, and contact lenses.
- Before the patient leaves for the hospital, make them spend at least 30–60 minutes in the shower.[14]
- Carry the chemical's MSDS sheet to the hospital with the patient.
- Avoid using neutralizing agents.

If there is involvement of the eyes:

- Use the eye wash station to completely flush your eyes.
- Remove your contact lenses and keep your eyelid open while using water to cleanse.
- Never employ an agent that neutralizes.

Once the Patient Reaches the Hospital

In the emergency, take the history preferably from the patient; if not possible, the accompanying person(s) can give the history. It is important to know the mode of burn and any associated injuries so that treatment can be instituted accordingly.

History

- *Type of burn*:
  - Thermal:
    - Scald
    - Flame
    - Contact
    - Flash
  - Nonthermal:
    - Electric
    - Chemical
    - Radiation
- Duration of exposure or contact with a hot object.
- In case of chemical burns, the concentration of the offending agent should also be known, the type of chemical (acid, base, etc.), and whether it was ingested or only dermal exposure should also be known.
- In case of an electric burn, one should know whether it was an electric flash or high- or low-voltage contact electric burn.

  The next important thing to know is whether the patient had any fall from a height or whether any heavy object has fallen on the patient (common in case of steel industry) in case of a hot furnace blast in which the patient sustains flame burns as well as soft-tissue and bony injury as well **(Figs. 12A to C)**.
- Another important point is to know whether water has been used to extinguish the flames or cool down the skin surface or to wash off the chemical from the skin surface as it definitely reduces the depth of burn.

After taking history, the patient should be thoroughly examined to know:

- The airway and circulation status
- Extent and depth of burn
- Presence of any head injury or spinal injury which takes priority over burn treatment
- Any ocular exposure (especially in chemical or electric flash burn)
- Presence of any long bone fracture

Treatment in an Emergency Room

- Ensure airway patency and breathing.
- Establish a good intravenous line and start IV infusion with Ringer lactate.
- Intravenous analgesics and/or sedation (if a head injury is ruled out).
- Stabilize fracture(s) with splint.
- If chemical burn, then thorough washing with running tap water must be done for at least 30 minutes to 1 hour and further confirmation for whether adequate washing has been done is by litmus paper if available.
- CT scan for head injury and spinal injury should be done.
- ECG should be done if there is history of electric current injury.

After this, the patient should be transferred to the burn ward. In the burn ward, the patient should be examined in detail.

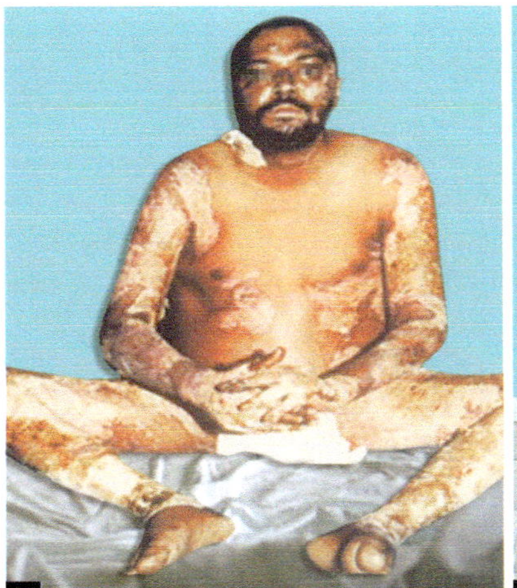

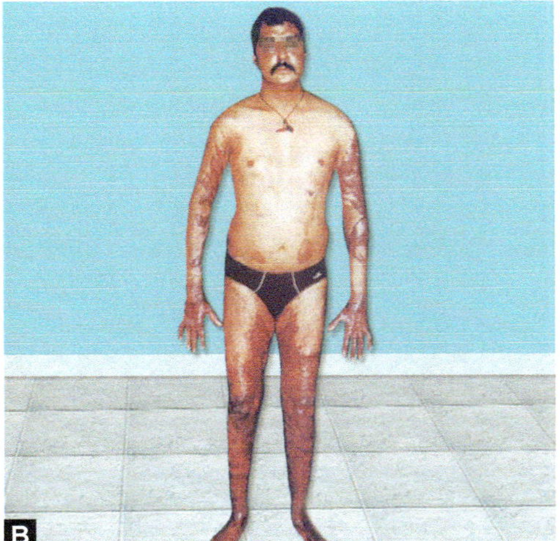

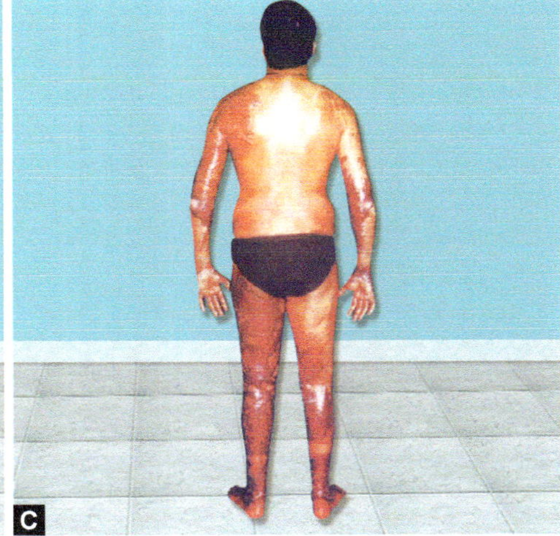

FIGS. 12A TO C: (A) 80% of the flame burns are sustained during a hot furnace blast; (B) Same patient after complete healing from the front; (C) Same patient from the back showing hypertrophic scarring in the lower limbs and upper limbs.

History is taken again in detail. Any history of an associated illness, such as diabetes mellitus, hypertension, ischemic heart disease, etc., must be taken as this affects the prognosis. In female patients, a history of pregnancy and lactation must be taken. Physical examination should be done in detail again to know the extent and depth of the burn and any other associated injury.

If good intravenous access has not been already set up in the emergency room, it must be started now.

The patient should be catheterized. Analgesics and/or sedatives should be given.

If the patient has any associated inhalation injury, bronchodilators and oxygen by mask should be given. If these measures do not suffice, endotracheal intubation or tracheostomy can be done. Intravenous fluids should be given using the Parkland formula or modified Brooke formula aiming to keep the urine output at 0.5–1 mL/hour/kg. In electric burn, more intravenous fluids (as much as 6–7 mL/kg/% burn) are required to flush out the pigments released by damage to RBC or muscles. If needed, mannitol can be given to increase urine output.

Once the patient is stabilized with sufficient intravenous fluids and analgesics and the urine output is satisfactory, the wound should now be dressed and the investigations sent.

Investigations

Routine: Complete hemogram, biochemistry (urea, sugar, creatinine, electrolytes, etc.), serum protein and albumin level and sometimes serum transferrin level tests are done if available. In case of electric burn, samples for serum creatinine phosphokinase and lactic dehydrogenase should also be sent.

If required, serum bilirubin, serum glutamic oxaloacetic transaminase (SGOT), serum glutamate pyruvate transaminase (SGPT), alkaline phosphatase, etc., should be sent, especially in chemical burns. In tribal areas and in certain communities like Sahu in Chhattisgarh, sickling test must be done routinely, and if required, complete Hb electrophoresis should be done.

Blood grouping should be done routinely.

ECG should be done routinely in all electric burn patients and elderly patients.

X-ray chest should be done to rule out any hemothorax or pneumothorax in electric burn patients or in any other patient if required.

Radiography of spine and long bones should be done if there is history of fall.[15]

Computerized tomography and radiography of the skull should be done again to rule out head injury in suspected cases.[11]

Gastrografin contrast studies may be indicated for a suspected perforated viscera.

Wound Management

In case of thermal burns (scald, flame, contact, flash, etc.), wound is first washed thoroughly with any soapy solution (Surgiscrub or Savlon) to remove all dirt or grease, etc. All blisters are punctured; large blisters should be debrided. The wound should be washed with saline or distilled water.

Second-degree superficial and deep dermal burn wounds are dressed with antimicrobial creams and nonadherent and absorbent dressings. Skin substitutes may be used depending on their availability in a particular hospital.

Various biological dressings available in India are amniotic membrane, collagen, etc. Integra[16] which is a double-layered biological dressing (outer Silastic epidermis and inner artificial dermis) is available but very costly. Other skin substitutes like porcine skin and cadaver skin are not easily available for use in India.

Biological dressings reduce the number of dressings, thereby reducing the workload on the burn team. Other important advantages of biological dressings are that they reduce evaporative water loss from the denuded body surface, thereby reducing fluid requirement, reducing pain as the exposed nerve endings are covered, and also reducing the need for antibiotics by preventing bacterial invasion of the wound.

Sometimes, in second-degree deep dermal burns the biological dressing is rejected. Still wound healing is enhanced as initial prevention of wound desiccation (because of evaporative loss), and bacterial invasion prevents conversion of second-degree deep dermal wounds into third-degree burns. After the initial biological dressing, the wound is opened after 48 hours and reviewed. If the dressing is adherent and patient is stable, he/she can be discharged with advice to come for outpatient treatment.

If burns are very extensive, especially in circumferential burns, biological dressings become too costly and we opt for conventional dressings. Again for the same reason because the biological dressing does not adhere, it is not used for third-degree burns.

We go for conventional dressing in extensive circumferential burns and in third-degree burns. After cleaning with Surgiscrub and saline, a final wash with 5% povidone iodine lotion is done (optional) and then dressing is done with 1% silver sulfadiazine ointment. The author uses silver sulfadiazine ointment mixed with 30% *aloe vera* juice for dressing in their setup. It is known that silver sulfadiazine inhibits the wound epithelization[17] and *aloe vera* enhances epithelization by increasing wound circulation and enhancing collagen formation.[18]

Aloe vera acts as an antimicrobial also as it prevents bacterial growth. Ointment like mafenide acetate is very good for burn wound as it has very good penetration of eschar, but it is not available in India and is also very toxic.[19] Other ointments like povidone iodine, nitrofurazone, Neosporin, etc., are also in use, but they are better used for small wounds as their antimicrobial spectrum is very limited.

For extensive burns, silver sulfadiazine is the best.[20]

In third-degree circumferential burns, escharotomy should be done once the patient is adequately resuscitated as distal circulation may be compromised or in case of burns of the trunk, respiration may be compromised.

In electrical burns, fasciotomy must be done immediately.[11] Other resuscitative measures are the same as for thermal burns.

Chemical Burns

The management of chemical burns differs a little from other burns.[14,21,22]

Management Guidelines for Chemical Burns

- Assess the ABCs (breathing, circulation, and airway).
- Begin the cleansing process:
  - Ensure the safety of the medical staff.
  - Take off all clothing (undress to gain access).
  - Remove or debride all solid chemical particles.
  - Examine web spaces, nails, and hair for chemical accumulation.
  - Use a green soap solution (10% isopropyl alcohol and liquid soap) to remove any caked chemicals.
- Take history:
  - Chemical kind and concentration
  - Exposure type and length
  - Concomitant traumatic injuries
  - Current medical conditions
  - Immunization against tetanus and allergies
- Physical examination:
  - Ingestion-related exposure can cause stridor, esophageal edema, the usage of auxiliary muscles, and other symptoms.
  - Exposed skin: Dimensions, depth, position, circumferential burns, etc.
  - Exposure of the eyes
  - Acuity of vision
  - Periorbital injuries
- If the chemical agent's composition is unknown, an alkali or acid can be determined using the litmus paper test **(Fig. 13)**.

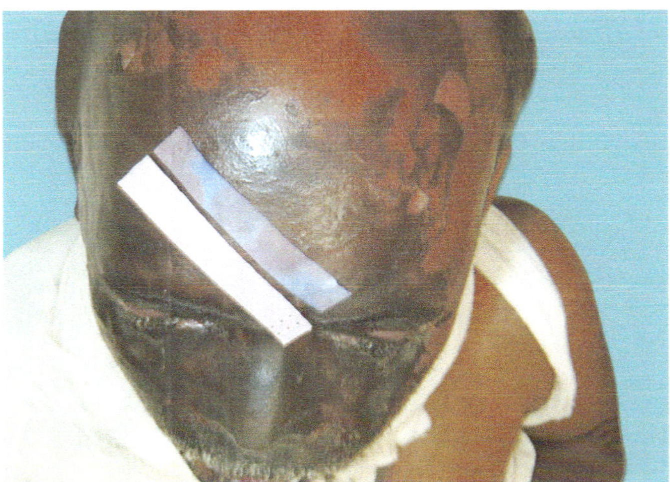

FIG. 13: Litmus paper test to identify the chemical (blue litmus turning red indicated acid and red paper turning blue indicated alkali).

- If necessary, begin therapy with certain antidotes (but only after an initial thorough irrigation with water).
- Determine the hospitalization requirements.
- Use pH or litmus paper to check the efficiency of the irrigation; if the pH is not neutral, irrigate for an extra hour (dilution is the remedy to chemical pollution).

Caustic Ingestions

Emptying the stomach is not advised. Activated charcoal is ineffective and can cause issues for an upcoming endoscopy. In case when there is any kind of airway compromise, dilution with milk or water is not advised. Milk could get in the way of a later endoscopy. Water is safe. Certain chemicals, such as sodium hydroxide or sulfuric acid-based drain cleaners, release heat when diluted with water. A considerable amount of fluid (250–500 mL) can be diluted to reduce the amount of heat generated locally.

- Do not attempt to neutralize the caustic agent. Neutralizing the caustic agent may generate excessive heat from the exothermic reaction of neutralization.

Endoscopy for Ingestions

- Perform esophagoscopy and gastroscopy on all symptomatic patients as well as on asymptomatic patients who have a history of considerable ingestions of substances that could result in serious harm.
- There is a poor correlation between esophagoscopy results and indications and symptoms. Between 2 and 15% of patients with esophageal injuries do not have mouth burns.
- Burn findings can be categorized as transmural, transmucosal, or superficial.

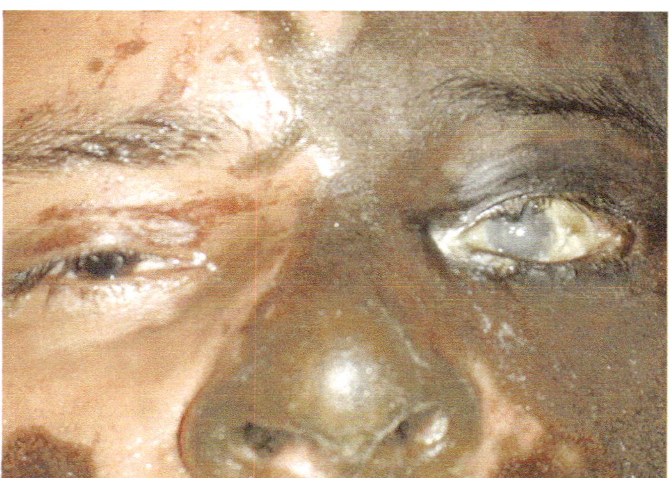

FIG. 14: Ocular chemical burns showing complete corneal opacification.

- The results of esophagoscopy are used to direct further care. Full-thickness or circumferential burns are linked to the development of strictures in the future. It is debatable whether or not to continue the endoscopic examination past the initial site of damage.
- Gastric and esophageal burns may cause strictures to occur.

Ocular Exposures to Chemicals[23]

- A pH of at least 7.2, but ideally 7.4, should be attained for the eye wash in order to accomplish decontamination.
- If pH paper is unavailable, decontaminating using 1–2 L of irrigation fluid over a 30- to 60-minute period is a sufficient substitute.
- Ocular burns may cause the cornea to become opaque and cause total blindness **(Fig. 14)**.
- Chemical burn patients should be admitted to the hospital for almost the same reasons as other burn patients, such as:
    - Patients at high risk (concurrent diseases)
    - Burns on the hand, foot, face, eye, or perineum
    - Burns covering more than 15% of the body's surface
    - Deep burns (second- or third-degree deep dermis)
    - Burns with compounds that are hazardous to the system as a whole

SPECIFIC AGENTS

In case of an industrial setting, the causative agent is usually known. The following list of chemicals is not definitive but it provides an inventory of the most common agents to cause chemical burns.

Acetic Acid

Acetic acid is a protoplasmic poison. Glacial acetic acid which is nearly 100% pure is the usual offender. Vinegar, a 5% solution of acetic acid, is usually benign unless scalding hot.

Alkali (Strong)

Caustic alkali burns are caused by a variety of chemical substances. Sodium hydroxide, lime, and potassium hydroxide are the most frequent substances that can cause chemical damage. Infants and toddlers can sustain injuries accidentally. Three things contribute to the mechanism that causes these alkali damages:

- Saponification of fat causes fatty tissue to lose its function with increased damage due to heat reaction.
- Extraction of considerable water from cells causes damage because of an alkali's hygroscopic nature.
- Alkalis dissolve and unite with the proteins of the tissues to form alkaline proteinates, which are soluble and contain OH ions, and these ions cause further chemical reactions which initiate deeper injury of the tissues.

Alkalis have the same deep penetration capability as other chemical burns, which can result in excruciating pain. In order to begin treatment, the causative material must be eliminated as soon as possible by washing with a lot of water.

Washing is presumed to cause dilution and elimination of a chemical substance, attenuation of the chemical reaction, and suppression of any raised tissue metabolism to have an anti-inflammatory action, to suppress the hygroscopic action, and to return skin pH levels to normal. In lime burns, the dry lime must be brushed away before washing in order to minimize the production of heat.

It is very difficult to determine the depth of tissue damage on admission to a hospital because chemical burns are different from thermal burns. Because the corrosive material blackens the skin, rapidly converting it to a firmly adherent, firm, dry eschar, a true assessment of the depth of an injury can only be made in retrospect as spontaneous healing or nonhealing occurs.

Postalkali exposure eye injury is very common. Damage is related to the pH: the higher the pH, the greater the damage to the eye, with the most significant injury occurring around pH 11–11.5. Alkali penetrates quickly and with little resistance, saponifies plasma membranes, denatures collagen, and causes vascular thrombosis in the conjunctiva, the episclera, and even the anterior uvea. Very small volumes of alkali material can cause significant damage. Repetitive attempts to remove the chemical agent with the hands or insufficient eye cleaning may exacerbate such harm. The protocol calls for topical anesthetics to be used first, then extensive irrigation, induction of cycloplegia, and mydriasis as soon as feasible. Antibiotics such as gentamicin and chloramphenicol are effective. Topically cysteine, a collagenase inhibitor, is applied every 2 hours in order to prevent perforation. Topical steroids are applied four times a day after complete epithelization has taken place.

Assorted Acids

Strong protoplasmic toxins include tungstic, picric, sulfosalicylic, trichloroacetic, and cresylic acids. They create hard eschars that might protect the underlying tissue from harm. Tannic acid has been used in the past as a treatment for thermal injury. These acids are absorbable and cause metabolic symptoms and are both renal and hepatic toxic. Most have pungent, suffocating odors and have wide industrial usage.

Cement

Cement is really an alkali but warrants a separate mention as it differs in many ways. When mixed with water, sand, and gravel, it becomes more abrasive and is known as concrete. Injuries are not infrequently found in construction workers and do-it-yourself enthusiasts.[24] Cement (calcium oxide) penetrates clothing and reacts with sweat and an exothermic reaction takes place. If the dry powder is not exposed to moisture, it becomes desiccation-prone. It is highly hygroscopic. Calcium hydroxide is produced when calcium oxide is hydrated. A wound worsens similar to a strong alkali. The hydroxyl ion is the key component that causes damage to the skin.[25] A victim may not know until many hours later that he has sustained burns beneath the garments. The course of treatment entails washing the afflicted region with soap and water and removing any contaminated garments. Surgical excision is probably necessary because these wounds are frequently deeper than they seem.

Chromic Acid

Chromic acid is a strong oxidizing agent that is used to clean other metals. In a strong sulfuric acid solution, chromic trioxide (CrO_3) is the active ingredient. Examining a sample reveals it to be a viscous, smelly yellow liquid. Blisters, ulcers, and protein coagulation are all brought on by skin contact. Ingestion causes gastroenteritis, which quickly worsens and causes unconsciousness, vertigo, cramping in the muscles, and collapse of the peripheral arteries. This is connected to glycosuria and is succeeded by nephritis. Between 5 and 10 g is the fatal dose. Lavage with water is the first step in treating contact areas since it dilutes the acid. Washing with a dilute solution of sodium hyposulfite followed by rinsing with a buffered phosphate solution is the treatment of choice and should be available if this agent is in common use (70 g monobasic potassium phosphate and 180 g dibasic sodium phosphate to 850 mL of water). Systemic manifestations are to be treated with Dimercaprol 4 mg/kg by deep intramuscular injection every 4 hours for 2 days, followed by 2–4 mg/kg daily for about a week along with support for the failing organ system.

Formic Acid

Dermal damage is rare, even though this organic acid is frequently used for hay preservatives and industrial descaling.[26] Because cutaneous absorption from the damaged area can produce metabolic acidosis, intravascular hemolysis, hemoglobinurea, renal failure, and pulmonary consequences, including acute respiratory distress syndrome (ARDS), all patients injured by formic acid should be hospitalized, even if only for observation. Vomiting and abdominal pain are usually common and although the cause is unknown, necrotizing pancreatitis has been described as a complication of formic acid ingestion. However, elevated serum amylase has not been reported in formic acid poisoning. Acidosis should be corrected with intravenous sodium bicarbonate. Minor hemolysis requires no treatment, but diuresis with mannitol is recommended where hemolysis occurs after deep burns. Where extensive absorption of formic acid has occurred, hemodialysis should be considered. The wound has a greenish hue and is followed within 48 hours by gross edema and blister formation. Wounds tend to be deeper than they initially appear and are best treated by surgical excision.

Hydrocarbons

Petrol burns are seen in patients trapped under vehicles following road traffic accidents. The solvent properties of hydrocarbons promote cell membrane injury and dissolution of lipids, resulting in skin necrosis. Symptoms present with erythema and blistering. Burns tend to be superficial and heal spontaneously;[27] grafting is usually not necessary although full-thickness burns do occur. If absorbed systemically, toxicity can cause respiratory depression. If ignited deep thermal injury is common.

The use of lead compounds to enhance performance qualities may complicate exposure to petrol. Fuel exposure may result in significant lead absorption and eventual brain damage. In this sense, tetraethyl lead is more hazardous than elemental lead.

Toxic consequences from ingesting and inhalation are common issues from the contact effects of petrol and other light petroleum compounds, such as kerosene. The patient frequently experiences major multisystem complications in addition to skin burn such as organ system failure. Similar to the effects of ethanol in descaling, inhaling or absorbing petrol can cause ataxia, mental disorientation, and slurred speech. Petrol vapor concentrations too high might cause a coma or even death. The petrol snifter was once significantly more frequent, but it is now much less so.

When intense exercise or stressful circumstances follow inhalation, there is a risk of sudden mortality due to cardiovascular problems. In some situations, the cause of death is severe spontaneous cardiac arrhythmias. The petroleum distillate's potential for toxicity appears to rise with catecholamine release.

Renal injury from petrol absorption includes renal tubular acidosis and glomerulonephritis. Hydrocarbon hepatitis is typically a transient lesion with no long-term consequences, arising from vascular endothelial injury.

The first step in treating a petrol immersion burn is to take off all clothing and washing the affected areas of the skin with low-pressure water irrigation for at least an hour. Admitted to the hospital, the patient needs to be monitored for a minimum of 24 hours. Serum lead levels should be measured and if the lead level is more than 30–40 ng/100 mL, therapy should be started. In some cases, calcium EDTA and dimercaprol (British anti-Lewisite) combined with penicillamine therapy for 15–20 days have proven effective.

Hydrofluoric Acid Burns

Sulfuric acid and fluorospar are allowed to combine in heated ovens to produce HF acid, a colorless liquid or vapor. An English glassworker created HF acid for the first time in 1720.[20] It begins as a gas, gets refined, and eventually condenses into a liquid state. Aqueous solutions that have concentrations higher than around 50% will fume. Compared to hydrochloric acid, HF acid is 1,000 times less dissociated and is a weak acid. It indicates that HF acid is capable of being absorbed or passing through the skin without splitting into its component ions, fluoride, and hydrogen.

Hydrofluoric acid finds applications as an etching agent in the glass and semiconductor industries, as well as in the manufacturing of diverse plastic products and in the nuclear industry as a uranium solvent. A lot of rust removers have HF acid in them. The glass or semiconductor industries appear to be the primary sources of HF acid burns.

Hydrofluoric acid, even in low concentrations, causes significant tissue damage.[28] Moreover, a 50% concentration of HF acid solution causes instantaneous pain and tissue damage. Less than 20% of solutions may not show symptoms for up to 24 hours after exposure; however, solutions of intermediate strength may show symptoms for up to 8 hours. The skin and all mucous membranes, including those of the digestive and respiratory systems, are potential entry points for fluoride ions into the body.

Every calcium-dependent activity in the cell membrane is disrupted by the fluoride ion. The skin and subcutaneous tissues experience liquefaction necrosis as a result of this cell membrane degradation. Because they are soluble, the ions that HF acid produces seep into the tissues and cause ongoing damage. In addition to being a biological toxin, fluoride ions also stop glycolysis, which results in cell death.

The fluoride ions need to be inactivated while the salts are still functional. In the absence of targeted therapy, the harm worsens and may even be lethal. Fluoride ions combine with calcium and magnesium ions to generate insoluble salts. The remaining salts are all soluble and totally dissociate, enabling the ions to keep diffusing into the tissues.

$$HF = H^+ + F^- \text{ (Toxic)}$$

The area has to be heavily flooded at low pressure with water as soon as it has been exposed. To reduce the chance of additional contamination, the worker should take off all clothing and shoes before entering the shower. Topical magnesium oxide ointment or calcium chloride/calcium gluconate solutions can be used to fix the residual fluoride ions in insoluble salts after the area has been submerged in water for at least half an hour. Calcium seems to have the most potential for treating HF acid skin burns:

$$Ca^{++} + F^- = CaF_2 \text{ (nontoxic)}$$

Additionally, some authorities advise using quaternary ammonia compounds such as Zephiran or Hibiclens. The impact of these ammonia compounds on skin toxicity from fluoride is questionable. Moreover, they could have a tendency to irritate delicate skin, such as the face.

Initial Presentation

Pain at the exposure location is typically the first symptom to appear. There can be edema and localized erythema. Everyone who has experienced the agony describes it as unbearable, especially after being exposed to solutions with a concentration of more than 20%. It is also common to describe the pain as profound, throbbing, or searing. For alleviation, regional nerve blocks can be necessary.

Systemic fluoride poisoning has been fatally caused by exposure to concentrated HF acid over as small a skin area as 2.5% of total body surface area (TBSA).

Blanching follows erythema and edema in the course of the damage. Bullae indicate a more serious burn that has to be treated aggressively. A severely necrotic area may appear, followed by tissue sloughing and a wound that heals slowly. Severe decalcification and bone damage may be observed in extreme situations. Hydrofluoric acid burns have caused systemic hydrofluorosis with subsequent death.

Initial Treatment

In the event that skin damage is evident, even in the form of erythema, fluoride ions have penetrated the skin and need to be neutralized. Assuming that all spills are polluted and that the patient would have an injury if treatment is not received is usually acceptable and safe. The supplier has to make sure that there is sufficient protection against this agent accessible and being deployed before moving further. As a bare minimum, gloves and an apron made of butyl rubber or nitryl are used. Covers for the shoes of the provider reduce "tracking" and shoe contamination. To prevent spills, all contaminated bedding and clothes should be put in large plastic rubbish bags with clear labels.

While the materials and additional preparations are being made, the area should be thoroughly rinsed with running water. Fluoride-containing fluids should be sucked out of all bullae and vesicles. It is important to take precautions to avoid getting aspirated on any other skin area. Next, the lesions need to be debrided.

Local Infiltrating Therapy

10% calcium gluconate is injected into the burn to bind the fluoride ions following debridement. For every square centimeter of tissue injury, an intradermal injection of approximately 0.5 mL of solution is recommended.[29] To bind ions that may have already moved to the burn's margins, the injection is prolonged around 0.5 cm into those areas. An injection site is gradually penetrated with a 27–30-gauge needle to lessen discomfort. In most cases, the injection of calcium gluconate relieves pain effectively. Sadly, each injection of calcium chloride can only contain 0.5 cc of the substance. This significantly reduces the quantity of calcium that can be therapeutically injected in a single session. If the pain returns, further fluoride ion migration occurs, necessitating another injection.

Intra-arterial Injection

Compared to injection into the burned area, intra-arterial calcium may offer better tissue distribution and less tissue distention. It goes without saying that the distribution system should hold the vascular catheter. Burns to the tips of the fingers may be relieved by an arterial injection of calcium without causing loss of the distal finger or nail. Over the course of 4 hours, the calcium may be delivered as either gluconate or chloride. More calcium may be administered if the patient complains of ongoing pain. Since systemic calcium toxicity limits the concentration of calcium salts, intravenous calcium delivery has not proven useful.

Eye Injuries

When HF acid solution or vapor gets into the eyes, it damages them more severely than other acids at comparable concentrations. The liquefaction necrosis and deeper penetration of HF acid render it more harmful to the eyes. The first line of treatment for eye burns is to immediately and heavily rinse the affected eye. A Morgan contact irrigating lens could be perfect for this if one is available. Tetracaine or other ocular anesthetic treatments can reduce eyelid spasms. After this irrigation, drops containing 1% calcium gluconate solution in isotonic sodium chloride can be infused every 2–3 hours. Some employees believe that the sole therapeutic benefits come from water irrigation, isotonic saline solutions, or magnesium chloride solutions.

Other therapies that have been used on the skin have been associated with increased rates of ocular injuries. An ophthalmologist's prompt consultation is essential.

Dressings

Following the calcium injection, dressings with either calcium or magnesium oxide may be applied to the affected area. Although they are less costly and simpler to get, dressings containing magnesium oxide are not as effective as those containing calcium. Soaks with calcium chloride can also be utilized. While other authors suggest 2.5% calcium gluconate in a gel vehicle, further clinical research is necessary before endorsing this more expensive course of treatment. A cheap substitute could be a mixture of 2.5–5.0% calcium gluconate in K-Y jelly.

To find out if there is any more damage, the wound needs to be checked often. A new examination and injection are necessary when discomfort returns. Re-examining a fluoride burn at 24-hour intervals is recommended regardless of its size or appearance.

Hydrofluoric acid has a high penetration rate and can quickly dissolve the matrix and nail bed underneath. The painful process of calcium ion infiltration into the subungual regions can lead to vascular impairment in the narrow space that exists between the nail and the nail bed. Under regional anesthesia, the afflicted nail must typically be removed when HF acid burns involve ungual regions. After an accident, nail removal promotes healing.

Steroids and early surgical lesion removal have been suggested as treatments in the past. While surgical therapy may result in unnecessary mutilation, steroids have not demonstrated any therapeutic effects.

Complications

Significant systemic absorption of fluoride ions may be linked to skin burns caused by HF acid. Because fluoride ions create poorly soluble calcium fluoride complexes, they can lead to systemic hypocalcemia and decalcification of the bones. Fluoride-induced abrupt mortality has been linked to this sharp decline in serum calcium levels.

Usually, uncontrollable ventricular fibrillation is the cause of mortality; however, standard intravenous calcium dosages have little effect on this dysrhythmia.[30] Numerous writers have documented that treating hypocalcemia with large dosages of calcium salts can be helpful. It is common for this severe hypocalcemia to be unrelated to tetany.

According to some authors, a deadly hyperkalemia is brought on by potassium leakage from cells harmed by fluoride. Quinidine has been shown to inhibit the calcium-dependent channels responsible for this hyperkalemia in dogs. Quinidine has not been studied in fluoride-toxic people with ventricular dysrhythmias, hypocalcemia, or hyperkalemia. Nonetheless, quinidine might be suitable for these particular patients given the inadequate response to current treatments.

The patient has to be admitted to the hospital and monitored for a minimum of 24 hours if there is any indication of systemic fluorosis or if there is a chance of an inhalation damage. Serial serum calcium levels, electrolytes, renal function testing, and liver function studies should all be monitored in these patients.

Nitric Acid Burns

Nitric acid is a significant chemical that is used in the production of fertilizer, metal refining, engraving, and electroplating. It is a potent oxidizer and acid that can nitrate organic molecules.[31]

The injured site's yellowish discoloration serves as a diagnostic indication. This yellowish color is indicative of chemical damage brought on by exposure to nitric acid.[32] Acids lead to thrombus development in the lesion's microvasculature and coagulation necrosis of the tissues **(Fig. 15)**. After just 5 seconds of contact, superficial burns happen, and full-thickness burns happen after 30 seconds.[31]

By combining with complex proteins (xanthoproteic reaction) and creating a yellow substance called xanthoproteic acid, skin contact with nitric acid causes distinctive yellow-to-brown stained wounds that may accumulate eschar and demarcate differently than thermal burns.[33]

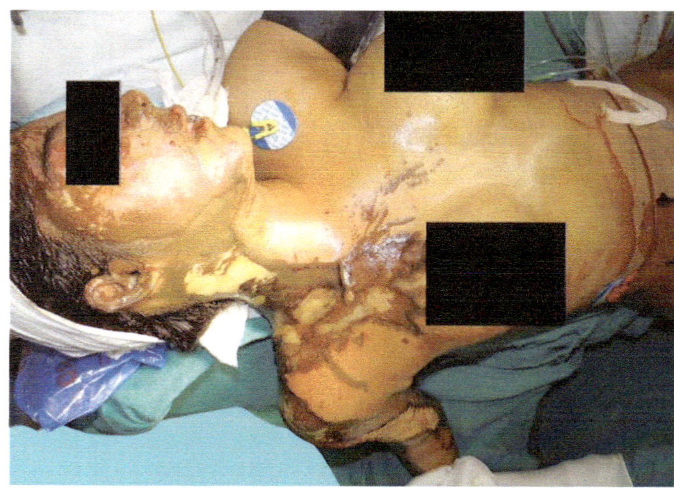

FIG. 15: Patient with nitric acid burns. We can see characteristic yellowish discoloration of the skin at the injury site.

Management is irrigation of the wound until complete washout of the chemical, and further treatment is similar to other corrosive burns.

Elemental Sodium, Potassium, and Lithium Burns

Sodium, potassium, and, to a lesser extent, lithium spontaneously ignite when in contact with water, including water vapor in the air or on the skin **(Fig. 8)**. Using water to irrigate these burns only intensifies the combustion effects. When these metals combine with water, sodium, potassium, and lithium hydroxides are formed. These are among the strongest of alkalis and are capable of causing severe caustic burns.

Water and oxygen must be removed from the region in order to put out these burning metals. The fire can be put out using sand or a class D fire extinguisher. To protect the metal from moisture, the area needs to be covered with oil once the fire is put out, such as cooking or mineral oil. To preserve healthy tissues, small metal fragments should be extracted by debridement. Surgical removal is necessary for embedded fragments. The region needs to be irrigated with water using the same methods as for an alkali burn after debridement to make sure all pieces are gone.

Light Metals

Water should be avoided for extinguishing burning light metal fragments as the hydroxides and hydrogen gases that are produced cause further harm when water is added to hot metals. Particularly injurious are burning fragments of elemental magnesium, which produces magnesium oxide. If the pieces of magnesium are not removed, the small ulcers that form slowly enlarge and become extensive lesions. After these fragments of burning metal are removed, the resultant wound must be treated as alkali burns.

Phosphorus Burns

When white phosphorus comes into contact with air, it spontaneously ignites. It is a transparent, waxy substance. It is often kept submerged in water, and around 44°C it turns liquid. White phosphorus is a component of insecticides and rodent poisons, and it is employed in the manufacture of fireworks and military weapons.[34] The most prevalent kind of phosphorus in chemical burns is white phosphorus **(Fig. 9)**. The fuming, crystalline mass of phosphorous pentachloride has a strong odor and is yellowish white in color. It is extensively employed as dehydrating, chlorinating, and catalyst. White phosphorus explosions are characterized by the production of dense clouds of white smoke that smell strongly of garlic and burning droplets of white phosphorus that are hurled around extensively. The burning fragments of phosphorus mostly harm tissue by heat, although they can also inflict injuries from fast-moving projectiles. Phosphorus oxidizes to phosphoric acid, which can harm both the skin and the lungs, producing smoke. Certain "tracer" bullets include a significant amount of white phosphorous. This can result in the absorption of phosphorus fragments that have been retained following a phosphorus-based shell explosion or a tracer bullet wound.

White phosphorus is readily absorbed from phosphorus particles pushed into the subcutaneous lipid tissues, or if consumed via the gastrointestinal tract since it is extremely fat-soluble. Hepatotoxicity and renal impairment are the two most frequent systemic consequences, although blood phosphorus and calcium levels are frequently altered. Bradycardia, T-wave abnormalities, ST segment depression, and QT interval lengthening are also observed in the ECG. Fortunately, sudden mortality is not common; however, it has been documented in patients with inverted calcium-phosphorus ratios.[35] Patients with large wounds should be watched for abnormalities in their electrocardiogram and for changes in their serum levels of calcium and phosphorus. Regular assessments of blood urea nitrogen (BUN), creatinine, serum phosphorus, and liver enzymes are recommended when there is a suspicion of systemic absorption **(Fig. 16)**.

The bits of flaming white phosphorous are put in water to put it out. Both surface- and clothing-embedded pollutants should be removed right away. In order to stop additional burning, the emergency medical crew should cover the burned regions with damp towels during transport. The Israeli and American militaries advise the same procedure for the transfer of patients who have been burned by white phosphorus. Irrigation can aid in the removal of surface particles, but it is ineffective against particles that blast impacts have driven deeply into tissue.

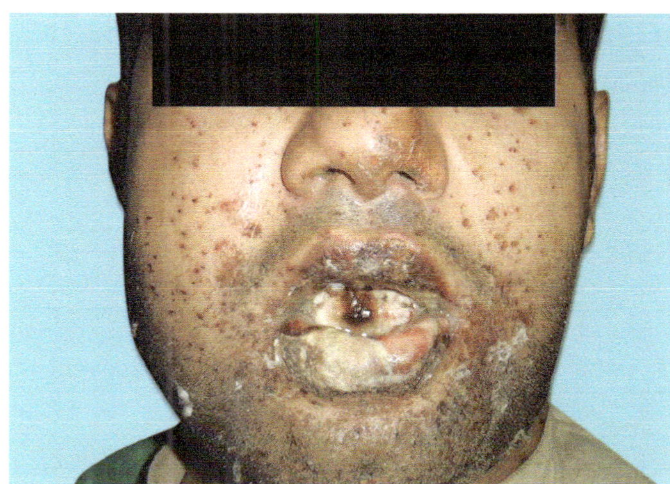

FIG. 16: Patient with explosive phosphorus burns. We can see multiple small burns around the mouth due to projectile particles.

A solution containing 1% copper sulfate can then be used to clean the wound. Phosphorus and copper sulfate solution mix to generate copper phosphate, easily recognized as black particles. Debridement of these dark fragments is not difficult. Particles that are not debrided are absorbed, which has systemic implications. This is a contentious step; some researchers believe it is unnecessary and can even be harmful to the patient. Without doubt, no additional copper sulfate solution is required after debridement is finished.

Long-term usage of the copper sulfate solution should be avoided due to the possibility of systemic copper poisoning. Hepatic necrosis, hematuria, oliguria, vomiting, diarrhea, and circulatory collapse are some of the symptoms of systemic copper poisoning. It is believed that copper inhibits the erythrocyte hexose monophosphate shunt, which causes hemolysis. Hemolysis akin to that observed in G6PD-deficient disease is the consequence of this. The wound can be irrigated with a solution of 5% sodium bicarbonate and 3% copper sulfate suspended in 1% hydroxyethyl cellulose to reduce copper absorption. Any type of wet treatment containing copper sulfate should never be used on an open wound. After debridement, a large volume of water is applied to the wound in order to flush out the copper salts.

Unfortunately, applying this gel did not reduce animal mortality in Eldad and Simon's trials.

Other researchers rinse the wound with sodium bicarbonate to counteract the phosphoric acid's effects. Additionally, there was no discernible drop in mortality in the experimental model as a result.

White phosphorus injuries have been linked to metabolic disturbances. It is reported that there is hyperphosphatemia, hypocalcemia, and irregular ECG. Bradycardia, nonspecific ST-T wave abnormalities, and QT interval lengthening are among the electrocardiographic abnormalities.

Sulfur Mustard Gas

A vesicant gas mainly utilized in combat is sulfur mustard. It shares a strong kinship with the cytotoxic nitrogen mustard chemicals that are administered as chemotherapy for cancer. There are various designations for sulfur mustard: H, HD in the US military classification system, mustard, mustard gas, or even Yperite (referring to the 1915 battle of Ypres, the site of the first known chemical warfare).

Mustard's extremely reactive and unstable "onium" molecules are responsible for its hazardous reactions, which also lead to DNA disintegration, alkylation of DNA purine bases (guanine and adenine), and suppression of cellular glycolysis.[36]

The clinical effects of sulfur-mustard exposure occur after inhalational or contact with skin or eye. After exposure, there is a latent period of 4–12 hours before the onset of symptoms.

Effects on skin are classified as mild, moderate, or severe. Mild injury presents as erythema, edema, and first-degree burns. Moderate injury is like severe edema and vesication. Severe injury causes areas of necrosis with spreading vesication.

Inhalation of sulfur-mustard aerosol or vapor can lead to respiratory failure and death. After a delay of several hours, victims suffer tracheobronchitis with symptoms, such as chest pressure, hacking cough, sore throat, and hoarseness.

Sinusitis, sinus pain, increasing cough, and tachypnea develop as symptoms progress over the next 12 hours. Bronchospasm and bronchiolar obstruction by sloughed epithelium and secretions can be expected. Severe exposures lead to hemorrhagic pulmonary edema, secondary pneumonia, and respiratory failure after 24–48 hours.

Chronic pulmonary effects after acute, severe mustard inhalation include chronic bronchitis, bronchiectasis, nonspecific bronchial hyperreactivity (reactive airway dysfunction syndrome), and emphysema.

Injuries to eye can be classified as mild, moderate, or severe. Mild injury causes erythema, edema, lacrimation, and discomfort. Moderate injury leads to severe pain, blepharospasm, edema of conjunctiva and eyelids, iritis, and temporary blindness. Severe exposure leads to permanent blindness.

High-dose exposure produces systemic toxicity like bone marrow suppression and gastrointestinal effects like diarrhea and gastrointestinal bleeding.[37]

Treatment is immediate irrigation of exposed areas like skin or eyes with copious amounts of saline or water. All clothing, jewelry, and leather should be removed. Skin can be decontaminated chemically using agents that produce "free" chlorine, which inactivates sulfur mustard.[38] Examples of such agents are chloramine powder and dilute (0.5%) hypochlorite solution (standard 5% chlorine bleach diluted, 1:10). There is no specific antidote. Experimental studies showed increased survival, and fewer pathological organ effects were noted in rats who were administered parenteral doses of sodium thiosulfate (3,000 mg/kg), vitamin E (20 mg/kg), or dexamethasone (8 mg/kg) within 15 minutes of exposure.[39]

Phenol Burns

A highly reactive and caustic contact toxin, phenol is an aromatic acid alcohol. Phenols have been employed in industry as the basis for organic polymers and plastics, as well as bactericidal agents. It is also utilized as a wood preservative in the form of creosote.

Lister utilized phenols as antiseptics for the first time in 1867, and their effects on tissues have been well investigated. Phenol is quickly absorbed through the skin surface in both liquid and vapor forms. The lungs can easily absorb phenol fumes. Significant skin absorption can lead to harmful consequences on the central nervous system (CNS) and cardiovascular system from the exposure. Among them are:

- CNS depression
- Hypotension
- Intravascular hemolysis
- Pulmonary edema
- Shock
- Death

A severe fulminant CNS depression accompanied by a coma, hypothermia, loss of vasomotor tone, and respiratory arrest is the most typical sign of systemic phenol poisoning. After skin contact, loss of consciousness is frequently observed within 30 minutes. This CNS presentation is often accompanied by cardiopulmonary collapse, which is caused by phenol's cardiac-depressive properties. Phenol as little (as 0.625 mg/kg) has been shown to be fatal in animal experiments.

Initial pain from phenol skin burns is followed by numbness when the nerve terminals become anesthetized. After that the skin turns white and an eschar develops over the burned region over several hours.

Highly concentrated phenols quickly cause a white slough that eventually transforms into an that is either copper- or greenish-black in color. The absorption is temporarily delayed by coagulation necrosis of the dermis.

Therapy needs to start right away. Eliminate any liquid that may be on the skin before cleaning the infected area. For this, swabs, gauze pads, or even clothes are appropriate. Removal of phenol is done preferably by polyethylene glycol or glycerol if former is not available. Liquid removal should not wait for the availability of these products.

Certain experts advise against the use of water irrigation. When phenol burns are severe, the necrotic tissues may serve as a transient barrier to prevent water from seeping into the deeper layers of the burn. Additionally, the phenol may be diluted by the water, allowing for quicker skin penetration.

Water irrigation works well for phenol burns, but undiluted polyethylene glycol 300 or 400 wipes work faster and remove phenols from the skin.[40] Glycerol and alcohols also work well for eliminating phenols. Facial burns and eye injuries can be safely irrigated with polyethylene glycol solution since it does not irritate the surrounding tissues.

Alcohol Burns

Isopropyl alcohol is a disinfectant that is frequently used in hospital environments as well as for household and commercial cleaning. It is linked to skin burns in babies and young children. The skin's desertification is assumed to be the mechanism of action. The concentration of alcohol, the length of the exposure, and the state of the skin all affect the degree of burn. The most vulnerable are premature babies. Burns happen most frequently in places where pressure builds up and alcohol can collect such as the nappy region.

Coal Tar Burns (Figs. 17 and 18)

Coal tar or bitumen is used for making roads and roofs. They are composed of different aliphatic, aromatic, and heterocyclic compounds. They are used in a molten form at very high temperatures (292°C). When the skin comes in contact with bitumen, it rapidly cools down and adheres tightly to the skin. The heat contained within this layer of

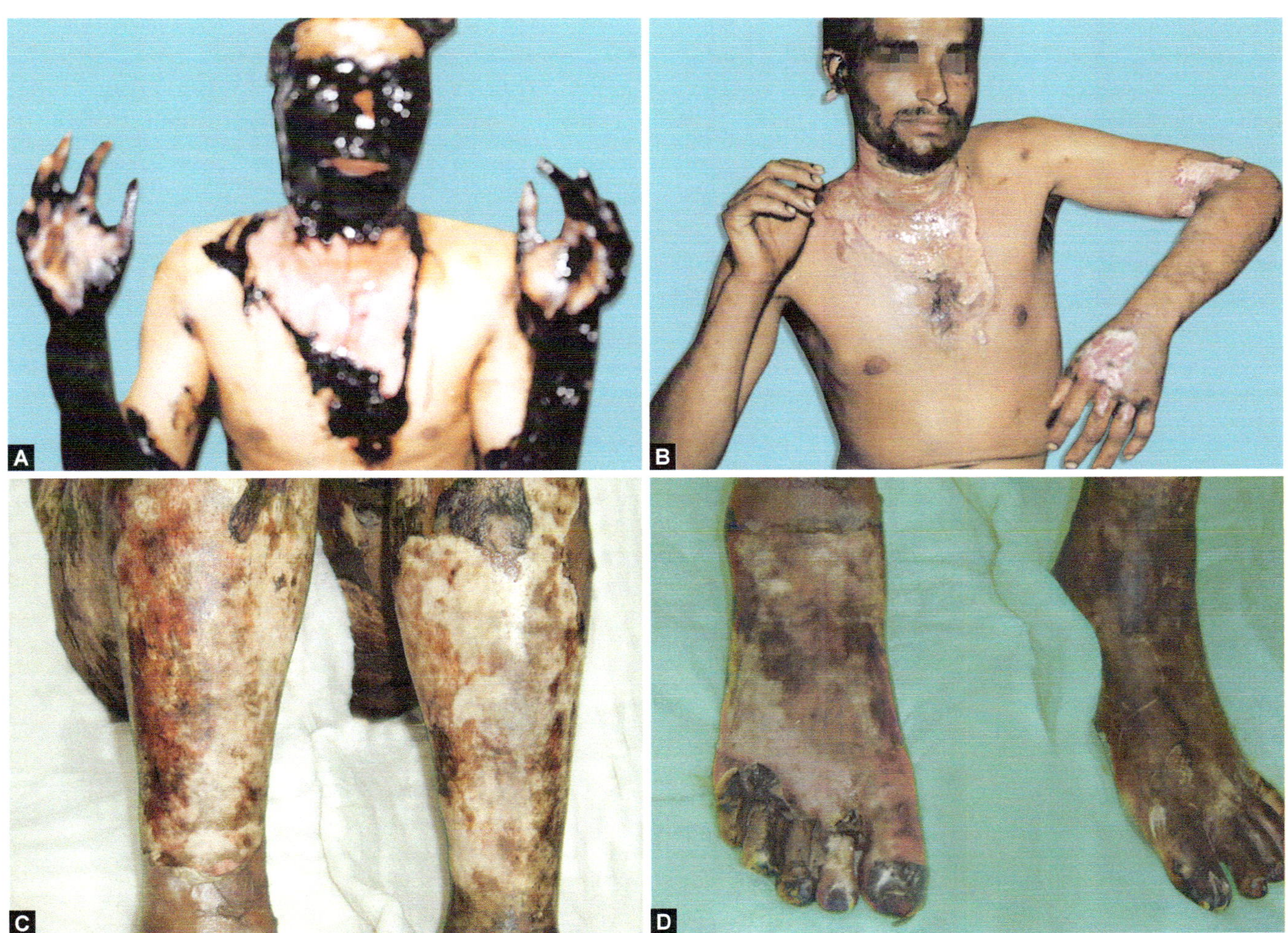

FIGS. 17A TO D: (A) Coal tar burns involving face, chest, and both arms; (B) Same patient with completely healed face, arms, and chest in 10 days indicating superficial burns; (C) Same patient's legs with deep burns due to coal tar; (D) Same patient's feet with deep burns.

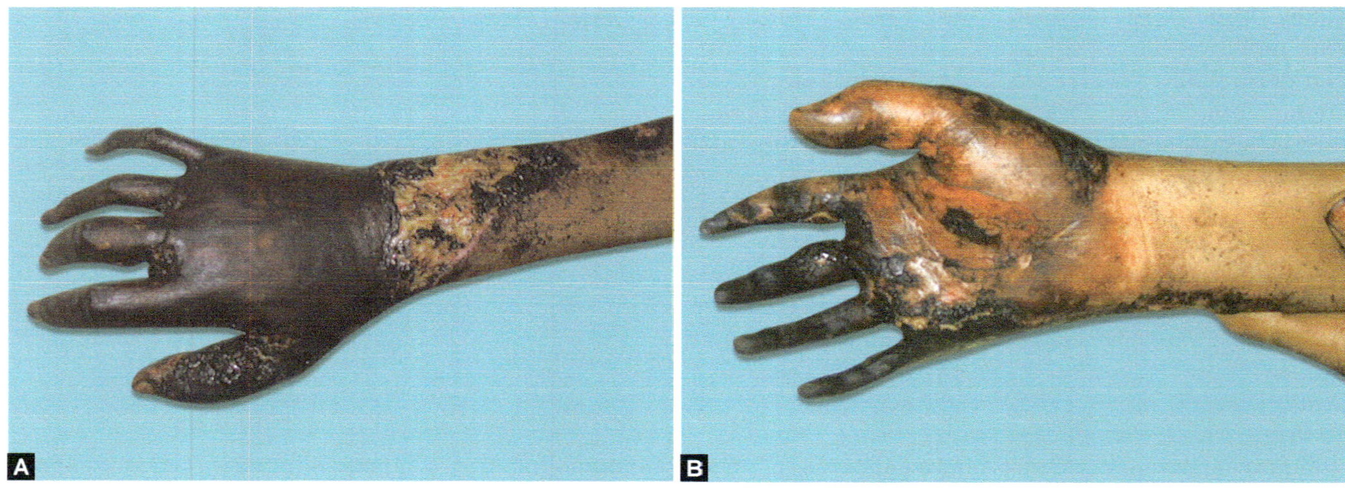

FIGS. 18A AND B: (A) Patient with deep burns of hands due to coal tar; (B) Same hand—palmar aspect.

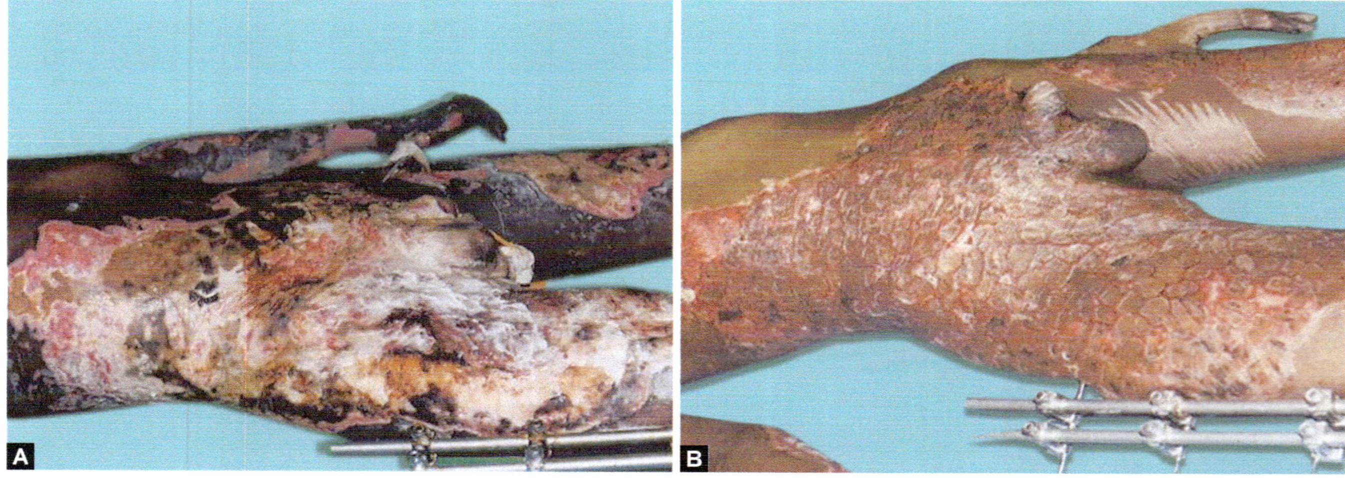

FIGS. 19A AND B: (A) Deep burns of the lower half of the body and arms with crush injury of thigh due to fall of a hot metal box; (B) Same patient with completely healed wounds after grafting.

tar can continue to damage the underlying skin and cause deeper burns if not acted upon very quickly. However, if an attempt is made to peel off the bitumen, it can cause further damage to the epidermis to which it bonds tightly. In case of small areas, the tar is best left as such because the skin under it is usually sterilized by heat, and the layer of tar acts as a "dressing" under which the skin heals spontaneously and the tar separates slowly in 2–3 weeks.

It is advisable to cool the skin with water for 30 minutes as a first-aid measure to limit the damage to the skin. For extensive areas or if the patient's face or limbs are involved circumferentially, the tar can be safely removed by wiping with swabs soaked in cooking oil or fat or butter, or paraffin oil. It can be a time-consuming and messy procedure and may not remove the entire material. The remaining bitumen can be trimmed away as it separates spontaneously over 3 weeks as the skin heals.

Many organic solvents, such as carbon tetrachloride, kerosene, and petrol, can readily dissolve bitumen, but there is always a danger of the solvent causing chemical damage to the skin or being absorbed through the skin and poisoning the patient.

Molten Plastic Burns

Burns with molten plastic are seen in the plastic industry and like coal tar tend to adhere to the skin and may produce deep burns. It has to be removed surgically only.

Hot Metal Burns (Figs. 19 and 20)

Molten metal burns are seen in men working in furnace, molders, and casters in the iron, steel, brass, or aluminum industries. Since iron and steel have very high melting points (approaching 1500°C), the molten iron and steel usually produce full-thickness burns. Aluminum has a lower melting point comparatively (650°C); it produces deep dermal burns. Sometimes, if the temperatures are very high as it falls directly from the furnace onto a body part such as the dorsum of the foot, the molten metal may even penetrate through and through like a bullet wound.

Majority of these burns are due to accidental stumbling of the worker into a molten metal container or due to an explosion in the furnace. The main reason for the explosion is water getting into the molten metal accidentally following which the molten metal splatters onto the workers' body parts or clothes which catch fire. The more common body part involved is the feet as it may trickle down from the trousers inside the boots.

Molten metals typically produce full-thickness burns which demand primary full-thickness excision and grafting for best results. Molten aluminum burns may be deep dermal, and in these cases, tangential excision and grafting suffice. Some of the burns in which bones get exposed may require flap cover.

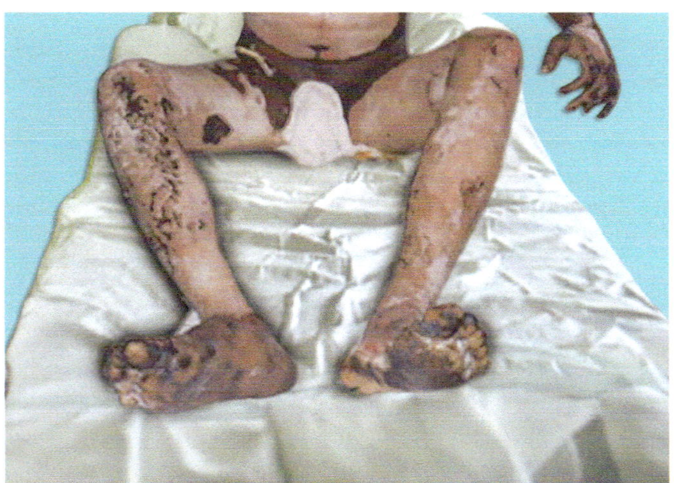

FIG. 20: Deep burns due to hot coal dust.

SURGICAL TREATMENT IN CHEMICAL AND INDUSTRIAL BURNS

Small deep burns sustained from hot metal or slag are very common, especially in the steel industry. Though they are usually too small to cause serious threats to life or limb, they cause a loss of huge man-hours.[41] These small deep burns are best treated by excision of slough and skin grafting at the earliest under local anesthesia.

For moderate burns and full-thickness burns of face, early excision and skin grafting is the treatment of choice. The patient should be taken for surgery after 48–72 hours after the patient is well resuscitated and adequate blood is arranged. Early excision and grafting are reserved only for those cases, which are full-thickness burns **(Figs. 21A and B)**. In case the burn injury is extensive involving subcutaneous tissues, excision will continue till the subfascial plane **(Fig. 22)**.

If the burns are of mixed nature or if there is any doubt regarding the depth, it is better to wait for 2 weeks as by that time partial-thickness burns start healing **(Fig. 23)**. This reduces the area requiring grafting, and thereby the blood transfusions required are also reduced. In extensive burns also because of the paucity of the donor area, delayed excision and grafting (in the 3rd week postburn) is the treatment of choice, as by this time the second-degree superficial and some third-degree deep burns heal. Healed second-degree superficial areas can be utilized for harvesting skin grafts in addition to the small available

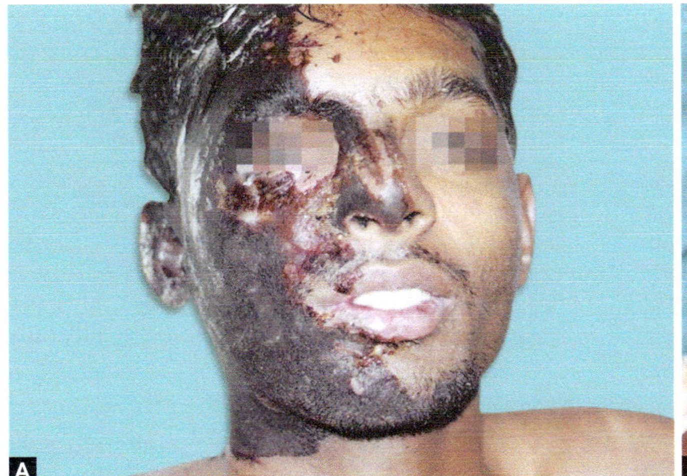

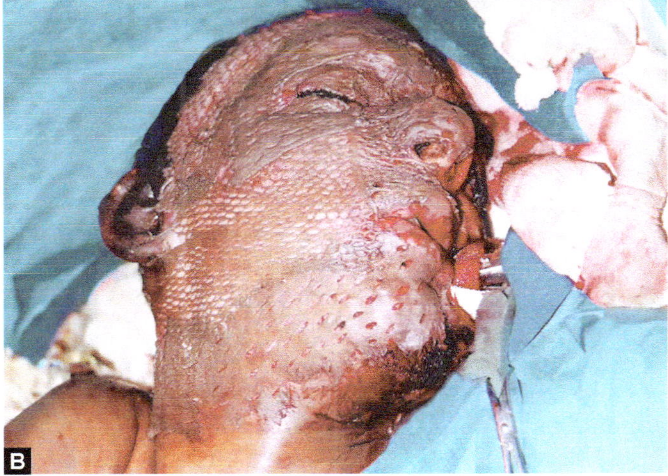

FIGS. 21A AND B: (A) Full-thickness chemical burns involving the face; (B) Full-thickness chemical burns involving the face where early excision and split-thickness grafting were done.

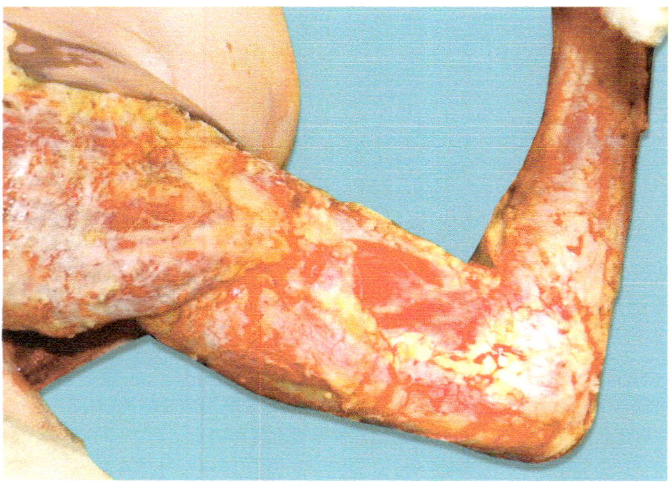

FIG. 22: Chemical burns involving deep subcutaneous tissue where subfascial excision was done.

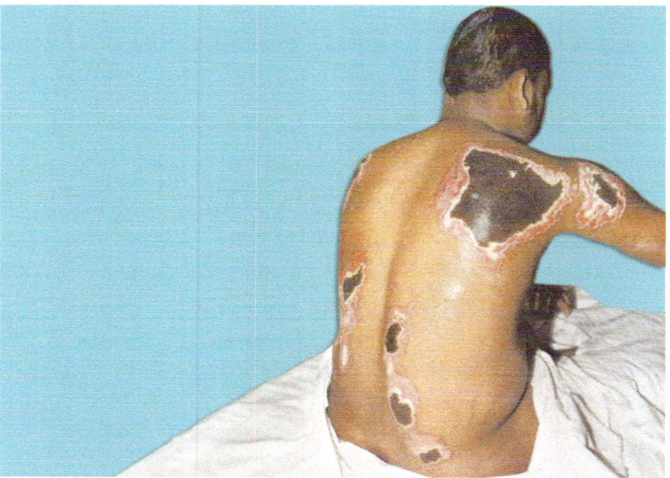

FIG. 23: Deep acid burns of the back showing separation of eschar in the middle and healing of superficial burn from the periphery.

donor area in extensive burns. In metal burns with crush injuries also, it is better to delay the grafting until the 3rd postburn week as the polytrauma is to be taken care of first **(Figs. 19A and B)**.

We like to take the patient for grafting in the 3rd week postburn. Usually, by this time, the partial-thickness burns have either healed or they are in the healing phase.

We prefer to give antibiotics as per the wound culture sensitivity reports to take care of both gram-positive and gram-negative bacteria. Antibiotics are started a day prior to surgery and continued till 5th postoperative day when the primary dressing is done. Subsequently, injectable antibiotics are stopped and switched over to oral antibiotics for another 3–5 days, if required. After the first dressing, subsequent dressings are done every alternate day or as per requirement till the wounds heal. Accordingly, the patient is asked to take a bath around 11th to 14th postoperative day.

Subsequently, the patient is asked to do massage of the grafted and donor areas with a corticosteroid ointment twice a day. Physiotherapy, which is a continuous ongoing process, is continued during the recovery phase. After massage and physiotherapy, the patient is asked to use either pressure bandage or pressure garments. After 2–3 weeks, corticosteroid ointment is replaced with bland oils or creams. The duration varies in individual cases (4–6 months). Plain coconut oil massage is continued till the scar matures (1–2 years). If there is extensive hypertrophy, it is advisable to use silicon gel sheet-lined pressure garments. For smaller hypertrophic areas, intralesional triamcinolone injections are very effective at 4-week interval.

Surgical Procedure

Usually, thin split-thickness grafts are preferred. Donor areas are simply dressed using Vaseline gauze, dry gauze, cotton, and pressure bandage in that order. Readymade available collagen sheets are used for donor areas, which are in the near vicinity of burn wounds (in patients where separate donor areas like leg, thigh, or back are not available). Donor dressings are not changed. They are opened after 11–14 days, when the patient is asked to take a bath. In extensive burns when grafting is to be done in multiple sittings, the same donor area can be used for graft harvesting after 3 weeks. In the authors unit, burn wound is injected with saline adrenaline and gentamicin for proper hemostasis in the beginning at least 10 minutes prior to excision (1 ampoule adrenaline and 80 mg of gentamicin are added to 500 mL of saline). 5 mL of this solution is injected every 5 cm^2 area. If the patient is sensitive to adrenaline or the anesthetist has some objections, adrenaline 1 ampoule is added to 1,000 mL of saline. While one surgeon harvests skin graft, another one prepares the burn wound. The operating nurse prepares the graft for application by meshing it in a ratio of 1:2. We do not spread the meshed graft to its fullest unless the available graft is much less. The burn wound is excised tangentially using Watson's skin grafting knife or a silver knife (for small areas) till a healthy bleeding surface is reached. After the excision of slough, the bleeding surface is covered with wet saline-soaked gauze pieces and pressure is applied. Any big bleeder is cauterized. If bleeding is not controlled by these methods, we sometimes use hemostatic solution-soaked gauze pieces on the bleeding surface and wait for 5 minutes. A meshed graft is then applied over these raw surfaces. Pressure is again applied with wet gauze to remove any clots beneath the graft. The wound is covered with a very thin layer of Vaseline gauze. Over this, four to six layers of thick povidone iodine solution-soaked gauze are applied. These gauzes are squeezed nicely before application and they help to soak any discharge from the wound. Over this, dry gauze and then gamgee pads are applied. Pressure bandage is then applied and plaster of Paris splints are used for immobilizing the grafted area. Subsequent dressing changes are done as mentioned earlier.

Summary of Treatment Measures for Specific Chemical Burns

- *Irrigation with water*: Hydroxides of potassium, sodium, barium, calcium, etc.; carbohydrates; phenol; HF acid; dichromate salts; tungstic acid, picric acid, trichloroacetic acid, formic acid; sulfosalicylic acid; potassium permanganate; dimethyl sulfoxide (DMSO); sodium hypochlorite; petrol; and cantharides, lyes, and alkalis.
- *Calcium salt irrigation or injection*: Hydrofluoric acid.
- *Cover burn with oil*: Sodium metal, lithium metal, potassium metal, and mustard gas.
- *Cover with water*: Phosphorous metal.

Special Measures for Certain Chemicals

- *Sodium, potassium, and lithium metals*: Pieces must be excised.
- *Phenol:* Polyethylene glycol wipes.
- *White phosphorus*: Copper sulfate irrigation.
- *Alkyl mercury agent*: Debride and remove vesicle fluid.

REFERENCES

1. Centers for Disease Control and Prevention (CDC). Occupational burns among restaurant workers—Colorado and Minnesota. MMWR. 1993;42:713-6.
2. Sunder S, Bharat R. Industrial burns in Jamshedpur, India: Epidemiology, prevention and first aid. Burns. 1998;24(5):444-7.
3. Mozingo DW, Smith AA, McManus WF, Pruitt BA Jr, Mason AD Jr. Chemical Burns. J Trauma. 1988;28:642-7.
4. Pruitt B A Jr, Mason A D Jr, Goodwin CW. Epidemiology of burn injury and demography of burn care facilities. In: Gann DS (Ed), Problems in General Surgery, Vol. 7, No. 2, Philadelphia: JB Lippincott; 1990. pp. 235-51.
5. Rossignol AM, Locke JA, Boyle CM, Burke JF. Epidemiology of work-related burn injuries in Massachusetts requiring hospitalization. J Trauma. 1986;26:1097-101.
6. Renz BM, Sherman R. Automobile carburetors- and radiator-related burns. J Burn Care Rehabil. 1992;1:414-42.
7. Eighth Annual Flammable Fabrics Report. Washington, DC: Consumer Product Safety Commission; 1980.
8. Milner SM, Rylah LTA, Nguyen TT, Redelmeier RJ, Pierre EJ, Herndon DN. Chemical injury. In: Herndon DN, Jones JH (Eds), Total Burn Care. Philadelphia: W B Saunders; 1999.
9. Mellor SG, Rice P, Cooper GJ. Vesicant burns. Br J Plast Surg. 1991;44:434-7.
10. Jelenko C 3rd. Chemicals that burn. J Trauma. 1974;14(1):65-72.
11. Robson MC, Smith DJ. Care of thermally injured victim. In: Jurkiewicz MJ, Krizek TJ, Mathes SJ, Ariyan S (Eds). Plastic Surgery: Principles and Practice. St Louis: C V Mosby Company; 1990. pp. 1355-410.
12. "Beyond the Road" Chemical Skin Burn, Charles Stewart.
13. Bromberg BF, Song IC, Walden RH. Hydrotherapy of chemical burn. Plast Reconstr Surg. 1965;35:85-95.
14. Leonard LG, Scheulen JJ, Munster AM. Chemical burns: Effect of prompt first aid. J Trauma. 1982;22:420-3.
15. Baxter CR. Present concepts in the management of major electrical injuries. Surg Clin North Am. 1970;50(6):1401-18.
16. Heimbach D, Luterman A, Burke J, Cram A, Herndon D, Hunt J, et al. Artificial dermis for major burn. Ann Surg. 1988;208:313-20.
17. McCauley RL, Linares HA, Pelligrini V. et al. In vitro toxicity of topical burn therapy. Drugs. 1990;40;364-73.
18. Maenthaisong R, Chaiyakunapruk N, Niruntraporn S, Kongkaew C. The efficacy of aloe vera used for burn wound healing: A systemic review. Burns. 2007;33:713-8.
19. White MG, Asch MJ. Acid base effects of topical mafenide acetate in the burn patients. Arch Surg. 1984;119:183-8.
20. Flood S. Hydrofluoric acid burns. Am Fam Physician. 1988;37(3):178-82.
21. Currerie PW, Asch MJ, Pruitt BA. The treatment of chemical burns: Specialized diagnostic, therapeutic and prognostic considerations. J Trauma. 1970;10:634-42.OP CIT.
22. Sawhney CP, Kaushish R. Acid and alkali burns: Considerations in their management. Burns. 1989;15:132-5.
23. Kunkel DB. Burning issues: Acids and alkalies. Skin and eye exposures. Emerg Med. 1984;165-72.
24. Fisher AA. Cement burns resulting in necrotic ulcers due to kneeling on wet cement. Cutis. 1979;23:272-4.
25. Pike J, Patterson A, Arons MS. Chemistry of cement burns: Pathogenesis and treatment. J Burn Care Rehabil. 1988;9:258-60.
26. Sigurdsson J, Bjornsson A, Gudmundsson ST. Formic acid burns: local and systemic effects, report of a case. Burns. 1983;9: 358-61.
27. Hunter GA. Chemical burns of the skin after contact with petrol. Br J Plast Surg.1968;28:337-41.
28. Division of Industrial Hygiene, National Institute of health. Hydrofluoric acid burn. Ind Med. 1943;12:634.
29. Dibbell DG, Iverson RE, Jones W, Laub DR, Madison MS. Hydrofluoric acid burns of the hand. J Bone Joint Surg Am.1970;52:931-6.
30. McIvor M, Cummings C, Mower M, Wenk RE, Lustgarten JA, Baltazar RF, et al. Sudden cardiac death from acute fluoride intoxication: the role of potassium. Ann Emerg Med. 1987;16:777-81.
31. Çelik E, Eroglu S, Dinçer M, Karacaog lan N. Nitric acid burns (case report). Istanbul, Turkey: Uzunismail AHaydarpas a Numune Education and Research Hospital Department of Plastic and Reconstructive Surgery; 2020.

32. Greenberg MI. The diagnosis: nitric acid burn. Emerg Med News. 2002;24(2):32.
33. Kolios L, Striepling E, Kolios G, Rudolf KD, Dresing K, Dörges J, et al. The nitric acid burn trauma of the skin. J Plast Reconstr Aesthet Surg. 2010;63(4):e358-63.
34. Summerlin WT, Walder AI, Moncrief JA. White phosphorus burns and massive haemolysis. J Trauma. 1967;7:476-84.
35. Bowen TE, Wheeler TJ, Nelson TG. Sudden death after phosphorus burns: Experimental observations of hypocalcaemia, hyperphosphemia and electrocardiographic abnormalities following production of a standard white phosphorus burn. Ann Surg. 1971;174:389-95.
36. Willems JL. Clinical management of mustard gas casualties. Ann Med Milit (Belg). 1989;3(suppl):1-61.
37. Borak J, Sidell FR. Agents of chemical warfare: Sulfur mustard. Ann Emerg Med March. 1992;21:303-8.
38. Koslow EE. Decontamination. NBC Defense Technol Intl. 1987;1:28-30.
39. Vojvodic V, Milosavljevic Z, Boskovic B, Bojanić N. The protective effect of different drugs in rats poisoned by sulfur and nitrogen mustards. Fund Appl Toxicol. 1985;5:160-8.
40. Brown VKH, Box VL, Simpson BJ. Decontamination procedures for skin exposed to phenolic substances. Arch Environ Health. 1975;30:1-6.
41. Sarma BP. Epidemiology and man days loss in burn injuries amongst workers in an oil industry. Burn. 2001;27:475-80.

CHAPTER

23 Radiation Burns Injuries

BC Shankar, Suvashis Dash, Lukesh Patil

INTRODUCTION

Radiation is a form of energy in motion through space or matter. It can be present in particulate form (particle) or wave form (electromagnetic waves). If the radiation can cause removal of bound electron from the atom, it is called ionizing radiation.[1] The particulate form of radiation has mass as well as energy. This particle may be neutral or may possess charge. Alpha particles, beta particles, neutrons, and protons are different examples of the particulate form of radiation. The waveform of radiation neither has mass nor charge. So, this waveform travels as pockets of energy called photons. X-rays, gamma rays, and visible lights are some of the examples of waveform of radiation.[2]

After witnessing the force of nuclear weapons first-hand, people started to understand the dangers of radiation and how it may cause harm. The 1945 bombings of Hiroshima and Nagasaki taught us many crucial lessons. One was that mortality was directly affected by closeness to the detonation; at 0.6 miles from ground zero, the incidence of fatalities was 86%; at 0.6–1.6 miles, it dropped to 27%; and at 1.6–3.1 miles, it was 2%. Furthermore, the first 20 days saw the highest death rate. 68,000 of the 122,338 deaths at Hiroshima happened during this period. 118,613 of the 197,743 survivors were unharmed, and 79,130 had injuries. 90% of those hurt in Hiroshima are thought to have had burns, 83% to have severe injuries, and 37% with radiation injuries.[3]

Since then, there have been many accidents in a variety of contexts, including a nuclear reactor accident, teletherapy equipment theft, and radioactive source theft, all of which have resulted in radiation burns and deaths of several persons.[4,5] Radiation burns though rare are a possibility due to the growing usage of radiation in many industries, including power generation, agriculture, medicine, and industry. Understanding the treatment of damage resulting from radiation exposure is therefore required.

The International Nuclear and Radiation Event Scale (INES) is used for signifying level of radiation disaster and to communicate safety significance in these cases. The events are rated from 1 to 7, seven being the highest.[6] Both Chernobyl (erstwhile USSR) and Fukushima (in Japan) Disasters were labeled as level 7 on INES while Mayapuri disaster (in New Delhi) was labeled as level 4.[6]

TYPES OF EXPOSURE

Radiation exposure can be categorized as:

- Accidental
- Medical (when used as diagnostic or therapeutic modalities)
- War activity

Accident

Radiological materials are used in several different industries. Technical failures, natural disasters, accidental spillage, or manhandling can lead to accidental exposure of radioactive substances. It can be nuclear when it involves nuclear fission especially in a nuclear reactor, e.g., Chernobyl in 1986 and Fukushima in 2011. While a radiological accident, on the other hand, involves a release of ionizing radiation [X-ray equipment or sealed sources like Cobalt 60 (60 Co), Cesium137 (137 Cs), or Iridium 192 (192 Ir) in teletherapy equipment, industrial radiography cameras, or irradiators] or discharge of radioactive materials (unsealed sources used in nuclear medicine and scientific research) into the environment, e.g., Goiania (Brazil) 1987, Mayapuri in 2010.[3,6]

Medical Modalities

Radiological isotopes are used in several medical modalities such as, diagnostic—cumulative effect of diagnostic modalities including computed tomography and C-arm. *Therapeutic*: Radiotherapy used in cancer treatment is a known cause of cutaneous syndrome as well as other variants of acute radiation syndrome (ARS). Another example is stereotactic neurosurgery where radionecrosis is the most common complication associated with it. *Academic and scientific uses*—in different academic institutions for learning and experiments.

Industrial uses: It is used for disinfection on large-scale basis, removal of toxic pollutants, preparation of different products, e.g., nonstick cookware.[7-9]

War Activity

Nuclear bomb and other radioactive war weapons, e.g., radiological dispersal device or dirty bombs, tactical nuclear weapons.[8,9]

BASICS OF RADIATION

Radioactive materials emit energy in the form of alpha (α) particles, beta (β) particles, and gamma (γ) rays. This radiation may interact with matter and give rise to the emission of X-rays and neutron particles. Certain machines operated at high voltages can generate X-rays and neutrons. The shorter wavelength of the neutrons or X-rays gives them a higher energy and ability to penetrate matter.[10-12]

Beta (β) particles are emitted by radionuclides such as hydrogen-3 (3H) and phosphorus-32 (32P) and neutron particles in general travel more slowly than β particles, but being heavier they consequently have higher energy.[12,13]

As radiation travels through human tissue, it collides and interacts with the component atoms and molecules resulting in the atom or molecule to be altered and becoming an ion. The radiation leaves a trail of ionized atoms and molecules in its course.[10]

Alpha (α) particles are heavy particles (nuclei of Helium atom) and carry a positive charge. They can travel for a few centimeter in air or about 50 microns (μm) in human soft tissue and can be easily stopped by a thin sheet of paper. Thus, they do not even penetrate the outer horny layer of skin and, therefore, do not cause any external radiation damage. However, they can cause great damage if they get incorporated in the body following inhalation, ingestion, or through open wounds due to the intense ionization given by them.[13,14]

Beta (β) particles are light particles (electrons) and can travel several meters in air and about a cm in tissues and can be stopped by a thin sheet of aluminum or 1 cm of plastic. As they deposit their energy in a smaller thickness of tissue, they can cause greater damage to the superficial layers of the skin giving rise to burns.[13,14]

Gamma (γ) and X-rays have a range of many meters in air and many centimeter in tissues and eventually pass through a human body and can be attenuated by about 20 cm of concrete. As they penetrate deeper into the body, they cause harm to the deeper structures and vital organs, including the bone marrow, giving rise to systemic effects of "acute radiation syndrome (ARS)" apart from causing skin damage.

Neutrons interact with atoms and molecules in complex ways causing ionization indirectly through the charged particles (α, β, and γ) they release upon interaction. They have a range of many meters in air and many centimeter in the tissues and eventually get absorbed or pass through the human body **(Table 1)**.[15]

RADIATION BIOLOGY

Effect of Radiation Exposure on Cell

Ionizing radiation can have a direct action on the DNA within the cell by breaking the bonds between the atoms. Indirectly, ionization of water molecules produces free radicals which can attack the coded genetic information in the cell nucleus, disrupting the cell's chemistry and function or physically rupturing membranes containing the digestive enzymes. Natural repair mechanisms

TABLE 1: Characteristics of different types of radiation.

Type of radiation	Relative mass in amu (atomic mass unit) and charge	Range in air	Absorber material which can be used as a shield
Alpha	4 amu; (+2)	Few centimeters	Paper
Beta	Negligible; (−1)	Few meters	Plastic or aluminum
Gamma	Zero; (0)	Very large	Lead, water, or concrete
Neutrons	1 amu; (0)	Very large	Cadmium or boron for thermal neutrons
			Paraffin followed by cadmium or boron for fast neutrons

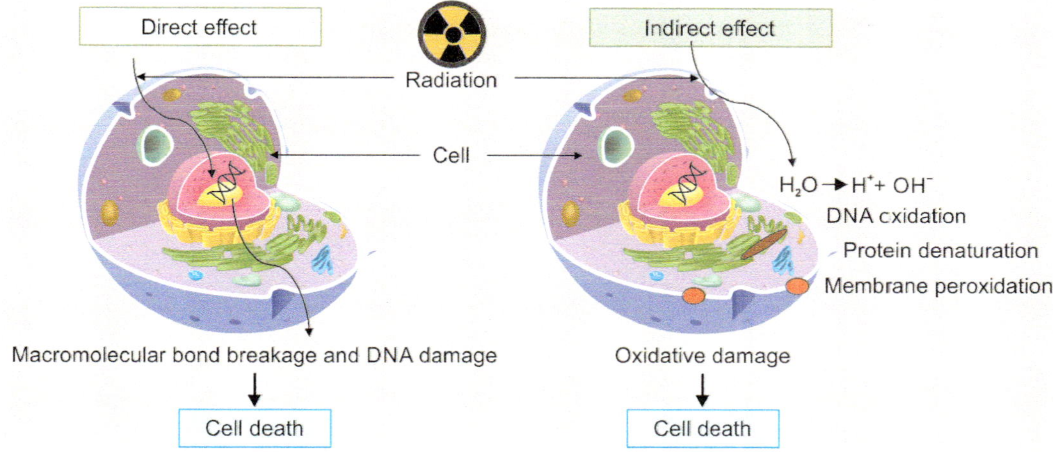

FIG. 1: Biological effect of radiation on cell.

can limit the damage and improve the cell's chance of survival. However, if the repair is incomplete, the cell may become incapable of dividing and may eventually die or may behave abnormally leading to development of cancers **(Fig. 1)**.[16,17]

The sensitivities of different tissues of the body are different, being the highest in lymphocytes, the fast dividing cells of the bone marrow, and the cells lining the intestinal villi. The nerve tissue, by contrast, is the most radioresistant tissue.

Deterministic Effects

The short-term or relatively early effects of exposure to ionizing radiation are called deterministic effects because, essentially, the radiation dose "determines" the effect. There are also other factors that help to determine radiation effects: total dose, dose rate, volume of tissue irradiated, type and quality of the radiation, presence of other disease conditions, concomitant physical trauma and/or thermal burns, and individual susceptibility.[17,18]

Stochastic Effects

Stochastic effects of radiation exposure are effects that occur by chance. An example of a stochastic effect is carcinogenesis and others are mentioned in **Box 1**. As the dose is increased, the likelihood that cancer will develop increases.[17,18]

BOX 1 **Stochastic effects.**

- Carcinogenesis
- Genetic abnormalities
- Infertility
- Cataract
- Vascular fibroatrophy
- Thyroid dysfunction

Exposure or Irradiation versus Contamination

An exposed or irradiated patient cannot contaminate others, equipment, or facilities. On the other hand, if something or someone has radioactive materials physically in them (internally contaminated) or on them (external contamination), they can cause contamination of others.

RADIATION UNITS

The unit of radiation dose is defined as energy absorbed per unit mass of matter with which radiation reacts (measured in Joules/kg). The SI unit of the absorbed dose is Gray (Gy), the earlier unit for which was rad (1 Gy = 100 rad).

Equivalent Dose or Dose Equivalent

The method for equating the biologic effect and longer-term risk from exposure to the various kinds of ionizing radiation is called equivalent dose.

The biological damage (cell killing, transformation, and chromosomal damage) caused by different radiations may vary and hence a quantity called "Relative Biological Effectiveness (RBE)" was introduced. The ICRP (International Commission for Radiation Protection) has recommended a quantity called "Quality factor (Q)" or "Radiation weighting factor (WR)" to find the dose equivalent **(Table 2)**.

The dose equivalent is derived by multiplying the dose with the radiation weighting factor. The SI unit for dose equivalent is Sievert (Sv), the earlier unit for which was rem (1 Sv = 100 rem).

Median Lethal Dose 50/60 (LD50/60)

The LD50/60 is the acute dose of ionizing radiation that will cause the death of 50% of a human population within 60 days without medical treatment. This radiation dose is of the order of 3.5–4.5 Gy (350–450 rad).

RADIATION INJURIES

Radiation injuries may manifest as a localized or whole body exposure or as external deposition or incorporation (internal contamination) of radioactive material in the body. The effects may be dependent on the dose and type of radiation received and the area of the body involved.

TABLE 2: Radiation weighting factor for different radiations.

Type of radiation	Radiation weighting factor (WR)
Gamma	1
Beta	1
X-rays	1
Alpha	20
Heavy ions	20
Neutrons	5 to 20 depending on the energy of the neutrons
Protons	5

Careful history and early clinical findings may guide the treating physician.[19,20]

ACUTE RADIATION SYNDROME

Whole-body Exposure

A single acute high-dose (≥1 Gy) exposure of penetrating radiation like radiation or X-rays to the major portion of the body can give rise to a clinical entity of "acute radiation syndrome (ARS)". The condition is heralded by a prodromal phase which may be marked by nausea, vomiting (hematopoietic involvement), diarrhea (gastrointestinal involvement), prostration, hypotension (cardiovascular involvement), ataxia, and convulsions (central nervous system involvement) in increasing order of severity. The time of onset and severity may give an indication of the system involved **(Tables 3 to 5)**.[14,15,19,20]

The prodromal period may be followed by a latent period of 2–3 weeks during which the person may feel better (at higher doses the latent period may be absent) only to be followed by a stage of manifest illness.

Acute radiation syndrome may be classified according to the system most affected as:

- *Hematopoietic syndrome (1–10 Gy)*: The injury to bone marrow results in thrombocytopenia and granulocytopenia with resultant hemorrhages and infections needing blood component therapy and treatment of opportunistic infections. Hematopoietic growth factors—G-CSF (granulocyte colony-stimulating factor), rhGM-CSF (recombinant human granulocyte macrophage colony-stimulating factor), and rhIL6

TABLE 3: Dose–effect relation after acute whole-body radiation from gamma rays or X-rays.

Whole-body absorbed dose	Effect
0.05 Gy	No symptoms
0.15 Gy	No symptoms, but possible chromosomal aberrations in cultured peripheral-blood lymphocytes
0.5 Gy	No symptoms (minor decreases in white-cell and platelet counts in a few persons)
1 Gy	Nausea and vomiting in approximately 10% of persons within 48 hour after exposure
2 Gy	Nausea and vomiting in approximately 50% of persons within 24 hour, with marked decreases in white-cell and platelet counts
4 Gy	Nausea and vomiting in 90% of persons within 12 hour, and diarrhea in 10% within 8 hour; 50% mortality in the absence of medical treatment
6 Gy	100% mortality within 30 days due to bone marrow failure in the absence of medical treatment
10 Gy	Approximate dose that is survivable with the best medical therapy available
>10–30 Gy	Nausea and vomiting in all persons in <5 minutes; severe gastrointestinal damage; death likely in 2–3 weeks in the absence of treatment
>30 Gy	Cardiovascular collapse and central nervous system damage, with death in 24–72 hours

Source: Data are from Gusev et al.[21]

TABLE 4: Skin changes after single acute localized exposure.

Absorbed dose	Change
3–4 Gy	Epilation in 2–3 weeks
10–15 Gy	Threshold for erythema; appears 18–20 days after exposure at lower doses but may appear within a few hours at higher doses
20 Gy	Moist desquamation with possible ulceration
25 Gy	Ulceration with slow healing
30–50 Gy	Blistering and necrosis at 3 weeks
100 Gy	Blistering and necrosis at 1–2 weeks

Source: Data are from Gusev et al.[21]

TABLE 5: Time of onset of clinical signs of skin injury—depending on the dose received.

Stage/Symptoms	Dose range (Gy)	Time of onset (days)
Erythema (transient)	3	Hours to days
Erythema (fixed)	6–10	14–21
Epilation	>3	14–18
Dry desquamation	8–12	25–30
Moist desquamation	15–20	20–28
Blister formation	15–25	15–25
Ulceration (within skin)	>20	14–21
Necrosis (deeper penetration)	>25	>21
Gangrene	>30	

Source: Data are from Gusev et al.[21]

(recombinant human interleukin-6) have been used to stimulate the residual bone marrow. Doses >9 Gy may require a bone marrow transplant (BMT) or peripheral blood stem cell transplant (PBSCT).[14,15]

- *Gastrointestinal syndrome (10–20 Gy)*: The injury to intestinal mucosal stem cells gives rise to death due to severe diarrhea, electrolyte disturbances, and sepsis.[14,15]
- *Cardiovascular syndrome (>30 Gy) and central nervous system (CNS) syndrome (>30–50 Gy)*: The hypotension and cerebral edema and injury to various other vital organs result and only terminal care remains possible.[14,15]

Localized Exposure

Handling of highly radioactive sources (e.g., placing a hand in the beam of industrial radiography camera) may give rise to a very high dose locally. However, the torso being spared, the dose may not give rise to symptoms of whole-body exposure or ARS and the systemic manifestations may be absent. The signs of radiation burn may take several days to appear. The vascular insufficiency caused by endarteritis obliterans may result in breaking down of previously healed skin **(Tables 4 and 5)**.[14,15,22]

INVESTIGATIONS

For Dose Estimation

History of exposure to radiation in the form of X-rays or gamma rays from teletherapy/industrial radiography source may be elicited. Absence of contact with corrosives, heat, or insect bites should arouse suspicion of a radiation injury.[23,24]

Physical Dosimetry

- If the person has a personal thermoluminescent dosimeter (TLD), it should be collected and sent for reading to give an indication about the dose received by the person.
- *Accident reconstruction*: A detailed history of the accident should be recorded. The exposure geometry which includes activity of the source, the distance from the source, and the approximate time of exposure can give an idea of the dose received by the person.
- The use of electron spin resonance method can be helpful to estimate the dose incurred. This can be used with samples such as dental enamel, clothes, buttons, earrings, or any organic substance exposed to radiation.

Biological Dosimetry

- 6 hourly peripheral blood counts for absolute lymphocyte counts when plotted on a graph called "Andrew's nomogram" give an accurate indication of the dose.
- Chromosomal analysis of cultured lymphocytes
- *Semen analysis*: Estimation of sperm counts immediately after exposure (as a baseline reading) and 40–60 days thereafter
- Slit-lamp examination of eyes

Investigative Modalities for Assessing the Severity of Cutaneous Radiation Injury

- *Serial color photographs*: Even a detailed description is not enough to give a proper indication about the progress of the lesion as a function of time. While assessing the damage, serial color photographs (calibrated by using a piece of white paper) may be valuable.

- *Ultrasound (7.5–20 MHz B-scan sonography)*: A 20-MHz probe is used for evaluating epidermis, dermis, and subcutaneous fat tissue up to the depth of 10 mm, whereas a 7.5-MHz probe can be used for evaluation of dermis, subcutaneous fat tissue, muscle fascia, and musculature. It is also useful for assessing the depth of ulcers and the extent of radiation fibrosis.
- Vascular scintigraphy is a radioisotopic method in which 99mTc pertechnetate is injected intravenously to record the vascular circulation.
- Computed tomography (CT) scan for assessing damage to deeper structures.
- *Magnetic resonance imaging (MRI)*: This noninvasive investigation can reveal fluid in the tissues (because of inflammation, edema, or necrosis). The extent of ulcer can be estimated as also the extent of necrotic tissue, and this can influence the decision about conducting a conservative necrectomy or a more radical amputation.
- *Thermography*: The heat emitted by the skin is directly dependent on the surface temperature of the skin, which in turn is dependent on the cutaneous vascularity. Significantly lower skin temperatures are seen in necrosis. The different techniques available are liquid crystal contact thermography, infrared and microwave telethermovision.
- *Capillary microscopy*: The capillaries of the stratum papillare can be evaluated by using this noninvasive method, the capillaries of the nail fold of the fingers or toes being dilated in the manifest stage whereas they are few and smaller in the chronic phase of cutaneous syndrome.
- Profilometry
- *Histology*: In the manifest stage, dilated blood vessels, edema, and neutrophilic and eosinophilic infiltration are observed whereas the chronic/late stage is set apart by epidermal atrophy/hypertrophy, dermal fibrosis, dilated blood and lymphatic vessels, pigmentary changes like hypo-/hyperpigmentation, and a deficit of hair follicles. Investigations required for effective treatment are:
  - Peripheral blood counts
  - Bacterial culture and antibiotic sensitivity tests

TREATMENT

Initial Management of Radiation Casualties

There are some general rules for management of radiation casualties. Most importantly, the morbidity and mortality from ionizing radiation injuries increase dramatically in the face of physical trauma, thermal burns, and other significant medical conditions. Therefore, unstable medical and surgical conditions should be stabilized before radiological issues increase to any level of significance. Effects can be minimized by controlling contamination, removal of victims from contaminated environments, and removal of contaminated clothing.[14,15]

Internal Decontamination

General principles of management of internal contamination include the following: reduce absorption and internal deposition; enhance elimination or excretion; and begin treatment as soon as a credible and significant dose has been determined **(Table 6)**.

As the cutaneous injury may be associated with ARS, the following care may be required:[13-15]

- *Supportive care*:
  - *Antiemetics*:
    - Antihistamines (dimenhydrinate): Poor efficacy
    - Serotonin selective 5-HT_3 receptor antagonists (e.g., ondansetron, tropisetron, and granisetron): High effectiveness
    - Dopamine-D2 receptor antagonists (e.g., metoclopramide): Good efficacy
  - *Analgesics*:
    - Analgesics (paracetamol)
    - Nonsteroidal anti-inflammatory drugs (ibuprofen, diclofenac, and meloxicam). Aspirin is avoided as it can cause bleeding in thrombocytopenia.

TABLE 6: Modalities to decrease internal contamination.

Method	Example
Reduce and/or inhibit absorption	• Activated charcoal • Bronchoalveolar lavage
Block uptake	Oral stable iodine to saturate the metabolic processes of radioiodine incorporation into the thyroid hormone
Isotopic dilution	Forced diuresis with IV fluids for 3H (or tritium, the radioactive isotope of hydrogen)
Reduction of absorption	Ion exchange resins orally [e.g., Prussian blue or ferric (III) hexacyanoferrate (II) for internalization of radiocesium, radiothallium, or nonradioactive thallium]
Alter chemistry of the substance	Barium sulfate or aluminum-containing antacids orally for ingested radiostrontium to result in strontium sulfate, which will be eliminated in the feces
Chelate	Diethylenetriaminepentaacetic acid (DTPA)

  - Opiates (codeine, tramadol, pethidine, morphine, and buprenorphine in increasing order of effectiveness). These may be combined with antiemetics to offset the emesis caused by opiates.
- *Nutrition*: Severe nausea may necessitate use of parenteral nutrition in the form of prefabricated solutions or total parenteral nutrition through a central venous line.
- *Antibiotics, antifungals, and antivirals*: In case of associated ARS with attendant leukopenia and thrombocytopenia, infection of the respiratory tract, mucous membranes, skin ulcers, and internal organs can take place. Mostly, these infections are a result of preexisting endogenous organisms. This has to be adequately countered by use of oral drug combinations such as metronidazole and ciprofloxacin for sterilization of the gut. Antibiotics can be administered as per the results of the antibiotic sensitivity tests. Empirically, broad-spectrum penicillins combined with third-generation cephalosporins or carbapenems alone can be given. If there is evidence of an infection not responding to antibiotics, antifungals like fluconazole should be considered. Antivirals like acyclovir or ganciclovir may have to be employed in herpes simplex or cytomegalovirus infections respectively.

- *Skin treatment*:
  - *Anti-inflammatory cream*: Linoleic acid cream
  - Nonatrophogenic local steroid/systemic steroid (equivalent to prednisolone 0.5–1.0 mg/kg body weight)
  - Analgesics (as above)
  - *Nonsedative mast-cell stabilizer*: Loratadine
  - Antibiotic creams/systemic antibiotics
  - Heparin
  - Argon laser for ablation of telangiectasias
  - Lioxasol cream increases cell proliferative activity in the skin
  - Tretinoin cream
  - Topical/systemic superoxide dismutase (SOD)
  - Systemic pentoxifylline
  - Systemic alpha-tocopherol
  - Systemic proteinase inhibitors like aprotininum (Gordox)
  - Systemic interferon gamma
  - Topical tetrachlorodecaoxide (TCDO)
  - Solcoseryl gel has regenerative properties
  - Actovegin is obtained by ultrafiltration of calf blood. It contains inositol phospho-oligosaccharides (IPOs), which are known to increase uptake and utilization of oxygen by hypoxic tissues and cells by promoting mitochondrial respiratory function, decreasing the formation of lactate, and in turn, protecting hypoxic tissue.
  - Hydrocolloid dressings
  - Topical thrombocytic growth factors
  - Semisynthetic skin equivalent: Integra

The various degrees of radiation burns described are as follows:

Erythema and dry desquamation: Treatment is purely symptomatic. Severe erythema associated with edema is treated with lotions or sprays containing hydrocortisone to relieve the symptoms. Tight clothing should not be worn over the affected part.

Moist desquamation needs daily sterile protective dressings and bathing of the affected skin in antiseptic solutions. Antibiotic creams can also be used to prevent bacterial infections.

Ulceration requires isolation of the limb in a sterile environment. Daily dressing and bathing of the ulcer in antiseptic solutions is recommended. Analgesics or stronger opioids may be necessary. Topical or systemic antibiotic therapy should be considered if secondary infection is suspected or verified by bacterial culture.

Necrosis needs excision followed by skin grafts or other types of skin cover. Unless the underlying vasculature is intact, skin grafting may not be possible and a myocutaneous flap or pedicle flap may be required. Surgery in the form of ulcerectomy, necrectomy, and amputation may be needed, the extent, timing, and type of surgical intervention being determined on a case-to-case basis as the lesion progresses.

Indications for amputation depend on the following determinants:

- Intractable pain
- Size and location of the injury
- Degree of control of infection
- Very severe destruction of underlying tissues with vascular damage
- Value of the part

Not only does the latent period for development of signs and symptoms but also the intensity and duration of lesions depend on the dose and the type of radiation received. Thus, at a high dose (>100 Gy), the manifestations may develop early (within a week), whereas with a low dose, they may take weeks to develop.

CUTANEOUS RADIATION SYNDROME (FIGS. 2 TO 5)

The basal cells of the epidermis, including those cells situated within the canal of the hair follicle are the cells, which are damaged resulting in denudation of the epidermis resulting in manifestations of cutaneous radiation injury syndrome (CRI). The erythema is a result of dilatation of superficial blood vessels due to an inflammatory reaction **(Table 7)**.[25]

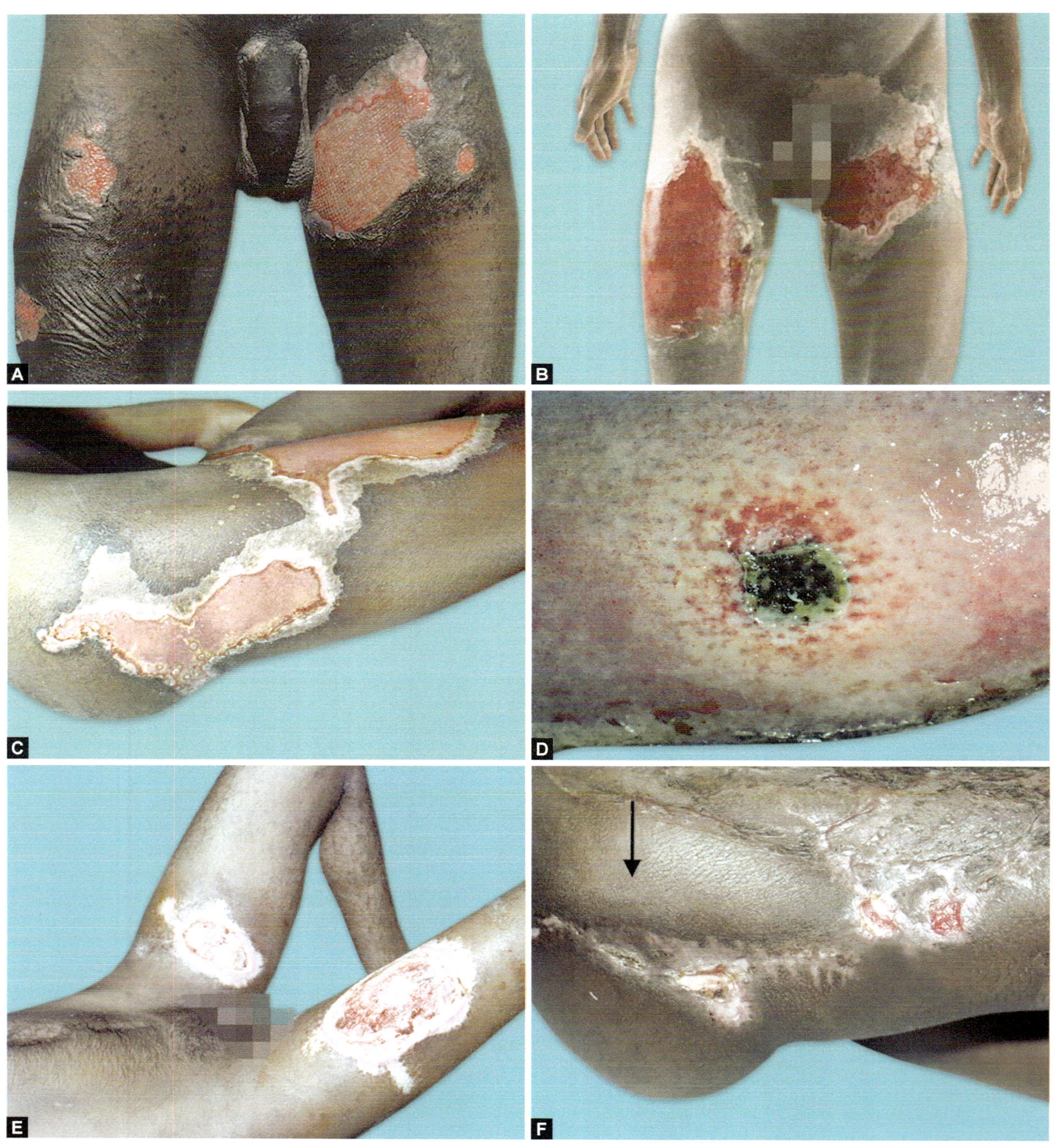

FIGS. 2A TO I: *Continued*

Continued

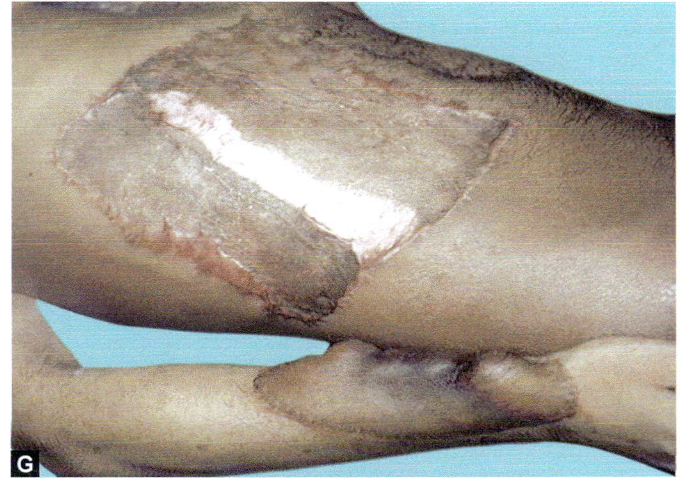

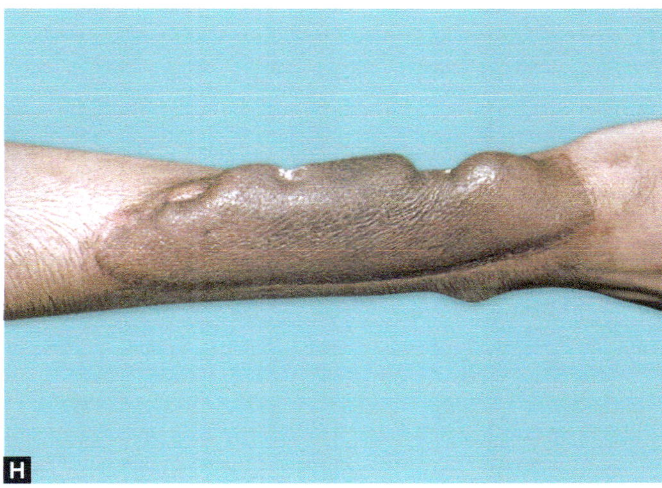

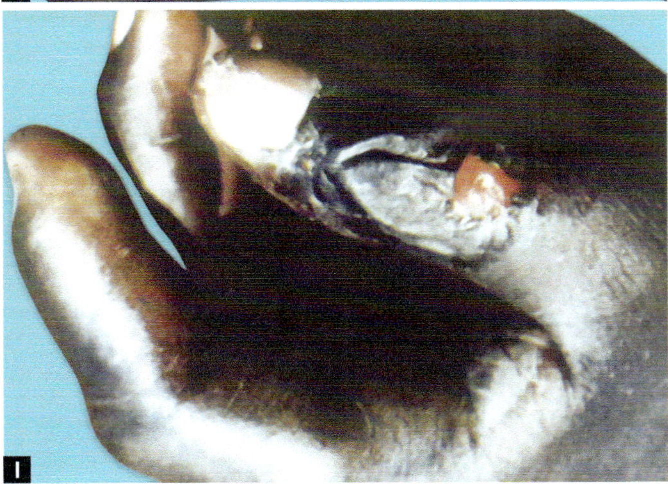

FIGS. 2A TO I: (A) Evolution of cutaneous radiation syndrome following accidental exposure to an industrial radiographic device showing fixed erythema and blistering 4 weeks postexposure. Erythema is best appreciated in fair skinned individuals. The transient erythema cannot be appreciated in the dark skinned. In the dark skinned, fixed erythema appears darkly pigmented. (B) Ulceration 5 weeks postexposure. (C) Ulceration and partial healing 6 weeks postexposure. (D) Ulceration with central necrosis 8 weeks postexposure. (E) Same wound 14 weeks postexposure showing deepening of ulceration up to the fascia and muscle. (F) Even after 9 months with surgical cover few areas of ulceration still remain. (G) Same patient with abdominal flap cover following radiation burn wound over forearm. (H) Close up view of the flap on forearm. (I) Acute radiation burn of left hand following a 20 Gy exposure to a Co-60 source.

Grading

Grade 1

Prodromal stage may start with itching and a brief transient erythema usually subsiding within 36 hours of exposure. True erythema (a second wave of erythema also referred to as fixed erythema) appears around 5 days postexposure and lasts a few weeks. Damage to sweat and sebaceous glands may give rise to dry, scaly desquamation of the skin in 20–30 days, which resolves within a few weeks.

Treatment: Outpatient care—
- Topical anti-inflammatory, antiproliferative, and nonanthropogenic glucocorticoids
- Systemic nonsedative antihistamines

Investigations: Ultrasound to determine changes in thickness of the skin and basal thermography may show hyperthermic and hypothermic areas, which can serve as a reference for long-term follow-up.

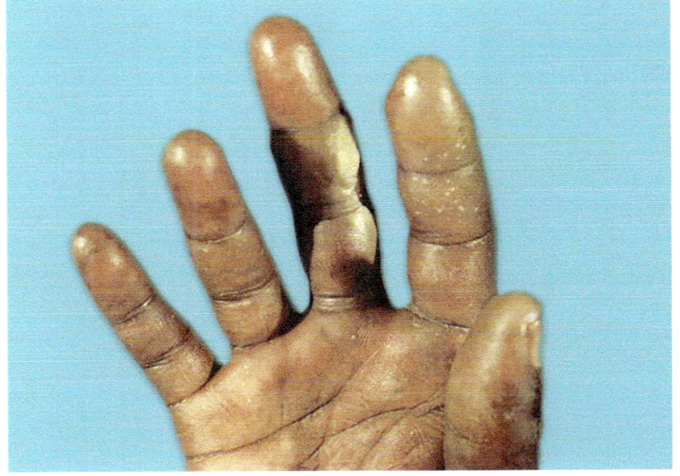

FIG. 3: Hand exposed to a radiographic unit showing changes in middle finger and thumb 6 weeks after exposure.

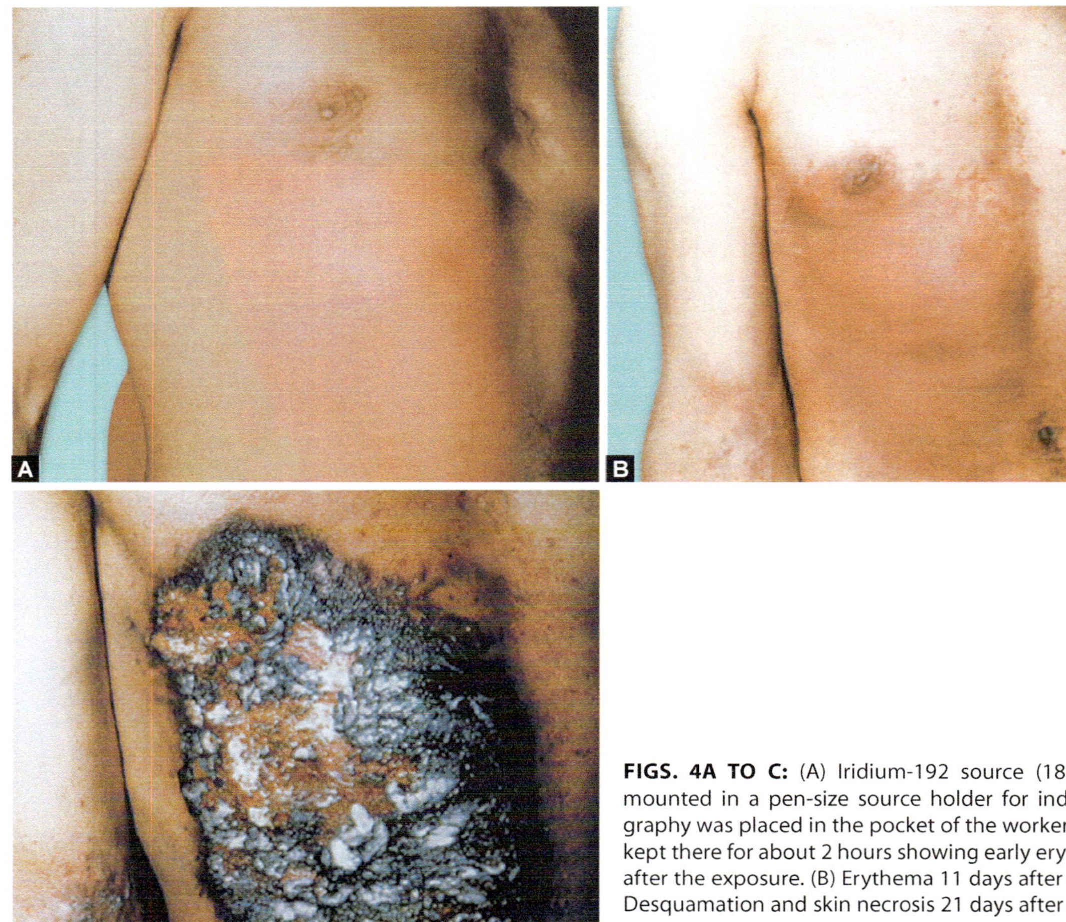

FIGS. 4A TO C: (A) Iridium-192 source (185 GBq, 5 Ci) mounted in a pen-size source holder for industrial radiography was placed in the pocket of the worker's overall and kept there for about 2 hours showing early erythema 5 days after the exposure. (B) Erythema 11 days after exposure. (C) Desquamation and skin necrosis 21 days after exposure.

Courtesy: From How to recognize and initially respond to an accidental radiation injury (pamphlet), IAEA, Vienna, Austria, 2000.

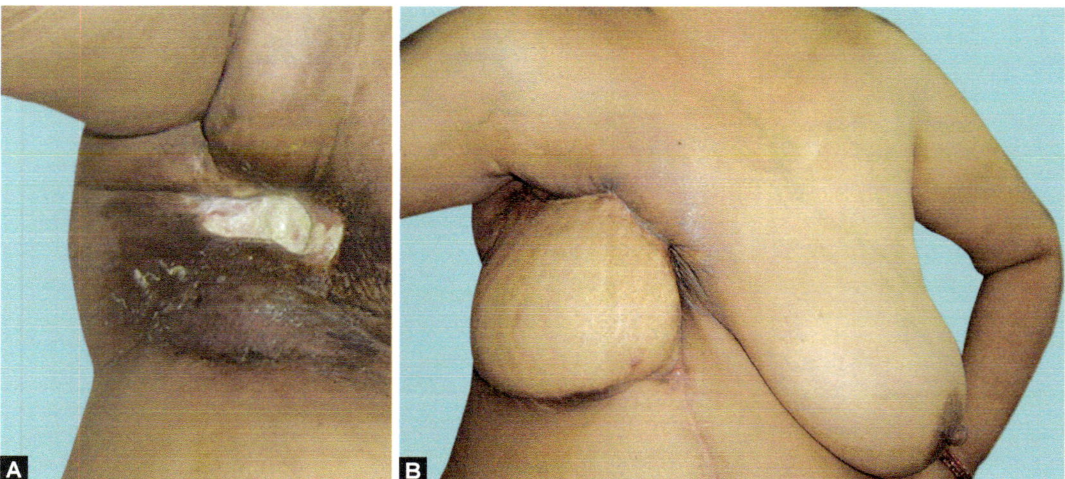

FIGS. 5A AND B: (A) Nonhealing ulcer on right chest following radiotherapy given postmastectomy. (B) TRAM flap done for cover of the same defect.

(TRAM: transverse rectus abdominis muscle)

Courtesy: Editor

TABLE 7: Grades of cutaneous radiation injury (CRI).[25]

Grade	Skin dose*	Prodromal stage	Latent stage	Manifest illness stage	Third wave of erythema†	Recovery	Late effects
I	>2 Gy (200 rads)‡	1–2 days postexposure or not seen	No injury evident for 2–5 weeks postexposure§	• 2–5 weeks postexposure, lasting 20–30 days: redness of skin, slight edema, possible increased pigmentation • 6–7 weeks postexposure, dry desquamation	Not seen	Complete healing expected 28–40 days after dry desquamation (3–6 months postexposure)	• Possible slight skin atrophy • Possible skin cancer decades after exposure
II	>15 Gy (1,500 rads)	6–24 hours postexposure with immediate sensation exposure of heat lasting 1–2 days	No injury evident for 1–3 weeks postexposure	• 1–3 weeks postexposure; redness of skin, sense of heat, edema, skin may turn brown • 5–6 weeks postexposure, edema of subcutaneous tissues and blisters with moist desquamation • Possible epithelialization later	• 10–16 weeks postexposure, injury of blood vessels, edema, and increasing pain • Epilation may subside, but new ulcers and necrotic changes are possible	Healing depends on size of injury and the possibility of more cycles of erythema	• Possible skin atrophy or ulcer recurrence • Possible telangiectasia (up to 10 years postexposure) • Possible skin cancer decades after exposure
III	> 40 Gy (4,000 rads)	4–24 hours postexposure, with immediate pain or tingling lasting 1–2 days	None or less than 2 weeks	• 1–2 weeks postexposure: redness of skin, blisters, sense of heat, slight edema, possible increased pigmentation • Followed by erosions and ulceration as well as severe pain	• 10–16 weeks post-exposure: Injury of blood vessels, edema, new ulcers, and increasing pain • Possible necrosis	Can involve ulcers that are extremely difficult to treat and that can require months to years to heal fully	• Possible skin atrophy, depig-mentation, constant ulcer recurrence, or deformity • Possible occlusion of small vessels with subsequent disturbances in the blood supply, destruction of the lymphatic network, regional lymphostasis, and increasing fibrosis and sclerosis of the connective tissue • Possible telangiectasia • Possible skin cancer decades after exposure
IV	>550 Gy (55,000 rads)	Occurs minutes to hours postexposure, with immediate pain or tingling, accompanied by swelling	None	• 1–4 days postexposure accompanied by blisters • Early ischemia (tissue turns white, then dark blue or black with substantial pain) in most severe cases • Tissue becomes necrotic within 2 weeks following exposure, accompanied by substantial pain	Does not occur due to necrosis of skin in the affected area	Recovery possible following amputation of severely affected areas and possible skin grafts	• Continued plastic surgery may be required over several years • Possible skin cancer decades after exposure

*Absorbed dose to at least 10 cm^2 of the basal cell layer of the skin.
†Especially with beta exposure.
‡The Gray (Gy) is a unit of absorbed dose and reflects an amount of energy deposited in a mass of tissue (1 Gy = 100 rads).
§Skins of the face, chest, and neck have a shorter latent phase than the skin of the palms of the hands and the skin of the feet.

Grade 2

Skin surface affected <10% body surface. This phase consists of blisters which generally form around 4 weeks postexposure and can result in moist desquamation which can even occur without prior blisters due to depletion of epidermal stem cells. This may be associated with transient hair loss (around 2 weeks).

Treatment: Outpatient care—
- Topical anti-inflammatory, antiproliferative, and non-atrophogenic glucocorticoids
- Systemic nonsedative antihistamines
- Linoleic acid creams
- Puncture of blisters
- Nonadherent dressings
- Prevention of infections as per antibiotic sensitivity tests

Investigations: 20-MHz sonography to determine changes in thickness of the skin.

Thermography to detect hyperthermic and hypothermic areas as a reference for regular follow-ups.

Grade 3

Skin surface affected 10–40% body surface. This phase consists of severe swelling, which is caused by increased vascular permeability and loss of fluids in the third space. Blisters form around 5 days postexposure resulting in ulcer or necrosis. Recovery may follow. However, it is incomplete and the sequelae may be alopecia, fibrosis, contractures, pigment changes, increased vulnerability to trauma, and repeated breakdown of healed areas.

Treatment:
- Inpatient care
- Topical antibacterial agents
- Linoleic acid creams
- Systemic anti-inflammatory, antiproliferative, non-atrophogenic glucocorticoids to reduce edema
- Analgesia
- Aspiration of fluid from blisters
- Debridement of necrotic tissues
- Nonadherent dressings
- Prevention of infections as per antibiotic sensitivity tests

Investigations:
- 7.5-MHz sonography to determine changes in thickness of the skin
- Doppler ultrasound to assess damage to underlying larger vessels
- Sonography to assess the depth of the lesion
- MRI to detect damage to underlying muscles

Surgery may be required in the form of full-thickness skin grafts/flaps.

Grade 4

Skin surface affected >40% body surface. This phase consists of severe damage to not only epidermis and dermis but also to subcutaneous tissues, underlying muscles, and perhaps bones. This is associated with severe swelling, which is caused by increased vascular permeability and loss of fluids in the third space. Bullae form within a few days postexposure and can result in acute necrosis. Recovery is unlikely and leaves deficits like alopecia, fibrosis, contractures, pigment changes and increased vulnerability to trauma, thermal and pressure changes, subcutaneous sclerosis, and keratosis. Amputation of extremities may have to be considered.

Because of the extensive exposure, there may be associated ARS with resultant granulocytopenia (causing opportunistic infections) and thrombocytopenia (causing hemorrhages).

Treatment:
- Inpatient intensive care
- Topical antibacterial agents
- Linoleic acid creams
- Systemic anti-inflammatory, antiproliferative, non-atrophic glucocorticoids to reduce edema
- Analgesia
- Aspiration of fluid from bullae
- Debridement of necrotic tissues
- Necrectomy and full-thickness skin graft
- Amputation
- Prevention and treatment of infections as per antibiotic sensitivity tests

Investigations:
- 7.5-MHz sonography to determine changes in thickness of the skin
- Doppler ultrasound to assess damage to underlying larger vessels
- Sonography to assess the depth of the lesion
- MRI to detect deeper damage to underlying muscles

The percentage of the surface area of burns can be calculated by the rule of nine. The fluid and electrolyte/colloid requirements vary according to the extent of burns. It is simpler to calculate the fluid requirement for partial burns wherein various formulae used in thermal burns may serve as a useful guide for maintenance of fluid and electrolyte balance. However, in case of whole body burns with concomitant ARS and also in deep burns as a result of irradiation, the hemodynamic stability needs measurement of central venous pressure (CVP), electrolytes, renal profile, and associated management of ARS as mentioned earlier.

The management of radiation burns needs a team of:

- Physician trained in handling radiation injuries
- Health physicist to help arrive at the dose received and to ascertain the type of radiation (β, γ) using various dosimetry techniques
- Hematologist (for management of ARS) when radiation burns are associated with partial or whole-body exposure
- Plastic and reconstructive surgeon

Unlike thermal, chemical, or other forms of burns injuries, there are no physical symptoms at the time of exposure to radiation sources. The full extent of tissue damage can take a few days, weeks, and even years to evolve and hence early decision regarding the type of surgical intervention has to be avoided. The only early intervention would be in the form of maintenance of fluid, electrolyte balance, and life-saving measures.

SURGICAL MANAGEMENT

Surgical management depends on:

- Type of burns (β and γ)
- The extent of surface area of burns
- The depth of burns

So overall the surgery has three phases:

1. Initial damage control surgery (1–2 days)
2. Reparative surgery (2 days to 2 months)
3. Reconstructive surgery > 2 months

Guiding principles:

- Meticulous debridement
- Extensive wound lavage
- Avoid early surgical wound closure by suturing
- Full-thickness graft better than split thickness graft

Because there is a well-organized radiation safety system in place for both humans and machinery, the global accident rate for atomic power reactors is incredibly low. Most burn accidents are reported involving industrial radiography, and a small number are related to radiological procedures in the medical field, such as tele-radiotherapy, where the patient unintentionally meets an exposed source, and interventional radiography where there is a failure to follow routine maintenance and calibration checks.[14,15]

First-degree burns heal with conservative treatment spontaneously just as in the case of thermal burns. However, the recovery may take a longer time. Extensive second-degree burns may require split thickness skin grafting to reduce the morbidity and to expedite healing. Third- or fourth-degree burns (γ, X-rays) require investigations directed at the vascular viability of the affected tissues and procedures such as local flap, myocutaneous and neurovascular flaps must be employed. Deep burns adjacent to torso and limbs have a potential to cause associated injury to hollow viscera (bladder, intestines, etc.) and to the underlying bone giving rise to radionecrosis requiring additional major surgical procedures for fecal and urinary fistulae thus carrying a high mortality and poor outcome. First-degree burns, like thermal burns, heal on their own with conservative care. Still, it can take longer to heal. Split thickness skin grafting may be necessary for extensive second-degree burns in order to lower morbidity and hasten recovery. Investigations into the vascular viability of the damaged tissues are necessary for burns of the third or fourth degree and techniques like rotation flap, myocutaneous flap, and neurovascular flap must be used. Deep burns that are close to the torso and limbs may result in damage to the hollow viscera (bladder, intestines, etc.) and the underlying bone, which may lead to radionecrosis and the need for additional major surgical procedures to treat fecal and urinary fistulae. This can have a fatal consequence. Given how common hand injuries are, especially those involving the digits, special attention needs to be given to them. Adding a hand surgeon to the team of specialists to aid with repair, care, and recovery would be essential. Making a prompt choice on amputation—partial or total—would lower the risk of morbidity for those hurt.

It is possible for late sequelae such as radiation fibrosis and squamous cell carcinoma of skin to emerge even after recovery.[15,16]

Radionuclide decorporation drugs and products have been developed by DRDO, India for the management of radiation and nuclear injuries **(Table 8)**.

RADIATION PROTECTION PROGRAMS

Radiation protection involves restriction of exposure or potential exposure. This may be achieved by:

- Engineering controls employing reducing the time of operation, increasing the distance from the source by use of remote handling operations, and provision of good shielding and suitable containment to prevent the spread of unsealed radioactive materials to restrict external exposure.
- Administrative methods such as documented procedures, good working practices, adequate supervision, and restricted exposure times.
- Personal protective equipment such as lead aprons for work with X-rays, laboratory wear, and industrial suits to protect against body contamination and devices such as respiratory protective equipment.

The radiation protection program works on the philosophy of ALARA (As Low As Reasonably Achievable) and contributes by preventing accidents which cause acute exposures with resultant deterministic effects and also by reducing routine exposures and the risks of stochastic effects.[11,27]

Personal dosimeters are worn by individual employees and the actual doses received are measured. Personal air samplers (PAS) can measure the air activity that might contribute to an internal dose. Organ and whole-body monitoring for internal exposure and biological assessments of intakes of radioactivity are used to determine internal doses.[28]

It is important to note that everybody who deals with intervention radiological and therapeutic procedures, e.g., those undertaken by urologist, cardiologist, or orthopedicians should compulsorily use TLD (thermo-luminescent protection dosimeter) badges and stay out of the field of radiation as far as possible to prevent delayed radiation response.[29]

THE RADIOLOGICAL TRIAGE AND TREATMENT FLOW (FLOWCHART 1)

The radiation triage is done either for irradiation or for radiological contamination. Time of onset of vomiting is a reliable symptom for establishing clinical radiation dose

TABLE 8: Radionuclide decorporation drugs and products as developed by DRDO.[26]

Drugs	Use
Potassium iodate tablet (85 mg)	• Oral decorporation agent specifically for radioiodine I^{131} • Enhances radioiodine excretion from body
Zn-DTPA injection	Decorporating agent suitable for bivalent radioactive cations
Alendronate tablet (1 mg)	Oral decorporation agent and treatment agent specifically for uranium
Prussian blue tablets and capsules (500 mg)	Oral decorporation agent for radiocesium Cs^{137}, radiothallium Tl^{201}
Alginic acid tablet (350 mg)	• Decorporation agent • Specifically useful for radiocesium and radiothallium
EDTA tablet (100 mg)	Decorporation of radioactive heavy metals, i.e., lead, mercury uranium, americium, and strontium
EDTA injection	Decorporating agent suitable for bivalent metallic cations
EDTA eye drops/gel	For chelation of radioactivity in eye exposure

(DRDO: Defence Research and Development Organization; EDTA: ethylenediaminetetraacetic acid)

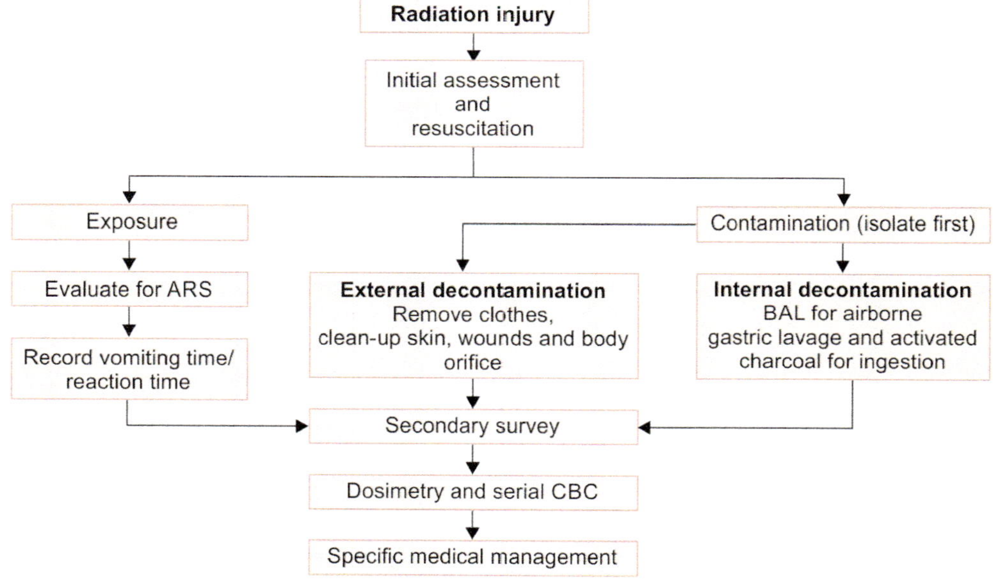

FLOWCHART 1: The radiological triage and treatment.

(ARS: acute radiation syndrome; CBC: complete blood count; BAL: bronchoalveolar lavage)

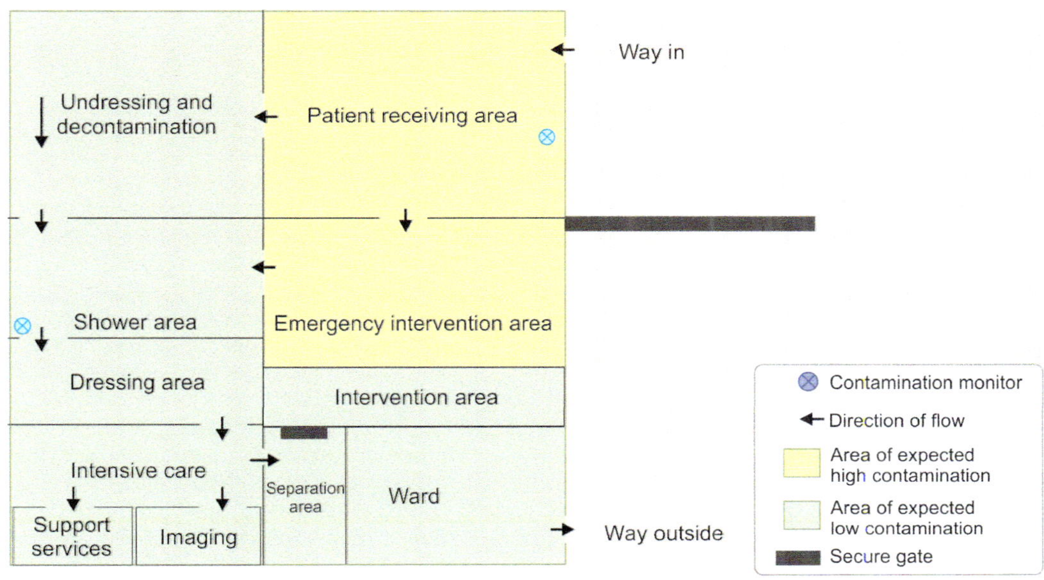

FIG. 6: The emergency reception area plan and patient flow.

received. For radiological contamination, a dosimeter is used and treated accordingly.

THE EMERGENCY RECEPTION AREA PLAN AND PATIENT FLOW (FIG. 6)

The radiation injury treatment area or CBRNE center should be a separate facility with designated areas, movements, and planned protocol for patient flow.

SUMMARY

Radiation burns is one of the rare causes of burn injuries which requires timely detection and management. It is now gaining importance in view of radiation being used for therapeutic purpose for cancer treatment. Conservative management usually helps in most of the cases but surgical treatment in the form of meticulous debridement and flap cover is required in some of the cases.

REFERENCES

1. Weisstein EW. "Radiation". Eric Weisstein's World of Physics. Wolfram Research. [online] Available from https://scienceworld.wolfram.com/physics/Radiation.html. [Last accessed May, 2024]
2. Centers for Disease Control and Prevention. (2015). The Electromagnetic Spectrum: An Overview. [online] Available from https://www.cdc.gov/radiation-health/about/electromagnetic-spectrum.html. [Last accessed May, 2024]
3. ICAN. Hiroshima and Nagasaki bombings. [online] Available from https://www.icanw.org/hiroshima_and_nagasaki_bombings. [Last accessed May, 2024]
4. International Atomic Energy Agency. Accident Reports. [online] Available from https://www.iaea.org/topics/accident-reports. [Last accessed May, 2024]
5. Centers for Disease Control and Prevention. Radiation Accidents. [online] Available from https://www.atsdr.cdc.gov/ToxProfiles/tp149-c4.pdf. [Last accessed May, 2024]
6. International Atomic Energy Agency. International Nuclear and Radiological Event Scale. [online] Available from https://www.iaea.org/resources/databases/international-nuclear-and-radiological-event-scale#:~:text=The%20International%20Nuclear%20and%20Radiological,that%20occur%20within%20their%20territory. [Last accessed May, 2024]
7. United States Environmental Protection Agency. Radiation Used in Nuclear Medicine. [online] Available from https://www.epa.gov/radtown/radiation-used-nuclear-medicine#:~:text=Nuclear%20medicine%20procedures%20help%20detect,to%20shrink%20or%20destroy%20it. [Last accessed May, 2024]
8. United States Nuclear Regulatory Commission. Uses of Radiation. [online] Available from https://www.nrc.gov/about-nrc/radiation/around-us/uses-radiation.html. [Last accessed May, 2024]
9. Occupational Safety and Health Administration. Radiological Dispersal Devices (RDD) / Dirty Bombs. [online] Available from https://www.osha.gov/radiological-dispersal-devices#:~:text=Radiological%20dispersal%20devices%20(RDD)%2C,such%20as%20multiple%20city%2Dblocks. [Last accessed May, 2024]

10. International Atomic Energy Agency. Practical Radiation Technical Manual: Individual Monitoring. Vienna: International Atomic Energy Agency; 2004.
11. International Atomic Energy Agency. Practical Radiation Technical Manual: Health effects and medical surveillance. Vienna: International Atomic Energy Agency; 2004.
12. International Atomic Energy Agency. Practical Radiation Technical Manual: Personal Protective Equipment. Vienna: International Atomic Energy Agency; 2004.
13. International Atomic Energy Agency. Medical management of persons Internally contaminated with Radionuclides in a nuclear or radiological emergency: A manual for medical personnel. Vienna: International Atomic Energy Agency; 2018.
14. Koenig KL, Goans RE, Hatchett RJ, Mettler Jr FA, Schumacher TA, Noji EK, et al. Medical Treatment of Radiological Casualties: Current Concepts. Ann of Emerg Med. 2005;45(6):643-52.
15. Coleman CN, Casagrande R, Hick JL, Weinstock DM, Bader JL, Chang E, et al. Triage and Treatment tools for Use in a Scarce Resources: Crisis standards of care setting following a nuclear detonation. Disaster Med Pub Health Prep. 2011;5 Suppll:S1l1-21.
16. International Atomic Energy Agency. (2010). Radiation Biology: A Handbook for Teachers and Students. [online] Available from https://www-pub.iaea.org/MTCD/Publications/PDF/TCS-42_web.pdf. [Last accessed May, 2024]
17. Hall EJ, Giaccia AJ. Radiobiology for the radiologist, 7th edition. Philadelphia: Lippincott Williams & Wilkins; 2012.
18. Shadad AK, Sullivan FJ, Martin JD, Egan LJ. Gastrointestinal radiation injury: Prevention and treatment. World J Gstroenterol. 2013;19(2):199-208.
19. Atomic Energy Regulatory Board. (1990). AERB Safety Guide - Medical Management of Persons Exposed in Radiation Accidents. [online] Available from https://www.aerb.gov.in/storage/uploads/documents/regdocn4jR6.pdf. [Last accessed May, 2024]
20. Atomic Energy Regulatory Board. (1989). AERB Safety Manual—Handbook of Medical Management of Persons Exposed in Radiation Accidents. [online] Available from https://www.aerb.gov.in/storage/uploads/documents/regdoci9Usx.pdf. [Last accessed May, 2024]
21. Gusev IA, Guskova AK, Mettler FA Jr. Medical Management of Radiation Accidents, 2nd edition. New York: CRC Press Inc.; 2001.
22. Fiedner TM, Friesecke I, Beyrer K. (2001). Medical Management of Radiation Accidents: Manual on the Acute Radiation Syndrome. [online] Available from https://oparu.uni-ulm.de/server/api/core/bitstreams/fdda72b2-e0ba-41ad-a398-2e836206d34f/content.
23. Radiation Emergency Medical Management. 8 Categories of Radiation Dosimeters for Dose and Exposure Monitoring and Worker Safety. [online] Available from https://remm.hhs.gov/radiation-dosimeters-dose-monitoring-worker-safety.htm. [Last accessed May, 2024]
24. International Atomic Energy Agency. Radiation Dosimetry. [online] Available from https://www.iaea.org/resources/hhc/medical-physics/radiotherapy/dosimetry. [Last accessed May, 2024]
25. Centers for Disease Control and Prevention. Cutaneous Radiation Injury: Fact Sheet for Physicians. [online] Available from https://emergency.cdc.gov/radiation/pdf/criphysicianfactsheet.pdf. [Last accessed May, 2024]
26. DRDO. Radiation Protection Products. [online] Available from https://www.drdo.gov.in/radiation-protection-products#:~:text=Using%20innovative%20aspects%20of%20medicine,conventional%20formulation)%20within%20three%20days. [Last accessed May, 2024]
27. International Atomic Energy Agency, World Health Organization. (1998). Safety Reports Series No. 2—Diagnosis and Treatment of Radiation Injuries. [online] Available from https://www-pub.iaea.org/mtcd/publications/pdf/p040_scr.pdf. [Last accessed May, 2024] .
28. International Atomic Energy Agency. How to recognize and initially respond to an accidental radiation injury (pamphlet). Vienna: International Atomic Energy Agency; 2000.
29. Chambers JA, Long JN. Radiation injury and the hand surgeon. J Hand Surg Am. 2008;33(4):601-11.

CHAPTER

24

Friction Burns

Karoon Agrawal, Mula Rohit Babu

INTRODUCTION

Historically, fire was produced by friction between two stones. The Olympic lamp was lit by rubbing stones and this tradition is still followed. Friction can generate a large amount of heat, so much, so that it can melt stones and burn meteors in space. When rockets and spaceships enter the earth's atmosphere, there is a danger of their burning due to the extreme heat produced by friction with the atmospheric air.[1] The greatly talked-about Discovery space shuttle accident in which India-born astronaut Kalpana Chawla was killed along with other colleagues is an example of the high magnitude of heat generated due to friction in space.

Burns due to friction are very often, not reported and are overlooked in our practice as well as in literature. This is probably because in the majority of patients, friction causes partial-thickness burn in a small body surface area which is ignored. Usually, it is associated with mechanical injury, which may be more severe than the burns. Whenever there is friction between two objects, the relatively delicate object bears the brunt of the mechanical trauma in the form of abrasion, laceration, or avulsion. Hence, most often, the burn takes a backseat and the mechanical injury becomes the priority.

PATHOGENESIS

Friction is generated as mechanical energy when two surfaces rub against one another, out of which at least one is moving. The kinetic energy is converted into thermal energy or heat. When the delicate body surface comes in contact with this heat energy, it causes burn. As it is always associated with kinetic energy, friction burn and mechanical injury are seen together in various combinations and proportions.

The quantity of energy produced following friction is determined by the coefficient of friction which depends mainly upon the material of the surface causing friction; for example, stainless steel has a very low friction coefficient as compared to rubber on a pavement. Similarly, when a part of the human body rubs against any hard object, the high coefficient of friction produces a large amount of heat energy causing body surface burn.

EPIDEMIOLOGY

Epidemiological studies of friction burns are difficult. Majority of these studies available in the literature are hospital-based, which have their inherent deficiencies. To know the correct incidence, community-based studies are required which are neither available nor feasible. Trying to quantitate the reported cases of friction burn is only the tip of the iceberg. A vast majority of these cases are ignored or managed with first aid or household care. Only relatively major burns or burns associated with other trauma report to the hospital, hence, the fallacy of the reported incidence and degree of burn reported due to friction.

In a retrospective epidemiological study on childhood burns conducted in New Zealand in 1981, 14% of children had friction burns, and it was the third most common burn after scalds (40%) and contact burns (20%).[2]

In an epidemiological study from Ahmedabad, India, 60 patients with friction burns were reported over a period of 2 years. Majority of the patients were males in the 21–30-year age group. The lower limb was affected in the majority of patients due to roadside accidents. Split-thickness skin graft was required in 41.7% of the patients and a flap cover was performed in 10% of the patients.[3]

In an review of 1,211 American children younger than 6 years over a period of 6 years, there were 48 patients (4%) with friction burns because of household treadmills

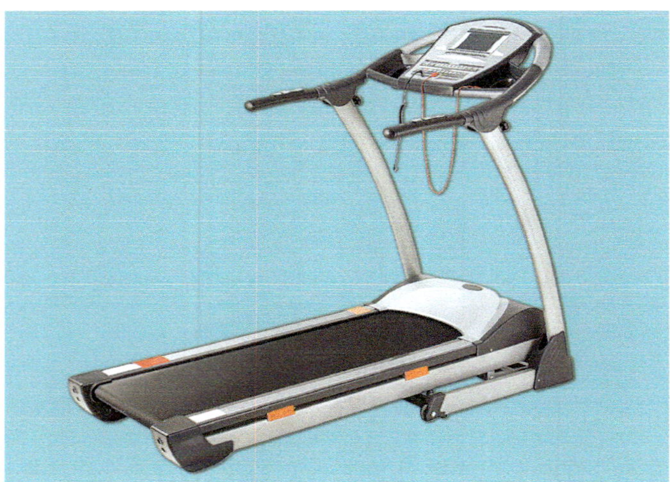

FIG. 1: A photograph of a household treadmill for exercising.

(Fig. 1). The palmar surface of the hand was the most common site.[4] Maguine et al. reported 10 patients of treadmill-related friction burn over a period of 4 years.[5]

In a similar retrospective study from Korea, records of 25 children with treadmill-induced friction burns were analyzed. Friction burns constituted 1.4% of the total number of pediatric burn injury. All lesions affected the hands and forearms. Most injuries affected the volar surface.[6]

The database of patients over 20 years from Brisbane and Queensland was analyzed. Out of 4,523 patients admitted to the hospital, friction burn constituted 1%.[7]

ETIOLOGY

A friction burn is a nonconventional burn injury and is not reported to the hospital unless it is unusually large or else associated with other injuries. The etiological factors are very interesting and worth enlisting here **(Table 1)**.

In an Indian epidemiological study of 60 friction burn patients, road traffic accidents constituted 93% and the rest were equally contributed by falls and sports.[3]

Sports activities are the most common cause of friction burn. These are usually small, superficial, and localized injuries, which are mostly managed on the spot and hence not recorded in hospital statistics. These can occur while skidding over synthetic turf. Rope seems to be a common etiological factor in rope-based sports, such as rope climbing, water skidding, and tug of war. Running causes burns over soles, especially if one runs barefoot or with ill-fitting shoes. Aerobic dancing causes burns over the soles. The water slides in water sports cause burns due to friction against the railing and the floor of the slides, especially if the flow of water is inadequate.[8]

TABLE 1: List of etiological factors of friction burn.

Sports	• Skidding over turf • Rope-based sports[8] • Barefoot trekking[12] • Water slides • Aerobic dancing
Road traffic accidents	• Car tire friction[13] • Bicycle spoke[15-18] • Loose clothing getting caught • In automobile[25]
Household and industrial machines	• Treadmill[4-7,9-11] • Child activates the machine • Accidentally an unsupervised child comes in contact with the moving belt • Washing machine[2] • Domestic vacuum cleaner[12] • Rolling belt in industries and agriculture
Medical equipment	• Tourniquet applied over bare skin[19] • Reaming of bone[20]
Miscellaneous	As a part of pathomimia[25]

Increased popularity of physical fitness in modern society has brought many mechanized equipment into our homes. The presence of such equipment at home increases the hazard of friction burn of the hands in young children.[4-7,9-11] A review of 1,211 pediatric patients of less than 6 years from the USA revealed treadmill friction injuries in 48 (4%) patients. The mean burnt area reported was 0.5%, mostly over the volar surface of the hand.[4] In another study, 14 injuries in nine patients were recorded. The average age of the children was 3–4 years.[10] Another American study reported six treadmill-related hand friction burns at an average age of 31 months. These were mostly on the palmar aspect of the fingers.[9]

Till now, all the friction burn reports were from American centers. In a retrospective study, treadmill injury from Korea constituted 1.4% of all pediatric burn admissions. The mean age was 3.9 $\pm$ 3.2 years. This indicates the spread of treadmill-related pediatric friction burn to other countries.

There are two ways by which a child can get friction burn due to treadmills at home: One is when a child activates the machine in the absence of an adult, and second, when a child accidentally comes in contact with the moving belt of the treadmill causing trauma and friction.[10]

In children, portable vacuum cleaners, a result of recent technological advancements, emerged as one of the causes of friction burns. Vacuum cleaner injuries occur as the bristles of the brush bar move up to 90 rotations/second against the surface of the child's skin, thus causing frictional burns. Walsh et al. reported 288 children who have sustained friction burn injuries to their hands and feet due to vacuum cleaners in Manchester, UK.[12]

In children, most commonly the nondominant side is involved because the child tends to take support with the dominant hand while reaching the object.

Roadside accidents are a cause of a large number of friction burns, especially in hospital-based studies. Al-Qattan reported 25 cases of car tyre friction injuries of foot in children. These injuries occurred while trying to stop the car.[13] In an Indian study, the incidence of friction burn reported due to road traffic accidents was as high as 93.33% **(Fig. 2)**.[3]

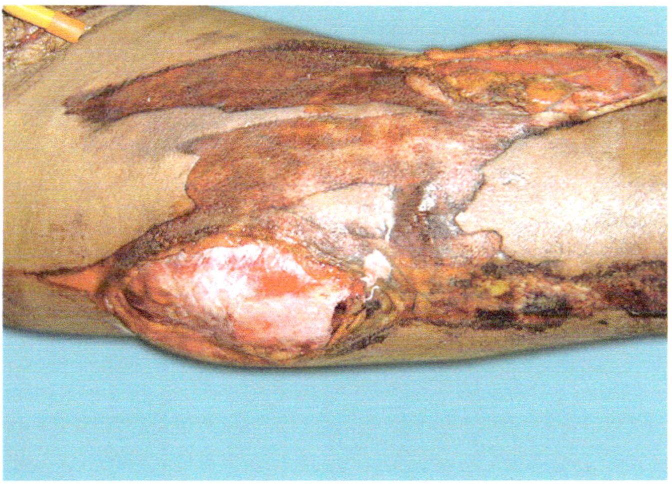

FIG. 2: A large full-thickness burn over the thigh following friction with the truck tire. The presence of thick eschar indicates the occurrence of deep burn due to friction. There is evidence of avulsion injury laterally.

In a study from Japan, 26% of their patients with lower limb trauma caused by bicycle spoke injuries were abrasion and friction burn from the shearing effects of the spokes causing partial- to full-thickness skin defect.[14] Occasionally, the friction burn may be severe enough to cause full-thickness loss of the chest wall.[15]

Modern technology brings some unexpected problems with it. Airbags are an effective and a well-accepted safety device that reduce the impact of motor vehicle accidents and the morbidity and mortality associated with them. Rapid deceleration due to an impact causes the ignition of sodium azide cartridge, thereby releasing nitrogen to inflate the nylon rubber bag. Most of the airbags inflate in 0.01 second at a speed of >160 km/h **(Figs. 3A and B)**[16]. Physical contact with rapidly inflating airbags causes friction burns. Also, direct thermal burns from high-temperature gases, indirect injuries due to the melting of clothing, or chemical burns due to direct contact are possible with airbags.[17,18]

There are many other interesting etiological factors causing friction burn reported in the literature. These are caused by common machines used in day-to-day life and are commonly ignored. There are reports of friction burn caused by washing machine wringers **(Fig. 4)**.[2]

Among the medical equipment, a tourniquet applied over the thigh without padding causes friction burn,[19] the reaming of bone[20] significantly increases the temperature inside the bone, use of power drills without proper insulation will increase the surrounding bone and soft-tissue temperatures > 100°C causing thermal necrosis of bone and soft tissues,[21] most commonly used in orthognathic surgery, maxillofacial surgery, orthopedic procedures, and dental implants and procedures. Even cosmetic procedures such as liposuction can also cause friction burns at the port sites due to vigorous to and fro movement of the suction cannula.[22]

Rolling belts in industries are hazardous as these cause friction burns. Loose clothes around the body may

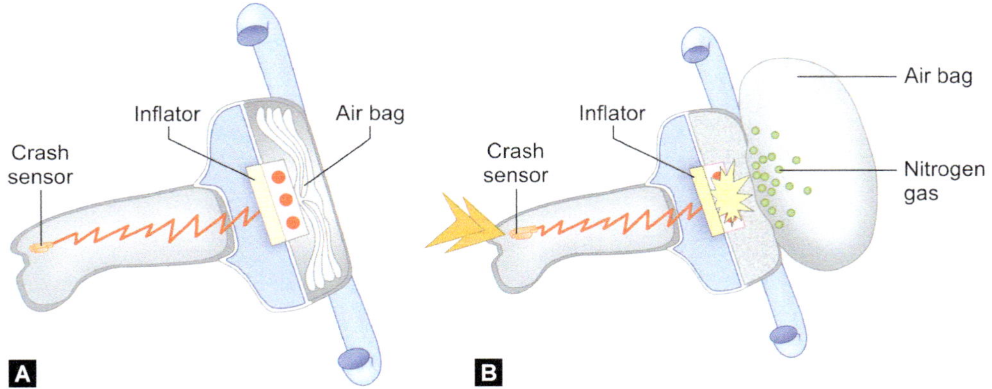

FIGS. 3A AND B: (A) A line diagram showing the inflation of car airbag after impact; (B) The airbag inflates with nitrogen after the crash sensor activates the inflator.

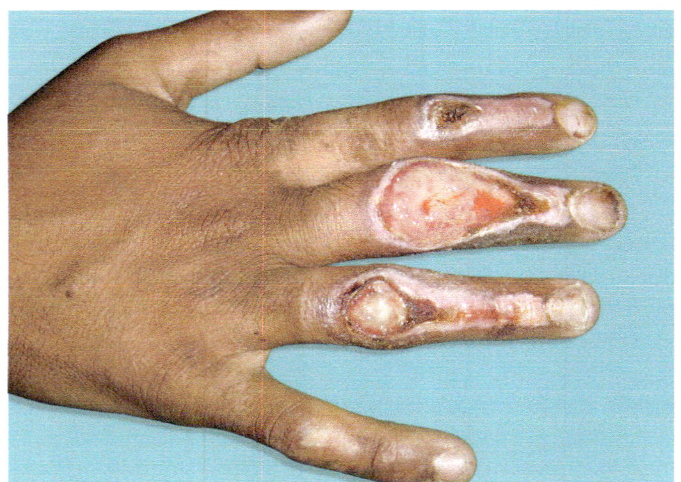

FIG. 4: Friction burns over the dorsum of fingers because of the hand coming in the pressing machine, showing full-thickness loss in the center surrounded by a zone of partial-thickness skin loss.

get caught in a revolving machine or in automobiles and can snare the neck or other parts of the body. In a freak accident, a 17-year-old girl had friction burn over the neck due to her "Chunni" (also called "dupatta"),[23] a traditional Indian clothing, wrapped around the neck, being caught in a three-wheeler auto wheel. Barefoot mountain trekking can cause friction/frost burn.[24]

Friction blisters may be a manifestation of pathomimia, which can be produced by nails, razors, blades, cigarettes, chemicals, etc.[25] These are not true friction burns, but resemble them; hence, we should be aware of them.[22]

Apart from these etiological factors, environmental factors play a very important role in the occurrence of and in determining the degree of friction burn. In the summer season, the incidence and magnitude of friction burns are more. Inadequate clothing in summer also increases the risk. Less than 10% of friction burns occurr during winters, due to multiple layers of thick clothing. On the other hand, the incidence was higher in summer because of inadequate clothing such as use of shorts and thin flimsy shirts.

TYPE OF BURNS

The burns inflicted with friction are mostly minor and superficial **(Figs. 3 and 4)**. However, there are a few reports of deeper friction burns too.[3,14] In an Indian study of 60 burn patients, 31.66% had first-degree **(Fig. 5)**, 20% had second-degree **(Figs. 6 to 8)**, and 48.33% had third-degree burns **(Figs. 9 and 10)**.[3] This is a hospital-based study, hence, a large number of more severe burns. The majority of small, superficial, first- and second-degree burns may have taken treatment at home or from general practitoners and hence not reported.

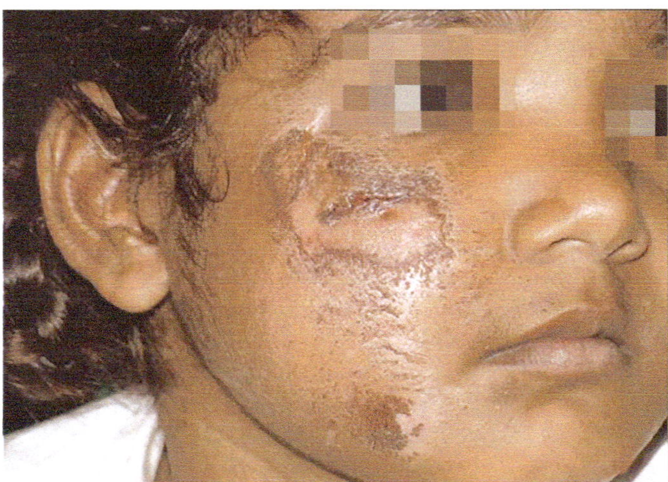

FIG. 5: A typical superficial friction burn over the face after a roadside accident in a child.

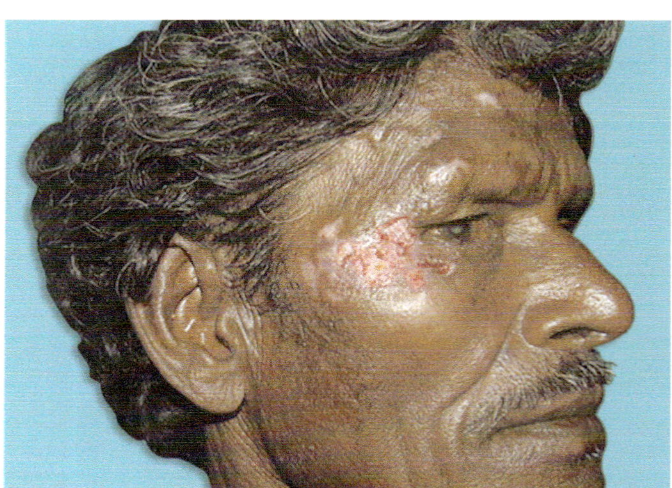

FIG. 6: A deep partial-thickness friction burn over the right zygomatic region following a roadside accident requiring closure of the wound by grafting.

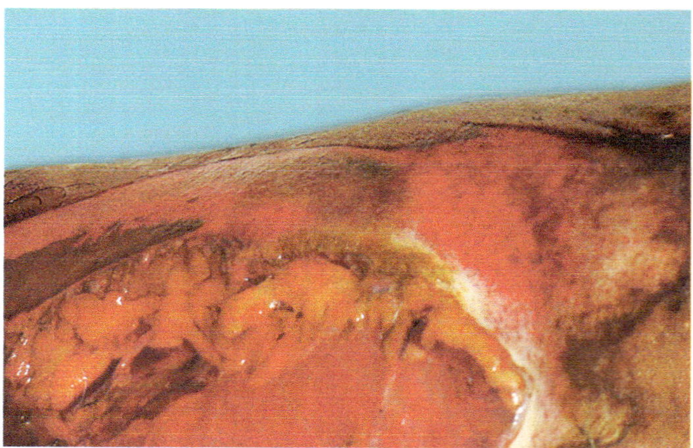

FIG. 7: Deep friction burns with associated avulsion injury in the thigh of a young man following a road traffic accident.

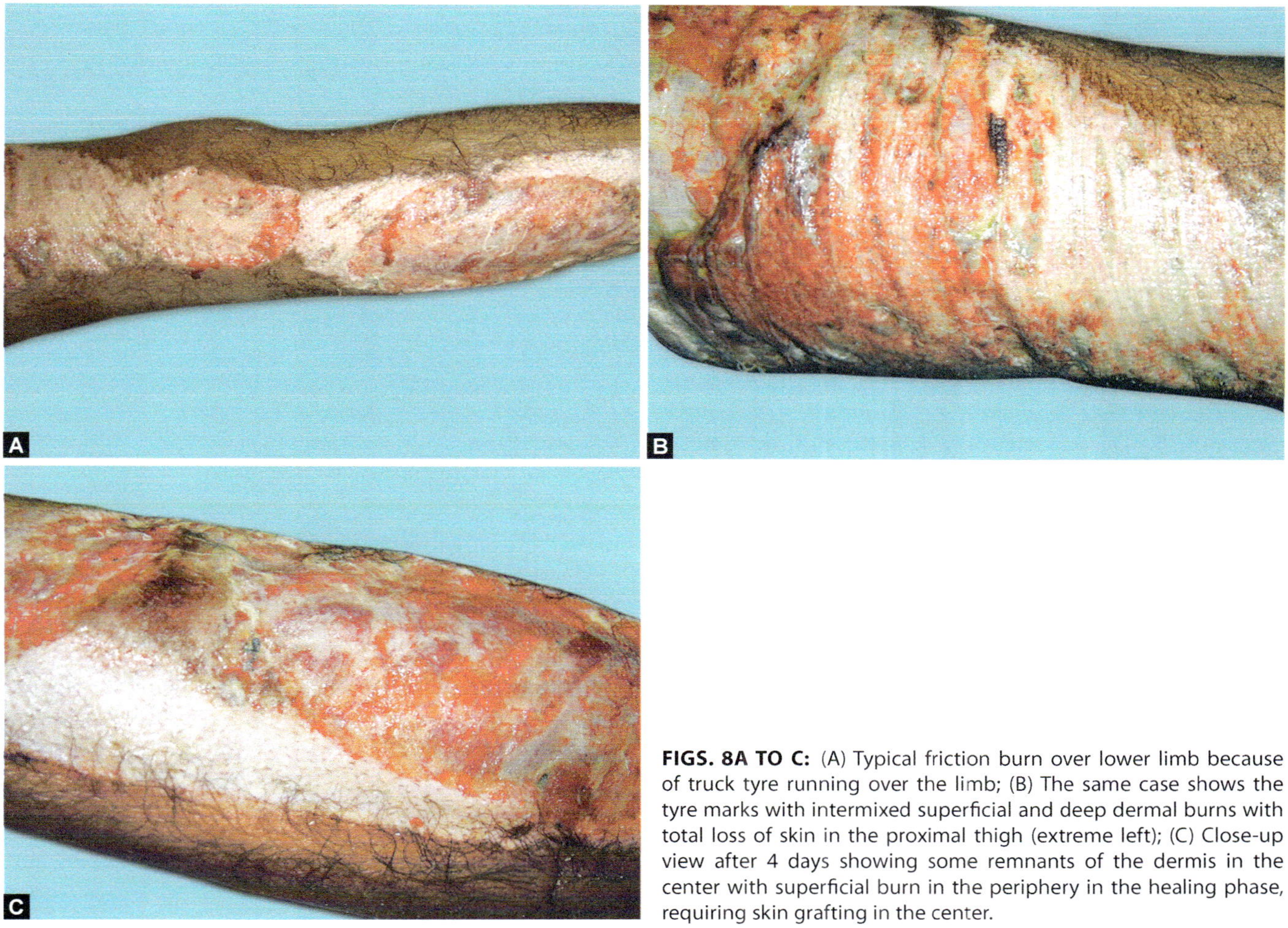

FIGS. 8A TO C: (A) Typical friction burn over lower limb because of truck tyre running over the limb; (B) The same case shows the tyre marks with intermixed superficial and deep dermal burns with total loss of skin in the proximal thigh (extreme left); (C) Close-up view after 4 days showing some remnants of the dermis in the center with superficial burn in the periphery in the healing phase, requiring skin grafting in the center.

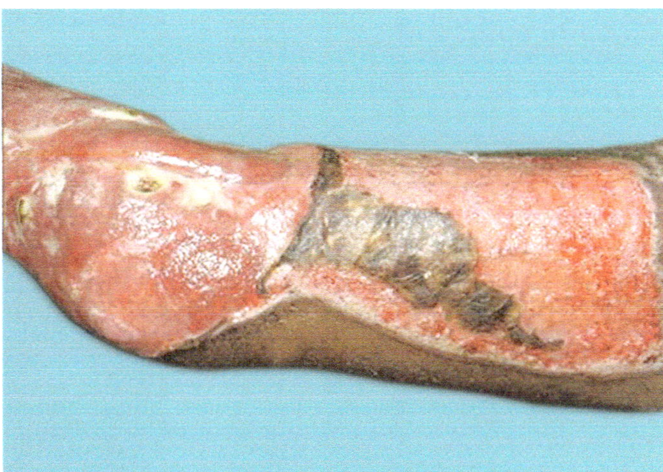

FIG. 9: A large full-thickness burn over thigh following friction with the truck tire. The presence of thick eschar indicates deep burn due to friction. There is evidence of avulsion distally.

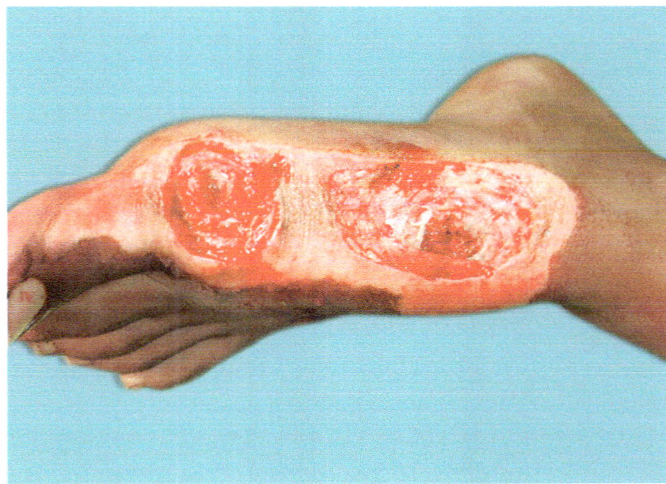

FIG. 10: Full-thickness friction burn over the dorsum of the foot by a car tyre running over it.

Majority of the accidental friction burns in children take place at home. Although the burn is small, it should be taken seriously in children.

MANAGEMENT

Management is simple and straightforward because of the limited extent of burns in the majority of patients. The principles of management of friction burns are the same as for thermal burns. Majority of the friction burns are managed as minor burns with tetanus prophylaxis, local wound care, topical antimicrobials, and analgesics. Sometimes, it requires surgical management with tangential excision and split-thickness skin grafting. In treadmill-related injuries, 46% of children with friction burns had full-thickness burns requiring surgical management.[5] In another study, 33% of treadmill-related friction burn cases required skin grafting.[9] Major friction burns are associated with other injuries which should be managed simultaneously. In an Indian study, 35% had hand fractures, 10% had head injury, and 5% had associated tendon and nerve injury.[3]

Majority of the airbag friction burns are minor and partial thickness and do not require hospitalization.[18] Though the majority of airbag lesions are minor, a correct diagnosis of the type of burn is necessary as it may be a friction or chemical burn or mechanical trauma. Based on the type of trauma, the appropriate treatment is instituted. The benefit of airbags far outweighs the risks of the burns, and hence are acceptable.

In the Indian study, 41.66% required split-thickness skin graft **(Fig. 11)** and 10% required major flap procedures **(Figs. 12A to C)**.[3] A full-thickness defect of the chest wall has been reported requiring multiple flap reconstructions.[15]

Early recognition and appropriate management result in excellent functional outcomes with minimum morbidity.

PREVENTION

Majority of unreported and reported friction burns occur during sports and routine activities, and hence, these may not be totally preventable in a large number of cases. However, appropriate preventive habits, prevention of roadside accidents, and specific precautions observed while dealing with etiological factors may reduce the incidence of friction burns.

Benever et al. predicted that the incidence of friction burn injury with treadmill-like domestic machines is likely to increase in the future unless protective modification of exercise machines is done.[9] Additional safety measures, warning labels, and parental education can prevent friction burns due to domestic and industrial causes.

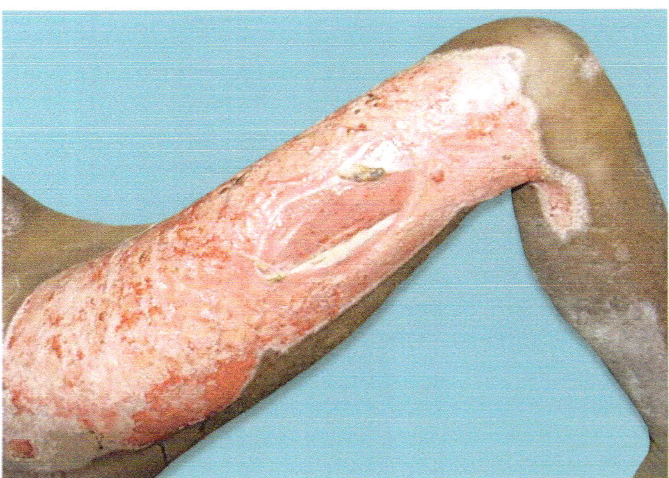

FIG. 11: Combination of friction burn and avulsion due to roadside accident. The proximal and distal parts of the raw areas are following the separation of eschar. The central area with exposed muscle is due to associated avulsion injury. These areas can be covered with split-skin grafts alone.

Proper use of seat belts through the shoulder and lap reduces the overall injury to the car passengers. The airbag friction burn is also less when the riders have their seat belts on.

The use of closed-loop and open internal cooling systems while using power drills regulates the temperature of the surrounding bone and soft tissue, thus preventing frictional burns, which leads to osteonecrosis, and decreased regenerative capacity of bone, which leads to loosening of implants. Closed-loop cooling systems are those in which coolant courses through tubules and tunnels incorporated into the drill bit or bur itself and back through a central heat exchanger. Thermal energy generated at the machining face heats the coolant through a mechanism of conduction, thereby preventing an increase in the temperature of the bone to above a critical level. In open cooling systems, fluid courses through tubules in the drill but exits through openings at the cutting tip, thereby absorbing heat but also providing some lubrication in the process of cutting.[22]

Friction burns during liposuction can be prevented by making the port site bigger, reducing the power of the liposuction, using lubricating gels at the cannula port site, excising the cannula port site edges routinely before closing, and using a small patch of Tegaderm over the cannula site to avoid friction burns.[23]

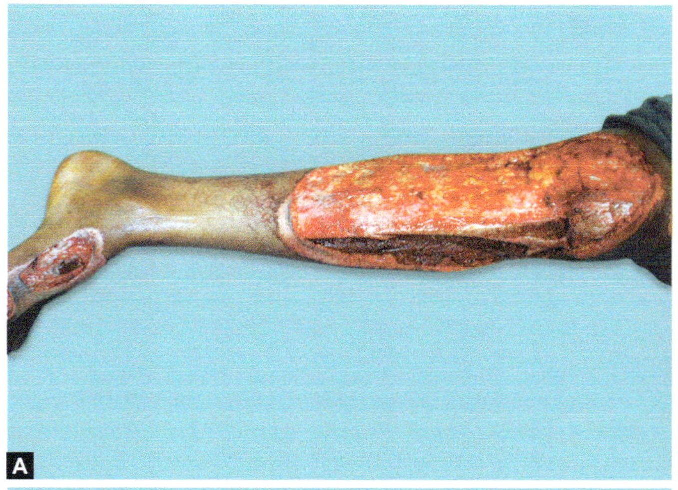

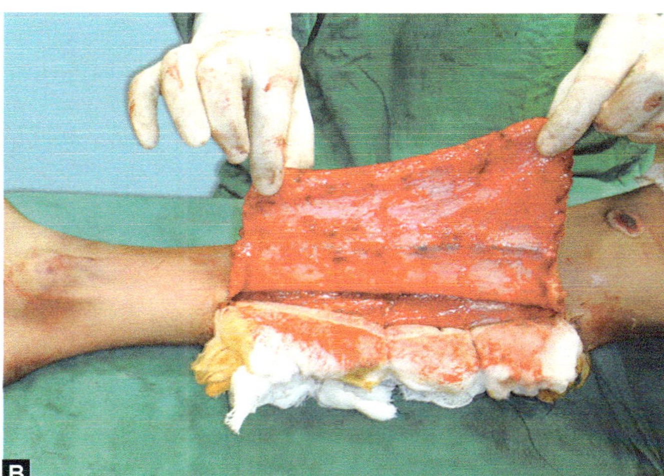

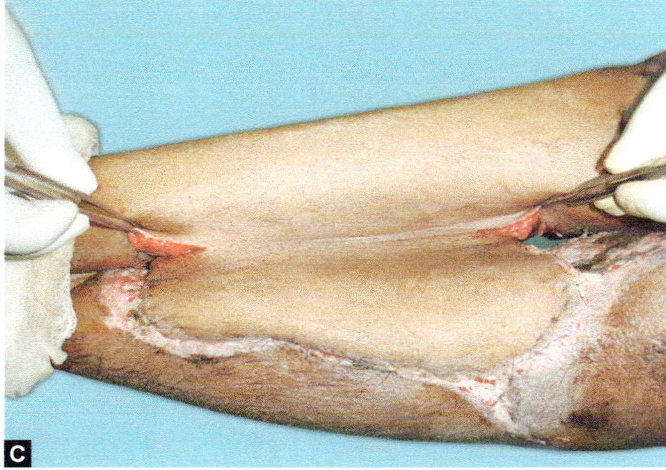

FIGS. 12A TO C: (A) Exposed tibia after removal of thick eschar following deep friction burn over the leg in a road traffic accident; (B) Fasciocutaneous flap raised from the opposite leg for cover; (C) Crossleg flap covering the same defect completely.

SUMMARY

The friction burn is an interesting trauma associated with day-to-day active life. One has to accept the occurrence of friction burn as a part of life. Modern gadgets have become a part of today's lifestyle, which may increase the possibilities of friction burn. There are a few areas where preventive measures and a watchful lifestyle may significantly reduce the incidence of friction burn.

REFERENCES

1. www.answers.com/topic/spacecraft-structure?cat=technology.
2. Langley J, Tobin P. Childhood burns. N Z Med J. 1983;96(739):681-4.
3. Agrawal A, Vora HJ, Raibagkar SC. Friction burn: Epidemiology and prevention. Indian J Burns. 2006;14(1):20-22.
4. Collier ML, Ward RS, Saffle JR, Edelman LS, Morris SE, Lundy C. Home treadmill friction injuries: A five-year review. J Burn Care Rehabil. 2004;25(5):441-4.
5. Maguine P, Palmieri TL, Greenhalgh DG. Treadmills: A preventable source of pediatric friction burn injuries. J Burn Care Rehabil. 2004;25(2):201-4.
6. Han T, Han K, Kim J, Lee G, Choi J, Lee J, et al. Pediatric hand injury induced by treadmill. Burns. 2005;31(7):906-9.
7. Pegg SP. Burn epidemiology in the Brisbane and Queensland area. Burns. 2005;31(Suppl 1):S27-31.
8. Wright JB. Wild water rapid burns. Br J Sports Med. 1995;2993:208-9.
9. Benever GT, Moriarty KP, Sachs BF, Courtney RA, Konefal SH Jr, Barbeau L. Pediatric hand treadmill injuries. J Craniofac Surg. 2003;14(4):487-90.
10. Borschel GH, Wolter KG, Cederna PS, Franklin GA. Acute management of exercise treadmill-associated injuries in children. J Trauma. 2003;55(1):130-4.
11. Marshall J. Lourie GM. Pediatric hand friction burn injuries secondary to treadmills. J Pediatr Orthop. 2003;23(3):407-9.
12. Walsh K, Osman-Elabd M, Sheikh M, Soueid A. Vacuum cleaner friction injuries in paediatrics. A 10 year review looking at national trends. Burns. 2022;48(4):1013-8.

13. Al-Qattan MM. Car-tyre friction injuries of the foot in children. Burns. 2000;26(4):399-408.
14. Mine R, Fukui M, Nishimura G. Bicycle spoke injuries in the lower extremity. Plast Reconstr Surg. 2000;106(7):1501-6.
15. Ono I, Tateshita T. Reconstruction of a full-thickness defect of the chest wall caused by friction burn using a combined myocutaneous flap of teres major and latissimus dorsi muscles. Burns. 2001;27(3):283-8.
16. Baruchin AM, Jakim I, Rosenberg L, Nahlieli O. On burn injuries related to airbag deployment. Burns. 1999;25:49-52.
17. Ulrich D, Noah EM, Fuchs P, Pullua N. Burn injuries caused by air bag deployment. Burns. 2001;27(2):196-9.
18. Corazza M, Trincone S, Virgili A. Effects of airbag deployment: lesions, epidemiology and management. Am J Clin Dermatol. 2004;595:295-300.
19. Choudhary S, Koshy C, Ahmed J, Evans J. Friction burns to thigh caused by tourniquet if applied over bare limb skin. Br J Plast Surg. 1998;51(2):142-3.
20. Giannoudis PV, Snowden S, Matthews SJ, Smye SW, Smith RM. Friction burns within the tibia during reaming. Are they affected by the use of a tourniquet? J Bone Joint Surg Br. 2002;84(4):492-6.
21. Bertollo N, Walsh WR. Drilling of bone: Practicality, limitations and complications associated with surgical drill-bits. In: Klika V (Ed). Biomechanics in Applications. InTech Open. DOI: 10.5772/20931.
22. Jayakumar R, Kumaran S, Kishore P, Guild AJ. A simple technique to prevent friction burns in liposuction. J Plast Reconstr Aesthet Surg. 2009;62(5):579.
23. Mehrotra S, Nanda V, Chittoria R, Ksharma R. "Chunni burn": A rare mode of clothing-induced friction burn. Plast Reconstr Surg. 2004;114(1):282-3.
24. Mahahan AL, Regan PJ. Tolls of a trek up Croagh Patrick: A case of friction/frost burns to the feet. Burns. 2004;30(3):283-5.
25. Brehmer-Andersson E, Goransson K. Friction blisters as a manifestation of pathomimia. Acta Derm Venereol. 1975;55(1):65-71.

CHAPTER

25

Fireworks and Firecracker Injuries

Aakanksha Goel, Arun Goel, Sameek Bhattacharya

INTRODUCTION AND HISTORY

Fire, which changed the face of human civilization, has been man's fascination since its discovery. Among the modalities of its use, ranging from highly beneficial to highly destructive, fire has been central to numerous occasions of celebration. Its initial uses must have been limited to illumination only and then for decorative purposes. Later on, with the evolution of ordnance technology, the art of manufacturing and setting off of fireworks was developed. Fireworks are an aesthetic arrangement of various fire producing elements with an audio-visual imagery changing from moment to moment. Pyrotechnic compositions are usually based on organic or inorganic chemical oxidizers and fuels to produce visual, thermal, audible, and mechanical effects such as light, loud noise, smoke, motion, color, and floating matter. The first three are especially important. The word "pyrotechnics" (synonymous with "fireworks") originated from Greek. They are produced not only for entertainment by the lay public but also for military and industrial use where pyrotechnic mixtures are used for demolition work and they comprise ammunition or signaling and illuminating items.

The earliest documentation of "fireworks" is from ancient city Liuyang, China during Han dynasties (200 BC) which dates even before the discovery of gunpowder. Burning of green bamboo stems by throwing them into fire, led to an expansion of trapped air resulting in a loud bang. This was believed to disperse evil spirits. The bursting bamboo or "pao chuk" in Chinese, were part of Lunar New Year celebrations and other festivities for about a thousand years till gunpowder was invented during Sui and Tang dynasties (600–900 AD) and flourished during Song dynasty (960–1279 AD). The precursor to the discovery of gunpowder was a chance finding of a sulfurous mixture by Chinese alchemists during the course of their experiments, which burst into illuminating flame on burning. "Hao Yao" or fire dung as they called it were packed in bamboo tubes and burned as firecrackers.

The knowledge of pyrotechnics reached the West in 1200 AD when Marco Polo brought the Chinese know-how to Italy. The Italians added an aesthetic dimension to the fireworks by adding metal powder to gunpowder in order to produce colorful sparkles. With further advances in chemistry, some more metal salts were added to produce multicolored pyrotechnic-effects.

While firecrackers originated in China, they made their way into India through trade and military contact and dates back to Mughal times. Some historians point out that the knowledge of materials used to make firecrackers existed in India as far back as 300 BC. Pyrotechnic shows were part of royal entertainment in many medieval Indian kingdoms during festivals and weddings. Others believe Chinese pyrotechnic formulas were brought to India around 14th century AD with several changes being made later.

The first fireworks factory in modern India was established in early 20th century. In 1923, Nadar brothers from Sivakasi, Tamil Nadu went to Kolkata in search of job, worked there in a match factory and returned back home to start a match factory. In 1940, an amendment in the Explosives Act made the manufacture of some types of fireworks legal. They seized the opportunity and started the first fireworks factory in the little town of Sivakasi soon transforming it into a hub for this industry, with supplies to whole of India even today.[1,2] In 1980, there were 189 factories in Sivakasi which increased to around 1,070 registered firecracker manufacturing companies in 2020 with 8 lakh people being directly and indirectly employed by them. Approximately 70% of the firecrackers and matches produced in India are from Sivakasi.

Presently, fireworks/firecrackers are billions of dollars industry in the world giving employment to millions from manufacturing to retail sale. China is the largest manufacturer and exporter in the world.

FIREWORKS/FIRECRACKERS SCENARIO IN MODERN TIMES

In modern times, social events such as marriage, religious functions and state functions, e.g., Independence day all involve display of fireworks and bursting of firecrackers. So much so that even fireworks competitions are organized at a number of places in the world, e.g., the prestigious annual Montreal Fireworks Festival in Canada and World Pyro Olympics held in Manila, Philippines. The latter is one of the largest and most intense international fireworks competitions organized over a period of 5 days. Many major cities around the globe begin their New Year with fireworks and firecrackers. The opening and closing ceremonies of various Olympiads are marked by great fireworks displays.

Use of fireworks/firecrackers on festivals is universal all over the world, be it a highly developed or underdeveloped nation. In India, their widespread and large-scale use during Diwali ("festival of lights") is unparalleled in the world. Diwali is celebrated to mark the victorious return of Shri Ram (an incarnation of Shri Vishnu, a Hindu God) to his kingdom in Ayodhya after killing the evil Ravan, the demon king of Lanka (now Sri Lanka). During this festive night of victory of good over evil, the houses are adorned with small earthen oil lamps, candles, and colorful electric lights. After offering the prayers, the entire family participates in the bursting of firecrackers. 20 days preceding Diwali, Dussehra is celebrated by burning the towering effigies of Ravan, his brother Kumbhakaran and son Meghnaad. These are packed with massive amounts of various types of firecrackers and fireworks and this public display is watched by thousands of onlookers in every locality. Diwali is now celebrated with firecrackers in several major countries of Southeast Asia, Europe, and even USA on a grand scale because of large migrated population of Indian origin. Sikhs also celebrate "Gurpurab" with bursting of crackers.

Thrissur Pooram, a two-century old festival to mark the end of caste supremacy is celebrated in Kerala, southern India. The festivities are attended by millions of people from across the state and even international visitors. The spectacular fireworks display, biggest in India, starts in the early hours (02:30 hours IST) and lasts for 3–4 hours. In India, marriages and even victory in international cricket matches, whether played in or out of country, are celebrated by cricket fans at home by bursting crackers. With the passage of time, the celebrations of these occasions have gained gigantic proportions. Promotors of the industry have given a further buoyance to this fervor.

Hari Raya Puasa, marking the culmination of "Ramadan", the holy month of fasting is celebrated in Malayasia by Muslims. Shab-e-Barat in Pakistan and Halloween season in Ireland and elsewhere are all celebrated with fireworks and firecrackers. In England, the firecrackers (also known as "bangers")/fireworks are traditionally set off on "Bonfire night" or "Guy Fawkes night" (5th November). In France, they are used around Bastille Day (14th July). As in India, these are available throughout the year in several Mediterranean countries such as Spain and Malta.

The firecrackers have also been known for their use to exorcise evil spirits with their loud sound. They are even utilized by farmers as a modality to scare away wild animals and birds from farms.

EPIDEMIOLOGY

Fireworks/firecrackers are used worldwide to express festive mood. They have become a source of recreation for people all over the world breaking the barriers of varied cultures, religion, literacy, urban-rural, rich-poor, developed-underdeveloped, etc. At the same time, they are a menace as well, as is evident from research papers being published from centers across the globe, be it Asia, Australia, Europe, America, South Africa, Russia, or Israel.[3-7] The epidemiological profile of injuries caused by them is unique to a region. Globally, the burden of these injuries shows a wide variation and depends on:

- The number of days at a stretch, month, and season during the which the celebrations occur.
- Whether related to a religion, sports event, or a national day
- The type of fireworks/firecrackers available and used
- Legislation with respect to them and extent of its effective implementation
- Education and prosperity of the people

Thus, statistical comparisons between two countries or even within two regions in any large country are definitely inappropriate. India is a geographically vast country with 140 crore population. Differences amongst various study results are bound to occur. Tandon et al.[8] saw a total of 1,373 patients in a major burn center in Delhi during the three consecutive days during Diwali from 2002 to 2010. There was an increasing trend in number of patients (111 in 2002 vs. 251 in 2010). Sarma[9] from Guwahati also found an increasing trend in number of patients during Diwali. Puri et al.[10] from Mumbai treated 157 cases from 1997 to 2006, 92 cases in first 3 years retrospectively, and 65 cases in subsequent 7 years, prospectively. They concluded that the decreased incidence was due to increased awareness by various campaigns.

Mohan A et al.[11] found that 4,436 individuals attended accident and emergency in England because of fireworks/firecrackers injury in 2018, a figure that has more than doubled from 2,141 seen in 2010 and are increasing in severity as well.

By virtue of their inherent aggressiveness, the males handle fireworks/firecrackers more and account for majority of victims. Most of the victims are children below 15 years of age and young adults. In India, especially in Delhi, "*Anar*" has been incriminated in majority of cases followed by other firecrackers.[12] A study from Ahmedabad reports firecrackers followed by igniting of powder taken out from firecrackers, rockets, and "*Anar*" as the most common causes.[13] Sparklers and ground spinners are relatively safer as compared to "*Anar*", rockets, and bombs. Practices such as trying continuously to ignite a cracker "refusing" to burn or reigniting half lit crackers is a common cause of injury. Use of protective eyewear during the festive season (even by bystanders) although advocated, is not followed.[14]

Globally, a decrease in fireworks/firecracker injuries has been attributed to a positive impact of legislation, which includes strong restrictive measures to use firecrackers privately, ongoing educational campaigns as well as assistance in promoting public performances in exchange for private use of firecrackers. In US where the firecrackers followed by sparklers are the leading causes of injury, the number of cases dropped by nearly 30% over an 11-year period from 2000 to 2010.[15] Adolescents from 10 to 19 years of age and three times more males as compared to females were injured during this period. Although no national data is available for India, the figures must be far higher considering the magnitude of their use almost whole of the year, larger population, scant safety consciousness, and poor regard for abiding by the laws.

Kalita et al.[16] received 106 patients during Diwali in a 5-year period from 2016 to 2020 at a tertiary care hospital in Guwahati, Assam. Due to the COVID-19 crisis and national lockdown and strict protocols, there were only two male and no female patients in the year 2020. 46% were males < 19 years of age.

Tamil Nadu reports the highest number of trauma victims from India, many of which are firecracker related. A tertiary care center in Vellore, South India reported having seen 13,604 patients of all types of trauma over a 2-year period up to December 2018. Out of these, 92 (0.7%) were firecracker injuries.[17]

During a 2-year period of study related to Diwali period, 30 patients with firecracker-induced eye injuries were seen in a tertiary care center in Kolkata. There was a male preponderance of 3:1, with all <15 years of age and 50% between 6 and 10 years.[18] Similarly, 49 patients with these injuries seen by a tertiary care eye hospital in southern India had 40 males and 50% were <15 years of age. Also, half of the victims were bystanders.[19] The percentage of bystanders in a study from Germany conducted over a 10-year period was almost 75% (113/149 patients).[20] Shiuey et al.[21] presented the data of almost two decades from USA and blamed bottle rockets to be the worst offender, disproportionately causing the most severe ocular trauma, including ruptured globe.

TYPES OF FIREWORKS/FIRECRACKERS

The new age pyrotechnic devices are broadly classified as fireworks and explosive firecrackers. A firework is a low explosive pyrotechnic device used primarily for aesthetic illumination and entertainment in the form of light, sparkles, and floaters, noise being secondary. They are generally large items used during celebrations at a community level and ignited only by professional workers, e.g., during Dussehra celebrations, beginning, and culmination of Olympic games, pyrotechnic competitions etc. A firecracker, on the other hand, is a relatively higher explosive device designed primarily to produce noise in the form of a loud bang with visual effect being incidental. They are generally smaller in size than professional items and are used by the public (consumer) themselves including small children during Diwali/other religious celebrations, winning of sports events, beginning of New year, etc.

The fireworks/firecracker can also be classified as to where they perform, ground level (e.g., "*phooljhari*") or aerial (e.g., rockets). In the latter case, they need incorporation of a mechanism for propulsion. Basically, both fireworks and firecrackers are explosives wrapped in heavy paper casing with a long fuse to ignite.

The various types of firecrackers available are:

- *Phooljhari or "sparkler"* (**Fig. 1**): Apart from enjoying its own sparkles, it is commonly used in lighting most of the other firecrackers. It consists of a metal stick with one-half covered with pyrotechnic compounds and the other half acts as a handle.
- *Anar or "fountain" or "flowerpetal"* (**Fig. 2**): It emerges as a big sparkling fountain of fire when lit. In addition, "*Anar*" is unique to our country and many people make its crude form at home, which poses grave risk while preparing as well as igniting them.

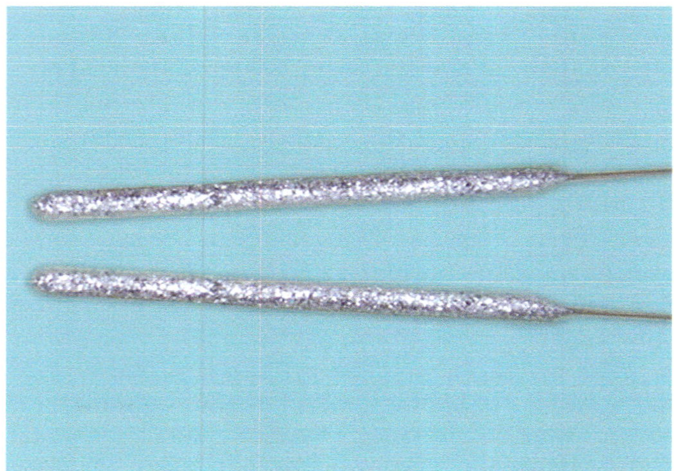

FIG. 1: *Phooljhari.*

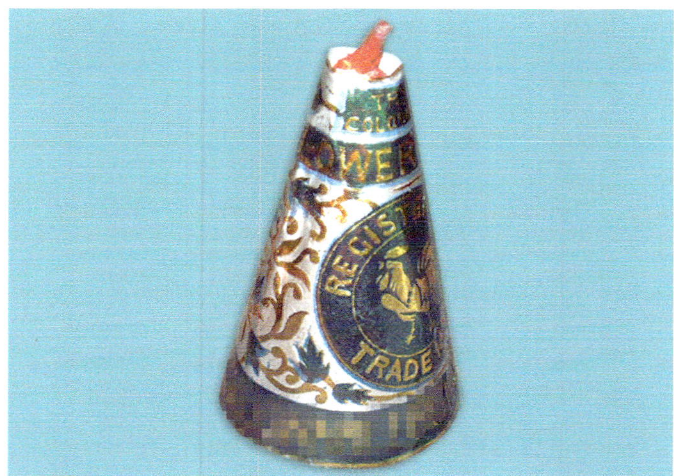

FIG. 2: *Anar.*

- *Zameen chakri or ground spinner* **(Fig. 3)**: It is a spinning circle of fire with sparks coming out of it.
- *Rocket* **(Fig. 4A)**: As the name suggests, when fired, it goes toward the sky and bursts into myriad of colors and designs. They may prove dangerous if they are misdirected accidentally and change their course and enter into residential buildings. They may be responsible for major fires after landing on inflammable material instead of going up in the air and bursting in the sky.
- *Bombs* **(Figs. 4B to D)** are available in various sizes and intensity. On bursting, they produce a lot of noise. The largest ones may even rupture the ear drum due to their intense blast wave. Many people tie a large number of them in series so that the noise continues for some time in multiple outbursts till all the bombs explode. Some others ignite them in their hand and throw away just before it explodes. All these are highly dangerous practices leading to a lot of injuries.

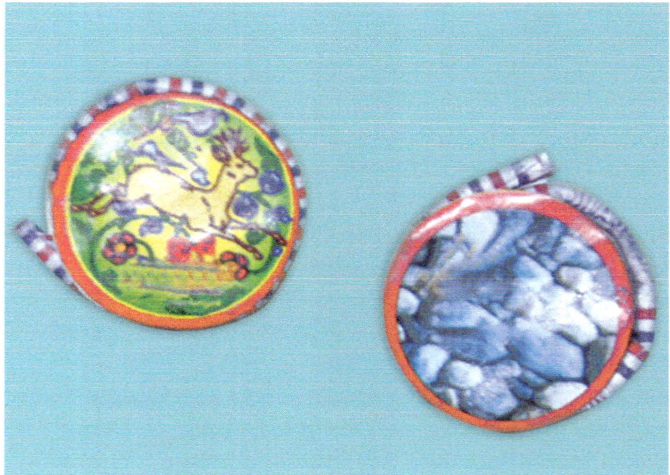

FIG. 3: *Zameen chakri.*

- *Miscellaneous*: "Snake" consists of an innocuous looking small black tablet (size of a medicinal tablet) which when ignited enlarges in the form of a long snake emitting a lot of smoke.

Fireworks/Firecrackers Cause Injuries and Damage in the Following Circumstances

During Production

Fireworks industry is well known for its hazardous nature.[22] Right from the site of manufacturing through storage, transportation and final retail sale, the risk to life and property is very high. In India, as elsewhere, one has to obtain a license from the government authorities and comply with the rules and regulations laid therein, to manufacture, store, and sell fireworks/firecrackers. Unfortunately, there is mushrooming of illegal factories even in residential and thickly populated areas. Flouting of safety norms is more of a routine rather than an exception. Firecrackers are mostly hand made in smaller places in highly unsafe conditions with precarious infrastructure. Most workers are illiterate poor young males and females and even children and many of them are from the same family in order to augment their income.[1] Safety is the last word in priorities for these unfortunate workers.[23] When these factories catch fire, there is not only loss of life but the adjoining houses also catch fire and collapse with loss of property. Thus, most deaths are seen in people who are themselves not enjoying the firecracker bursting but rather involved in production, transport and storage. Many unscrupulous vendors hide firecrackers in places where fruits or other items are sold without any safety precautions. Many of

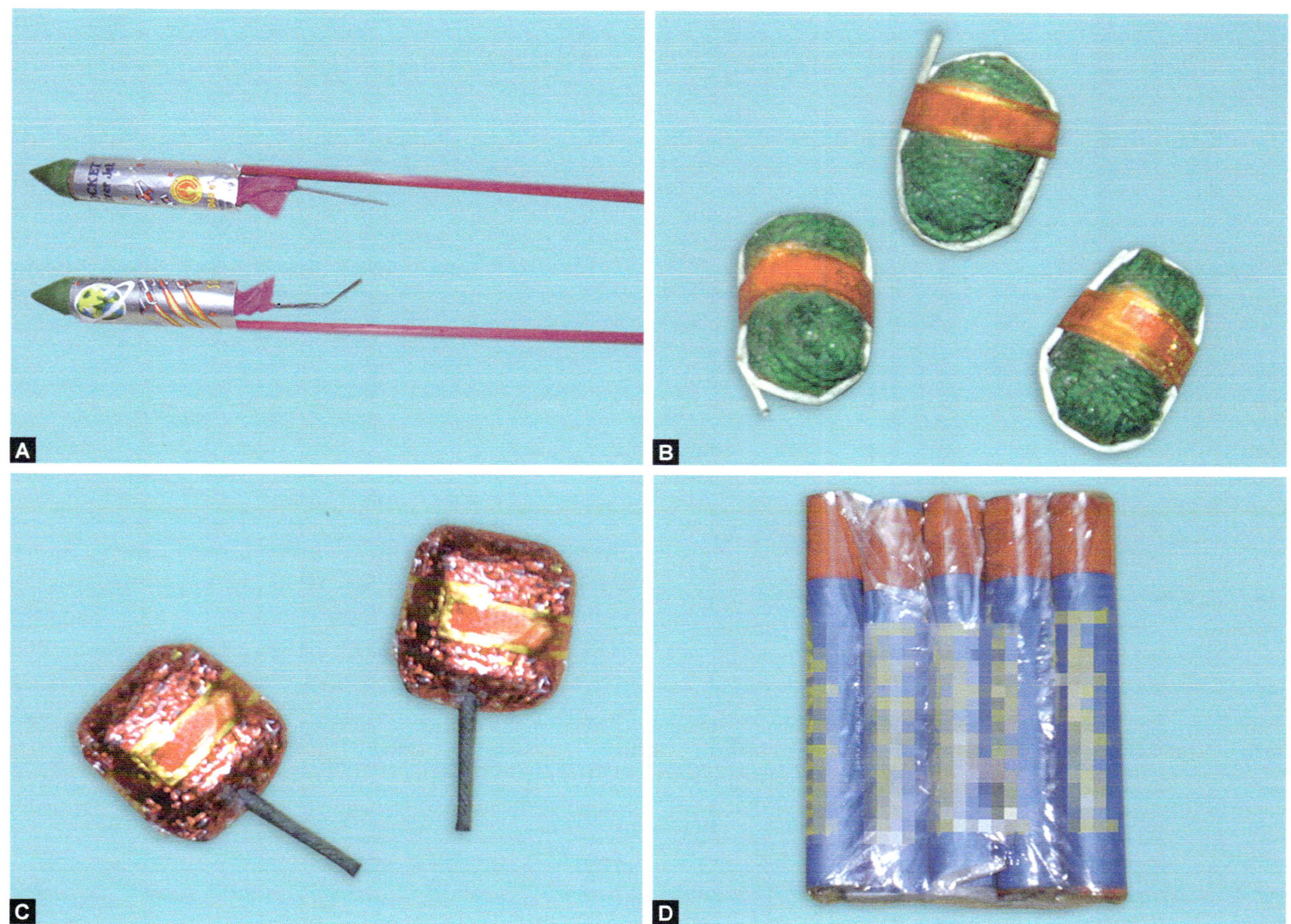

FIGS. 4A TO D: (A) Rockets; (B to D) Bombs.

these items have not undergone quality control and are sold very cheap. Once these poor-quality products reach the hands of general public, they frequently malfunction leading to burns and other injuries.

Incidents of accidents, sometimes in the form of disasters, are quite common in Sivakasi.[1] In 1991, 39 people were killed and 65 others were injured in a factory fire. In July 2009, >40 people were killed due to mishap in a firecracker unit. Similarly, blast and fire accident in 2012 killed 40 while >70 were injured (burns and other injuries). About 50 sheds in the factory were also gutted. In February 2024, a massive blast and fire took place in an illegal cracker manufacturing factory in Madhya Pradesh. More than a dozen people died, almost 200 were injured while >50 houses were damaged. Apart from accidents due to firecrackers getting ignited unintentionally, child labor is also an important issue plaguing this industry. Inadequate training of workers and supervisors involved in production and marketing is commonly blamed. The children in these industries also suffer from various diseases due to exposure to harmful chemicals present in the air.[2]

Storage

Once out of factory, these products, whether produced under license or not, are sometimes stored illegally in thickly populated and unlicensed areas and godowns with great risk of catching fire.

More than 110 people were killed and almost 400 were injured (>40 seriously) during fireworks display at Puttingal temple in Kollam, Kerala in 2016. This place is about 200 km from Sivakashi. A competitive display of fireworks was being held as part of the temple festival when a spark triggered by fireworks fell on the building storing fireworks/firecrackers, resulting in a huge explosion at around 3.30 AM. The massive impact was felt even 1 km away with building on the temple premises completely collapsed and around 150 houses surrounding the temple were badly damaged. Several spectators were blown to pieces. Some died due to injuries in collapse of buildings while others had burns and many were killed due to the stampede which followed.

Retail Sale

During festive season like Diwali, a number of shops come up in every small neighborhood selling crackers in open spaces as if they are innocuous items, again endangering the shoppers.

Improper and Unsafe Use of Fireworks/ Firecrackers by End Users (Figs. 5A and B)

This is the most common cause of morbidity during various festivities and accounts for the majority of patients visiting emergency services.

- Simultaneous igniting of multiple crackers/sparklers
- Igniting "bombs" and "*anar*" in hand in an act of bravado
- Bowing over a firecracker while trying to light it.
- Unsupervised bursting of firecrackers by small children. Young children have no knowledge of dangers of firecrackers just as they have no road sense. While labeled instructions cannot be read in dark, they are not read even in the best of light.[24]
- Trying to find out the cause of nonbursting of a cracker by picking up a "dud" which has failed to go off in expected time or trying to reignite it and it explodes in hand.
- Collection of the combustible powder out of a number of semiburnt crackers and burning them in a heap.
- Throwing lighted crackers on onlookers or a passerby
- Firecrackers exploding earlier or later than expected
- Errant flight paths of "rocket" and spinner
- Sparks or debris from fireworks/firecrackers initiating a house on fire
- Trying to make crude crackers (e.g., "*anar*") at home
- Bursting cheap quality crackers
- Insufficient open space
- Ladies wearing loose flowing dresses made of synthetic, highly inflammable material during marriage functions in congested, narrow streets with vehicles, children surrounding the site at close range as onlookers is a big recipe for disaster. The make-shift "pandals" (*tents*) are also made of inflammable cloth.
- Firecracker exploding in boy's trouser pocket. The clothes may start a fire.

CLINICAL FEATURES OF FIREWORKS/ FIRECRACKERS INJURY

The spectrum of injuries and harmful effects due to fireworks/firecracker use is very vast and diverse. Although for purpose of description, these are discussed under various headings as below, any individual patient can have more than one type of injury and area of body involvement.

Thermal Burns

Burns are the most common type of injuries sustained by end users due to firecrackers and affect the hands **(Figs. 6 to 10)** and face **(Figs. 11 to 15)** including ocular adnexa. The extent of burn as related to body surface area is generally small. Also, they are generally not more than superficial dermal in depth. However, any part of the body may get burnt especially when clothes catch fire during their use and may become even critical in extent and full

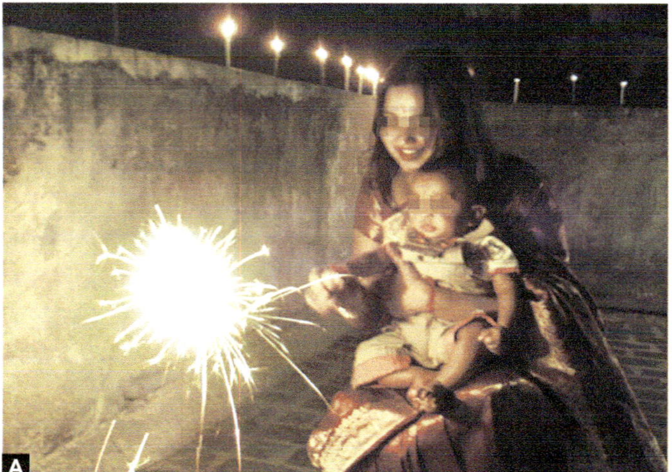
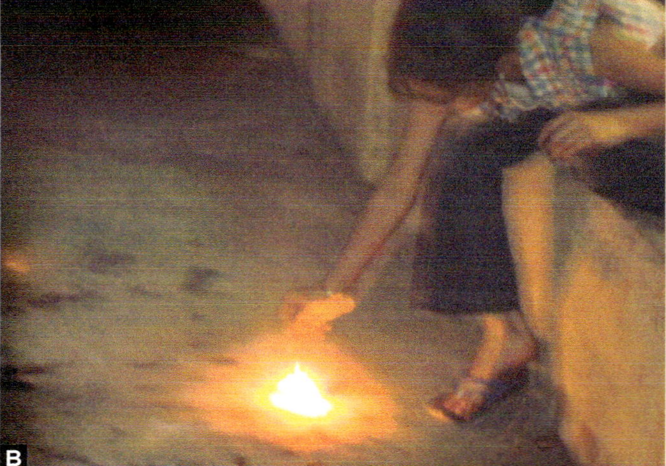

FIGS. 5A AND B: (A) Unsafe use of "*phooljhari*" by adults wearing synthetic clothes and holding a child in the arms. (B) Unsafe use of "*zameen chakri*" by a child who is likely to get burns of feet.

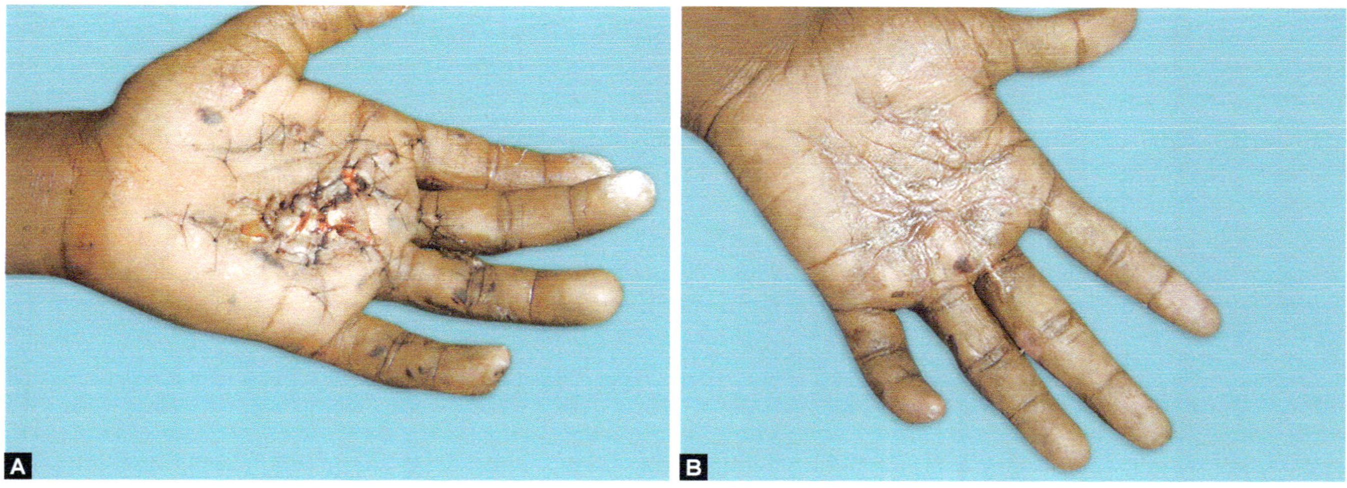

FIGS. 6A AND B: Explosion of "*anar*" in hand causing (A) laceration with burns with stitched wounds. (B) Healed.

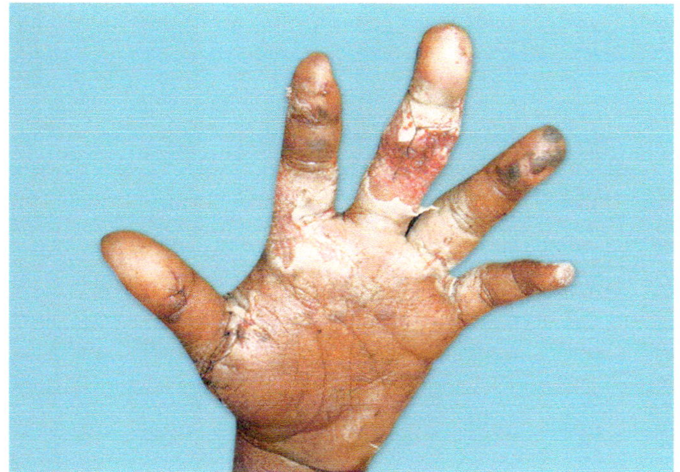

FIG. 7: Laceration of first web space with burns.

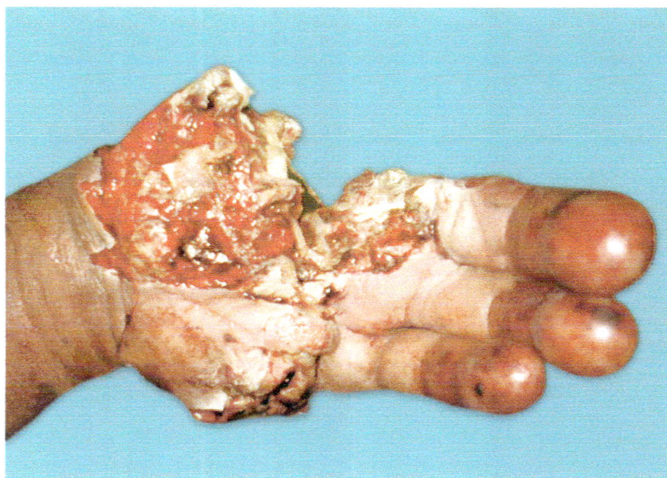

FIG. 8: Massive lacerations with avulsions and amputations of thumb and finger due to bomb exploding in hand.

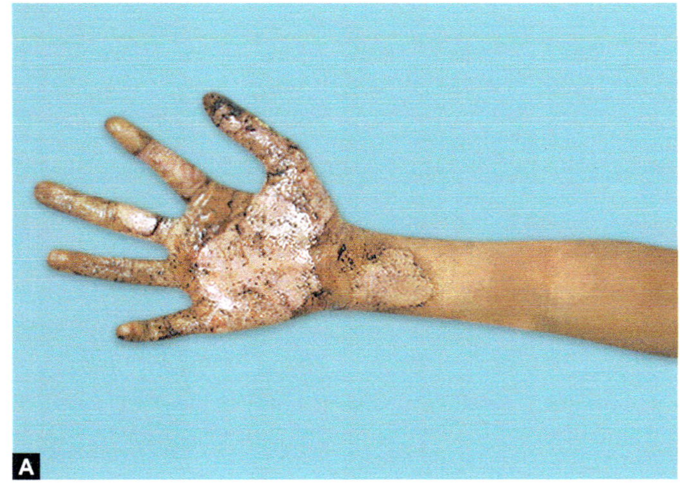

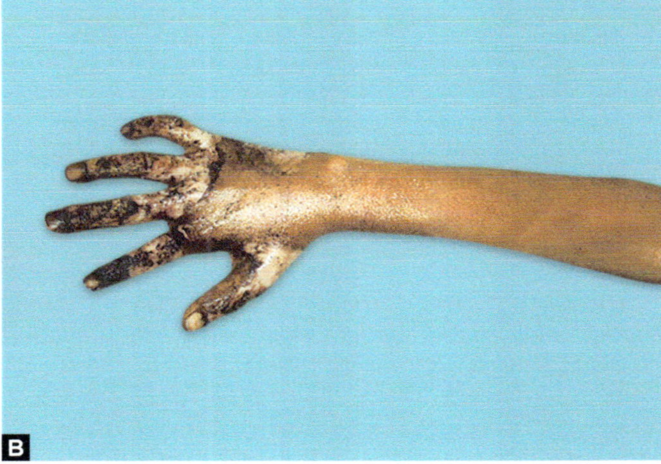

FIGS. 9A TO D: *Continued*

Continued

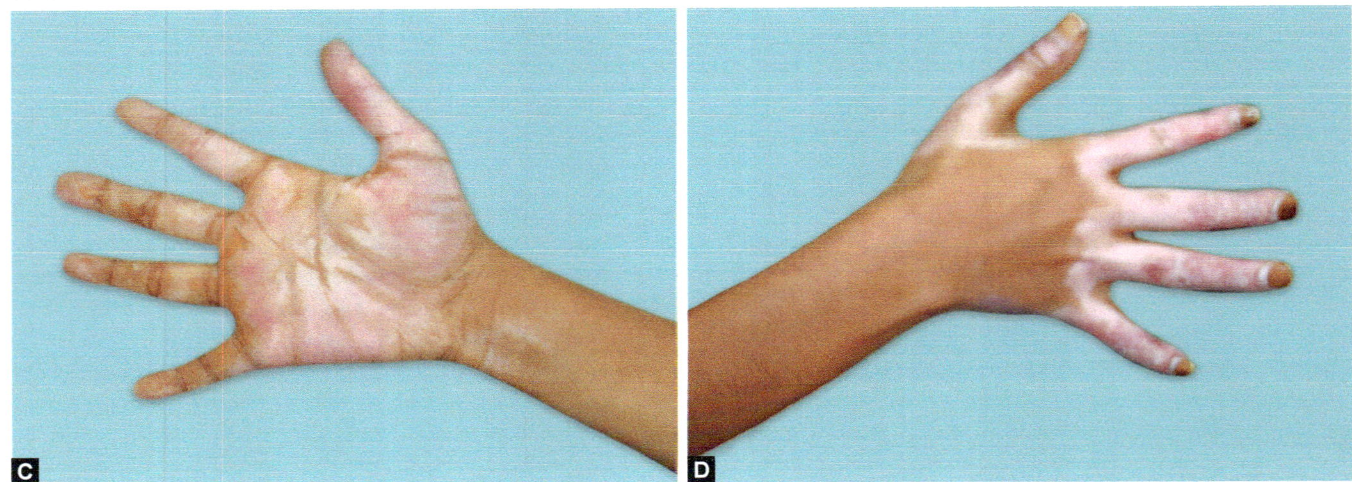

FIGS. 9A TO D: Burn due to cracker. Healed after conservative treatment. Please note the application of "*Ratanjyot*" (indigenous medicine) used in some parts of our country for faster healing.

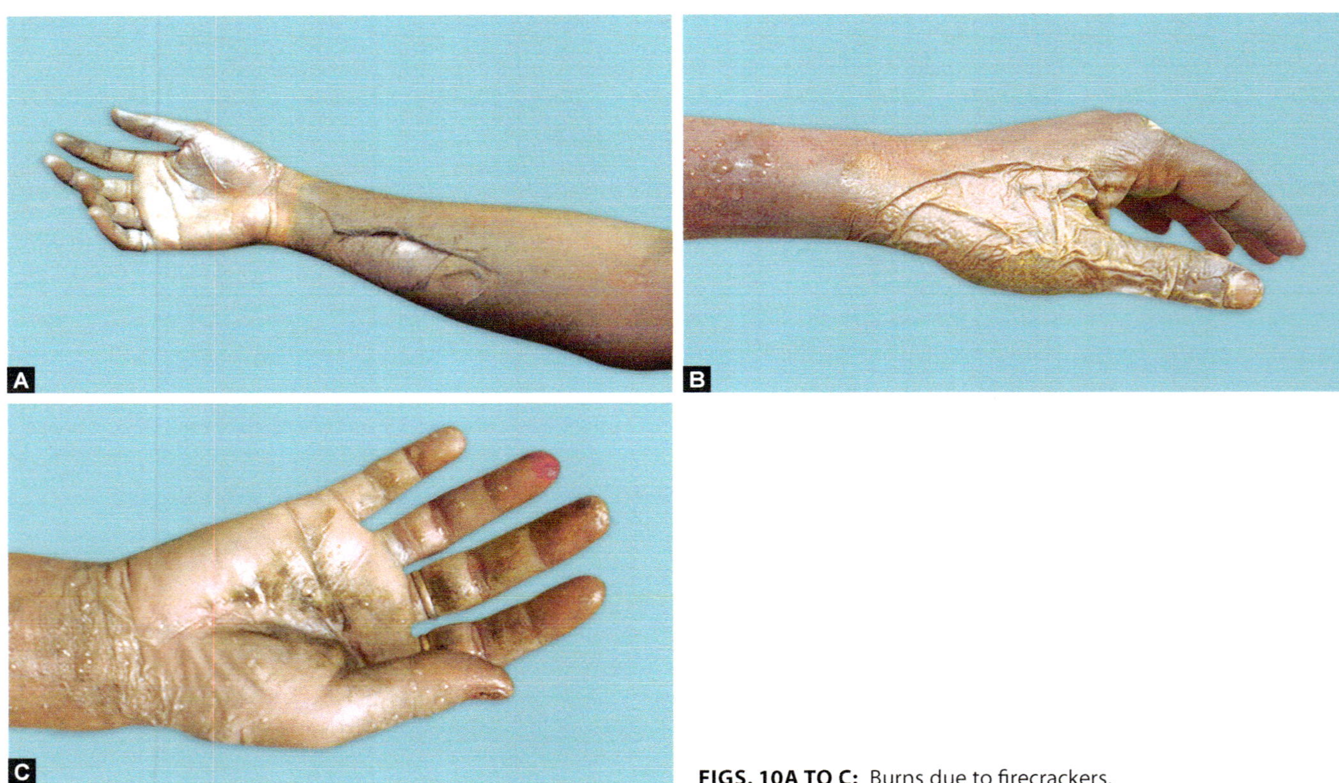

FIGS. 10A TO C: Burns due to firecrackers.

thickness in depth. The feet may get burnt by stepping on the hot sparkles from "*phooljhari*" or "*zameen chakri*" **(Fig. 5B)**. The injuries can be due to flash, flame, contact, and blast. Decorative fireworks are more likely to cause major cutaneous burns as compared to firecrackers. Flash burns are usually caused by crackers like "*anar*", "*chakri*", and sparklers and may affect bystanders and unsuspecting passersby as well.

Injuries of the Ocular Globe and Adnexa[25-29]

Facial burns can be complicated by injury to eyeball and ocular adnexa. They account for some of the most disabling firecracker-related injuries and form an important indication for admission to hospital. Bombs, flowerpots, rockets, and sparkles are found to be the cause of ocular injury in almost 90% of patients. Again,

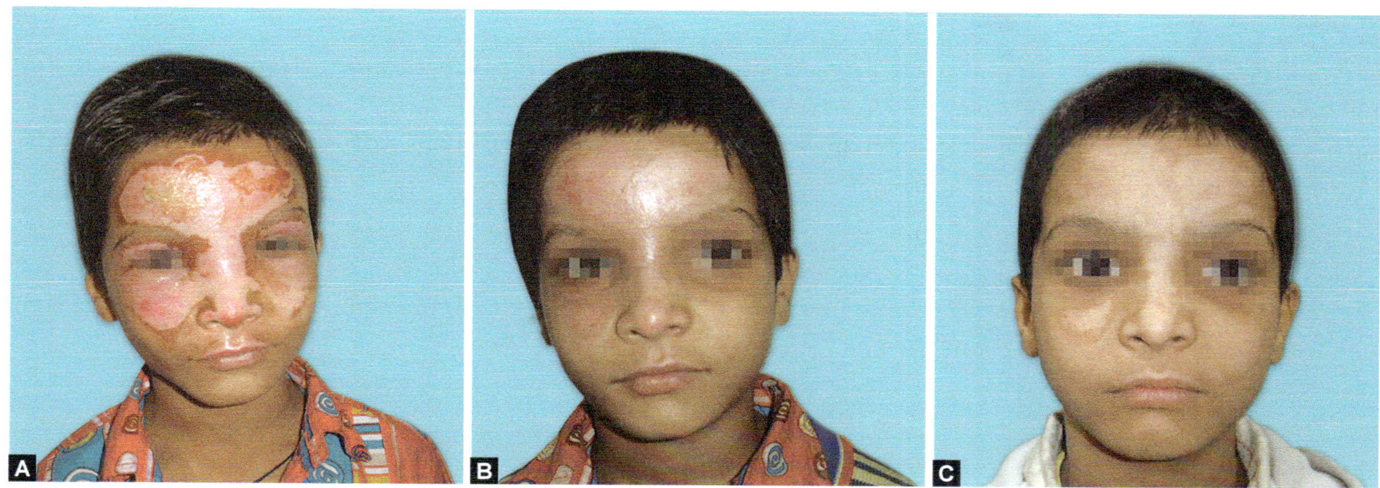

FIGS. 11A TO C: Superficial burns of face due to cracker injury being managed conservatively; healed.

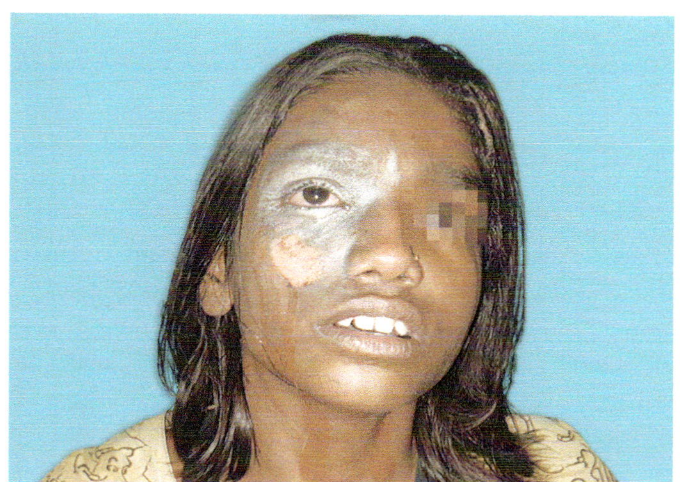

FIG. 12: Cracker injuries to face and right eye.

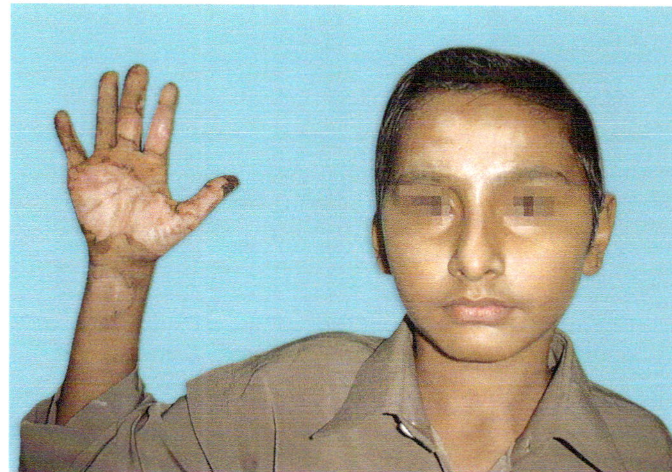

FIG. 14: Cracker injury to hand and face, a usual combination.

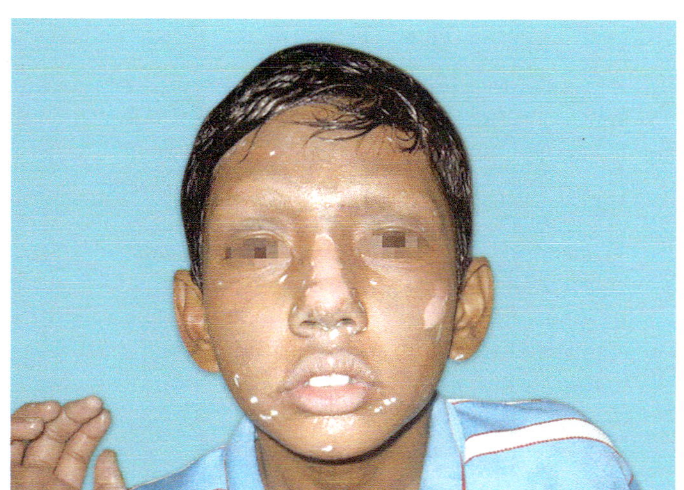

FIG. 13: Cracker injuries to face.

three-fourths of patients are male probably because they are more inclined to show "bravado" and present in streets. The periocular burns are present in all the cases while corneal involvement occurs in three-fourths of victims.[30] While negligent and risky behavior, curious nature, and nonanticipation of danger with lack of adult supervision are very important causes of injury in children from 5 to 15 years of age, onlookers, or even passersby also become victims.

The severity of eye trauma can range from minor superficial conjunctival foreign body to most major injury requiring multiple surgical interventions and still ending up in permanent partial or total loss of vision. They include:

- Eyelid burn/laceration/ hematoma
- Conjunctival burn/contusion/foreign body, scleral tears

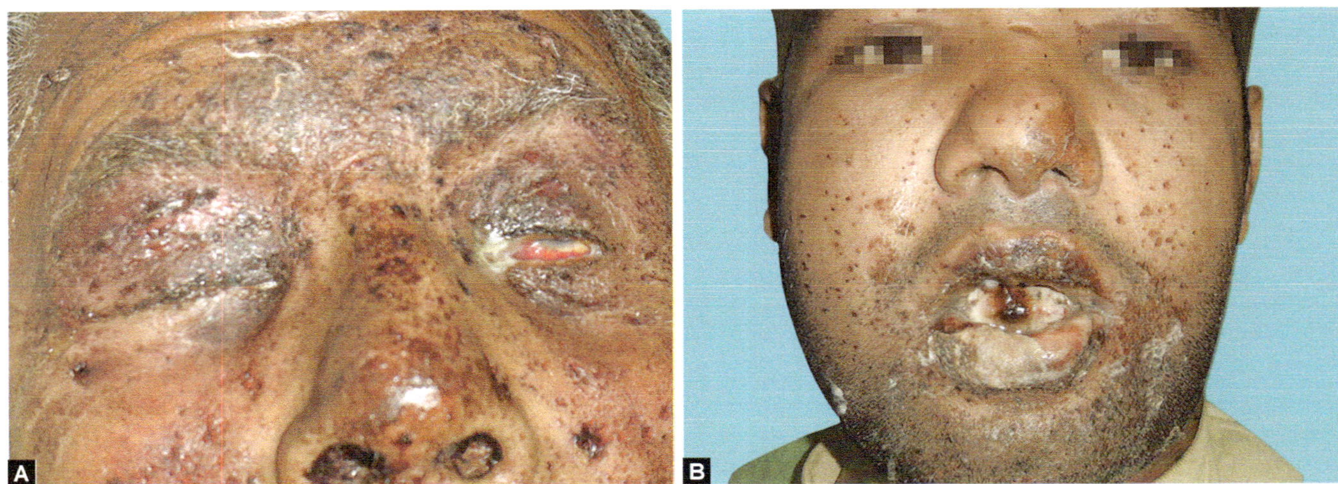

FIGS. 15A AND B: Cracker injuries to face with cracker powder causing tattooing.

- Corneal burn/contusion/foreign body, perforation, or hyphema
- Traumatic cataract
- Rupture of iris sphincter or even globe
- Vitreous/macular hemorrhage
- Retinal edema, retinal detachment, etc.

Since the firecracker-induced ocular injury almost always occurs in addition to burn injuries of face and other parts of the body, all such patients are bound to reach a burn surgeon first. The management of these ocular injuries is beyond the realm of a burn surgeon and certainly requires the intervention of an ophthalmologist. The responsibility of coordinating with an eye specialist right from the patient's first presentation in burn emergency, thus falls on the burn specialist.

Blast Injuries of the Hand (Figs. 6A to 8 and 16)

Along with the major thermal burns sustained due to a fire started by use of fireworks/firecrackers and ocular injuries, blast injury of the hands is the most important and common cause necessitating hospital admission. These injuries, quite common in warfare, are frequently seen by burn surgeons treating civilians and range from superficial lacerations of skin of hand to a mangled hand where skin, muscle, and neurovascular bundles are completely shattered, multiple bones fractured with even amputations at several levels or even whole of hand.[31-37] Thus, these injuries represent a surgical emergency for a reconstructive hand surgeon and as a rule requires prolonged hospital stay and multiple operative interventions. They may still end in amputations, stiffness, and permanent functional and cosmetic impairment. The radial side of the hand is most commonly affected.

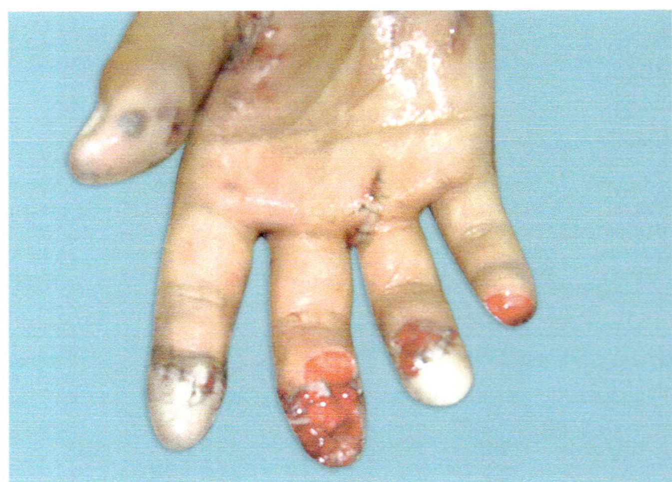

FIG. 16: Blast injury of hand due to firecracker leading to multiple lacerations and loss of soft tissue in the fingertips—managed by reposition of tissue and local advancement flaps and skin grafting.

The thenar and first web space soft-tissue losses show that the exploding firecracker was held by the victim in the prehension grip.[38] The central rays are comparatively spared but hypothenar ray may also be injured. These injuries are not only due to explosion pressure but also due to particulate matter driven into the tissues. Presence of white phosphorus particles embedded into the tissues causes a lot of pain and tattooing. The shock wave from the exploding firecracker causes cavitation of the muscles of the thenar ray and the blast energy then propagates proximally along the flexor tendons. Within the tight confines of the carpal tunnel, there occurs a concentrated dissipation of this energy.[39] There may be even complete mangling of hand with loss of digits. There can be multiple fractures of bones of hand with loss of skin.

The victim is usually the one who was bursting the cracker, most commonly a bomb or "*anar*". The self-propelling rockets are also known to cause severe damage if they are misdirected accidentally.

Air Quality and Atmospheric Pollution

Fireworks/firecrackers are one of the most unusual sources of pollution in atmosphere although these episodes are for short periods of time only. The bursting of firecrackers during Diwali, events like New Year Day, winning of international cricket and other matches etc., occurs simultaneously by almost the whole of the population in India within a short span of 8–10 hours. With time, these celebrations are increasing in magnitude because of growing affluence of the people, especially in larger cities which are densely populated as well. All firecrackers contain toxic metals and other substances which release toxic gases and fine particulate matter in the atmosphere upon burning, leading to severe health and environmental hazards. Gases like SO_2, NO_2, and black carbon (BC) particulates are emitted by fireworks/firecrackers and generate dense clouds of smoke. Even in the absence of precursors and sunlight, O_3 has been found. There is a strong relationship between them and numerous adverse health effects including reproductive and developmental effects such as increased risk of preterm birth.[40,41] Inhalation of smoke from fireworks/firecrackers may lead to acute eosinophilic pneumonia. Heavy metals that are very harmful to human health are also emitted in large volumes. Perchlorates are teratogenic and can affect thyroid functions adversely. Consequent to the dense cloud of smoke, reduction in visibility also takes place. Speed of dispersion of smoke depends upon the meteorological conditions of the area.

A number of studies have been done in various countries to look for impact of fireworks/firecrackers on airborne particles. All show an increase in air pollution during their use on large scale.[42,43] A number of studies have been done in our country as well to study the changes in the atmospheric conditions during Diwali days in various major cities/regions of India.[44-49] There are also reports of short-term rise of PM10 loadings by many folds. The concentrations of PM10, SO_2, and NO_x have been reported to be 5.7, 6.6, and 2.7 times higher respectively on Diwali day as compared to on a routine day in Lucknow, India.[50] As the firecrackers mainly contain potassium nitrate, ammonium nitrate, charcoal, and sulfur, higher concentration of K^+, Mg_2^+, SO_4^2, NH_4^+, and NO_3^- has been observed. Hirai et al.[51] found that inhalation of smoke from fireworks/firecrackers causes cough, fever, and dyspnea and leads to acute eosinophilic pneumonia.

Noise Pollution and Deafness

In addition to fire-related mishaps, the firecrackers are also a source of noise pollution and adversely affect millions of people. While there has been much ado about air pollution, a high level of concern also needs to be drawn to the harmful effects of firecracker induced noise pollution.[52-54] Infants and small children do get frightened on hearing the sudden loud sounds produced. Elderly and ill are also not comfortable with them. Increase in the sound levels can lead to temporary or permanent hearing loss, restlessness, sleep disturbances and even high blood pressure, nausea and stress-related illnesses, and lost productivity. Also, many people tend to use loudspeakers and loud musical instruments, etc., during the festivities adding to the overall level of noise pollution.[55]

In some bombs, the sound level produced is >100 decibels (dB). This is known to cause damage to the tympanic membrane leading to temporary deafness which recovers in 7–10 days. If the sound level is >140 dB, permanent deafness can result. To avoid this, the governmental regulations do not allow bombs with >80 dB to be manufactured. A noise level beyond 125 dB is equivalent to take-off of an air force jet. The government limits noise level to 55 dB in daytime and 45 dB at night for residential areas. The Central Pollution Control Board (CPCB) of India and the Ministry of Environment, Forests and Climate Change (MoEF and CC) prohibits the manufacture, sale and use of firecrackers breaching the noise limits of 125 dB (AI) or 145 $dB(C)_{pk}$ tested at 4 m distance from the point of bursting.[56]

Respiratory Illnesses Produced/Precipitated by Smoke Pollution in the Environment

Fireworks/firecrackers can also cause respiratory problems such as allergic bronchitis, bronchial asthma, sinusitis, rhinitis, pneumonia, and laryngitis. A lot of smoke is produced and precipitates the attacks of asthma in susceptible people. The byproducts of combustion contain various toxic and nontoxic chemicals which can cause inhalational injury. Thus, signs and symptoms of respiratory tract injury must be looked for in burns in closed spaces due to firecrackers.

Miscellaneous

A number of people die due to collapse of buildings and may sustain head injuries and fractures of bones, etc. Crackers also contribute to "smog" which is a mixture of smoke and fog. This reduces visibility leading to road traffic accidents. The light and sound of crackers also scares and tortures the birds and pet and stray animals because their ears have greater sensitivity as compared to humans. Some mischievous and rogue people even mess with the poor strays during such times. They tie firecrackers to their tail and ignite for fun, not realizing what it costs to the poor animals. The birds also get impacted badly. The bright light can disorient or blind them.

MANAGEMENT

Not >10% of the firecracker injury victims require admission. Patients are generally treated on outpatient basis. However, the moderate to extensive burn injuries due to clothes catching fire need to be admitted. Patients coming with ocular injuries, blast injuries of hand, and facial burns with edema require admission.

Management of a burn patient in general and wound care in particular is the same as for any other minor or major thermal burn which has been elaborated elsewhere in several chapters of this book. All burn wounds must be thoroughly washed with saline to remove foreign bodies before dressing. Cracker injuries to face may lead to permanent tattooing, if not taken care of well.

Blast injuries of the hand need a fast and carefully planned approach for treatment. There may be isolated skin lacerations to devastating injuries necessitating amputations and staged reconstructions including microsurgical tissue transfers over a prolonged period of time. A detailed clinical examination initially in the emergency room but sometimes exploration only under anesthesia without and with tourniquet will reveal the extent of injury and help in further management. X-ray skiagrams, both anteroposterior and lateral views, need to be done before the victim is shifted to operation theatre.

For lacerations of the hand, suturing is done to reposition the tissues back to as normal as possible. Meticulous debridement is done with removal of all the devitalized tissues and particulate matter.[57] Firecrackers commonly fracture the thumb bones and destabilize its carpometacarpal joint. It requires fixation of fractures generally with K-wires.[32,33] In case the bones and neurovascular structures are exposed, various pedicled, distant flaps, and rarely free flaps have to be considered. The most commonly used flap is the groin flap. The first web space needs special consideration as a bad adduction contracture may result, requiring secondary reconstructive procedures, in case not prevented. Severe mutilating blast injuries of the hand may need amputations at appropriate levels. The principles of "spare part surgery" must be remembered before throwing any amputated part(s) into the dustbin.

The patients of ocular injuries require thorough and copious irrigation of the eyes with normal saline. Particulate matter and soot particles including phosphorus and other foreign bodies have to be removed manually under local topical/general anesthesia followed by saline irrigation again and Fluorescein staining done to look for corneal involvement. pH is monitored before and after.

While every patient with ocular trauma undergoes thorough clinical examination, selected cases require slit lamp examination, intraocular pressure, ocular B-scan ultrasonography, gonioscopy, fundus photography, X-ray, and CT scan of the orbit to rule out intraocular/intraorbital foreign body or orbital fractures.[58,59] Visual acuity is also checked at the time of first examination and finally after complete recovery. >85% patients have unilateral injury. Surgical intervention is required in one-fourth of cases. Sclerocorneal tears need to be sutured, if required. Evisceration of the affected eye may be required in extreme cases. Antibiotic eye drops, lubricating solutions and ointments, and cycloplegic eye drops are prescribed. Systemic antibiotics and anti-inflammatory drugs and other adjuvant drugs may have to be prescribed.

All patients who complain of diminished hearing need to be examined by an otologist who gets audiometry and other tests done and advises appropriate treatment.[55] Use of green crackers which have lesser dB noise production, watching crackers bursting from a greater distance and use of ear plugs are some of the options at an individual level to reduce harmful effects of noise.

PREVENTION

For the last several decades, it is well known that bursting of fireworks/firecrackers leads to millions of burns and other injuries and deaths every year apart from atmospheric and noise pollution and destruction of property and consequent economic losses. They are a major source of preventable trauma and a worldwide menace. A retrospective study over 15 years from 2000 to 2015 found that consumer fireworks/firecrackers usage leads to a number of life-altering injuries annually.[60]

From time to time, many medical associations and environmentalists all over the world approach the authorities for the enactment/modification of laws to ban/limit their production and sale. Several governments have tried to ban them but none has succeeded completely and permanently. This is because of the pressure of a large, ever-increasing size of this industry providing livelihood to millions of people and the socio-religious nature of the festivals. A total ban on fireworks/firecrackers is even counterproductive.[61] In fact, it promotes the development of illegal manufacture and sale without informing end users about the potential dangers. Such illicit products, obviously devoid of standard safety features pose greater risk, ultimately lifting of ban allowing restricted use. Homemade fireworks/firecrackers are always illegal and thus should not be used.

In Singapore, a partial ban on firecrackers was imposed in 1970 and converted to complete ban in 1972. However, in 2003 firecrackers were allowed to be set off during festival seasons under controlled conditions by Singapore Tourism Board. Similarly, in United States in 1973, the National Society for the Prevention of Blindness proposed to The US Consumer Product Safety Commission (responsible for regulating fireworks under Government Act) a total ban on the sale of firecrackers for personal use and a temporary ban was imposed. Despite this ban having the support of American Academy of Pediatrics, American Public Health Association and National Fire Protection Association, etc., the ban had to be lifted the same year. At present, although these are not illegal in US, there are strict regulations regarding their sale, possession, and use. Unfortunately, the laws vary widely from one state to another and even one county to another.[56,62,63]

Dutch Safety Board, an independent authority for the government, found New Year Eve as the most dangerous event in Netherlands and recommended prohibition of some specific firecrackers for private use.[64] Some selected devices are sold for one day in a year.[65] Despite all the efforts by the government legislation and enforcement, illegal firecrackers are readily available and injuries occur outside legal period.[66]

Various studies are being conducted and published from all parts of the world and from various regions of large countries, collecting data, and trends over several years or decades as information for the respective governments to revise their policies with respect to firecrackers.[67]

Unfortunately, contradictive legislation exists where in one country explosives are banned and aerials allowed (e.g., South Africa and New Zealand) and in another country, aerial devices are banned and explosives allowed (e.g., Norway). Even within a single country, the laws may be different in different states. As a medical community, it is our responsibility to collect and supply data on the health risks of consumer fireworks/firecrackers and feed the government agencies on their legislation with evidence-based arguments.[68]

The fireworks/firecrackers are deeply ingrained in the Indian psyche and sociocultural fabric. Their sale is largely unrestricted in India and people including small children have access to a variety of firecrackers.

Green Firecrackers

In 2017, Supreme Court of India banned firecrackers in Delhi. This led to a loss of 1,000 crores rupees of business to the firecracker industry leading to a loss of employment to a very large number of workers. Consequent to this, the National Environmental and Engineering Research Institute (NEERI) [under the aegis of Council for Scientific and Industrial Research (CSIR)] developed what are known as "green crackers or ecofriendly" crackers in 2018.[69] In 2020, National Green Tribunal of India banned the sale and use of conventional firecrackers in the National Capital Region. Stated simply, the green crackers cause lesser air and noise pollution (100–130 dB vs. 160–200 dB) than the crackers manufactured and available earlier. Barium nitrate, magnesium, and arsenic were replaced by potassium nitrate, aluminum, and carbon in green crackers. At present, the green crackers can be legally manufactured only by those manufacturers who have signed agreements with CSIR and obtained license.

The green crackers have the following advantages:

- Reduction in air smoke pollution
- Reduction in toxic chemicals pollution
- Reduction in noise pollution

They do have the following shortcomings:

- There is no reduction in risk of getting burnt by the end user and fire-related incidents.
- Even so-called green firecrackers do emit toxic chemicals.
- There is extreme shortage of these crackers because of permission being given only to a few large manufacturers by CSIR.
- Increased risk of manufacture and sale of spurious products and difficulty in their identification with consequent greater risk of injuries
- Higher cost to the public at large
- Complete absence of small-scale and cottage industry and last but not the least
- No alternatives have been suggested for the livelihood of the thousands of crores of rupees industry feeding lakhs of people and their families directly or indirectly (increased unemployment).

A green logo and quick response (QR) coding system have been devised to distinguish green crackers from standard ones.

Not only green, but another concept toward a cleaner environment being tested by CSIR-CEERI in Pilani, Rajasthan is called E-crackers or electric crackers.

Recommendations to Prevent/Minimize Fireworks/Firecracker-related Injuries

A number of recommendations have been made to prevent/minimize fireworks/firecracker-related injuries. The most important consideration is the recognition by the general public as well as the authorities to the fact that these innocuous looking toys in various shapes and sizes covered in attractive, multicolored paper have the full potential of harm as we relate with the military combat ammunitions. Hence, the laws with respect to their manufacture, quality control, transportation, storage, retail sale, and finally use by the lay public must be stringent, modified/upgraded from time to time and strictly enforced. These rules also require obtaining a license for the intended activity (e.g., manufacture or retail sale, etc.) from the appropriate governmental agencies. Unfortunately, the failure to strictly implement the rules and regulations is the biggest cause of mishaps in our vast country.

Over the last few decades, with sustained education of school children about the harm caused by firecrackers coupled with the slogan, "say "NO" to crackers", the incidence of these injuries has declined. In Safdarjung Hospital, New Delhi, one of the largest burn care facilities in India, the number of patients presenting to Burns Casualty on Diwali night has fallen to 131 in 2008 from over 400 cases in1991 (authors' personal unpublished data) despite a manifold increase in the city population.

As far as possible, there should be a community display of fireworks in open areas by professional persons during festivals and celebrations. The display site should be a large, flat, and open area. There must not be any electric wires, huts, and houses with combustible material lying on rooftop so common in Indian scenario, railways, fuel tanks, etc., which might initiate fire. Individual use of crackers by one and all should be discouraged.

Firecrackers are a significant cause of partial or total permanent blindness with children being especially vulnerable. Hence, all precautions should be taken to ensure their safety by the adults. Public awareness programs by ophthalmologists using media and public lectures, etc., along with activities at school level, government, and nongovernment organizations should help in decreasing this preventable blindness.

A number of unsafe practices at end user level have already been enumerated above and one must avoid them. Some other precautions to be observed are listed below:

- Ensure that passersby are out of range and onlookers are warned before lighting fireworks/firecrackers.
- While firing rockets, ensure that it is upright in a stable bottle.
- Keep one or two buckets of water available in the area where crackers are burst. In case of any mishap, they come handy not only to cool the burnt area but also to extinguish any fire (remember the logo, "pour water on burns," "every fire is small to begin with").
- Wear tight fitting thick cotton dresses. Avoid loose flowing synthetic dresses.
- Store firecrackers in a safe place, until they are needed, away from risk of fire.
- Always use a long "phooljhari" or a candle to ignite crackers keeping the elbow joint straight to maximize the distance between cracker and the body.
- Do not apply oil, toothpaste, or any other homemade remedies/ointment on burnt areas.
- Do not panic and drive recklessly while transporting the victim to medical services. A delay of 1 hour or so does not matter.

SUMMARY

The fireworks/firecrackers are more than two millennia old and have become synonymous with festive mood across the people of the world. They are associated with personal and religious functions, national state functions, New Year's Day of various countries, sports events, etc. They are billions of dollar industry providing employment and livelihood to millions of people. They are also associated with large short- and long-term morbidity and even mortality apart from economic losses and loss to property. The only solution to its minimization is strict enforcement of laws related to them and precautions being observed by the end user as a total ban on their manufacture is not possible. Various studies conducted in different countries have demonstrated time and again the positive effect of such measures. The festivals are occasions of joy and fireworks/firecrackers are an enjoyable spectacle. They must not be turned into "unfortunate dates" to be remembered for the rest of one's life.

REFERENCES

1. Ajith S, Sivapragasam C, Arumugaprabu V. A review on hazards and their consequences in firework industries. SN Appl. Sci. 2019;1:120.
2. Wikipedia. (2024). Sivakasi. [online] Available from https://en.wikipedia.org/wiki/Sivakasi [Last accessed May, 2024].
3. Smith GA, Knapp JF, Barnett TM, Shields BJ. The rockets' red glare, the bombs bursting in air: Fireworks-related injuries to children. Pediatrics.1996;98:1-9.
4. Bagri N, Saha A, Chandelia S, Dubey NK, Bhatt A, Rai A, et al. Fireworks injuries in children: A prospective study during the festival of lights. Emerg Med Australas. 2013;25(5):452-6.
5. Wang C, Zhao R, Du W-L, Ning FG, Zhang AZ. Firework injuries at a major trauma and burn center: a five-year prospective study. Burns. 2014;40:305-10.
6. Smittenberg MN, Lungelow D, Rode H, B van As A, Millar AJW. Can fireworks-related injuries to children during festivities be prevented? S Afr Med J. 2010;100:525-8.

7. Nizamoglu M, Frew Q, Tan A, Band H, band B, Barnes D, et al. The 10-year experience of firework injuries treated at a UK regional burns and plastic surgery unit. Ann Burns Fire Disasters. 2018;31(1):13-6.
8. Tandon R, Agrawal K, Narayan RP, Tiwari VK, Prakash V, Kumar S, et al. Firecracker injuries during Diwali festival: The epidemiology and impact of legislation in Delhi. Indian J Plast Surg. 2012;45:97-101.
9. Sarma BP. Epidemiology, treatment and preventive strategy in Diwali-related burns. Indian J Burns. 2012;20:42-5.
10. Puri V, Mahendru S, Rana R, Deshpande M. Firework injuries: a ten-year study. J Plast Reconstr Aesthet Surg. 2009;62(9): 1103-11.
11. Mohan A, Nolan GS, Jain A. Firework-related blast injury to the hand and treatment algorithm. BMJ Case Rep. 2019;12:e231804.
12. Mohan D, Varghese M. Fireworks cast a shadow on India's festival of lights. World Health Forum. 1990;11:323-26.
13. Mehta DR, Suri MP, Patel CK, Agrawal AB, Vora HJ, Raibagkar SC. Firework Injuries-Epidemiology and Prevention. Indian J of Burns. 2004;12:48-50.
14. Rosenthal AR, Oakley G. Firework related ocular injury. J R Soc Med. 1988;81(10):559-60.
15. Moore JX, McGwin G, Griffin RL. The epidemiology of firework-related injuries in the United States: 2000–2010. Injury. 2014; 45(11):1704-9.
16. Kalita K, Gurindagunta SV. Fire-cracker burn injuries during Diwali, a seasonal and preventable epidemic. Indian J Burns. 2021;29:70-5.
17. Sethy A, Saha S, Hazra D, Abhilash KP. A retrospective study on clinical profile of patients with firecracker-related injury presenting to the emergency department of a tertiary care center in South India. Curr Med Issues. 2020;18:1-6.
18. Chakraborti C, Majumdar S, Gayen S. Profile of firecracker injuries of the eye during Diwali: A tertiary eye-care center study. Med J DY Patil Vidyapeeth. 2019;12:415-8.
19. Patel R, Mukherjee B. Crash & Burn: Ocular Injuries due to Fireworks. Semin Ophthalmol. 2016;31:243-8.
20. Unterlauft JD, Rehak M, Wiedemann P, Meier P. Firework-related eye trauma in Germany. Curr Eye Res. 2018;43(12):1522-8.
21. Shiuey EJ, Kolomeyer AM, Kolomeyer NN. Assessment of firework-related ocular injury in the US. JAMA Ophthalmol. 2020;138(6):618-23.
22. Katoria D, Mehta D, Sehgal D, Kumar S. A Review of Risks to Workers Associated with Fireworks Industry. Int J Environ Engineer Manag. 2013;4(3):259-64.
23. Jegatheesan K, Selvakumar M, Kalaivani K. Quality of work life of workers in fireworks industry–A study with reference to Tamil Nadu. Int J Sci Technol Manag. 2017;6(2):287-97.
24. Jackson D. Injuries from fireworks. Br Med J. 1961;2(5261):1184-7.
25. Jeyabal P, Davies L, Rousselot A, Agrawal R. Fireworks: boon or bane to our eyes? Int Ophthalmol. 2019;39(10):2407-11.
26. Kumar R, Puttanna M, Sriprakash KS, Sujatha Rathod BL, Prabhakaran VC. Firecracker eye injuries during Deepavali festival: a case series. Indian J Ophthalmol. 2010;58(2):157-9.
27. Kuhn F, Morris R, Witherspoon CD, Mann L, Mester V, Módis L, et al. Serious fireworks-related eye injuries. Ophthal Epidemiol. 2000;7(2):139-48.
28. Frimmel S, Faber DJT, Wubbels RJ, Kniestedt C, Paridaens D. Type, severity, management and outcome of ocular and adnexal firework-related injuries: the Rotterdam experience. Acta Ophthalmol. 2018;96:607-15.
29. John D, Philip SS, Mittal R, John SS, Paul P. Spectrum of ocular firework injuries in children: A 5-year retrospective study during a festive season in Southern India. Indian J Ophthalmol. 2015;63:843-6.
30. Gupta H, Gupta P, Tyagi R, Gupta M. Analysis of ocular trauma due to firecracker injury in oculoplasty clinic at a tertiary care hospital of North India. Int J Ocul Oncol Oculoplasty. 2019;5(4):251-5.
31. Adhikari S, Bandyopadhyay T, Sarkar T, Saha JK. Blast injuries to the hand: Pathomechanics, patterns, and treatment. J Emerg Trauma Shock. 2013;6:29-36.
32. Hazani R, Buntic RF, Brooks D. Patterns in blast injuries to the hand. Hand (NY). 2009;4(1):44-9.
33. Otene CI, Emeagui NK, Obu GO, Odikpo BO, Otene CO, Ikubor JE. Blast injuries to the hand from celebrations gone wrong – a series of disabling injuries from firecrackers. Int J Forensic Med Invest. 2016;2(1)36-40.
34. Ortiz R, Ozkan S, Chen NC, Eberlin KR. Firework Injuries of the Hand: An Analysis of Treatment and Health Care Utilization Hand (NY). 2020;15(6):831-6.
35. Ng ZY, Shamrock A, Chen D, Dodds SD, Chim H. Patterns of Complex Carpal Injuries in the Hand from Fireworks. J Hand Microsurg 2018;10:93-100.
36. Al-Qattan MM, Al-Tamimi AS. Localized hand burns with or without concurrent blast injuries from fireworks. Burns. 2009; 35(3):425-9.
37. Sandvall BK, Keys KA, Friedrich JB. Severe hand injuries from fireworks: injury patterns, outcomes and fireworks types. J Hand Surg Am. 2017;42:385.e1-385.e8.
38. Hahn P, Brederlau J, Krimmer H, Lanz U. Explosion injuries of the hand. Spatial relationship and injury pattern. J Hand Surg Br. 1996;21(6):785-7.
39. Philipson MR, Southern SJ. The blast component of firework injuries-not to be underestimated. Injury, Int J Care Injured. 2004;35:1042-3.
40. Liu S, Krewski D, Shi Y, Chen Y, Burnett RT. Association between gaseous ambient air pollutants and adverse pregnancy outcomes in Vancouver, Canada. Environ Health Perspect. 2003; 111(14):1773-8.
41. Curtis L, Rea W, Smith-Willis P, Fenyves E, Pan Y. Adverse health effects of outdoor air pollutants. Environ Int. 2006;32(6):815-30.
42. Vecchi R, Bernardoni V, Cricchio D D'Alessandro A, Fermo P, Lucarelli F, et al. The impact of fireworks on airborne particles. Atmospheric Environment. 2008;42(6):1121-32
43. Singh A, Pant P, Pope FD. Air quality during and after festivals: Aerosol concentrations, composition and health effects. Atmos Res. 2019;227:220-32.
44. Khaiwal R, Kumar S, Mor S. Long-term assessment of firework emissions and air quality during Diwali festival and impact of 2020 fireworks ban on air quality over the states of Indo Gangetic Plains airshed in India. Atmospheric Environment. 2022;285.
45. Yerramsetti VS, Sharma AR, Navlur NG. Rapolu V, Dhulipala NSKC, Sinha PR. The impact assessment of Diwali fireworks emissions on the air quality of a tropical urban site, Hyderabad, India, during three consecutive years. Environ Monit Assess.2013;185: 7309-25.
46. Chatterjee A, Sarkar C, Adak A. Mukherjee U, Ghosh SK, Raha S. Ambient Air Quality during Diwali Festival over Kolkata–A Mega-City in India. Aerosol and Air Quality Research, 2013;13: 1133–44.

47. Agrawal A, Vinay K, Upadhyay VK, Sachdeva K. Study of aerosol behavior on the basis of morphological characteristics during festival events in India. Atmospheric Environment. 2011; 45(21):3640-4.
48. Deka P, Hoque RR. Diwali Fireworks: Early Signs of Impact on PM10 Properties of Rural Brahmaputra Valley Aerosol and Air Quality Research. 2014;14:1752-62.
49. Rao PS, Gajghate DG, Gavane AG, Suryawanshi P, Chauhan C, Mishra S, et al. Air quality status during Diwali festival of India: a case study. Bull Environ Contam Toxicol. 2012;89: 376-9.
50. Barman SC, Singh R, Negi MP, Bhargava SK. Ambient air quality of Lucknow City (India) during use of fireworks on Diwali Festival. Environ Monit Assess. 2008;37(1-3):495-504.
51. Hirai K, Yamazaki Y, Okada K, Furuta S, Kubo K. Acute eosinophilic pneumonia associated with smoke from fireworks. Intern Med (Japan). 2000;39:401-3.
52. Gupta D, Vishwakarma SK. Toy weapons and firecrackers: a source of hearing loss. Laryngoscope.1989;99:330-4.
53. Smoorenburg GF. Risk of noise-induced hearing loss following exposure to Chinese firecrackers. Audiology. 1993;32(6): 333-43.
54. Liao YH, Young YH. Inner ear damage by firecracker trauma. Audiol Neurotol. 2018;23:116-21.
55. Le TN, Straatman LV, Lea J, Westerberg B. Current insights in noise-induced hearing loss: a literature review of the underlying mechanism, pathophysiology, asymmetry, and management options. J Otolaryngol Head Neck Surg. 2017;46(1):41.
56. Lokhande SK, Garg N, Jain MC, Rayalu S. Evaluation and analysis of firecrackers noise: Measurement Uncertainty, legal noise regulations and noise induced hearing loss. Applied Acoustics. 2000;186:108462.
57. Saucedo JM, Vedder NB. Firework-related injuries of the hand. J Hand Surg Am. 2015;40(2):383-7.
58. Tomar M, Sharma G, Tuli R, Sharma RK. Firecracker-related ocular injuries during Diwali festival season in a tertiary care center in Northern India. International Medicine 2020;2(1):20-7.
59. Parija S, Chakraborty K, Ravikumar SR. Firework related ocular injuries in Eastern IndiaA clinicoepidemiological analysis. Indian J Ophthalmol. 2021;69:3538-44.
60. Read DJ, Bradbury R, Yeboah E. Firework-related injury in the Top End: A 16-year review. ANZ J Surg. 2017;87(12):1030-4.
61. Matheron AS, Hendriks S, Facca S, Liverneaux PA. Hand injuries due to firework devices: A series of 58 cases. Chirurgie de la Main. 2014;33(2):124-9.
62. Serra Lopez VM, Cheema AN, Gray BL, Pirruccio K, Kazmers NH. Epidemiology of Fireworks-Related Injuries to the Upper Extremity in the United States From 2011 to 2017. J Hand Surg Glob Online. 2020;2(3):117-20.
63. Canner JK, Haider AH, Selvarajah S, Xuan Hui MPH, Wang H, et al. US emergency department visits for fireworks injuries, 2006–2010. J Surg Res. 2014;190(1):305-11.
64. Van Yperen DT, Van Lieshout EMM, Dijkshoorn JN, Vlies CHVD, Verhofstad MHJ. Injuries, treatment, and impairment caused by different types of fireworks; results of a ten-year multicenter retrospective cohort study. Scandinavian J Trauma, Resusc Emerg Med. 2021;29:1-9.
65. Martín-Alberca C, García-Ruiz C. Analytical techniques for the analysis of consumer fireworks. Trends Anal Chem. 2014;56: 27-36.
66. Van de Kar AL, Eijffinger EM, Lapid O, van der Horst CM, de Haart M. An exploratory study of the impact of firecracker-induced hand injuries on adolescents and their parents. Euro J Plastic Surg. 2022:45:159-68.
67. Chaparro-Narváez P, Cotes-Cantillo K, Castañeda-Orjuela C, Hoz-Restrepo FDL. Injuries due to fireworks use: A surveillance data analysis in Colombia, 2008–2013. Burns. 2016;43(1):149-56.
68. Wisse RP, Bijlsma WR, Stilma JS. Ocular firework trauma: A systematic review on incidence, severity, outcome and prevention. Br J Ophthalmol. 2010;94:1586-91.
69. CSIR- National Environment Engineering Research Institute (NEERI). (2024). Green Crackers. [online] Available from https://www.neeri.res.in/abouts/details/green-crackers#googtrans(en|en) [Last accessed May, 2024).

SECTION

5

Burns of Special Sites

CHAPTER 26

Facial Burns

PS Bhandari, Aakanksha Goel, Arun Goel

INTRODUCTION

Burns of the face (including head and neck), hands and perineum (including external genitalia) have always been considered as "burns of special sites". As elsewhere, the face is also a composite structure of bone, muscles, nerves, fat, blood vessels, skin, and other tissues. Thus, one may like to ask as to what is so special about the face. The fact is that the face is much more than the sum of its tissues.

It is a functional, dynamic, and aesthetic region playing an important role in formal introduction, interaction, and communication with the rest of the world. It is the physical basis of self-image. Shilder defined body image as "the picture of our body which we form in our mind," or "the way in which our body appears to ourselves."[1] Body ideal is how an individual desires to appear. Any facial disfigurement or deformity that alters body image, leads to a great psychological trauma. The face with all its facial expressions is a mirror of the person's personality and thoughts. Many afflicted may choose to hide from public gaze and remain confined to four walls of their house. The victim becomes crippled both socially and psychologically. The root cause of patient's distress lies in the pressure a modern society puts to confirm to an ideal appearance. Any deviation leads to diminished value and stigmatization. Most of the scars in the body can be hidden by clothing and other means but facial scars are visible at first sight. One has to consider in a balanced way what all a plastic surgeon's intervention can offer for physical improvement of postburn facial disfigurement. Such patients also require supportive counseling. McGrouther has termed facial disfigurement as "the last bastion of discrimination."[2] A scarless, beautiful face is peer's envy, owner's pride. Indeed, beauty is skin deep only.

The Courts of law in India considers permanent facial disfigurement as a grievous hurt, keeping them at par with several other injuries, one of which is emasculation.

Apart from aesthetic reasons, face is the seat of sensory organs and aerodigestive orifices. There are various specialized structures such as eyes, mouth, nose, and ears which are critical to function and survival. Respiratory burns may threaten the very survival of a victim.

ETIOLOGY

Facial burns affect all age groups **(Figs. 1 and 2)**. As elsewhere, they can also be caused by dry or wet heat (thermal), electricity (high or low voltage; flash or contact), various chemicals, and radiation. Thermal burns are most common. Almost all the patients of flame burns have facial involvement to a lesser or greater extent.

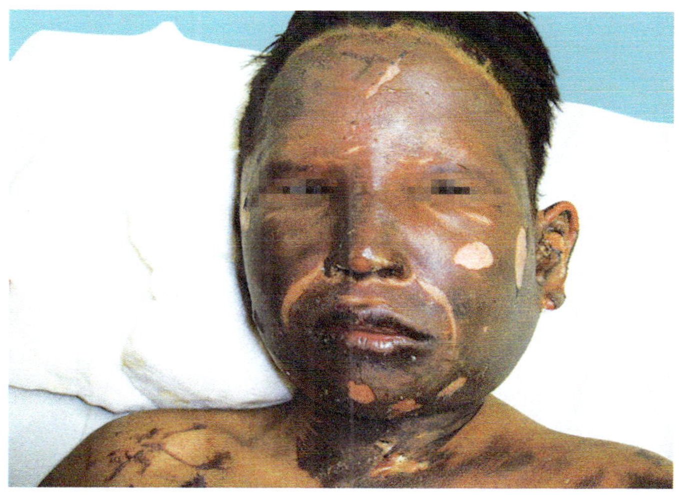

FIG. 1: Superficial burns of the face which are best treated by only conservative management—exposure treatment.

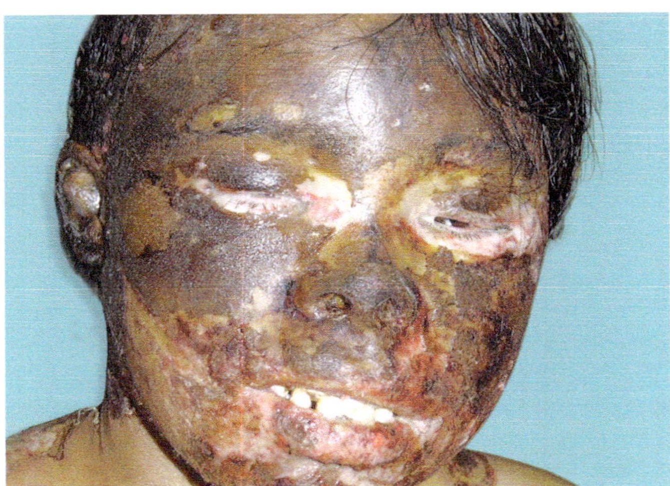

FIG. 2: Deep burns of the face which require surgical intervention for faster healing and to give good results.

Burns due to spillage of hot liquids is very common in small children. Steam burns of face are quite common in our kitchens apart from industries using boilers. Being exposed part of body, it is almost always involved in electrical flash burns and firecracker/fireworks injuries. Most of these burns are second-degree superficial dermal. Conversely, since the face is almost always an uncovered part of the body, any hot liquid or chemical coming in contact with face is immediately shaken off reflexly or else wiped off or trickles down with minimal duration of contact period. This is in contrast to usually covered areas where the removal of clothes with hot liquids or chemicals takes time increasing the contact period, in turn increasing the depth. Some of the deepest thermal burns are seen in epilepsy when the victim falls over a hot object in kitchen during a seizure attack and remains unconscious and unattended for a long time. Similar extremely deep burns involving even calvarium or deeper muscles of neck are seen in contact burns due to high-tension wires. Burns due to "chewing" of live electrical wire and leading to full thickness necrosis of angle of mouth along with adjacent upper and lower lips is seen in very small children. Contact electrical burns of scalp/calvarium often present with cataract after a few months. Homicidal acid burns (vitriolage) seen in our country, as a rule, involve face because the very intent of the culprit is to disfigure the face of the victim. They are one of the most important reasons for permanent loss of vision apart from causing one of the worst forms of disfigurement. Chemical burns are also seen following accidental ingestion and may be even suicidal or homicidal. Radiation burns have become rare because of improved technology of delivering radiation and alternate better methods of managing malignancies of cheek. Radiation necrosis of mandible with orocutaneous fistula was often seen earlier. Inhalation burns due to fires occurring in closed spaces [e.g., in modern centrally air-conditioned high-rise offices, shopping malls, and even hospital intensive care unit (ICUs)] and inhaling products of combustion and other toxic chemicals are being increasingly seen. Burns due to bursting of pressure kerosene stove can be associated with inhalation injury due to kerosene vapors.

GENERAL MANAGEMENT[3,4]

Burns of face (head and neck) rarely occur in isolation and vary from relatively minor insults to severe debilitating injuries. They need evaluation and management in the context of total body surface area (TBSA) burns of the patient as a whole, i.e., primary and secondary survey as per advanced trauma life support (ATLS) guidelines. For all these patients, first consideration to look for is, whether the air passages or the eyes have been burnt. In case of associated respiratory burn, it should be given the first priority and be treated accordingly (refer to Chapter 11 on respiratory tract injury). Burns of the face, especially thermal, are commonly associated with massive swelling of the head and neck due to looseness and rich vascular supply of tissues. There can be disproportionate loss of fluid as compared to other sites, with edema reaching its maximum in 72 hours, especially in second-degree burns. This may warrant intravenous fluid replacement more than the amount calculated as per TBSA burnt. At times, in third-degree full thickness burns, the swelling may not be apparent due to tough unyielding eschar. The edema fluid spreads and collects in the deeper tissues of the neck and may press upon the upper respiratory tract leading to obstruction of pharyngolarynx necessitating endotracheal intubation or even a tracheostomy in extreme cases. This means that it is possible that the victim is able to breath normally at the time of admission but may soon go downhill. They may need escharotomy of neck and chest (if involved in full thickness circumferential burn with tight constricting eschar) for decompression and improved respiration. There may be difficulty in swallowing or throwing out vomitus as well with risk of inhaling it. It is preferable to insert a Ryle's tube before edema makes this simple procedure difficult. The endotracheal tube and nasogastric tube should be fixed in such a way that they do not cause pressure necrosis locally. The eyes may be closed (due to periorbital edema) and hence need examination as soon as possible before edema makes the assessment almost impossible. Thus, help of an intensivist/pulmonologist and ophthalmologist, has to be sought early in many of such cases, immediately after the patient comes under one's care. Patients with facial burns should be nursed in head elevated position as this reduces edema by increasing the venous return and also helps in breathing by facilitating diaphragmatic excursion.

The patient is assessed as a whole with respect to extent and depth of burn. Apart from the initial depth of burn, it is the better standards of treatment of the burned face in the acute stage that decides the improved overall aesthetic and functional outcome. Treatment of facial burns in acute stage is controversial as there is no consensus amongst burn specialists regarding the type of treatment (conservative or excisional), timing of surgical intervention, the technique to be used, etc. Traditionally, facial burns have been treated conservatively for following reasons:

- Difficulty in evaluating the depth of facial burn injury.
- Excellent blood supply of head and neck region makes the burn heal faster and almost resistant to infection. However, saliva and food eaten may cause contamination and infection of facial wound.
- Presence of increased number of sweat and sebaceous glands ensures faster and spontaneous re-epithelialization of partial-thickness burns and faster separation of eschar in full-thickness burns. In males, the roots of a large number of hair follicles in beard and moustache region go deeper into dermis and subcutaneous tissues and survive and supply keratinocytes even in deep dermal burns for faster healing. Their deeper locations make them withstand the onslaught of burn injury.
- Full-thickness burns of face are uncommon and other associated injuries must be attended to first because of their life-threatening nature.
- Excessive bleeding during early tangential excision.
- One must remember that the muscles of facial expression are attached to overlying dermis and radical debridement may even excise the muscles, seriously affecting the facial expression.
- Last but not the least, excision of subcutaneous fat may lead to severe contour deformity.

The goal of facial burn wound management, as elsewhere, is to heal them in minimum period of time to avoid scars. Thus, they have been broadly classified into two types, one which heal within 3 weeks of time and those which take longer. While the former heals with or without minimal scarring, the latter often leads to hypertrophic scar formation and contraction, and usually requires surgical intervention **(Fig. 3)**. Unfortunately, there is no objective measurement which can predict whether a facial burn will heal of its own or will require surgical intervention. This is because the appearance of burn wound changes with time and also after application of

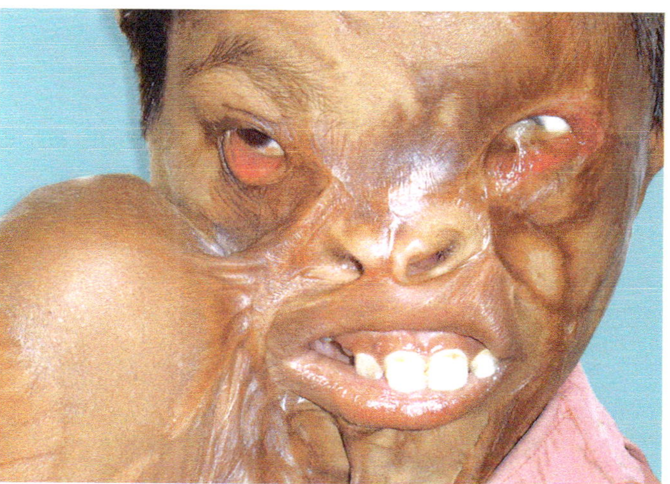

FIG. 3: Neglected facial burns in which wounds healed by severe scarring and contraction—severe contraction of neck with ectropion of lids and lips and left eye corneal loss and nose deformity. These cases are very difficult to manage for correction of all the deformities. *Courtesy:* Editor.

various antimicrobial creams/ointments. Furthermore, a given anatomical depth of burn may not heal in a nonhair-bearing area whereas it may heal reasonably well in a hair-bearing area in a male.

Conservative management of facial burns can be either by exposure technique or closed technique though the former is more commonly followed. The burned area is cleansed gently with mild antibacterial soap and normal saline. The hair in the burnt area and around, which try to stick on burnt areas due to oozing from wound, should preferably be clipped short or combed and kept away with hair pins. Mild debridement can be done but sharp debridement should be avoided as it is often difficult to determine the exact depth of injury. Flash or scalds usually result in superficial partial-thickness burn. Because of rich vascularity, there is a lot of oozing from the burn wound. This fluid forms a thick crust on drying. It can develop cracks due to dryness and may bleed or serve as a culture medium for bacteria. An antibiotic ointment should be applied to the burn wound to maintain a moist environment, prevent bacterial growth and crust formation. Paraffin gauze may also be applied **(Fig. 4)**. It keeps the crust soft and prevents it from cracking and bleeding until healing. It also prevents any increase in depth of burn wound. Eyes must be protected from the topical ointment applied on the face by leaving a periorbital margin uncovered by the ointment or alternatively applying an ophthalmic antibiotic ointment over the face so that it does not harm the eye. All this is followed on daily basis. Second-degree superficial dermal

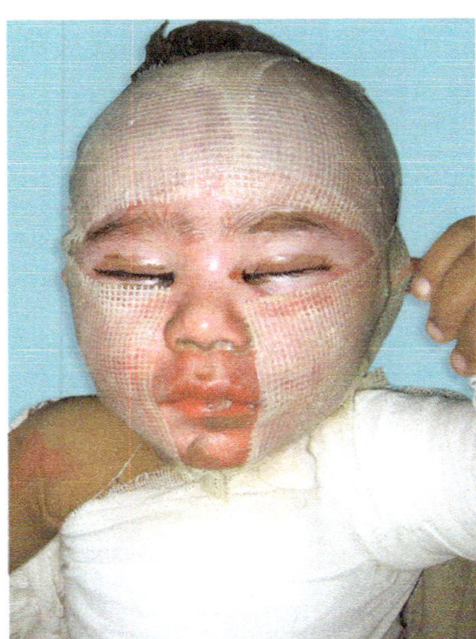

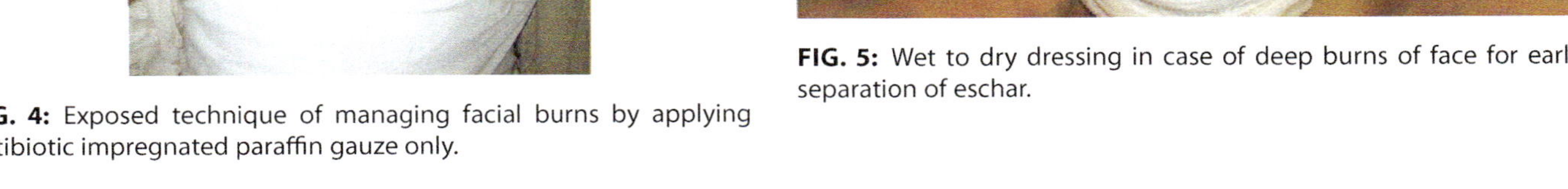

FIG. 4: Exposed technique of managing facial burns by applying antibiotic impregnated paraffin gauze only.

FIG. 5: Wet to dry dressing in case of deep burns of face for early separation of eschar.

burns heal in <3 weeks. However, deep dermal burns may take up to 6 weeks to heal but with severe hypertrophic scarring and even severe contractures. Chemical burns of the face are best treated by leaving the wound open and dry as the wound epithelializes rapidly under the eschar and the eschar separates by itself.

The conservative management by closed technique is followed when the burns are very limited and dressings can easily be applied without any hinderance to oral cavity, eyes, and nostrils. It consists of application of nonstick paraffin gauze, antimicrobial cream or ointment, multiple layers of absorbent gauze, Gamgee pads, and bandage. If available, biological dressings or skin substitutes may be used to expedite the healing and need for dressing change is also lessened.[5] Burns of the pinna need closed method only for their optimal management (discussed later). The healed areas should be gently washed daily and kept lubricated to prevent drying up.

Historically, even apparently full-thickness burns of face have been managed conservatively by dressings, allowing for spontaneous eschar separation, and formation of healthy granulation tissue underneath. This takes around 3 weeks. This raw area is then split skin grafted. Topical antimicrobial creams/ointments should be replaced by wet to dry dressings with saline (or povidone-iodine solution) impregnated gauze after it becomes clear (usually by 2 weeks) that the burn is deeper and will need skin grafting for its closure. It helps in superficial debridement of necrotic tissues. These dressings are applied wet over the wound after placement of a layer of nonstick paraffin gauze and are removed

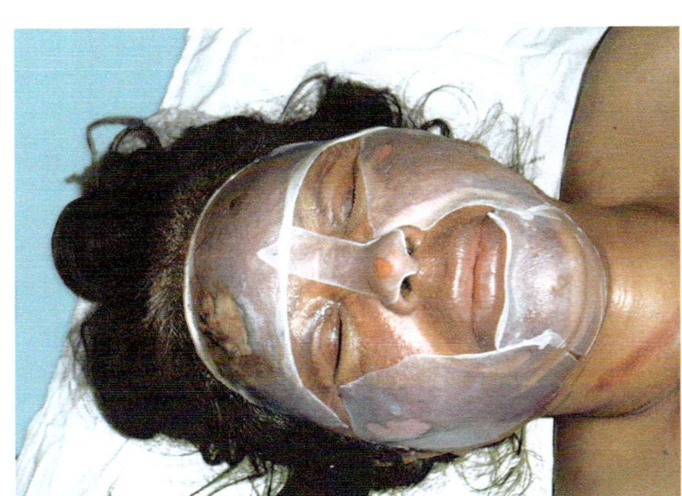

FIG. 6: Collagen application on facial burns.

only when dry **(Fig. 5)**. Necrotic debris gets attached to the dry dressing and on removal, the necrotic tissue also comes out with the dressing. Direct application of gauze to wound is not only painful but also causes severe pain every time the dressing is changed. It can also damage any regenerating neoepithelium. This should continue till the appearance of granulation tissue. Biological dressings and skin substitutes can be used **(Fig. 6)**. Various hydrogels, hydrocolloids, and alginates-based dressings are available. Human amnion and homograft can also be used. They help in formation of healthy granulation tissue, early wound closure, and shorten the period before grafting. Surgical debridement of obviously necrotic and

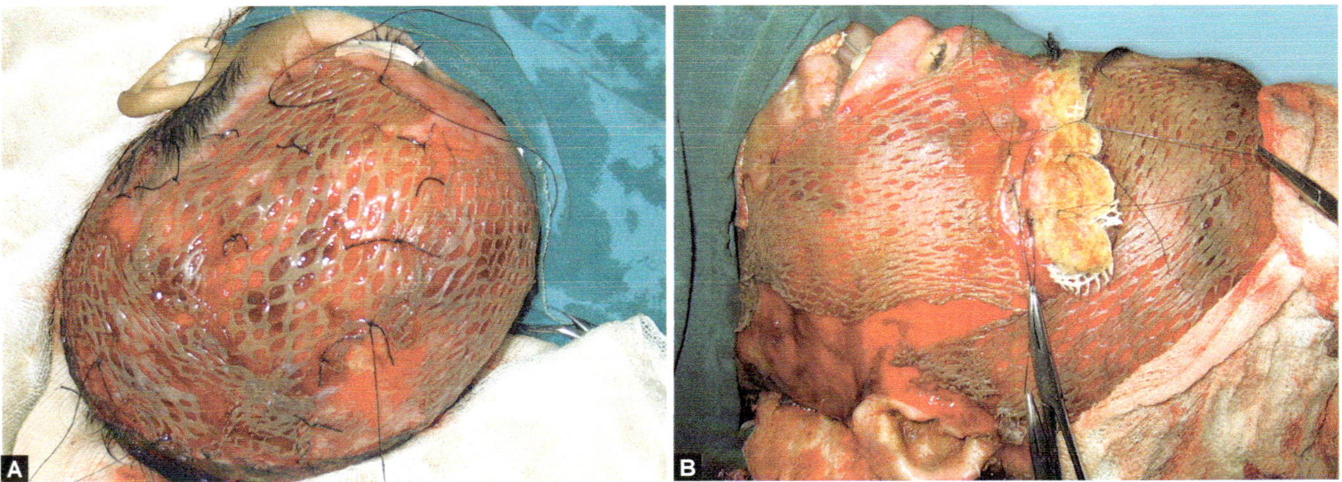

FIGS. 7A AND B: (A) Postburn raw areas of scalp grafted once the granulation is healthy. (B) Split skin graft applied to the raw area of face following deep burn. Graft meshed because of excessive bleeding from the wounds. Lids also released to correct the exposed eye.

loose tissue can also be done by forceps and scissors. When the granulation tissue is healthy and microbial culture-sensitivity reports of wound congenial for graft "take", it is covered with sheets of split thickness skin grafts. Meshed grafts are rarely, if ever, recommended unless the surface is bleeding profusely and there is risk of hematoma formation under the graft **(Figs. 7A and B)**. When the patient is taken up for grafting of raw areas, if any ectropion is developing in the eyelids, they can be released at the same sitting, thus, preventing any damage to the cornea.

Several authors have reported gratifying results after tangential excision and grafting of facial burn within 3–5 days of burn injury in selected patients where the burn wound is unlikely to heal within 21 days. Full thickness burns have also been treated by early excision and skin grafting with good results **(Figs. 8A and B)**.[6,7] One must remember that excisional surgery on face should be done only by surgeons who are doing it routinely for all other areas also and not by anyone doing once in a while.

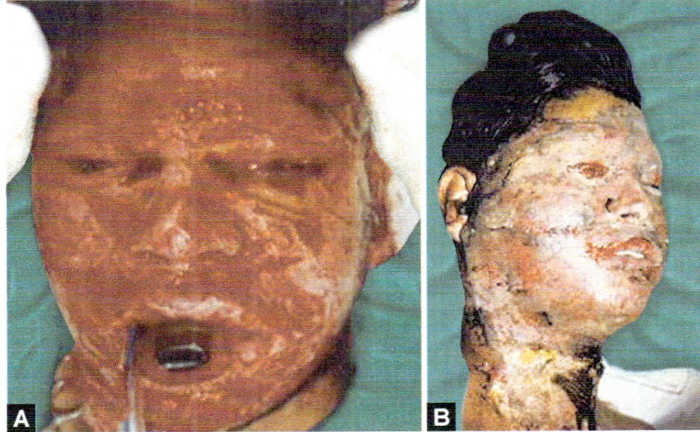

FIGS. 8A AND B: (A) Preoperative picture of early tangential excision of deep burns of face. (B) Postoperative picture of same patient with full "take" of skin graft over the excised area.

Patients with spontaneously healed partial-thickness burns and with full-thickness burns where grafting has been done are advised to avoid exposure to sunlight to prevent hyperpigmentation for at least 6–12 months following burn injury till the scars are mature. Sunscreen lotions [with sun protection factor (SPF) > 30] should be applied apart from other physical measures like umbrella, etc. if they need to move out during the sun. Because of loose and mobile nature of tissues in the face, postburn contractures after healing and grafting are common after facial burns. Patients should be advised to do regular massage of the spontaneously healed and skin grafted areas with bland oils and creams. There is a great risk of hypertrophy in the wounds that heal in >3 weeks and it should be prevented by use of pressure garments (face mask) 24 hours a day till scar maturation **(Figs. 9A and B)**. Splints, e.g., cervical collar, may be worn to prevent/minimize development of contracture neck. Conservative management of facial burn may, sometimes, lead to a poor aesthetic result, especially in deep dermal and full-thickness burns. They may need improvement after scar maturation using one or more of the wide array of reconstructive options at the disposal of a plastic surgeon.

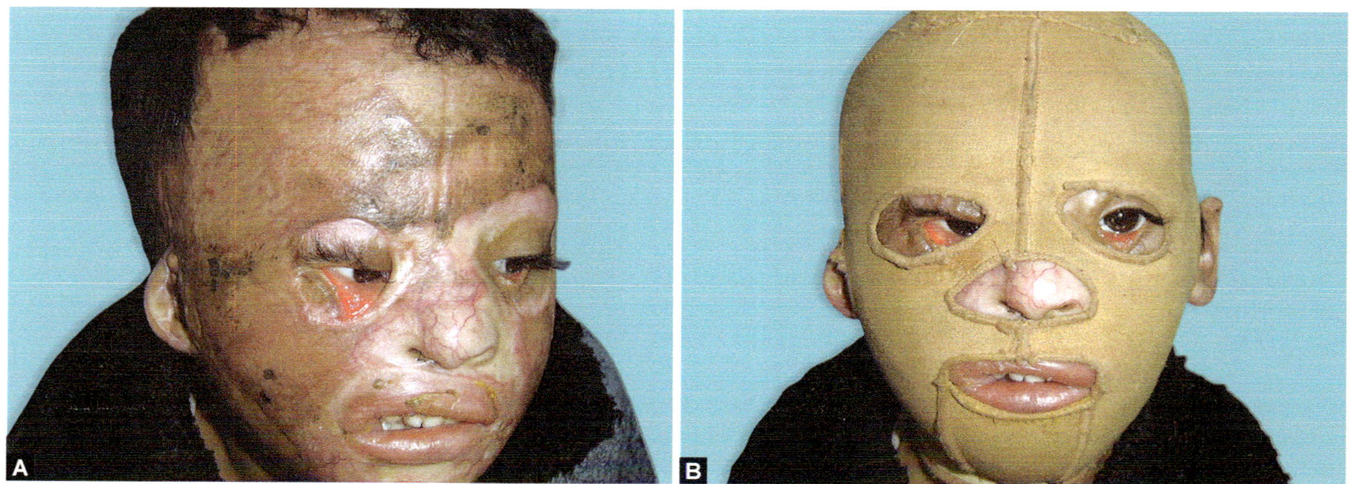

FIGS. 9A AND B: (A) Postoperative picture of skin grafted postburn raw areas of face. (B) Pressure garment in the form of a tailormade mask to be worn over the face for preventing hypertrophy of scars.

MANAGEMENT OF BURNS OF DIFFERENT PARTS OF THE FACE

Nose[8-10]

Nose is the most prominent and central part of face and is involved in almost all cases of facial burns. It is composed of three basic elements, namely (1) mucosal lining, (2) skeletal framework (cartilaginous and bony), and (3) external skin cover. The skin is quite thin in middle one-third, comparatively thicker in upper one-third and thickest and sebaceous in lower one-third of nose. It is the skin cover which is mostly burnt and destroyed in burns with distortion of cartilaginous framework being secondary. Mucosal lining is usually intact except at the nostril margins or in extensively burnt cases. Healing scars may cause stenosis of nostrils leading to airway obstruction apart from cosmetic disfigurement and deformity. Nasal burns are managed conservatively because excisional surgery may give a skeletonized look to nose.

The nostrils should be carefully cleaned several times daily and a thin film of antimicrobial ointment should be applied with a cotton applicator for lubrication to prevent crust formation which can compromise breathing. In case of deep burns, there can be severe stenosis of the nostrils. This can be prevented by using customized nostril splints for long periods of time. In case the nostrils are already stenosed, they can be widened by various methods which can be skin graft based or local tissue rearrangement or local flap based. The aim of reconstruction is restoration of function (to increase efficiency of nasal breathing) and aesthetics of nose. Release and application of thick split skin graft is a simple procedure but requires prolonged postoperative splintage to prevent restenosis.[11] Repeated release may still be required because of graft/scar contraction. Composite chondrocutaneous grafts from the auricle may be used. Unpredictable survival is their biggest limitation. Multiple W-plasty flaps can be designed on the external and internal surfaces of the stenosed nostril and the staggered flaps are interdigitated.[12] A similar procedure is "Starplasty", in which two incisions perpendicular to each other are given in skin and mucosa to raise four skin flaps and four mucosal flaps. The skin and mucosal flaps are then interposed with each other in the form of a "Star" to achieve a good nostril opening[13] **(Figs. 10A to C)**. The main advantage of these operations is that the interposed flaps break the scar line, preventing/minimizing chances of restenosis. Postoperative splintage is not required. Flaps from the perialar region may need to be raised and transposed into nostril to add to its circumference.

Scars on the dorsum of whole of nose can be thinly excised and resurfaced with a single sheet of thick split/full thickness skin graft or else with an expanded forehead flap **(Figs. 11A to C)**. If entire nose is destroyed, the forehead flap is used to reconstruct the nose in stages, with costal cartilage for support, if required. However, forehead skin is usually not available, being itself involved in burn. Distant flaps may therefore be needed. While lining can be restored with turn down flaps or nasolabial flaps, cover is provided with arm tube (multistaged but pedicled) (refer to Chapter on "Postburn Sequelae and their Management") or free radial forearm flap, sometimes used as a prelaminated flap.

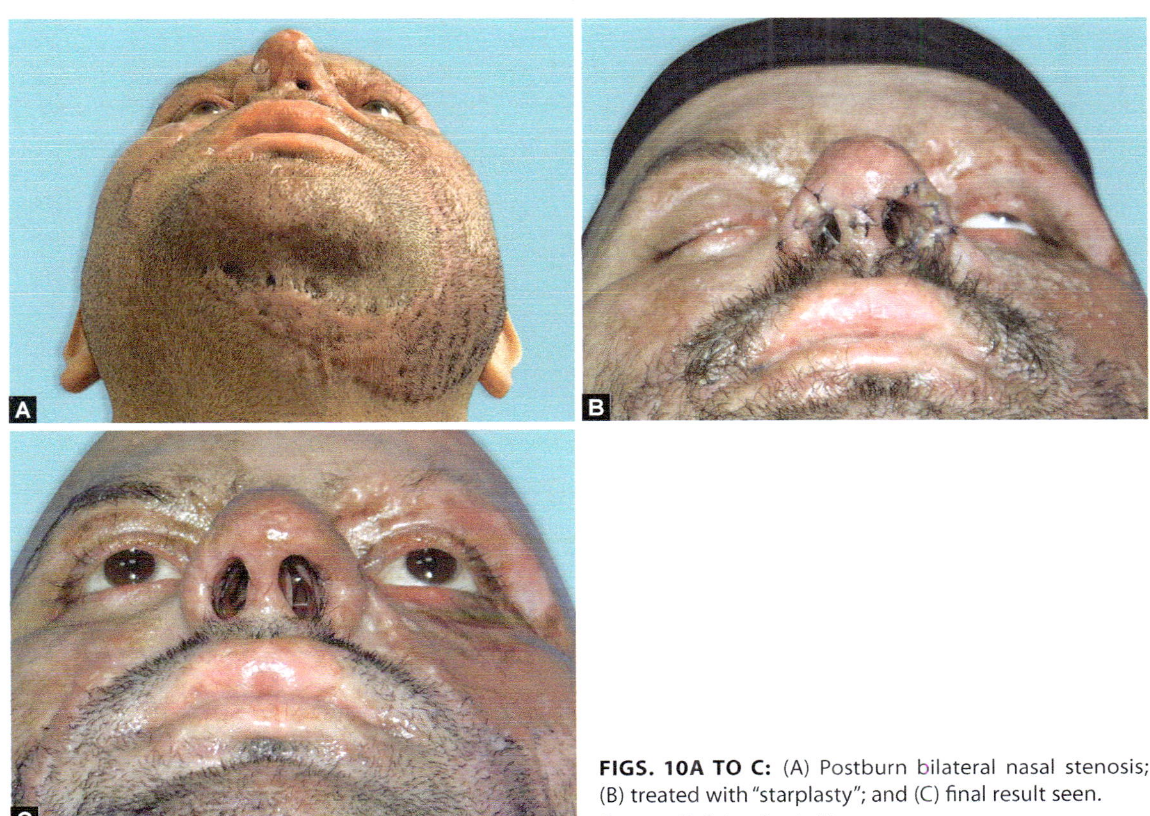

FIGS. 10A TO C: (A) Postburn bilateral nasal stenosis; (B) treated with "starplasty"; and (C) final result seen.
Courtesy: Dr Sujata Sarabahi.

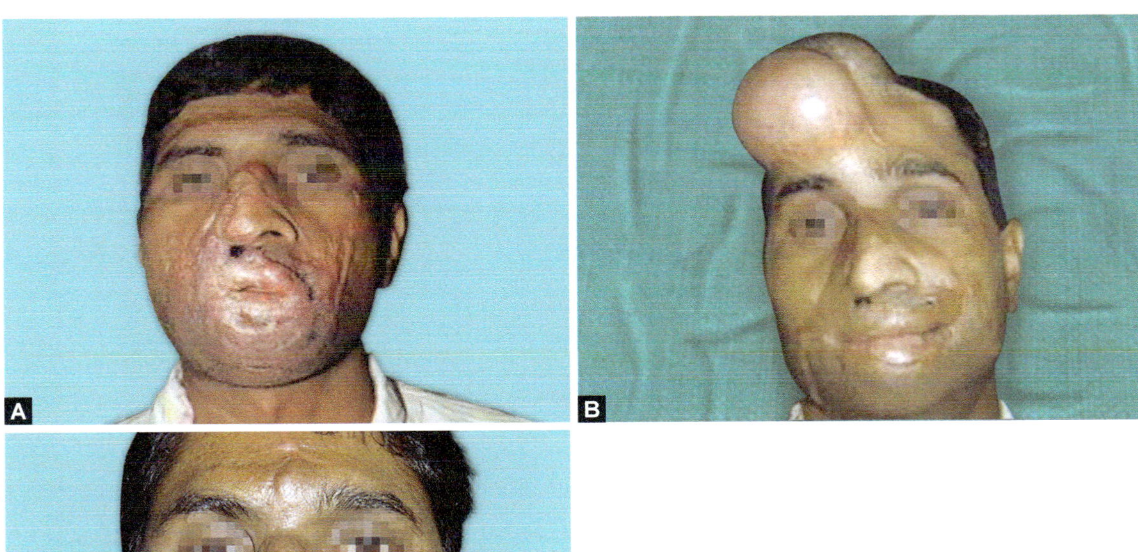

FIGS. 11A TO C: (A) Postacid burn hypertrophic scarring with stenosed right nostril and severe microstomia. (B) Release of microstomia and excision of hypertrophic scar and coverage of lower lip and chin with expanded neck flaps and nose and upper lip with skin graft. Second stage tissue expander placed in forehead and scalp for reconstructing nose and upper lip. (C) Reconstructed nose and upper lip with expanded forehead and scalp flap.

Eye and its Adnexa[14]

Burn injuries to the eyeball itself are rare in thermal injuries due to protective mechanism of blink reflex and reflex protective movement of the head at the time of injury. Nevertheless, in all patients of facial burn, corneal injury must be ruled out by thorough clinical examination. Examination by an ophthalmologist must be done early because, if delayed, subsequent periorbital edema makes the assessment almost impossible. Occasionally, cloudiness of cornea is observed with flash injuries which clear out in the next few days.

In chemical burns, the eyelids cannot close promptly because of the rapid splashing of the harmful liquid and thus, injuries of eyeball and ocular adnexa are common **(Figs. 12A to D)**. All chemical burns of the eye are a potential threat to vision **(Fig. 13)**. There is photophobia, lacrimation, pain, and diminished vision. A foreign body sensation in the eye is suggestive of corneal injury and must be ruled out or confirmed by fluorescein test. The actual damage depends upon the volume of the chemical, its concentration, its duration of contact, and the unique property of some chemicals. In acid burns, immediately after its contact with tissues of the eye, there is coagulative necrosis due to tissue protein precipitation and formation of a pseudomembrane (or eschar) which may prevent further permeation into deeper layers of tissues and protect the cornea. The acids are proton donors, release hydrogen ions and bring the pH down to as low as 0. Alkalis are more dangerous than acids. The hydroxyl (OH) ions rapidly penetrate the cornea, producing corneal ulceration with potential for phthisis bulbi (liquefactive necrosis). Ammonia can penetrate to the interior of globe within 30 seconds. The hydroxide ions cause saponification of fatty acid component of plasma

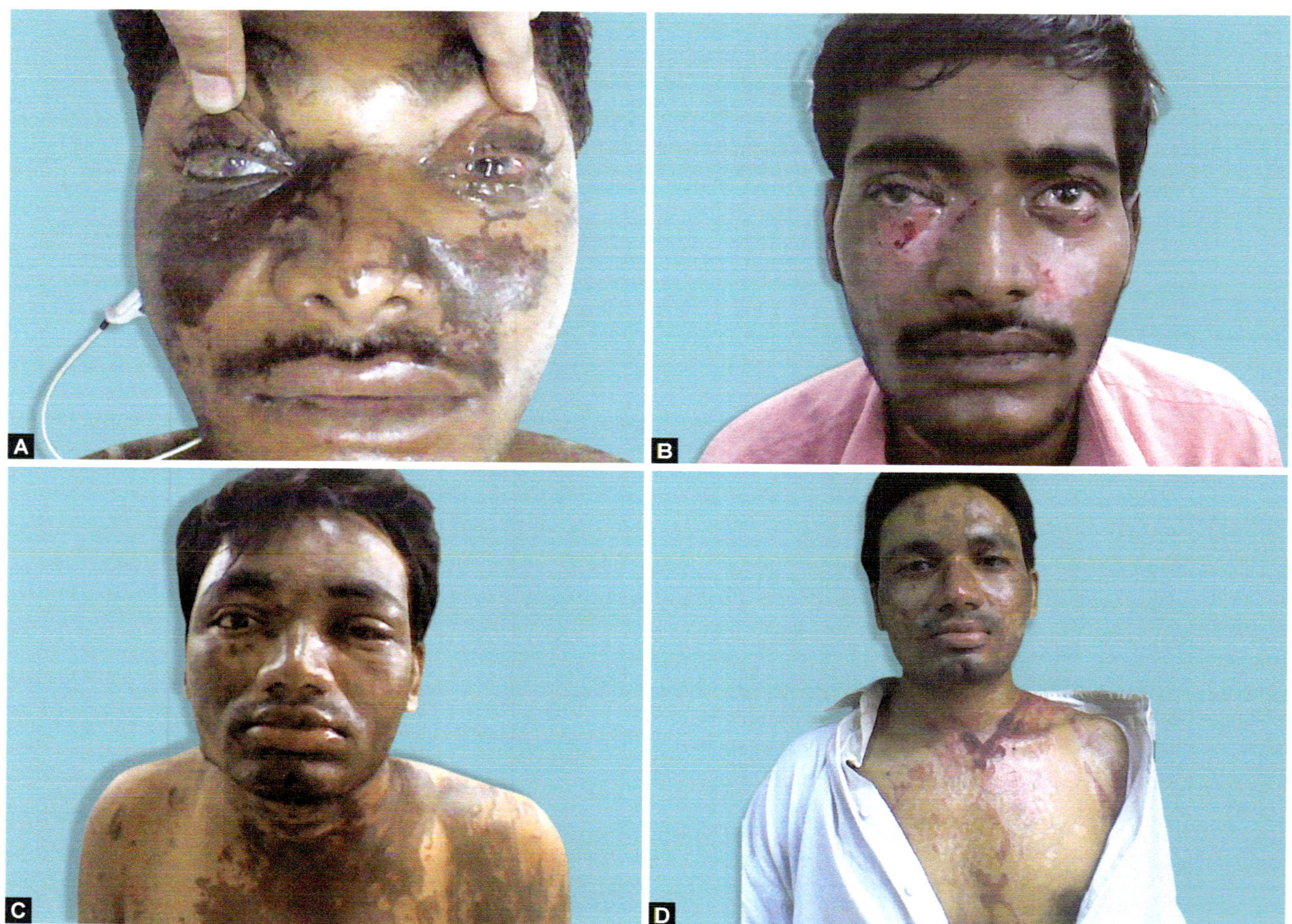

FIGS. 12A TO D: (A) Superficial dermal chemical burns of face involving the eyes. (B) 10 days later almost healed wounds after leaving the wounds and eschar separated by itself as the wounds healed. (C) Another patient with extensive mixed burns due to chemical injury. (D) 1 month later completely healed areas after leaving the wounds exposed with only antibiotic ointment application.

membrane resulting in cell disruption and death. They denature collagen and cause vascular thrombosis in the vessels of the conjunctiva, episclera, and anterior uvea leading to globe appearing white. The cations are responsible for penetration of specific alkali. Burns caused by phosphorus demand careful removal of all the particles. Damage is caused by a high or a low pH and by collagenases released by damaged epithelial cells and granulocytes. Lime burns are notorious with a persistent pH of 11–11.5 due to particles lodged in the conjunctival sac that are not irrigated away easily.

In chemical injuries, irrigation of the eye with copious amounts of normal saline is done to minimize the damage to the eye. Ideally, this should be initiated immediately at the scene of injury with even tap water and should continue till the arrival of the patient in the emergency department where it can be replaced by normal saline. Litmus paper is useful in knowing that a neutral pH has been achieved. Specific diluent for a particular agent is not required because of the potential for exothermic reaction and the delay in its procurement. Subsequent care of the eye focuses on maintenance of adequate lubrication to prevent corneal desiccation. Cornea should be frequently evaluated. A corneal abrasion may progress to ulceration and ultimately perforation and loss of vision. If a corneal injury is present, topical antibiotic drops and atropine (a mydriatic agent, 1% ointment or solution) should be started to prevent ciliary spasm and iridocyclitic adhesions. Ointments should be put repeatedly to prevent adhesions from forming between conjunctival surfaces. All corneal injuries should be covered (patched). Intense periorbital edema in the early postoperative period serves the same purpose. Subsequently, if lid retraction occurs, specific methods to prevent corneal exposure are necessary. Examples include scleral lens, antibiotic ointment, or some surgical intervention.

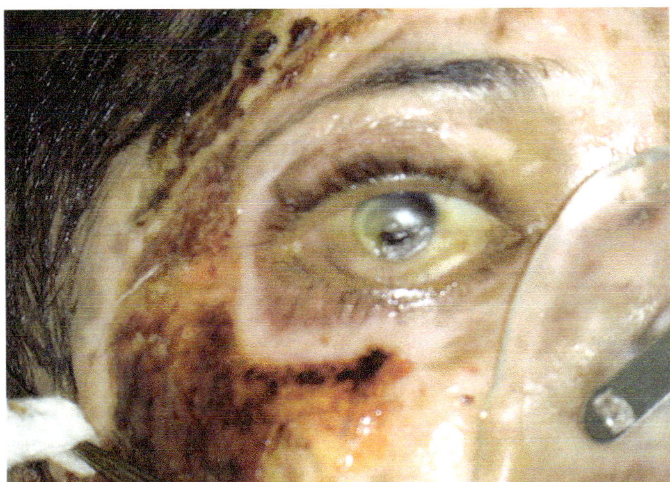

FIG. 13: Corneal ulceration/impending perforation.

Tarsorrhaphy, surgical fusion of upper and lower eyelids, is one of the means to close the eye. Two techniques have generally been advocated to achieve adherence of the eyelid margins, the apposition technique and the "tongue in groove" technique. In apposition technique, the epithelium of margins of both the eyelids is surgically removed and the eyelids are sutured together with the help of bolster sutures to prevent scarring of eyelids. The other, "tongue in groove" technique, ensures a stronger union between the two lid margins. However, the use of tarsorrhaphy in the acute management of eyelid burns is controversial. Most workers do not favor this operation. This is because the action of eyelids itself pulls them apart with cutting off of the sutures and damage to lid margin. This significant distortion of lid margins jeopardizes any future reconstruction. Thus, it is not only ineffective but also produces complications which are difficult to manage.

When most of the skin of both eyelids and lid margins is destroyed significantly, masquerade procedure is used to protect the eye **(Figs. 14A to D)**. Here, conjunctival flaps are developed by dissecting conjunctiva from surrounding tissues and used to cover and protect the eyes. After suturing the flaps together with absorbable sutures, it is covered with split thickness skin graft.

If timely debridement and grafting for deep burns of eyelids is not done, they tend to heal with contraction leading to ectropion of the lids. In full thickness chemical burns, the eschar may be excised and skin graft applied. To prevent corneal damage from exposure, the ectropion of the lids should be released early even if the scars are not mature **(Figs. 15A to C)**. Ideally, the upper lids should be released first and grafted with intermediate thickness skin graft followed by release of the lower lids. In case of severe ectropion, repeated release may be required if surrounding skin of face is also scarred and still contracting because of immature scars **(Fig. 16)**.

External Ear[15-18]

The pinna enjoys a special place in the society all over the world. Women use a wide range of jewelry to enhance its beauty. Even males adorn their ear with a variety of ornaments. It is a very sophisticated morphological structure in itself. Because of its very small area with respect to TBSA and limited functional significance (except to support a pair of spectacles) and survival of the patient being more important, management of a burnt ear often gets neglected. Burns of pinna may lead to a permanent cosmetic deformity, if not cared for properly. The skin covering the anterolateral surface of cartilage is

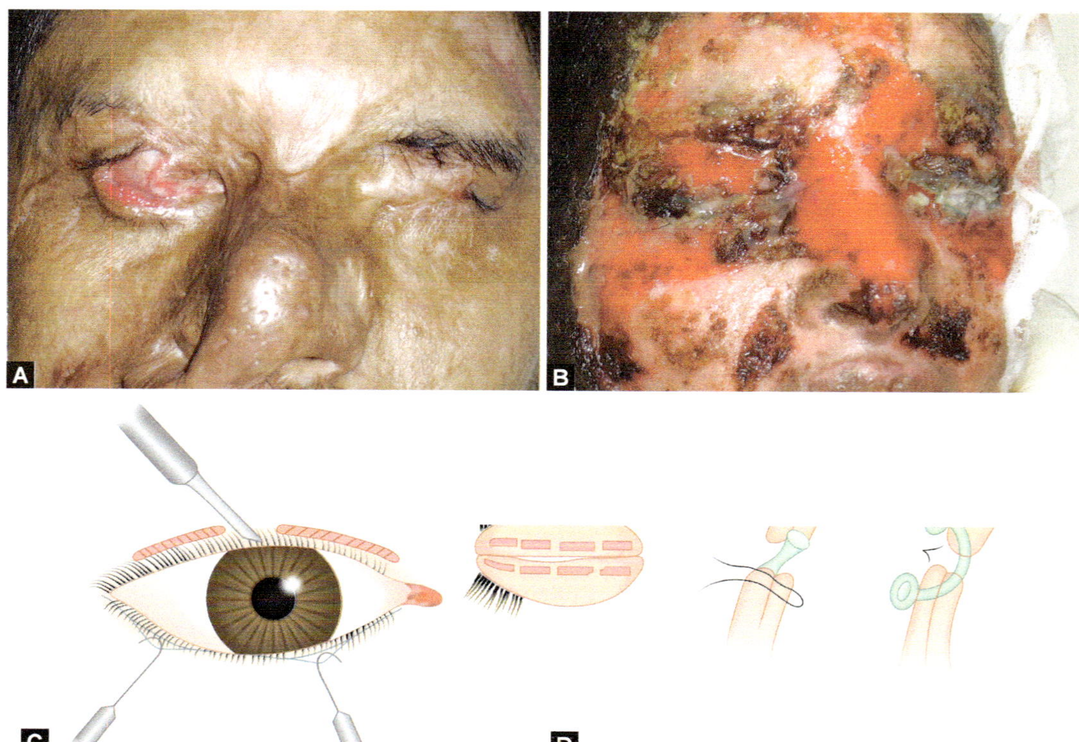

FIGS. 14A TO D: (A) Symblepharon in right eye and in left eye total loss of both lids for which upper and lower conjunctiva was mobilized, sutured over exposed cornea, and skin graft applied over it. (B) Deep burns of the lids with retraction of lids exposing the cornea—temporary tarsorrhaphy done in both eyes and raw area was later grafted after debriding the dead skin over the lids. (C and D) Line diagram to show the technique of tarsorrhaphy.

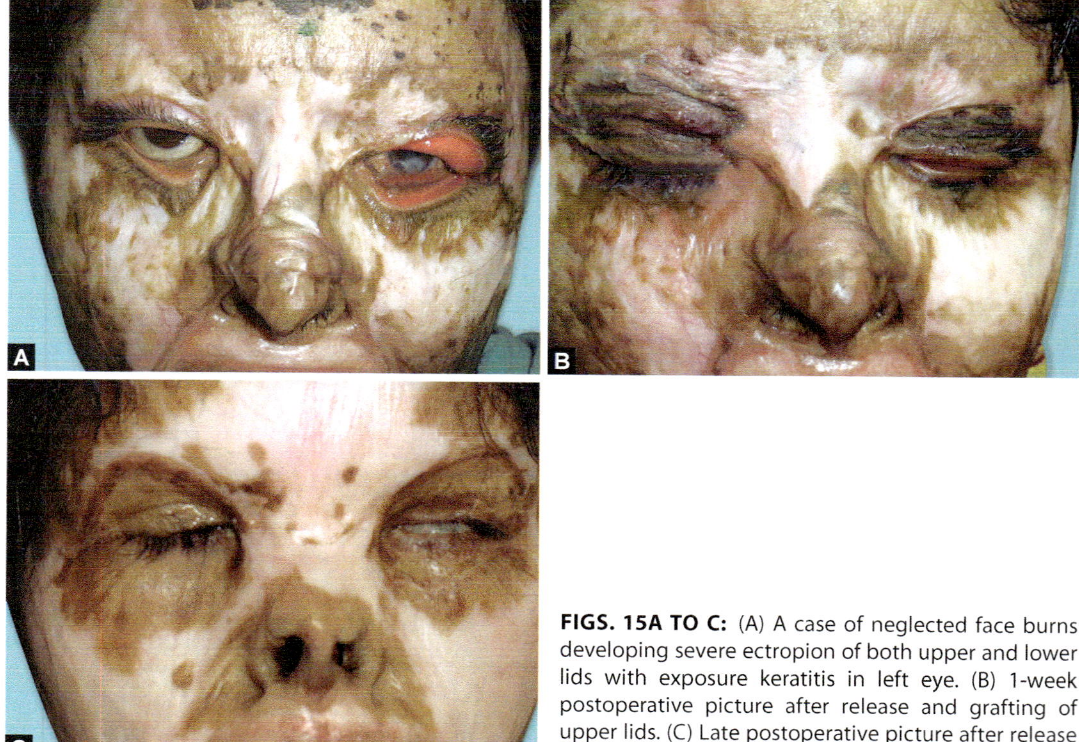

FIGS. 15A TO C: (A) A case of neglected face burns developing severe ectropion of both upper and lower lids with exposure keratitis in left eye. (B) 1-week postoperative picture after release and grafting of upper lids. (C) Late postoperative picture after release of all four lids with well-settled grafts.

thin, adherent, and nonprotective to underlying cartilage and is very easily damaged from thermal injury **(Fig. 17A)**. Posteromedial aspect of ear is covered by thicker layer of subcutaneous tissue and skin which give some protection to the underlying cartilage. Cartilaginous framework of pinna has no intrinsic blood supply and intact perichondrium gets its nourishment by diffusion from the surrounding soft tissues.

External ears are particularly vulnerable to thermal injury of facial burns due to their prominent location on both sides of the face. They may get damaged if the skin burns are so deep that it no longer supplies nourishment to cartilage or else the cartilage itself may be burnt. They may also be damaged because of suppurative chondritis leading to necrosis and dissolution of cartilage. This loss of supporting structure ultimately results in deformity of the ear. All cases of burned ear must be treated aggressively to prevent this complication.

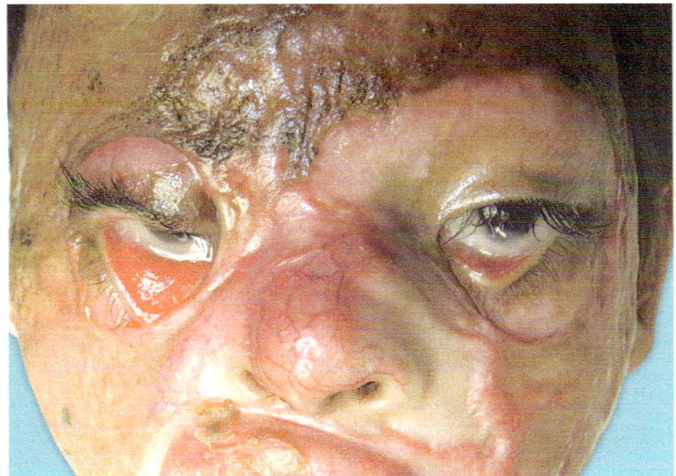

FIG. 16: Severe ectropion of both lower lids with immature scars in the surrounding face. Leading to persistent watering from the eyes and exposure of conjunctiva and lower cornea. Requires early release with grafting and may even need rerelease because of contraction of the surrounding immature scar.

The disfigurements and deformities following thermal injury show a whole spectrum from minor irregularities of helical rim to severe hypertrophy of skin to partial or even total destruction of external ear. Because of the poor quality and quantity of skin in the auricular region in a healed postburn patient, total ear reconstruction is a daunting task. Every attempt should be made to prevent a deformity. Majority of pinna burns are superficial dermal and heal without surgical intervention. To avoid pressure which can harm the burnt pinna by decreasing blood supply, pillows should not be used under the head and the patient is also not allowed to lie on either side. A "donut" can be kept under the head to keep the head lifted up without the ears touching it **(Fig. 17B)**. Application of topical antimicrobial cream/ointment and avoidance of pressure helps in preventing the development of chondritis/pressure necrosis in deeper ear burns. Mafenide cream is the most effective topical agent used in burns of pinna because of its ability to penetrate eschar. When a contour dressing is done, a minimal pressure should be applied while bandaging. With this wound care, the swelling subsides and partial-thickness burn heals. If perichondrium is preserved, it will "take" the graft. If cartilage is exposed in a small area, it can be debrided and split thickness skin grafting can be done over the viable soft tissues underneath. In a large area of full

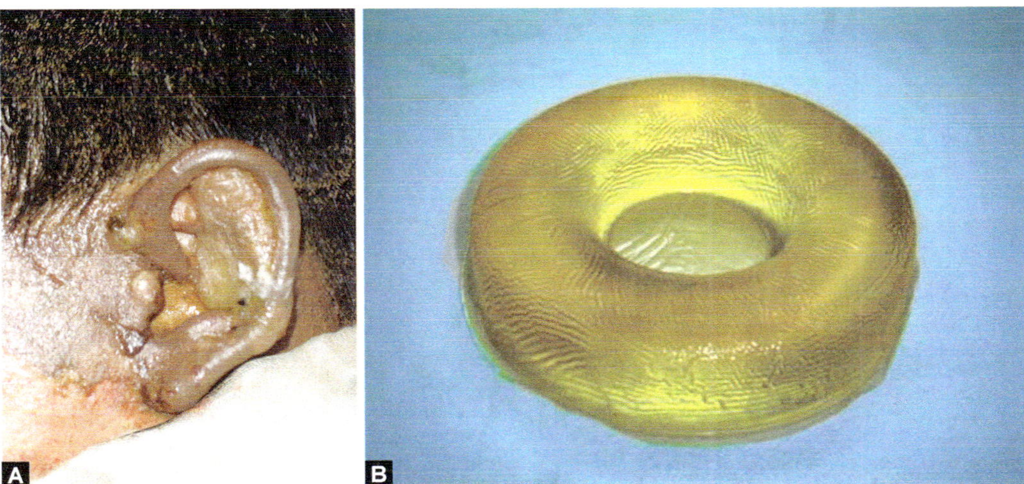

FIGS. 17A AND B: (A) Acute ear burns showing how the thin skin over the anterolateral surface of the ear gets blistered and lifted off the underlying cartilage, thus impairing the blood supply to it. This can be prevented by early contoured dressing of the burned ear. (B)"Donut" used for ear burns.

thickness burn where perichondrium has been damaged leading to exposure of cartilage, some form of vascularized coverage is necessary to salvage the remaining cartilage. Unfortunately, local surrounding tissues cannot be used as they are also involved in severe burns. Regional or distant flaps have been described to cover the exposed cartilage. These include the temporoparietal fascial flap, which is a thin, pliable and very versatile flap and is the best choice for coverage of exposed auricular cartilage **(Figs. 18A to E)**. The authors believe that this best option should not be exhausted for primary coverage of exposed cartilage in less than the best situation. Additionally, the

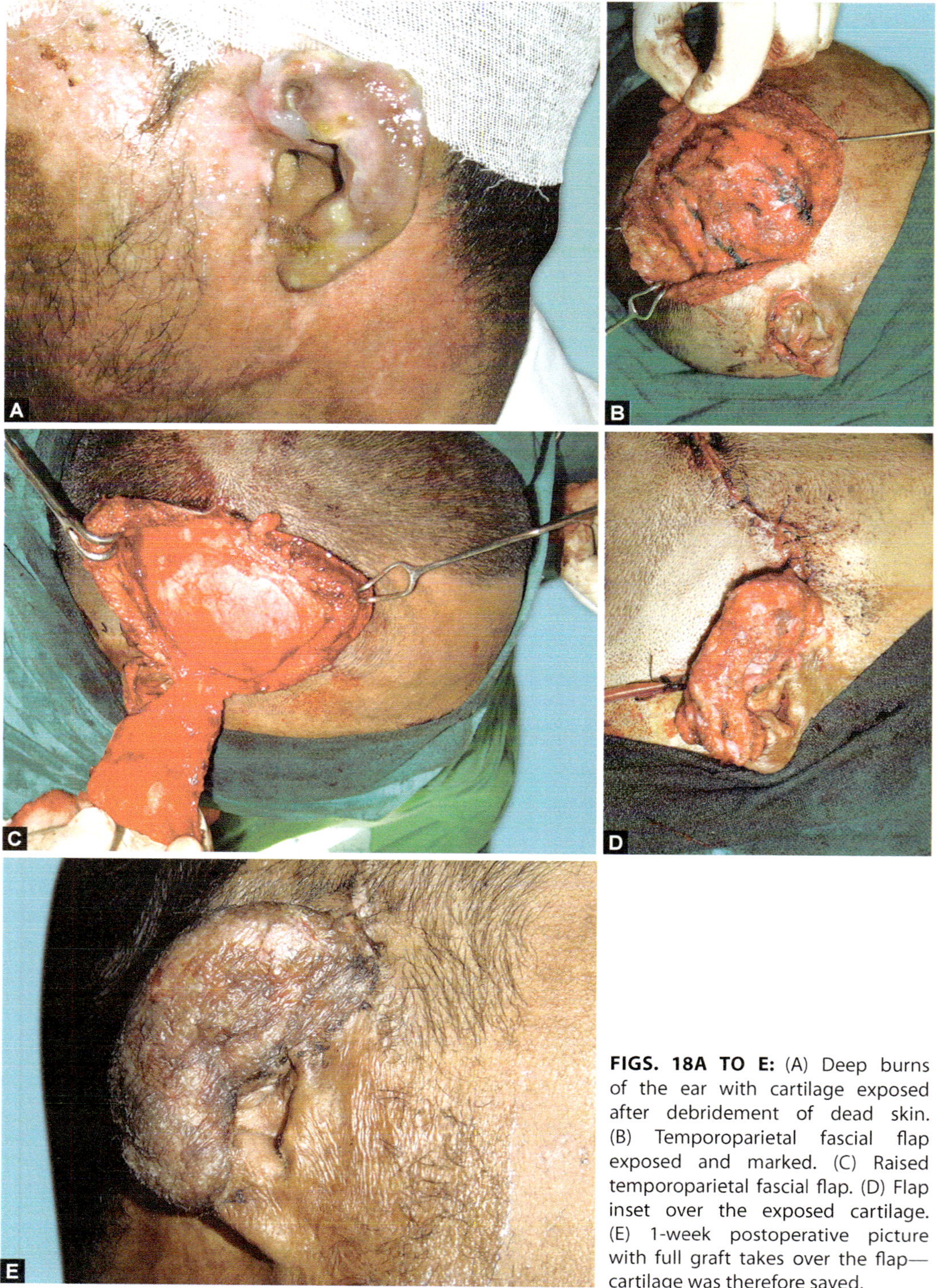

FIGS. 18A TO E: (A) Deep burns of the ear with cartilage exposed after debridement of dead skin. (B) Temporoparietal fascial flap exposed and marked. (C) Raised temporoparietal fascial flap. (D) Flap inset over the exposed cartilage. (E) 1-week postoperative picture with full graft takes over the flap—cartilage was therefore saved.

original ear cartilage (as compared to costochondral graft framework) may not withstand the forces of secondary contraction of split skin graft, which is applied over the temporoparietal fascia, defeating the purpose. Post-auricular fascia, if not damaged by burn, is another option to provide cover to the exposed cartilage.

Acute suppurative chondritis is the most dreaded complication of burns of the pinna because of the severe throbbing pain in the ear, not relieved by analgesics. McIndoe (1983) described the severity of this continuous intolerable pain as one which "reduced strong men to weeping broken wrecks".[19] It is rapid in onset with tenderness and erythematous swelling of the pinna. The cephaloconchal angle is increased which is considered diagnostic. Early diagnosis is essential to achieve the best results. It can develop even 4–5 weeks after the burn **(Figs. 19A to G)**. The common organisms responsible are *Pseudomonas aeruginosa* and *Staphylococcus aureus*. The

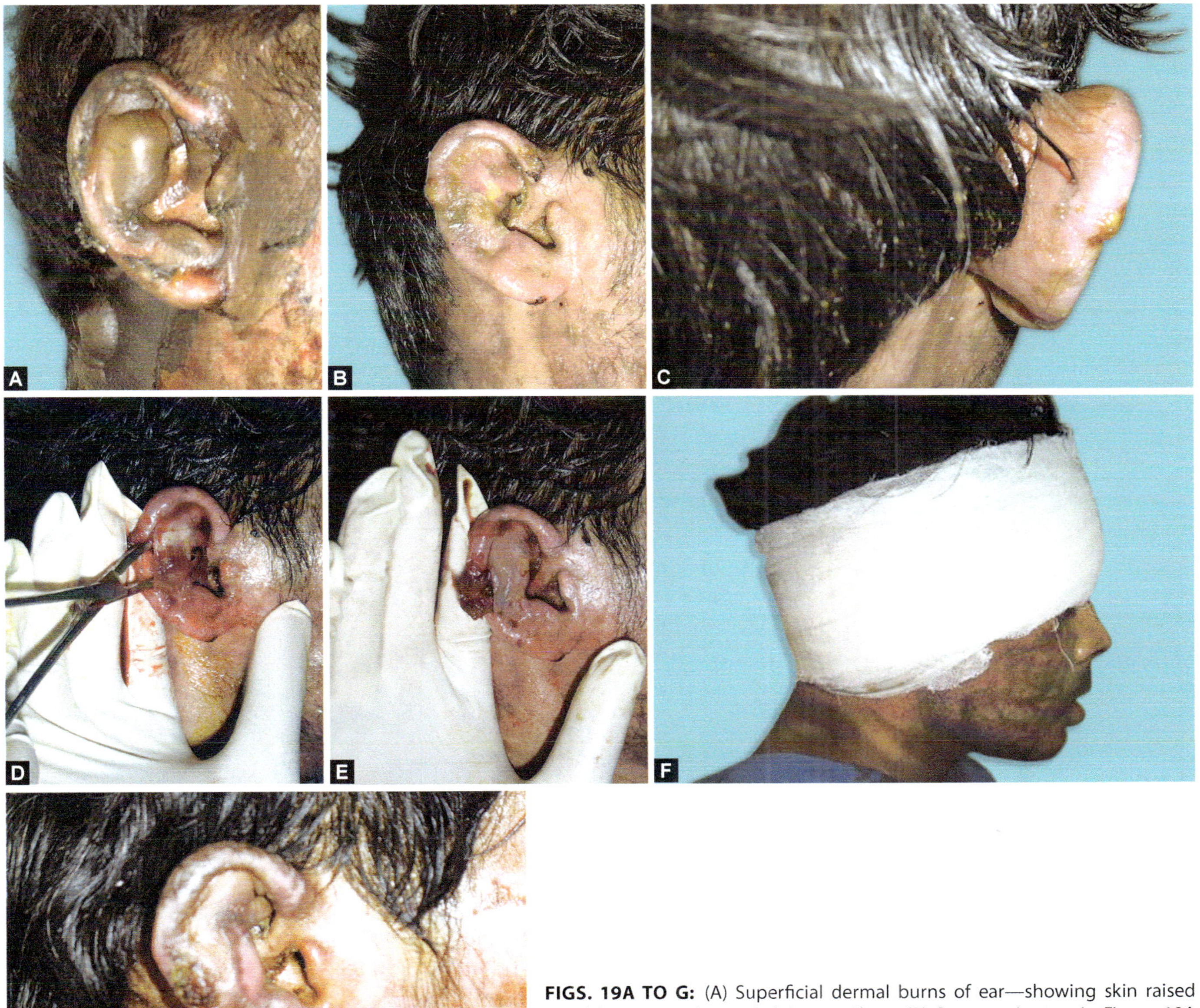

FIGS. 19A TO G: (A) Superficial dermal burns of ear—showing skin raised as a blister over the underlying cartilage. (B) Same patient as in Figure 19A neglected and developed chondritis and chondral abscess indicated by the erythema, swelling, severe pain, and tenderness. (C) Increased cephaloconchal angle diagnostic of chondritis. (D) Incision given in the rim and pus drained and loose and dead cartilage if any removed. (E) Cavity packed. (F) Contoured dressing over the treated ear. (G) Same ear after 1 month with well-maintained contours and minimal deformity.

treatment consists of a bivalving incision along the helical rim that splits the ear into anterolateral and posteromedial skin flaps. All the infected and necrotic cartilages are excised and the bivalved ear packed with fine mesh gauze impregnated with antibacterial cream. A contour dressing with fluffed gauze is done with gentle pressure. The dressing should be changed after 24 hours and any leftover necrotic cartilage, which may become the cause of continued suppuration, is excised. Dressings are continued till the wound heals. The extent of loss of cartilage determines the severity of auricular deformity. In a major or complete loss, what remains is a crumpled-up mass of skin.

In a postburn ear deformity, very often, the skin around the auricular region is burned and scarred and hence, not available for draping of the framework. Reconstruction of ear is usually accomplished by autogenous costal cartilage framework or commercially available implants (e.g., porous polyethylene, Silastic, etc.) and temporoparietal fascial flap cover. In cases where majority of the cartilage is intact but deformed, the ear can be reconstructed by using local flaps from postauricular region without adding any cartilage framework **(Figs. 20 and 21)**. Some cases with extensive local scarring may need reconstruction using free radial forearm flap and costal cartilage in the form of a prelaminated flap.

Perioral Region[20-22]

In extensive facial burns, lips and mouth are commonly involved. In all cases of perioral burns, orodental care should be given to the patients after every meal by the nursing staff and/or by the family member of the patient or by the patient himself/herself. The care includes daily inspection of the mouth to look for any sign(s) and symptoms of fungal infection. Treatment should be started immediately before it becomes severe enough to prevent feeding of the patient and healing of the wound. Lips are frequently burnt and antibiotic ointment should be applied to soften the crust and prevent cracking and bleeding until they heal. After every meal lubrication by ointment should continue to prevent crusting.

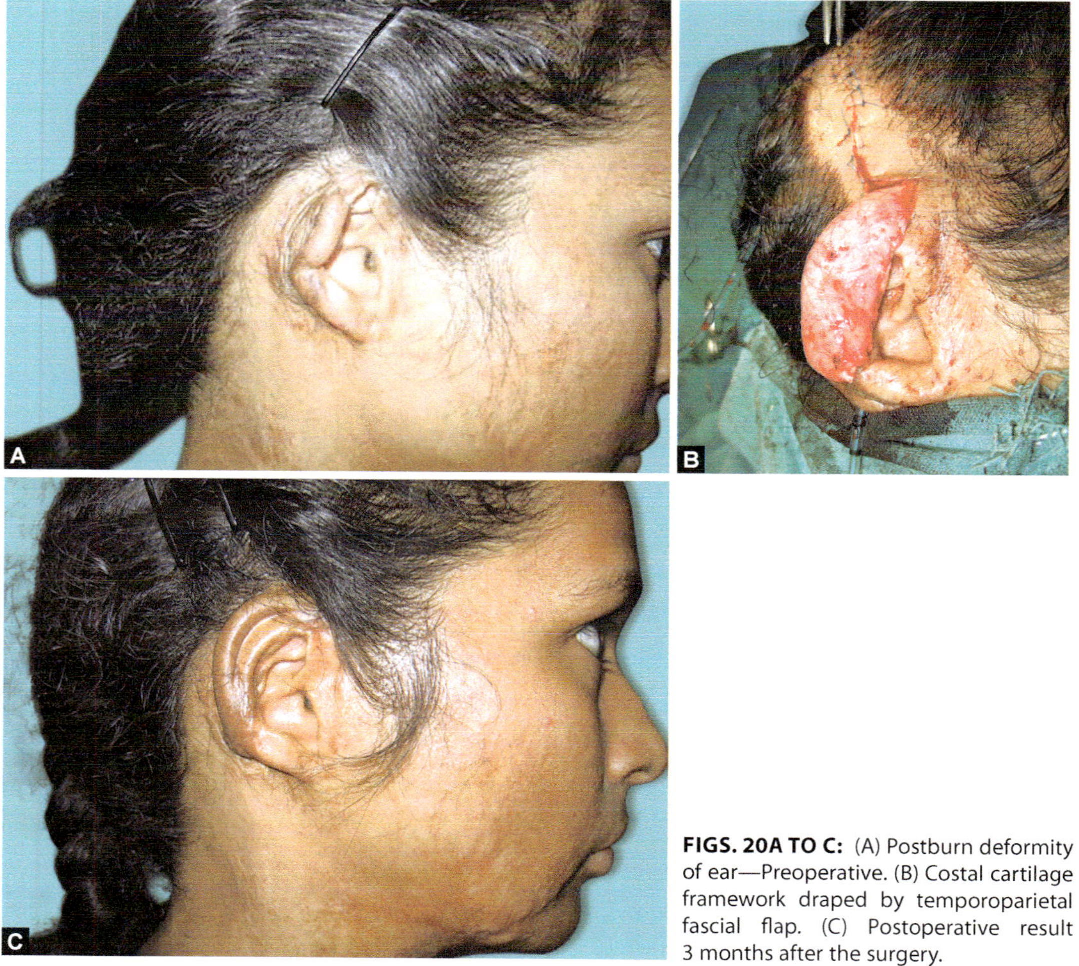

FIGS. 20A TO C: (A) Postburn deformity of ear—Preoperative. (B) Costal cartilage framework draped by temporoparietal fascial flap. (C) Postoperative result 3 months after the surgery.

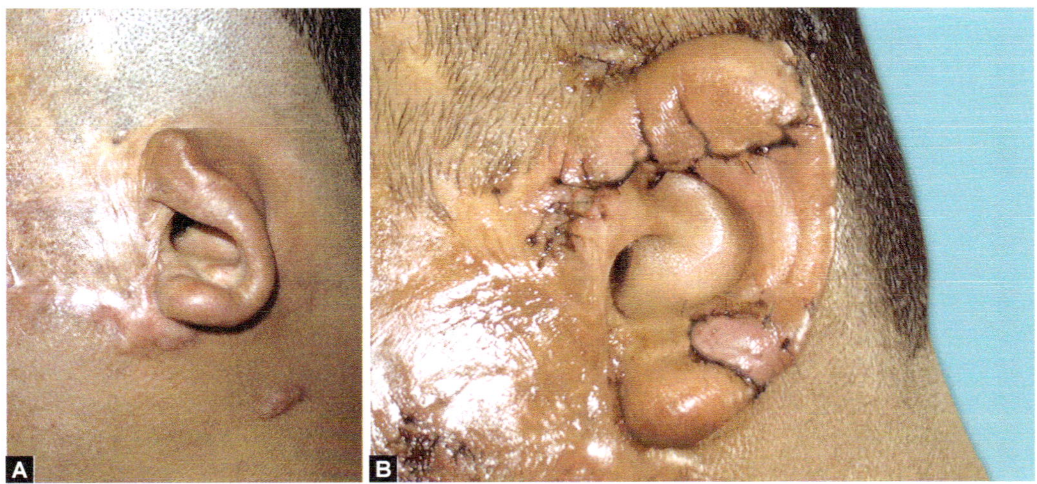

FIGS. 21A AND B: (A) Postburn ear deformity with constricting effect due to loss of helical rim cartilage. (B) Ear reconstruction done after releasing the constricted ear with postauricular flaps.

Isolated burns of lip and mouth due to electrical contact are common in toddlers and small children. They typically result from an inquisitive child biting/sucking on a "live" wire. These are usually domestic voltage injuries. The saliva (rich in electrolytes) lowers the resistance to current flow and an arc is produced with local temperature rising to 3000°C. The latter chars the area in contact, usually angle of mouth and adjoining upper and lower lips, gums, and adjoining bone and teeth buds. The current flows out through the same wire (contact burn in series). Anterior tongue may also be involved. The resistance of moist oral mucosa, approximately 100 ohms/cm^2, is very small as compared to thoroughly wet skin (10,000 ohm/cm^2). Sometimes, the current exits the body to ground from the child's wet diapers, feet or buttocks involving the heart in its pathway and may prove fatal (contact burn in parallel). It may be difficult to assess the depth and extent of injury at the initial examination. The initial appearance of the burnt area is that of painless, grayish white, coagulated lesion with surrounding erythema and swelling. Generally, there is no respiratory problem. There is drooling of saliva and food. Commonly, full thickness of lip and cheek (skin, muscle, and mucosa) is damaged. The eschar gradually sloughs out leaving an ulcer with granulation tissue in its bed which heals by contraction leading to microstomia. Microstomia is severe because of sphincteric action of orbicularis oris muscle. Orodental hygiene, eating, speech, and facial expression are all affected.

There is controversy whether primary excision should be done or else left for 10–12 days or so to allow edema to subside and develop a clear demarcation of the zone of injury as well as granulation tissue. The former may end up in excising tissues whose viability is doubtful at initial examination but may eventually survive. In the latter, only definitely nonviable tissues are debrided. It must be remembered that facial structures are highly specialized, difficult to restore to preinjury status and elective reconstructive surgery is more likely to give a better result than early intervention on edematous and infected tissues. However, there is a risk of secondary hemorrhage due to blow-out of the labial artery in the waiting period. Its possibility and the technique of control by pressing the vessel between finger and thumb must be taught to the parents of the child, especially if the child is discharged from in-patient care before this period. All patients of perioral burn must be prescribed an oral splint during the period of scar maturation. In minor burns, the oral splints can avoid the need for surgery while in moderate-to-severe burns the splint can minimize deformity. In some severe cases, an earlier intervention, before scar maturation may be needed. A wide variety of splints have been described and the help of a prosthodontist is a must.[19] If splints are not used, the resultant contracture (microstomia) may need a difficult reconstructive surgery as well as intubation by the anesthetist. In mild-to-moderate cases, one may wait for scar maturation before definitive treatment.

Scalp[23-25]

Management of scalp wounds at the time of burn is governed by depth and extent of injury. Presence of hair on the scalp in most patients does provide some protection to it from thermal injury. These burns can be divided into two categories depending upon whether scalp is burned alone or even calvarium is also involved. Because of a very rich blood supply and high density of hair follicles,

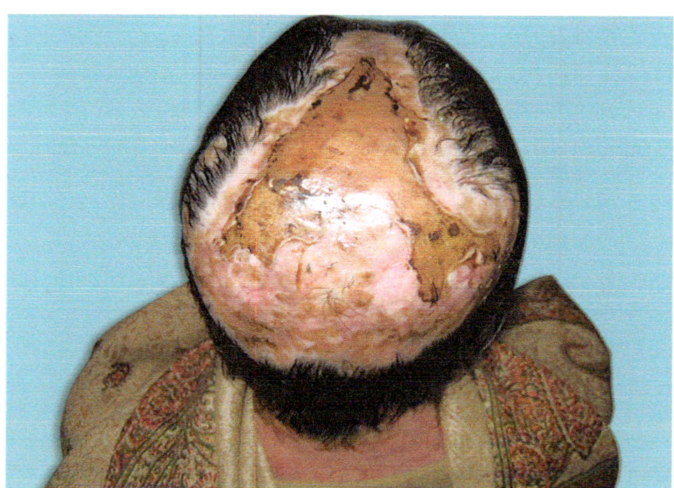

FIG. 22: Postburn raw area scalp covered with split skin graft.

even a second-degree deep dermal burn is likely to heal of its own. This means that most of the scalp burn wounds require conservative treatment only. Although, it is expected that this will save a number of hair follicles but a severe scarring itself may damage the roots of hair follicles ultimately leading to alopecia. Full-thickness burns when managed conservatively lead to formation of granulation tissue over the pericranium which can be split skin grafted **(Fig. 22)**. In these cases, it is of utmost importance that the viable pericranium is not allowed to dry.

Full-thickness burns of scalp exposing the bone without viable pericranium or where it has dried up usually require a vascularized flap cover because skin graft does not "take" over bare bone without pericranium. There are two ways of managing these patients. The exposed and devitalized outer table of calvarial bone is chiseled out exposing the bleeding diploe. This is either immediately split skin grafted or the wound is covered with moist dressings till the development of granulation tissue (5 days approximately). The well vascularized diploe provides an excellent bed for skin grafting. Immediate grafting runs the risk of poor graft "take" because of bleeding. Delayed application ensures complete graft "take". This option is satisfactory for smaller areas. These patients may desire provision of hair bearing scalp once the patient recovers completely from burn injury and the scars and grafts have matured.

Some workers make multiple burr holes, 3–4 mm apart in the outer table to promote the development of granulation tissue from diploe. Granulation tissue comes out through these holes, spreads over the exposed bone, and becomes confluent ultimately providing a bed to accept a skin graft. This practice is to be discouraged as it takes a very long time. Also, it buries the bone which sometimes goes on coming out as small pieces of sequestrum (discharging sinus) over a very prolonged period.

The second option consists of providing a flap cover immediately. Larger areas are better handled with this technique. The flap may be local **(Figs. 23A to D)** or distant microvascular free flap. Debridement of all non-viable soft tissue and devitalized bone is done. There is a controversy regarding the amount of bony debridement in full thickness burn of scalp. This is because the bare calvarium, if covered by vascularized flap, is considered to act as a bone graft in situ with the expectation of its invasion by osteoblasts from surrounding bone. However, grossly infected and necrotic bone needs to be debrided (as is possible in patients presenting very late) lest it continues as a discharging sinus till whole of the sequestrum comes out. In the latter case, the flap is elevated, all dead necrotic bone/sequestrum is excised and flap replaced. The aim in such cases is avoiding the need for calvarial reconstruction for full-thickness bone defect. The local flap used should ideally be planned in such a way that there is no secondary defect requiring coverage with skin graft. This is because multiple cuts in scalp skin jeopardize the future tissue expansion for definitive reconstruction of the scalp for complete hair restoration. Thus, a rotation flap, single or double, or its modification is better than a transposition flap. A variety of free flaps, such as latissimus dorsi muscle or omentum with skin graft, radial artery forearm, and parascapular or anterolateral thigh flaps have been used to provide cover. The advantage of skin flap is that it may serve as a base for hair grafting procedure later, if the patient desires and sufficient unburnt scalp is available to act as donor. In patients with skin grafts, this type of hair restoration is not possible.

Electrical contact burns of scalp are notorious for causing burns which involve the scalp as well as cranium. Both the tables may be burnt along with even dura and brain. There may be direct contact of electrical wire with the scalp or else it may be a part of "exit" wound. These patients do require provision of flap cover after thorough debridement with immediate or delayed calvarial reconstruction after the patient stabilizes. Such patients are also likely to develop cataract over a period of several months.

Once all the wounds of the patient have healed, grafts and scars matured, many patients do wish to get hair restoration for alopecic areas. A variety of options are available from primary excision to serial excision for smaller areas to local rotation flaps to tissue expansion for <50% alopecic area. For scattered areas hair grafting by one of the modern techniques may be an option. It can also be used over skin flaps used to cover scalp in acute stage. For very extensive areas local delayed flaps to restore anterior hairline may be the aim while a wig may be the last resort.

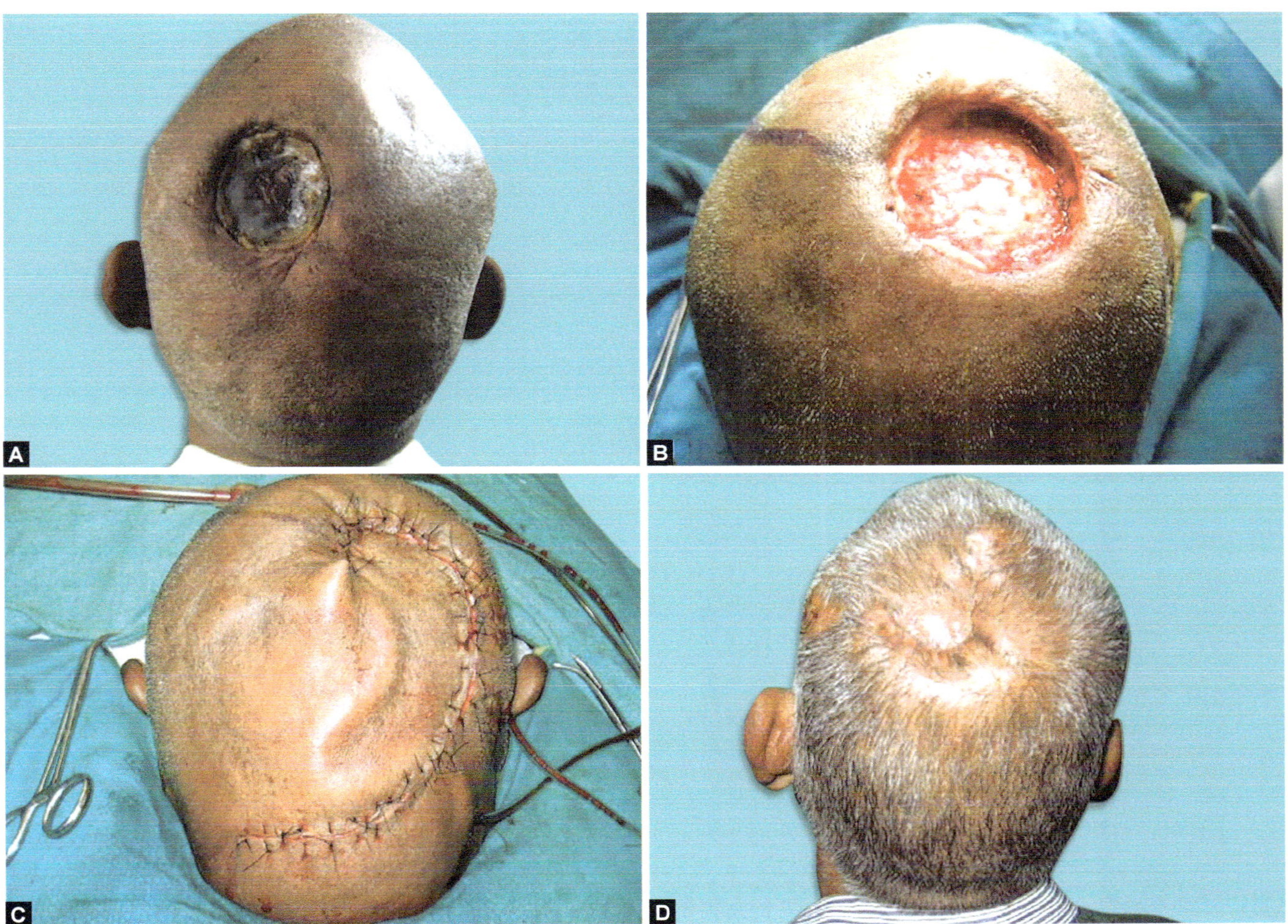

FIGS. 23A TO D: (A) Postburn full thickness defect of scalp involving calvarium following electrical injury. (B) After debridement—preoperative. (C) After coverage by rotation flap; (D) Postoperative result—well healed flap.

Eyebrows[26]

Very commonly, facial burns involve the eyebrows. The eyebrows are very important not only for facial aesthetics but also for their role in emotional expression of a person. They should never be excised in acute stage even in apparently full-thickness burns or in a situation of early postburn alopecia. To restore the normal appearance of eyebrow is extremely difficult and hence, conservative management should be adopted. Regrowth of hair in eyebrow is unpredictable and can occur several months after injury. It is because hair follicles are situated very deep in the dermis and even in the subcutaneous tissues and hence, survive in deep burns. Their growth is very slow and thus, may reappear after a long period of time. Partial hair loss within the eyebrow can be managed by excision of alopecic areas and primary closure. Reconstruction of eyebrows can be done by several techniques including one of the modern hair transplantation techniques (as is commonly being done for male pattern baldness) from scalp and pedicled temporoparietal island flap based on temporal branch of superficial temporal artery **(Figs. 24A to C)**. In both these interventions, periodic trimming of hair by the patient is required. If the defects are minor and opposite eyebrow normal, hair can be harvested from it. The advantages of hair transplantation procedures are that they can be done under local anesthesia, may be repeated easily, if required and direction of hair can be adjusted. However, they need the presence of reasonably thick tissues over the recipient area. In patients with complete loss of eyebrow(s), the operative procedure should be contemplated only after the surrounding scars have matured and stabilized to avoid any change in position. Till such time, patient is advised to use eyebrow pencil. Some patients may be contented with continuation of its use and may opt out of surgical restoration.

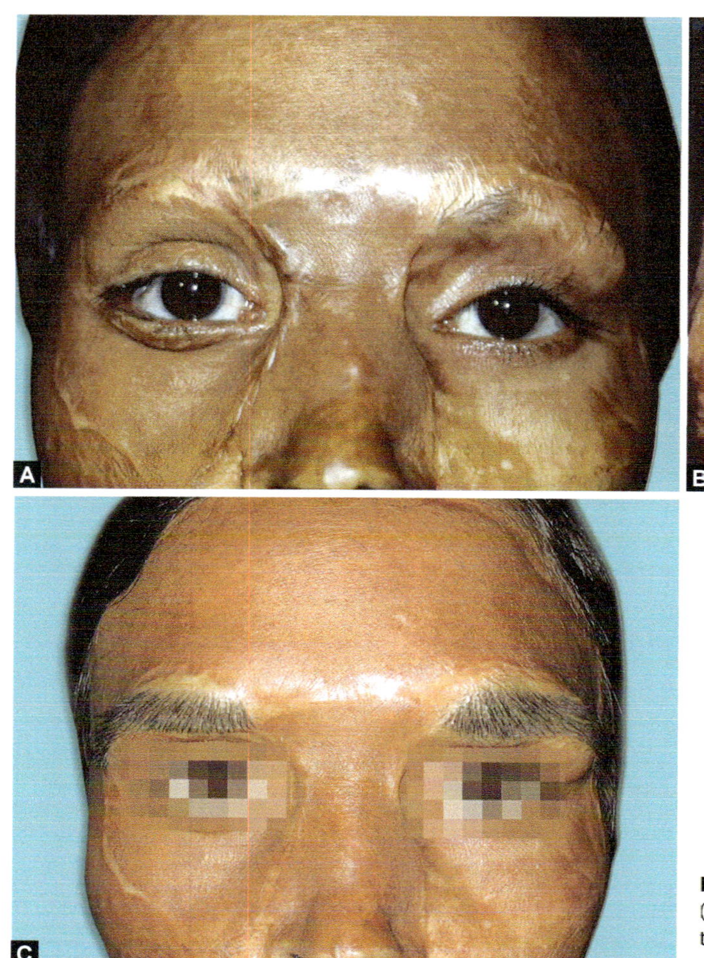

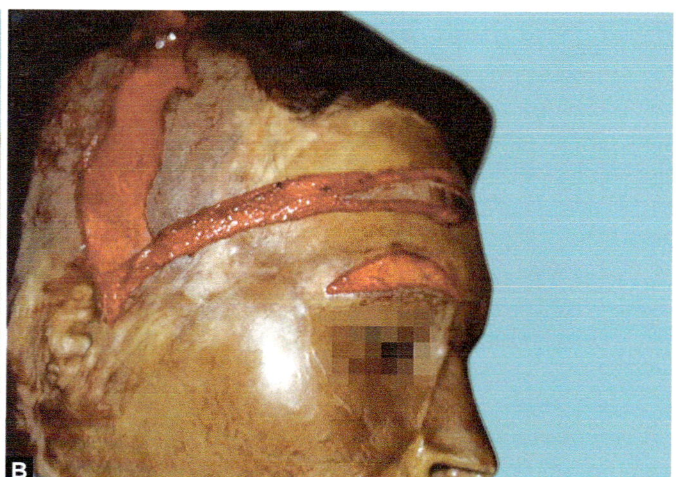

FIGS. 24A TO C: (A) Postburn loss of bilateral eyebrows. (B) Hair bearing island flap based on temporal branch of superficial temporal artery. (C) Postoperative result after reconstruction of both eyebrows by superficial temporal artery flap.

POSTBURN FACIAL SCARRING

Postburn facial disfigurement is devastating not only for those with extensive involvement but also for even smaller areas. The patient wishes to get rid of it at any cost. This is seen in the massive turnover in quantity as well as money involved in scar removing creams sold over the counter. Additionally, patients visit and consult multiple number of plastic surgeons in search of the one who says that all the scars can be erased. For scarred facial structures, whole of plastic surgeon's armamentaria, from primary excision and closure to free microvascular flaps, have been used. Thick split thickness skin graft, full thickness skin graft, and various types of flaps are commonly used to improve aesthetic look of the burn patient. Tissue expansion is a good option to transfer normal skin to the scarred areas. Laser therapy has also been used.

Alloplastic face transplantation is also a possibility now.[27-29] It may be expected to not only improve the appearance but also to provide a remedy to the prejudice and discrimination attached to this stigma. However, when a surgeon and the patient think of alloplastic face transplant as an option, one must compare the risks and benefits of this innovative procedure with known risks and benefits of autogenous facial reconstruction. As on today, following alloplastic face transplantation, the possibility of life-threatening consequences of immunosuppression, the likelihood of graft rejection and/or graft failure appears more than the gain of receiving a normal face as compared to a surgically reconstructed face with autogenous tissues. Additionally, it does change the face completely, which may not be recognized as one's own by the recipient. Risks are too high when compared with the relative gain of normal facial appearance versus a reconstructed face. At present, use of autologous tissues can only take care of millions of postburn patients who visit the plastic surgery services.

SUMMARY

Face, including head and neck, is a dynamic, functional, and aesthetic region having an important role in breathing, eating, formal interaction, and communication with world. Facial burns affect all age groups from infancy to old age. They can be caused by heat, electricity, various chemicals, and radiation. They may be isolated but are usually part of extensive burns and thus, need evaluation and management in the context of TBSA burns of the patient as a whole. Traditionally, facial burns have been treated conservatively for several reasons, most important being the excellent blood supply of the region and consequently faster spontaneous healing. Presence of inhalational injury and injury to the eye need to be assessed and taken care of first of all. Reconstruction of nose, pinna, eyelids and eyebrows and scalp is difficult and appropriate care in the acute stage diminishes the need for multiple surgical interventions later.

REFERENCES

1. Sainsbury DC. Body image and facial burns. Adv Skin Wound Care. 2009;22(1):39-44;quiz 45-6.
2. McGrouther DA. Facial disfigurement. BMJ. 1997;314(7086):991.
3. Greenhalgh DG. Management of facial burns. Burns Trauma. 2020;8:tkaa023.
4. Wong S, Melin A, Reilly D. Head and Neck Reconstruction. Clin Plast Surg. 2017;44(4):845-56.
5. Saffle JR. Closure of the excised burn wound: temporary skin substitutes. Clin Plast Surg. 2009;36(4):627-41.
6. Friedstat JS, Klein MB. Acute management of facial burns. Clin Plast Surg. 2009;36(4):653-60.
7. Mosier MJ, Gibran NS. Surgical excision of the burn wound. Clin Plast Surg. 2009;36(4):617-25.
8. Prousskaia E, El-Muttardi N, Philp B, Dziewulski P, Shelley OP. Treatment of nasal burns: Analysis of 150 cases. Ann Burns Fire Disasters. 2015;28(2):121-7.
9. Bouguila J, Ho Quoc C, Viard R, Brun A, Voulliaume D, Comparin JP, et al. Nose burns: 4-dimensional analysis. Eur Ann Otorhinolaryngol Head Neck Dis. 2017;134(5):333-7.
10. al-Qattan MM, Robertson GA. Acquired nostril stenosis. Ann Plast Surg. 1991;27(4):382-6.
11. Daya M. Nostril stenosis corrected by release and serial stenting. J Plast Reconstr Aesthet Surg. 2009;62(8):1012-9.
12. Stallings JO, Sessions DG. Stenosis of the nostril-repair by triplanar W-plasty. Arch Otolaryngol. 1971;93:525-30.
13. Tiwari VK, Sarabahi S. Starplasty: An ideal method for correction of occluded external nares following burns. J Plast Reconstr Aesthet Surg. 2006;59(10):1105-9.
14. Sarabahi S, Kanchna K. Management of ocular and periocular burns. Indian J Burns. 2014;22:22-32.
15. Bhandari PS. Total ear reconstruction in post burn deformity. Burns. 1998;24(7):661-70.
16. Guo P, Jiang H, Yang Q, He L, Lin L, Pan B. Burned Ear reconstruction using a superficial temporal fascia flap. Ear Nose Throat J. 2021;100(10_suppl):1134S-38S.
17. Bos EJ, Doerga P, Breugem CC, van Zuijlen PP. The burned ear; possibilities and challenges in framework reconstruction and coverage. Burns. 2016;42(7):1387-95.
18. Sarabahi S. Management of ear burns. Indian J Burns. 2012;20(1):11-7.
19. McIndoe AH. Total reconstruction of the burned face. The Bradshaw Lecture 1958. Br J Plast Surg. 1983;36(4):410-20.
20. Baig N, Parasrampuria N, Yeshwante B, Tated G. Electrical injuries of the oral cavity: A menace to mankind. Indian J Health Sci. 2015;8:11-7.
21. Yeroshalmi F, Sidoti EJ Jr, Adamo AK, Lieberman BL, Badner VM. Oral electrical burns in children-a model of multidisciplinary care. J Burn Care Res. 2011;32(2):e25-30.
22. Thomas SS. Electrical burns of the mouth: Still searching for an answer. Burns. 1996;22(2):137-40.
23. Srivastava JL, Biswas G, Narayan RP, Goel A. Chronically exposed calvarium following electrical burns. Burns. 1993;19(2):138-41.
24. Sittitavornwong S, Morlandt ABP. Reconstruction of the Scalp, Calvarium, and Frontal Sinus. Oral Maxillofac Surg Clin North Am. 2013;25(2):105-29.
25. Golpanian S, Kassira W, Habal MB, Thaller SR. Treatment options for exposed calvarium due to trauma and burns. J Craniofac Surg. 2017;28(2):318-24.
26. Klingbeil KD, Fertig R. Eyebrow and eyelash hair transplantation: A systematic review. J Clin Aesthet Dermatol. 2018;11(6): 21-30.
27. Bharadia D, Sinha I, Pomahac B. Role of facial vascularized composite allotransplantation in burn patients. Clin Plastic Surg. 2017;44(4):857-64.
28. Shokri T, Saadi R, Wang W, Reddy L, Ducic Y. Facial transplantation: complications, outcomes, and long-term management strategies. Semin Plast Surg. 2020;34(4):245-53.
29. Vyas K, Bakri K, Gibreel W, Cotofana S, Amer H, Mardini S. Facial transplantation. Facial Plast Surg Clin North Am. 2022;30(2): 255-69.

CHAPTER

27 Hand Burns

S Raja Sabapathy

INTRODUCTION

Optimal hand function has a very positive impact on the quality of life of a postburn patient. This assumes considerable importance because the ultimate integration of the burn patient back into society depends upon the functional status of the hands to carry out the daily activities and make an independent living. Tredget[1] found that in patients with a mean total body surface area (TBSA) burn of 15%, 54% of the patients' sustained burns of the hand and upper extremity. Sheridan[2] analyzed the outcome of 1,047 acutely burned hands in 659 patients treated over a 10-year period. They found that in patients with superficial burns, 97% had normal hand function while in those with deep dermal and full-thickness injuries requiring surgery, only 81% regained normal hand function. Although only 9% of those with injuries involving the extensor mechanism, joint capsule, or bone had normal functional outcomes, 90% were able to perform activities of daily living independently. This high percentage of good function is achieved when hand burns are properly assessed at presentation and timely surgical intervention is done for those who need it. If the opportunity is missed, the result is a bad, scarred hand with severe contractures which are difficult to correct **(Figs. 1A and B)**. It is a preventable complication. The purpose of this chapter is to guide the surgeon to meet the specific demands of the burn injured hand and obtain the best possible outcome.

ACUTE HAND BURNS

Anatomical Considerations

The palm of the hand is covered with thick glabrous skin which is attached to the bone by fibrous septa. The

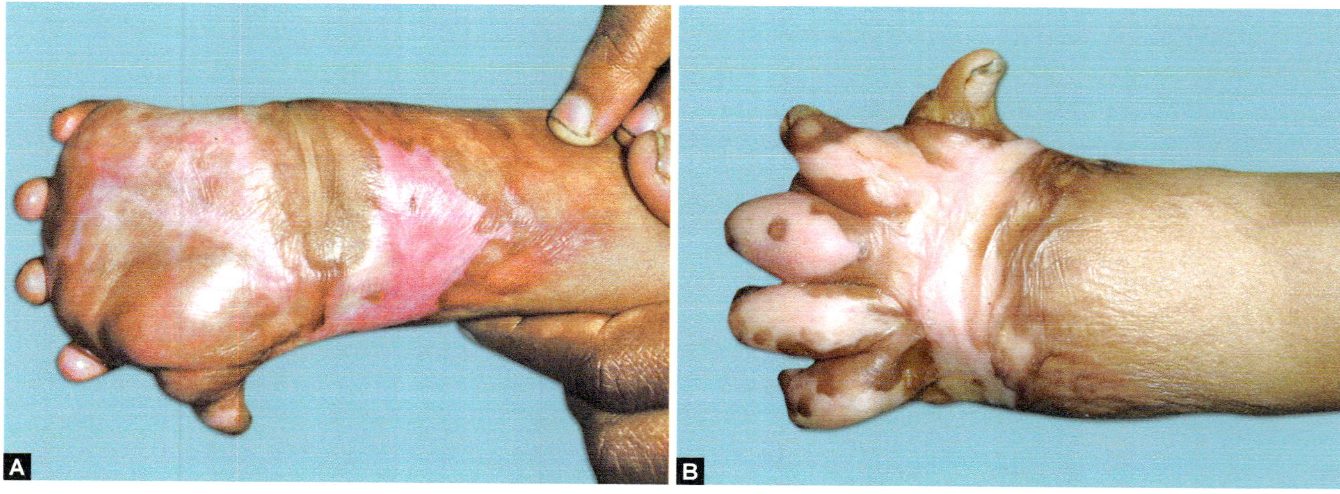

FIGS. 1A AND B: An 18-month-old child who sustained flame burns to the dorsum of the hand with severe contractures due to allowing the deep burns to heal spontaneously.

dorsal surface is covered with thin skin, loosely attached to the underlying structures. Postburn edema causes significant swelling on the dorsum which leads to unphysiological joint positions. On the other hand, on the palmar aspect, although the edema may not be apparent, it can lead to severe physiological disturbances by causing pressure on the vessels in the palm and the median nerve in the carpal tunnel. The swelling in the palm can cause arterial insufficiency while the swelling on the dorsum can compromise the venous return. The combination results in compartment syndrome of the intrinsic muscles.

The collateral ligaments are taut when the metacarpophalangeal (MCP) joints are in full flexion and the interphalangeal (IP) joints are in extension. This is the ideal position of immobilization of these joints after injury. If stiffness occurs with the MCP joints in extension and the IP joints in flexion, the contracted collateral ligaments of the MCP joints and the volar plate of the proximal interphalangeal (PIP) joints resist correction. The joints of hand form a system of intercalated joints wherein the distal joint takes up the deformity opposite to that of the proximal joint. The wrist joint is the key. If not splinted, the joints take up the position of maximum comfort which is exactly the opposite of what is ideal for function. In the stage of edema, if the hand is unsupported, the wrist gets flexed, the MCP joints become hyperextended and the PIP joints become flexed **(Figs. 2A and B)**. If the central slip gets attenuated or the dorsal skin over the PIP joint becomes thin, the stage is

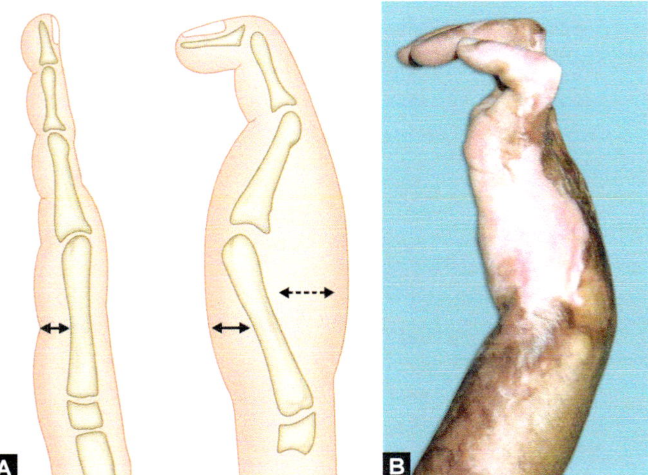

FIGS. 2A AND B: (A) The edema of the acute stage of the burns occurs predominantly on the dorsum of the hand due to the loose tissue on the dorsum. This results in hyperextension of metacarpophalangeal (MCP) joints. (B) If the joints are not properly splinted in the acute stage, this typical deformity of wrist flexion, MCP hyperextension and interphalangeal (IP) joint flexion occurs. This is an avoidable disaster which is difficult to correct.

set for the development of the boutonnière deformity. Alternatively, if the intrinsic muscles suffer from compartment syndrome, swan neck deformity develops in the fingers and first web contracture occurs. The optimum treatment of a burnt hand revolves around keeping the joints in the position of optimum function, regularly making the joints go through the full range of movement while achieving healing of the wound as early as possible.

Assessment

It is advisable to admit all cases of hand burns with the exception of very minor ones. This is because, should a complication occur, the morbidity produced far outweighs the cost and efforts involved in in-patient treatment.

If the hands are burnt as part of a major burn injury, the general management of the patient should rightfully deserve all the attention. Whatever be the total percentage of burns, a preliminary examination of the affected hand is done. One should look for associated injuries like hand and finger amputations, fractures, and dislocations. The depth of burns is assessed. Second-degree superficial dermal burns are pink, moist and painful, and blanch on pressure. Blisters are considered to be characteristic of superficial burns. Deep dermal burns are waxy white in appearance. Full-thickness burns are obvious by the thick leathery skin, appearance of thrombosed subcutaneous veins through the skin and absence of pain to pin prick. Assessing ends of extremes is easy but assessing deeper partial-thickness burns can be difficult. Newer technologies like laser Doppler flowmeter, intravenous fluorescein and ultrasound have been tried but traditional clinical assessment remains unsurpassed by new technology.[3] If the area does not blanch on pressure and is dull to pin prick, then probably it is a deep partial thickness injury. The areas in question must be marked in a drawing and attached to the case records. This must be done before the application of topical antimicrobials, as otherwise the assessment may become difficult later.

In circumferential full-thickness burns and deep partial-thickness burns, the edema can cause circulatory compromise. Ultrasound recordings, pulse oximetry, photoelectric plethysmography have been tried but escharotomy must be performed on clinical grounds. Significant increase in survival of fingers has been found following lateral digital escharotomy compared with those not decompressed.[4] If the hand starts feeling cold and palmar arch pulse disappears on Doppler, it is better to decompress the part. Escharotomy has to start proximally in the arm depending upon the involvement. If proximal escharotomy does not make the fingers warm, it has to be continued to the hand and digits. In the digits, it is done on the ulnar side of the index, middle, ring, and

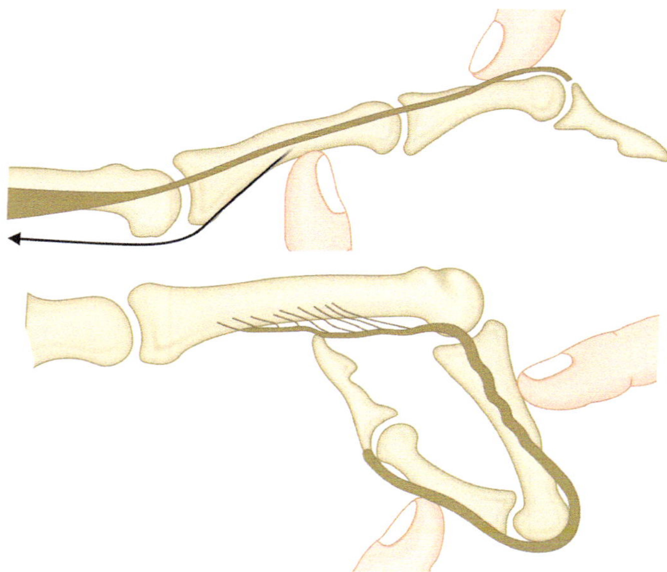

FIG. 3: Intrinsic tightness test (Finochietto–Bunnell). When intrinsics are tight, it becomes difficult to flex the proximal interphalangeal (PIP) joint with the metacarpophalangeal (MCP) joint hyperextended. If this is positive, then the intrinsics have to be released. When the MCP joint is in extension, the contracted interosseous muscles impede flexion of the PIP joint because of the traction exerted on the extensors. Flexion of the MCP joint relaxes the extensors and flexion becomes possible at the PIP joint.

little fingers and the incision can be carried proximally into the dorsum of the hand. For the thumb, the initial incision is on the radial side. Escharotomy is done with fine cautery and some patients may need anesthesia. Hemostasis must be carefully secured after release.

The edema may mask the onset of compartment syndrome of the intrinsic muscles. High levels of suspicion are necessary. The Finochietto intrinsic tightness test must be done **(Fig. 3)**. The MCP joint is passively extended and when in that position the PIP joint is passively flexed. Presence of good resistance is an indication for the release of the intrinsic muscles. This requires anesthesia. The escharotomy incisions can be used to release the intrinsic compartments and usually in such instances the carpal tunnel and the Guyon canal are also decompressed. If during initial examination or after a few hours the sensation in the fingertip is blunted, it is better to do carpal and Guyon canal decompression. If nerve compression is the predominant problem, claw hand deformity results **(Figs. 4A to J)**. If intrinsic muscle contracture is the main issue, swan neck deformity results.

Initial Management

Once assessment of the depth of injury is made and recorded and the need for decompression is taken care of, the hand is dressed with moist nonadherent dressings. Dry dressings and exposure method are not recommended for hand burns. The hand is dressed with topical antimicrobials like silver sulfadiazine 1% cream. After dressing, the hand is immobilized with a splint with the wrist in mild dorsiflexion, the MCP joints in about 70° of flexion and the IP joints in extension. Between two dressings, the hand should be put through possible range of movement at least twice a day. In the initial stage, the dressings may need to be done daily and the movements must be started on Day 1, even in critically ill patients.

If the depth of burns is assessed as superficial, the wound can be dressed, splinted, and left as such for 4–5 days. An earlier dressing change may be indicated in case there is soakage of dressing, or the patient complains of undue pain, fever, or foul smell/discharge, etc. Very frequent dressing changes in such cases disturb the healing epithelium and may increase the chances of infection. Another method for the management of superficial burns is to smear the hand with silver sulfadiazine and place the hand inside a sterile surgical glove and allow continuous movement. The glove can be replaced when it gets soiled. Good healing with absence of contracture has been shown by this technique.[5]

If one is unsure of the depth of burns or if the dressings get extensively soaked, the wound is redressed. Lack of adherence of the dressings to the wound is considered another indication of deep burns.[6] At all times, the hand is diligently splinted in functional position and early motion exercises started. The hand is kept elevated and in a splint at all times except when the patient is on therapy. By about 3–5 days, the wound can be reassessed, and decision made for continuation of conservative management or operative intervention.

EARLY SURGERY FOR BURNS OF HAND

Early surgery for a burnt hand must be done for second-degree deep dermal, third-degree full thickness, or in the fourth-degree burns when underlying tendons, bone or joints are also involved. In second-degree deep dermal burns, the aim is to obtain near normal function, while in the deeper degree burns the aim is to maximize the restoration of function.

Tangential Excision

Early tangential excision and coverage of burns initiated by Janzekovic (1970)[7] is a milestone in burn care **(Figs. 5A to J)**. She applied the principles of debridement learnt in trauma to burn care. She found that not all deep dermal burns healed primarily with

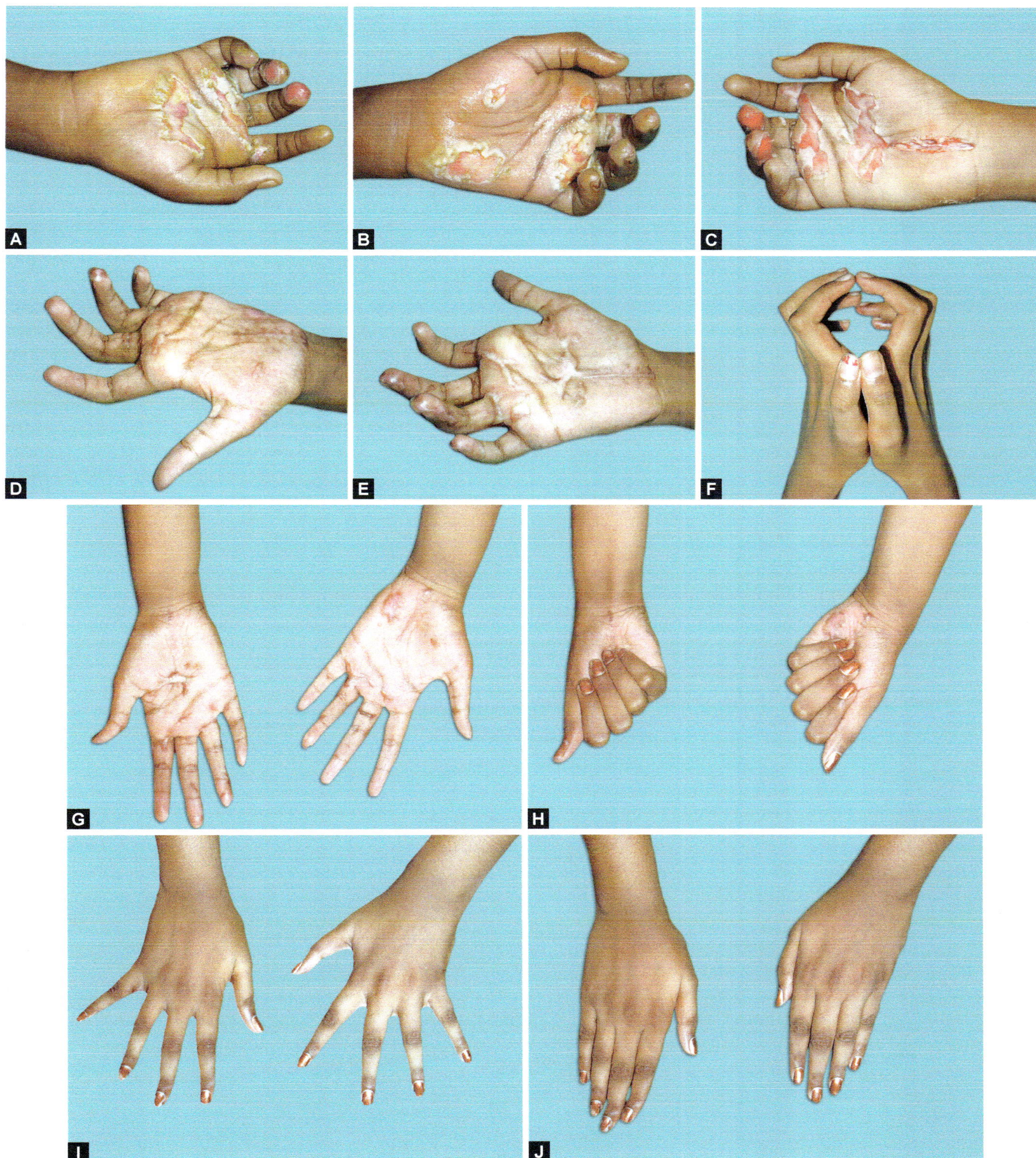

FIGS. 4A TO J: A 12-year-old girl with electrical burns of both hands admitted after 14 hours of injury. She had numbness in all the fingertips (A and B). Carpal tunnel and Guyon's canal decompression was done in both the hands (C). Despite this, the patient developed complete intrinsic paralysis in both hands (D to F). The intrinsics recovered in 3 months time (G to J). If the nerves are not decompressed in time, patients usually end up with gross deficit.

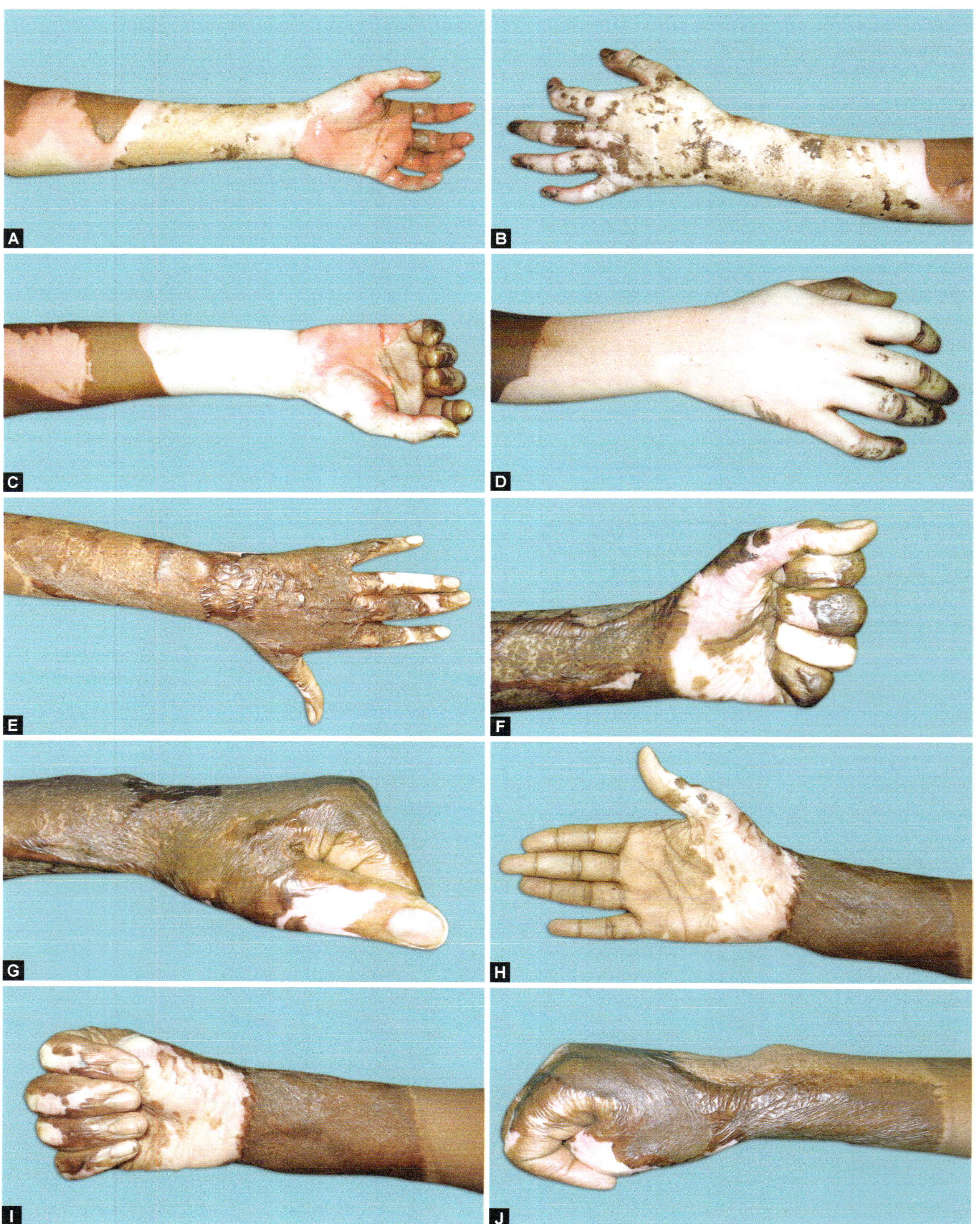

FIGS. 5A TO J: Deep dermal flame burns involving both hands (A to D). Patient had tangential excision of the burns and skin grafting. Good functional results have been seen during follow-up (E to J).

good outcomes. If the burnt nonviable part of the dermis got infected, it was converted to a full thickness burn. Janzekovic proposed shaving off the dead superficial component of the dermis before infection sets in and cover it up with a thin split thickness skin graft so that the native unburnt dermis could be saved. It is done around 4 days postburn when the patient has recovered from the burn shock phase or earlier if the patient is fit. The burnt surface is successively shaved with a skin grafting knife, set to cut a thin slice, until fine punctuate bleeding is encountered as the tips of the vertical dermal capillaries are shaved off. This is done under tourniquet. Without tourniquet the blood loss can be heavy and inadequate excision can result due to the oozing of blood from some areas obscuring full excision. With experience it is possible to define the correct level of excision while working under tourniquet. The tourniquet is deflated and completeness of excision confirmed. If there are small patches left over, the tourniquet is reinflated and excision is done. Between the sites of dermal bleeding, dermal collagen is exposed and some epithelium remains viable in the deep skin adnexae. This surface needs a skin graft applied immediately so that it does not dry out. Grafts survive by picking up a blood supply from the capillary loops which have been transected. The intervening dermis becomes incorporated beneath the graft. Healing is faster and better esthetic and functional results are achieved because the deeper dermis of the native skin is saved. To prevent the problem of hematoma formation beneath the graft, tourniquet is released after shaving and all brisk bleeding points are coagulated till it is felt that the fine ooze can be controlled with pressure. When all brisk bleeding points have been coagulated, the tourniquet is inflated again, grafts applied, gentle compression dressing given and then the tourniquet is released. If there is doubt about hemostasis, the first dressing can be done at 48 hours to drain any subgraft collection.

It is ideal to apply a split thickness sheet graft with a thin layer of dermis (0.010–0.012 inches thickness) to cover the raw areas **(Figs. 6A and B)**. 1:1.5 meshing of the skin graft can be done, but it should not be expanded. In tangential excision, thick grafts and meshed grafts must not be applied. They give a poor cosmetic result.[8] Remnants of epithelium which grow after graft "take" may produce small inclusion cysts on the surface for some months. As the cysts appear beneath the thin skin graft, they can be decompressed and they settle well. In the tangential excision technique, the area shaved must always be covered with graft either immediately or at least within 2 hours. Skin allografts from the skin bank or the many available dermal regeneration templates can be used. If left uncovered, the exposed dermis desiccates and the deep dermal burns get converted into a full-thickness injury. The technique involves blood loss and hence should always be done under tourniquet. Blood loss is not a problem when surgery for hand burns is done under tourniquet.

Tangential excision requires correct choice of patient, availability of blood and blood products, infrastructure, and skill. It is suitable for experienced personnel. While the conventional teaching of an upper limit of TBSA excised at one sitting of 10–15% is practiced in many centers, established burn care centers have gone in for total burn excision of all deep and deep dermal burns with good success. For others, the safer option is the conservative management with dressings and grafting the raw areas at the earliest.

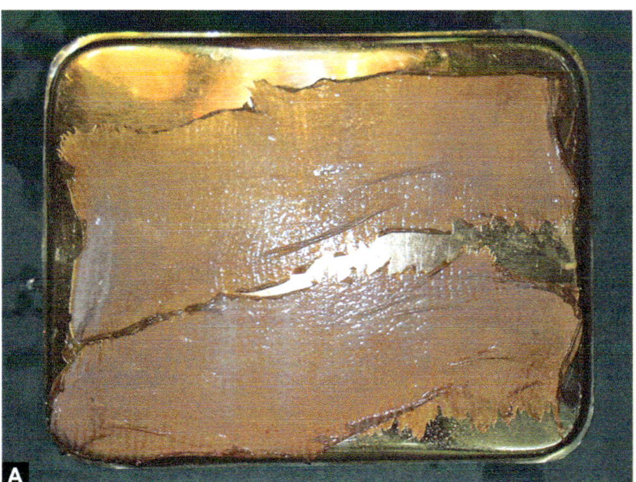

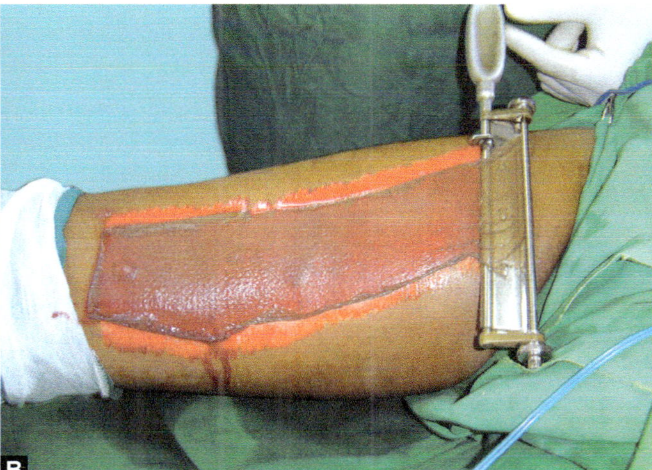

FIGS. 6A AND B: When early tangential excision of burns is done, the raw area must be immediately covered with thin graft. Figures show the recommended thickness of the graft.

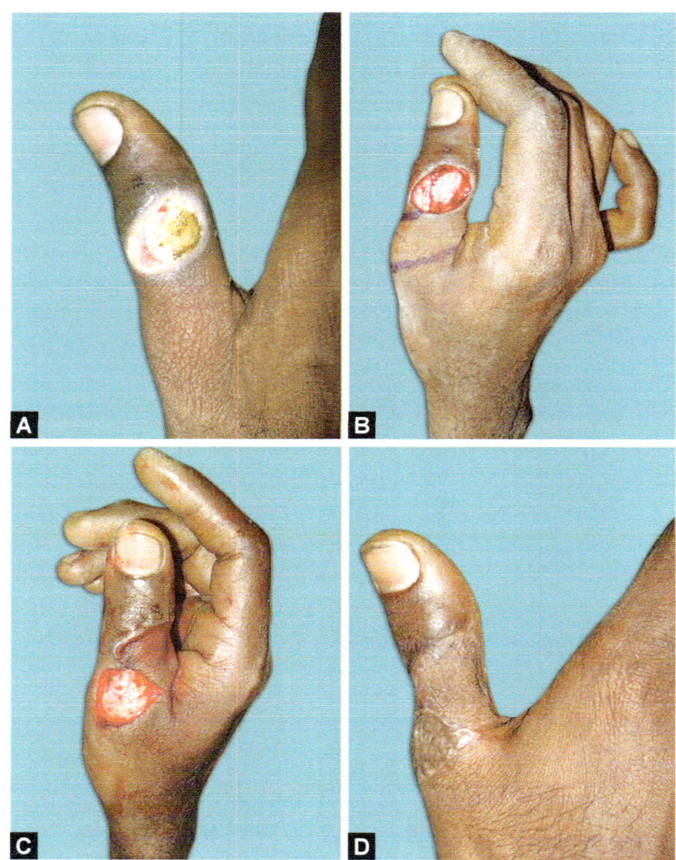

FIGS. 7A TO D: Localized deep burns of the hand can be excised primarily and covered with local flaps.

In tangential excision, a layer of viable dermis must be left behind to be covered with thin skin graft. It must not be confused with excision of the burns done for full-thickness injuries which is dealt with later. Tangential excision is good for deep dermal burns involving the dorsum of the hand. It is generally not used for the palm.

Excision of Burns

When the injured area is limited, definitely full thickness and the general condition of the patient permits, the burn wound can be excised and skin cover is provided. In hand burns, it is usually applicable to limited area full-thickness burns overlying joints, tendons, and bone **(Figs. 7A to D)**. In such circumstances if allowed to take the natural course, the necrosing burnt area will be complicated by infection and loss of critical tissue. Early excision and flap cover in such circumstances help to salvage critical structures. In burns of upper limb, it is better to limit this excision to such instances. When done for wide areas of the forearm and arm, the level of excision has to be up to the deep fascia. Mere excision of the full thickness skin will expose the subcutaneous fat which may not be a good bed for the survival of the split skin graft. In such cases of full-thickness burns, it is better to excise to up to fascia and graft.

BOX 1 Jebsen's[10] objective test criteria.

- Writing words as quickly and clearly as possible with dominant and nondominant hands
- Turning over five 3 × 5-inch index cards (simulated page turning)
- *Picking up small common objects*: Asked to pick up a coin and paperclip, placed on a desk
- *Simulated feeding*: Had to pick up peas from a plate with a teaspoon and bring it to his/her mouth
- *Stacking checkers*: A stack had to be made with five small wooden checkers, placed in front of the patient
- *Picking up large light objects*: The patient was asked to pick up an empty can with a diameter of 10 cm
- *Picking up large heavy objects*: The patient was asked to pick up a full can (600 g) with a diameter of 10 cm

Timing of Surgery

To obtain a better understanding of the parameters involved in the long-term functional outcome of hand burns a retrospective study was performed by VanZuijlen et al. on 88 consecutive patients with hand burns (143 hands).[9] Patients were followed for 12 months. Hand function was assessed by seven objective test criteria (7-OTC) described by Jebsen **(Box 1)**.[10] Five parameters were found to have a significant predictive value for long-term hand function. In order of predictive value, these were finger amputations, age at admission, impaired autograft "take", the full thickness hand burn surface area and the full thickness total body burn surface area. No relationship was found between the postburn day of operation and the long-term hand function. This finding is inconsistent with the consensus that functional outcome is improved by early excision and grafting. While provision of early cover to the hand burns is beneficial, in a patient with major burns general measures and coverage of large segment raw area take priority. It is the opinion of this author that hand function is well preserved when burns of uncertain depth are treated expectantly, followed by selective debridement and grafting. Advantages include reduced blood loss, no loss of vital tissue and a reduction of the need for donor sites.

If a diagnosis of full-thickness burn of the hand is certain, early primary excision and grafting are advocated. If diagnosis is a clear deep dermal second-degree burns of the dorsum of the hand and fingers, tangential excision and grafting are done within 4–5 days. Rehabilitation is commenced as early as possible and the length of hospital stay is reduced. If the assessment of burn depth is difficult, the operation can be postponed to prevent excision of vital tissues allowing those areas with partial-thickness burns to heal spontaneously. A "wait and see" approach to hand burns of uncertain depth is valid. The function of the hand will not be adversely affected by delayed surgical treatment in those patients with extensive burns in whom early large area wound closure takes priority.[9] The aim is to achieve skin cover to the hand within 2–3 weeks from injury before infection sets in. However, till wound healing is achieved, the hand has to be splinted in the functional position and range of movement exercises have to be provided. After grafting, if there are areas of graft losses, re-grafting of the areas is important. Allowing healing by secondary intention results in poor outcome.

FLAP COVER TO THE DEEP BURNS OF THE HAND

In fourth degree burns, it is wiser to resort to early flap cover than just rely on positioning the joints. Various local, regional pedicle flaps like radial and posterior interosseous flaps, distant pedicle flaps, and free flaps have been used to cover postburn raw areas **(Figs. 8A to J)**. Any of them can provide good result provided care is taken to keep the joints in functional position during flap transfer. Critical to the success of flap transfer is debridement of the area. The base has to be debrided to viable depth and the wound margins excised to good viable skin. This is crucial for success, for otherwise the flap detaches and slips off from the edges. A vascular flap cannot make the dead burned tissues in the base alive.

It is rare for palmar side to need flap cover. Palmar skin is thick and during most injuries the palm escapes

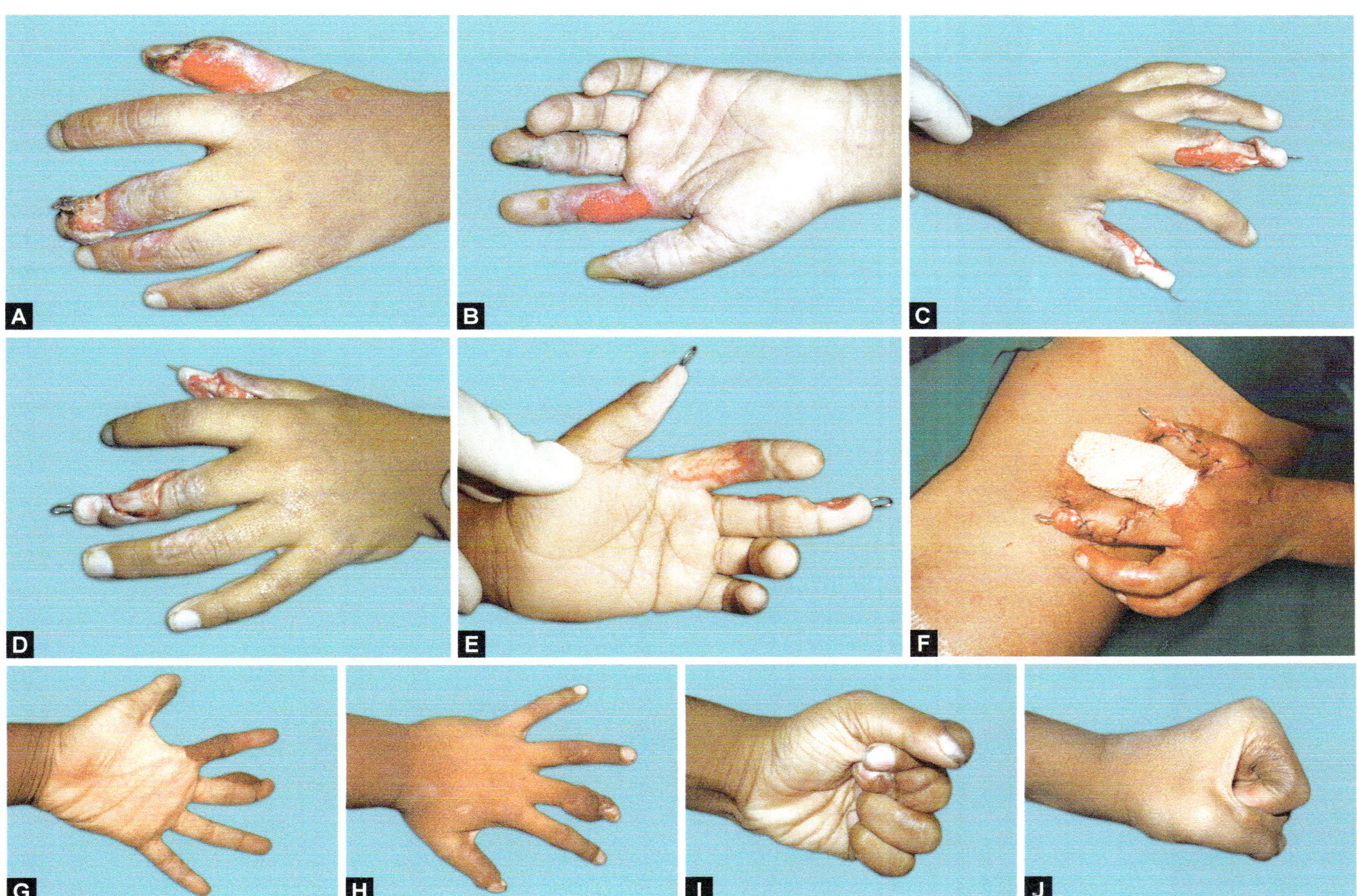

FIGS. 8A TO J: A 3-year-old child was brought 3 weeks after electrical burns to the hand involving the thumb, index, and middle fingers (A to C). The wounds were radically debrided and the bones stabilized by K-wire (D to F). Small abdominal flaps were given to the thumb and middle finger and the index raw area skin grafted (G). Good functional result achieved (H to J).

deep burns because of the clenched fist position during injury. Deep palmar burns usually require flap reconstruction only when there is associated flexor tendon exposure or loss. Skin grafting is preferred because it produces the fixity and resistance necessary for satisfactory grip **(Figs. 9A to E)**. As with all hand burns it is essential to ensure total "take" of the graft. When flap cover is required for the palm it has to be thin. Bulky flaps give a sense of fullness in the hand and prevent gripping of objects.

Reconstruction of severely burned fourth-degree hand burns: Circumferential fourth-degree burns may need amputation. In all other burn injuries, all effort must be

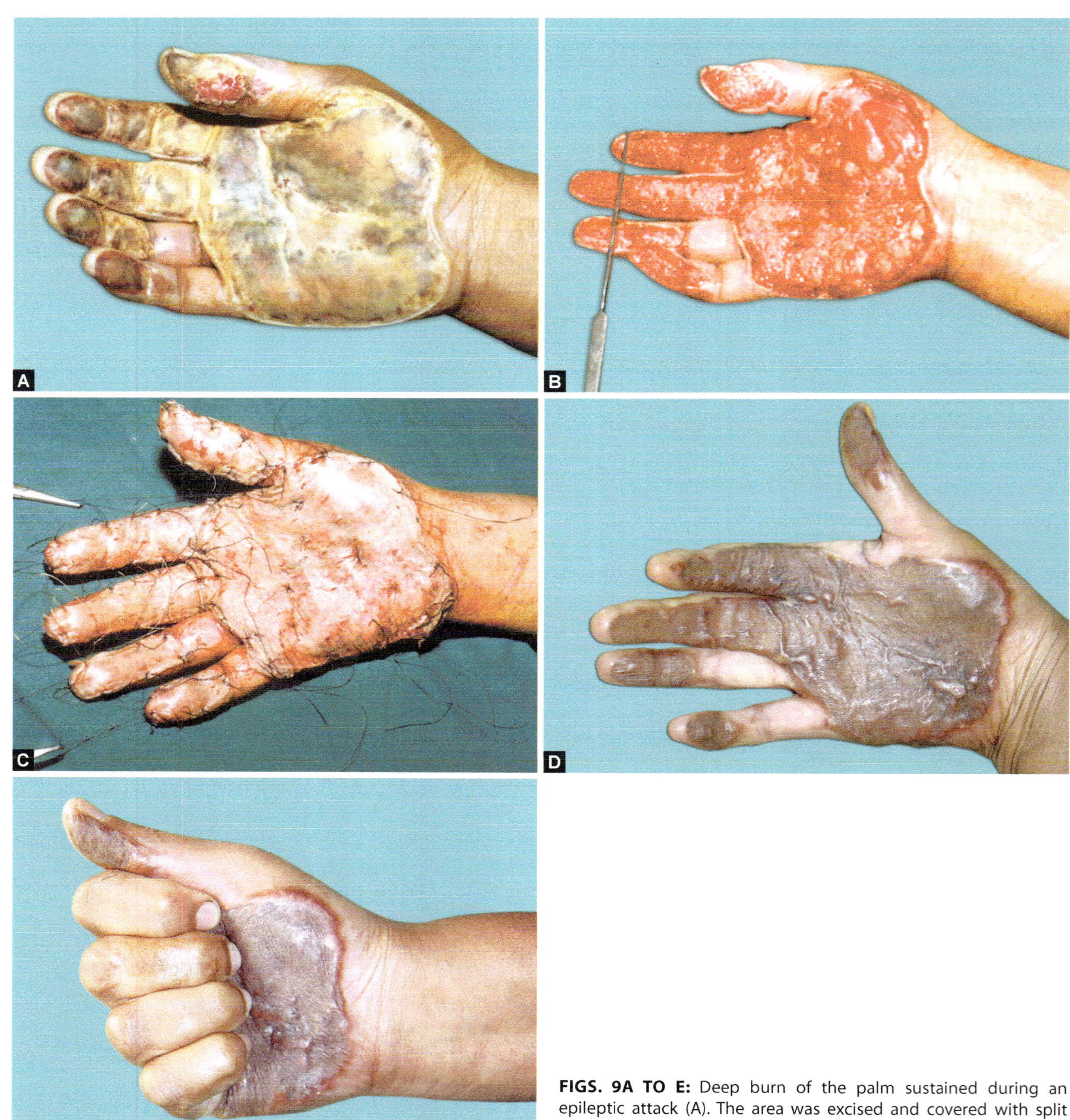

FIGS. 9A TO E: Deep burn of the palm sustained during an epileptic attack (A). The area was excised and covered with split skin graft (B and C). Good after care with compression garment and massage gave satisfactory outcome (D and E).

made to save available length of the hand. A very common pattern of injury is very deep dorsal injury exposing burned bone with viable volar side **(Figs. 10A to 11K)**. Advances in flap cover and microsurgery can make these hands functional. Early flap cover rather than simple K wire stabilization is advocated for salvage of these hands.[11]

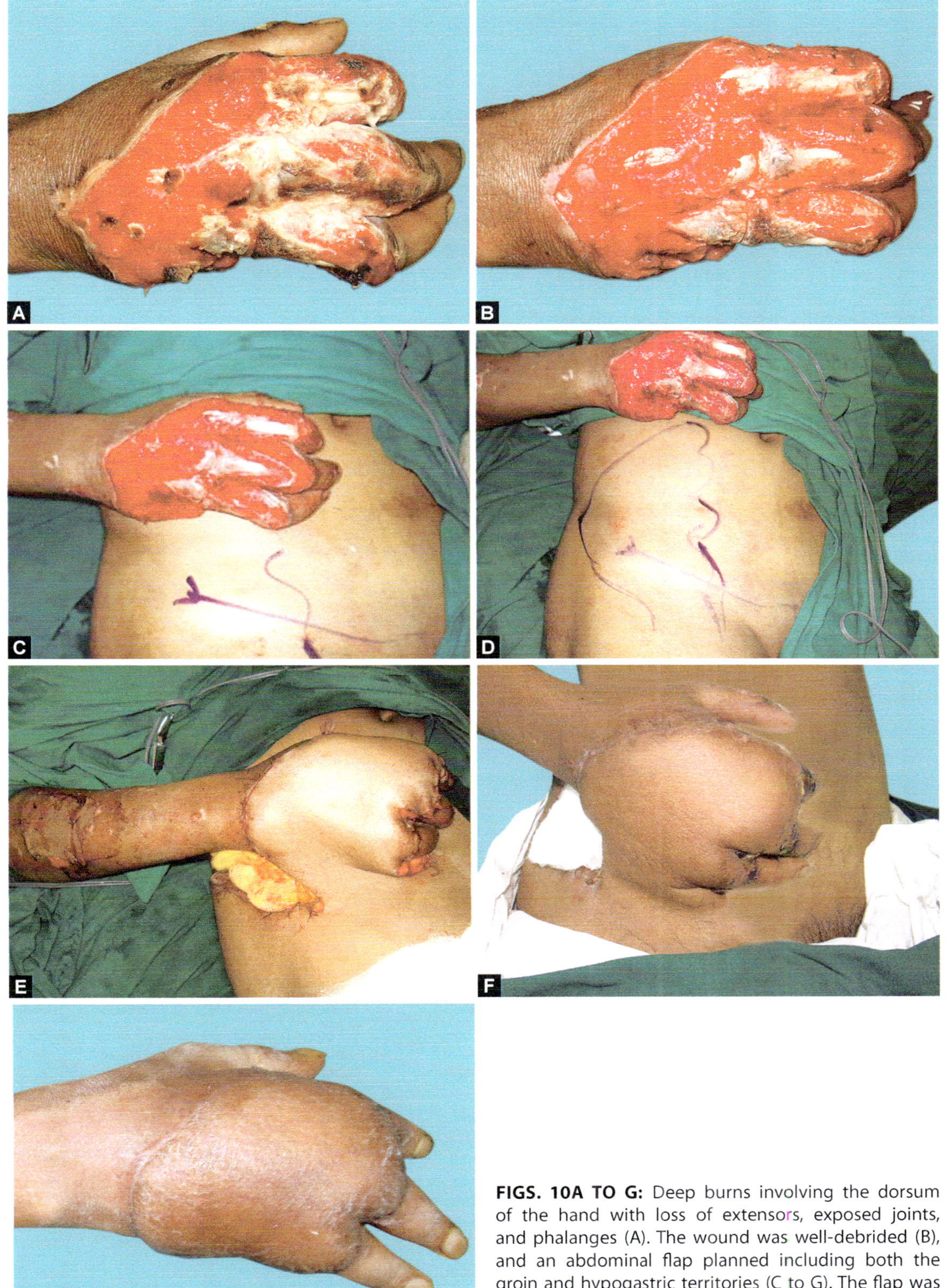

FIGS. 10A TO G: Deep burns involving the dorsum of the hand with loss of extensors, exposed joints, and phalanges (A). The wound was well-debrided (B), and an abdominal flap planned including both the groin and hypogastric territories (C to G). The flap was subsequently thinned. He had reasonable function of the hand even without extensor tendon reconstruction.

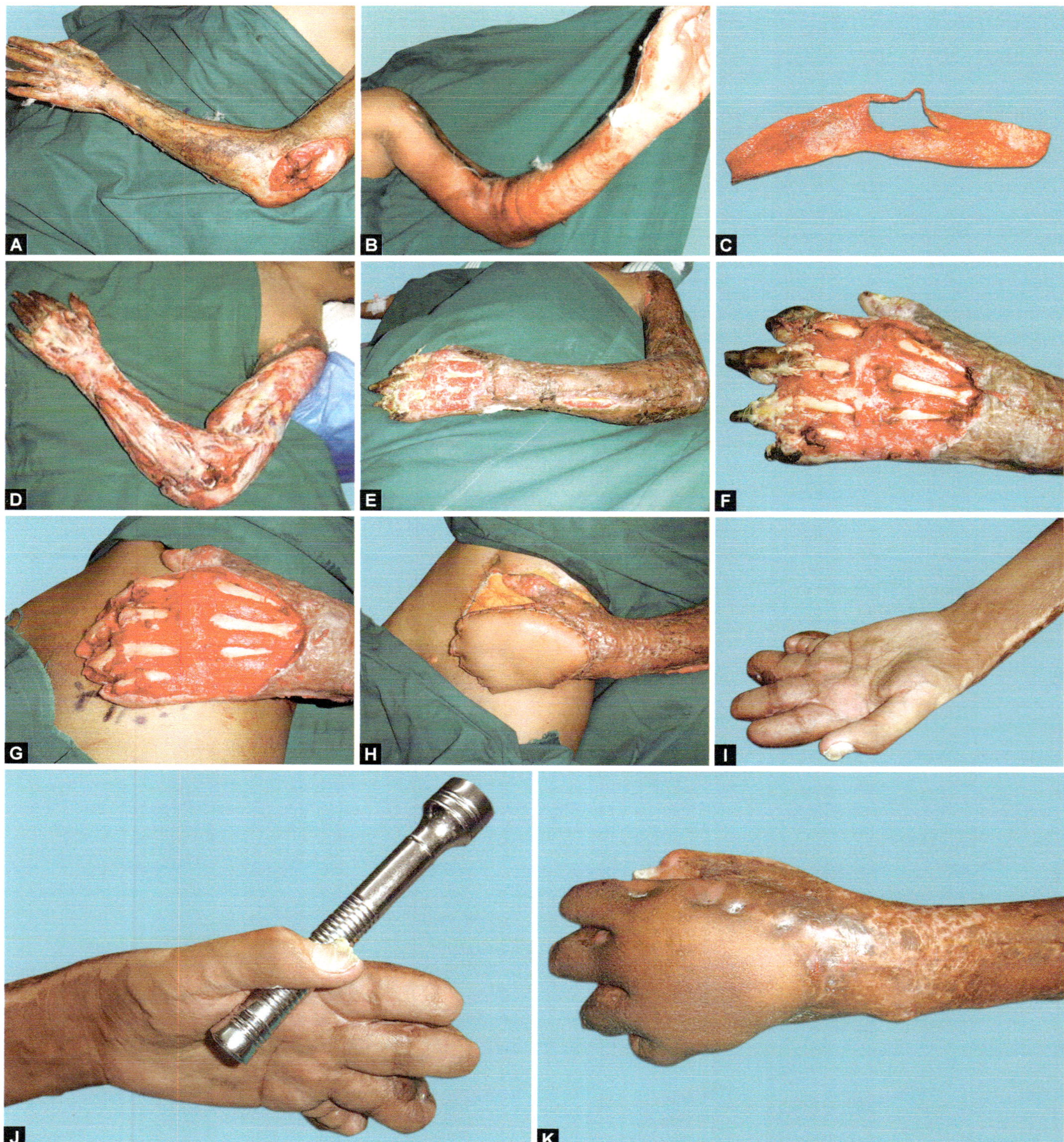

FIGS. 11A TO K: Fourth-degree burns of the dorsum of the hand, forearm, and arm with relative sparing of the volar side in an industrial accident (A and B). The dead skin was excised (C), which revealed the damage to the muscles (D). The wound was serially debrided and the arm and forearm were grafted. The hand was subsequently debrided and covered with a groin flap to achieve a satisfactory functional outcome (E to K).

AFTERCARE OF BURNED HANDS

Totally healed burned hand is a good platform to start rehabilitation. Even small areas of unhealed wounds give rise to inflammation, need regular dressing, are painful, and make the patient uncooperative for rehabilitation schedules.

The aim is to minimize the edema, increase the range of movement, and prevent scar hypertrophy. Daily supervised physiotherapy is essential.

The value of pressure to prevent hypertrophy of scar was advocated by Parks[12] and Larson.[13] They advocated continuous controlled pressure above the capillary pressure. Custom-made compression garments are prescribed and the patient is made to wear it at all times other than at the time of exercises. They must be worn for at least 6 months. These are most effective in the early stages and hypertrophic scar is responsive to pressure in the first 3 months **(Figs. 12A to H)**. For this reason, it is emphasized that the endpoint of acute burn management of the hand is to get stable healing of all the wounds. Patient compliance with pressure garments is not good if they are worn over dressed wounds. The bleeding from the wound and the pain deter them from wearing the pressure garment and ranging of the joints. Hence, it is our practice to readmit the patients even when there is a small area of skin loss and re-graft to get good stable healing. It is common for contractures to occur in the web. One of the effective ways to prevent it is to roll the micropore plaster, place it in the web, and hold it by tapes **(Fig. 13)**.

Perkins[14] initiated the use of silicone gel in scar for controlling hypertrophic burn scars. Probably they act by decreasing the evaporation of water from the skin and maintaining the optimum hydration of the stratum corneum. Like pressure garments it also has to be

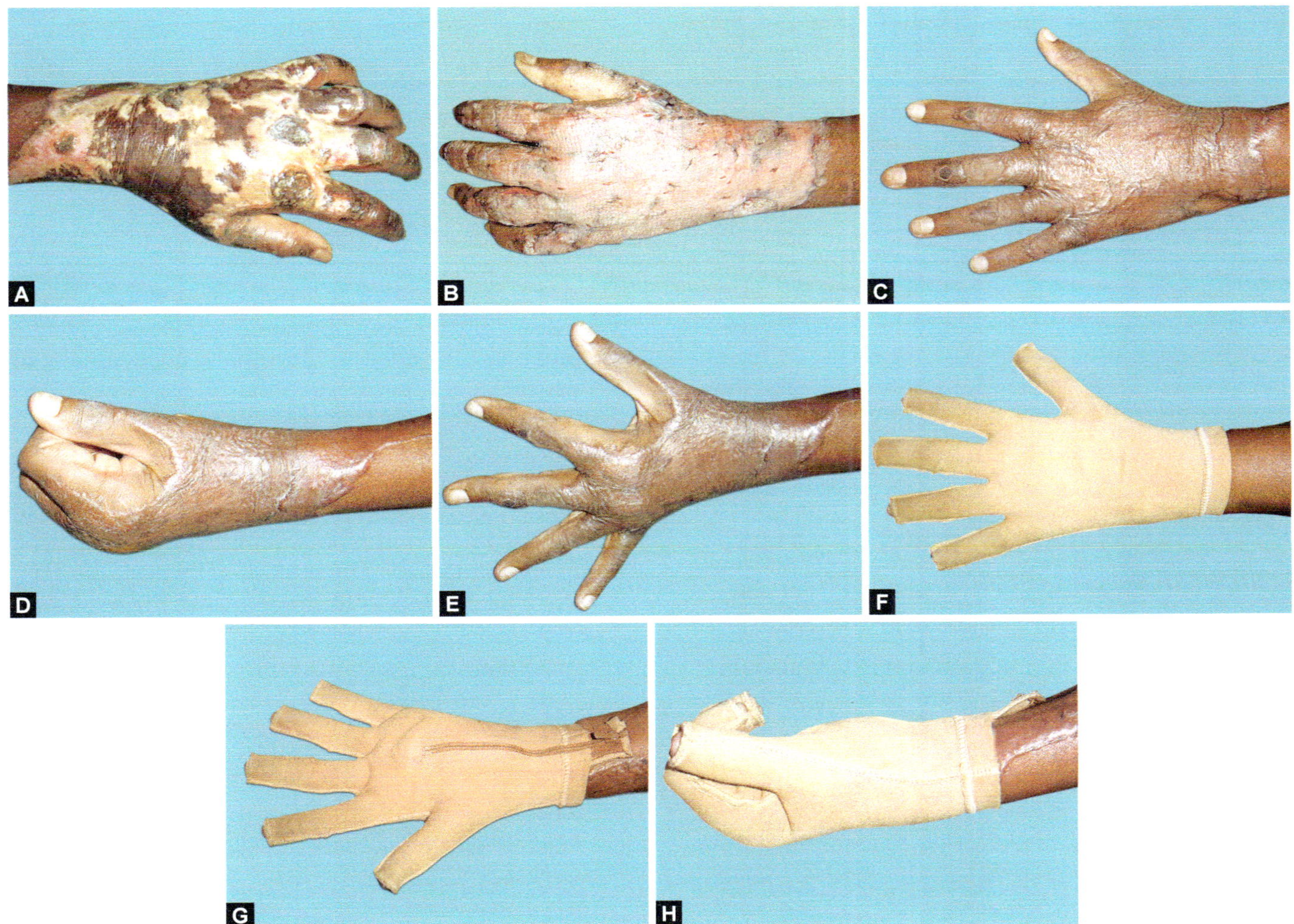

FIGS. 12A TO H: A deep dermal burn of the dorsum of the hand treated by early tangential excision (A and B). The grafts settle well and yield good results (C to E). When followed up with custom-made compression garments (F to H).

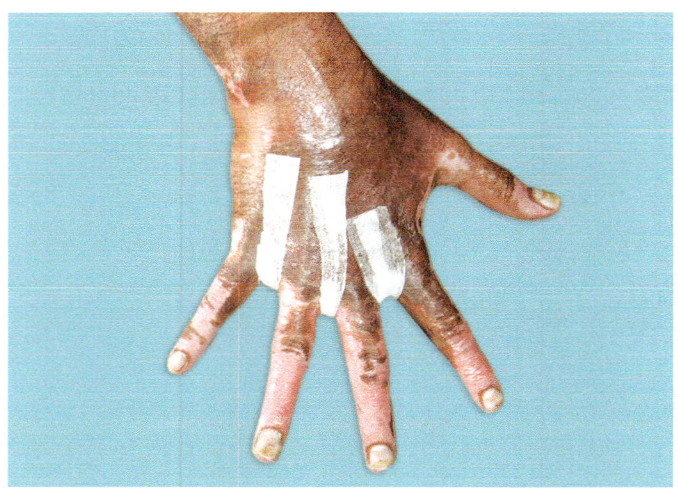

FIG. 13: To prevent web creep after grafting of the web spaces, compression is needed. It can be obtained by placing a rolled micropore plaster retained by a tape.

applied for a few months. Silicone gel application allows early pain-free movements of stiff joints. When applied over healed skin grafts it prevents contraction of the grafts and when applied over hypertrophic scars, the scars soften and make them more amenable to pressure therapy. It is the practice of the author to use both silicone gel sheet and pressure garment together whenever possible to get optimum results. Silicone product improvement has been done and now it is available in a tube as a gel. It has the advantage of easier application in areas of varying contour and patients find it easier to comply. Equally, good results have been claimed.[15]

It is to be emphasized that prime consideration in the prevention of hypertrophic scar and contracture is to obtain early and complete healing of the burn wound in the hand.

POSTBURN HAND DEFORMITIES AND THEIR MANAGEMENT

Complications of hand burns are due to poor wound healing, namely hypopigmented scars, hypertrophic scars, and joint contractures. They cause both functional and esthetic problems. At Ganga Hospital, we apply the following principles when we manage postburn contractures of the hand.[16]

- While reconstructing a burnt hand, the burn surgeon must concentrate on restoring function rather than just on increasing the range of movement of individual joints.

  Surgery on the burnt hand must restore pinch, the ability to grasp large objects and the power grip. This is obtained when the thumb pulp meets the pulp of other fingers, the hand has adequate first web space and the musculotendinous units function to provide adequate power. Surgical procedures must be chosen to achieve these rather than aiming for an increase in the range of movement in each individual joint. For example, it might be an advantage to have a PIP joint arthrodesed in good functional position than to perform complicated procedures to restore movement in a bad boutonnière deformity.
- When a hand is severely involved, first choose the set of procedures that will bring the maximum benefit to the patient.

  It is usual for a severe burn contracture to undergo a series of procedures to obtain the ultimate functional result, but the first procedure must produce a perceivable improvement in function. Early restoration of independence in the use of the hand will boost the morale and encourage the patient to adhere to postoperative protocols and take up subsequent procedures.

  When contractures occur at multiple joints, correction usually starts from proximal to distal unless the proximal deformities are minor.
- Function is very important, but a burn surgeon must also constantly think of the esthetic aspect of reconstruction of a burned hand.

  The hand is a part that is always exposed and constantly reminds the patient that he is different. An esthetically acceptable reconstruction helps him or her to easily integrate back into the society. The statement by Guy Foucher that "hand surgery is also esthetic surgery" has never been truer than in the treatment of burned hands.[3]
- Assess the deformity in each tissue component to make the treatment plan.

  Burn deformities occur secondary to skin loss. But, deformity correction involves not only correcting the skin loss but also the secondary changes that have occurred in the musculotendinous units and joints. They usually are the limiting factors for deformity correction. Evaluate the deformity in each of the components of skin, tendons, joints, and bones while making the treatment plan.
- Correction of the deformity depends on the excision of the scar tissue and correcting the deforming forces than on the type of skin cover provided.

  Most deformity correction would need skin replacement. Mere replacement of the burn scar with skin graft or a flap will not correct the burn deformity. The deformity must first be corrected and then the defect planned for soft-tissue cover. The correction achieved on the table is the maximum that can be achieved.

- Timing of surgery is crucial to get a good outcome in deformity correction. It is better to perform the surgery when there is tissue equilibrium, as shown by a reduction of the induration and the scars becoming pale.

  While it holds good for most instances, the author prefers early correction of deformities in children, since the scar causes severe contractures and dislocation of joints.
- Physiotherapy, splinting, and scar control measures are important to achieve good outcome.

All these principles will apply to the correction of any burn deformity in some way or the other.

McCauley[17] proposed a classification system which correlates the severity of burn contractures to hand function **(Box 2)**. Technical considerations as they apply to the release of various contractures are detailed below.

Metacarpophalangeal joint contractures: The MCP joint contracture can be in extension or in flexion. A well-functioning MCP joint along with a good first web are the cornerstones for obtaining good function in the hand. When releasing extension contracture an assessment is made about the type of skin cover needed. If flap cover is to be provided, an incision can be made over the MCP joints to obtain release. Otherwise, a transverse incision is made 2 cm proximal to the joint line and flap raised. After contracture release, the distal skin migrates to cover the joint while skin graft is applied proximally **(Figs. 14A to D)**. Collateral ligament release and pericapsular dissection may be needed to obtain full release. Two major problems exist in MCP joint extension contractures which need attention. One, the contracted collateral ligament needs release (capsulotomy). Second, a pocket needs to be created on the volar side for the base of the proximal phalanx to slide down the head of the metacarpal. For capsulotomy, the capsule is entered by making an incision over the extensors and with gentle sweep of a No. 11 blade the contracted collateral ligament is incised. When released, it is possible to flex the proximal phalanx but without the pocket in the volar side, the joint subluxates **(Figs. 15A to C)**. This needs to be taken care of. By a combination of usage of curved scissors and curved dissectors, the adhesions on the volar aspect of the MCP joint are released. Proper translation of the base of the proximal phalanx over the articular surface of the head of the metacarpal is confirmed both clinically and radiologically. If there is resistance for maintaining the position, the joint should be pinned and most often, flap cover is required in such cases.

BOX 2	McCauley's[17] classification of burn scar contractures in hand.
Grade I	Symptomatic tightness but no limitation in range of motion, normal architecture
Grade II	Mild decrease in range of motion without significant impact on activities of daily living, no distortion of normal architecture
Grade III	Functional deficit noted, with early changes in normal architecture of hand
Grade IV	Loss of hand function with significant distortion of normal architecture of the hand
	Subset classification for Grade III and IV contractures—A: Flexion contractures; B: Extension contractures; C: Combination of flexion and extension contractures

Extension contracture of the MCP joints is frequently associated with flexion contracture of the IP joints. Release of the MCP joint may make the finger-tips bury into the palm. Usually, it is difficult to correct all the contractures at the same time and this temporary problem has to be explained to the patient beforehand. If the PIP joint contracture needs volar release, it is done in another sitting. For some cases, arthrodesis of the PIP joint may be the chosen option and, in that case, both the MCP and the PIP joint releases can be done at the same time.

Proximal interphalangeal joint problems: Although regaining of movement in all the joints is the aim of every hand surgeon, in burned hands particularly at the PIP joints, arthrodesis may be one of the common operations resorted to. This is because of the original damage to the extensor apparatus that occurred at the time of injury or subsequently due to edema, poor positioning of the joint, and loss of skin over the PIP joint. It is best to prevent the problem since an established PIP joint contracture is resistant to treatment. In the acute situation, the PIP joints are splinted in extension. If there appears to be a risk of skin loss over the joint, an oblique K-wire is passed through the joint to keep it in extension. This reduces the stress on the skin. It may heal or else granulate enough to be covered with skin graft. This step may prevent loss of extensor tendons and joint exposure. This is a crucial step in the care of hand burns. Otherwise, the central slip ruptures and the lateral bands slide down resulting in a boutonnière deformity. If the joint is exposed, early debridement and cover with local flap are tried. If not, distant flaps have to be resorted to. In isolated hand burns, this is practical, but if this problem occurs in a major burn, the joint may be lost in debridement and the wound heals with the finger shortened.

Boutonnière deformity is due to the attenuation or rupture of the central slip and the sliding volarward of

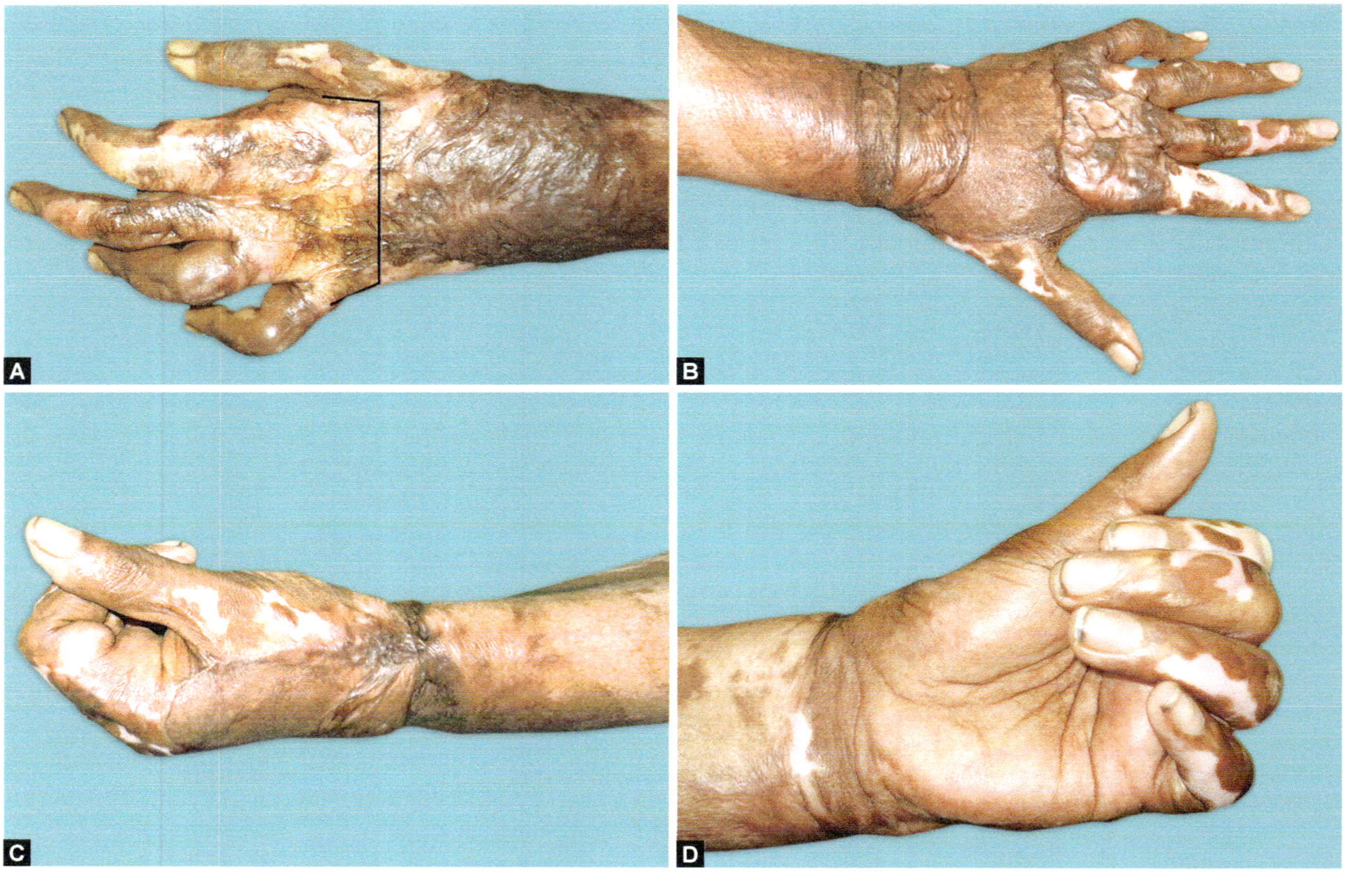

FIGS. 14A TO D: For the release of dorsal contractures, an incision as in the figure will slide the distal flap to cover the joint after release. Joint release can also be done under the flap. If the release process does not expose critical structures, skin graft may be applied to the raw areas.

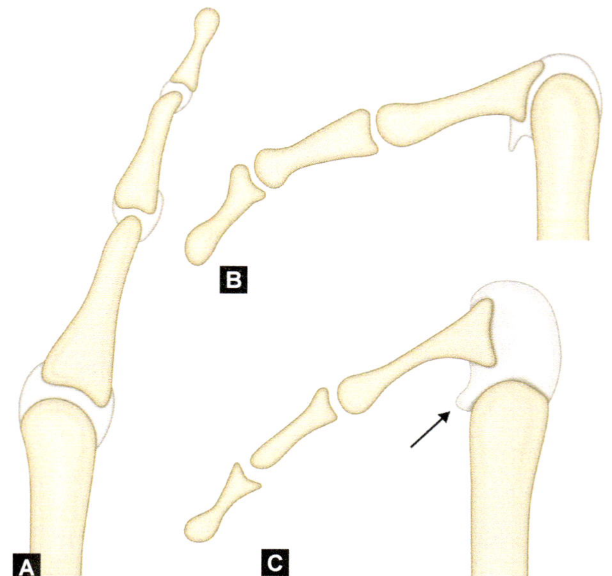

FIGS. 15A TO C: During the release of the hyperextension contracture of the metacarpophalangeal (MCP) joints of the fingers, it is important to clear the tissues on the volar aspect of the head of the metacarpal and create a pocket (A and B). Otherwise, the joint subluxates (C) and if pinned in that position, the contracture will recur.

the lateral bands. The deformity has two components—flexion at the PIP joint and extension at the distal interphalangeal (DIP) joint **(Figs. 16A and B)**. If a boutonnière deformity is passively correctable, the PIP joint is splinted in extension and the patient is encouraged to flex the DIP joint. The flexion of the DIP joint, in turn, makes the lateral bands slide up dorsal to the axis of PIP joint movement. Therapy is very important in boutonnière deformity correction and no surgery is likely to succeed unless both the components of the deformity are passively correctable. If passively correctable and the dorsal skin overlying the PIP joint is of good quality, correction can be attempted by reinserting the central slip, freeing the lateral bands from the volar side and plicating them dorsally. The limiting factor is the skin condition over the joint which usually is of poor quality. So, arthrodesis of the PIP joint is the commonly advocated procedure.

The aim of arthrodesis of the PIP joint is to bring the joint in a position so that it can achieve good contact with the thumb pulp. If stable fingers achieve pulp to pulp contact with the thumb, the hand becomes functional. To this end, the recommended angle of arthrodesis of the PIP joints are 25–35° for index, 30–40° for middle,

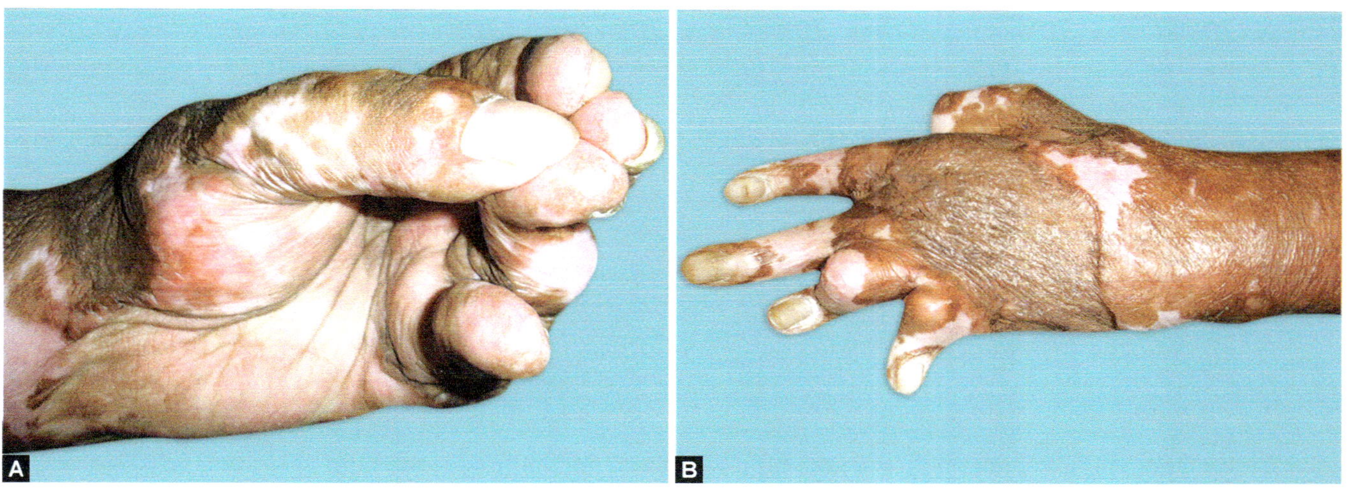

FIGS. 16A AND B: Boutonnière deformity in the ring finger. Correction is difficult because of poor quality skin on the dorsum in spite of the deformity function is preserved in most cases.

35–45° for ring, and 40–50° for little finger. This angle may be varied according to the length of the finger and the movement possible in the thumb and fingers. Technically, a few points are worth noting. It is better to access a severely flexed joint by a gentle curvilinear incision than a longitudinal incision. When a hyperflexed joint is arthrodesed, secondary to bone shortening which is part of the procedure, a longitudinal incision may open up into a diamond making closure difficult. A local flap may then become necessary for wound closure. After incision, skin flaps are carefully raised and the joint entered by making a longitudinal incision in the midline. The collateral ligaments are divided by a gentle sweep of No. 11 blade along the sides and the two articular surfaces are brought out to view. To obtain the correct angle of arthrodesis, one of the components is transected transversely and the other at the recommended angle of arthrodesis. The author finds this easier than trying to adjust the angle on both sides. K wires are used for stabilization. The bone is osteoporotic and fixation has to be done by single pass of K wires. As the fingers are immobilized, even a single oblique K wire is sufficient. The K wires are retained for a minimum period of 4 weeks and if the skin condition is good the wire may be retained for 6 weeks. The MCP joints are mobilized during this period.

Distal interphalangeal joint problems: Deep dorsal burns over the DIP joint cause attrition rupture of the extensor insertion resulting in a mallet finger. This can also, secondarily, lead to swan neck deformity. Mallet finger and swan neck deformities are functionally more disabling than boutonnière deformity. Due to the poor quality of the skin overlying the joint, tendon reconstructions are usually not possible. Arthrodesis of the joint in 0–5° flexion is done by wedge resection of the articular surfaces. Performed early, it may prevent the development of swan neck deformity. In burns, the swan neck deformity is more often due to scar hypertrophy and contracture of the dorsal skin of the fingers. In these situations, incision release of the hypertrophic scar in two places preferably over the proximal and middle phalanx and grafting the residual raw areas is very useful. When the hyperextension at the PIP joint is addressed and the DIP joint remains flexed, the deformity becomes nonfunctional. The DIP joint then needs to be arthrodesed in 0–5°.

Webspace problems—First web contracture: The problems of contracture of the first web are different from the contracture of other webspaces. While web contractures in the fingers affect the individual mobility of the fingers and the ability to spread, first web contracture affects the span of the hand. It reduces the working space of the hand and is functionally more crippling.

In the acute phase, the general tendency of the thumb is to lie in an adducted and extended position. Left as such, the narrowing of the first web occurs and thenar muscles and joints get stuck in that position. The contracture may be due to the tight skin or may be associated with intrinsic contracture and joint contracture. If it is due to the skin only, the contracture can be corrected by Z plasty or its various modifications **(Figs. 17A to D)**. Frequently, it needs further release, and in such situations, the author prefers to extend the dorsal limb of the skin incision proximally to access the deeper structures. The fascia over the interosseous and the adductor is incised. The Z-plasty flaps are transposed. This provides good skin in the web and the defect on the dorsal aspect of the

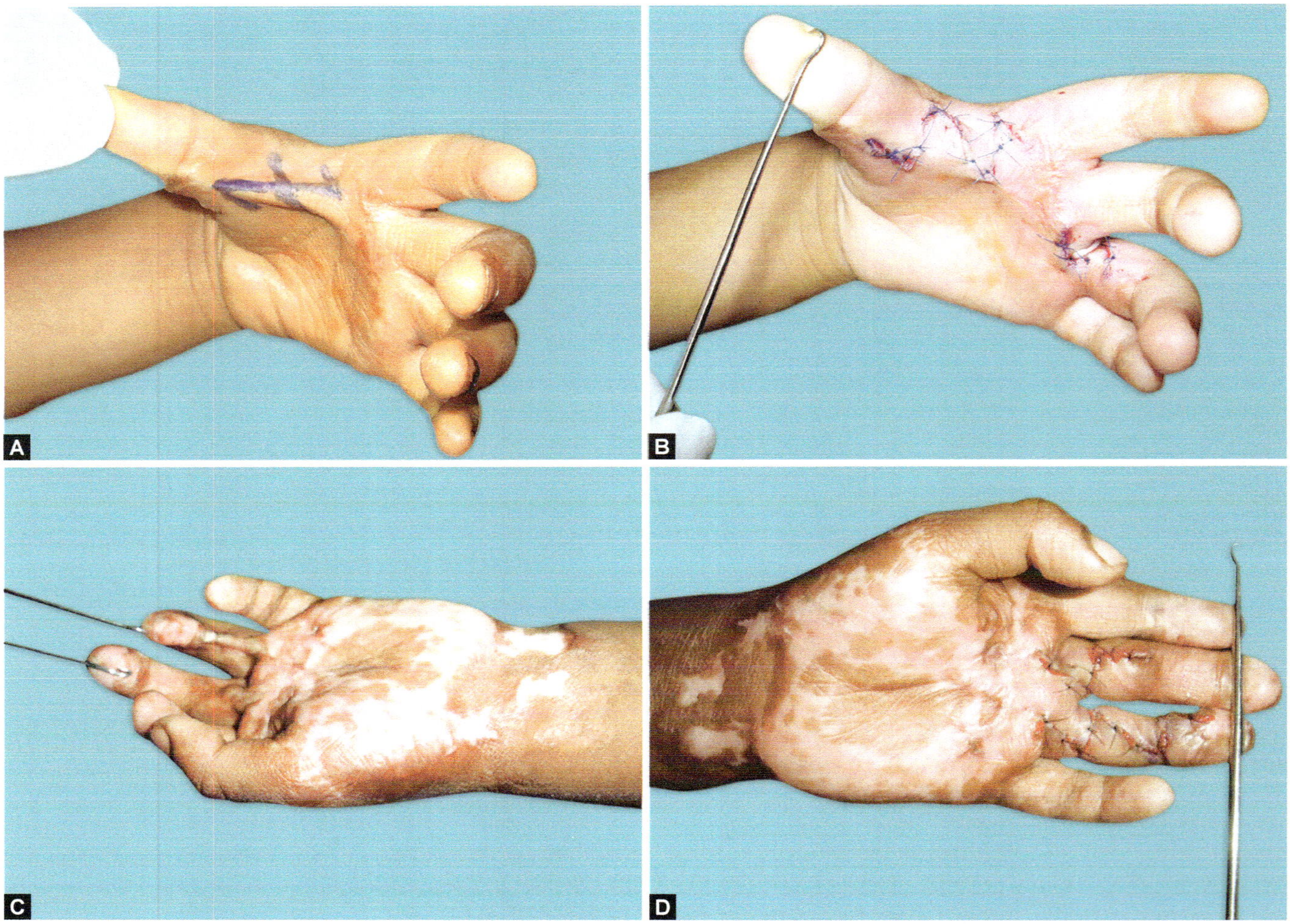

FIGS. 17A TO D: Z-plasty and its modifications are good for the release of band contractures (A and B). When done in the fingers, bigger Zs are better than small flaps (C and D).

web is skin grafted **(Fig. 18)**. If the contracture is more severe, the first dorsal interosseous muscle is released from its origin at the first metacarpal and the adductor pollicis origin is shaved off from the third metacarpal. This enables them to retain their blood and nerve supply. The badly contracted first web needs further release at the first carpometacarpal (CMC) joint. Only then, the web opens up. While doing this, one has to be careful not to damage the radial artery which passes from dorsal to the volar side close to the joint. The released web is maintained by a K-wire spacer and a flap cover is provided. As the local flaps are generally not available, a posterior interosseous flap or a distant groin flap has to be used **(Figs. 19A to J)**.

Postburn syndactylization of fingers: Fingers may need syndactyly correction or correction of the web creep. Minor web contractures can be corrected by Z plasties—four flap technique or V-M plasty. For a long time, the author is using the square flap technique which is also

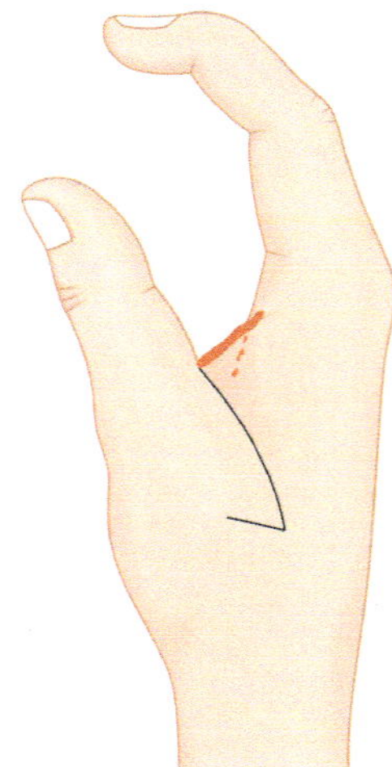

FIG. 18: For release of the first webspace, a Z-plasty incision extended on the dorsum gives good exposure. The transposed Z flaps cover the web and the raw area may be covered with graft. In addition, the proximal incision is extended transversely toward the volar side to enable the thumb to oppose.

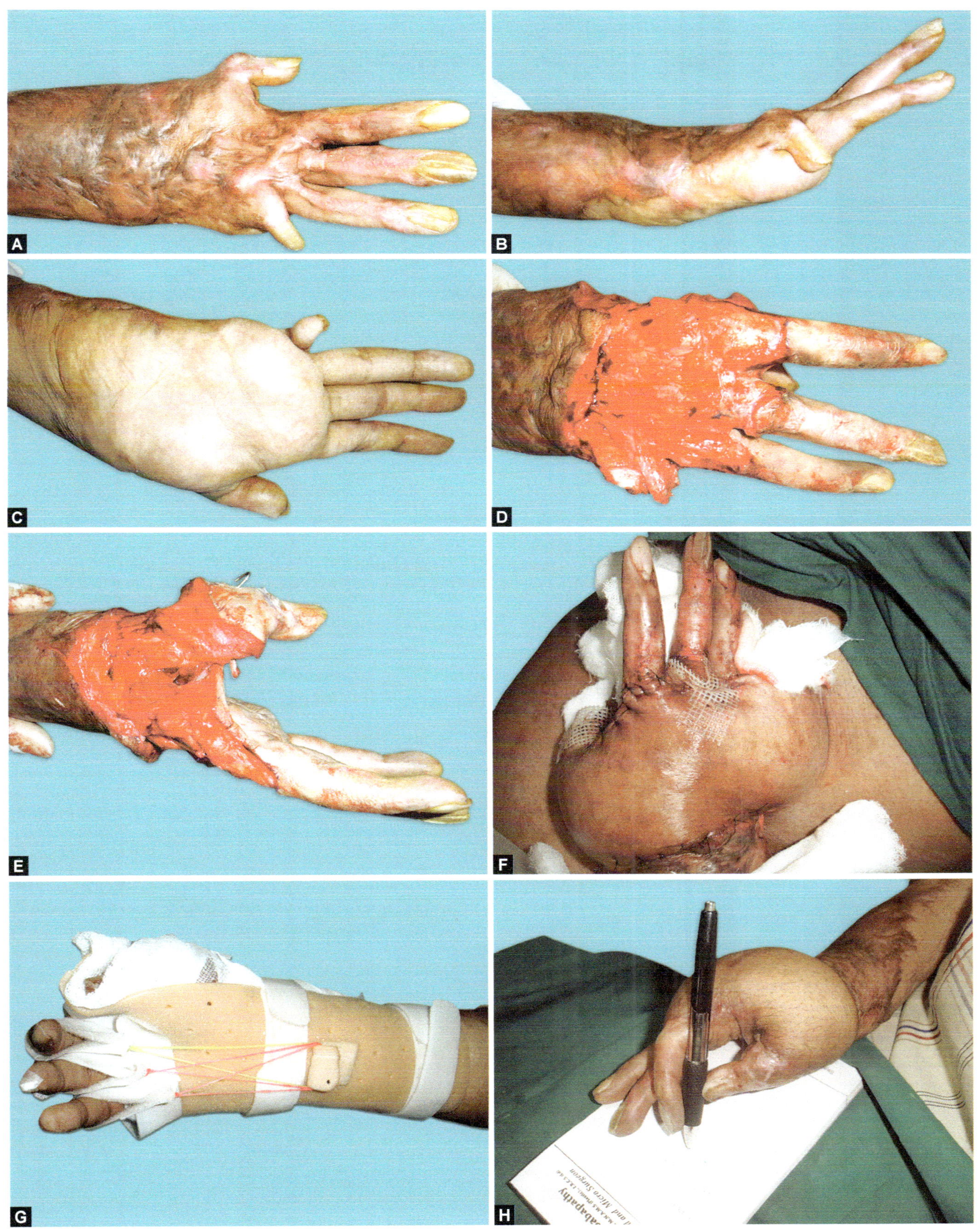

FIGS. 19A TO J: *Continued*

Continued

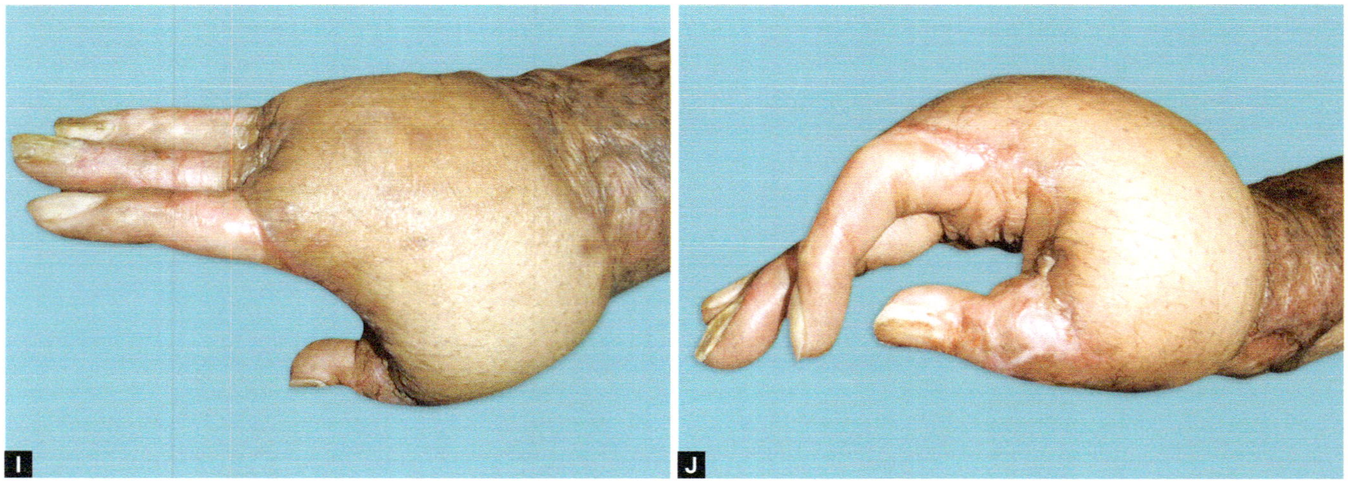

FIGS. 19A TO J: A severe contracture of the hand (A to C). Release requires complete excision of all scar tissue (D). Creating a good first web is important for function and is retained by a K wire (E). A groin flap cover is given (F), and aggressive physiotherapy is essential (G). Satisfactory functional outcome can be achieved (H to J).

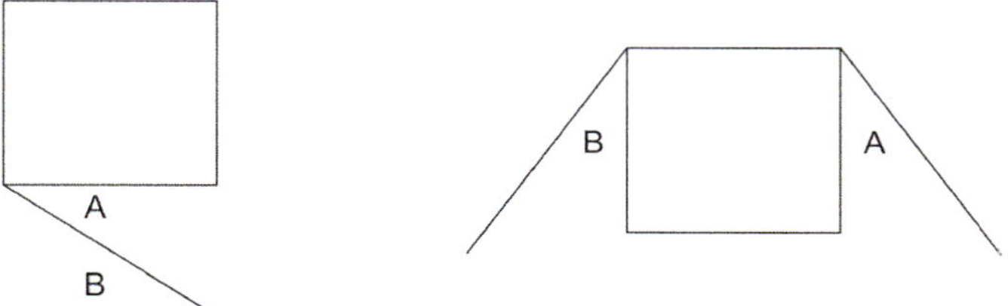

FIG. 20: Square flap technique for deepening of the web.

useful for more severe syndactylization **(Fig. 20)**. It is important to achieve good primary healing of the wounds after surgery so that pressure garments and silicone gel compression therapy can be instituted early. Physical therapy is the cornerstone for the prevention of web creep.

Volar contractures: Contracture of the volar aspect of the fingers is more common than that of the palm. Little finger is more often affected and more severely than other fingers and correction is also more difficult. Incision release is done for these contractures and the resulting raw areas are preferentially covered with full thickness skin grafts. Sometimes the volar plate and the joint capsule need release. In such situations, the joint needs stabilization with a K-wire till the skin cover settles. Limiting factor for release is distal vascularity. After obtaining the release possible, the tourniquet is released and vascularity of the fingertip is checked. If it is slow to pick up, the joint is gradually flexed to the extent where the fingertip turns pink and the joint is fixed at that level. Checking the vascularity of the fingertip is important at the completion of contracture release and in the immediate postoperative period. If joint release is done or the flexors and the nerves are exposed, it is preferable to provide flap cover. Cross finger-flap is a common flap used in this situation **(Figs. 21A to C)**. The author has a low threshold for using flaps on the volar aspect of the fingers after contracture release. In marginal situations, if skin graft is applied over the flexor sheath and digital neurovascular bundles, the graft may be expected to "take". In the event of recurrent contracture during revision surgery, chances of injury to the digital neurovascular bundles are very high.

Color of the skin graft on the volar aspect of the fingers is a cause of concern for some patients. If the raw area to be covered is small, palmar graft from the hypothenar eminence is a good source for a better color match; other sources are grafts from the instep area of the foot. The morbidity at the donor sites and the limited area of skin available are factors against their common use. Skin grafts, in course of time, become supple and the patient's acceptability increases with time.

Amputations: Finger and hand amputations occur in circumferential fourth-degree burns and in major electrical burns injury. While it is unavoidable in such situations, amputations must not be allowed to occur due to infective complications. Functionality of the hand depends upon the capability of the thumb stump to meet the tips of fingers. Length of the remaining fingers, the depth and the span of the first web are the limiting criteria of function. Following salvage procedures are possible.

Phalangization is one of the early procedures recommended for the reconstruction of the mitten hand. This involves deepening of the first web, receding the

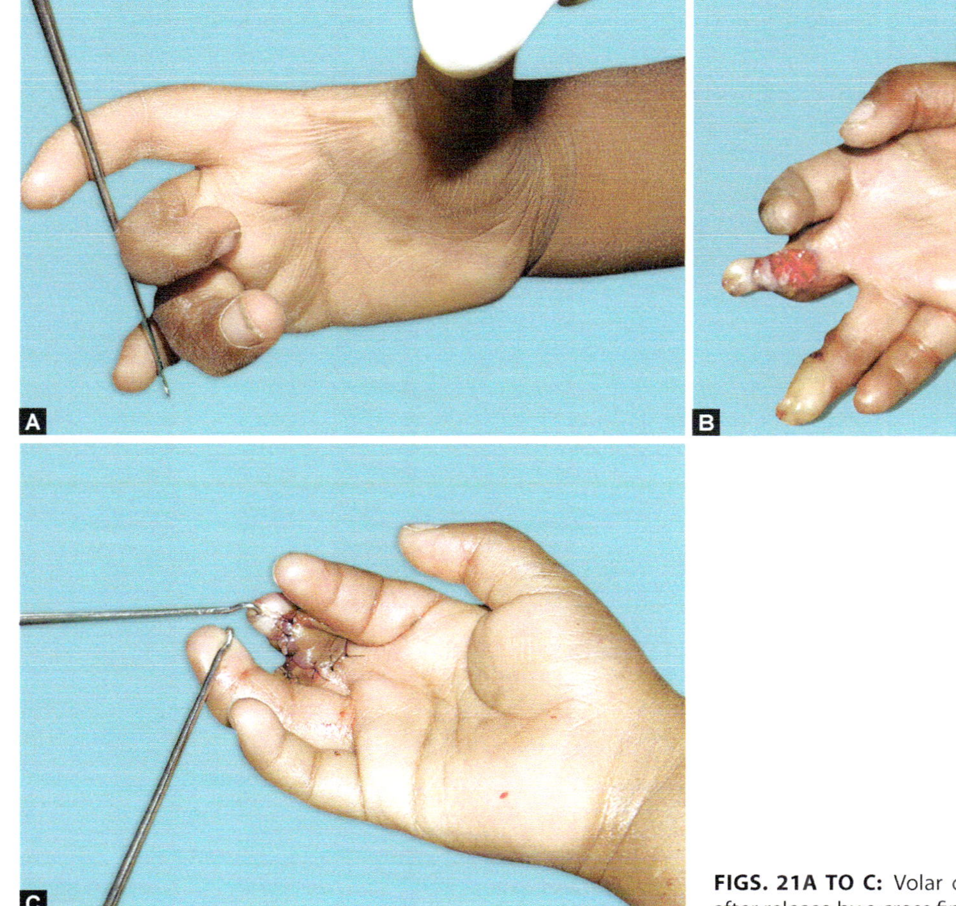

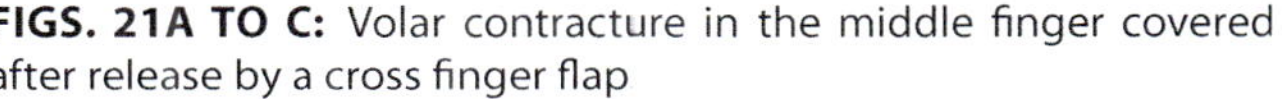

FIGS. 21A TO C: Volar contracture in the middle finger covered after release by a cross finger flap

adductor insertion proximally, and excising the index ray remnant. There is an increase in the first webspace at the expense of the palm width. This is succeeded by *Pollicization* wherein the index ray remnant is transferred over the thumb stump.[18] This is a technically demanding procedure particularly if the web skin is intact. If the index stump has some sensate volar skin, it is transferred with the nerve. In both techniques, the result depends upon the intact thenar musculature and the length of the remaining stumps. The third alternative is *distraction lengthening* of the stumps. If the whole of the first metacarpal is intact, distraction lengthening as first advocated by Matev may be done. Subperiosteal transverse osteotomy is done in the middle third of the first metacarpal and distraction of 25 mm can be achieved. Skin quality must be good both at the stump and in the line of the pins. Otherwise, prior flap cover is advised.

Advent of microsurgery has increased the options for reconstruction. The most valuable is *toe transfer*. This procedure gives a good functional and cosmetic result in one stage. This is the best possible reconstruction in isolated thumb and finger losses due to electrical burns and workplace burn injuries. In children, it has the added advantage of retaining the growth potential **(Figs. 22A to G)**.

The last alternative is *osteoplastic thumb reconstruction*. Though the literature is abounding with articles against it, the author finds it as a very valuable technique for a person who is unwilling to sacrifice the toe. When done well, the results of osteoplastic thumb reconstruction match in function with other types of reconstruction.[19] Osteoplastic thumb reconstruction must be used only if there is a potential for performing the neurovascular island flap to provide sensation. Otherwise, bone resorption rate is high. This is a limiting factor in the use of this technique in postburn reconstruction.

Dermal Substitute

Skin substitutes are commonly used in the reconstruction of burn contractures. They were primarily intended to treat acute burns. The current indications for dermal

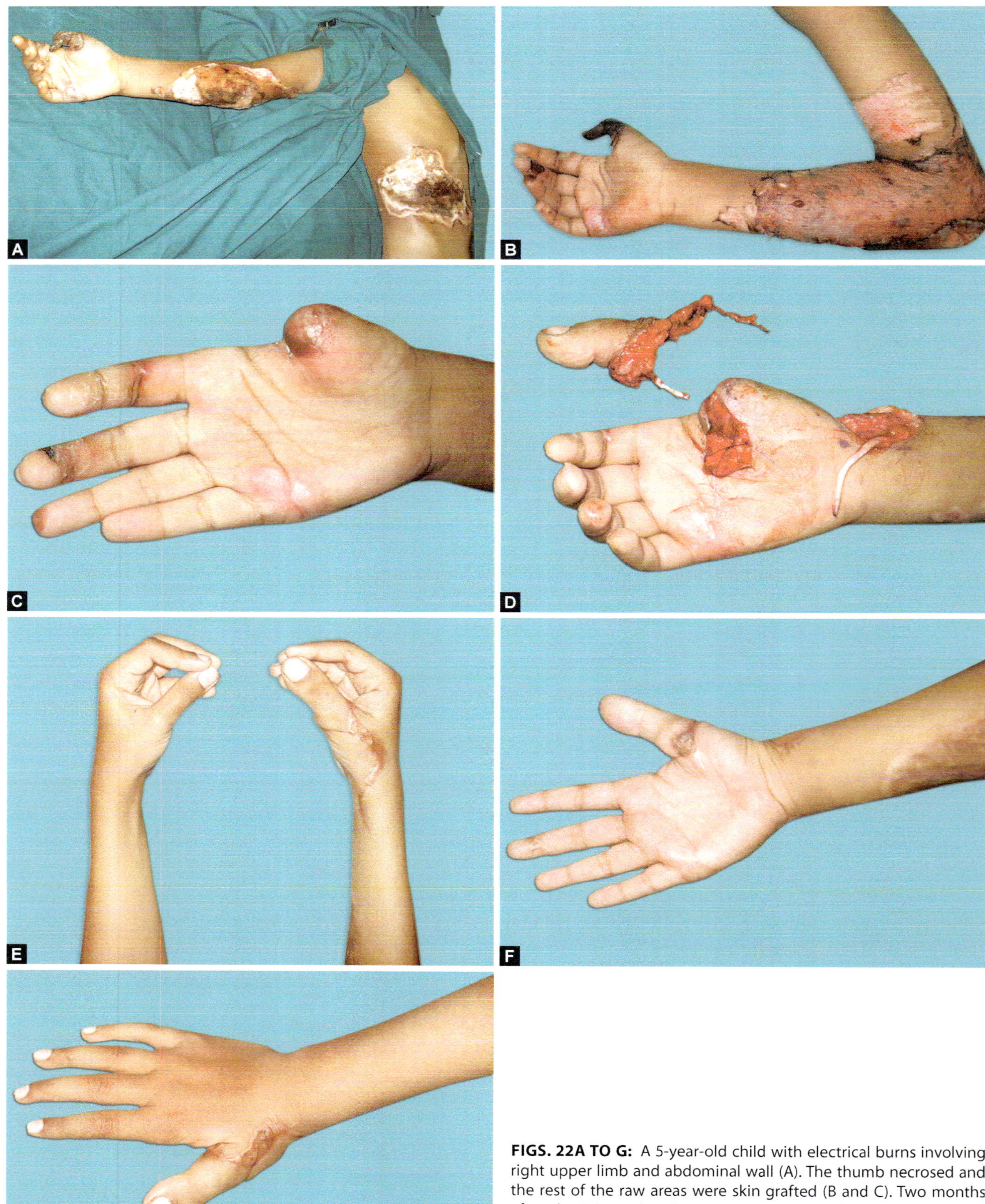

FIGS. 22A TO G: A 5-year-old child with electrical burns involving right upper limb and abdominal wall (A). The thumb necrosed and the rest of the raw areas were skin grafted (B and C). Two months after the injury, thumb reconstruction was done with great toe transfer (D), with excellent functional result (E to G).

skin substitutes include both acute (such as deep partial or full-thickness burns) and chronic post burn sequelae (such as hypertrophic scars and scar contractures).[20] The dermal scaffolds consist of an outer and an inner layer similar to that of the epidermis and dermis of the skin. The outer layer prevents water and protein loss and acts as a bacterial barrier. The inner layer provides the strength, mechanical resistance, and the elasticity to the skin. The main advantage of skin substitutes is that they offer an additional layer of dermis, making the skin more elastic and softer. They may also prevent using flaps to cover the raw areas, which may need multiple procedures that can be technically challenging and bulky. The first stage is debridement of the wound and application of skin substitutes. 2–3 weeks later, the outer silicon layer is removed and is covered by a thin-split thickness skin graft. During this period, cells migrate into the dermal matrix, resulting in new blood vessel formation and collagen production throughout the matrix. Once the skin substitute is fully integrated, the sealing membrane is removed, leaving a new vascularized dermal layer. The skin substitute must be applied only to defects that are not infected, and strict hemostasis has been done. Although it can be used over dry tendons and bones, the tendons and bones should not be infected. The skin substitute should have close immobile contact with the bed, and hence, quilting sutures/staples and tie-over dressings might be needed to achieve this. Small holes can be made in the skin substitutes to remove any collection between the substitute and the bed. Substitutes such as Matriderm® and recently Integra®, which are 1 mm thick, can be applied as a one-step procedure. Matriderm® consists of bovine collagen and bovine elastin. They act as a scaffold through which the cells proliferate and then accept the skin graft. The advantage of a single application is that it can be applied just once, preventing multiple surgeries, and a thicker dermis is obtained compared to a regular skin graft. One should not contemplate using substitutes if one has to do a secondary procedure like a tendon transfer for the hand later on, as secondary procedures are extremely difficult to do underneath. In this aspect, flaps are a far better choice. There can be graft loss, especially with infection and when hemostasis is not maintained well.

After burn wounds have been debrided or contracture released, autologous skin grafts are used to give skin coverage. Skin grafts usually contract, causing the reconstruction to be suboptimal. Revision surgery might be required due to the cosmetic deformity, the development of adherent scars, and recurrent scar contractures. The amount of dermis at the wound site is inversely correlated with scarring and contracture formation.[21,22] Therefore, it can be assumed that a thinner skin graft carrying less dermis would be more susceptible to contracture and scarring than a thicker graft. However, due to donor-site morbidity or availability, utilizing a thick split-thickness or full-thickness skin graft is not always feasible. The use of skin substitute to supplement or replace the dermis at the wound sites improve the cosmetic and functional outcomes. Hands treated with the dermal regeneration template fare better in terms of skin elasticity and active range of motion than wounds with skin grafts alone.[23] The majority of patients (88%) had satisfactory hand function, full range of articular motion, good skin pliability, and ideal cosmetic outcomes.[24] The composite graft is stable after 5–7 days in the case of a single-staged dermal regeneration template combined with skin grafting, enabling an early start to physical therapy. The risk of joint stiffness increases if a two-staged dermal regeneration template is used since the hand must be immobilized for up to 2 weeks before a skin graft can be applied.

REHABILITATION ISSUES IN HAND BURNS

Helms[25] studied the time to return to work following hand burns in 70 patients in relation to several variables. (1) TBSA burned, (2) Hand burned, (3) Grafting, (4) Patient's age, and (5) Occupational category. When assessed at 8 months, 74% had returned to work. The best predictor of time to return to work was TBSA burned, followed by "grafting" and the "hand burned". No significant differences or predictors were found for patient's age, occupational category or between nonburn hand trauma patients in prior reports.

The sight and condition of the burnt hand is frightening to the conscious burn patients. It produces doubts and fears about their future in the workplace and possible dependence on others for day-to-day existence. Along with good treatment, presence of reassuring physicians and therapists goes a long way to allay the fears and boost confidence in the patient. It encourages them to comply with the exacting schedules of physiotherapy and look up to a good future.

SUMMARY

Regaining optimal hand function and aesthetics have a great effect on the quality of life of an individual after a burn injury. Burns of hand are very common and can be due to heat, electricity, various chemicals, and radiation. They may be isolated but are usually part of extensive burns. A large number of delicate joints, musculotendinous units, ligaments, and nerves along with specialized skin of palmer aspect allow an individual to carry out day-to-day activities with ease. A burn injury can alter the tendons and joint balance and immobilization in inappropriate positions leads to stiffness, and loss of function. Escharotomy and fasciotomy are very commonly needed than elsewhere in the body to preserve the vascularity. Any delay may lead to gangrene or fibrosis. Electrical burns and firecracker injuries may end up in amputations. Thus, the burns of hand comprise a special category where complete range of motion of all joints and a functioning hand is of greater importance than just achieving a healed wound. Early excisional surgery and physiotherapy have a great role in the management of hand burns.

REFERENCES

1. Tredget E. Management of the acutely burned upper extremity. Hand Clin. 2000;16:187-202.
2. Sheridan RL, Hurley J, Smith MA, Ryan CM, Bondoc CC, Quinby WC, et al. The acutely burned hand: Management and outcome based on a ten-year experience with 1047 acute hand burns. J Trauma. 1995;38:406-11.
3. Foucher G, Smith D. Acute care and reconstructive management of hand burns. Curr Opin Orthopaed. 1995;7:2-9.
4. Sykes PJ. Severe Burns of the Hand: A Practical Guide to their Management. J Hand Surg. 1991;16B:6-12.
5. Sykes PJ, Bailey BN. Treatment of hand burns with occlusive bags: A comparison of 3 methods. Burns. 1976;2:162-8.
6. Falcone PA, Edstrom LE. Decision making in the acute thermal hand burn: An algorithm for treatment. Hand Clin. 1990;6:233-8.
7. Janzekovic Z. A new concept of the early excision and immediate grafting of burns. J Trauma. 1970;10:1103-8.
8. Hunt JL, Sato R, Baxter CR. Early Tangential Excision and Immediate Mesh Autografting of Deep Dermal Hand Burns. Ann Surg. 1979;189:147-51.
9. VanZuijlen PPM, Kreis RW, Vloemans AFPM, Groenevelt F, Mackie DP. The prognostic factors regarding long-term functional outcome of full thickness hand burns. Burns. 1999;25:709-14.
10. Jebsen RH. An objective and standardized test of hand function. Arch Phys Med Rehabil. 1969;50:311-9.
11. Nuchtem JG, Engrav LH, Nakamura DY, Dutcher KA, Heimbach DM, Veder NB. Treatment of fourth-degree hand burns. J Burn Care Rehabil. 1995;16:36-42.
12. Parks DH, Baur PS, Larson DL. Late problems in burns. Clin Plast Surg. 1977;4:547-60.
13. Larson DL, Abston S, Willis B, Linares H, Dobrkovsky M, Evans EB, et al. Contracture and scar formation in the burn patient. Clin Plast Surg. 1974;1:653-66.
14. Perkins K, Davey RB, Wallis KA. Silicone gel: a new treatment for burn scars and contractures. Burns. 1982;9:205-13.
15. Mustoe TA. Evolution of Silicone Therapy and Mechanism of action in Scar management. Aesth Plast Surg. 2008;32:82-92.
16. Sabapathy SR, Bajantri B, Bharathi RR. Management of post burn hand deformities. Indian J Plast Surg. 2010;43(Suppl):S72-9.
17. McCauley RL. Reconstruction of the paediatric burned hand. Hand Clin. 2000;16:249-59.
18. May JW, Donelan MB, Toth BA, Wall J. Thumb reconstruction in the burned hand by advancement pollicization of the second ray remnant. J Hand Surg. 1984;9:484-89.
19. Sabapathy SR, Venkatramani H, Bharathi RR. Functional Evaluation of Great Toe Transfer and Osteoplastic Technique for Thumb Reconstruction in the Same Individual. J Hand Surg. 2003;28B:405-8.
20. Dantzer E, Queruel P, Salinier L, Palmier B, Quinot JF. Dermal regeneration template for deep hand burns: clinical utility for both early grafting and reconstructive surgery. Br J Plast Surg. 2003;56(8):764-74.
21. Corps BV. The effect of graft thickness, donor site, and graft bed on graft thickness in the hooded rat. Br J Plast Surg. 1969;22:125-33.
22. Klein L, Rudolph R. 3 H-collagen turnover in skin grafts. Surg Gynecol Obstet. 1972;135:49-57.
23. Frame JD, Still J, Lakhel-LeCoadou A, Carstens MH, Lorenz C, Orlet H, et al. Use of dermal regeneration template in contracture release procedures: a multicenter evaluation. Plast Reconstr Surg. 2004;113(5):1330-8.
24. Cuadra A, Correa G, Roa R, Piñeros JL, Norambuena H, Searle S, et al. Functional results of burned hands treated with Integra®. J Plast Reconstr Aesthet Surg. 2012;65(2):228-34.
25. Helms PA, Wlaker SC, Peyton SA. Return to work following hand burns. Arch Phys Med Rehabil. 1986;67:297-8.

CHAPTER 28

Burns of Perineum and External Genitalia

Deepak Nanda, Mula Rohit Babu

INTRODUCTION

The perineum is protected by a deep furrow between the thighs so it usually gets spared from burns and other injuries. Burns of the perineum and external genitalia occur in patients with extensive burns although isolated injuries are not uncommon. According to Lund and Browder's chart for body surface-area estimation, only 1% of the total body surface has been allocated to external genitalia and perineum. However, the American Burns Association has classified burns of this region as major burns similar to those of face and hand. Burns in these areas can result in great psychological trauma which is disproportionate to the percentage area of the total body surface involved.

Michielsen et al.[1] found an incidence of 2.7% for burns involving genitalia and perineum out of more than 4,200 patients admitted over a period of 15 years. One-fourth of them were children with a preponderance of males (2.4:1). Angel et al.,[2] reporting from Shriners Hospital (Texas) catering to children only, found 76 patients out of a total of more than 2,300 over a period of 10 years, having burns of this region, again with boys outnumbering girls by 1.5-1. A study by Chicago Burn Center[3] indicates that out of 1,600 patients admitted for burns, 93 patients had involvement of genitalia and perineum (5.8%). In India, a study was conducted and out of 503 patients admitted, those who sustained burns involving the perineum were 51 (10.1%). Males are three times more commonly affected than females.[4] Majority of cases were from rural areas. Another study from Japan[5] found that the percentage of patients with involvement of genitalia and perineum was higher about 21.5%. The severity of burn injury to external genitalia was higher in males for obvious anatomical reasons.

ETIOLOGY AND PATHOGENESIS

The most common cause of perineal burns is hot liquids or scalds which varied from 55 to 85%.[1,2,6] The second most common cause was flame burns accounting for 24%, 30%, and 7%, respectively in these studies. Other common causes are electrical contact and flash burns and chemical burns. Some rare causes of burns of the perineum and genitalia have been enumerated, such as alkali leak into a baby diaper, ignition of collected spirit-based cleaning agent on a plastic sheet by diathermy, involvement of the area by blasts injuries and during brachytherapy for prostatic malignancy **(Box 1)**.

In India, an earthen-made stove, called "*chullah,*" is used in which wood is used as fuel, and kerosene stoves are commonly used in rural areas. In addition to that, women wear loose clothes such as sari, dupattas, etc. While cooking, spilling of kerosene on them from a burning stove or explosion of such stoves is associated with these types of burns. Gupta et al.,[7] reported an epidemic in Rajasthan of burns caused by using kerosene mixed with petrol in pressure stoves. Surface level cooking practices, with the females in our country squatting or kneeling in front of the kerosene pump or "*chullah,*" expose the

BOX 1 Epidemiology.

- Incidence of perineal and external genitalia burns varies from 2.7 to 21.5% from center to center[1-5]
- These burns usually occur as a part of extensive, large area burns
- Males outnumber females in both incidence and severity because of social lifestyle and anatomical reasons[4,5]

perineum as it is unprotected by the thighs, thus making it vulnerable in the event of a disaster. Also, the perineum is easily exposed to these hot liquids when spilled or a boiling vessel is tipped over in this position **(Box 2)**.

The burns of the perineum and external genitalia involve people of all ages from infancy to elderly (86 years). Studies from the USA have suggested child abuse where the "ring sign" is supposed to be pathognomonic, and these children are usually branded for life. In the study from Japan, "sitz bath" has been blamed for burns of perineum in old people, especially during the winter months when these baths are a custom **(Figs. 1A and B)**.

Abdel-Razek[8] reported cases of rare isolated chemical burns of genitalia and perineum from King Saud Hospital. These burns constituted about 3.4% of total burns at his center. They were due to sulfuric acid used for cleaning water closet which was accidentally used to wash genitalia as an initial step of performing the ritual of "WUDU" before praying in Islam. Sulfuric acid and its precursor, sulfuric trioxide, are strong acids and desiccants which cause coagulative necrosis of the parts involved. These burns are either second-degree deep dermal or third-degree full thickness, the latter being more common **(Fig. 2)**.

In Kashmir and Himachal Pradesh, because of extreme weather conditions during winter, people of low socioeconomic strata, particularly in villages, use "Kangri", a very economical source of heat to keep themselves warm in the extreme cold weather.[8] They usually place it between the medial aspects of the thighs and lower abdomen.[9] Due to very close proximity, the perineum, genitalia, and medial aspects of thighs are usually susceptible to burns whenever the Kangri tips over.

Most chemical burns of the perineum are caused by accidental or unintentional contact with a chemical agent at the workplace. There are limited case reports on genital chemical burns.[8,9] Genital burns due to topical use of medications, such as imiquimod, podophyllin, or trichloroacetic acid which are used to treat genital warts, are reported in the literature.[10]

Rare cases of genitalia and perineal burns have been reported due to fireworks during Guy Fawkes Nights, and a case has been reported where a mentally depressed woman inserted a rocket two inches into her vagina and ignited it while trying to commit suicide.[11]

Burns due to scalds are usually second-degree burns **(Fig. 3)**. Out of these, superficial dermal are 1.5–2 times more common than deep dermal injuries. Third-degree or full-thickness burns constitute a small proportion only. Flame burns are usually deeper as compared to scalds **(Fig. 4)** while high-voltage electrical contact burns may lead to full-thickness burns of the perineum and partial or total loss of external genitalia **(Fig. 5)**. Scalds are more

BOX 2 Etiology.

- Scalds are the most common cause of perineal burns in children
- Flame and chemical burns are the most common cause in adults
- In Indian rural communities, cooking using *"Chullah"* and kerosene burning stove is one of the most common cause of perineal burns[4]
- Rarely caused by brachytherapy for prostate cancer, topical imiquimod, podophyllin, or trichloroacetic acid[11]

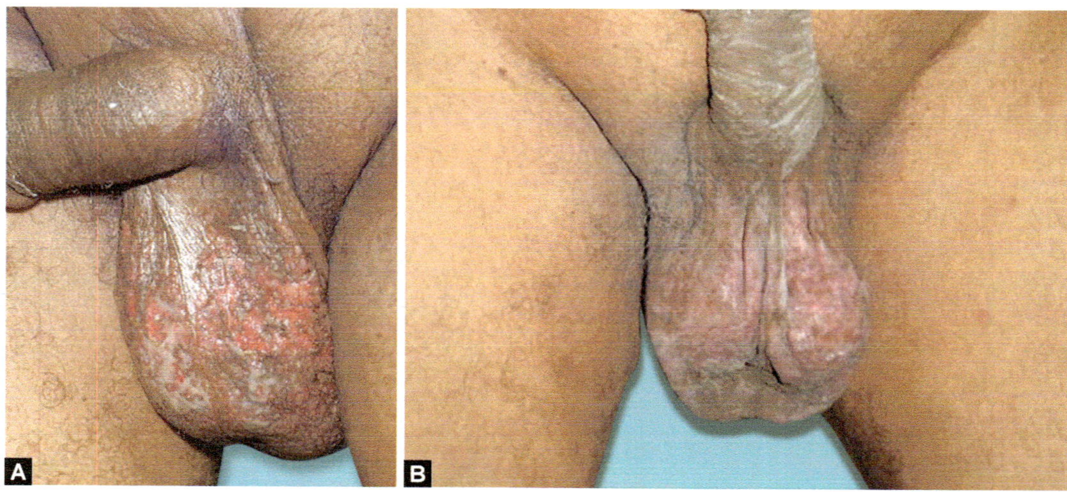

FIGS. 1A AND B: (A) Accidental superficial burns of scrotum and perineum by concentrated potassium permanganate during sitz bath; (B) Same patient after 1 week with healed areas showing hypopigmentation.

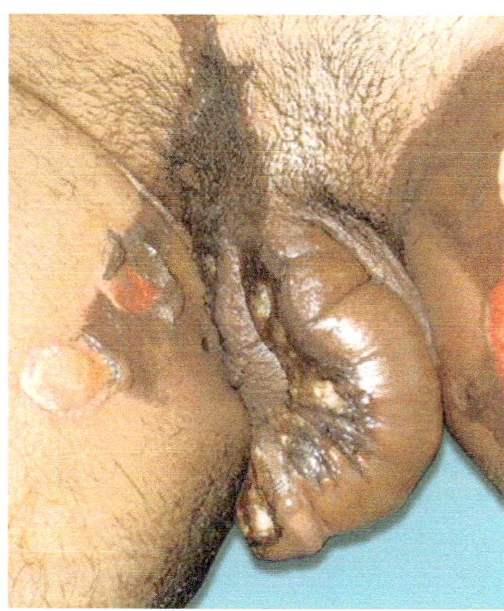

FIG. 2: Accidental acid burns showing the track of acid trickling down from the abdomen toward the perineum with deep burns over one side of the penis causing lateral curvature with edema of penile skin.

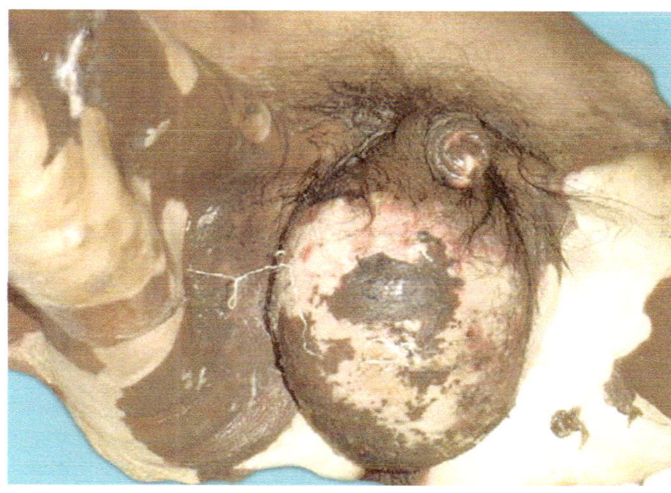

FIG. 4: Deep dermal thermal burns of scrotum and thighs.

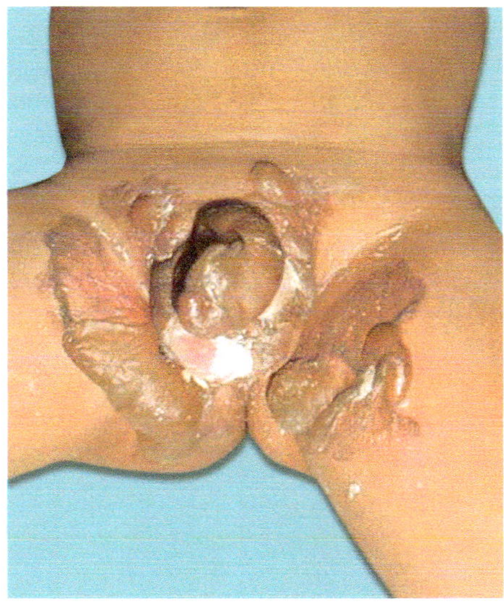

FIG. 3: A 10-year-old child with scalds of the perineum leading to superficial dermal burns with blister formation.

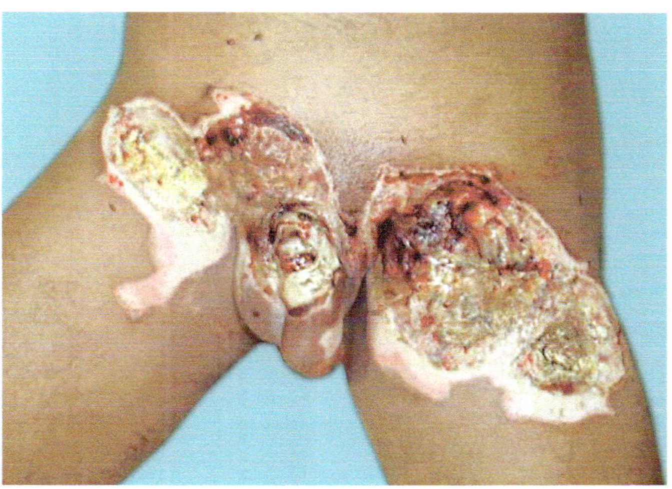

FIG. 5: Electrical contact injury causing full-thickness burns in the lower half of the penis and scrotum and in the groin causing exposure of femoral vessels on the left side. Foley's catheterization is possible in such cases.

common in children below 2 years of age, while flame burns are more common in the older age groups. The psychological consequences of these injuries cannot be ignored. Repeated examination of the private anatomical areas tends to affect modesty as well as self-respect. Fear of sexual dysfunction and unattractiveness leads to depression. About 25% of adult patients complain of loss of libido and orgasmic dysfunction.[3]

MANAGEMENT DURING ACUTE STAGE (BOX 3)

Acute cases are managed by two different schools of thought, namely conservative and aggressive; the former advice only dressing of the involved area with antimicrobials so that bacterial count is kept below 10^5 microorganisms/g of tissue and wait for the wounds to heal while the latter advocate early excision and resurfacing. What is generally followed in most centers is that superficial burns are managed conservatively or nonoperatively with topical antimicrobials; small deep wounds of perineum are also treated conservatively as on healing, they tend to contract and close rapidly by secondary intention. Eschar debridement and bacterial balance of $<10^5$ microorganisms/g of tissue should be maintained.

Urinary and Fecal Diversion

Urinary diversion is usually required; catheterization may be sufficient in most cases but suprapubic cystostomy may be required rarely **(Figs. 6A and B)**. Catheterization is usually required for about 2 weeks as most of the wounds heal by this time. Foley catheter has the additional advantages of preventing meatal stenosis and ammoniacal dermatitis. But catheterization is not without complications, namely urinary tract infection, urethral strictures following trauma during insertion, and bladder stones. Rare complications, such as prostatic abscess, renal abscess, periurethral abscess, epididymo-orchitis, and even urethral sloughing, have been reported, especially when catheterization has been prolonged. Thus, catheterization is required but should be minimized and monitored.

BOX 3 Management of acute burns.

- Urinary diversion done with Foley's catheterization as it prevents meatal stenosis and ammonical dermatitis
- Diversion colostomy is the last option or done in cases where anal sphincter involvement is present causing stool incontinence
- Allograft is preferred in patients who are unstable
- Open method of dressing is preferred and graft should be typically meshed
- Early mobilization, splinting in abducted position, active and passive exercises, and pressure garments with special inserts prevent contractures

Fecal diversions have been abandoned in most places but a study from Japan suggested temporary diverting colostomy for very old patients with perineal burns **(Figs. 7A and B)**.[5] Superficial perianal and buttock wounds can be managed with topical care and cleansing. Diarrhea should be avoided. If patients can tolerate, it is better to nurse them in the prone or lateral decubitus position.

Deep perianal and buttock wounds are managed with excision and grafting at the time of the first-prone procedure. Autograft is usually preferred. However, in patients with high revised Baux score initially wounds may be covered with allograft to minimize the risk of autograft loss. Bolster dressing to the wounds with a "Montgomery strap" (suture placed in an interrupted fashion and tied to create an eyelet through which umbilical tape can be passed) and tie-over bolster dressing is done to allow easier dressing changes after soiling. If there is an adequate margin of the normal skin surrounding the anus, using negative pressure wound therapy (NPWT) is a good option because it provides stabilization and protection from fecal contents and hence, prevents graft contamination.

If the burns are severe with the involvement of the anus or if the patient has incontinence secondary to the sphincter injury, diverting colostomy should be performed prior to any wound management.[12]

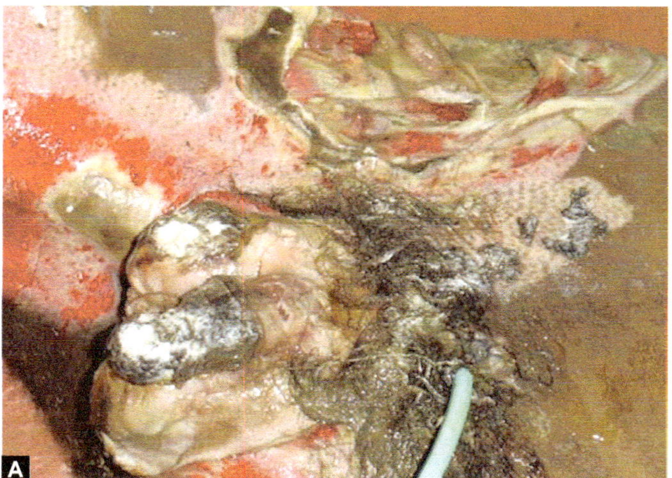

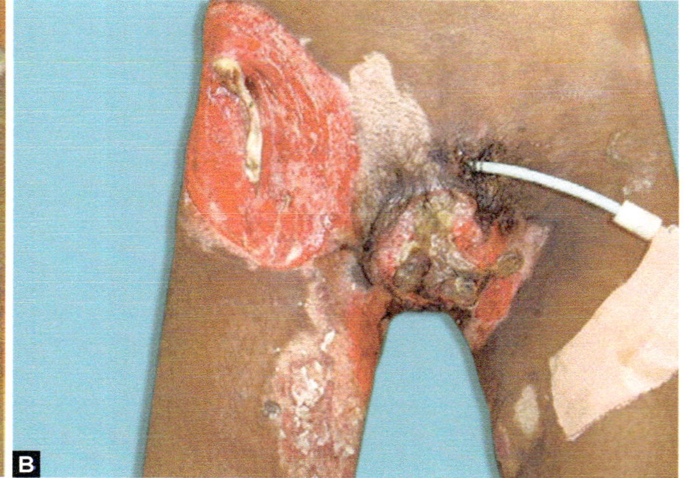

FIGS. 6A AND B: (A) Electrical contact burns in the perineum showing necrosed penis and scrotum with suprapubic cystostomy; (B) Same patient with total loss of penis and both testes.

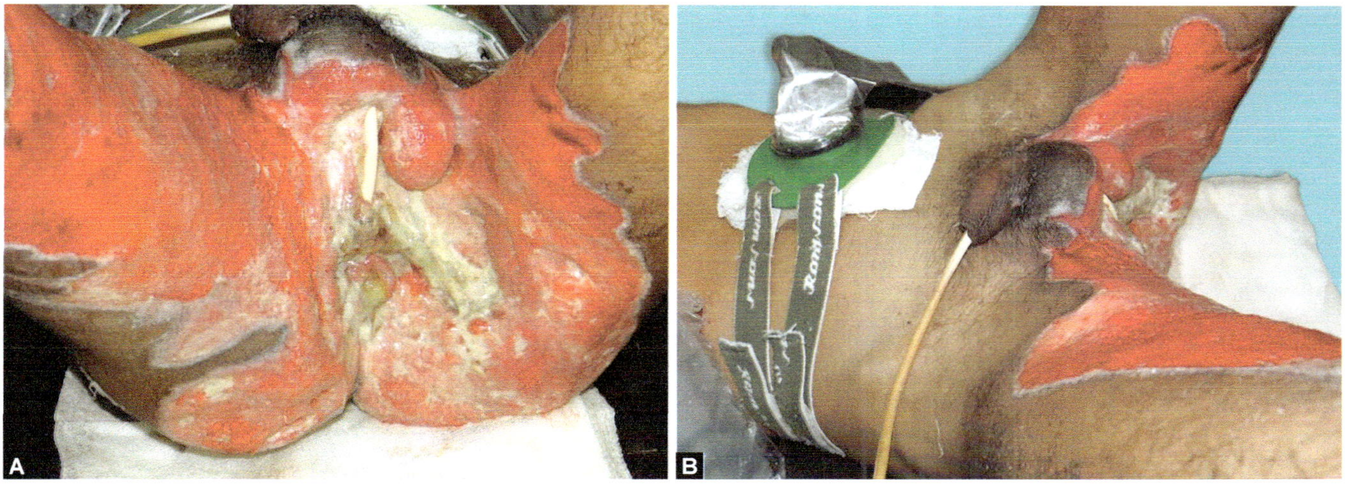

FIGS. 7A AND B: (A) Patient with severe perineal burns with involvement of anal sphincter; (B) Colostomy is done in the same patient for wound management.

Prevention of Infection

Autogenous infection of these areas is usually common due to proximity of the anus, particularly with *Pseudomonas aeruginosa*. Infection is dangerous as it destroys epithelial cells to convert partial-thickness burns into full-thickness burns, and also creates problems for graft "take."

Wound Management

Second-degree superficial wounds of genitalia and perineum of both sexes and all ages are treated by exposure and application of silver sulfadiazine or other antimicrobial drugs. Other substances, such as potassium permanganate and sodium bicarbonate, have been used but their efficacy is not proven. Daily baths and showers help in keeping the bacterial flora under control and separating the slough. Most partial-thickness burns heal satisfactorily and even small full-thickness burns can be managed by this method. Conservative management includes debridement of loose slough and application of topical antimicrobials. Broad-spectrum parenteral antibiotics also form an integral part of the treatment plan. An open method of dressing is usually advocated as the perineum and genitalia are difficult to dress. Most of the wounds heal satisfactorily by this method, although a few may require secondary surgery for contracture release. Early mobilization is advocated for prevention of contractures. Deeper the wounds, more frequent the surgical intervention.

For larger deep wounds, surgical removal of devitalized tissue by tangential excision and skin grafting of the resultant wound is the mainstay of management. Some authors believe that one should wait until eschar separates to maximize tissue preservation before one goes for grafting. Tissue preservation in this area is important, as specialized tissue of this area is difficult to reconstruct. In the perineum, the graft should preferably be meshed in order to accommodate the irregular contour, but expansion is not really required. Perioperative management of the graft is very important **(Figs. 8A and B)**.

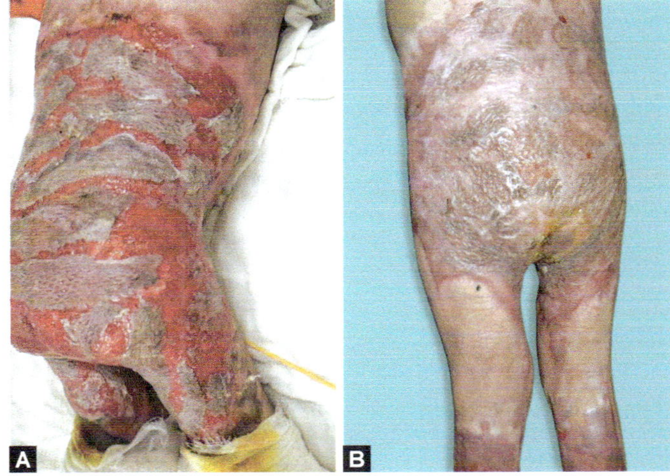

FIGS. 8A AND B: (A) Perineal burns in a child; (B) Managed with homograft and then autograft leading to severe anal opening stenosis and perineal contracture which required colostomy before release of contracture.

The grafts require well-vascularized bed with bacteriological balance. It requires stabilization with sutures, staples, or fibrin glue. Postoperative shearing has to be prevented where a nylon mesh over the graft is helpful. Use of air ripple beds, nursing in prone position, and minimization of fecal soiling decrease wound infection and graft loss. It has been observed that flame burns require more surgical intervention than scalds as the former are deeper. In one study, only 20% of scalds were classified as second-degree deep or third-degree, whereas in contrast, 66% of flame burns were in the same category.

When testes are involved, the burns are obviously full thickness as these are protected by skin, dartos, tunica vaginalis, and cremasteric reflex. In such cases, usually the thin penile skin also is involved and does not survive. Early surgical intervention by excision followed by resurfacing with skin grafts is beneficial. Decompression of penis by escharotomy should be done for full-thickness burns of the phallus when vascular compromise is suspected. Excision and grafting are done as soon as possible, but efforts should be made to spare the dartos which has a rich venous network. If this can be preserved, the problems of distal swelling, wound contraction, and subsequent contracture can be eliminated. The laxity of penile skin enables about one-fourth of the circumference to be excised and primarily closed. This can be a useful method when burns affect only the dorsum of the penis. Unmeshed grafts are preferable for better esthetic appearance. Circumcision discarding non-burned penile skin is forbidden as it might be required for later reconstruction. Acute circumcision is indicated only for full-thickness burns of the prepuce. When testes are exposed, they can be sutured together for stability and covered with partial-thickness skin graft. Intrinsic contractures of the penis, scrotum, or vulva are rare, but extrinsic contracture or webbing across the perineum and groin are more common **(Flowchart 1)**.

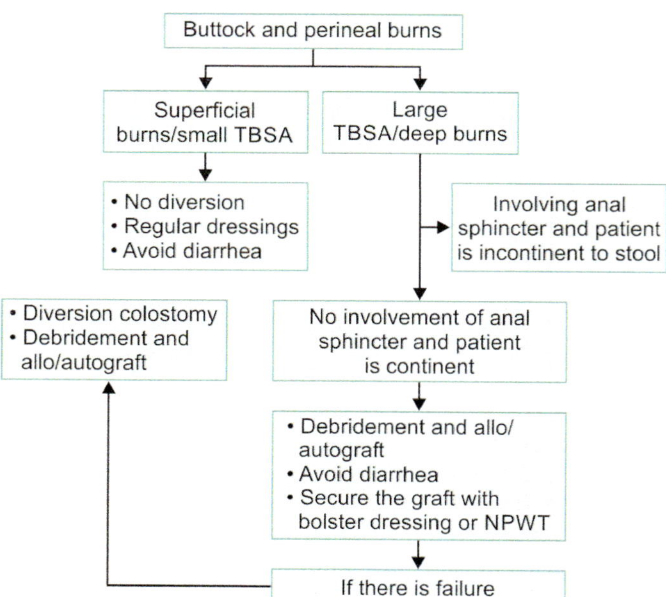

FLOWCHART 1: Algorithm for management of perineal burns. (NPWT: negative pressure wound therapy; TBSA: total body surface area)

Prevention of Contractures

To prevent contractures, lower limbs should be in an abducted position during the wound healing period with a spreading bar or wedge splinting. Active and passive exercises for hip joints and pressure garments with special inserts are also important in the prevention of contractures.

MANAGEMENT OF PERINEAL BURN CONTRACTURES/RECONSTRUCTION[13-16]

Gottlieb and Saunders[3] have classified burn scar deformities of the perineum into quantitative and qualitative types.

Quantitative types are those in which there is loss of skin surface and/or functional tissues, for example, most contractures. Qualitative scars are those which have altered skin texture, hypo/hyperpigmentation, and changes in pliability. Although quantitative contractures are more disabling functionally, the reconstruction of qualitative ones is more difficult, a challenge that should not be neglected as it can lead to problems of sexuality. Perineal burn contractures have also been described as scar bands between the medial thighs crossing the area between genitalia and anus **(Fig. 9)** or a band extending from the proximal medial thigh to the perineum **(Fig. 10A)** or a band in the suprapubic area extending to the root of the penis, causing dorsal contracture of the penis **(Figs. 11A and B)**.

In spite of early surgical intervention and early mobilization, perineal contractures do occur in a small percentage of patients. These numbers are higher in places where education levels are low and patient follow-up is poor. Linear contractures can usually be treated

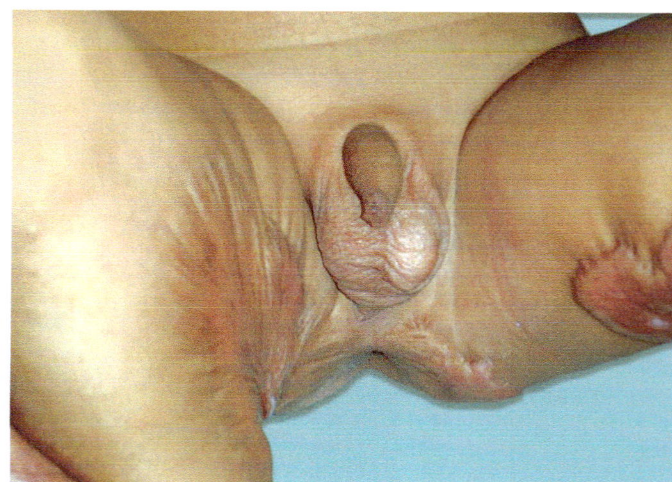

FIG. 9: A child with postburn contracture of perineum.

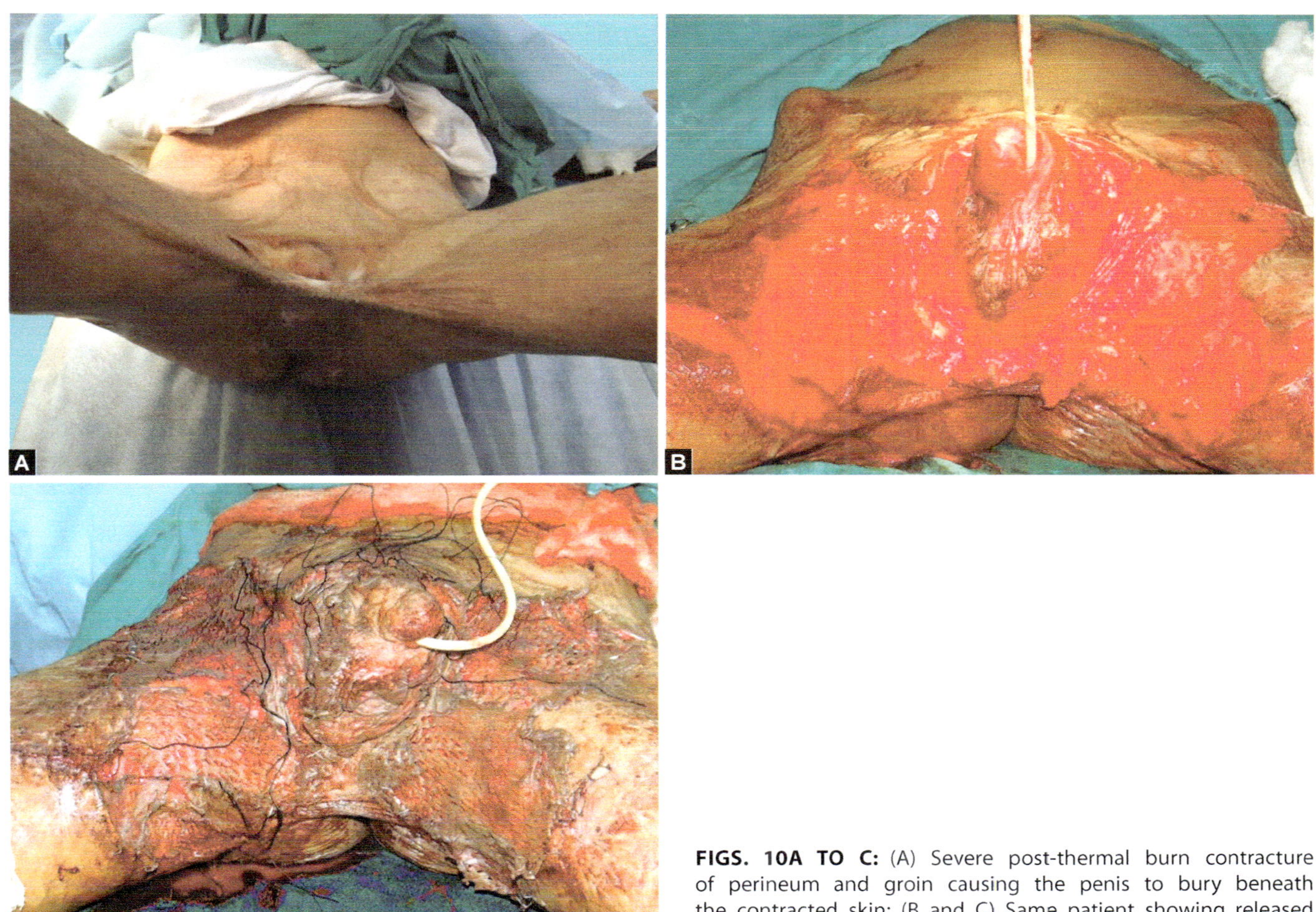

FIGS. 10A TO C: (A) Severe post-thermal burn contracture of perineum and groin causing the penis to bury beneath the contracted skin; (B and C) Same patient showing released contracture followed by skin grafting.

FIGS. 11A AND B: (A) Postburn scarring of the suprapubic area extending to the root of the penis causing dorsal contracture of the penis; (B) Same patient in lateral view showing the dorsal contracture of the penis. The patient had difficulty during micturition as the stream of urine was directed horizontally. The patient required a dorsal release at the root of the penis.

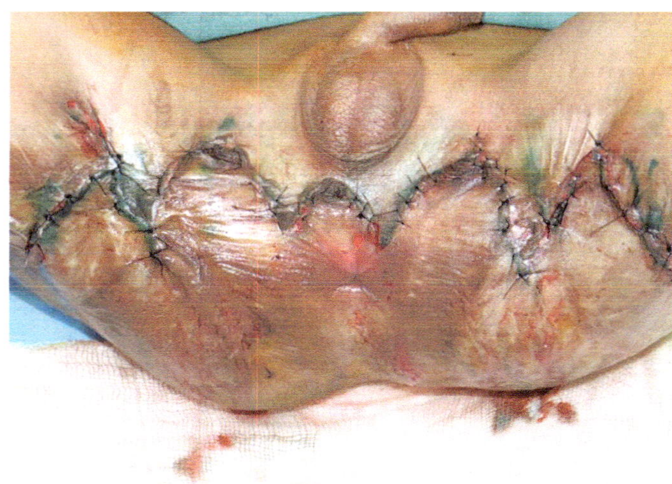

FIG. 12: Perineal contracture released with multiple Y-V advancement flaps.

with single Z-plasty, multiple Z-plasty **(Fig. 12)**, or its variants. Scar excision and closure, with local rotation, and transposition flaps are other methods of dealing with small contractures. Larger contractures need to be released and grafted **(Figs. 10B and C)**. Grafting of both thighs, leaving the intervening portion intact, as advocated in double release or bipedicled release for elbow and popliteal fossa, can be done. If the lower abdomen is spared, this skin can be brought down to avoid skin grafting in the suprapubic area. It is a good method but is rarely applicable as in most cases of burns of genitalia and perineum which require surgery, the lower abdomen is also burnt. When the undesirable scar is not extensive and the adjacent skin is normal and adequate, tissue expansion is an option. It allows one to get qualitatively normal skin without any donor site deformity. However, expanders in the perineal area are fraught with dangers. High incidence of infection and exposure is seen. Patients find it very cumbersome to sit, move around, and perform their normal daily activities with the bulges of the expanders. However, when the expanders are successful, they produce the best results. Alternatively, full-thickness skin donor sites are expanded and used for better cosmetic results.

Postoperative rehabilitation includes massage, stretching and leg abduction exercises, maintenance of abducted position with spreading bar splint, and regular usage of pressure garments for 3–6 months. Postoperative rehabilitation did not appear to influence recurrence which has been reported to be as high as 20%.

Indications for surgery are decreased range of motion and leg abduction. The ideal time for contracture release is after the scar has matured fully. This can take from 6 months to 2 years. An exception to this rule is when the patient needs relief from a severe functional disability.

Intrinsic contracture of the penis results from injury and secondary scarring of dartos, Bucks fascia, tunica, or corpora. Small scars limited to dartos or Bucks fascia can be treated with incision or excision. More severe deficiency needs excision followed by reconstruction with dermal graft and covered by Byar's or any other local flap. If there is scarring of the urethral meatus, dilatation may be enough for mild cases. Z-plasty and other interdigitating flaps are reserved for more severe cases.

Total reconstruction of the penis was started with tube pedicle flaps, which gave way to the axial pattern flaps and muscle flaps, which have now been replaced by state-of-the-art neurosensory fasciocutaneous free flaps. The best results have been obtained by the neurosensory radial forearm flap which can offer both erogenous and protective sensation with prosthesis for erectile function. Other methods which have been used include bilateral gracilis muscle flap and rectus abdominis muscle flap. The girth provided by the flap should be adequate to contain both the neourethra and the prosthesis. Subtotal penile loss is treated the same way, adding the flap to the preserved portion of corpora and urethra.

Vulvar injuries are rare but when they occur they might lead to webbing which compromises normal sexual activity and causes difficulty in micturition. If adjacent tissues are healthy and pliable, Z-plasty, local transposition flaps, or V-Y advancement flaps can be done. Basically, flaps from normal tissue are used to break up the scar contracture line. If the surrounding skin is scarred, the contractures must be released and split skin grafted.

Extensive burns involving buttocks can sometimes result in perianal stenosis or hooding, which can impede fecal evacuation. These patients, on closer examination, may reveal entrapped unburned tissue. This can be released by incising the burnt tissue from the perineal body to the coccyx through the stenotic orifice and everting the unburned tissue away from the anus. Lateral excisions of bands of burnt skin allow recreation of gluteal folds.

Repeated discussions concerning realistic expectations regarding appearance, sexual function, and reconstructive options are important. This should be started early in the acute phase and continued throughout the treatment period till reconstruction is complete. Discussions regarding the nature of deformity, surgical improvement, various available options, and realistic expectations of both the patient and surgeon are critical.

SUMMARY

- Isolated perineal and genital burns are rare. They are usually seen in patients who have sustained a large percentage of burns, more than 40%.
- Superficial burns are treated conservatively, while deeper wounds need excision and resurfacing.
- Burns involving deep anus or sphincter with incontinence need fecal diversion via colostomy.
- Full-thickness burns need reconstructive procedures.
- Urinary diversion with catheter is usually required but fecal diversion is not done.
- Perineal contractures are a rare complication.
- Indications for surgery include decreased leg abduction as well as urinary and bowel complications.
- Surgery for perineal contractures usually requires simple methods such as local flaps and skin grafts, and complicated procedures are reserved for reconstruction of genitalia.
- Local flaps are superior to skin grafts, which should be used only when local tissues are unavailable.
- Aggressive rehabilitative techniques help in preventing recurrences.

REFERENCES

1. Michielsen D, Van Hee R, Neetens C, Lafaire C, and Peeters R. Burns to the genitalia and the perineum. J Urol. 1998;159:418-9.
2. Angel C, Shu T, French D, Orihueta E, Lukefahr J, Herndon DN. Genital and perineal burns in children: 10 years of experience at a major burn center. J Pediatr Surg. 2002;37(1):99-103.
3. Gottlieb LJ, Saunders JN. Perineal burns In: Achauer BM (Ed). Burns Reconstruction. New York: Thieme Medical Publishers Inc.; 1991. pp. 165-82 (Chapter 13).
4. Baba PUF, Shah RA, Rasool A, Kaul A, Wani AH. Perineal burns: Epidemiology, severity factors, management issues and outcome. Burns Open. 2022;6:97-104.
5. Nakazawa H, Ito H, Morioka K, Kikuchi Y, Honda T, Isago T. The use of temporary diverting colostomy to manage elderly individuals with extensive perineal burns. Burns. 2002;28:595-9.
6. Michielsen D, Van Hee R, Neetens C, Lafaire C, Peeters R. Burns to the genitals and the perineum in children. Br J Urol. 1996;78:940-1.
7. Gupta M, Bansal M, Gupta A, Goil P. The kerosene tragedy of 1994, an unusual epidemic of burns: Epidemiological aspects and management of patients. Burns. 1996;22:3-9.
8. Abdel-Razek SM. Isolated chemical burns to the genitalia. Ann Burns Fire Disasters. 2006;19(3):148-52.
9. Demir Z, Eroglu A, Celebioglu S. An interesting case of chemical burn injury of the genital and perianal region caused by hydrochloric acid exposure. Burns. 2003;29(2):175-7.
10. Givens ML, Rivera W. Genital burns from home use of podophyllin. Burns. 2005;31:394-5.
11. Weiler-Mithoff EM, Hassall ME, Burd DA. Burns of the female genitalia and perineum. Burns. 1996;22:390-5.
12. Merchant N, Boudana D, Willoughby L, Lin JJ, Rehou S, Shahrokhi S, et al. Management of adult patients with buttock and perineal burns: The Ross Tilley Burn Centre experience. J Trauma Acute Care Surg. 2014;77(4):640-8.
13. Bandi G, Santucci RA. J Trauma, Injury, Infection Crit Care. 2004;56:1368-69.
14. Pisarski GP, Greenhalgh DG, Warden GD. The management of perineal contractures in children with burns. J Burn Care Rehabil. 1994;15(3):256-9.
15. Sawhney CP. Management of burn contractures of the perineum. Plast Reconstr Surg. 1983;72(6):841-2.
16. Bangma ChrH, van der Molen ABM, Boxma H. Burns to the perineum and genitalia: management, results and function of the thermally injured perineum in a five year review. Eur J Plast Surg. 1995;18:111-4.

CHAPTER

29

Pediatric Burns

Harish Chellani, Sugandha Arya, Raghav Rajesh Mago

"A child is not just a small adult, but a person who is ever more devastated by the burn injury, and who is less able to respond to it."

—Lindsey T.A. Rylah, 199

INTRODUCTION

In the pediatric age group, as is true for adults, a burn injury is the second most important cause of trauma-related deaths, ranking after motor vehicular accidents only. Globally, infants have the highest death rates from burns. The rate of pediatric deaths from burns is currently over seven times higher in low- and middle-income countries than in high-income countries.[1] Pediatric burns are more prevalent in developing countries due to lack of supervision. Besides causing death, many children survive burns only to have lifelong disfigurement, loss of function, and physical deformity, leading to psychological sequelae initially for the parents and later for the victims. Burns are the third leading cause of death in children aged 1–9 years.[1] In India, pediatric burns account for 17–25% of total burn admissions.[2] Approximately, 90% of burns are caused by household accidents. The actual incidence of burn injuries in India is lacking for which a National Burn Registry is necessary.

MODE OF INJURY

Most of the burns in children occur in the child's own house. The age of the child and his environment suggest subgroups of children at risk for burn injury.[1] The infants and toddlers <2 years of age are frequently burned. An important factor leading to burns even in neonates is overcrowding in a small house, where a small area in the room serves as kitchen (with floor level cooking). While the mother is out earning money at work, the victim is taken care of by his or her siblings, who are no more than 5 or 6 years old. When cluster of thatched huts (*"jhuggis"*) catch fire and small children are either sleeping alone or unable to save themselves, infants and young children are the only ones who suffer injuries **(Figs. 1A and B)**.

Moreover, children out of curiosity actively search for and manipulate their physical environment. Scald burns are the most common type of thermal injury in children. They usually suffer scalds by pulling down or knocking hot liquids on to themselves. Immersion scalds can occur when a child steps into a tub of hot water or stumbles onto a container of hot milk or cooked food **(Figs. 2 and 3)**.

Children also feel a temptation to experiment with match boxes. Fireworks during Diwali and other festivals are a major cause of burns in children **(Fig. 4)**. Adults in our country often gather old, worn-out car tires and wooden sticks during the winter and light them to stay warm. It is common for children to mimic adults, which can cause burns.

Electrical burns in children are generally caused by domestic voltage electric current which is 220 volts in India. Usually, a toddler chews an electric cable and suffers a disfiguring third-degree of the lips and cheek burns **(Fig. 5)**.[2]

An electrical injury might result by child sticking his finger or an item like a metallic hairpin into an electric socket. Perineal scalds **(Fig. 6)** and acid burns are very common in children. Strong acids and alkalis that are frequently kept improperly and are used to clean domestic toilets and drains can result in chemical burns.

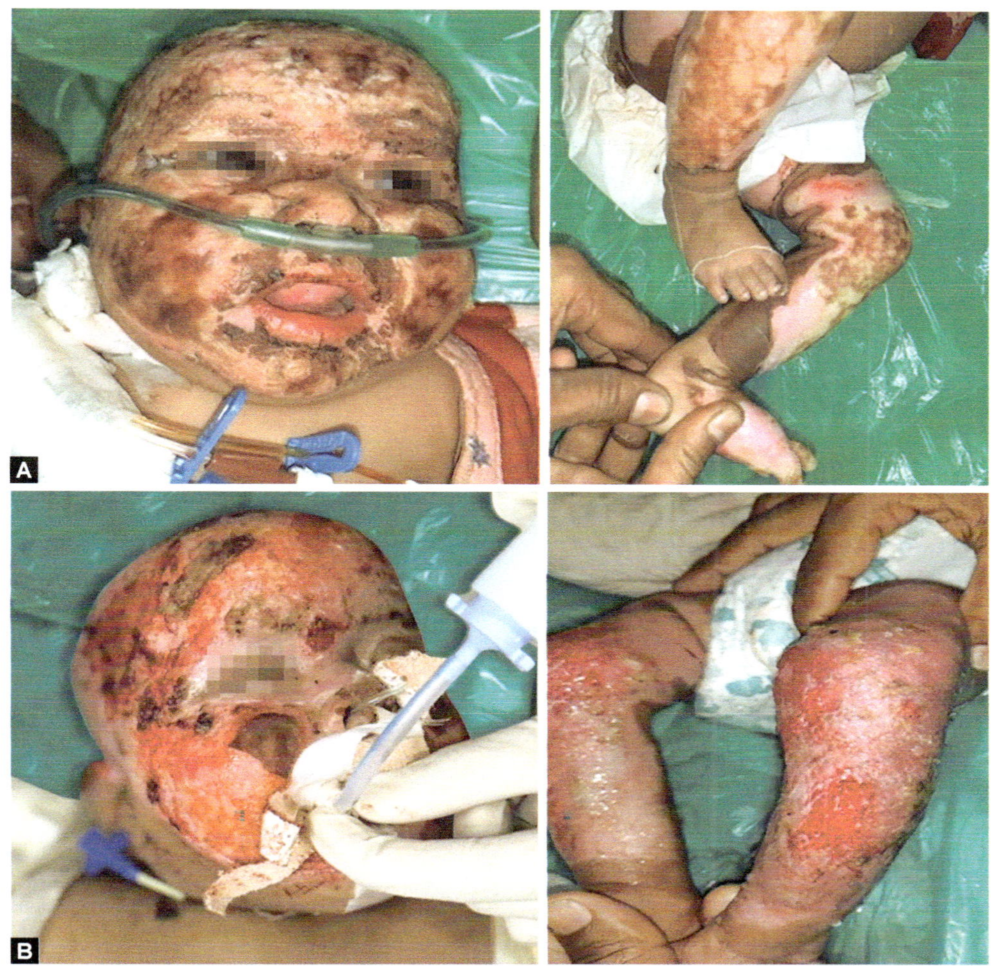

FIGS. 1A AND B: (A) A 6-month-old infant with 35% full-thickness burns sustained accidentally in a *"jhuggi"* fire when the child was left unattended by the mother; (B) 2 weeks postburn picture of the same patient showing eschar separating and wounds starting to granulate from underneath.

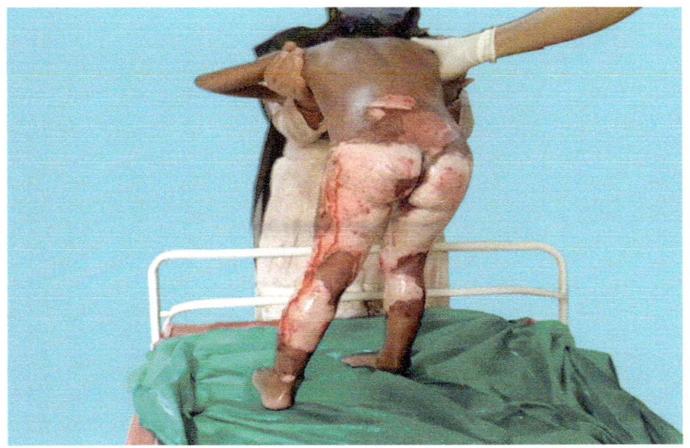

FIG. 2: A 3½-year-old child with 20% scalds due to child stumbling into a container of hot milk.

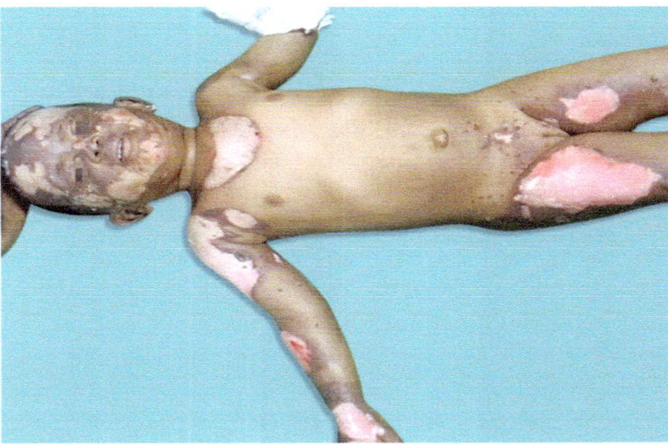

FIG. 3: Another child with 20% superficial dermal scalds due to hot water bucket falling on her.

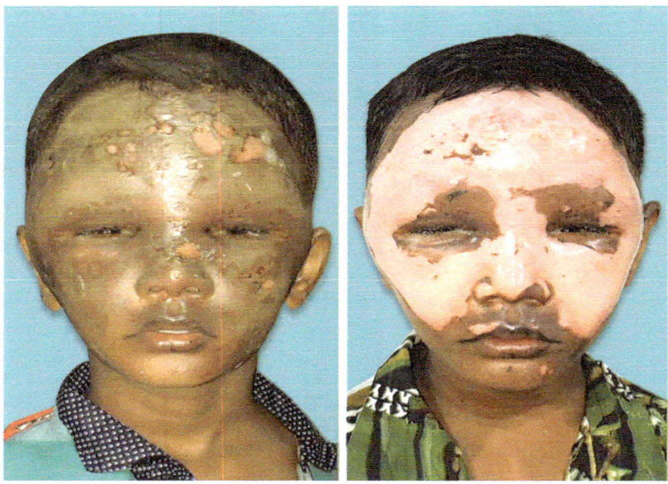
FIG. 4: A 7-year-old child sustained facial burns involving the forehead, cheek, and ear from bursting crackers.

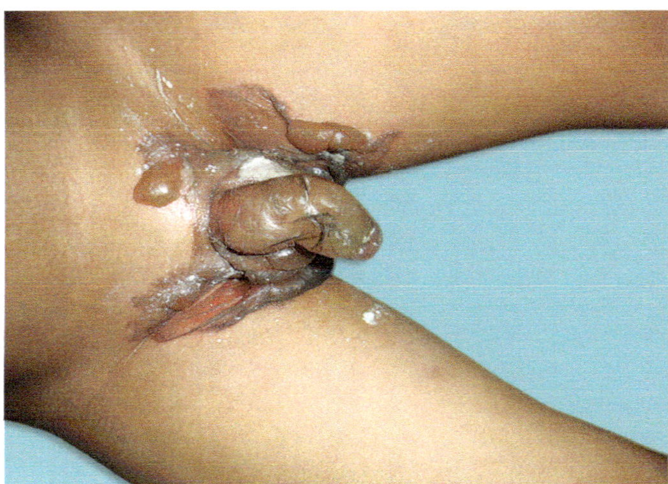
FIG. 6: Perineal scalds because of spilling of hot tea from a cup lying on the table, when the child pulled down the tablecloth.

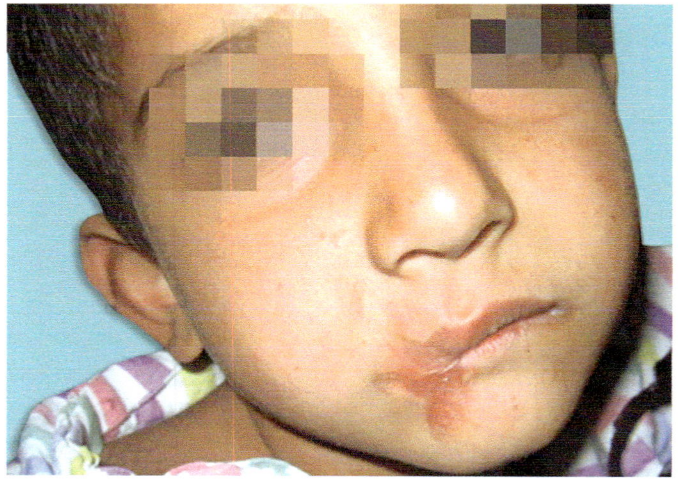
FIG. 5: Postburn microstomia following electric burn sustained by a 4-year-old child while chewing on an electric cord.

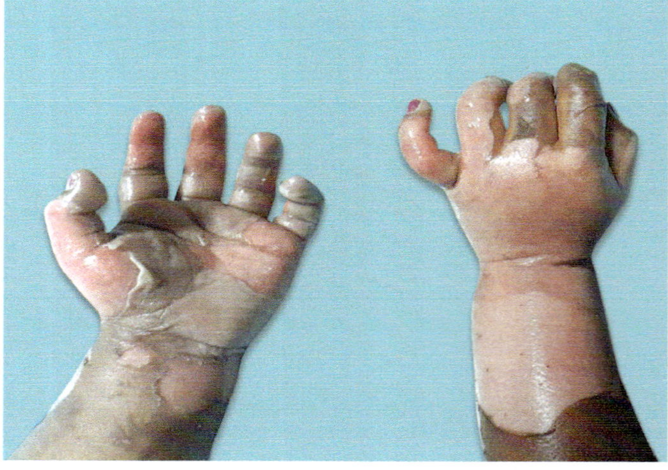
FIG. 7: A case of child abuse with deep partial-thickness burn of the left hand after her hand was forcefully dipped into hot water.

A very small percentage of pediatric burns are due to homicide and child abuse in India, although they are more frequently reported from developed countries **(Fig. 7)**.

PATHOPHYSIOLOGY

Understanding the pathophysiology and sequalae of burn is crucial for managing hemodynamic and multi-organ failure in children. A system-by-system approach to the pediatric burn patient provides the framework for delivering comprehensive care.

- *Cardiovascular system:* Children experience a greater challenge in maintaining the balance of their cardiovascular system and fluid balance, which can impact their response to hypovolemia and subsequent fluid resuscitation following burns. Infants, in particular, rely heavily on their heart rate to increase their cardiac output, and rates as high as 220 beats/min are seen in hypovolemic infants following burns. This compensatory mechanism is easily exhausted making infants more vulnerable to burn shock. Normal heart rates of children are higher than that of adults **(Table 1)**. This helps in meeting the substantially higher metabolic requirements of an infant. The blood pressure is also on the lower side in infants and children, and it increases with age because of the corresponding increase in systemic vascular resistance.
- *Renal:* In children, the renal blood flow and glomerular filtration (GF) rate are lower with delayed maturation and tubular function, and it does not reach adult

TABLE 1: Normal heart rate and blood pressure in children.

Age group	Heart rate (beats/min)	Blood pressure (systolic/ diastolic) (mm Hg)
Newborn	140	65/45
1 year	110	75/50
3 years	100	90/60
8 years	90	95/65
10 years	80	100/70

levels until after they are between 9 and 12 months of age. The osmolar concentrating capacity is also about half that of an adult during this period, and the water load is managed inefficiently. They are likely to retain a significant amount of the fluid load given as part of burn resuscitation during the first few weeks of life. The syndrome of inappropriate antidiuretic hormone secretion (SIADH) is associated with the acute phase of burns. The elevated antidiuretic hormone levels result in the conservation of water and high sodium excretion, causing dilutional hyponatremia and water overload leading to convulsions.[3] It has also been observed that during the acute phase of burn illness, there is an upregulation of acetylcholine receptors and their proliferation to extrajunctional locations. Therefore, it is unsafe to administer succinylcholine to patients who have burn injuries more than 24 hours after the injury while doing surgical interventions. The anesthetist also must be made aware of it as this can result in life-threatening hyperkalemia and cardiac arrest.[4]

- *Immune:* Nonspecific downregulation of immune response occurs and a variety of vasoactive mediators, catecholamines, and inflammatory markers are released with an elevation of circulating cytokines such as tumor necrosis factor alpha (TNF-α) and interferon-gamma (INF-γ).[5] This development is a manifestation of the systemic inflammatory release syndrome (SIRS), which is common after burn injury. The SIRS criteria include an elevation in heart rate, increased body temperature and respiratory rates, and a surge in circulating white blood cells. This effect on the body is directly proportional to the magnitude of the burn. That is, the greater the depth of injury and the greater the surface area affected, the larger the systemic response.
- *Neurologic*: Carbon monoxide (CO) poisoning or associated head injury may cause decreased cerebral perfusion due to hypoxia. CO has over 200 times the affinity of oxygen for hemoglobin. Prolonged smoke exposure causes elevated blood levels of CO, which become increasingly toxic, leading to profound hypoxic brain damage, seizures, jerky movements, and brain death. While headache, nausea, and vomiting are the most common presenting symptoms in children, the most common symptom in infants is altered consciousness.[6]
- *Respiratory system:* From a respiratory standpoint, burn injury results in a complicated picture, with initial management focused on securing a potentially edematous airway and the management of acute respiratory distress syndrome (ARDS).
- *Gastrointestinal system:* The initial goal of the therapy is to protect the stomach from mucosal injury and dysfunction with bacterial translocation across the gut and avoid severe intra-abdominal complications, such as abdominal compartment syndrome and nonocclusive mesenteric ischemia. With regard to mucosal injury, antacids, H2-blockers, and proton-pump inhibitors provide adequate protection to prevent stress ulcers. Abdominal compartment syndrome can best be avoided by careful initial fluid resuscitation and monitoring of abdominal girth and urine output.[7] A pediatric patient with a significant burn must be protected from stress ulcers. Bowel function often is impaired and can be a consequence of narcotics used for pain control and will present with constipation. This needs to be addressed once enteral nutrition has been established. Agents like bisacodyl or glycerine suppositories can also be used to relieve constipation.
- *Hematologic system*: The pediatric burn patient with a burn >20% total body surface area (TBSA) is at risk for anemia and disseminated intravascular coagulation (DIC). Anemia can occur in the setting of an aggressive fluid resuscitation regimen but is also commonly seen during the excision or autografting phase of burn care. DIC is seen in larger burns where sepsis is a consideration. Prolonged prothrombin time (PT), prolonged partial thromboplastin time (PTT), low fibrinogen, and elevated D-dimer are markers of disease.

TEMPERATURE REGULATION

A child is not merely a small adult. Children react differently from adults to thermal trauma, both in their local reactions and systemic responses. One of the most important features of infants is their larger surface area relative to weight when compared with older children and adults. The evaporative water losses and hence the heat losses are greater for children compared to adults because of their larger surface area.[8] The temperature regulatory mechanisms in children is also different in different age groups. For infants <6 months of age, the body temperature is usually regulated by a nonshivering thermogenic response wherein the stores of brown fat are catabolized under the influence of norepinephrine.[9] Since this process utilizes large amounts of oxygen, prolonged hypothermia can lead to excess lactate production leading to acidosis. After 6 months of age, children are able to shiver, but more body heat is still lost as their surface area per unit body weight is larger than that of adults.

The First Aid and Prehospital Care

First aid is carried out by parents, other relatives, or any other person present at the site of the accident, most commonly at the house of the child or neighbor.

- The priority is to stop the burning. The patient must be separated from the burning source. If clothes catch fire: Instructions to the victim should be—Stop where you are. Drop to the ground, lay flat with your legs out straight, and cover your eyes and mouth with your hands. Roll over and over and back and forth until the flames are out **(Fig. 8)**.[10]
- For thermal burns, the burned area is cooled immediately with tap water (preferably running water) to bring the burning skin to normal body temperature. Very cold water or ice should not be used as this can lead to hypothermia.
- For electrical burns, the offending source should be removed from the victim with a nonconducting object made of wood or rubber.
- In chemical injuries, the agent should be diluted with copious irrigation, not immersion.
- Rings, bracelets, or watches, etc., should be removed from the affected area as they may cause tightness or constriction when edema occurs.

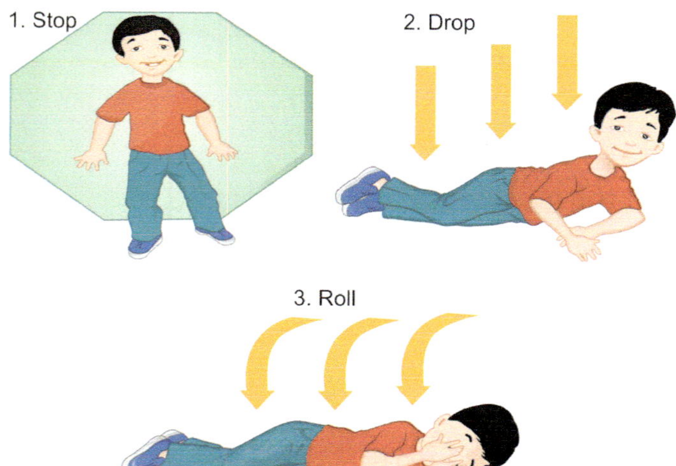

FIG. 8: Fire safety instructions to the victim.

- After cooling, remove the clothing from the burned area. However, do not try to pull out clothing that is stuck to the skin. This may cause more harm.
- A cold compress such as a towel soaked in cold water may be soothing over the burned area. This can be applied after the initial cooling.
- Before going to the hospital, cover the burned area with a clean sheet to prevent contamination and hypothermia.
- Paracetamol or ibuprofen syrup may be given to decrease pain.
- To ensure that determining the depth of the burns is not compromised, no topical treatment should be applied to the burned region.

Indications for Admission to Hospital

The indications to admit a child to a burn care facility are as follows[11]:

- *Extent of the burn*: Children with >10% burns
- *Areas involved*: Involvement of face, neck, both hands, both feet, or perineum
- *Types of burn*: Children with electrical or chemical burns, third-degree burns of >5%
- *Associated injuries*: If burns are associated with soft tissue trauma or head injury, fractures, etc.
- Inhalation burns
- *Social problems*: If there is suspected child abuse or neglect, self-inflicted burns, poor guardianship at home regarding wound care, or psychological problems present, ambulatory management may not be desirable.

Initial Assessment and Management

Nearly, 10% of all burns have concomitant trauma.[12] These should be suspected, diagnosed, and managed following the guidelines of advanced trauma life support (ATLS) and advanced burn life support (ABLS),[13] which suggest following a primary survey followed by a detailed secondary survey.[14]

C-spine Precaution

Protect the cervical spine with cervical spine motion restriction if there is associated trauma.

Airway Assessment

The pediatric airway is funnel shaped with the narrowest portion of the airway being at the level of the cricoid with a diameter is 4 mm (as opposed to 8 mm in an adult). Thus, with 1 mm edema, resistance will increase 16X **(Fig. 9)**. A small amount of narrowing due to edema

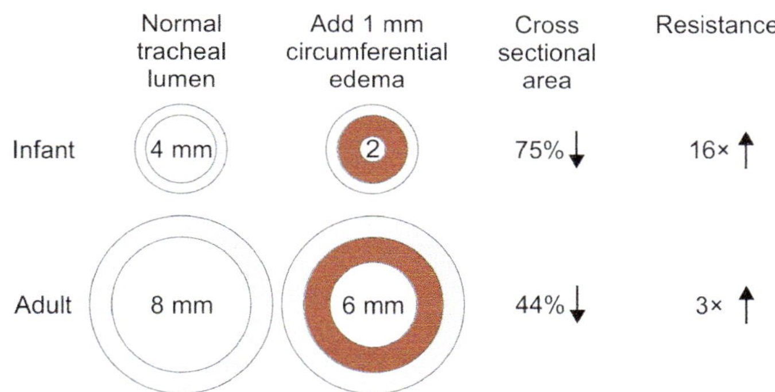

FIG. 9: Tracheal lumen differences between an adult and infant.

or inflammation caused by burns in the already small pediatric airway can have severe consequences on respiratory function.[15]

Indications for early intubation:

- *Signs of airway obstruction*: Hoarseness, stridor, accessory respiratory muscle use, and sternal retraction
- Extent of the burn (TBSA burn >40–50%)
- Extensive and deep facial burns
- Burns inside the mouth
- Significant edema or risk for edema
- Difficulty in swallowing
- *Signs of respiratory compromise*: Inability to clear secretions, respiratory fatigue, poor oxygenation, or ventilation
- Decreased level of consciousness where airway protective reflexes are impaired
- Anticipated patient transfer of large burn with airway issue without qualified personnel to intubate en route

INHALATIONAL INJURY

Pediatric patients require a lower threshold for intubation because of the possibility of airway edema developing quickly. The duration of smoke exposure, temperature of the inhaled smoke, and composition of the smoke are determinants of severity of injury.[16] Inhalation injury is a composite of multiple insults, including supraglottic thermal injury, subglottic airway and alveolar poisoning, and systemic poisoning from absorbed small molecule toxins. The clinical diagnosis of inhalation injury rests upon a high index of clinical suspicion and observations.[17] The warning signs of airway burn/inhalation injury include:

- Inspiratory stridor and breathing difficulty
- Hoarseness, change in voice
- With or without carbonaceous (black) sputum, brassy cough
- Singed nasal hairs or facial swelling

The alarming signs of oropharyngeal burn include:

- The presence of soot in the mouth
- Intraoral edema and erythema
- Significant neck burn

Supraglottic Injury

The supra glottis is typically the primary site of thermal injury, because air has a low heat capacity and the upper airway efficiently dissipates heat. Additionally, the glottis acts as a protective mechanism by closing to prevent heat from reaching the infraglottic area. Injury to the supraglottic structures can lead to edema, which can obstruct the upper airway and compromise ventilation. This obstruction can rapidly worsen during resuscitation in the presence of burn edema.[18]

Subglottic Injury

Injury below the glottis, aside from inhaled steam, is primarily caused by the inhalation of irritants and harmful chemicals found in smoke that enter the lungs. The main pathophysiologic changes that occur after inhalation injury in the subglottic region include airway mucosal hyperemia, bronchospasm, and the formation of airway casts due to fibrinous exudation and blood clots. Other changes include mucosal sloughing and the formation of thick mucus that cannot be cleared due to impaired mucociliary escalator function, which ultimately leads to impaired gas exchange in the distal airways.[19] This can result in ventilation/perfusion (V/Q) mismatching, intrapulmonary shunting, and compromised oxygenation.[20] Acute lung injury is the usual sequelae followed by ARDS as the potential terminal endpoint of subglottic inhalational injury leading to acute respiratory failure which is commonly followed by multisystem organ failure and death.[21] Clinical manifestations of ARDS include pulmonary edema, inability to ventilate and eliminate carbon dioxide, and severe arterial hypoxemia.

Systemic Injury

Systemic injury occurs when the soluble products of combustion which are often present in smoke, particularly when the combustible is plastic, such as CO and cyanide, are inhaled and enter the blood causing hypoxia. Normal COHb levels are generally below 3%. As levels increase above 10%, symptoms such as headache and lethargy become common. At 30% and above, these symptoms are supervened by dizziness, nausea, and impaired vision, and unconsciousness develops at levels between 40 and 50%; 60% and above is frequently associated with death.[22] Children are more vulnerable to CO poisoning because of their increased metabolic demand

and their inability to vocalize symptoms or recognize a dangerous exposure whereas newborn infants are more vulnerable to CO poisoning because of the persistence of fetal hemoglobin.

Management

Supraglottic Injury

The primary treatment for a supraglottic inhalation injury compromising the airway is orotracheal, nasotracheal intubation, or tracheostomy who present with respiratory distress or hypoxemia or with signs of upper airway compromise, such as mucosal edema, erythema, stridor, or hoarseness on vocalization which is also consistent with supraglottic injury **(Figs. 10A and B)**.

The patient should receive 100% humidified oxygen through nonrebreather mask (NRBM) or high-flow nasal cannula (HFNC) which effectively provides temperature and humidity-controlled gas to the nasopharynx to prevent secretions from thickening. The head of the bed should be elevated 45° to reduce supraglottic edema and minimize the pressure exerted by the intra-abdominal structures when the patient is lying flat.[23]

Subglottic Injury

Management is directed at the principal pathophysiologic alterations, such as mucosal hyperemia and edema, bronchospasm, expectoration of mucous and casts, and improving V/Q ratio. Patients with inhalation injury require more intravenous fluid for resuscitation than predicted by resuscitation formulae keeping the urine target output up to 1–2 mL/kg/h. Bronchoalveolar lavage of lung segments is done using normal saline to flush the contaminant materials and casts from the lung until the fluid runs clear. However, some casts may be lodged in the alveoli, which makes it difficult to remove using bronchoalveolar lavage; hence, removal of these obstructive casts by medical intervention is vital. Breaking down airway casts and augmenting expectoration comprise the core of managing subglottic inhalation injury. Fibrin casts are broken down with nebulized heparin, which prevents coagulation of transudated plasma leaking from injured pulmonary capillaries.[24] Sloughed mucosa, mucus portions of casts are flushed away by nebulization with n-acetylcysteine acting as a mucolytic agent and permitting expectoration.[25] Bronchospasm is treated with nebulized bronchodilators like albuterol sulfate with or without nebulized epinephrine, which produces immediate effects, provoking bronchodilation, and reducing airway pressure. We at our unit follow aggressive airway toileting which is the recommended burn injury protocol by the American Burn Association:

- N-acetylcysteine (20% aerosolized solution): 3 mL
- Heparin aerosolized solution (10,000 unit(s)/mL): 1 mL
- Albuterol sulfate aerosolized solution (2.5 mg/0.5 mL): 0.5 mL

Given every 2 hours alternately for the first 7 days postinhalation injury. This inhalation protocol continues even after extubation in patients who initially required mechanical ventilation. Our unit's additive approach in patients with inhalation burns includes:

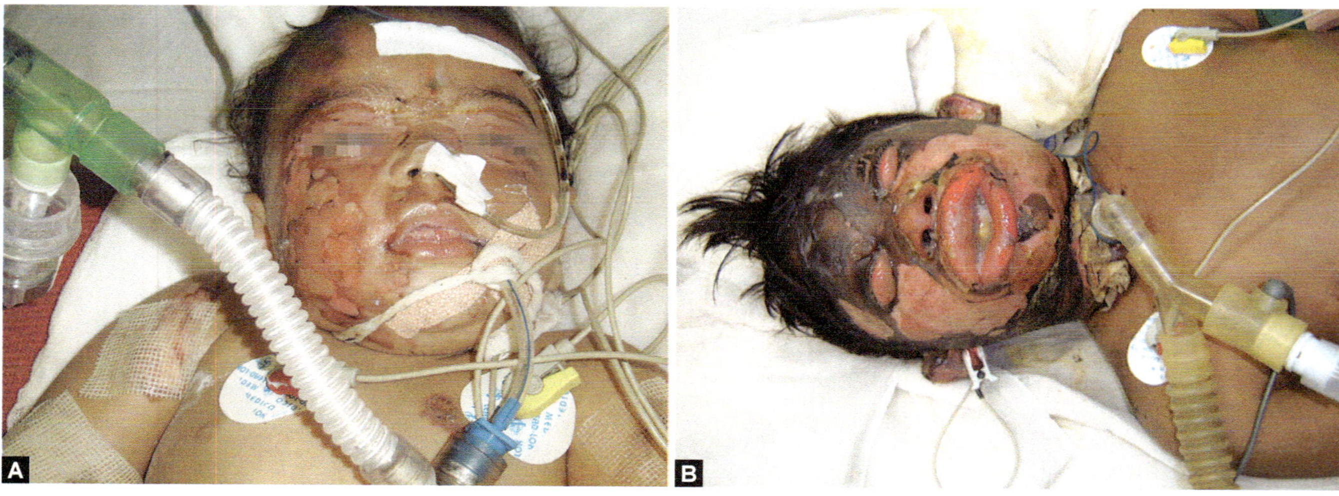

FIGS. 10A AND B: (A) The patient intubated for mechanical ventilation even though the child sustained only 10% scald with hot tea following which the caretaker poured a bucket full of water on his face and the child aspirated hot tea and water both leading to aspiration pneumonitis; (B) Another child with 10% facial burns with smoke inhalation injury requiring tracheostomy for ventilation.

- Supervise the patient performing percussive and coughing techniques and deep breathing exercises every 2 hours.
- Turn the patient side to side every 2 hours for postural drainage.
- Administer chest physiotherapy every 2 hours by chest percussion and vibration such as high-frequency chest wall oscillation.[26]
- Perform nasotracheal suctioning as needed with normal saline.
- Encourage early ambulation with the use of DVT pump/air mattress.
- If the patient does show signs of lung infiltrates and increased broncho vascular markings as in most cases of inhalational injury after 48 hours, our unit uses adjunctive therapy with aerosolized colistin 1000,000 units every 8 hours to prevent nosocomial pneumonia.[27]

Ventilator management is centered on a tidal volume between 6 and 8 mL/kg of predicted body weight ensuring sufficient oxygenation, ventilation, optimizing expectoration, and limiting harm such as ventilator-induced injury through excessive pressure causing tension pneumothorax and ARDS. The use of both volume and pressure-cycled modes is widespread, but there is ongoing debate regarding the optimal ventilator mode for inhalation injury. According to a survey, pressure support ventilation, and volume-assist control modes were the most frequently reported initial modes used in burn patients.[28] A study comparing pediatric inhalation injury patients on high-frequency percussive ventilation (HFPV) versus conventional ventilation indicated that patients in the HFPV group had fewer cases of pneumonia, lower peak inspiratory pressure, and decreased work of breathing.[29,30]

Systemic

Treatment for CO and cyanide intoxication is essential or else, it can cause systemic toxicity. When carboxyhemoglobin (COHb) levels exceed 10%, 100% humidified oxygen should be administered. With humidified oxygen, the half-life of the COHb t(1/2) is reduced to 74 ± 25 minutes from 4 to 6 hours till the levels reduce to <10%. Measurement of COHb on ABG and, CO oximetric studies can quantify CO quickly which is to be done every 4 hours.

Treating cyanide poisoning can be an indirect therapy for CO intoxication because of the synergistic toxicities of the molecules, thereby shortening the duration of oxygen administration. Hydroxocobalamin, the precursor of vitamin B12, is a safe treatment with few side effects. Other drugs like sulfur donors such as sodium thiosulfate and sodium nitrate accentuate the conversion of cyanide to thiocyanate, reducing its toxicity are also used but hydroxocobalamin is the preferred drug to treat cyanide intoxication.[31]

TABLE 2: Normal resting respiratory rates in children.

Age	Normal resting respiratory rates (breaths/min)
Newborn	30–60
1–6 months	30–50
6–12 months	24–46
1–4 years	20–30
4–6 years	20–25
6–12 years	16–20
>12 years	12–16

BREATHING

Pediatric respiratory rates vary according to age (infants naturally breathe slightly faster than older children), so age-related respirate rates must be kept in mind as mentioned in **Table 2** to understand ideal rate.[32]

It is crucial to recognize the unique respiratory features of neonates and infants, such as their underdeveloped respiratory control and ineffecient respiratory muscles. Recognizing and comprehending the distinct respiratory characteristics observed is imperative especially in:

- Circumferential full-thickness burns
- Blast injuries can cause tension pneumothorax, lung contusions
- Chemicals (plastic) can cause a chemical pneumonitis
- CO poisoning

Management

- Chest auscultation with respiratory movement, breath sounds, and rate with depth to be evaluated.
- If inhalation injury is suspected, start 100% humidified oxygen through NRBM.[33]
- If breathing seems to be compromised because of tight circumferential trunk burns then escharotomy is needed for adequate expansion as shown in **Figure 11**.

CIRCULATORY SYSTEM

Children have smaller circulating volume when compared to adults and require a greater degree of accuracy when replacing.

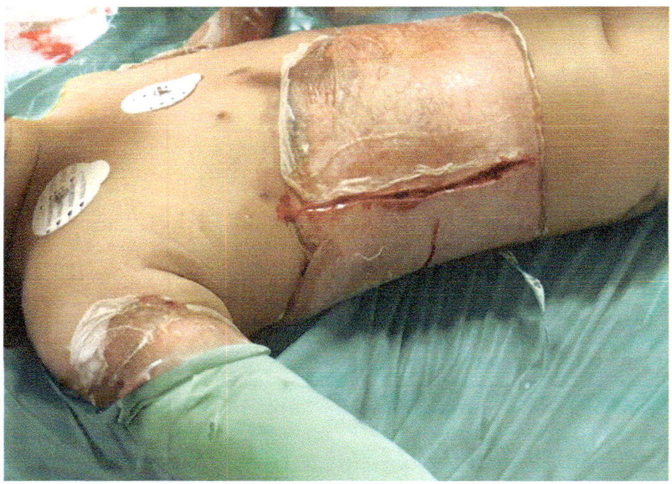

FIG. 11: Escharotomy done in a 6-year-old who sustained circumferential flame burns over trunk.

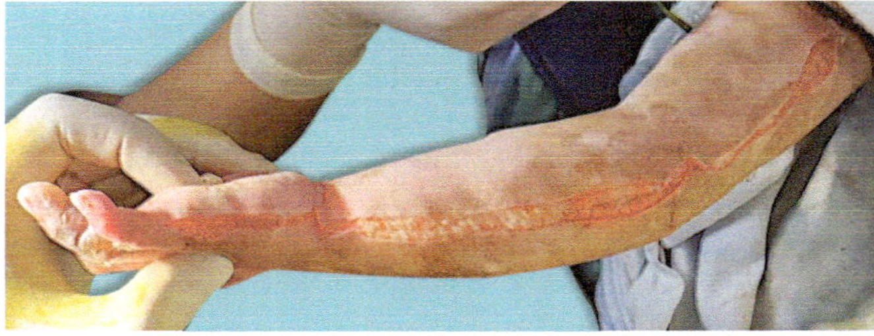

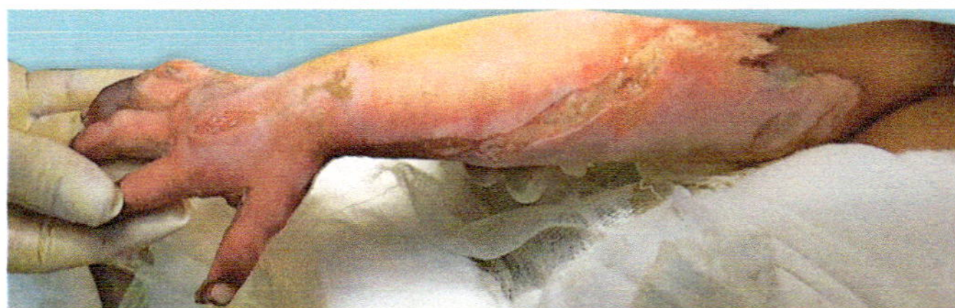

FIG. 12: A 7-year-old sustained full-thickness circumferential burns over both upper limbs with compartment syndrome, feeble pulses, and escharotomy done.

They also have greater insensible and burn related fluid losses and hence hypotension is a *late sign of shock in pediatric patients.*

Examination

- Check for peripheral pulses at the brachial or femoral artery.
- Blood pressure and heart rate are age related and must be checked and recorded **(Table 1)**. Abnormal cardiac rhythms may be due to electrical injuries.
- If early shock is present, consider causes other than the burn, like potential sources of internal bleeding.
- In case of circumferential burns, check peripheral perfusion and look for 7 P's—*P*allor, *P*ain, *P*ulseless-ness, *P*oikilothermia, *P*aresthesia, *P*rogression of ischemia, and *P*aralysis.
- Escharotomy/fasciotomy is to be performed if progression of ischemia is observed as shown in **Figure 12**.

Management

- Intravenous access with two large-bore intravenous lines and send blood for cross-matching and baseline investigations.
- Catheterize the patient with Foley's catheter with uroflow meter to accurately measure hourly output.
- The patient will benefit from central venous cannulation for reliable access for a tailored fluid resuscitation plan. Monitoring central venous pressure and urine output are helpful in assessing the goal-directed fluid therapy.
- Unburned skin is usually preferred for venous access but if not available, burned skin is preferred to cut-down procedure.
- Hypothermia is prevented by providing blanket, closed dressing, warming up fluids prior to administration and encouraging mother to cuddle baby to provide warmth.
- Peripheral I/IV lines must be changed every 5 days and central line every 10 days.

DISABILITY

- Assessment is done by determining the neurological state either using AVPU scale (awake, verbal, pain and unresponsive) or GCS scoring to assess a patient's level of consciousness.
- Patient with burns is initially alert and oriented. If not, consider shock, hypoxemia, CO poisoning, and also analgesia influence on awareness have to be taken into consideration and assessed.
- Associated head injury must be noted and managed by taking a neurosurgical consultation into account.
- While assessing the level of consciousness *do not ever forget* to measure *glucose levels.*

EXPOSURE

- *Maintain core body temperature and prevent hypothermia*: Cover the patient with a sterile sheet and a blanket to keep warm or use radiant heaters.
- Remove all burned clothes, fully expose the patient to assess the extent of injury in terms of TBSA% that is affected by the burn injury, and gauge the burn depth and surface.
- Remove all jewelry, nail paints, and ritual threads.
- Examine for signs of abuse and any suspicion of nonaccidental burns.

SECONDARY SURVEY

History Taking

In the secondary survey, a detailed history, cause of burn (scald/electric/chemical/radiation/friction), and head-to-toe examination are involved. Detail of resuscitation from referring health centre is taken—with respect to what medications have been given, what dressing material has been used, and what line of management has been followed for the patient.

BURN EVALUATION

Before definitive wound care commences, a protocol for rapid assessment of the injury and resuscitative measures to be taken is formulated.

Assessment

Total body surface area burned, expressed as a percentage, is one of the most important aspects of the initial care of a burn victim. It determines whether transfer to a burn center is necessary as well as the need for, and amount of, intravenous fluid resuscitation. The burn injury should be assessed for:

- Percentage of TBSA involved
- Depth
- Location
- Any associated injuries

Estimation of Burn Size

Lund and Browder's Chart

The percentage of body surface area (BSA) involved can be readily assessed by standard Lund and Browder chart[34] **(Table 3)**, which is an accurate technique for assessing the percentage of burn surface area in children.

In children, the head is proportionately a larger contributor to TBSA, while the lower limbs contribute less as compared to adults. The head and neck comprise 19% of the total surface area in an infant. With each year, the surface area decreases by 1% till 10 years of age, when it is like that of an adult. Similarly, each lower limb constitutes 13% of the surface area of the body in an infant and it increases by 0.5% per year till 10 years of age when it almost matches that of an adult (18%).[35]

Another simple formula that can correct for differences in BSA in children is, to subtract child's age in years from 12 and the resulting number is added to the figure for adult head and neck or subtracted from the figure for both lower limbs. *Example*: At 8 years, the head and neck constitute 9 + (12 – 8) = 13% of TBSA. At 8 years, both lower limbs constitute 36 – (12 – 8) = 32% of TBSA, that is, 16% for each lower limb.

TABLE 3: Lund and Browder's chart showing changes in body surface area (%) with age.

Area	Birth to 1 year	1–4 years	5–9 years	10–14 years	15 years	Adult
Head	19	17	13	11	9	7
Neck	2	2	2	2	2	2
Anterior trunk	13	13	13	13	13	13
Posterior trunk	13	13	13	13	13	13
Right buttock	2.5	2.5	2.5	2.5	2.5	2.5
Left buttock	2.5	2.5	2.5	2.5	2.5	2.5
Genitalia	1	1	1	1	1	1
Right upper arm	4	4	4	4	4	4
Left upper arm	4	4	4	4	4	4
Right lower arm	3	3	3	3	3	3
Left lower arm	3	3	3	3	3	3
Right hand	2.5	2.5	2.5	2.5	2.5	2.5
Left hand	2.5	2.5	2.5	2.5	2.5	2.5
Right thigh	5.5	6.5	8	8.5	9	9.5
Left thigh	5.5	6.5	8	8.5	9	9.5
Right leg	5	5	5.5	6	6.5	7
Left leg	5	5	5.5	6	6.5	7
Right foot	3.5	3.5	3.5	3.5	3.5	3.5
Left foot	3.5	3.5	3.5	3.5	3.5	3.5
Total	100	100	100	100	100	100

Wallace's Rule of "Nine"

The "Rule of Nines" divides the body surface into areas of 9% or multiples of 9%, with the exception that the perineum is estimated at 1%. This allows the extent of the burn to be estimated with reproducible accuracy.

According to this:

- *Head and neck*: 9% TBSA (9 × 1)
- *Upper limbs*: 9% TBSA (9 × 2)
- *Anterior trunk*: 18% TBSA (9 × 2)
- *Posterior trunk*: 18% TBSA (9 × 2)
- *Lower limbs*: 18% TBSA (9 × 2 × 2)
- *Perineum and external genitalia*: 1% TBSA
- Total = 100%

Children have different BSA proportions; hence, pediatric rule of nines is used by adjusting for age by taking 1% TBSA from the head and adding ½% TBSA to each leg for each year of life after 1 year until 10 years

(**Fig. 13**). In children over 12 years, burn wounds are estimated by the formula used in adults.[36]

Rule of "Five"

Lynch and Blocker developed a formula for estimating the extent of burns in children.[37] It works very well in infants where the head and neck, anterior and posterior aspects of the trunk are 20% each and each limb constitutes 10%. For older children, this is slightly modified. The head, posterior trunk, and lower limbs are 15% each, the anterior trunk is 20% and each upper limb is 10%.

Rule of Palm or Hand

The palmar surface of a person's hand indicates 1% TBSA for all age groups. This is helpful in evaluating scattered burned regions. Only second-degree burns or greater should be included in the TBSA burned for burns management. Scald of the scalp is not usually visible, especially in children 3 years and above, so if you notice burned hair or for that matter even burned ears suspicion for scalp burns is to be raised and evaluated closely, and shaving of the scalp is to be done for further evaluation and treatment.

Overestimation of Burn Wound

In children, the burn size is often overestimated by referrers from referral hospitals by up to 30% TBSA, while underestimation was up to 13% TBSA.[38] Various reasons can be there but regardless of the method used, it is difficult especially when a child is crying, when there is confusion about skin redness, or when erythema is suspected instead of a second-degree burn. Furthermore, a crying and uncooperative, painful child and anxious, scared parents can distract healthcare workers and force them to make quick decisions and calculations that may lead to errors.[39] It has also been shown that burn size estimation by burn surgeons over telemedicine correlates closely with inaccurate estimation.[40]

Estimation of Burn Depth (Figs. 14 to 17)

The burn depth estimation is discussed in detail elsewhere in this volume. During infancy, the epidermis is loosely connected to the dermis. As a result, blisters form more readily in burns in infants. The stratum corneum layer of the epidermis is thinner in children so scalds cause deeper burns in children compared to adults. The amount of sebum and sweat production in an infant's skin is also less than that in older children and adults. Due to all these reasons, a child's skin is susceptible to

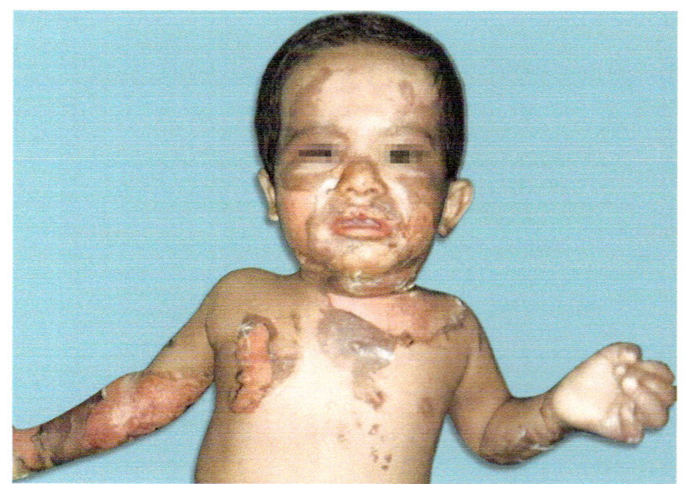

FIG. 14: Accidental superficial dermal burns of the face in a toddler.

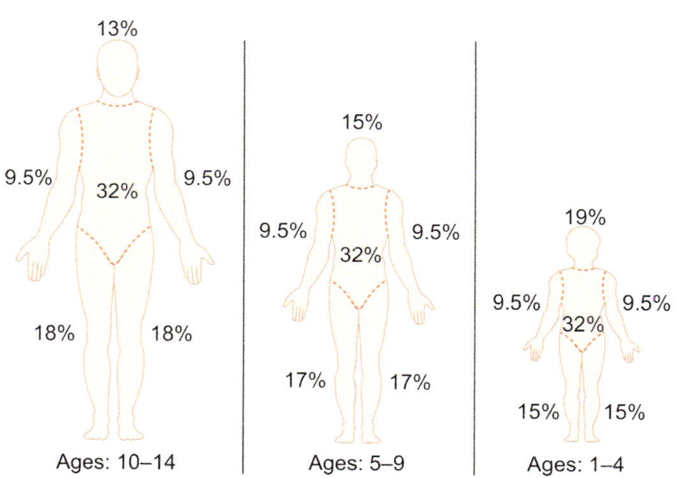

FIG. 13: Rule of nine.

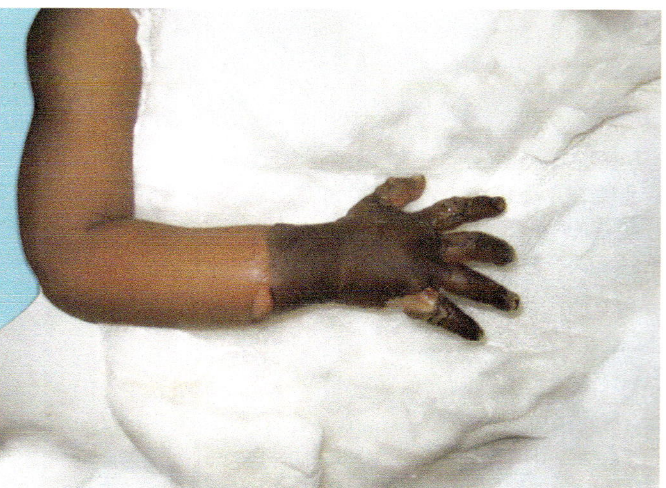

FIG. 15: Full-thickness burns of the hand and distal forearm of a child.

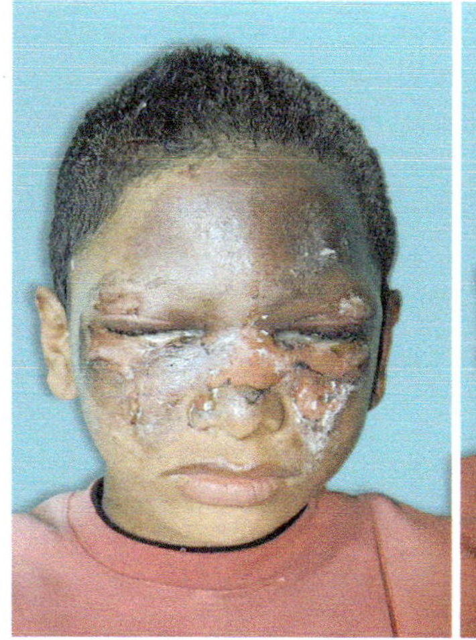
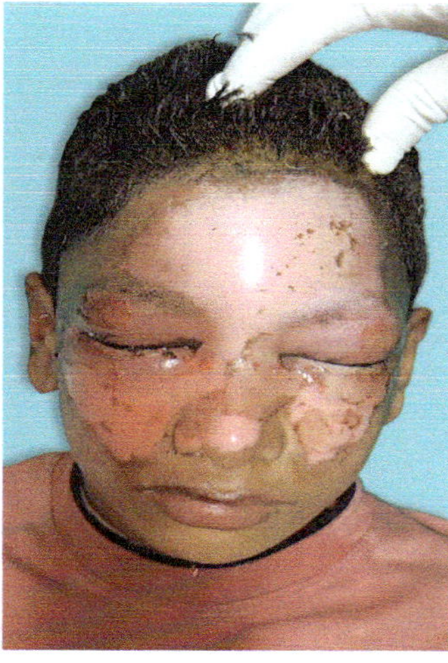

FIG. 16: Second-degree flame burns of the face by burning cracker powder.

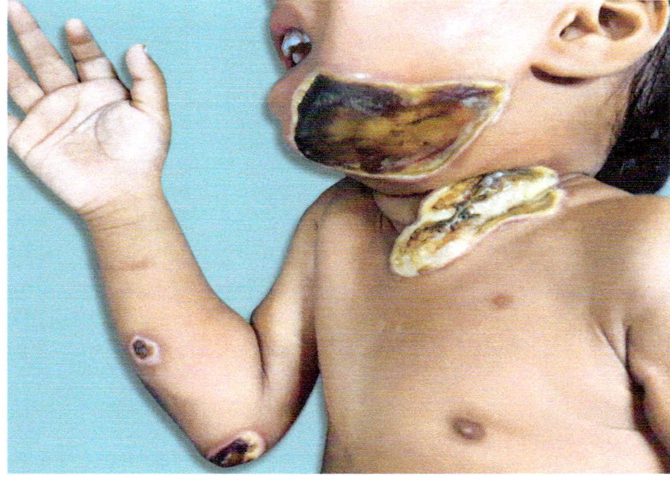

FIG. 17: Another child with deep dermal or deep second-degree burns on the face and forearm.

greater damage by heat and chemicals even if exposure is for a short duration.

Many burn wounds which initially appear superficial may eventually turn out to be deeper and may require skin grafting. A scald injury which looks bright red and is taken as a superficial burn in an adult may turn out to be full-thickness burn in young children.

A severe burn is one that covers greater than 15% of the BSA or involves the face or perineum. Second-degree and third-degree burns of the hands or feet, as well as circumferential burns of the extremities, are also classified as severe. Inhalation injuries resulting in bronchospasm and impaired pulmonary function must be considered as severe burns.

Fluid Management

Goal-directed fluid resuscitation is of utmost importance. Many fluid resuscitation regimens have been advocated over the last 50 years. Pruitt et al.[41] recommended 3 mL/kg/% burn surface area as a resuscitation formula for thermally injured children. Baxter reported 4 mL/kg/% BSA for fluid calculation[42] while Warden et al.[43] recommended a mean fluid requirement of 5.8 mL/kg/% BSA for children. For minor burns, oral hydration may be acceptable, but children will require fluid resuscitation for burns as small as 10–20% BSA because of their limited physiological reserve, there is systemic edema, which develops at 4 hours and continues until 36 hours after injury. Various studies have demonstrated that children with burns <30% area require less fluid/kg/% burn than those with >30% burns.[7,8] Prompt resuscitation is critical in pediatric patients due to their small circulating blood volumes. There is also a need to standardize resuscitation protocols in pediatric age group as there are many protocols in the literature. Delays in resuscitation can result in increased complications and increased mortality.

No single formula can be adhered to strictly in the management of a burned child. The most important fact underlying this decision is not to overload the vascular system and at the same time not to under-resuscitate the child. Similar to adults, a formulaic approach, adapted based on physiological endpoints, is advocated. Pediatric-specific formulae are available. These incorporate physiological differences in the pediatric patient.

The most used formula is the Parkland formula, measured in milliliters.[44] This is 4 mL/kg × TBSA% burns over a 24 hours period without any additional daily maintenance fluid. Half the total is given over the first 8 hours from the time of burn, and half over the following 16 hours. The fluid calculated as per these formulae in infants, especially with smaller burns may not suffice as it may not even meet the total daily requirement. For example, in a 10 kg child with 20% burns the daily fluid requirement is 1000 mL. However, the amount of resuscitation fluid calculated for the same using the Parkland formula (4 × 20 × 10) comes to only 800 mL in the first 24 hours. This results in gross under-resuscitation of the patient. Therefore, the daily maintenance fluid has to be added to these formulae in the form of dextrose saline. This is given as N/2 saline with 2.5% dextrose or N/4 saline with 3.75% dextrose according to the age of the child (for <2 months of age N/5 or N/6; 2 months to 5 years, N/4 and for 5–12 years, N/3 or N/2). The addition of dextrose decreases the incidence of hypoglycemia in infants in the first

24 hours. On the other hand, in extensive burns in children, the Parkland/Baxter formula is again unsatisfactory as the amount of fluid calculated is very high. There is no restriction to the percentage of burn area to be included. For example, a 10 kg child with 80% burns would be predicted to require 10 × 80 × 4 = 3,200 mL fluid in the first 24 hours, although the daily fluid requirement for the same patient is only 1000 mL.

This large amount of Ringer's lactate, if given to the child, can result in fluid overload and resultant hyponatremia can precipitate convulsions in children. Therefore, a formula with a ceiling of 50% TBSA is essential along with the addition of daily fluid requirement. For this purpose, modified Brooke's formula satisfies all the requirements and is followed in our burn unit as well.

According to modified Brooke's formula, the first 24 hours requirement is calculated as follows:

2 mL × weight in kg × % BSA burned + daily maintenance

The fluid of choice is crystalloid, namely Ringer's lactate is used as the first-line fluid replacement in burn resuscitation, and an appropriate urine output remains the main goal of resuscitation.

Daily maintenance fluid is given in the form of N/2 dextrose saline (0.45% NS with 2.5% dextrose) or N/4 dextrose saline (0.23% NS with 3.75% dextrose) and is calculated as per the weight of the child **(Table 4)**.

Half of this fluid is given in the first 8 hours and the second half in the next 16 hours. In the second 24 hours, the formula recommended for use is 1 mL/kg/% BSA burned of Ringer's lactate + daily maintenance (same as above). According to Cincinnati-Shriners, the first 24 hours requirement is as follows: 4 mL × weight (kg) × %BSA burned + baseline requirements (1,500 mL/m^2 total body surface) and the fluid used is Ringer's lactate with 5% dextrose as required. The *administration instructions are* 50% of the volume in the first 8 hours postburn (0–8 hours) and 5% dextrose, sodium, potassium, and albumin solutions to be considered according to serum level for the next 24–48 hours.

In our unit, we follow the following fluid protocol as given in **Table 5**. Note that 24 hours is calculated from the time of the burn.

TABLE 4: Daily maintenance therapy in children.

Weight of child	Daily maintenance fluid (mL/kg/day)
0–10 kg	100 mL/kg
10–20 kg	1,000 mL + 50 mL/kg for every 1 kg above 10
More than 20 kg	1,500 mL + 20 mL/kg for every 1 kg above 20 kg

Burn Arrival Situations

- If arrival is <8 hours from the time of burn: The calculated fluid is to be infused in the remaining hours of the first 8 hours.
- If arrival is >8 hours: Give all the calculated fluid in the next 16 hours.
- Lastly if presented >24 hours late which is usually the case in our unit, we start maintenance fluids according to weight and maintain urine output at 1 mL/kg/h.
- *Note: If the patient has already received fluid before referral, then that amount of fluid must be subtracted from the calculated fluid amount.*

The decision to use colloids or crystalloids is controversial. The rationale for giving crystalloids in the form of Ringer's lactate and avoiding colloids in the first 24 hours is that following burns, it is the plasma which is lost from the intravascular compartment into extravascular space because of increased capillary permeability. Since Ringer's lactate is equivalent to plasma without proteins, it restores the intravascular pressure without adding to the loss of proteins into extravascular space. Colloids, on the other hand, add to the loss of high molecular weight molecules from the vascular compartment to extravascular space till such time that the capillary permeability is increased, usually between 18 and 24 hours. By 48 hours postburn, the permeability is restored to normal, the leaked-out proteins cannot be reabsorbed back into the circulation easily. This increases the chances of pulmonary edema and peripheral edema persisting for a very long time with deleterious effects on the GF, coagulation, and cardiac function.[45,46] Baxter showed that colloids probably do not exert any measurable expansion of plasma over and above that exerted by Ringer's lactate till the second postburn day.[42]

Martin et al. compared patients receiving only colloid-based fluids in the first 24 hours and those

TABLE 5: Fluid protocol at our unit.

First 24 hours	3cc × body weight × % of burns (RL) + Maintenance DNS
Next 24 hours	2cc × body weight × % of burns + Maintenance DNS or as required to maintain urine output • 0.5 mL/kg/% of burns colloids • Potassium supplementation as per requirement
After 48 hours	Give fluids titrated to urine output and electrolytes

receiving a combination of colloids and crystalloids and reported that the only colloid regimen used much less fluid during resuscitation with much-reduced rates of ARDS, hypoalbuminemia, and sodium disturbances but more peripheral and pulmonary edema and renal impairment.[47]

So, the consensus is that in the first 24 hours, only if the fluid requirement is very high as in extensive pediatric burns, colloids can be added to crystalloids in the regimen. In massive burns, if only large volumes of crystalloids are given, the intravascular volume is expanded but the plasma oncotic pressures are not restored as they are devoid of proteins. On the other hand, the plasma oncotic pressure is restored faster with colloids because they contain high molecular weight molecules. Crystalloids in large amounts dilute the remaining proteins further in the intravascular space thus decreasing the oncotic pressure as well. As a certain level of oncotic pressure is essential to maintain GF, any further decrease in this pressure will affect the GF and thus decrease the urine output, which should be increasing. This gives a false impression that fluid resuscitation is inadequate and by default more crystalloids may be infused to increase urine output, resulting in volume overload without improving the oncotic pressure. In such circumstances, infusion of colloids is required to improve plasma oncotic pressure and increase GF.

In the second 24 hours postburn, many centers prefer to add colloids to their fluid regimen.[47,48] In our unit, we use colloids after 24 hours which are given in the form of 5% albumin or fresh frozen plasma in a volume of 0.3–0.5 mL/kg/% BSA burned.

Since the routine formulae are exclusively weight-based, and in children there is no linear relationship between weight and surface area, there are problems of under and overresuscitation in pediatric age group. To overcome this, studies have shown the benefits of using Galveston formula based on BSA calculated from the height and weight of the child from standard nomograms.[49,50] According to this formula, the amount of fluid administered in the first 24 hours is calculated as 5,000 mL/m^2 BSA burn + 2,000 mL/m^2 BSA, with half the volume given in in the first 8 hours and the second half in the next 16 hours. This has not yet been standardized and is not being used worldwide.

Monitoring of Fluid Resuscitation

The best way to monitor the adequacy of fluid resuscitation is by measuring pulmonary capillary wedge pressure. Since this is not routinely practicable in a clinical setting, hourly urine output measurement is the most practical and easily done to know the adequacy of resuscitation.

TABLE 6: Required urine output according to age.

Age of child	Urine output
0–2 years	10–20 mL/h
2–5 years	20–30 mL/h
Above 5 years	30–50 mL/h

The physiologic goal is maintaining urine output of at least 1 mL/kg body weight/h. During the first 48 hours, adequate urine output is considered as given in **Table 6**.

The concept of "fluid creep" has been identified, which refers to the situation where patients are given a significantly larger quantity of fluids than what is calculated, without considering the volumes of medications like antibiotics and electrolyte replacements such as magnesium. It is important to note that excessive resuscitation with intravenous fluids can be harmful and may lead to complications, such as ARDS, multiorgan dysfunction, abdominal and limb compartment syndrome, and cerebral edema.[51] Hence, a close watch is maintained on serum electrolyte levels because of rapid fluid and electrolyte shifts in burned children. Using the endpoints of resuscitation and hydration and measuring hourly central venous pressure, doing timely ABGs, IVC monitoring can help to avoid over and underresuscitation-related complications. Some commonly used clinical endpoints are:

- Intact sensorium
- Normothermia
- *Age-appropriate hemodynamics*: The child's pulse, respiratory rate, and blood pressure are also monitored closely.
- Sustained urine output
- Minimal systemic acidosis, base deficit <2

Intravenous fluids are progressively decreased and stopped starting on the third day when the child is weaned off them. Urinary volumes considerably surpass the total amount of fluid consumed orally and intravenously once capillary permeability is restored. This is because fluid from the extracellular compartment returns to the intravascular compartment.

Children with partial-thickness burns that cover <15% of the body surface may be given oral fluids in the form of milk or other clear liquids, but carbonated beverages should be avoided as they may contribute to gastric dilatation and vomiting.

Adjunctive Management

- *Nasogastric tube*: Aim for an early postburn enteral feeding.
- Very early intestinal feeding, that is, it begins in the first 6–12 hours after an injury that allows for

the preservation of intestinal lymphoid tissue and stimulation of gastrointestinal motility and blood circulation to safeguard against intestinal hypoperfusion. It also has the effect of lowering stress hormone levels, hypermetabolic response, increased immunoglobulin production, reduction in inflammation, and reduced risk of malnutrition and lack of energy. Feeds are started at the rate of 10 mL/h, and the quantity can be increased by 10 mL/h every 6 hours to reach a maximum of 3 mL/kg/h.

- Each feed is preceded by NG aspiration and Ryles tube must be changed every 21 days. In the case of extensive burns, especially toddlers and infants who find it difficult to chew and masticate the food, liquid food, which is specifically prepared and given in small, measured quantities. This is recommended for all children with burns of 10% in the case of infants and 15% or more of BSA for toddlers.
- *Urinary catheter:* It is routinely inserted in all patients with above 10% burns in the case of infants and 15% or more of BSA for toddlers to monitor hourly urine output and should be changed every 5 days.
- *H2 receptor antagonists:* Children with burns requiring admission should be given proton-pump inhibitors (e.g., lansoprazole) and antacids for prophylaxis against gastroduodenal erosions and ulcerations (curling ulcers).
- *Tetanus prophylaxis*: Tetanus toxoid is administered for prophylaxis against tetanus along standard recommended lines. With the great emphasis by the Government of India on immunizing children against many diseases in the first year of life, tetanus being one of them, many children may be already immunized at the time of burn. In children not properly immunized, passive protection is also provided with 250 units of tetanus immunoglobulin.
- *Analgesia and sedation*: The dynamic and evolving nature of pain means that background, breakthrough, procedural, and postoperative pain all need to be taken care for. For children with minor burns being treated on an outpatient basis, paracetamol (10–15 mg/kg every 6 hours) alone or its combination with ibuprofen can be used, although NSAIDs must be used cautiously in those with severe burn injuries as the incidence of adverse effects (including renal toxicity, gastric ulceration, and antiplatelet effects) may preclude their use in many cases. For major burns, infusion of opioids (injection tramadol) as a solution for infusion may be required. Playing animation movies on the television to distract while dressing helps a lot and reduces analgesic requirements **(Fig. 18)**.

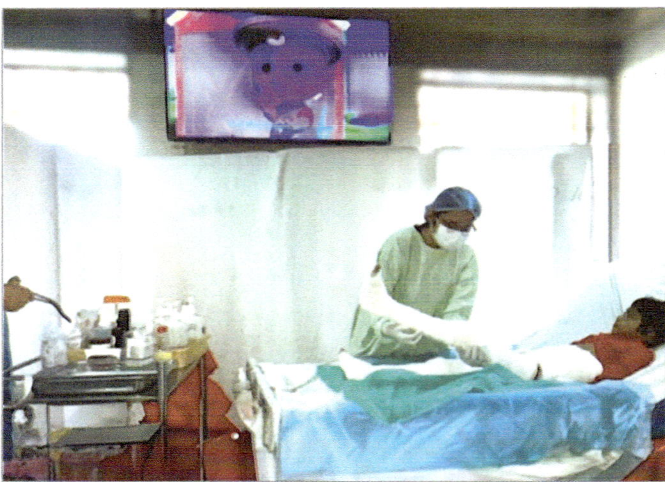

FIG. 18: Playing animation movies while doing daily dressings in the burn ward.

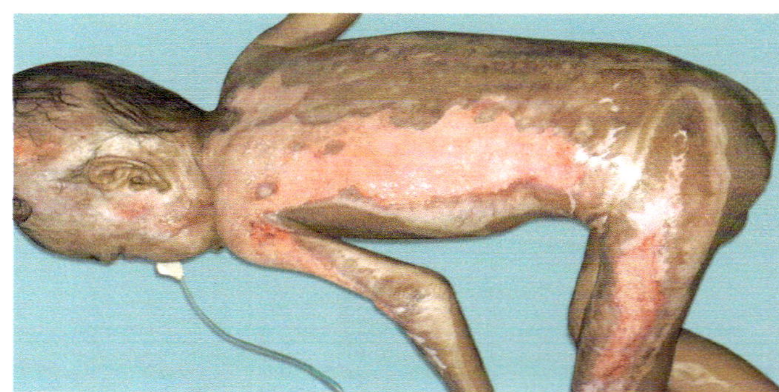

FIG. 19: Infant with 20% postburn raw area with severe anemia. Wounds show unhealthy pale granulation tissue. Requires building up with blood transfusion and nutrition till wounds are prepared for grafting.

- *Blood transfusion*: These are not required in the first 48 hours unless the child is anemic. It may be required later to maintain hematocrit between 35 and 40% and a hemoglobin level of >10 g/dL **(Fig. 19)**.

Systemic Antibiotics

Numerous endogenous and exogenous bacteria may thrive in the big, warm, wet, and protein-rich habitat that burn wounds provide. The weakened immune system of children who have burns makes them more prone to infection. Sepsis is therefore the main reason why burn victims die. Prophylactic systemic antibiotic usage on a regular basis, however, is not advised as it promotes the quick emergence of resistance bacteria.

The burn wound is routinely monitored bacteriologically using surface swab cultures. Infection is identified

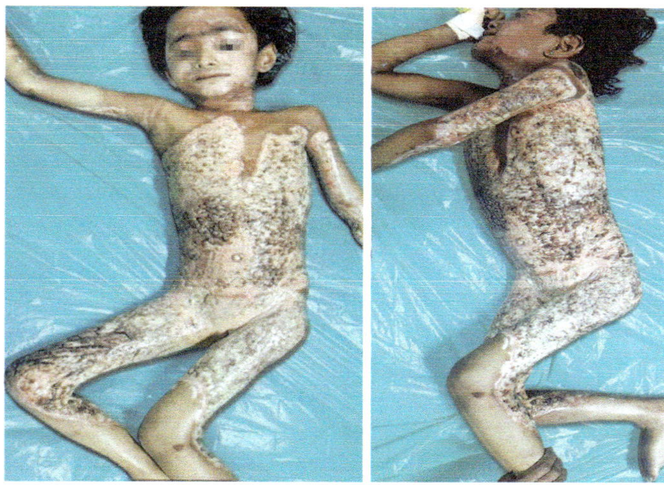

FIG. 20: A 2-year-old child with burn wound sepsis due to *Pseudomonas.*

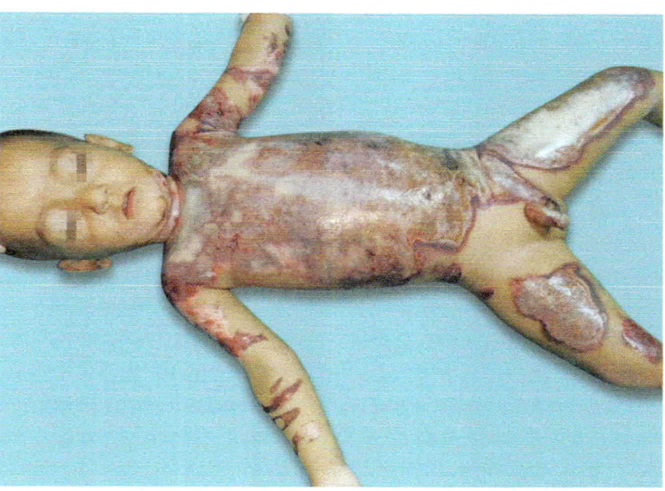

FIG. 21: Child sustaining full-thickness flame burns with typical gram-negative sepsis.

when there is an invasion of adjacent healthy tissue or when there are more than 105 bacteria per gram of tissue in burn wound biopsies. These procedures have been used to quantify the number of bacteria in the wound. Black or purple necrotic patches developing in the wound and bleeding in the sub-eschar fat are local indicators of burn wound sepsis. Bacteria generally isolated from the burn wounds are *Pseudomonas, Klebsiella, Staphylococcus aureus, Streptococcus faecalis, Proteus,* and *E. coli.* A change in the wound's status, the presence of fever or hypothermia, altered sensorium, tachycardia, tachypnea, abdominal distension, diarrhea, and oliguria are clinical indicators of septicemia, even if there is not a specific clinical sign for it. While leukocytosis and fever are signs of infection, hypothermia, and leucopenia can also be signs of sepsis in children who have been burned.

For burn sepsis, systemic antibiotics are the mainstay of treatment **(Figs. 20 and 21)**. The detected bacteria are treated with the appropriate antibiotic if the culture and sensitivity data are available. If not, antibiotics are begun empirically in wide spectrum combinations (such as aminoglycosides and cephalosporins) while waiting for culture data. The first indication of sepsis prompts the administration of antibiotics at maximal therapeutic dosages, which are only discontinued after around 7 days.[52]

Toxic shock syndrome (TSS) is a rare complication of an infected burn and can be life-threatening caused by a bacterial toxin. The most common causative organisms are *Staphylococcus aureus* and *Streptococcus pyogenes* (PS1) (Group A *Streptococcus*). It is mostly seen in young children aged 1–5 years, 2–5 days after a burn injury. Burns are initially sterile. Colonization of burn wounds with bacteria known to produce toxins (*Staphylococcus aureus* and *Streptococcus*) occurs after 1–2 days. Antibody protection against TSST-1 increases with age; of adults in their fourth decade, 90–95% have antibodies compared with 70% in early adulthood, and <30% in those under 5 years of age.[53] At birth passive immunity, lasting for 3–6 months, is conferred by the mother. Antibodies are also present in breast milk, so infants are partially protected showing that the prevalence of protective antibodies is high in newborns, declines until 2 years, and then gradually increased with age, showing low antibody titers against TSST-1 with burns colonized with *Staphylococcus* are at chances of developing TSS.[54]

Signs/symptoms of TSS are:
- Shock (tachycardia, hypotension)
- Fever > 38.9°C
- Erythematous rash
- Diarrhea and vomiting
- Lethargy
- Irritability

Treatment includes active resuscitation with IV fluids, IV antibiotic clindamycin, and provision of passive immunity against TSST-1 with fresh frozen plasma or intravenous polyspecific immunoglobulin G (IVIG) as adjunctive therapy in neutralizing cytokines.

Nutrition

Nutrition plays an integral part in the treatment of a pediatric burn patient. Adequate energy and protein intake are required to meet the increased metabolic demands of the hypermetabolic state of the burn injury as well as normal growth and development. Prompt initiation of nutritional support is crucial and is associated with a reduction in the length of hospitalization. The enteral route is preferred for nutritional support and is generally available. Oral feeding is instituted within 24 hours to meet the predicted caloric requirements. Freshly prepared meals are administered through a nasogastric tube if the youngster is incapable of taking them orally. If the child is having diarrhea, vomiting, or malabsorption, parenteral nutrition or supplements are required. Amino acid solutions and emulsified fats are combined with a 10–20% dextrose solution for parenteral feeding. The daily caloric requirements in children can be estimated by the following formulae:

- *Curreri's formula:*[55] 60 kcal/kg body weight + 35 kcal/% burn
- *Carjaval's formula:*[56] 2200 kcal/m^2 of burned area + 1,800 kcal/m^2 BSA

Along with calories, an adequate amount of protein is given which is important to improve resistance and survival. One of the formulae suggested for estimating protein requirements in a burned patient is 3 g/kg + 1 g for every 1% of BSA burned. No >4 g/kg protein should be provided. Fats are a concentrated source of energy, but excessive intake of fat has been associated with many complications. 5–15% of nonprotein calories should be provided as fats and the rest as carbohydrates. Whether taken orally or administered intravenously, dietary supplements containing vitamins and trace minerals, such as zinc, copper, chromium, and molybdenum are crucial for wound healing.

Butter milk diet (BMD) is provided to all burn patients consisting of 1 liter curd which acts as probiotic, 4 bananas that have binding properties, fiber and caloric value, four eggs which are a source of protein, and 50 g of sugar for taste and calories, all together having a total calorie count of 1,760 kcal with a total volume of 1,760 mL, protein 60 g and carbohydrates of 340 g. Fats constitute the most significant nutritional source of energy for which we add medium-chain triglycerides oil as a supplement in infants and children below 5 years.

Management of the Burn Wound

Burn wounds in children are best treated by dressings as the child will be able to move around and play more easily after he is out of the resuscitation phase. Perineal burns are a difficult area to treat in children. For this paraffin gauze dressing with topical antimicrobial cream can be applied directly on the nappy and the nappy can be changed as frequently as required.

DRESSING PROTOCOL

Microorganisms proliferate rapidly in burn wounds, especially in those severe enough to impair immune function. Topical antimicrobials have an important role to play. They delay the interval between injury and colonization and maintain low levels of the wound flora. Three agents have proven efficacy for major burns viz., 1% silver sulfadiazine cream, 0.5% silver nitrate solution, and 11.1% mafenide acetate cream. Traditional dressings, such as chlorhexidine gauze and silver sulfadiazine **(Fig. 22)**, can cause leukopenia and also do not effectively penetrate the eschar.[57] Whereas modern wound dressings which are comprising of hydrocolloids, hydrofiber, alginates, silver nanocrystalline, and polyurethane, fulfill many of the essential criteria of an ideal dressing **(Fig. 23)**. Use of silver-impregnated modern dressings

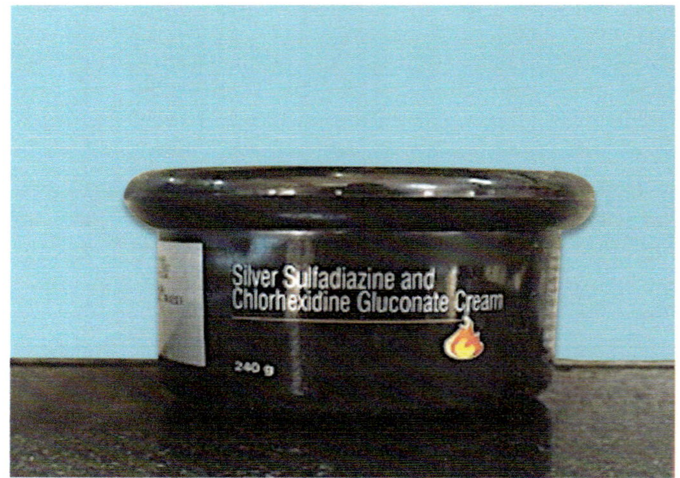

FIG. 22: Silver sulfadiazine with chlorhexidine cream.

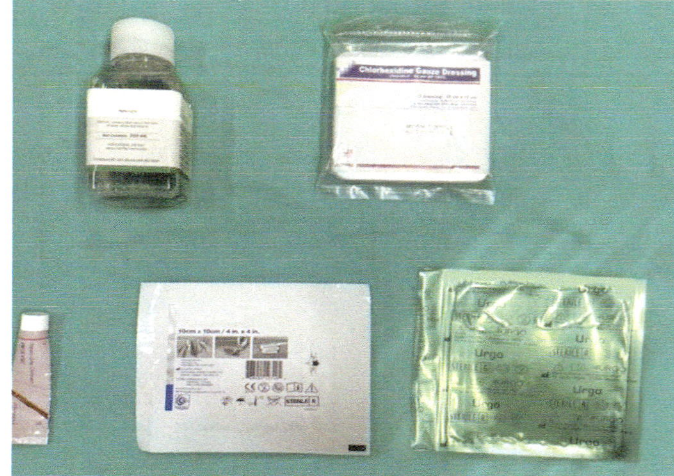

FIG. 23: Modern silver-based wound dressings.

has now become more widespread in both general hospitals and specialized burn centers.

Superficial burns are treated with regular dressings and local wound care until epithelialization occurs. They can also be treated by covering the denuded wound with allograft, xenograft, or synthetic materials available commercially.

Collagen dressings have been found to be very helpful in superficial burns as they decrease pain and evaporative losses, seal the wound from the environment, make the child more comfortable, and encourage early healing **(Figs. 24 and 25)**.

In the case of full-thickness burns planning of the excision of extensive surface burns is the one of most challenging aspects of burn care. When, how, and in how many stages excision must be performed all have to be determined. The decision depends on several factors, including patient hemodynamic stability, the existence of concomitant injuries, pulmonary considerations, and availability of resources.[58] Children with deep dermal burns particularly benefit from early excision **(Figs. 26A and B)** and grafting as it reduces morbidity, allows early recovery, reduces length of hospital stay and number of dressings, facilitates early mobilization,

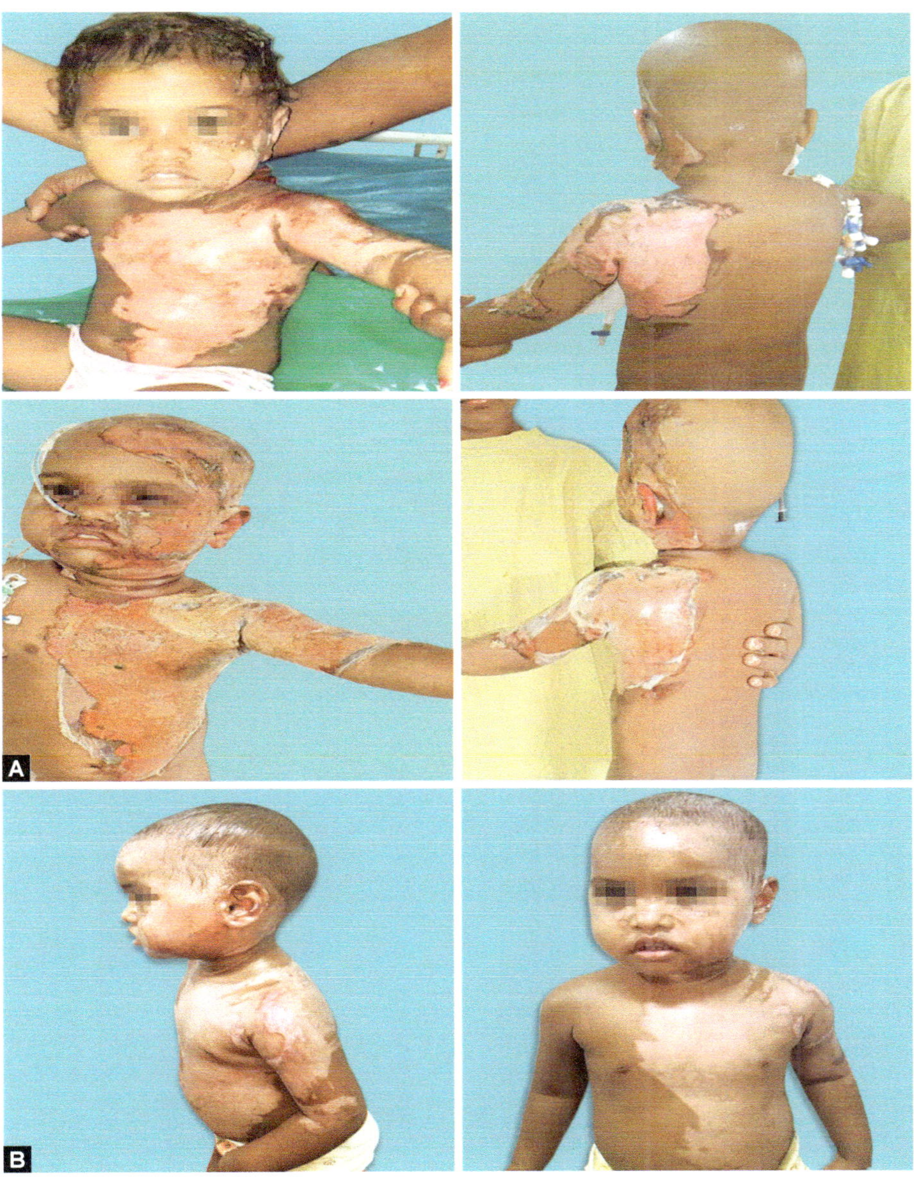

FIGS. 24A AND B: (A) Child with extensive superficial to deep dermal burns due to spillage of hot ghee dressed with wet collagen dressing; (B) Same patient with healed areas in 14 days.

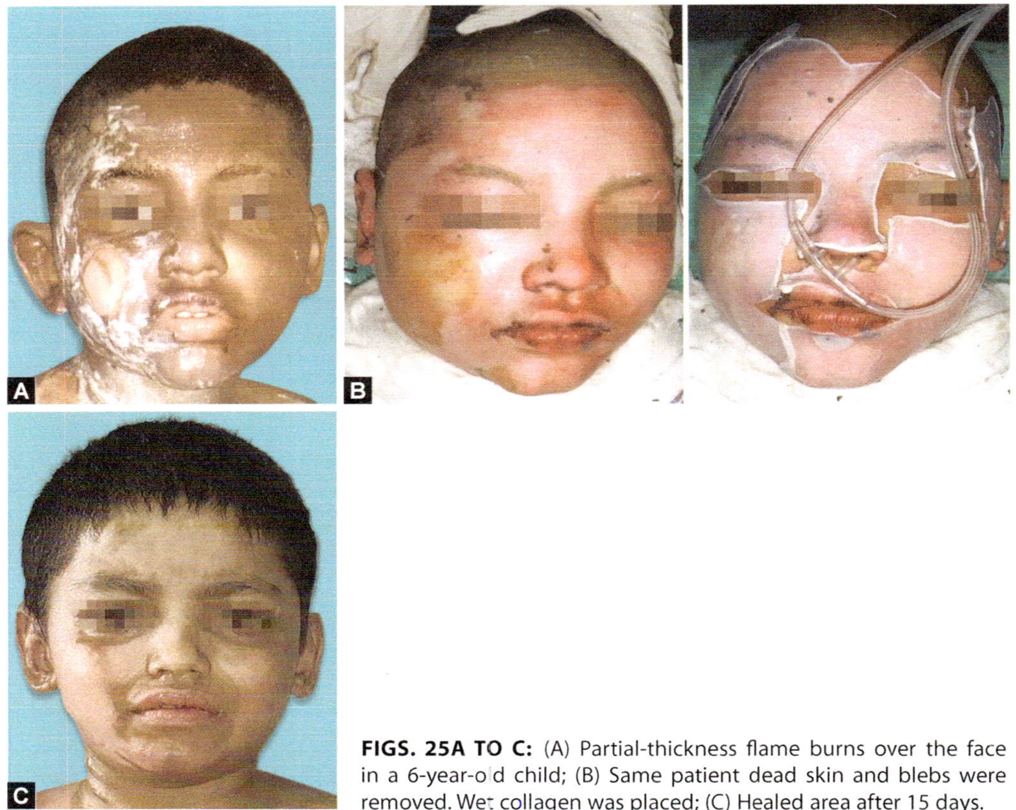

FIGS. 25A TO C: (A) Partial-thickness flame burns over the face in a 6-year-old child; (B) Same patient dead skin and blebs were removed. Wet collagen was placed; (C) Healed area after 15 days.

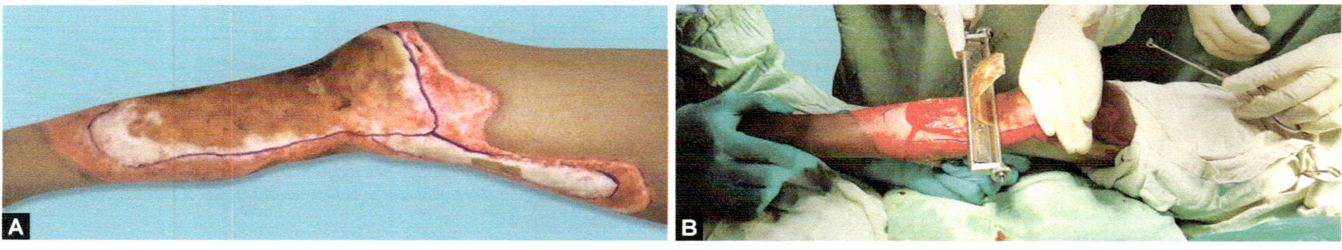

FIGS. 26A AND B: (A) Mapping the area to be excised in the case of full-thickness flame burn; (B) Early tangential excision of the eschar.

and thus lessens the psychological trauma at such a young age.

The goal is to remove all devitalized tissue and prepare the wound for skin grafting early enough up to 72 hours postburn. The prerequisites for early excision are mentioned in **Box 1**.

To reduce blood loss, tourniquet control, 1 in 2 lakh epinephrine-soaked sponges, and infiltration of tumescent fluid (1:5 lakh epinephrine in 1000 cc saline) are used; the area left behind should bleed uniformly and no thrombosed vessels should be visible after excision. Another important fact to be kept in mind during excision in the pediatric age group is that the dermis is very thin. A true tangential excision leaving behind viable dermis can be difficult at times and may turn out that excision has gone till subcutaneous fat leading to marked cosmetic deformities later on.[59]

BOX 1 Prerequisites for early excision.

- Hemodynamically stable
- Operative time < 2 hours
- 2 units of PRC in hand
- < 20 % of TBSA excised in one sitting
- Adequate donor site/allograft availability
- Spaced apart (every 2 or 3 days)
- Good intensive care backup

(PRC: packed red cell; TBSA: total body surface area)

Hydrotherapy with water-jet debridement device has demonstrated several benefits, including improved precision and control of debridement of a full-thickness burn as well as decreased blood loss **(Fig. 27)**. It is a valuable tool to maximize preservation of the dermis prior to skin grafting in the pediatric burn population.[60]

An overview of the wound management of pediatric burn patients is shown in **(Flowchart 1)**.

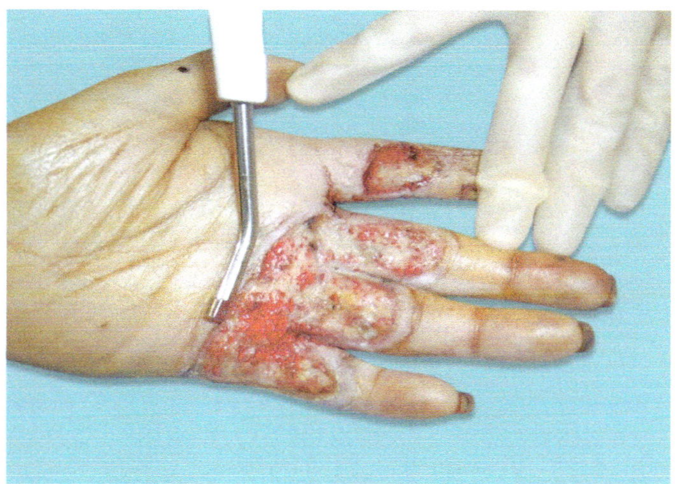

FIG. 27: The hydrosurgery device being used to debride the fingers in a case of bike silencer burn.

In the case of extensive deep burns in which the patient cannot be taken up for early excision and grafting, the patient is treated by conservative management in the form of regular dressings till the eschar separates and the wound starts granulating **(Figs. 28A and B)**. In case there is deficiency of donor areas because of extensive wounds or in chronic neglected cases where the patient is cachexic and not a favorable candidate for autografting, the raw areas can be covered with homograft till such time that the area can be covered by autograft in stages. The best way is to apply alternate sheets of autograft and homograft. In such cases, it is found that as the autograft starts spreading by epithelialization from the margins, the homograft starts separating automatically. But more commonly, it becomes necessary to excise the homograft like amniotic membrane before 2 weeks and replace them with autografts **(Figs. 29 and 30)**. This intervening 2–3-week period allows exceptionally good anabolic recovery of the child, improving not only the condition of the wounds but also the general condition of the patient.

Because of the paucity of epidermal appendages, the healing by epithelialization in the case of deep dermal burns is much less in young children compared to the older children and adults, and usually they heal by

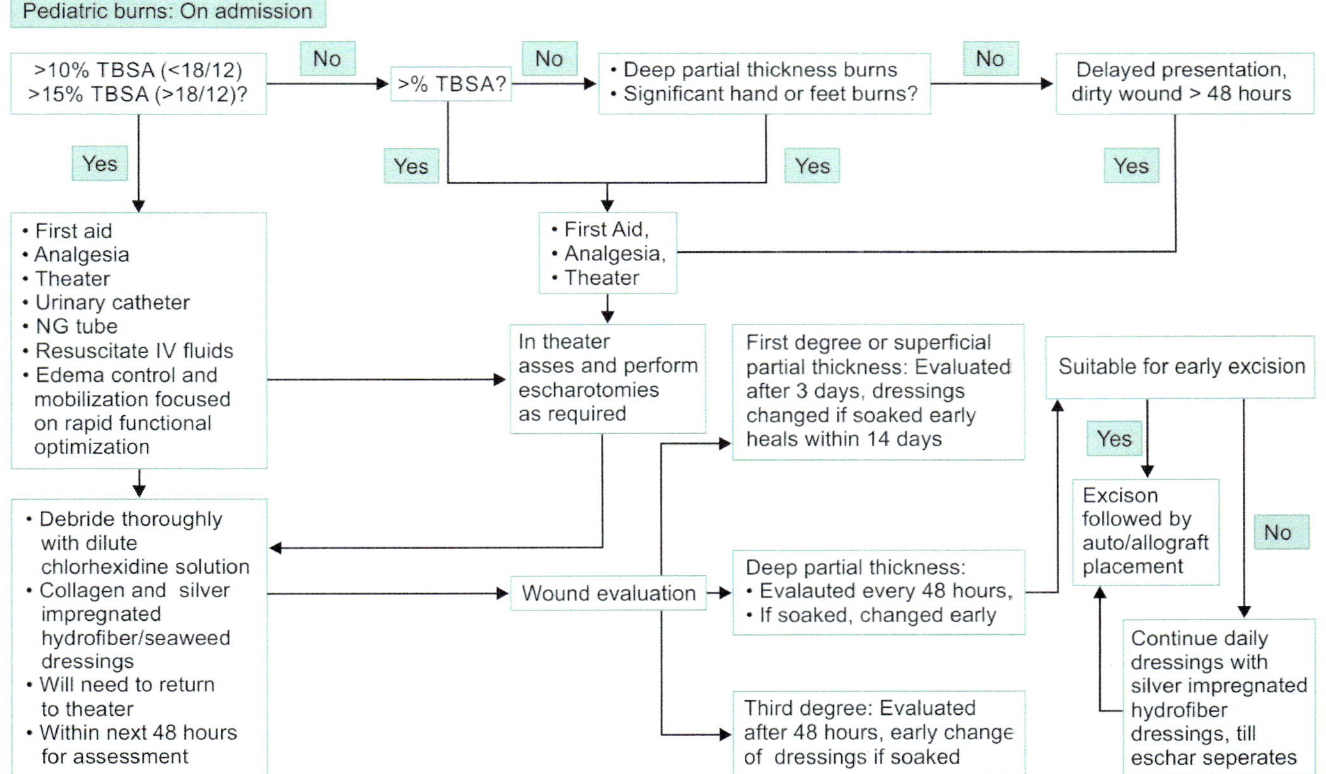

FLOWCHART 1: Step by step management of pediatric burn wound management.

(IV: intravenous; NG tube: nasogastric tube; TBSA: total body surface area)

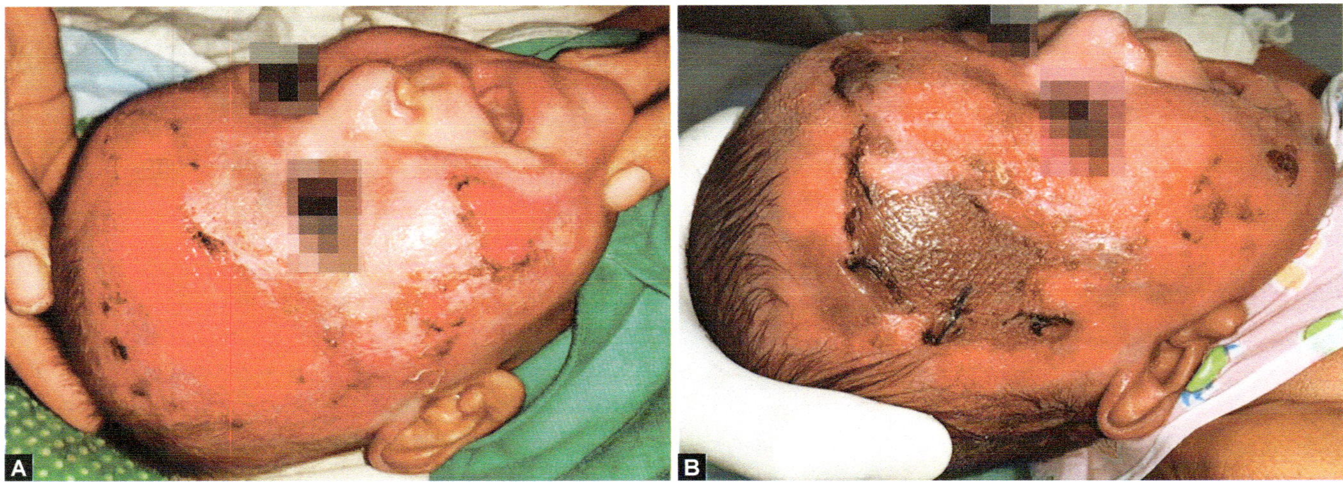

FIGS. 28A AND B: (A) Deep partial-thickness flame burns on the face where eschars were subjected to chemical debridement which separated slowly, with well-granulated wound underneath, split-thickness skin graft applied; (B) Well-settled graft with a completely healed wound over the face.

migration of epithelium from the edges and contracture formation. In children <1 year of age, the usual tendency is to keep the limbs in an attitude of flexion so that at times the wounds heal by the formation of flexion contractures. All these contractures should be prevented; hence, early closure of wounds is of prime importance usually within 21 days.

COMPLICATIONS

The most common complications of burns are wound infection and respiratory complications, which are leading causes of death in burned children. Gastrointestinal complications are also common and include gastric ulceration (stress ulcer–Curling's ulcer), pancreatitis, enterocolitis, and superior mesenteric artery syndrome. Adequate fluid resuscitation is the most effective means of prevention. Large surface area burns may cause hemolysis and electrical burns may cause muscle necrosis which lead to hemoglobinuria and myoglobinuria respectively. Most often ignored are psychological sequelae because of disfigurement and loss of function.

SUPPORTIVE MANAGEMENT

Thus, burn injury management should not focus only on the immediate treatment. Long-term outcomes and the required rehabilitation that burn victims must go through should be given equal if not more attention.[36]

Physiotherapy

A severe burn, in addition to disfiguring scarring and debilitating contractures, results in a hypermetabolic and catabolic state characterized by increases in resting energy expenditure (REE), tachycardia, insulin resistance, negative muscle protein balance, decrease in bone mass, and growth delay.[35] Aims of chest physiotherapy in the acute stage in pediatric burns patients are as follows:

- To maintain good air entry bilaterally in the lungs
- To prevent secretions in large and small airways
- To facilitate airway clearance by removing secretions if the patient has developed airway obstruction because of secretions.

The techniques given to achieve the above goals include the following: **(Fig. 31)**

- Deep breathing exercises with emphasis on segmental breathing with coughing
- Spirometry or flutter every 6 hourly
- Expiratory breathing exercises with pursed lip breathing
- Thoracic mobility exercises
- Postural drainage techniques with humidification/nebulization

Psychological Support

Children and young people who experience a burn face many hardships, which should be acknowledged by clinical care teams in the journey toward recovery. Factors that improve the mental health and well-being of children and young people who sustain a burn injury should be promoted, such as mental health and social support, the promotion of adaptive coping mechanisms, and meeting the needs of the family as a whole. Ultimately, the implementation of trauma-focused, family-centered interventions is crucial for the

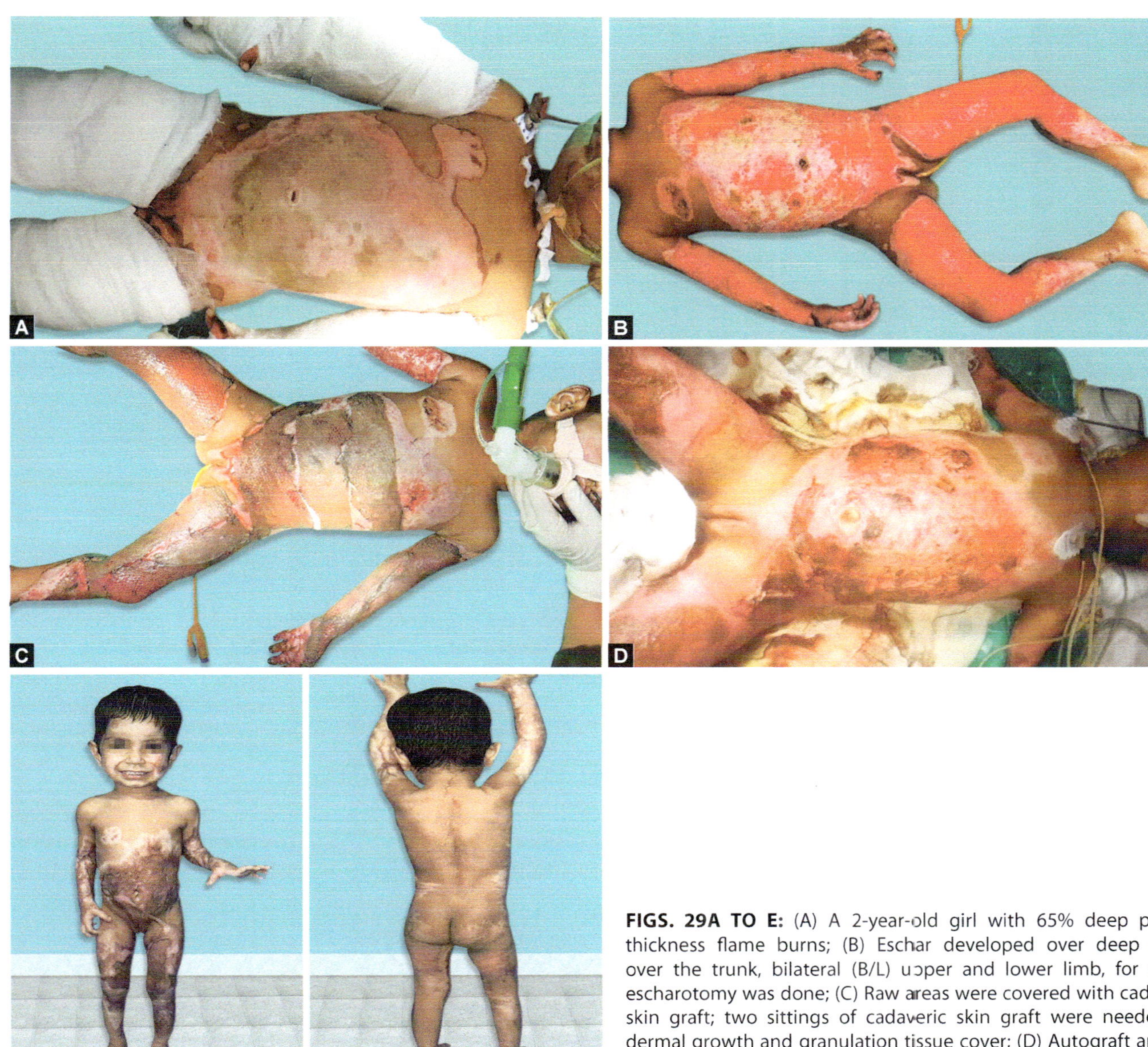

FIGS. 29A TO E: (A) A 2-year-old girl with 65% deep partial-thickness flame burns; (B) Eschar developed over deep burns over the trunk, bilateral (B/L) upper and lower limb, for which escharotomy was done; (C) Raw areas were covered with cadaveric skin graft; two sittings of cadaveric skin graft were needed for dermal growth and granulation tissue cover; (D) Autograft applied after removing homograft; (E) Same child with completely healed areas after one and a half months

psychosocial recovery of pediatric burn survivors. We at our unit encourage purposeful playing activity for mobilization rather than conventional physiotherapy and occupational therapy in order to improve the mental health and compliance of a burn survivor **(Figs. 32 and 33)**.

PROGNOSIS

Many factors affect the prognosis in a burned child. Mortality in pediatric burns is affected by three main risk factors: Inhalational injury, burn size of >30%, and age of <4 years.[47] The presence of inhalational injury doubles the mortality rate. Management of extensive burns is extremely expensive and often prolonged. The poor socioeconomic status is certainly a contributing factor in increasing morbidity and mortality.

PREVENTION

If adults take extra precautions and do not leave the children alone, burns in children may be prevented. From a very young age (possibly as early as two years old), we should teach kids to be cautious about hot liquids, fire, and electricity. Since immersion scalds are very common while giving a bath to the child, especially in winter, it is important for parents to ensure not to leave the hot water bucket unattended and mix hot water into cold water while preparing for a child's bath and not vice versa. Firecrackers should be burst only under the supervision of adults. Electrical outlets must be placed higher up and out of small children's reach. Strong alkalis and acids should be kept out of children's reach in homes. General public can benefit from increased awareness campaigns carried out by schools, television, and other media. In India, strict enforcement of laws to prevent burns in childhood are not there resulting in a very high incidence of burns. In developed countries like the UK, there are a number of Acts, such as "The Children and Young Persons Act,1914," "Heating Appliances Act, 1971," and Night Dresses for Children's Act, 1962, to safeguard against burns in children.

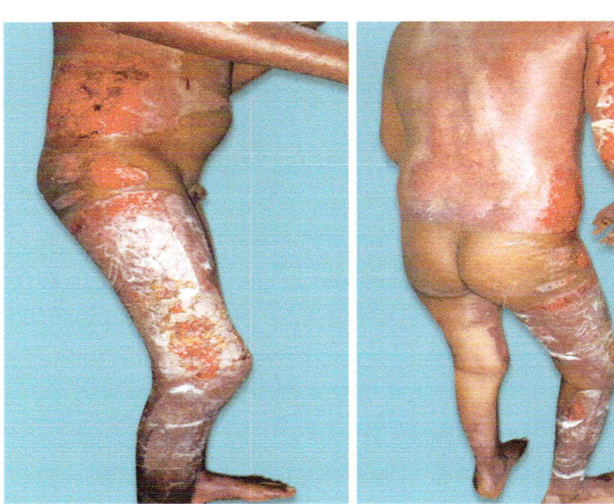

FIG. 30: Amniotic membrane dressings applied in flame burn patients when wounds started granulating, preventing evaporative water loss and formation of dermal bed.

RECENT ADVANCES

Progressive improvement in the understanding of the pathophysiology of burn injury, advancements in critical care, and rapid development of biotechnology assure high expectations regarding future advancements in burn care.

Hypercatabolic Response in Pediatric Burn Patients

Various pharmacological strategies to suppress or reduce hypermetabolism—which is frequent in burned patients—have been demonstrated to be effective.

- *Insulin*: Apart from its primary function of preventing hyperglycemia, insulin has been found to have other positive effects. It can decrease the concentration of proinflammatory cytokines, increase levels of anti-inflammatory cytokines, and reduce acute phase proteins.[61] Furthermore, administering insulin to children has been shown to result in a decreased need for albumin to maintain the required levels.[62] Treatment of burn victims with insulin may act directly to achieve anti-inflammatory and anti-catabolic effects, not simply through the lowering of the serum glucose,[63] although strict glucose control is critical with an objective to maintain mean glucose levels <110–140 mg/dL.
- *Propranolol*: Burn treatment can be effectively managed with this anticatabolic therapy, which effectively counteracts the excessive presence of circulating catecholamines. This treatment is specifically recommended for patients with a TBSA >20%.[64]
- *Oxandrolone*: This is a testosterone analog used in combination with propranolol in burn patients

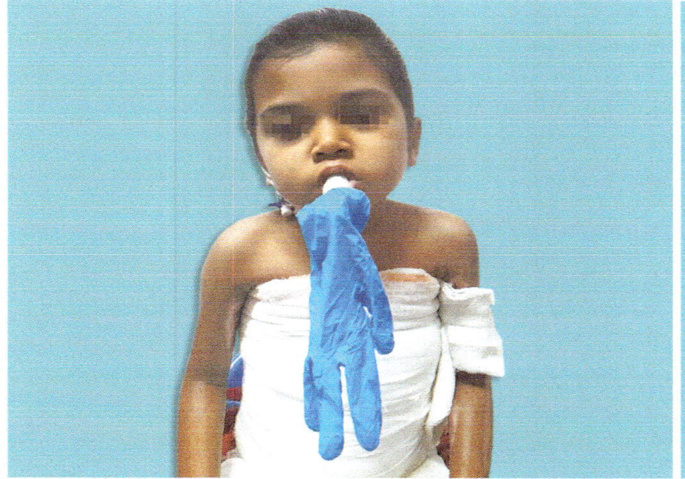

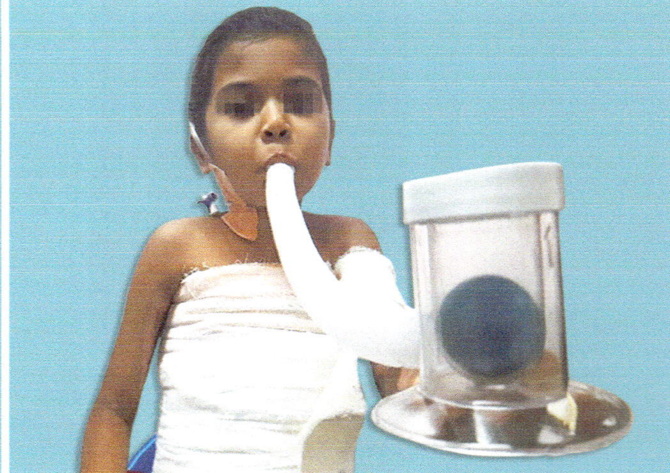

FIG. 31: Balloon bladder and incentive spirometry exercises performed by 6-year-old child, 35% flame burns.

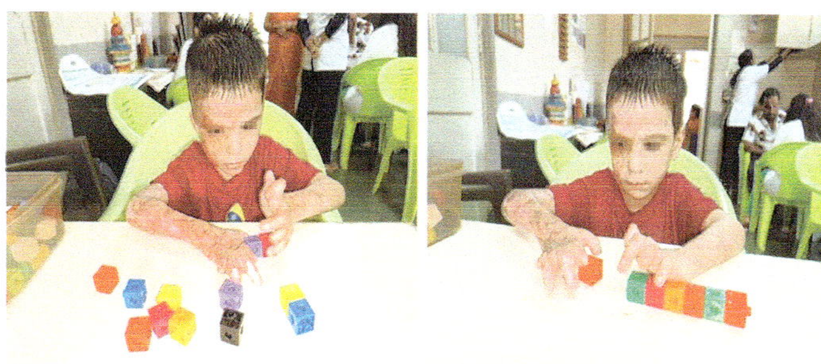
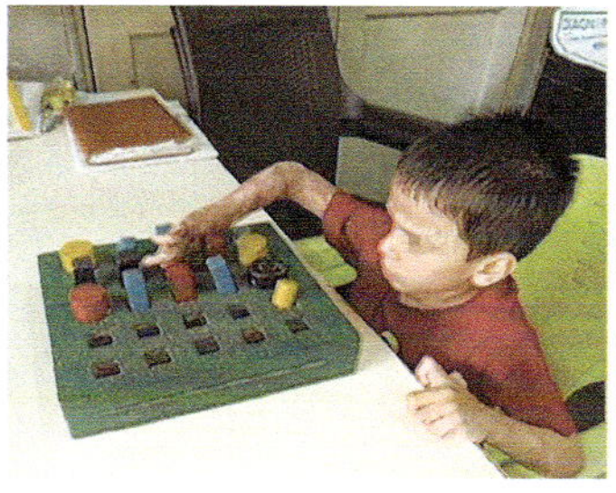
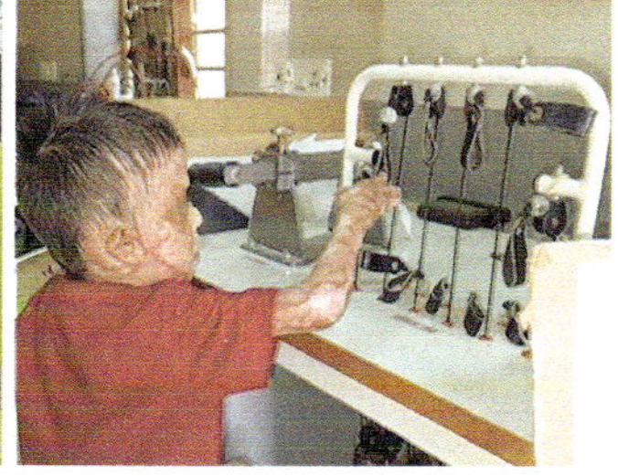

FIG. 32: A 4-year-old child, 40% accidental flame burn in a purposeful playing activity providing occupational therapy.

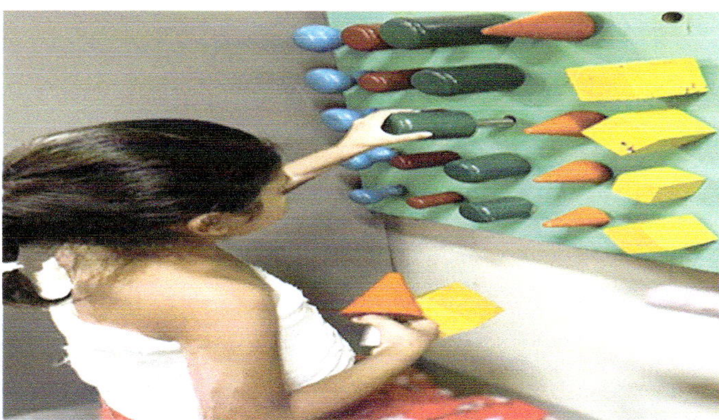

FIG. 33: Specially designed splints and activity box to help mobilization exercises in a playful manner.

with a TBSA >30% and has been demonstrated to be beneficial with accelerated muscle recovery, reduce hypertrophic scarring, and was associated with improved physical abilities and emotional well-being.[65]

- Other anabolic agents still under development include metformin, IGF-1 combined with IGFBP-3, GLP-1, and PPAR-γ agonists.

Biomarkers

Biomarkers have the potential to reveal insights into normal biological processes and have been extensively studied in the context of burns. Researchers have identified markers that are associated with clinical outcomes like sepsis, scarring, and long-term co-morbidities. In the case of pediatric burns, specific biomarkers are being investigated to achieve these outcomes such as the following:

- *Procalcitonin (PCT)*: Several studies have established PCT as a highly characterized biomarker that plays a vital role in predicting sepsis. It can also be utilized as a diagnostic and prognostic marker in pediatric burn patients, assisting in the detection of infections in patients with significant underlying inflammation.[66]
- *Cytokine TNF-α and interleukin 6 (IL-6)*: The levels of cytokines TNF-α and IL-6 can be utilized to forecast the outcome of patients with sepsis. In response to a burn stimulus, the body exhibits an elevated production of TNF-α and IL-6, which can be detected soon after the burn. As complications from burn-related infections arise, the levels of these cytokines continue to rise in the blood and can serve as a reliable prognostic factor for mortality and are closely linked to the clinical outcome.[67]
- *Basic fibroblast growth factor (bFGF)*: This particular element is intricately involved in the repair and regeneration of tissue. A recent study investigated the effects of applying bFGF topically on scar formation in children, and the findings revealed improved healing outcomes. Further research is currently being conducted to gain a deeper understanding of the specific role that bFGF plays in the healing process of burn wounds in pediatric cases.[68]
- *Growth hormone (GH)*: The stimulation of insulin-like growth factor (IGF) is the primary function of GH, which is involved in growth and metabolism. However, GH levels are reduced in burn patients. To accelerate healing and reduce hospital stays in children with burns covering >40% of their TBSA, recombinant human growth hormone (RHGH) is administered exogenously. Although its use during the acute phase is controversial, long-term administration during the chronic phase (within the first 12 months postburn) has been associated with fewer complications and sustained effectiveness.[69]

SUMMARY

Burns in children leave lifelong scars which cause enormous stress for both the child and his parents as they affect their development not only physically but mentally as well. Burn management in the pediatric age group can be a great challenge because physiologically, the skin and organ systems are immature and cannot tolerate stress like an adult, and therefore, they respond differently to thermal injury. Emotionally, children are again immature and incapable of handling pain and disfigurement associated with burn. The burn wound management and the surgical approach to pediatric patients, therefore, varies according to the depth and extent of burns. Both the child's family and the treating doctor have an important role to play in the eventual outcome of the child who comes out successfully from the physical trauma of burns. The public must be made aware of how to prevent burn injuries in children and what measures should be taken in case an unfortunate event takes place. Media, especially television, has a great role to play where the invited burn specialists teach the public about it.

REFERENCES

1. Reed JL, Pomerantz WJ. Emergency management of pediatric burns. Pediatr Emerg Care. 2005;21:118-29.
2. Ahuja RB, Bhattacharya S. An analysis of 11,196 burn admissions and evaluation of conservative management technique. Burns. 2002;28:555-61.
3. Schneider DF, Dobrowolsky A, Shakir IA, Sinacore JM, Mosier MJ, Gamelli RL. Predicting acute kidney injury among burn patients in the 21st century: A classification and regression tree analysis. J Burn Care Res. 2012;33:242-51.
4. Osta WA, El-Osta MA, Pezhman EA, Raad RA, Ferguson K, McKelvey GM, et al. Nicotinic acetylcholine receptor gene expression is altered in burn patients. Anesth Analg. 2010;110: 1355-9.
5. Ali SN, O'Toole G, Tyler M. Milk bottle burns. J Burn Care Rehabil. 2004;25:461-2.
6. Hampson NB, Dunn SL. UHMCS/CDC CO Poisoning Surveillance Group. Symptoms of carbon monoxide poisoning do not correlate with the initial carboxyhemoglobin level. Undersea Hyperb Med. 2012;39(2):657-65.
7. Streit S, Hebra A. Abdominal compartment syndrome in a three-year-old child following a severe burn injury. J Ped Surg Case Rep. 2013;1(7):177-9.
8. Garcia-Souto M, Dabnichki P. Core and local skin temperature: 3–24 months old toddlers and comparison to adults. Build Environ. 2016;104:286-95.
9. Anderson GS, Mekjavic IB. Thermoregulatory responses of circum pubertal children. Eur J Appl Physiol Occup Physiol. 1996;74(5):404-10.
10. Schottke D, Chiefs IaOF. Fundamentals of Fire Fighter Skills. Sadbury, MA, USA: Jones & Bartlett Publishers; 2014.
11. Sharma RK, Parashar A. Special considerations in paediatric burn patients. Indian J Plast Surg. 2010;43(Suppl):S43-50.
12. Wong L, Spence RJ. Escharotomy and fasciotomy of the burned upper extremity. Hand Clin. 2000;16(2):165-74, vii.
13. Advanced Trauma Life Support for Doctors (ATLS). Chicago: American College of Surgeons (ACS); 1997.
14. American Burn Association. Advanced Burn Life Support, Chicago, IL: American Burn Association; 2007.
15. Harless J, Ramaiah R, Bhananker SM. Pediatric airway management. Int J Crit Illn Inj Sci. 2014;4(1):65-70.
16. Moylan JA, Chan CK. Inhalation injury--an increasing problem. Ann Surg. 1978;188(1):34-7.
17. Kimura R, Traber LD, Herndon DN, Linares HA, Lubbesmeyer HJ, Traber DL. Increasing duration of smoke exposure induces more severe lung injury in sheep. J Appl Physiol (1985). 1988; 64(3):1107-13.
18. Moritz AR, Henriques FC, McLean R. The effects of inhaled heat on the air passages and lungs: An experimental investigation. Am J Pathol. 1945;21(2):311-31.
19. Nakae H, Tanaka H, Inaba H. Failure to clear casts and secretions following inhalation injury can be dangerous: Report of a case. Burns. 2001;27(2):189-91.
20. Dries DJ, Endorf FW. Inhalation injury: Epidemiology, pathology, treatment strategies. Scand J Trauma Resusc Emerg Med. 2013;21:31.
21. Matthay MA, Ware LB, Zimmerman GA. The acute respiratory distress syndrome. J Clin Invest. 2012;122(8):2731-40.
22. Prockop LD, Chichkova RI. Carbon monoxide intoxication: An updated review. J Neurol Sci. 2007;262:122-30.
23. Branson RD, Gentile MA. Is humidification always necessary during noninvasive ventilation in the hospital? Respiratory Care. 2010;55(2):209-16.
24. Cox CS Jr, Zwischenberger JB, Traber DL, Traber LD, Haque AK, Herndon DN. Heparin improves oxygenation and minimizes barotrauma after severe smoke inhalation in an ovine model. Surg Gynecol Obstet. 1993;176(4):339-49.
25. McIntire A, Harris SA, Whitten JA, Fritschle-Hilliard AC, Foster DR, Sood R, et al. Outcomes following the use of nebulized heparin for inhalation injury (HIHI Study). J Burn Care and Res.: Official Publication of the American Burn Association. 2016;38(1):1.
26. Koga T, Kawazu T, Iwashita K, Yahata R. Pulmonary hyperinflation and respiratory distress following solvent aspiration in a patient with asthma: Expectoration of bronchial casts and clinical improvement with high-frequency chest wall oscillation. Respir Care. 2004;49(11):1335-8.
27. Michalopoulos A, Kasiakou SK, Mastora Z, Rellos K, Kapaskelis AM, Falagas ME. Aerosolized colistin for the treatment of nosocomial pneumonia due to multidrug-resistant Gram-negative bacteria in patients without cystic fibrosis. Crit Care. 2005;9(1):R53-9.
28. Chung KK, Rhie RY, Lundy JB, Cartotto R, Henderson E, Pressman MA, et al. A survey of mechanical ventilator practices across burn centers in North America. J Burn Care Res. 2016; 37:e131.
29. Lucangelo U, Fontanesi L, Antonaglia V, Pellis T, Berlot G, Liguori G, et al. High frequency percussive ventilation (HFPV). Principles and Technique. Minerva Anestesiol. 2003;69:841-51.
30. Cortiella J, Mlcak R, Herndon D. High frequency percussive ventilation in pediatric patients with inhalation injury. J Burn Care Rehabil. 1999;20:232-5.
31. Hardman JG, Limbird LE, Gilman AG (Eds). Goodman & Gilman's The Pharmacological Basis of Therapeutics, 10th edition. New York: McGraw-Hill; 2001.
32. Saikia D, Mahanta B. Cardiovascular and respiratory physiology in children. Indian J Anaesth. 2019;63(9):690-7.
33. Batool S, Garg R. Appropriate use of oxygen delivery devices. Open Anesthesiol J. 2017;11(1):35-8.

34. Lund CC, Browder NC. The estimation of area of burns. Surg Gynecol Obstet. 1944;79:352-8.
35. Conway H. Management of burns in children. Am J Surg. 1964;107(3):537-43.
36. Knaysi GA, Crikelair GF, Cosman B. The rule of Nines: Its history and accuracy. Plast Reconstr Surg. 1968;41:560-63.
37. Lynch JB, Blocker V. The rule of five in estimation of extent of burn. In: Converse JM (Ed). Reconstructive Plastic Surgery, 1st edition. Philadelphia: WB Saunders Co. 1964; New York, p. 208.
38. Baartmans MGA, van Baar ME, Boxma H, Dokter J, Tibboel D, Nieuwenhuis MK. Accuracy of burn size assessment prior to arrival in Dutch burn centres and its consequences in children: A nationwide evaluation. Injury. 2012;43(9):1451-6.
39. Swords DS, Hadley ED, Swett KR, Pranikoff T. Total body surface area overestimation at referring institutions in children transferred to a burn center. Am Surg. 2015;81:56.
40. Saffle JR, Edelman L, Theurer L, Morris SE, Cochran A. Telemedicine evaluation of acute burns is accurate and cost-effective. J Trauma. 2009;67(2):358-65.
41. Pruitt BA, Jr. Advances in fluid therapy and the early care of the burn patient. World J Surg. 1978;2:139-50.
42. Baxter CR. Problems and complications of burn shock resuscitation. Surg Clin North Am. 1978;58:1313-22.
43. Merrell SW, Saffle JR, Sullivan JJ, Navar PD, Kravitz M, Warden GD, et al. Fluid resuscitation in thermally injured children. Am J Surg. 1986;152:664-9.
44. Suman A, Owen J. Update on the management of burns in paediatrics. BJA Educ. 2020;20(3):103-10.
45. Bissoni RS, Holtgrave DR, Lawler F, Marley DS. Colloids versus crystalloids in fluid resuscitation: An analysis of randomized controlled trials. J Family Pract. 1991;32(4):387-90.
46. Gore DC, Dalton JM, Gehr TW. Colloid infusion reduces glomerular filtration in resuscitated burn victims. J Trauma: Injury Infect Crit Care. 1996;40(3):356-60.
47. Cocks AJ, O'Connell A, Martin H. Crystalloids, Colloids and kids: A review of pediatric burns in intensive care. Burns. 1998; 24:717-24.
48. Sheridan RL, Schnitzer JJ. Management of the high-risk pediatric burn patient. J Pediatric Surg. 2001;36(8):1308-12.
49. Nguyen TT, Gilpin DA, Meyer NA, Herndon DN. Current treatment of burned patients. Ann Surg. 1996;223(1):14-25.
50. Carvajal HF. A physiologic approach to fluid therapy in severely burned children. Surg Gynaecol Obstet. 1980;150:379-84.
51. Rogers AD, Karpelowsky J, Millar AJ, Argent A, Rode H. Fluid creep in major pediatric burns. Eur J Pediatr Surg. 2010;20: 133-8.
52. Brown AP, Khan K, Sinclair S. Bacterial toxicosis toxic shock syndrome as a contributor to mortality in children with burn injuries. Burns. 2003;29:733-38.
53. Davis TC, Griffin NK. The consequences of toxic shock syndrome in an 18-month-old boy with 20% scalds. J R Soc Med. 1996;89:115-6.
54. Vergeront JM, Stolz SJ, Crass BA, Nelson DB, Davis JP, Bergdoll MS. Prevalence of serum antibody to staphylococcal enterotoxin F among Wisconsin residents: Implications for toxic shock syndrome. J Infect Dis. 1983;148:692-8.
55. Curreri PW, Luterman A. Nutritional support of the burned patient. Surg Clin North Am. 1978;58:1151-6.
56. Hildreth M, Carjaval HF. Caloric requirements in burned children: A simple formula to estimate daily caloric requirements. J Burn Care Rehabil. 1982;3:78-80.
57. Manafo WW, Freedman B. Topical therapy for burns. Surg Clin North Am. 1987;67:133-45.
58. Tenenhaus M, Rennekampff HO. Burn surgery. Clin Plast Surg. 2007;34(4):697-715.
59. Cartotto R, Musgrave MA, Beveridge M, Fish J, Gomez M. Minimizing blood loss in burn surgery. J Trauma. 2000;49(6): 1034-9.
60. Kimble RM, Mott J, Joethy J. Versajet hydrosurgery system for the debridement of pediatric burns. Burns. 2008;34(2): 297-8.
61. Jeschke MG, Klein D, Herndon DN. Insulin treatment improves the systemic inflammatory reaction to severe trauma. Ann Surg. 2004;239(4):553-60.
62. Klein D, Schubert T, Horch RE, Jauch KW, Jeschke MG. Insulin treatment improves hepatic morphology and function through modulation of hepatic signals after severe trauma. Ann Surg. 2004;240(2):340-9.
63. Jeschke MG, Klein D, Thasler WE, Bolder U, Schlitt HJ, Jauch KW, Weiss TS. Insulin decreases inflammatory signal transcription factor expression in primary human liver cells after LPS challenge. Mol Med. 2008;14(1-2):11-9.
64. Jeschke MG, Finnerty CC, Kulp GA, Przkora R, Mlcak RP, Herndon DN. Combination of recombinant human growth hormone and propranolol decreases hypermetabolism and inflammation in children. Pediatr Crit Care Med. 2008;9:209-16.
65. Chao T, Porter C, Herndon DN, Siopi A, Ideker H, Mlcak RP, et al. Propranolol and oxandrolone therapy accelerated muscle recovery in burned children. Med Sci Sports Exerc. 2018;50(3): 427-35.
66. Koutroulis I, Loscalzo SM, Kratimenos P, Singh S, Weiner E, Syriopoulou V, et al. Clinical applications of procalcitonin in paediatrics: An advanced biomarker for inflammation and infection—can it also be used in trauma? Int Sch Res Notices. 2014;2014:286493.
67. Abdel-Hafez NM, Saleh Hassan Y, El-Metwally TH. A study on biomarkers, cytokines, and growth factors in children with burn injuries. Ann Burns Fire Disasters. 2007;20(2):89-100.
68. Akita S, Akino K, Imaizumi T, Tanaka K, Anraku K, Yano H, et al. The quality of paediatric burn scars is improved by early administration of basic fibroblast growth factor. J Burn Care Res. 2006;27:333-8.
69. Frohman LA. Growth hormone. In: Squire LR (Ed). Encyclopedia of Neuroscience. Oxford: Academic Press; 2009. pp. 993-8.

CHAPTER

30

Burns during Pregnancy

Shailesh Ranade, Akanksha Mohanty, Rekha Bharti

INTRODUCTION

Burns during pregnancy present a unique medical problem. Both mother and fetus are at great risk of fluid loss, hypoxemia, and sepsis. Most of the textbooks on obstetrics do not deal with burns in pregnancy, nor is the topic considered in depth in books devoted to the treatment of burns. In India and other countries where burns are present as a sociomedical problem, the incidence of burns in pregnancy is far more than that in the Western world.

INCIDENCE

The literature on burns during pregnancy is quite limited. However, the incidence calculated by the various authors in relation to the total number of female burn patients of reproductive age, does not appear to be low. The incidence in early pregnancy was unknown in past due to the absence of routine pregnancy testing on admission. Easy availability of pregnancy determination tests has increased the reporting of burns in pregnancy.

The highest incidence of burns during pregnancy has been reported from India. It has ranged from 7% as calculated by Akhtar[1] to 13.3% reported by Jain[2] and 15% reported by Prasanna.[3] Taylor[4] calculated an incidence of 7% while Amy[5] (1985) reported the incidence as 6.7%. Similar incidences have been reported by Gang[6] from Kuwait (7.8%) and Srivastava[7] (7.9%). Benmeir[8] from Israel reported an incidence of 0.6%. In a study from India it was observed that 18% women with burns in the reproductive age group were pregnant.[9]

ETIOLOGY

The etiology of burns in pregnancy does not vary from the general etiology of burns as a whole. A special mention is, however, required for burns in pregnancy in countries like India, where dowry and familial disputes in a joint family are common causes of suicidal and homicidal burns. These are wrongly reported as accidental burns due to false history given by the victim. Most of these patients are very severely burned and often have very high maternal and fetal mortality. Most of the studies have reported kerosene as the most common agent causing burns.[10]

PATHOPHYSIOLOGY OF BURNS IN PREGNANCY (FLOWCHART 1)

A pregnant burned patient presents the following additional pathophysiological changes:[11,12]

- Pregnant patients have a lower functional residual capacity (FRC) and are less able to compensate for hypoxia. Moreover, exposure to burns often puts

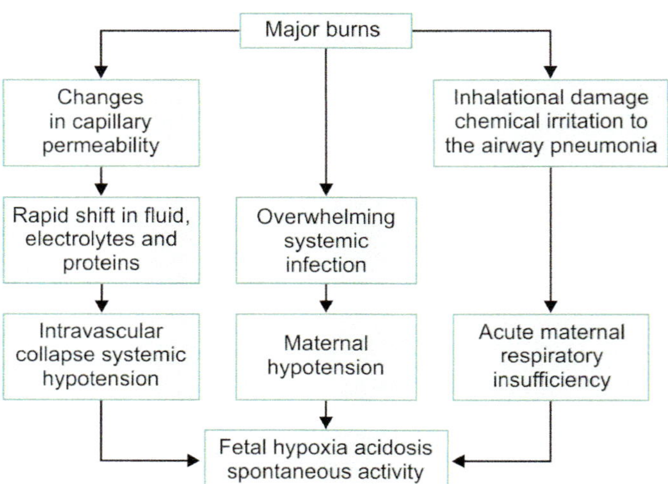

FLOWCHART 1: Pathophysiological changes in pregnant patients following major burns, affecting the fetus.

Courtesy: Rayburn, 1984.

the mother at risk for carbon monoxide inhalation. The fetus is especially susceptible to carbon monoxide poisoning because fetal hemoglobin has a higher affinity for carbon monoxide than maternal hemoglobin. Thus, carbon monoxide can easily lead to fetal hypoxia.

- *Effect of burns on uterine activity*: The onset of labor in a premature delivery shortly after a serious burn was in the past thought to be triggered by the endocrine function, especially by secretion of adrenocortical hormones related to stress. Later observations confirmed that minor burns had no effect on the course of pregnancy, while bums of at least 35% TBSA were capable of provoking early labor and the loss of the fetus following intrauterine death within a week of the burns.

Both spontaneous miscarriage and premature delivery were subsequently thought to be related to the synthesis and release of prostaglandins (responsible for early uterine contractions) from the skin in the burned area. Later, however, the correct importance was attributed both to maternal shock, which determines a considerable reduction in the uterine blood flow and causes fetal hypoxia and to pleuropulmonary complications, especially in cases of inhalation injuries with grave reduction of maternal pO_2 and consequently fetal hypoxia. Maternal acidosis may also play a role in inducing preterm delivery.[13] The fetus may be able to tolerate the early phases of maternal sepsis but is notably affected in the advanced phases, when the mother is decompensated and her cardiovascular system collapses. Thus, hypotension and acute respiratory insufficiency with septicemia can lead to complications in the fetus, even some time after the burn **(Flowchart 1)**.

As the maternal intravascular space is in a state of equilibrium with the amniotic liquid, the reduction of this liquid during serious hypovolemia can cause the intrauterine death of the fetus. The onset of spontaneous uterine contractions is also favored by the release from bacteria and the placenta of an enzyme, phospholipase A, which is necessary for the conversion of arachidonic acid into prostaglandin. It has recently been shown that there is a considerable reduction in plasma levels of 17b-estradiol in pregnant burned women who had either an abortion or a still birth in the first week post burn **(Figs. 1 and 2)**.

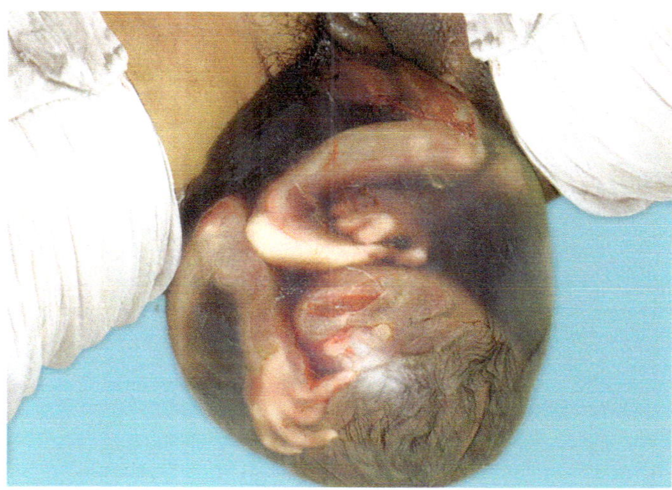

FIG. 1: Patient with 90% thermal burn and 7 months pregnancy aborted on the third day postburn spontaneously. Aborted fetus seen within intact membranes.

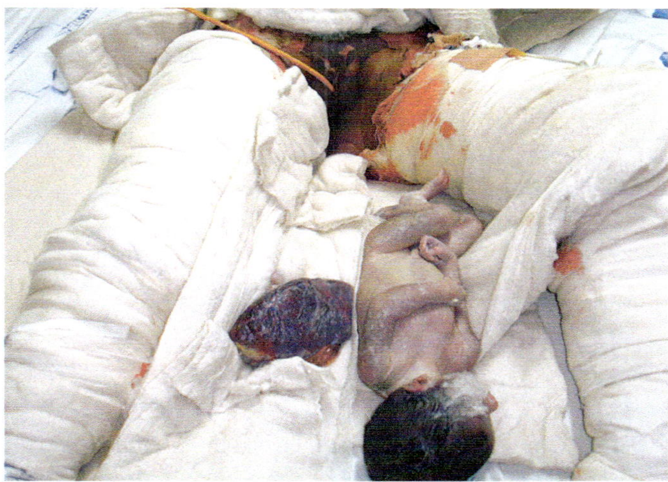

FIG. 2: A patient with 60% thermal burns and full-term pregnancy was induced within 48 hours to deliver a normal live baby.

MANAGEMENT OF BURNS AND ITS INFLUENCE ON THE COURSE OF PREGNANCY AND THE FETUS

Medical Treatment

Resuscitation treatment in the burned pregnant woman is no different from that in the non-pregnant burned woman. Women with more than 20 weeks' gestation should be nursed with left lateral tilt between 15 and 30 degrees for displacing gravid uterus to prevent aortocaval compression. In case cardiopulmonary resuscitation is required, chest compressions is given in supine position and lateral uterine displacement is maintained by either pushing uterus to left with one hand or pulling gravid uterus to right with both hands **(Fig. 3)**. In case woman is not revived within 4 minutes, decision for resuscitative hysterotomy should be taken and fetus should be delivered within 5 minutes to improve maternal and fetal outcome.[14] The prevention of hypovolemic shock by adequate early fluid resuscitation, therefore, requires that the uterine blood flow should be able to maintain fetus tissue pO_2

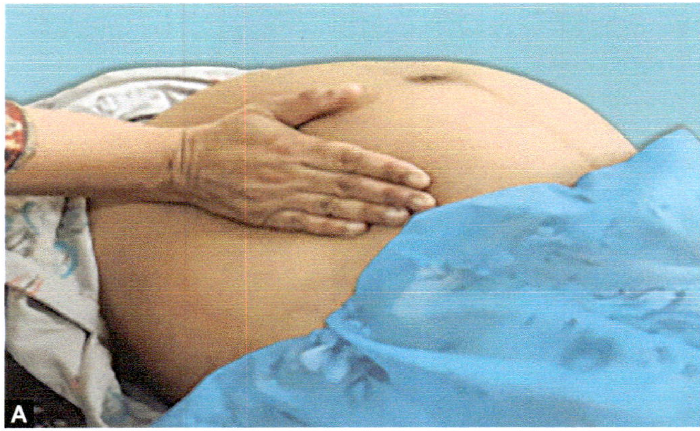

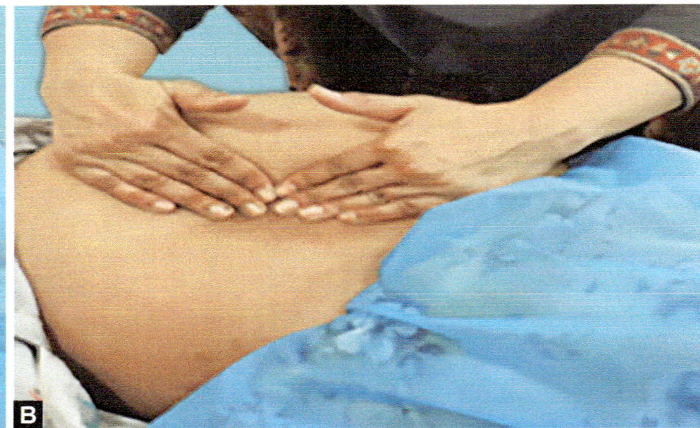

FIGS. 3A AND B: Left uterine displacement.

levels within the normal range. It has been recommended that a quantity of fluid should be administered that is sufficient to maintain the mother's blood pressure within the normal range and maintain urine output to 0.5–1.0 mL/kg body weight/h. The maintenance of arterial pressure levels at normal values is essential at all stages of the burn disease. Diuretics and antihypertensive drugs should, therefore, be avoided, whenever possible. Episodes of hypotension should also be avoided in the event of surgical operations. It is recommended that surgery should be performed with intraoperative maintenance of a minimum of 1 mL/kg body weight/h of urine volume and 100% oxygen saturation. Since extensive surface burns are frequently associated with an increased rate of arterial shunting and hypoxia, it becomes necessary to administer oxygen. A pregnant patient's oxygenation can often be improved by nursing her in a semi-sitting position. Maternal pO_2 values of less than 60 mm of Hg during the pleuropulmonary complications that are often secondary to inhalation injury have been considered critical. It has, therefore, been recommended that ventilatory support should be initiated as soon as possible. This is all the more necessary because inhaled carbon monoxide can also cross the placental barrier to compete for binding sites on fetal hemoglobin, provoking fetal cardiac edema and also affect cardiac development. The newer inventions in respiratory supportive care, like biphasic positive airway pressure (BIPAP) and continuous positive airway pressure (CPAP) ventilators have added a non-invasive method of ventilation as an option to standard ventilators. In cases of bronchopneumonia, it is necessary to use antibiotic treatment, if possible, by selecting drugs that the fetus can tolerate.

Wound Care

The local treatment of burns in pregnant women is not simple, because of the limitations imposed by the state of pregnancy.

- Sulfa drugs (silver sulfadiazine) are suspected of potential teratogenous activity if administered before the 14th week of pregnancy and of retarding growth, determining low birth weight if subsequently administered. Sulfa drugs administered near delivery may cause hyperbilirubinemia leading to kernicterus in the newborn.
- Povidone-iodine is widely used for burns cleansing. It must, however, be avoided during pregnancy since large amounts of iodine can be absorbed through the burn wound. Use of povidone-iodine is inadvisable in burns exceeding 20% total body surface area (TBSA) because the iodine passing through the placenta can be absorbed in sufficient quantities to affect thyroid functions and cause metabolic acidosis in fetus. It is, thus, clear that the state of pregnancy considerably reduces use of the commonest protocols for the topical treatment of burns.

Chloramphenicol, should be avoided throughout pregnancy since it is teratogenic if administered during the first period of pregnancy and responsible for neonatal pathology if used during the third trimester (Grey syndrome).

Gentamicin (ointment form) is an aminoglycoside capable of passing through the placenta after absorption through burned area. It can cause ototoxicity leading to vestibular and acoustic damage in fetus. In addition aminoglycosides are responsible for nephrotoxicity.

Rifamycin (for local application) is absolutely avoided during the last period of pregnancy because its interference with bilirubin metabolism can cause indirect hyperbilirubinemia with risk of kernicterus.

Even the local use of antibiotics that are normally administered systemically presents considerable difficulties.

The only antibiotics that can be considered safe in pregnancy are the penicillins and cephalosporins, while vancomycin, one of the most frequently used and most active antistaphylococcal drugs, is considered to be potentially teratogenic and ciprofloxacin may possibly damage articular cartilages in undeveloped organisms.

Tetracyclines are not widely used in burns but it should not be forgotten that they are contra-indicated during pregnancy because of their varying effects on fetal growth, bones, teeth and the immune system.

With regard to surgical procedures performed under anesthesia, it is important to avoid the use of ketamine, which increases the excitability of the myometrium because it is capable of triggering effective contractions. When the pregnancy is near term and delivery is imminent, ketamine may cause respiratory depression in the neonate.

It is preferable to keep the operative procedures as short as possible. During the period of anesthesia, it is important to maintain the oxygen saturation and blood pressure within normal limits throughout the procedure.

Surgical Treatment

Early, in view of the difficulties related to local medical treatment, early surgical treatment assumes vital importance. This is because early surgery facilitates healing of the wounds and thus improves prognosis of both mother and neonate. Early burn wound cover also minimizes septic complications and the need to administer antibiotics; in addition, it reduces the necessity of analgesic drugs.

The treatment for full-thickness burns comprises early tangential excision and split-thickness skin grafting 3–7 days postburn (but not more than 15–20% TBSA at one operation). The invention of biological skin substitutes has dramatically improved the management of second-degree burns. Processed animal collagen sheets (commercially available as Apocoll® and Kollagen®), Integra®, Biobrane® help in covering even very large burn wounds preventing the fluid loss, reducing pain, chances of wound infection and obviating the need of regular dressings.

Wounds over the abdomen and breast have to be treated first. Good early healing of the abdominal wound favors:

- Pain-free stretching of the abdominal skin during the developing pregnancy to term
- Abdominal obstetric supervision of the growing fetus
- Performance of cesarean section if required
- Early surgery of the breast wound prevents infection and sloughing of nipples and permits subsequent breastfeeding.

TABLE 1: Obstetric management in burned patients.[6,15,16]

Total percentage of burns	Age of gestation	Management
<30% TBSA	First trimester	No obstetric intervention, routine antenatal care
	Second trimester	No obstetric intervention, if in labor steroid cover after viability*
	Third trimester, <36 weeks	Conservative approach and monitoring of fetal heart rate, if in labor tocolytic therapy and steroid cover till 34 weeks
	Third trimester, >36 weeks	Induction of labor/cesarean section
30–50% TBSA	First trimester	Fetal monitoring by ultrasound 3–4 weeks
	Second trimester	Fetal monitoring every 3-4 weeks. Tocolytic therapy and steroid cover after viability*
	Third trimester, <36 weeks	Careful fetal heart rate, if in labor tocolytic therapy and steroid cover till 34 weeks, deliver within 48 hours
	Third trimester, >36 weeks	Deliver fetus within 48 hours (induction/cesarean)
50–70% TBSA	First trimester	No intervention
	Second trimester	No obstetric intervention, if in labor steroid cover after viability*
	Third trimester, if the baby is viable	Induce labor/cesarean section within 24 hours, steroid cover till 34 weeks
	Third trimester, intrauterine death	No active intervention up to 4 weeks/monitoring of thermocoagulation factors
>70% TBSA	First trimester	No intervention
	Second trimester	No intervention
	• Third trimester, If baby is viable	• Cesarean section as an emergency procedure at the earliest
	• Third trimester, intrauterine death	• No active intervention

**Viability*: After 24–26 weeks, depending on the nursery facility.

Obstetric Management of the Pregnant Woman with Burns (Table 1)

If it is known that a burned female is pregnant, it is important to establish as precisely as possible the exact stage of pregnancy at the time of the burn accident. This must be based upon the menstrual history and fetal ultrasound examination. The gestational period is in fact one of the factors determining obstetric procedures (no intervention, protection of pregnancy by tocolytic treatment, administration of steroids, induction and/or acceleration of labor). Other factors such as the severity of the burn and fetal viability must be confirmed immediately. Ultrasound examination helps in anatomical measurements to determine the age of fetus, biophysical measurements such as fetal muscle tone, limb motion and breathing patterns to know the wellbeing of fetus. In addition placental morphology, placental blood flow and amniotic fluid volume may be visualized in order to assess fetal health.

With regard to the stage of gestation, fetuses delivered before 24 weeks generally do not survive, while those delivered after 32 weeks do well with modern neonatal intensive care if born without hypoxia or birth trauma. The most difficult to manage are fetuses between 24 and 32 weeks' of gestational age, where ex-utero survival is difficult to predict. In such cases, therefore, when preterm labor occurs, tocolytic procedures are initiated.

In women with advanced state of pregnancy (second and third trimester) with more than 50% TBSA burns, it had an unfavorable effect unless delivery was immediate, as the burn created an unfavorable environment for the fetus. In burns less than 40% TBSA, pregnancy and its continuation had no effect on prognosis in the mother and every attempt had to be made to interrupt inception of labor if the fetus is too immature to survive. Maghsoudi et al. reported 100% maternal and fetal mortality in women with more than 40% TBSA.[17] However, in 39 women with burn in pregnancy, Rezavand et al. observed maternal mortality of 50% in women with >60% TBSA.[18]

Regarding the manner of delivery (vaginal route, cesarean section), spontaneous vaginal delivery is generally preferred, although obstetric considerations affect the choice of route and the timing of the delivery. Serial fetal sonography and fetal heart rate monitoring identify fetal stress at an early stage and may permit timely intervention, preventing intrauterine death. In a critically burned woman with a living and near-term pregnancy, fetal salvage by cesarean section appears justifiable.

When there are obstetric indications for a cesarean section, this can be performed even when the lower abdominal wall is part of the burned area.

Thus, a pregnant burned patient, especially when severely burned, is a big challenge for a burn surgeon. A comprehensive team effort involving a plastic surgeon, intensivist, obstetrician, neonatologist, anesthesiologist, chest physician, and well-trained nursing staff with other supportive departments can help in saving two lives at a time.

SUMMARY

Pregnancy-related burn management entails a complex interaction between maternal and fetal factors. After the mother is stabilized using airway management, breathing, and circulation (ABC) procedures, a thorough examination of the degree of the burns and the fetal health are conducted. The physiological changes that occur during pregnancy require careful consideration while adjusting fluid resuscitation to prevent overload. When treating pain, it is best to use safe analgesics rather than teratogenic ones. Regular dressing changes, topical antimicrobial agents (except from silver sulphadizines) that are safe to use during pregnancy, and prompt excision and grafting when required are all part of wound care. When fetal viability increases beyond 24 weeks' gestation, continuous fetal monitoring is crucial for evaluating heart rate and uterine contractions in viable pregnancies. When using medications, caution should be exercised to prevent teratogens, ensure that the right antibiotics are used, and get tetanus prophylaxis. Corticosteroids may be started if preterm labor is a risk. Nutritional support is critical, with increased caloric and protein needs, and adequate intake of vitamins and minerals essential for fetal development. Comprehensive care requires a multidisciplinary team approach comprising critical care specialists, anesthetists, neonatologists, obstetricians, and burn surgeons. Maternal stress and anxiety should be treated psychologically with counseling. Physical and occupational therapy specifically designed for the pregnant patient is part of the long-term care plan. Preference should be given to regional anesthetic where practical, and delivery mode and timing should be coordinated based on the severity of the burns, gestational age, and maternal-fetal status. When planning interventions, special attention is paid to the fetus's weight and gestational age because these characteristics have a significant impact on management measures. In order to maximize results for both the mother and the fetus, early and ongoing multidisciplinary collaboration is necessary for the effective management of burns during pregnancy.

REFERENCES

1. Akhtar MA, Mulawkar PM, Kulkarni HR. Burns in pregnancy: Effect on maternal and fetal outcomes. Bums. 1994;20:351-5.
2. Jain ML, Garg AK. Burns with pregnancy: A review of 25 cases. Burns. 1993;19:166-7.
3. Prasanna M, Singh K. Early burn wound excision in major bums with pregnancy: A preliminary report. Bums. 1996;22: 234-7.
4. Taylor JW, Plunkett GD, McManus WF, Pruitt BA Jr. Thermal injury during pregnancy. Obstet Gynecol. 1976;47:434-8.
5. Amy BW, McManus WF, Goodwin CW, Mason A Jr, Pruitt BA Jr. Thermal injury in the pregnant patient. Surg Gynecol Obstet. 1985;161:209-12.
6. Gang RK, Bajee J, Tahboub M. Management of thermal injury in pregnancy: An analysis of 16 patients. Burns. 1992;18:317-20.

7. Srivastava S, Bang RL. Bums during pregnancy. Burns. 1998;14: 228-32.
8. Benmeir P, Sagi A, Greber B, Bibi C, Hauben D, Rosenberg L, et al. Burns during pregnancy: Our experience. Burns. 1988;14:233-6.
9. Chandra G, Gaurav K, Kumar S, Yadav SK, Ranjan R, Nambiar M, et al. Burns during pregnancy: A retrospective analysis of 19 cases. Arch Int Surg. 2016;6:28-31.
10. Aghaie A, Lotfi B, Shaahmadi Z, Karami-Matin B, Ahmadi Jouybari T. Epidemiology of Maternal and Fetal's Burn in Iran: A Systematic Review and Meta-Analysis. Int J Pediatr. 2018;6(2):7219-40.
11. Rayburn W, Smith B, Feller I, Varner M, Cruikshank D. Major bums during pregnancy: Effect on fetal well-being. Obstet. Gynecol. 1984;63:392-5.
12. Napoli B, D'Arpa N, Masellis M, Graziano R. Burns in Pregnancy, Annals of Burns and Fire Disasters - vol. XIII – no. 1 - March 2000.
13. Kennedy BB, Baird SM, Troiano NH. Burn injuries and pregnancy. J Perinat Neonatal Nurs. 2008;22(1):21-30; quiz 31-2.
14. Lott C, Truhlář A, Alfonzo A, Barelli A, González-Salvado V, Hinkelbein J, et al. ERC Special Circumstances Writing Group Collaborators. European Resuscitation Council Guidelines 2021: Cardiac arrest in special circumstances. Resuscitation. 2021;161:152-219.
15. Mittal P, Kripa S, Ara A, Tiwari VK. Feto-maternal Outcomes in Pregnancies Complicated by Thermal Burns. J Obstet Gynaecol India. 2018;68(4):270-5.
16. Dijkerman ML, Breederveld-Walters ML, Pijpe A, Breederveld RS. Management and outcome of burn injuries during pregnancy: A systematic review and presentation of a comprehensive guideline. Burns. 2022;48(7):1544-60.
17. Maghsoudi H, Samnia R, Garadaghi A, Kianvar H. Burns in pregnancy. Burns. 2006;32:246-50.
18. Rezavand N, Seyedzadeh A, Soleymani A. Evaluation of maternal and foetal outcomes in pregnant women hospitalized in Kermanshah Hospitals, Iran, owing to burn injury, 2003-2008. Ann Burns Fire Disasters. 2012;25:196-9.

SECTION

6

General Management and Rehabilitation

CHAPTER

31 Multiple Organ Dysfunction Syndrome in Burns

Poonam Gupta, PK Verma

INTRODUCTION

Multiple organ dysfunction syndrome (MODS) can be defined as the development of acute and potentially reversible physiologic derangement involving two or more organ systems in a critically ill patient resulting from an uncontrolled inflammatory response to a potentially life-threatening physiologic insult that makes it impossible to maintain homeostasis without medical intervention. It can be triggered by multiple different and clinically diverse factors. The organ dysfunction may recover or can progress to organ failure and death.

HISTORICAL PERSPECTIVE

Our understanding of MODS can be parallel to advancements in combat injury resuscitation throughout the twentieth century. In the First World War, many soldiers succumbed to hemorrhagic shock due to wounds. By the Second World War, the use of whole blood transfusions by combat medics in the field reduced the incidence of wound shock but led to the emergence of post-traumatic renal failure as a significant issue. The Korean War saw a reduction in renal failure incidents, thanks to more aggressive fluid resuscitation strategies, which, in turn, led to the Vietnam War's challenge of post-traumatic acute hypoxemic respiratory failure, known as Da Nang lung. Innovations such as mechanical ventilation with positive end-expiratory pressure and renal dialysis not only extended the lives of critically ill patients, but also introduced new complications.[1] By the late sixties, researchers identified a new syndrome characterized by respiratory failure, hypotension, sepsis, and jaundice, often accompanied by hemorrhage from acute stress ulcers in the stomach.[2] One paper reported the failure of multiple organs in the postoperative period of ruptured aortic aneurysm.[3] Interestingly, a similar clinical picture was seen in diverse conditions like pancreatitis, peritonitis, bowel perforation, prolonged shock following valve replacement, and major burns by Baue in 1975.[4] It was termed "sequential system failure." In 1977, Eiseman, Beart, and Norton named it "multiple organ failure."[5] Fry and his colleagues in 1980 noticed that gram-negative sepsis was a common event that preceded multiple organ failure (MOF) due to the diverse causes. The lipopolysaccharide (LPS) was identified as the responsible bacterial endotoxin and from 1980 to 1985, empirical treatment of infection with antibiotics was the mainstay of therapy in MOF.[6] It was later realized that not all patients of MODS were due to infection and those dying of MODS did not always have a culture-proven infection.[7] MOF stems from an excessive inflammatory response triggered by either septic or nonseptic injuries. Meakins introduced the "two-hit" model for the development of MOF. This model proposed that an initial traumatic injury or shock (the first hit) primes neutrophils and macrophages for an amplified inflammatory response to a subsequent insult, such as a nosocomial infection (the second hit). The "two-hit" model clarified that early MODS is not associated with sepsis, whereas late MODS patients require a second insult to progress to organ failure.[8]

With the advances in supportive therapy/critical care and our increasing ability to keep severely ill patients' lives prolonged, so the consequent troubles in organ function occur, similar patterns of organ failures distant from the site of illness/injury were reported in patients with burns, pancreatitis, trauma, surgical hemorrhage, and abdominal sepsis. Currently, it is well known that almost any disease that initiates tissue injury has the potential of progressing to MODS. Even though many pathophysiological mechanisms to explain this have been put forth, the search for a common mechanism to the diverse etiologies of MODS is still elusive and the molecular basis for specific organ failure remains to be fully uncovered.

DEFINITION

Various terms like MOF, multiple systems organ failure (MSOF), or total organ failure have been used at different times to describe a phenomenon of "organ disease remote from the site of illness/injury."

The American College of Chest Physicians/Society of Critical Care Medicine (ACCP/SCCM) consensus conference in 1992 put forward the term "multiple organ dysfunction syndrome".[9] This term provides a distinction between "failure" and "dysfunction." The term "failure" is deemed unsatisfactory as it implies an outcome that is often irreversible, while "dysfunction" implies a wide range of organ severity and the dynamic nature of the disorder that may change over time. The evolution in understanding organ failure as an uninterrupted path has resulted in the creation of several scoring systems aimed at quantifying the severity of organ failure.[10] The term "syndrome" was introduced to describe a pattern of multiple physiological changes that likely share a common pathogenesis.

PATHOGENESIS

Severe/major burn injury evokes a systemic inflammatory response. Even though severe and extremely dysregulated inflammatory host response seems to be the main mechanism leading to the development of MODS, a multitude of other factors also contribute. The development of MODS can be best conceptualized as a highly complex and integrated process incorporating many different pathogenic processes that are highly interdependent. Dysfunction of a single organ may have cascade effects on other organs. Hence, the host response in MODS is highly interlinked, and the whole is far greater than the sum of its constituent parts.

An Overview

The current view for the development of MODS following burn injury involves systemic activation of the circulating immune cells, endothelium, and other cascades resulting in the release of inflammatory mediators. These proinflammatory mediators are released locally to combat foreign antigens, degrade necrotic tissues, and facilitate healing. Concurrently, anti-inflammatory mediators are also released to downgrade and contain the inflammatory process. The balance between the inflammatory and regulatory processes of the host response determines the ultimate outcome. If the balance between the two arms is controlled, regulated, and well maintained, it results in the resolution and restoration of tissue homeostasis. However, when this natural balance is disturbed or if the regulatory mechanisms fail to contain the response, the inflammatory mediators spread into the systemic circulation. Further recruitment and activation of leukocytes increase the inflammatory cascade excessively. This interplay of inflammatory and anti-inflammatory responses leads to tissue injury, multiple organ dysfunction, and, ultimately, death. In essence, when the immune response aimed at combating a localized infection fails to confine it, the resulting uncontrolled infection triggers a severe and inappropriate systemic inflammatory reaction. If this uncontrolled immune response is not promptly treated and managed, it can escalate to organ dysfunction.

The bodily reaction that a big or severe burn damage causes is what makes it unique.

Unlike sepsis or trauma, burns that affect more than 20% of the total body surface area (TBSA) cause an intensive pathophysiological response that can take up to 24–36 months to subside.[11] Any insult typically causes an inflammatory reaction to aid in the healing process. On the other hand, severe or substantial burns may cause a condition of widespread and dysregulated inflammation, which can lead to an intense inflammation that can cause systemic inflammatory response syndrome (SIRS), delayed healing, vascular endothelium dysfunction, and immunological suppression. Furthermore, a catabolic state is also induced by inflammation.[12]

This reaction, known as the hypermetabolic response, is nearly always present after burns, in terms of both severity and length.[12] Hyperdynamic circulation, enhanced body temperature regulation, proteolysis, glycolysis, lipolysis, increased resting energy expenditure, muscle atrophy, stimulated synthesis of acute-phase proteins, increased risk of organ failure, infections, and even death[13] are characteristics of this hypermetabolic state.

Various causes affect the host response **(Box 1)**.

Changes at the Cellular Level (Table 1 and Flowchart 1)

Damaged tissues produce endogenous damage-associated molecular patterns (DAMPs) (like double-stranded RNA and mitochondrial DNA) and exogenous pathogen-associated molecular patterns (PAMPs) (like LPS and peptidoglycans) as soon as a severe burn injury occurs. Innate immunity is triggered and inflammatory gene transcription is upregulated as a result of the interaction between these DAMPs and PAMPs and pattern-recognition receptors, such as toll-like receptors. The toll-like receptors facilitate signaling by the use of intracellular transcription pathways like nuclear factor κB (NF-κB). NF-κB, a transcription activator protein, is involved in the induction of several inflammatory mediators, including tumor necrosis factor α (TNF-α).[15] White blood cells in the damaged tissues are believed to be a major source of

BOX 1 Factors contributing to the host response.[14]

- *Patient factors*:
  - Age
  - Medical comorbidities (e.g., heart failure, kidney failure, cirrhosis of liver)
  - Drug or alcohol; intoxication
  - Genetic
- *Injury factors*:
  - Degree of burn
  - Percentage burnt area
  - Associated inhalational burn
  - Burns with trauma
  - Time of presentation to medical aid
- *Treatment factors*:
  - Shock
  - Volume of resuscitation fluids
  - Abdominal compartment syndrome
  - Units of blood transfused, its age
  - On ventilator
  - Fracture fixation
  - Fat embolus and sepsis

proinflammatory factors, which result in the damage of microvessels.[16]

The pathophysiology of burn injury involves a variety of cellular and molecular processes that can be broadly categorized into two stages: An initial proinflammatory stage and a subsequent immunosuppressive stage.[17]

Systemic Inflammatory Response Syndrome (Table 1 and Flowchart 1)

The beginning stage, known as the systemic inflammatory response syndrome, is mostly proinflammatory in character.[17,43] Macrophages and chemically active cytokines TNF-α and interleukin-6 (IL-6)[17,43] are the prominent elements in this phase.

- Macrophages are the primary source of proinflammatory mediators, such as prostaglandin E2, reactive nitrogen intermediates, IL-6, and TNF-α.[44] However, a few hours after burn damage, other immune cells, such as neutrophils and monocytes, are also activated.
- Apoptosis of numerous cell components is partially induced by TNF-α.[43] Furthermore, proapoptotic factors such as caspase-3 activity, Bcl-xl, and Bax exhibit

TABLE 1: Brief description of various inflammatory mediators/responses, cells, mechanisms, and pathogenic events involved in the development of MODS after burn injury.

Mediator/cells/ mechanism/ pathologic event	Description
PAMPs	PAMPs are usually microbial molecules that activate innate immunity and are recognized primarily through TLRs, and activate several signaling pathways (e.g., NF-κB)[18]
DAMPs	Released endogenously by the injured cell; activate the innate immunity; DAMPs include HMGB1, heat-shock proteins, uric acid, and DNA. HMGB1, a nuclear protein that binds to nucleosomes and promotes DNA bending, has been associated with SIRS and end-organ damage
HMGB-1	HMGB-1 is a molecule that facilitates the binding of inflammatory mediators to cells and acts as a nuclear cofactor that enhances the DNA transcription of many inflammatory mediators
TLRs	TLRs are transmembrane proteins present in most body cell types, which form the major pattern-recognition receptors that transduce signals in response to DAMPs and PAMPs resulting in the initiation of innate immune system responses, including NF-κB activation and proinflammatory cytokine production[19]
Pattern-recognition receptors	DAMPs/PAMPs trigger inflammatory responses when they interact with pattern-recognition receptors expressed by host cells in the cytoplasm (RLRs and NLRs20), in the endosome (TLRs), and on the cell surface (TLRs and CLRs)[20]
Cytokines	Proinflammatory cytokines (TNF-α, MIP, GM-CSF, IFN-γ, IL-1, IL-2, IL-6, IL-8, IL-17, IL-1β, etc.)[21] and anti-inflammatory cytokines (IL-4, IL-10, IL-13)[22] can be found in cytokines. Following burn damage, cytokines control the immune system, metabolism, and hemodynamic processes. When cytokines attach to particular cell receptors, intracellular signaling pathways are triggered, which in turn control gene transcription and affect the survival, proliferation, differentiation, and activity of immune cells. In addition, they control the synthesis and function of other cytokines, which can intensify or decrease the inflammatory response. One benefit is that burn victims experience immunological dysfunction in addition to hypermetabolism brought on by inflammatory cytokines. TNF-α stimulates the generation of reactive oxygen species, adipose catabolism, and the release of free fatty acids in individuals with thermal injuries, which leads to hypermetabolism.[23] In addition to TNF-α, IL-1β contributes to the hypermetabolic state because it interferes with insulin sensitivity (as explained). Anti-inflammatory cytokines (IL-4, IL-10, and IL-13) downregulate synthesis of the proinflammatory cytokines

Continued

Continued

Mediator/cells/ mechanism/ pathologic event	Description
IL-1β	It is a proinflammatory mediator, which is an antagonist to insulin sensitivity by causing downregulation of insulin receptor substrate-1 expression. This causes hyperglycemia and stress-induced diabetes leading to metabolic dysfunction and hypermetabolism in postburn period[24]
TNF-α	It is a proinflammatory cytokine. Its role includes:[24] • Amplify inflammation by mediator response • Cause apoptosis and repair the inflammatory injury • Increase the formation of ROS • Enhance adipose catabolism by increasing the lipolysis and the release of FFAs
Hypermetabolic state	Along with immunological dysfunction and a hypovolemic response, hypermetabolic state also contributes to MODS following burn injury; it is more common in severe burns (>20% TBSA) and can last for up to 3 years following the burns. Hypermetabolic state increases the rates of lipolysis, glycolysis, and proteolysis; this leads to weight loss and muscular atrophy, which can have a significant change on immunity and wound healing; numerous factors are linked to the mechanisms producing burn-induced hypermetabolism, such as: • *Proinflammatory cytokines*: ○ TNF-α enhances adipose catabolism by increasing the lipolysis and the release of FFAs ○ By downregulating the expression of insulin receptor substrate-1, IL-1β impairs insulin sensitivity and contributes to stress-induced diabetes and hyperglycemia, which occur before long-term metabolic dysfunction and hypermetabolism after burns[24] • *Stress hormones*: Catecholamines, insulin, and cortisol, among other stress hormones, operate on several target organs, such as adipose tissue, skeletal muscle, and liver, to produce pleiotropic hypermetabolic effects that enhance glucose metabolism, lipolysis, and proteolysis • *Mitochondria dysfunction*: Skeletal muscle mitochondria's uncoupling of oxidative phosphorylation leads to an increase in metabolic rate, which rather than producing ATP causes thermogenesis[25] • *Endoplasmic reticulum stress*: Pathologically induced hypermetabolism puts a heavy load on the ER and causes misfolded and unfolded proteins to build up inside the organelle. We refer to this process as ER stress • *Browning of WAT*: Brown adipose tissue, which is distinguished by increased lipolysis rates, is created when WAT is transformed into brown adipose tissue. After heat damage, an increase in WAT browning and the circulation of free fatty acids is linked to the hypermetabolic state.[26] Additionally, IL-6 and the mitochondrial uncoupling protein 1 can cause browning of WAT[27,28]
Histamine	The early stage of enhanced microvascular permeability that occurs right after a burn is caused by histamine. Venular endothelium cells contract in response to histamine, resulting in the temporary formation of massive endothelial gaps. Additionally, histamine can increase PC by venular contraction and arteriolar dilatation[29]
Catecholamines	Massive levels of catecholamines, adrenaline, and norepinephrine are released following a burn injury.[29] When paired with hypovolemia and lowered venous pressure from burn shock, these drugs activate the alpha 1 receptor on the arteriolar side of the microcapillaries, causing vasoconstriction and a tendency to lower capillary pressure. In nonresuscitated burn shock, decreased capillary pressure may restrict edema and cause interstitial fluid to reabsorb from nonburned skin, skeletal muscle, and visceral organs. Moreover, catecholamines may also partially block the increased capillary permeability brought on by bradykinin and histamine through their β-agonist activity
Oxygen radicals	Inflammation is a major function of oxygen radicals in burn shock. Following an inflammatory response or the reperfusion of ischemic tissue, active neutrophils generate and release superoxide anion (O-2) and hydrogen peroxide (H_2O_2). By causing harm to microvascular endothelial cells, these oxygen radicals have the potential to promote vascular permeability.[30,31] It has been discovered that free radicals promote wound healing and antibacterial activity. On one hand, the organism may suffer from oxidative stress brought on by the large-scale synthesis of oxygen radicals. On the other hand, the large creation of oxygen radicals and the resulting oxidative stress can have several detrimental effects on the organism. They impair cellular functions, oxidize lipids, and harm organ tissues—all of which are factors in MODS. Furthermore, the elevation of NF-κB transcription factor and peripheral vasodilatation may result from burn-related inducible NO synthase overexpression. Elevated oxygen radicals also trigger the production of inflammatory cytokines via a number of different routes. Most often, MODS associated with a burn injury is produced by an excess of ROS brought on by systemic inflammatory processes after burns[32,33]

Continued

Continued

Mediator/cells/ mechanism/ pathologic event	Description
Alteration in vascular permeability—role of the endothelium in response to burn injury	ECs line the inner surface of vessels and create a barrier from the tissue. Following inflammation, the gap junctions widen to form a leaky passage, which leads to defective function of the gap junctions. Numerous vascular-permeability-increasing mediators, such as reactive oxygen species, cytokines (platelet activating factor, tumor necrosis factor, etc.), and other inflammatory mediators (histamine, bradykinin, etc.), are released in response to burn injury, inflammation, and other traumatic injuries. EC is also activated by alterations in hemorheology, such as blood flow slowing down and leukocyte adherence to the vascular wall. These mediators increase contractile force through actin–myosin interaction and widen intercellular gaps, which allows the transflux of large molecules and leakage of mass fluid from vascular space. These mediators bind to their specific chemical receptors or mechanosensors, which activate multiple signal pathways through second messengers and protein kinases. This increases permeability and tissue edema.[34] Bradykinin is an effective vasoactive mediator that raises microvascular permeability and venular dilatation. It also has an effective vasoactive mediator that induces pain, smooth muscle contraction, enhanced microvascular permeability, and venular dilatation.[17] Therefore, the following factors may lead to aberrant blood flow distribution (after endothelial cell activation) leading to increased vascular permeability and excessive vasodilatation mediated by nitric oxide, blockage by microthrombi, platelets, or leukocyte aggregates, abnormal red cell deformity, endothelial cell edema, and hypoperfusion secondary to reduced cardiac output (i.e., reduced preload, myocardial depression, and reduced lusitropy)
Coagulopathy	Following major burns, coagulopathy occurs due to impaired fibrinolytic (by increased activity of plasminogen activator inhibitor type I) and natural anticoagulation systems (by activated protein C, antithrombin, and tissue factor pathway inhibitor). Factors responsible for this state include tissue hypoperfusion, acidemia, hypothermia, consumption and/or dilution of coagulation factors (because of fluid resuscitation, endothelial damage, and development of SIRS), and bleeding due to burn wound excision[35]
Coagulation cascade	Microvascular thrombosis is brought on by the coagulation cascade being activated, and recurrent episodes of ischemia and reperfusion are caused by fibrinolysis that follow. Thrombin and other coagulation system components are strong proinflammatory mediators that drive endothelial cells to produce adhesion molecules and activate neutrophils, which result in microvascular damage. The kallikrein–kininogen cascade is also triggered by coagulation, which adds to hypotension. NETs generated from dying neutrophils further aid in the production of thrombi. Tissue hypoperfusion brought on by thrombus formation is made worse by vasodilatation, hypotension, and decreased red-cell deformability[36,37]
Complement cascade	Inflammatory peptides are activated by systemic complement hyper-regulation brought on by burn injury:[21] • Proinflammatory peptides that cause lysis of the target cells at the end of the complement activation cascade are C3a, C3b, C4b (chemotaxis of leukocytes; degranulation of phagocytic cells, mast cells, and basophils; smooth muscle contraction and increased vascular permeability), and C5b-9, or membrane attack complex • Arachidonic acid metabolites, cytokines, and oxygen-free radicals are also produced when complement is activated
Apoptosis autophagy[38]	• In autophagy, damaged cells are disposed by phagocytosis including macromolecular structures. Autophagy helps in recovery from critical illness; dysfunction in autophagy leads to pathology
Necroptosis[38]	• Both necroptosis and apoptosis are important processes in cell death, although they usually elicit conflicting immunological reactions. While necroptotic death emits chemicals that encourage inflammation, apoptotic death typically results in immunologically quiet reactions
Pyroptosis[38]	• Apoptosis is an example of a highly controlled, noninflammatory process that proceeds in a systematic manner and does not damage nearby cells. Conversely, pyroptosis is a proinflammatory form of programmed cell death characterized by strong activation of inflammatory caspase after cell lysis. In conclusion, it seems that while autophagy might provide some defense against the emergence of MODS, pyroptosis and necroptosis might potentially be harmful
NF-κB	NF-κB is a cofactor that is involved in the transcription of genes that encode: • Inflammatory proteins • Apoptotic signaling pathways • Nitric oxide production It exists in the preformed state in cytoplasm and when activated, translocated to the nucleus. NF-κB levels increase when the disease is severe.[39]

Continued

Continued

Mediator/cells/ mechanism/ pathologic event	Description
Role of gastro-intestinal system	Blood flow to the colon reduces by over 60% of baseline following a thermal injury, and this reduction lasts for up to 4 hours. An extreme hyperinflammatory reaction could be brought on by bacterial translocation and loss of the intestinal barrier. The gut bacteria can spread to extraintestinal locations such as the liver, lungs, and mesenteric lymph nodes because of an increase in intestinal permeability brought on by hypoperfusion and the ensuing tissue inflammation and injury. Gastrointestinal failure may also be caused by the atrophy of the gut mucosa in the absence of intraluminal feeding. Additionally, it has been observed that the Enterobacteriaceae family has sharply increased in relative abundance compared to the usual flora (Bacteroidaceae, Lachnospiraceae, and Ruminococcaceae families) in stool samples from burn damage patients[14]
Blood transfusion	Blood products include proinflammatory cytokines and lipids and are immunoactive. They have an early immunosuppressive effect that raises the possibility of infection, MOF, and SARS. Furthermore, compared to transfusions using RBCs kept for shorter periods of time, the transfusion of stored RBCs older than 3 weeks soon after injury is associated with a greater rate of MOF.[40] Blood can still operate as a secondary hit even after leukodepletion because red blood cells still carry proinflammatory mediators. Furthermore, other blood constituents that are immunoactive include platelets, plasma, and coagulation factors[41]
Mechanical ventilation	Positive-pressure ventilation has the potential to cause mechanical lung injuries, such as barotrauma, atelectrauma, and volutrauma. It can also cause biotrauma, which releases inflammatory mediators from injured cells and draws in PMNs, as well as enhance pulmonary dysfunction.[42] Ischemia-reperfusion damage following burns is exacerbated by inadequate oxygen delivery. Through direct cell signaling, these inflammatory cytokines produced in the lung may seep into the systemic circulation, increasing the inflammatory state and leading to organ dysfunction[21]

(ATP: adenosine triphosphate; CLRs: C-type lectin receptors; DAMPs: damage-associated molecular patterns; ECs: endothelial cells; ER: endoplasmic reticulum; FFAs: free fatty acids; GM-CSF: granulocyte-macrophage colony-stimulating factor; HMGB1: high mobility group box protein-1; IFN-γ: interferon γ; IL: interleukin; MODS: multiple organ dysfunction syndrome; MOF: multiple -organ failure; NETs: neutrophil extracellular traps; NLRs20: nucleotide-binding oligomerization domain-like receptors; PAMPs: pathogen-associated molecular patterns; RBCs: red blood cells; RLRs: retinoic acid-inducible gene 1-like receptors; ROS: reactive oxygen species; SARS: systemic anti-inflammatory response syndrome; SIRS: systemic inflammatory response syndrome; TBSA: total body surface area; TLRs: toll-like receptors; TNF-α: tumor necrosis factor alpha; WAT: white adipose tissue)

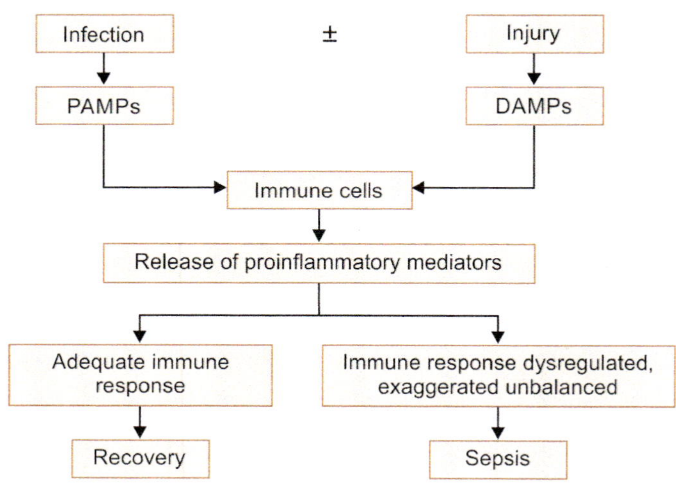

FLOWCHART 1: Host response to an infection/injury: Injury (via DAMPs) and infection (via PAMPs) can stimulate the same inflammatory reaction through the same receptors present on the surface of host immune cells.

(DAMPs: damage-associated molecular patterns; PAMPs: pathogen-associated molecular patterns)

elevated expression. Moreover, severe burn injuries frequently result in the death of organ cells, which can be brought on by a systemic inflammatory response triggered by severe burns. TNF-α activates monocytes and neutrophils and can stimulate the release of IL-1 and IL-643, among other proinflammatory mediators. Additionally, TNF-α is essential to the pathophysiology of an early shock state (fever and hypotension).

Acute-phase proteins and complement factor C5a are important elements that, in addition to inflammatory mediators, further intensify inflammatory activities during this stage. This stimulation of the coagulation system results in disseminated intravascular coagulopathy (DIC). Microvascular thrombosis is brought on by the coagulation cascade being activated, and fibrinolysis that follows causes recurrent episodes of ischemia and reperfusion. Thrombin and other coagulation system components are strong proinflammatory mediators that drive endothelial cells to produce adhesion molecules and activate neutrophils, which results in microvascular damage. Additionally, coagulation factors cause the kallikrein-kininogen cascade to be activated, which results in hypotension.

Additionally, persistent and deep hypermetabolism brought on by thermal injury results in the production of proinflammatory cytokine. This leads macrophages to produce more of these mediators[44] and forms superoxide anion, hydroxyl radical, hydrogen peroxide, and reactive oxygen and nitrogen species (RONS) including nitric oxide (NO) and peroxynitrite, which are examples of reactive oxygen species.[45]

Furthermore, generalized venular hyperpermeability is also induced by heat injury.

- The main function of this stage is to communicate the proper signals to the adaptive immunity cells in order to boost the immune responses and speed up the removal of pathogens.
- Early organ failure, sometimes known as inflammatory response failure, can occur during this early stage of burn injury.

Counter Anti-inflammatory Response Syndrome (Table 1 and Flowchart 1)

The majority of a burn injury's second phase is anti-inflammatory.[43] Helper Th-2 T cells and three main mediators—the cytokines IL-4/IL-10 and transforming growth factor (TGF)[43]—are necessary for this phase. This condition raises the risk of nosocomial infections due to a loss of delayed-type hypersensitivity (DTH) response and an incapacity to manage secondary pathogenic challenges.

Adaptive Immune Response[28]

Severe burns reduce the total number of T cells in addition to affecting the function of the innate immune system. On the other hand, Th-2 cells are more prevalent than Th-1 cells because of elevated amounts of IL-4 and IL-10.[46] The increase that occurs after burn injury is also attributed to the decreased levels of IL-2 and interferon.

One of the main causes of the inhibition of the adaptive immune response is the declining ratio of Th-1 to Th-2. Furthermore, following severe burn injury, the ratio of CD4-positive T helper cells to CD-8-positive T suppressor cells also decreases.[47]

Similarly, severe burn injuries that result in immunological dysregulation also tip the scales against regulatory T cells and helper T lymphocytes 17 (Th 17). Dysfunction of neutrophils and reduced macrophage phagocytosis take place. When the weakened changes in innate and adaptive immune responses are combined, the risk of infection, sepsis, and various organ dysfunction is increased.

Endothelial cell connections enlarge and gaps occur in response to inflammation, impairing barrier function.[17] Actin rearrangement that is dependent on actomyosin is the mechanism behind these vascular alterations.[17] The main causes of the systemic microvascular leakage seen in burns are these previously mentioned inflammatory mediators and the rise in vascular hydrostatic pressure brought on by channel dilatation.[17] Moreover, the burn damage site produces kinins, more precisely bradykinin.[15] Bradykinin is a potent vasoactive mediator that induces discomfort, smooth muscle spasm, enhanced microvascular permeability, and venular dilatation.[15]

Lipid mediators are additional significant mediators. These are important signaling molecules in the resolution of inflammation, particularly eicosanoid and "specialized proresolution lipid mediators," which are essential in controlling the inflammatory profile and encouraging the restoration of homeostasis after burn injury.[48] Increased tissue damage and persistent inflammation may result from their dysregulation.[48]

Systemic Effects

Disorders of one or more organ systems may be brought on by aberrant immune reactions manifested as systemic or localized inflammation. Almost every organ can be impacted. Nonetheless, the most commonly affected organ systems and those that exhibit clinical features include the respiratory, cardiovascular, hepatic, and neurological systems, as well as hematologic abnormalities.[49]

Cardiovascular System

Cuthbertson (1942) originally characterized the two distinct phases of the early systemic consequences of a significant burn injury that are generated by a cytokine-mediated inflammatory response: Burn shock (ebb) phase and hypermetabolic (flow) phase.[50,51] Increased microvascular permeability (from direct vascular thermal injury and release of inflammatory mediators),[15] intravascular fluid loss in the burned areas (and even in noninjured tissues with injuries covering more than 25%–30% of TBSA), and development of edema are the hallmarks of the initial hypodynamic ebb phase.[17] Hypoproteinemia occurs due to loss of proteins into the edema fluid from the injured skin surface.[15] These changes result in intravascular hypovolemia and a resultant hemoconcentration within the first 12–24 hours following injury.[15] Additional factors that lead to a shock state include depressed cardiac output [caused by loss of intravascular volume, direct myocardial depression, and increased pulmonary and systemic vascular resistance (SVR)] and increased SVR (caused by release of catecholamines, antidiuretic hormone, and hemoconcentration). The aim of care during this phase is resuscitation using intravenous fluids to preserve tissue and limit ischemia and inflammatory reactions. The pathophysiologic changes during the ebb phase are summarized in **Table 2**.

TABLE 2: A few important pathophysiological changes in the early (24–48) hours after major burn injury.[51]

Cardiovascular system	Renal system	Brain	Lungs—inhalation injury	Skin	Adrenal gland
• Tachycardia • ↓ Cardiac index • ↓Stroke volume • ↑PVR and SVR • ↑Hematocrit • ↓ SvO_2	• Oliguria • Myoglobinuria	• Altered mentation • ? Cerebral edema • ↑ Pain response • ↑ADH	• Pulmonary edema • Bronchospasm • Bronchorrhea • ARDS	• Nonblanching burned skin • Mottled clammy nonburned skin • Generalized edema in >25% body burn	• ↑Aldosterone • ↑ Cortisol

(ADH: antidiuretic hormone; ARDS: acute respiratory distress syndrome; PVR: pulmonary vascular resistance; SVR: systemic vascular resistance; SvO_2: venous desaturation)

TABLE 3: A few important pathophysiological changes during the hypermetabolic/hyperdynamic phase of burn (>48 hours after major burn injury).[51]

Cardiovascular system	Renal system	Brain	Lungs—inhalation injury	Liver	Bone marrow	Systemic inflammatory response
• Tachycardia • ↑ Cardiac index • ↓SVR • ↑ SvO_2 • Subclinical myocardial dysfunction	• ↑ GFR • ↓ Tubular function	• Altered mentation • ? Cerebral edema • ↑ Pain response	• Pulmonary edema • Bronchospasm • Bronchorrhea • ARDS • Pneumonia	• Altered metabolic function • ↑Blood flow • ↑Gluconeogenesis • ↓Coagulation factors	• ↓ Hematopoiesis • Anemia • Immunoparesis	• ↑O_2 consumption • ↑CO_2 production • Muscle catabolism • Insulin resistance • Persistence of generalized edema in > 25% body burn

(ARDS: acute respiratory distress syndrome; GFR: glomerular filtration rate; SVR: systemic vascular resistance)

About 24–72 hours following injury, a “hyperdynamic and hypermetabolic flow phase” starts.[51] This phase is marked by a decrease in peripheral vascular resistance, a rise in heart rate, and a decrease in vascular permeability, which leads to an increase in cardiac output[15] (which, 3–4 days after the burn, may exceed 1.5 times that of a nonburned condition). Furthermore, the metabolic rate rises to about three times the basal rate.[15,51]

The metabolic rate also increases to almost three times the basal rate. The hypermetabolic state following a burn injury can persist for up to 36 months after the initial damage.[11] Stress hormones such as catecholamines, glucocorticoids, and glucagon elevate peripheral insulin resistance, blood pressure, and the breakdown of proteins, lipids, and glycogen. Increased resting energy expenditure, elevated body temperature, loss of total body protein, muscle atrophy, increased acute-phase protein synthesis [including insulin-like growth factor 1 (IGF-1), which has anabolic effects], and ultimately increased organ catabolism linked to organ dysfunction and death are the end results. The pathophysiologic[11] changes that take place during the flow phase are summarized in **Table 3**.

Heart

Reduced diastolic compliance, delayed isovolemic relaxation, and diminished left ventricular systolic function can all be consequences of severe heat injury.[52,53] Increased left ventricular filling pressures and left heart failure are two outcomes of cardiac stress that may encourage extravascular fluid transport to the lungs. Venous congestion, a rise in right ventricular filling pressure, and right heart failure can all result from an increase in right ventricular workload.[53,54] The cause of cardiovascular dysfunction is often multifactorial and includes mitochondrial damage, catecholamine surge, and release of inflammatory mediators after burn injury. Macrophage migration inhibitor factor (MIF), an inflammatory cytokine, has been hypothesized to be related to late and prolonged cardiac dysfunction.[55]

Renal

Renal dysfunction or acute kidney injury (AKI) in MODS is reflected as oliguria despite adequate intravascular volume, rising creatinine, and fluid and electrolyte derangements. Acute kidney injury following thermal injury more likely occurs at two distinct time points: Initial

TABLE 4: Sequential (sepsis-related) organ failure assessment (SOFA) score.

	Score				
System	**0**	**1**	**2**	**3**	**4**
Respiration					
PaO_2/FiO_2, mm Hg (kPa)	≥400 (53.3)	<400 (53.3)	<300 (40)	<200 (26.7) with respiratory support	<100 (13.3) with respiratory support
Coagulation Platelets, $\times 10^3/\mu L$	≥150	<150	<100	<50	<20
Liver Bilirubin, mg/dL (µmol/L)	<1.2 (20)	1.2–1.9 (20–32)	2.0–5.9 (33–101)	6.0–11.9 (102–204)	>12.0 (204)
Cardiovascular	MAP ≥ 70 mm Hg	MAP <70 mm Hg	Dopamine < 5 or dobutamine (any dose)*	Dopamine 5.1–15 or epinephrine ≤0.1 or norepinephrine ≤0.1a	Dopamine > 15 or epinephrine >0.1 or norepinephrine >0.1*
Central nervous system (CNS)					
Glasgow Coma Scale score†	15	13–14	10–12	6–9	<6
Renal • Creatinine, mg/dL (µmol/L)	<1.2 (110)	1.2–1.9 (110–170)	2.0–3.4 (171–299)	3.5–4.9 (300–440)	>5.0 (440)
• Urine output, mL/day				<500	<200

*Catecholamine doses are given as µg/kg/min for at least 1 hour.

†Glasgow Coma Scale scores range from 3 to 15; higher score indicates better neurological function.

(FiO_2: fraction of inspired oxygen; MAP: mean arterial pressure; PaO_2: partial pressure of oxygen)

period of resuscitation (associated with early MODS and higher mortality risk) or late secondary to sepsis.[56]

The growing depth and extent of burn injuries are the main determinants of AKI. Myocardial depression and hypovolemia are contributing variables.[57] Early and sufficient fluid preservation and resuscitation are necessary to prevent early AKI.

Pressure inside the abdomen is another early risk factor. The acute-phase inflammatory response that follows a septic episode, such as vasodilation and a hypercoagulable condition, is the primary cause of the multifactorial late AKI.[5,17] These are some of the mechanisms and contributing factors:

- Sepsis-induced acute renal damage has been found to be strongly correlated with the levels of cytokines (IL-6, IL-10), as well as macrophage MIF.[58]
- The occlusion of tiny vessels may be the consequence of leukocytes interacting with activated endothelial cells.[49]
- Renal tubular cells may be precipitated and occluded by pigmenturia resulting from deep tissue injury.[57]
- Relative ischemia and microcirculatory dysfunction result from the activation of a hypercoagulable condition.[59]
- Intrarenal vasoconstriction due to neurohormonal activation.
- Various interventions in the intensive care unit (ICU) such as the use of nephrotoxic drugs and vasopressors.

Postburn AKI is more common in patients with advanced age, infection, need for mechanical ventilation, high APACHE II score, high Sequential Organ Failure Assessment (SOFA) score **(Table 4)**, inhalation damage, rhabdomyolysis, diabetes mellitus, high TBSA percent burnt, and surgery. AKI is linked to longer length of stay (LOS) and higher mortality in burn patients.[60,61]

Skeletal Muscle

The body's principal source of lean tissue and the major location where peripheral glucose is disposed of is the skeletal muscle. It is crucial for the control of metabolism.[25] The systemic catabolic consequences of burns frequently lead the muscles far from the burn site to be compromised in badly burned patients. The morbidity and mortality of patients are significantly impacted by this catabolic state of muscular loss. There are several mechanisms that underlie the wasting of muscle, including:

- Skeletal muscle serves as an endogenous amino acid reserve after a significant burn, supplying substrates for more urgent postburn processes such as acute-phase protein synthesis and skin deposition[17]
- Muscle mass loss caused by apoptosis or ubiquitin/proteasome-mediated protein degradation[62]

- Altered control of skeletal muscle mitochondrial coupling, resulting in greater heat production within the skeletal muscle[25]

Pulmonary

The characteristic abnormality of the lung in MODS is failure of gas exchange, reflected mainly in arterial hypoxemia with evolution to acute respiratory distress syndrome (ARDS). In persons with major burn injuries with large surface areas, inhalational injury is usually present.[63] Multiple pathologic factors contribute to impaired gas exchange.

- Airway obstruction can result from direct heat or steam injury to the upper airway, which can cause noticeable swelling of the face, tongue, epiglottis, and glottic opening.
- Tracheobronchial injury caused by inhaling chemicals in smoke results in decreased mucociliary transport, which in turn impairs the clearance of mucosal debris and bacteria.[17]
- The synthesis of surfactants may be lost, and mucosal debris may clog tiny airways, causing alveolar collapse and atelectasis.[51]
- In the absence of inhalation injury, severe cutaneous burns may affect the airway and the lungs by several mechanisms including increased capillary permeability and alveolar flooding due to inflammatory mediators, effects of fluid resuscitation, and infection.[51]
- Regional injury due to associated trauma.
- Oxygen consumption or oxygen transport mechanisms are hampered by breathing in cyanide or carbon monoxide, respectively.
- The implementation of ventilatory support, which may be necessary in the event of respiratory failure, may lead to mechanical lung injuries (barotrauma, atelectrauma, and volutrauma), trigger a localized inflammatory response, and cause biotrauma due to the release of inflammatory mediators from damaged cells. Additionally, the mechanical harm caused by positive-pressure ventilation and the localized inflammatory response mediated by circulating leukocytes may exacerbate pulmonary dysfunction.[21] The implementation of mechanical ventilation is regarded as the "second hit" in reality. An enormous pulmonary inflammatory response is triggered by the "second hit" of mechanical ventilation after the lung has been "primed" by an initial insult such as pneumonia, acid aspiration, or trauma. The release of immune mediators into the systemic circulation from the lung is one potential method. This phenomenon is associated with programmed cell death (apoptosis) in distal organs (such as kidney and colonic villi) and end-organ dysfunction (kidney), which is likely to cause MODS.[64]
- Lung injury repair results in fibrosis and hyaline membrane formation may lead to further hypoxemia, increased work of breathing, and features of late ARDS.

Gastrointestinal

The intestinal epithelium physically divides the intestinal lumen from the internal milieu. The mucous layer, intestinal epithelial cells, intercellular junctions, submucosal lamina propria, and other mechanical elements make up the intestinal barrier. Immunological elements include a multitude of immune-competent cells, such as lymphocytes, macrophages, dendritic cells, and plasma cells. Biological elements include resident intestinal bacteria like *Lactobacillus* and *Bifidobacterium*. Lastly, chemical elements include substances like gastric acid, bile, digestive enzymes, muramidase, and mucopolysaccharide, which can inhibit the adherence and colonization of bacteria.[65]

Severe burn injuries usually exhibit intestinal barrier dysfunction.[66] A number of factors, including postburn shock bacterial translocation, hypercatabolism, sepsis, multiple organ dysfunction syndrome, immune disturbances, neuroendocrine mediators, hypoxia/ischemia, complement activation, oxygen-free radicals, inflammatory mediators, proinflammatory cytokines, and other mediators released in the stress response, are linked to intestinal mechanical barrier dysfunction, which is associated with severe burn injuries.[67,68]

Furthermore, during sepsis and severe burn injury, alterations in gastrointestinal motility and nutritional absorption are also noted.[69] These manifest as decreased colonic absorption of water and sodium,[70] lower net absorption of water, electrolytes, and glucose from the jejunum,[71] and increased contractions and motility of the colon.[72] Electrolyte imbalances, dehydration, and diarrhea may result from these alterations. If these alterations are substantial, there may be a reduction in tissue perfusion and oxygen supply, which puts these patients at a higher risk of developing MODS. Last but not least, the risk of Curling's ulcer is increased by elevated stress hormone output.

In a study assessing the symptoms of gut dysfunction (diarrhea, vomiting/regurgitation, bowel distention, high gastric residual volume, absence of bowel sounds, and gastrointestinal bleeding), it was shown that not one of these factors was a reliable indicator of death on its own. However, among critically ill patients using mechanical ventilation, the risk of death increased thrice when three or more of these were present on the first day of the ICU.[73] Patients with burns and other diagnoses were included in the study.

HEPATIC

Alteration of liver function tests is extremely common following major burns. Hepatic dysfunction following severe burn injury is reflected in increased levels of aspartate aminotransferase (AST) and alanine aminotransferase (ALT) levels. Following burn injuries, these levels rise right away and are high for 4–6 weeks.[17] The ALT test is more sensitive and specific for hepatocyte injury, while the AST test can also be elevated in cases of cardiac arrest or muscle injury. Hepatocyte damage can be sensitively detected by both AST and ALT levels. These increases typically have a benign nature and go away on their own. Serum bilirubin elevation is less common but has greater detrimental effects. Patients with severe and long-lasting abnormalities of the liver enzymes, such as elevated bilirubin, typically have some burn-related complication, such as sepsis and their prognosis is uncertain.[74]

It has been established that liver damage is associated with a higher risk of hepatic edema formation. The weight and size of the liver rise dramatically in the first week following injury, peaking 2 weeks later.[75] Even at 12 months, the weight of the liver might still increase by 40–50% in comparison to the expected liver weight.[75]

Coagulation

Patients with severe burns frequently experience coagulopathy, which is linked to higher rates of morbidity and death.[35] Coagulopathy in patients with severe burns has a complex etiology. While endothelial damage, hypoperfusion, hypothermia (caused by either massive fluid therapy or loss of heat through evaporation from nonepithelialized areas), and aggressive fluid strategies used to avoid shock, which also may induce hypothermia, and the consumption or dilution of coagulation factors caused by surgical interventions are significant factors involved in the exacerbation or initiation of coagulopathy, burn-associated complications such as sepsis and bleeding from repeated wound excisions and other surgical procedures[76] are the primary causes of coagulopathy in the later phase.

Following burn injury, coagulopathy is characterized by deficiencies in natural anticoagulation as well as procoagulant and antifibrinolytic alterations.[77,78] Within 7 days following the burn, this hypercoagulable state frequently returns to more stable levels,[78] barring the emergence of a complication that also leads to coagulopathy. Patients with severe burns are also susceptible to thrombotic and embolic consequences. In addition to immobility, other factors implicated are the hypercoagulable state, multiple blood transfusions, and recurrent surgical procedures.[79] The degree of burn[80] increases the risk of thromboembolization.

Additionally, it has been seen that coagulopathy is linked to a higher death rate in patients with severe burns when it coexists with hypothermia and acidemia. Patients who arrive at the hospital with coagulopathy, hypothermia, and acidemia have a five-fold increased death rate compared to those who do not experience these three conditions.[81]

Neurological

The most readily recognizable manifestation of severe burn injury-induced neurological dysfunction is an altered level of consciousness. Agitation, disorientation, unusual posture, brief loss of consciousness, convulsions, and even shock are possible additional symptoms.[17] The most common factor for altered mentation is due to inhalational burn causing cellular hypoxia. During the early stage, hypoxia can be related to fire injuries, inhalation injury, and exposure to carbon monoxide intoxication and cyanide toxicity. Other causes contributing to the altered mental state include subclinical cerebral edema,[17] reduced cerebral perfusion pressure, metabolic alterations, fluid and electrolyte derangements, and the use of sedatives and analgesics.

Since burn victims are immunosuppressed, they are easily subjected to bacterial infections and sepsis-induced encephalopathy which may result in greater neurological deterioration. These patients with sepsis, MOF and prolonged hospital stay are at risk for critical illness neuropathy.

Clinical Measurement Systems

Defining MODS has been difficult as it can develop following a variety of mechanisms, both noninfectious and infectious. Patients with severe burn injury are in an immunocompromised state and are at an increased risk of developing various infectious complications. In reality, >60% of fatalities from infectious complications were linked to at least one related organ failure, and 15% of patients with burns had MOF, according to one autopsy report.[82] Every infective episode has the potential to be a "second hit," triggering an abnormal hyperinflammatory reaction that damages organs.

Moreover, criteria of SIRS, which were used to diagnose sepsis in the past, are no longer used for this purpose and more specifically are not applicable to patients with severe burn injury. The basal temperature of these patients is reset to 38.5°C, and they may experience tachycardia and tachypnea for several months. Leukocytosis is a poor indication of sepsis due to ongoing exposure to inflammatory mediators. Therefore, it has been suggested to diagnose sepsis in these patients based on other markers such as increased fluid demand, declining platelet counts over a 3-day period, abnormal mentation, poor oxygenation, and decreased renal function. As patients with major burns are in a condition of persistent systemic inflammatory stimulation, it is actually inappropriate to refer to them as SIRS patients.

Infection and Sepsis

Since sepsis is a prominent cause of problems in critical care units, choosing an appropriate definition and set of criteria is essential for the early identification and prediction of sepsis in burn patients. In order to determine the sensitivity of the sepsis criteria in burn patients, Yan and colleagues compared the new Sepsis-3 consensus definition[83] with the ABA definition (60%) and Mann-Salinas definition (20%). They found that, in comparison to the two criteria,[28,84] Sepsis-3 has a higher sensitivity (85%). Sepsis-3's primary contribution is its argument that sepsis is more specifically caused by multiple organ dysfunction than by inflammation. It remains challenging to ascertain if MODS is more sepsis-specific than inflammatory. Consequently, rather than using retrospective criteria, it has been suggested that sepsis be clinically evaluated, diagnosed, and recorded prospectively. Thus, the abovementioned indicators of infection or sepsis (increased fluid requirement, decreasing platelet counts over 3 days, altered mentation, worsening oxygenation, and impaired renal function) are nonspecific when taken into account alone; however, the presence of two or more of these factors in a burn patient with an underlying suspicion of infection should strongly raise concern for early signs of sepsis.[84]

The revised Sepsis-3 Consensus Definition, which was created in 2016, has been demonstrated to be the most accurate in predicting the beginning of sepsis in the group of burn patients, while being intended for use in the general ICU setting.[84]

Predictors of Severity and Mortality

Several factors contribute to the host response and have been discussed previously **(see Box 1)**. Significant predictors of mortality include older age, higher burned surface area, concomitant inhalational burns, full-thickness burns, and a higher abbreviated burn severity index (ABSI).[85]

Management

The prevention of MOF is likely to be more effective than its treatment.[86] Preventing the onset of MODS through therapies directed at modulating SIRS or blocking CARS is more likely to be of benefit than the efforts to treat MODS once established, when the treatment is largely supportive.[21] Priorities in the management of MODS are as follows.

Early Recognition of Illness

An early and accurate assessment of the severity of the burn injury and associated injuries, if any, is important as it determines all subsequent treatment decisions.[14] As noted in the various chapters of this book, the assessment methodology must include an organized, sequential evaluation of the primary and secondary surveys as well as a consideration of the necessity for additional consultation and potential transportation in order to maximize results at specialized facilities.

Patients should be screened for the already existing comorbidities including depression or any substance abuse, possibility of the need for early intubation in view of the presence of smoke inhalation injury, risk of developing complications such as acute kidney injury[87,88] and acute respiratory distress syndrome,[89] and possibility of the presence of multidrug-resistant micro-organisms (which will help in choosing an appropriate antimicrobial). Another important aspect of planning burn care is to predict mortality following burn injury using Baux score or the modified Baux score, which includes the presence or absence of inhalation injury.

Early Resuscitation

Fluid resuscitation is typically necessary for patients with burn sizes more than 20% TBSA, electrical injuries, smoke inhalation, or concurrent trauma.[14] Maintaining end-organ perfusion while minimizing resuscitation-related morbidity, such as compartment syndromes involving the extremities, abdomen, and/or orbital compartments that require emergency decompression to prevent cell death, is the aim of fluid resuscitation.

The rate should be based on a combination of various endpoints including a targeted urine output of 0.5 mL/kg/h for adults and 1 mL/kg/h for children, decreasing lactate levels and base deficit, mixed venous saturation > 70%, central venous pressure < 6 cm H_2O, cardiac index > 2.2 L/min/m^2, and mean arterial pressure of 65–70 mm Hg.[53] If one of these goals is not met, a fluid challenge or a variety of dynamic tests [such as passive leg raising (PLR), pulse pressure variation (PPV), and stroke volume variation (SVV)] should be used to assess fluid responsiveness. If the patient does not respond to fluids, administer norepinephrine, conduct an echocardiogram (ECHO), and look for signs of heart dysfunction. When a patient responds well to fluids, escalate the IV crystalloid dosage by 20% and reevaluate each goal every hour. If every target is met, reduce the IV crystalloid rate by 10% every hour and verify each goal on an hourly basis.[53] Prerenal causes (such as a drop in renal blood flow or renal perfusion pressure brought on by fluid depletion) or other causes of acute kidney injury in burn patients (such as hemolysis, rhabdomyolysis, inflammation and immune-related response, and intrarenal vasoconstriction brought on by neurohormonal activation) may also contribute to decreased urine output. Urine production is therefore not a trustworthy measure of the best course of resuscitation. On the other hand, oliguria can be caused by venous congestion associated with an increase in venous pressure as a result of either an increase in ventricular filling pressure or a drop in belly pressure. Moreover, hyperosmolarity brought on by hyperglycemia or an increase in the glomerular transcapillary fluid rate fraction may occur after a sudden drop in plasma albumin concentration.[53]

The fluid of choice is a balanced crystalloid; warmed Ringer's lactate solution is the most popular type. It has been recommended to perform "colloid rescue" utilizing other adjuncts such as albumin or plasma since the exclusive use of a crystalloid solution might lead to over-resuscitation, which is linked to the development of resuscitation-related morbidity.[90]

In severely burned patients who are dependent on vasopressors, the use of low-dose hydrocortisone may shorten the shock period by reducing capillary leakage and correcting adrenal insufficiency.[91]

The major objective of treating patients in shock is to eliminate circulating inflammatory mediators, which can be achieved by using additional adjunct therapies including therapeutic plasma exchange (TPE) and high-volume hemofiltration (HVHF) at dosages > 70 mL/kg/h.[92] Patients with severe burn injuries have demonstrated improved organ function, reversal of shock, shorter time to need for vasopressor treatment, decreased mortality, improved mean arterial blood pressure, increased urine output, and decreased lactate levels when using these adjunct therapies. These therapies need a lot of resources and are only offered in a few centers.

Early Definitive Treatment

Prompt Control of Infection

Treating infections (bacterial, fungal, and parasitic) is one of the definitive ways to contain SIRS and prevent it from progressing to MODS.

Even though burn injury patients are at an increased risk for developing severe infection (secondary to loss of the skin barrier as well as immunosuppression) from both common and nosocomial organisms, and burn wound sepsis is one of the common causes leading to MODS, increased LOS, and mortality, there is no role of prophylactic antibiotics in burn injury patients.[93] Systemic antimicrobial therapy is indicated only for patients with proven wound infection or sepsis.

Burn Wound Coverage

The gold standard treatment for burn wounds is early excision and skin grafting, which lowers the risk of burn wound sepsis and improves both mortality and morbidity by removing the biological nidus for infection and attenuating the hypermetabolic state.[94]

Supportive Care

Providing evidence-based supportive critical care has the goal of creating the best possible environment for wound healing during the post grafting phase.[14] It should address every facet of enhancing the circumstances around wound healing and comprise the following:

- One important aspect that affects burn patients' prognosis is hemodynamic support during the early stages (fluid resuscitation and sporadic vasopressor support), as previously mentioned, and continuing thereafter.[95] Both under- and over-resuscitation may have a negative outcome; therefore, maintaining an optimum balance is always a challenge in these patients.[53]
- Support for nutrition is essential to the treatment of burns. Major burn patients exhibit hypermetabolic states that are higher than those of any other disease condition.[96] Upon acute admission, these patients' resting metabolic rates (RMRs) can reach up to 180% of basal rates, and their daily caloric requirements can surpass 5,000 kcal. If left untreated, this can lead to immunological compromise, decreased healing capacity, and loss of lean body mass.[97]
- The benefits of intravenous support include a reduction in sepsis linked to gut permeability and clinical infection, as well as notably shorter hospital stays. It also helps maintain gut mucosal integrity and can lessen the increase in catabolic hormone secretion associated with burns.[98]
- Using pharmaceutical adjuncts, such as propranolol and oxandrolone, to lessen the effects of hypermetabolism and aid in the healing process. Effective pain management, early wound excision and closure, adequate nutritional support, and a few pharmaceutical adjuncts such as anabolic steroids, insulin, and propranolol are therapeutic techniques used to block or attenuate hypermetabolic reactions.
    - The main mediators of the hypermetabolic response after burns larger than 40% TBSA

are catecholamines and corticosteroids. After a burn, plasma levels of catecholamines and corticosteroids increase 10- to 50-fold and last for up to 9 months.

- Oxandrolone is an androgen receptor agonist that decreases weight loss, promotes muscle growth, boosts donor-site wound healing, and enhances muscle protein catabolism by promoting protein synthesis.[99,100] Compared to testosterone, it has substantially less virilizing activity, which makes it more appropriate for usage in women and young children. Additional advantages include better whole body mass, preservation of lean body mass, and shorter hospital stays and critical care.[101]
- Propranolol and other beta-adrenergic blockers reduce energy expenditure, restrict insulin resistance, stop muscle loss, and function as anti-inflammatory medications to suppress the catabolic consequences of a burn. However, because adrenergic antagonists carry a risk of cardiorespiratory instability, care must be taken while using them in an ICU. A recent systematic review was unable to demonstrate any benefits in terms of incidence of sepsis, length of hospital stay, or mortality.[102] Other researches, however, have shown decreased muscle catabolism and enhanced wound healing.[103] Additionally, propranolol lessens hepatic fatty infiltration, which is often brought on by enhanced peripheral lipolysis and modified substrate handling.[104,105]
- It is crucial to have proper pain management with the right dosage of opioids and adjuncts that spare the opioid. Postburn pain is excruciating, often difficult to manage, and associated with depression and anxiety.[106]
- The burn patient's metabolic rate rises in response to pain. These patients suffer from both continuing background discomfort and procedure-related (e.g., dressing changes, excision and grafting procedures, physical therapy, and line insertion) suffering.[51]
- A universal approach to the management of pain during ICU treatment is not possible. Pain management must be individualized, especially for very ill and typically unstable patients.
- While performing a surgical procedure, any infusion of sedatives and narcotics should not be stopped to maintain a steady state of effect. In fact, the rate of infusion should be increased or other drugs must be added to maintain effective intraoperative analgesia.[51]

Hypothermia prevention: Several strategies are employed to prevent and treat burn-related hypothermia. These strategies include increasing the room temperature in preclinical rescue vehicles, the operating room (OR), the ICU, staged excision and grafting, limiting the amount of time an operation takes if at all possible, and giving warm fluids.[107-109] Invasive warming devices (esophageal heat-exchange devices[110,111] or a warming device inserted into the inferior vena cava[112]) may be used if these alternatives are ineffective given the severity of the injury.

Preventing common complications that arise from hospitalization, such as venous thromboembolic complications, stress ulcers, and pneumonia, are associated with a ventilator, bloodstream infections from catheter use, and urinary tract infections from catheter use.

Nosocomial Infections

The most common nosocomial infections in ICUs are bloodstream infections related to intravascular catheters, urinary tract infections associated with catheters, post-traumatic intra-abdominal infections, and surgical site infections. By applying preventive methods appropriately and effectively, which can only be done at the bedside, they can be avoided. It is imperative to adhere to the fundamental guidelines for surveillance tactics, as well as general preventive measures including standard and isolation precautions and antibiotic use monitoring. In order to standardize the practice, regardless of location or person, specific practical procedures for infections associated with ICUs should be implemented. Regular documentation of actions should be documented as part of "bundle care".[113]

In ICUs, at minimum, the following two bundles ought to be used: Ventilator bundle[113] and central-line maintenance bundle.

- Burn patients with bloodstream infections have a five-fold mortality increase compared with burn patients who do not have a bloodstream infection.[113] The following steps may help prevent central line bloodstream infection (CLABSI):
  1. Daily review of line necessity
  2. Hand hygiene before manipulation of the intravenous (IV) system
  3. Daily inspection of the insertion site
  4. Catheter-site care
  5. Alcohol scrub of insertion hubs for 15 seconds before each use

Burn patients are among the groups at maximum risk for ventilator-associated pneumonia (VAP), and meticulous care must be taken to prevent VAP.

The ventilator bundles have the following steps:

1. Elevation of the head end of the bed between 30° and 40°
2. Mouth care with 1–2% chlorhexidine (6 hours)
3. Subglottic aspiration 1–2 hours
4. Daily sedation vacation
5. Daily assessment of readiness to wean
6. Daily spontaneous breathing trial
7. Peptic ulcer disease prophylaxis
8. Deep venous thrombosis prophylaxis

Thromboprophylaxis

Individuals who have sustained burns are more susceptible to venous thromboembolism (VTE). The endothelial damage, hypercoagulable condition, and stasis (Virchow's triad) linked to burn injury[114] are the primary causes of this tendency. Furthermore, this risk is multiplied by extended hospital stays, ventilator support, repeated surgeries, multiple central venous cannulations, and decreased mobility.[114] However, there is a small risk of bleeding problems and heparin-induced thrombocytopenia when administering heparin; this risk can be further decreased to 0.1% by utilizing low-molecular-weight heparin (LMWH). Given the significantly higher incidence of symptomatic VTE, it would seem that there are more advantages to VTE prophylaxis than disadvantages to not taking preventive action. For patients with acute burns, a greater dose of LMWH and regular antifactor Xa level monitoring are beneficial.[114] However, another study has questioned the effectiveness of chemoprophylaxis[115] concluding that chemoprophylaxis does not prevent VTEs.

Stress Ulcer Prophylaxis

All patients with major burn injury (>20% TBSA) should receive stress ulcer prophylaxis, which should continue through ICU stay.[116,117]

Consideration of Premorbid Disease

Managing a burn injury patient with a significant comorbidity such as heart failure or cirrhosis of liver or the one who develops renal failure due to different causes during resuscitation is always challenging. These patients cannot be managed with a standard protocol;[57] rather, all will require an individualized approach to resuscitation based on pathophysiology and the severity of the comorbidity, and the remaining functional reserves of the patient. Therefore, it is important to have previous knowledge of comorbidities and their severity, and the functional reserves of the patient. Early recognition and appropriate treatment are the primary basis of prevention and successful management of MODS.

Heart Failure

When a patient with preexisting heart failure sustains a severe burn injury, the hypovolemia and myocardial depression linked to acute burns are combined with their preexisting cardiac illness, creating a true acute-on-chronic failure scenario. Systolic dysfunction, diastolic dysfunction with raised diastolic tone, and dysrhythmias are the clinical markers of failing heart tissue. A neurohumoral response is triggered by a failing heart, activating the renin–angiotensin–aldosterone axis and raising baseline norepinephrine and sympathetic tone levels.[57]

These patients require serial ECHO and/or other means such as estimation of serum B-type natriuretic peptide, which correlates well with volume overload, in a serial manner to guide optimum resuscitation.[118] One of the best indicators of survival in heart failure is response to dobutamine. Because they are maximum endogenously stimulated and do not have any functional reserve left, individuals who do not enhance their cardiac output during dobutamine stimulation have a lower chance of surviving.[119]

To restore a sufficient left ventricular end-diastolic volume (LVEDV) and maintain a right atrial pressure of <8 mm Hg and a pulmonary artery occlusion pressure of <18 mm Hg, volume resuscitation must be carefully titrated. To accomplish these goals, angiotensin-converting enzyme (ACE) inhibitors, diuretics, and milrinone (a phosphodiesterase inhibitor), which acts similarly to dobutamine in increasing intracellular cyclic adenosine monophosphate (AMP), might be utilized as needed. Intra-aortic balloon counterpulsation (IABP) and continuous veno-venous hemodialysis (CVVH) are more sophisticated adjuncts to the failing myocardium in the presence of heat injury. These techniques reduce large intravascular volume variations and enable cautious fluid removal.[57]

Cirrhosis of Liver

Because of its fibrosis, scarring, and regenerating nodules, cirrhosis causes portal hypertension, which makes the liver's perfusion particularly sensitive to changes in volume. Hypovolemia can quickly lead to further ischemia and necrosis of the hepatocellular membrane. However, over-resuscitation with crystalloids can result in tight ascites, which can exacerbate intravascular volume loss and intra-abdominal hypertension during resuscitation.[57]

There is a clear correlation between the diagnosis of cirrhosis and death. Patients without cirrhosis had a death rate of 12.7% in patients with burn sizes between 10 and 50%, but patients with cirrhosis had an 83.3% mortality rate ($p < 0.001$).[120]

For these patients, resuscitation with albumin or fresh frozen plasma (FFP) is more suitable and less dependent on traditional crystalloid resuscitation techniques. Furthermore, these individuals frequently exhibit reduced levels of factors V, VII, and X (resulting from both malnourishment and reduced hepatic synthesis) as well as a dysfunction of gluconeogenesis. For these individuals, vitamin K therapy, FFP transfusions, and 10% glucose infusions are required. A thorough monitoring process is required for a successful result. These patients frequently exhibit decreased SVR and higher cardiac output, which are most likely caused by gut hormones and a decreased susceptibility of the splanchnic vasculature to catecholamines.[57,121] These patients do not respond well to measures such as cardiac output, mixed venous O_2 saturations, or SVR. The best information available to direct resuscitation in these patients comes from right atrial pressure and pulmonary artery occlusion pressures.

Renal Failure

Renal failure can occur in up to one-third of patients with severe burn injury. Of these, about 30% happen within the first 5 days after the burn, and the majority happen later in the burn course and are typically linked to sepsis.[122] 50–60% of severely ill patients die in hospitals due to acute renal failure.[123]

Renal failure can be caused directly or indirectly by hypoperfusion (resulting from hypovolemia and cardiac depression), systemic neurohumoral chemicals and cytokines, and pigmenturia. Preventing renal failure entails treating pigmenturia as it arises, avoiding any nephrotoxic substances, and providing optimal volume resuscitation.

The prognosis of an acute renal failure event, which is the number of days until renal function is restored or the rate of end-stage renal loss, can be monitored using clinical criteria such as risk, injury, failure, loss of kidney function, and end-stage kidney disease (RIFLE) or acute-kidney injury network (AKIN), as well as a variety of plasma and urine tests {a urine osmolality > 500, urine/plasma osmolality ratio > 2, a urinary sodium < 20 mEq/L, and a fractional excretion of sodium < 1 [FENA = (UNa/PNa)/UCr/PCr)] and newer markers like neutrophil gelatinase-associated lipocalin (NGAL), kidney-injury marker 1 (KIM-1), N-acetyl-β-D-glucosaminidase (NAG), cystatin-C, and interleukin (IL)-18} in the first 24 hours following the onset of symptoms.[57,124]

When there is no urine output to indicate the volume status, and there are clinical symptoms such as a systolic blood pressure of <90 mm Hg, agitation, and confusion, it makes sense to titrate resuscitative fluid. Alternatively, a Swan–Ganz catheter or any other device may be used.[57]

However, both too little (can cause renal failure) and too much (can start the process of fluid creep) fluid have the potential to negatively impact the outcome.

It is necessary to try to utilize substantial doses of intravenous diuretics to convert oliguric renal failure to nonoliguric renal failure if the diagnosis of acute tubular necrosis (ATN) is fairly established. While there is no proof that this may lessen the requirement for dialysis or cause renal function to recover quicker, it might facilitate the management of intravascular volume status and avoid the hypoxia linked to edema and pulmonary congestion. Acidosis and hyperkalemia, if they exist, need to be managed properly.

Finally, some people do require dialysis. Patients who have symptoms of systemic uremic syndrome, pulmonary edema, blood urea nitrogen (BUN) > 70 mg/dL, creatinine > 5 mg/dL, K^+ > 6 mEq/L, base excess < 15 mEq/L, or any combination of these, then dialysis may be considered. The same standards apply to patients who do not have burns. Individuals who meet these criteria should be dialyzed with intermittent hemodialysis for patients whose blood pressure is stable or with CVVH for patients whose marginal intravascular volume status prevents them from being able to tolerate the flow rates and fluid withdrawal rates of intermittent dialysis without experiencing significant hypotension.[57] Nonetheless, each patient's care will need to be customized.

Prior understanding of the risk factors of mortality owing to MOF may aid in risk classification and the initiation of early therapeutic measures, according to an earlier study conducted in a high-risk group of surgical patients. The study found that MOF was the leading cause of death and that it was correlated with age, increased serum lactate, diabetes, peritonitis, and unexpected surgery.[125]

Prevention of Secondary Insults

Several conditions can serve as secondary stimuli that precipitate organ dysfunction. They consist of blood transfusions, infections, early primary or re-operative surgery to remove necrotic tissue and drain abscess, positive-pressure ventilation during a subsequent operation, and abdominal compartment syndrome (ACS).[21] The ACS results in high ventilator pressures, decreased cardiac output, and impaired renal function.[126] Even though the physiologic effects of ACS usually reverse on decompression, the immunomodulatory effects may persist and have the potential to trigger MOF.[127]

The role of other precipitating stimuli has already been discussed in appropriate sections.

Adjunctive Therapies

Antioxidants

Severe burns lead to inflammation and production of free oxygen radicals from multiple, distinct sources. Through a variety of processes, these free oxygen radicals damage organ tissues, oxidize lipids, disrupt cellular function, and cause the generation of inflammatory cytokines, which in turn causes MODS.[128]

It has been suggested that antioxidants be used in addition to initial resuscitation therapy. Adjuvant high-dose ascorbic acid delivery (66 mg/kg/h) during the first 24 hours following burn injury considerably reduces fluid volume requirements (5.5 vs. 3.0 mL/kg/% TBSA; $p < 0.01$).[129] This was demonstrated in a randomized controlled study.

Adrenal Insufficiency and Corticosteroids

Following a significant burn, there is typically a strong inflammatory condition that may result in adrenal injury.[130] Adrenal insufficiency (AI) development appears to be linked to older age and higher TBSA burn. The diagnosis of AI significantly raises the probability of mortality following severe heat injury.[131] Consideration should be given to adrenal insufficiency in major burned patients experiencing circulatory-refractory shock.[130] In badly burned patients who are dependent on vasopressors, low-dose hydrocortisone may shorten the shock period by reducing capillary leakage and correcting adrenal insufficiency. The corticosteroid-treated group in a randomized controlled trial had a shorter median norepinephrine treatment time (57 vs. 120 hours; $p = 0.035$) than the placebo group, but there was no difference in mortality.[91] However, there is still debate over the effects of hydrocortisone therapy on the immune system and the likelihood of secondary infection in burn patients.[53]

INSULIN

A major element of the postburn hypermetabolic response, hyperglycemia is linked to a high rate of morbidity and death. It has been demonstrated that hyperglycemia impairs immunological function by changing the cytokine production of macrophages, which in turn causes a reduction in lymphocyte proliferation and a suppression of leukocyte bactericidal activity.[132] Elevated glucose levels further impair immune function; at glucose levels > 220 mg/dL, immunoglobulin glycosylation occurs, decreasing opsonic action.[132] In critically ill patients, survival and morbidity improve when blood glucose is < 110 g/dL.[132] Better wound healing is also linked to glucose management.[17] Continuous infusions of this anabolic peptide in severe burn patients not only promote wound healing and normoglycemia, but also stop muscle protein breakdown and preserve lean mass.[132,133] In addition to its anabolic effects, insulin has been shown to potentially neutralize the proinflammatory action of hyperglycemia, thus exhibiting anti-inflammatory effects.[134]

The ideal target glycemic range is uncertain. In general, till ideal blood glucose levels for the treatment of severely burned adult patients are defined, the daily average glucose level of 140 mg/dL should be maintained for at least 70% of the hospital admission.

Insulin resistance lasts in burn patients for at least 9 months after hospital release and may continue for 3 years or longer.[17] Given its side effect profile in the outpatient situation, metformin is a promising substitute for insulin and seems to have effects comparable to those of the hormone in severely injured patients.[132]

Ulinastatin

A urinary trypsin inhibitor called ulinastatin has been demonstrated to minimize AKI damage following burns[135] and may lower mortality in acute patients, particularly those with intermediate levels (40–80%) of burned BSA.[136] Ulinastatin can dramatically reduce renal interstitial damage and inhibit interstitial collagen deposition, although without having a statistically significant effect on BUN or serum creatinine levels.[135] The downregulation of ulinastatin on the TGF-β/Smad signaling pathways is probably the cause of its renoprotective activity.[137]

Role of Biomarkers

The primary risk factors for the development of sepsis are cases of burn site infection, hypovolemia, dysregulated inflammatory response, and hypermetabolism. Burn patients who have sepsis may proceed to septic shock[28]—sepsis with MODS—if they are not properly recognized and managed. Actually, if the patient survives the first 24 hours after the injury, MODS is the primary cause of death in serious burn patients.[138] Selecting a suitable definition and set of criteria for the early identification and prediction of sepsis in burn patients is especially crucial because of the high mortality rate associated with the condition.

Even though Sepsis-3 argues that multiple organ dysfunction is more sepsis-specific than inflammation[83] and suggests more accurate signs for detecting sepsis, such as renal dysfunction, increased fluid requirement, decreased platelet count, change in mental status, and declining pulmonary function,[138] it is still difficult to distinguish sepsis from SIRS because they have similar clinical manifestations in many areas. Thus, to better define, differentiate (sepsis from burn inflammation), and prognosticate burn sepsis, several biomarkers associated with burn sepsis have been studied and a few have proven their clinical utility in certain organs. These include the following: Kidney (NGAL), liver (glutamate/glutamine and cytokeratin-18[139]), heart (NT-pro-BNP, adrenomedullin, and pentraxin), and lung (pentraxin-3, IL-8, and IL-18). Procalcitonin, presepsin,[28] and C-reactive protein (CRP) are further predictors linked to burn sepsis. Furthermore, studies have investigated the potential function of a few pro- and anti-inflammatory (IL-6 and IL-10) and proinflammatory (IL-8 and IL-18) cytokines in the early diagnosis of sepsis after burn injury. Burn patients with sepsis showed greater levels of TNF-α and IL-6 values[140,141] than burn patients without any signs of sepsis. Another clinical study on burn victims[142] found a strong correlation between blood levels of IL-8 and sepsis in pediatric patients with elevated IL-81.[143] However, it appears that there is no single cytokine, which is good enough to predict the outcome.[139]

SUMMARY

Results from MODS seem to have become better over time. In particular, mortality has dropped in specialist burn care facilities that use strong antibiotics, forceful resuscitation, early enteral feeding, and early wound excision and covering. Though the pathogenesis of MODS is becoming better understood, solid prognostication method, preventive measures, or viable clinical treatments are yet to be developed.[38] A complex web of physiologic insults, such as injury, tissue ischemia, infection, host response, and several therapies required to sustain failing organ systems, come together to form MODS.[144] The clinical syndrome that results represents the state of a dynamic balance that exists between each of the component mediators. This is because there are numerous interdependent mediators involved, and the activity of one inducing the expression of others may amplify, inhibit, or otherwise modify the expression of the entire process. Comprehending the intricate relationship between many systems and the failure of organs is essential for formulating logical approaches to stop, alter, or manage the condition.[144] Many problems are still unresolved. For instance, tactics that work well at the beginning of the process might not work well later on when the pathophysiological process has changed. In a similar vein, tactics focused on one manifestation can have surprisingly unanticipated effects on others, and so forth.[144]

The speed at which new findings are emerging at the genetic, molecular, and cellular levels, however, suggests a more fundamental and as-yet-undiscovered common pathway that could offer a more tenable explanation for the wide range of triggers and occasionally persistent organ dysfunction.[38] With any luck, the knowledge so acquired will direct the precise identification and treatment of infection, SIRS, and MODS at various stages of the disease.

REFERENCES

1. Mizock BA. The multiple organ dysfunction syndrome. Dis Mon. 2009;55(8):476-526.
2. Skillman JJ, Bushnell LS, Goldman H, Silen W. Respiratory failure, hypotension, sepsis and jaundice. A clinical syndrome associated with lethal hemorrhage from acute stress ulceration of the stomach. Am J Surg. 1969;117:523-30.
3. Tilney NL, Baily GI, Morgan AP. Sequential system failure after rupture of abdominal aortic aneurysm. An unsolved problem in postoperative care. Ann Surg. 1973;178:117-22.
4. Baue AE. Multiple, progressive or sequential systems failure. Arch Surg. 1975;110:779-81
5. Eiseman B, Beart R, Norton L. Multiple organ failure. Surg Gynecol Obstet. 1977;44:323-6.
6. Fry DE, Pearlstein L, Fulton RL, Polk Jr HC. Multiple system organ failure. The role of uncontrolled infection. Arch Surg. 1980;115:136-40.
7. Goris RJA, te Boekhorst TPA, Nuytinck JKS, Gimbrère JS. Multiple-organ failure: Generalized autodestructive inflammation? Arch Surg. 1985;120:1109-15.
8. Meakins JL. Etiology of multiple organ failure. J Trauma. 1990;30:5165-6 (suppl).
9. American College of Chest Physicians/Society of Critical Care Medicine Consensus Conference Committee. Definitions for sepsis and organ failure and guidelines for the use of innovative therapies in sepsis. Crit Care Med. 1992;20:864-70.
10. Marshall JC, Cook DJ, Christou NV, Bernard GR, Sprung CL, Sibbald WJ. Multiple organ dysfunction score: A reliable descriptor of a complex clinical outcome. Crit Care Med. 1995;23(10):1638-52.
11. Jeschke MG, Gauglitz GG, Kulp GA, Finnerty CC, Williams FN, Kraft R, et al. Long-term persistance of the pathophysiologic response to severe burn injury. PLoS One. 2011;6(7):e21245.
12. Rowan MP, Cancio LC, Elster EA, Burmeister DM, Rose LF, Natesan S, et al. Burn wound healing and treatment: review and advancements. Crit Care. 2015;19:243.
13. Porter C, Tompkins RG, Finnerty CC, Sidossis LS, Suman OE, Herndon DN. The metabolic stress response to burn trauma: current understanding and therapies. Lancet. 2016;388:1417-26.
14. Jeschke MG, van Baar ME, Choudhry MA, Chung KK, Gibran NS, Logsetty S. Burn injury. Nat Rev Dis Primers. 2020;6(1):11.
15. Vaughn L, Beckel N. Severe burn injury, burn shock, and smoke inhalation injury in small animals. Part 1: burn classification and pathophysiology. J Vet Emerg Crit Care (San Antonio). 2012;22:179-86.
16. Bohr S, Patel SJ, Shen K, Vitalo AG, Brines M, Cerami A, et al. Alternative erythropoietin mediated signaling prevents

secondary microvascular thrombosis and inflammation within cutaneous burns. Proc Natl Acad Sci USA. 2013;110:3513-8.

17. Nielson CB, Duethman NC, Howard JM, Moncure M, Wood JG. Burns: Pathophysiology of systemic complications and current management. J Burn Care Res. 2017;38(1):e469-81.
18. Bianchi ME. DAMPs, PAMPs and alarmins: All we need to know about danger. J Leukoc Biol. 2006;81(1):1-5.
19. Arumugam TV, Okun E, Tang S-C, Thundyil J, Taylor SM, Woodruff TM. Toll-like receptors in ischemia-reperfusion injury. Shock. 2009; 32(1):4-16.
20. Takeuchi O, Akira S. Pattern recognition receptors and inflammation. Cell 2010;140:805-20.
21. Sauaia A, Moore FA, Moore EE. Postinjury inflammation and organ dysfunction. Crit Care Clin. 2017;33(1):167-91.
22. Giannoudis PV. Current concepts of the inflammatory response after major trauma: an update. Injury. 2003;34(6):397-404.
23. Houstis N, Rosen ED, Lander ES. Reactive oxygen species have a causal role in multiple forms of insulin resistance. Nature. 2006;440:944-8.
24. Auger C, Samadi O, Jeschke MG. The biochemical alterations underlying post-burn hypermetabolism. Biochim Biophys Acta Mol Basis Dis. 2017;1863:2633-44.
25. Porter C, Herndon DN, Børsheim E, Chao T, Reidy PT, Borack MS, et al. Uncoupled skeletal muscle mitochondria contribute to hypermetabolism in severely burned adults. Am J Physiol Endocrinol Metab. 2014;307:E462-7.
26. Abdullahi A, Jeschke MG. White adipose tissue browning: a double-edged sword. Trends Endocrinol Metab. 2016;27: 542-52.
27. Meier JA, Larner AC. Toward a new STATe: the role of STATs in mitochondrial function. Semin Immunol. 2014;26:20-8.
28. Zhang P, Zou B, Liou YC, Huang C. The pathogenesis and diagnosis of sepsis post burn injury. Burns Trauma. 2021;9:tkaa047.
29. Keck M, Herndon DH, Kamolz LP, Frey M, Jeschke MG. Pathophysiology of burns. Wien Med Wochenschr. 2009;159 (13-14):327-36.
30. Friedl HS, Till GO, Tentz O, Ward PA. Roles of histamine, complement and xanthine oxidase in thermal injury of skin. Am J Pathol. 1989;135:203-17.
31. Till GO, Guilds LS, Mahrougui M, Friedl HP, Trentz O, Ward PA. Role of xanthine oxidase in thermal injury of skin. Am J Pathol. 1989;135:195-202.
32. Biesalski HK, McGregor GP. Antioxidant therapy in critical care—Is the microcirculation the primary target? Crit Care Med. 2007;35:S577-83.
33. Motoyama T, Okamoto K, Kukita I, Hamaguchi M, Kinoshita Y, Ogawa H. Possible role of increased oxidant stress in multiple organ failure after systemic inflammatory response syndrome. Crit Care Med. 2003;31:1048-52.
34. Huang Q, Zhao M, Zhao K. Alteration of vascular permeability in burn injury. MedicalExpress (São Paulo, online). 2014;1(2):62-76.
35. Glas, GJ, Levi, M, Schultz, MJ. Coagulopathy and its management in patients with severe burns. J Thromb Haemost. 2016;14: 865-74.
36. Angus DC, van der Poll T. Severe sepsis and septic shock. N Engl J Med. 2013;369(9):840-51.
37. Levi M, van der Poll T. Inflammation and coagulation. Crit Care Med. 2010;38(Suppl):S26-S34.
38. Gourd NM, Nikitas N. Multiple organ dysfunction syndrome. J Intensive Care Med. 2020;35(12):1564-75.
39. Silliman CC, Moore EE, Johnson JL, Gonzalez RJ, Biffl WL. Transfusion of the injured patient: proceed with caution. Shock. 2004;21(4):291-9.
40. Zallen G, Moore EE, Ciesla DJ, Brown M, Biffl WL, Silliman CC. Stored red blood cells selectively activate human neutrophils to release IL-8 and secretory PLA2. Shock. 2000;13(1):29-33.
41. Johnson JL, Moore EE, Kashuk JL, Banerjee A, Cothren CC, Biffl WL, et al. Effect of blood products transfusion on the development of postinjury multiple organ failure. Arch Surg. 2010;145(10): 973-77.
42. Acute Respiratory Distress Syndrome Network; Brower RG, Matthay MA, Morris A, Schoenfeld D, Thompson BT, et al. Ventilation with lower tidal volumes as compared with traditional tidal volumes for acute lung injury and the acute respiratory distress syndrome. N Engl J Med. 2000;342(18): 1301-8.
43. Ravat F, Payre J, Peslages P, Fontaine M, Sens N. Burn: An inflammatory process. Pathol Biol (Paris). 2011;59:e63-72.
44. Schwacha MG. Macrophages and post-burn immune dysfunction. Burns. 2003;29:1-14.
45. Sehirli O, Sener E, Sener G, Cetinel S, Erzik C, Yeğen BC. Ghrelin improves burn-induced multiple organ injury by depressing neutrophil infiltration and the release of pro-inflammatory cytokines. Peptides. 2008;29:1231-40.
46. Gosain A, Gamelli RL. A primer in cytokines. J Burn Care Rehabil. 2005;26:7-12.
47. Burleson DG, Mason AD Jr, Pruitt BA Jr. Lymphoid subpopulation changes after thermal injury and thermal injury with infection in an experimental model. Ann Surg. 1988;207(2):208-12.
48. Fullerton JN, O'Brien AJ, Gilroy DW. Lipid mediators in immune dysfunction after severe inflammation. Trends Immunol. 2014;35(1):12-21.
49. Asim M, Amin F, El-Menyar A. Multiple organ dysfunction syndrome: Contemporary insights on the clinicopathological spectrum. Qatar Med J. 2020;2020(1):22.
50. Cuthbertson DP: Post-shock metabolic response. Lancet. 1942;239:433-7.
51. Bittner EA, Shank E, Woodson L, Martyn JA. Acute and perioperative care of the burn-injured patient. Anesthesiology. 2015;122(2):448-64.
52. Abu-Sittah GS, Sarhane KA, Dibo SA, Ibrahim A. Cardiovascular dysfunction in burns: Review of the literature. Ann Burns Fire Disasters. 2012;25:26-37.
53. Soussi S, Dépret F, Benyamina M, Legrand M. Early hemodynamic management of critically ill burn patients. Anesthesiology. 2018;129(3):583-9.
54. Maybauer MO, Asmussen S, Flatts DG, Fraser JF, Sanfilippo F, Maybauer DM. Transesophageal echocardiography in the management of burn patients. Burns. 2014;40:630-5.
55. Willis MS, Carlson DL, Dimaio JM, White MD, White DJ, Adams GA 4th, et al. Macrophage migration inhibitory factor mediates late cardiac dysfunction after burn injury. Am J Physiol Heart Circ Physiol. 2005;288:H795-804.
56. Fagan SP, Bilodeau ML, Goverman J. Burn Intensive Care. Surg Clin North Am. 2014;94:765-79.
57. Harrington DT. Complicated Burn Resuscitation. Crit Care Clin. 2016;32(4):577-86.
58. Zarbock A, Gomez H, Kellum JA. Sepsis-induced acute kidney injury revisited: pathophysiology, prevention and future therapies. Curr Opin Crit Care. 2014;20(6):588-95.

59. Holthoff JH, Wang Z, Seely KA, Gokden N, Mayeux PR. Resveratrol improves renal microcirculation, protects the tubular epithelium, and prolongs survival in a mouse model of sepsis-induced acute kidney injury. Kidney Int. 2012;81(4):370-8.
60. Wu G, Xiao Y, Wang C, Hong X, Sun Y, Ma B, et al. Risk factors for acute kidney injury in patients with burn injury: a meta-analysis and systematic review. J Burn Care Res. 2017;38:271-82.
61. Brusselaers N, Monstrey S, Colpaert K, Decruyenaere J, Blot SI, Hoste EA. Outcome of acute kidney injury in severe burns: a systematic review and meta-analysis. Intensive Care Med. 2010;36:915-25.
62. Hosokawa S, Koseki H, Nagashima M, Maeyama Y, Yomogida K, Mehr C, et al. Title efficacy of phosphodiesterase 5 inhibitor on distant burn-induced muscle autophagy, microcirculation, and survival rate. Am J Physiol Endocrinol Metab. 2013;304:E922-33.
63. Lemeshow S, Teres D, Klar J, Avrunin JS, Gehlbach SH, Rapoport J. Mortality Probability Models (MPM II) based on an international cohort of intensive care unit patients. JAMA. 1993;270(20): 2478-86.
64. Papathanassoglou ED, Moynihan JA, Ackerman MH. Does programmed cell death (apoptosis) play a role in the development of multiple organ dysfunction in critically ill patients? a review and a theoretical framework. Crit Care Med. 2000;28(2): 537-49.
65. He W, Wang Y, Wang P, Wang F. Intestinal barrier dysfunction in severe burn injury. Burn Trauma. 2019;7:24.
66. Peterson CY, Costantini TW, Loomis WH, Putnam JG, Wolf P, Bansal V, et al. Toll-like receptor-4 mediates intestinal barrier breakdown after thermal injury. Surg Infect. 2010;11(2):137-44.
67. Wang FJ. Research on intestinal tight junction barrier dysfunction should be emphasized in burn injury. Chin J Burns. 2010;26(5):331-3.
68. Audra C, Imran J, Madni T, Wolf SE. Nutrition and metabolism in burn patients. Burns Trauma. 2017;5:11.
69. Osterbur K, Mann FA, Kuroki K, DeClu A. Multiple organ dysfunction syndrome in humans and animals. J Vet Intern Med. 2014;28:1141-51.
70. Cullen JJ, Spates ST, Ephgrave KS, Hinkhouse MM. Endotoxin temporarily impairs canine colonic absorption of water and sodium. J Surg Res. 1998;74:34-8.
71. Cullen JJ, Caropreso DK, Ephgrave KS, Hemann LL, Hinkhouse MM. The effect of endotoxin on canine jejunal motility and transit. J Surg Res. 1997;67:54-7.
72. Spates ST, Cullen JJ, Ephgrave KS, Hinkhouse MM. Effect of endotoxin on canine colonic motility and transit. J Gastrointest Surg. 1998;2:391-8.
73. Reintam Blaser A, Poeze M, Malbrain ML, Björck M, Oudemans-van Straaten HM, Starkopf J, et al.; GastroIntestinal Failure Trial Group. Gastrointestinal symptoms during the first week of intensive care are associated with poor outcome: A prospective multicentre study. Intensive Care Med. 2013;39(5):899-909.
74. Price LA, Thombs B, Chen CL, Milner SM. Liver disease in burn injury: evidence from a national sample of 31,338 adult patients. J Burns Wounds. 2007;7:e1.
75. Jeschke MG, Micak RP, Finnerty CC, Herndon DN. Changes in liver function and size after a severe thermal injury. Shock. 2007;28:172-7.
76. Palmieri TL, Greenhalgh DG, Sen S. Prospective comparison of packed red blood cell-to-fresh frozen plasma transfusion ratio of 4:1 versus 1:1 during acute massive burn excision. J Trauma Acute Care Surg. 2013;74:76-83.
77. Garcia-Avello A, Lorente JA, Cesar-Perez J, Garcia-Frade LJ, Alvarado R, Arevalo JM, et al. Degree of hypercoagulability and hyperfibrinolysis is related to organ failure and prognosis after burn trauma. Thromb Res. 1998;89:59-64.
78. Kowal-Vern A, Gamelli RL, Walenga JM, Hoppensteadt D, Sharp-Pucci M, et al. The effect of burn wound size on hemostasis: a correlation of the hemostatic changes to the clinical state. J Trauma. 1992;33:50-6. [discussion 6-7]
79. Mullins F, Mian MA, Jenkins D, Brandigi C, Shaver JR, Friedman B, et al. Thromboembolic complications in burn patients and associated risk factors. J Burn Care Res. 2013;34:355-60.
80. Harrington DT, Mozingo DW, Cancio L, Bird P, Jordan B, Goodwin CW. Thermally injured patients are at significant risk for thromboembolic complications. J Trauma. 2001;50:495-9.
81. Sherren PB, Hussey J, Martin R, Kundishora T, Parker M, Emerson B. Lethal triad in severe burns. Burns. 2014;40:1492-6.
82. Gomez R, Murray CK, Hospenthal DR, Cancio LC, Renz EM, Holcomb JB, et al. Causes of mortality by autopsy findings of combat casualties and civilian patients admitted to a burn unit. J Am Coll Surg. 2009;208(3):348-54.
83. Singer M, Deutschman CS, Seymour CW, Shankar-Hari M, Annane D, Bauer M, et al. The third international consensus definitions for sepsis and septic shock (Sepsis-3). JAMA. 2016;315:801-10.
84. Yan J, Hill WF, Rehou S, Pinto R, Shahrokhi S, Jeschke MG. Sepsis criteria versus clinical diagnosis of sepsis in burn patients: A validation of current sepsis scores. Surgery. 2018;164(6): 1241-5.
85. Usmani A, Pipal DK, Bagla H, Verma V, Kumar P, Yadav S, et al. Prediction of mortality in acute thermal burn patients using the abbreviated burn severity index score: A single-center experience. Cureus. 2022;14(6):e26161.
86. Baue AE. What's in a name? An acronym or a response? Am J Surg. 1993;165:299-301.
87. Mosier MJ, Pham TN, Klein MB, Gibran NS, Arnoldo BD, Gamelli RL, et al. Early acute kidney injury predicts progressive renal dysfunction and higher mortality in severely burned adults. J Burn Care Res. 2010;31:83-92.
88. Kumar AB, Andrews W, Shi Y, Shotwell MS, Dennis S, Wanderer J, et al. Fluid resuscitation mediates the association between inhalational burn injury and acute kidney injury in the major burn population. J Crit Care. 2017;38:62-7.
89. Sine CR, Belenkiy SM, Buel AR, Waters JA, Lundy JB, Henderson JL, et al. Acute respiratory distress syndrome in burn patients. J Burn Care Res. 2016;37:e461-9.
90. Lawrence A, Faraklas I, Watkins H, Allen A, Cochran A, Morris S, et al. Colloid administration normalizes resuscitation ratio and ameliorates "fluid creep." J Burn Care Res. 2010;31:40-7.
91. Venet F, Plassais J, Textoris J, Cazalis MA, Pachot A, Bertin Maghit M, et al. Low dose hydrocortisone reduces norepinephrine duration in severe burn patients: A randomized clinical trial. Crit Care. 2015;19:21.
92. Neff LP, Allman JM, Holmes JH. The use of therapeutic plasma exchange (TPE) in the setting of refractory burn shock. Burns. 2010;36:372-8.
93. Barajas-Nava LA, López-Alcalde J, Roqué i Figuls M, Solà I, Bonfill Cosp X. Antibiotic prophylaxis for preventing burn wound infection. Cochrane Database Syst Rev. 2013;6(6):CD008738.
94. Nitzschke SL, Aden JK, Serio-Melvin ML, Shingleton SK, Chung KK, Waters JA, et al. Wound healing trajectories in burn patients and their impact on mortality. J Burn Care Res. 2014;35:474-9.

95. Arlati S, Storti E, Pradella V, Bucci L, Vitolo A, Pulici M. Decreased fluid volume to reduce organ damage: a new approach to burn shock resuscitation? A preliminary study. Resuscitation. 2007;72(3):371-8.
96. Williams FN, Branski LK, Jeschke MG, Herndon DN. What, how, and how much should patients with burns be fed? Surg Clin North Am. 2011;91(3):609-29.
97. Herndon DN, Tompkins RG. Support of the metabolic response to burn injury. Lancet. 2004;363(9424):1895-902.
98. McClave SA, Marsano LS, Lukan JK. Enteral access for nutritional support: rationale for utilization. J Clin Gastroenterol. 2002;35(3):209-13.
99. Gauglitz GG, Williams FN. Hypermetabolic response to moderate-to-severe burn injury and management. UpToDate. 2023:1-24.
100. Williams FN, Herndon DN, Jeschke MG. The hypermetabolic response to burn injury and interventions to modify this response. Clin Plast Surg. 2009;36(4):583-96.
101. Wolf SE, Edelman LS, Kemalyan N, Donison L, Cross J, Underwood M, et al. Effects of oxandrolone on outcome measures in the severely burned: A multicenter prospective randomized double-blind trial. J Burn Care Res. 2006;27(2):131-9.
102. Hassoun-Kheir N, Henig O, Avni T, Leibovici L, Paul M. The effect of β-blockers for burn patients on clinical outcomes: Systematic review and meta-analysis. J Intensive Care Med. 2021;36(8): 945-53.
103. Herndon DN, Hart DW, Wolf SE, Chinkes DL, Wolfe RR. Reversal of catabolism by beta-blockade after severe burns. N Engl J Med. 2001;345(17):1223-9.
104. Barret JP, Jeschke MG, Herndon DN. Fatty infiltration of the liver in severely burned pediatric patients: autopsy findings and clinical implications. J Trauma. 2001;51:736.
105. Aarsland A, Chinkes D, Wolfe RR, Barrow RE, Nelson SO, Pierre E, et al. Beta-blockade lowers peripheral lipolysis in burn patients receiving growth hormone. Rate of hepatic very low density lipoprotein triglyceride secretion remains unchanged. Ann Surg 1996;223:777.
106. Patterson DR, Tininenko J, Ptacek JT. Pain during burn hospitalization predicts long-term outcome. J Burn Care Res. 2006;27(5):719-26.
107. Warden GD, Saffle JR, Kravitz M. A two-stage technique for excision and grafting of burn wounds. J Trauma. 1982;22:98-103.
108. Pruskowski KA, Rizzo JA, Shields BA, Chan RK, Driscoll IR, Rowan MP, et al. A survey of temperature management practices among burn centers in North America. J Burn Care Res. 2018;39: 612-7.
109. Rode H, Brink C, Bester K, Coleman MP, Baisey T, Martinez R. A review of the peri-operative management of paediatric burns: Identifying adverse events. S Afr Med J. 2016;106:1114-9.
110. Williams D, Leslie G, Kyriazis D, O'Donovan B, Bowes J, Dingley J. Use of an esophageal heat exchanger to maintain core temperature during burn excisions and to attenuate pyrexia on the burns intensive care unit. Case Rep Anesthesiol. 2016;2016:7306341.
111. Mertin V, Most P, Busch M, Trojan S, Tapking C, Haug V, et al. Current understanding of thermo(dys)regulation in severe burn injury and the pathophysiological influence of hypermetabolism, adrenergic stress and hypothalamic regulation:a systematic review. Burns Trauma. 2022;10:tkac031.
112. Corallo JP, King B, Pizano LR, Namias N, Schulman CI. Core warming of a burn patient during excision to prevent hypothermia. Burns. 2008;34(3):418-20.
113. Mukhopadhyay C. Infection control in intensive care units. Indian J Respir Care. 2018;7:14-21.
114. Vermaak PV, D'Asta F, Provins J, Farr M, Wilson YT. Thromboprophylaxis in adult and paediatric burn patients: A survey of practice in the United Kingdom. Burns. 2019;45(6):1379-85.
115. Sikora S, Papp A. Venous thromboembolism in burn patients is not prevented by chemoprophylaxis. Burns. 2017;43(6):1330-4.
116. Cook DJ, Fuller HD, Guyatt GH, Marshall JC, Leasa D, Hall R, et al. Risk factors for gastrointestinal bleeding in critically ill patients. Canadian Critical Care Trials Group. N Engl J Med. 1994;330(6):377-81.
117. Choi YH, Lee JH, Shin JJ, Cho YS. A revised risk analysis of stress ulcers in burn patients receiving ulcer prophylaxis. Clin Exp Emerg Med. 2015;2(4):250-5.
118. Friese RS, Dineen S, Jennings A, Pruitt J, McBride D, Shafi S, et al. Serum B-type natriuretic peptide: a marker of fluid resuscitation after injury? J Trauma. 2007;62(6):1346-50.
119. Dubois-Rande JL, Merlet P, Roudot F, Benvenuti C, Adnot S, Hittinger L, et al. Beta adrenergic contractile reserve as a predictor of clinical outcome in patients with idiopathic dilated cardiomyopathy. Am Heart J. 1992;124(3):679-85.
120. Burns CJ, Chung KK, Aden JK, Lundy JB, Nitzschke SL, Renz EM. High risk but not always lethal: the effect of cirrhosis on thermally injured adults. J Burn Care Res. 2013;34(1):115-9.
121. Benoit JN, Granger DN. Splanchnic hemodynamics in chronic portal hypertension. Semin Liver Dis. 1986;6(4):287-98.
122. Holm C, Horbrand F, von Donnersmarck GH, Mühlbauer W. Acute renal failure in severely burned patients. Burns. 1999;25(2):171-8.
123. Uchino S, Kellum JA, Bellomo R, Doig GS, Morimatsu H, Morgera S, et al. Acute renal failure in critically ill patients: a multinational, multicenter study. JAMA. 2005;294(7):813-8.
124. Koyner JL, Garg AX, Thiessen-Philbrook H, Coca SG, Cantley LG, Peixoto A, et al. Adjudication of etiology of acute kidney injury: experience from the TRIBE-AKI multi-center study. BMC Nephrol. 2014;15:105.
125. Lobo SM, Rezende E, Knibel MF, Silva NB, Páramo JA, Nácul FE, et al. Early determinants of death due to multiple organ failure after noncardiac surgery in high-risk patients. Anesth Analg. 2011;112(4):877-83.
126. Madigan MC, Kemp CD, Johnson JC, Cotton BA. Secondary abdominal compartment syndrome after severe extremity injury: are early, aggressive fluid resuscitation strategies to blame? J Trauma. 2008;64(2):280-5.
127. Balogh Z, McKinley BA, Cox CSJ, Allen SJ, Cocanour CS, Kozar RA, et al. Abdominal compartment syndrome: The cause or effect of postinjury multiple organ failure. Shock. 2003;20(6):483-92.
128. Sterling JP, Lombardi VC. Decreasing the likelihood of multiple organ dysfunction syndrome in burn injury with early antioxidant treatment. Antioxidants (Basel). 2021;10(8):1192.
129. Tanaka H, Matsuda T, Miyagantani Y, Yukioka T, Matsuda H, Shimazaki S: Reduction of resuscitation fluid volumes in severely burned patients using ascorbic acid administration: A randomized, prospective study. Arch Surg. 2000;135:326-31.
130. Nácul FE, Jardim A, MacCord F, Penido C, Gomes MV. Hemodynamic instability secondary to adrenal insufficiency in a major burn patient. Burns. 2002;8(3):270-2.

131. Reiff DA, Harkins CL, McGwin G Jr, Cross JM, Rue LW 3rd. Risk factors associated with adrenal insufficiency in severely injured burn patients. J Burn Care Res. 2007;28(6):854-8.
132. Rojas Y, Finnerty CC, Radhakrishnan RS, Herndon DN. Burns: an update on current pharmacotherapy. Expert Opin Pharmacother. 2012;13:2485-94.
133. Ferrando AA, Chinkes DL, Wolf SE, Matin S, Herndon DN, Wolfe RR. A submaximal dose of insulin promotes net skeletal muscle protein synthesis in patients with severe burns. Ann Surg. 1999;229(1):11-8.
134. Jeschke MG, Klein D, Herndon DN. Insulin treatment improves the systemic inflammatory reaction to severe trauma. Ann Surg. 2004;239:553.
135. Ning XH, Ge XF, Cui Y, An HX. Ulinastatin inhibits unilateral ureteral obstruction-induced renal interstitial fibrosis in rats via transforming growth factor β (TGFβ)/Smad signalling pathways. Int Immunopharmacol. 2013;15:406-13.
136. Abhyankar SV, Vartak AM. Impact of ulinastatin on outcomes in acute burns patients. J Burn Care Res. 2018;39(1):109-16.
137. Li J, Li NP, Gu YF, Yang X, Lu XB, Cong JN, et al. Dynamic activity of NF-kappaB in multiple trauma patients and protective effects of ulinastatin. Chin J Traumatol. 2011;14(6):354-8.
138. Greenhalgh DG, Saffle JR, Holmes JH 4th, Gamelli RL, Palmieri TL, Horton JW, et al. American Burn Association consensus conference to define sepsis and infection in burns. J Burn Care Res. 2007;28:776-90.
139. El-Menyar A, Al Thani H, Zakaria El R, Zarour A, Tuma M, Abdul Rahman H, et al. Multiple Organ Dysfunction Syndrome (MODS): Is It Preventable or Inevitable? Int J Clin Med. 2012;3:722-30.
140. Abdel-Hafez NM, Saleh Hassan Y, El-Metwally TH. A study on biomarkers, cytokines, and growth factors in children with burn injuries. Ann Burns Fire Disasters. 2007;20:89-100.
141. Finnerty CC, Herndon DN, Przkora R, Pereira CT, Oliveira HM, Queiroz DM, et al. Cytokine expression profile over time in severely burned pediatric patients. Shock. 2006;26:13-9.
142. Kraft R, Herndon DN, Finnerty CC, Cox RA, Song J, Jeschke MG. Predictive value of IL-8 for sepsis and severe infections after burn injury: A clinical study. Shock. 2015;43:222-7.
143. Csontos C, Foldi V, Pálinkas L, Bogar L, Röth E, Weber G, et al. Time course of pro- and anti-inflammatory cytokine levels in patients with burns–prognostic value of interleukin-10. Burns. 2010;36:483-94.
144. Marshall JC. Inflammation, coagulopathy, and the pathogenesis of multiple organ dysfunction syndrome. Crit Care Med. 2001;29(7 Suppl):S99-106.

CHAPTER

32 Guidelines for Nutritional Management of the Burn Patient

Savita Arora, Komal Tripathi

INTRODUCTION

Burn injury is one of the most severe forms of injury. Aggressive nutritional support in severe burns is an essential lifesaving therapy which is as important as control of infection and early excision and skin grafting. Due to the presence of acute phase responses in a burn patient, a number of pathophysiological alterations develop, leading to hormonal imbalances, immunologic dysfunction, and severe circulatory disturbances. It may lead to excess loss of nitrogen, poor nutrition, increase in the metabolic rate, and immune deficiency. This leads to increased rate of infection, disturbance in wound healing, and increased duration of hospitalization and mortality.

Severe burn injury leads to a hypermetabolic response which can persist up to 24 months after injury. This is due to multiple inflammatory mediators including various catecholamines and hormones leading to increased catabolism, elevated resting energy expenditures, and multiorgan dysfunction.

This catabolic state leads to elevated nitrogen loss due to increased amino acid efflux from the skeletal muscles. The amino acid efflux occurs to accommodate increased demands for repair of tissues, production of acute phase proteins, cellular immunity, and gluconeogenesis. This leads to diminished lean body mass (LBM) which directly relates to outcome. Due to major fluid shifts and exudative losses, there is loss of micronutrients which are the key factors in wound healing.

Treatment of burn patients remains incomplete and is unsuccessful if proper nutrition is not given. With proper nutritional management, modulation of the inflammatory response becomes possible, leading to strengthening of immune status and promotion of burn wound healing. Adequate provision of micronutrients plays an important role in prevention of wound infections and boosting the immunity of the patient.

Diets rich in protein and energy are required to provide sufficient calories and protein to give metabolic support and minimize further loss of LBM.

Adjuvant therapies and immunomodulators can be given to modulate energy requirements and promote wound healing.

Loss in body weight in burn patients may have severe consequences. A 40% loss in the weight of the body or a loss of 30–50% of protein is associated with death, particularly if the loss is rapid as seen in extensive burns. A 30% loss in body weight may lead to severe infections. Wound healing is limited when weight loss exceeds >20% of the preburn values, while a 10% weight loss leads to immune dysfunction.[1]

Oral feeding is the preferred method of providing nutrition to a patient with small burns. In extensive burns, decisions have to be made carefully regarding the safety and aggressiveness of nutrient therapy.

PHYSIOLOGIC AND METABOLIC RESPONSES TO BURN INJURY

Burn injury leads to various physiologic and metabolic alterations in the body. Effective nutritional therapy in these patients requires a thorough understanding of these alterations. Nutritional practice in burn injury requires a multifaceted approach aimed at providing metabolic support while accommodating surgical and medical needs of the patients.

Metabolism after burn injury is mediated through hypothalamic and pituitary axis. There are three phases:

1. Ebb or the shock phase
2. Flow or the recovery phase, and
3. Anabolic phase

Nutritional care is modified and individualized according to these three stages.

Ebb or Shock Phase

Ebb or shock phase is usually a brief phase occurring immediately after burns, lasting up to 12–24 hours. There is a decrease in blood pressure and cardiac output, along with a reduction in body temperature and oxygen consumption.

The skin cover is lost in burn patients and there is increased capillary permeability which leads to loss of water and electrolytes predominantly sodium and also protein loss. There is a shift of body water, from extracellular spaces to the site of burn which adds to the continuous loss of fluids and electrolytes from the body. This capillary fluid shift leads to decrease in blood pressure with resultant hemoconcentration and reduction in urine output. Extracellular fluid losses lead to cellular dehydration. To balance this loss, intracellular water is drawn out. During the first 12–24 hours, patients with extensive burns need immediate fluid and electrolyte replacement. Therefore, a balanced salt solution such as Ringer's lactate is provided to counter hypovolemia and prevent metabolic acidosis.

A colloidal solution such as albumin or plasma is not effective at this stage as it passes into the extravascular fluids due to the increased capillary permeability which returns to normal only after the first day. During the initial period of resuscitation, no attempts are made to fulfill the requirements of protein and energy, as the entire focus is on prevention and reversal of shock by providing rapid and effective fluid and electrolyte therapy. Our goal is to maintain sufficient blood pressure and adequate hematocrit and urine output.

Flow or Recovery Phase

Following the restoration of circulating blood volume, patient enters the catabolic or flow phase. After 48–72 hours of burn injury, there is reabsorption of fluid and electrolytes into the general circulation and excretion of excess fluid **(Flowchart 1)**. From 5th to 12th day postburn, metabolism increases greatly and is characterized by abnormal substrate utilization, increased heat elimination, and weight loss. The magnitude of postburn hypermetabolism is proportional to the extent of the injury. Metabolic rate may be accentuated by intervening infection. Cardiac output and oxygen consumption are increased with significant increase in blood flow to the burn wound, which is necessary to provide adequate glucose substrate as an energy source for wound healing. The wound preferentially utilizes anaerobic glycolytic pathways which are inefficient for energy production.

Large open wounds, increased blood flow to the burn wound, and loss of cutaneous vasomotor reflexes for heat retention account for major heat loss via evaporation. This also leads to increased oxygen consumption. To prevent lethal cooling, the core temperature of burn patient is elevated. Wound evaporative losses are estimated by the following formula:

$$\text{Total body surface area (TBSA) m}^2 \times (25 + \%\text{ of burn}) = \text{water loss in mL/h}$$

Being an energy-consuming process, evaporation adds to energy loss. For example, a patient losing 86 mL of water/h by evaporation needs 1,200 kcal/day in addition to his/her energy requirement. The increase in basal metabolic rate (BMR) is brought about by increased secretion of catecholamines which stimulate the production of glucagon which promotes glycogenolysis and gluconeogenesis and suppresses the insulin release. Protein catabolism (proteolysis) occurs mainly in the skeletal muscles. Alamine and glutamine released from the muscles are transported to liver which disintegrates them into pyruvates and turns it into glucose (gluconeogenesis). Amino acids usually get wasted as gluconeogenesis exceeds the demand of cells. Enhanced lipolysis occurs to counter increased demand; this combined with impaired fat oxidation results in the futile recycling of free fatty acids (FAs) and triglycerides. There may be increased excretion of nitrogen (20–25% of total nitrogen loss is from burn wound exudates), potassium, phosphate, creatinine, magnesium, and zinc sulfate in urine. In addition, burn injury decreases endogenic anabolic activity. As a result, if a patient is not getting proper nutrition, wasting of the visceral proteins occurs and the muscle volume declines. Because of this, the body becomes incapable of adapting to the existing situation and is unable to economize the use of energy. With the onset of wound healing, the metabolic rate and the production of catecholamines return to normal levels and protein synthesis follows as the insulin glucagon molar ratio reverses after the wound is healed.

Anabolic Phase

During this period, the patient's hydration becomes adequate and the adverse reactions due to metabolic stress are brought under control. The patient is still hypermetabolic and the reserves of all the nutrients get depleted. Intensive nutritional support is required during anabolic phase to promote early recovery and proper rehabilitation. Adequate nutritional care during

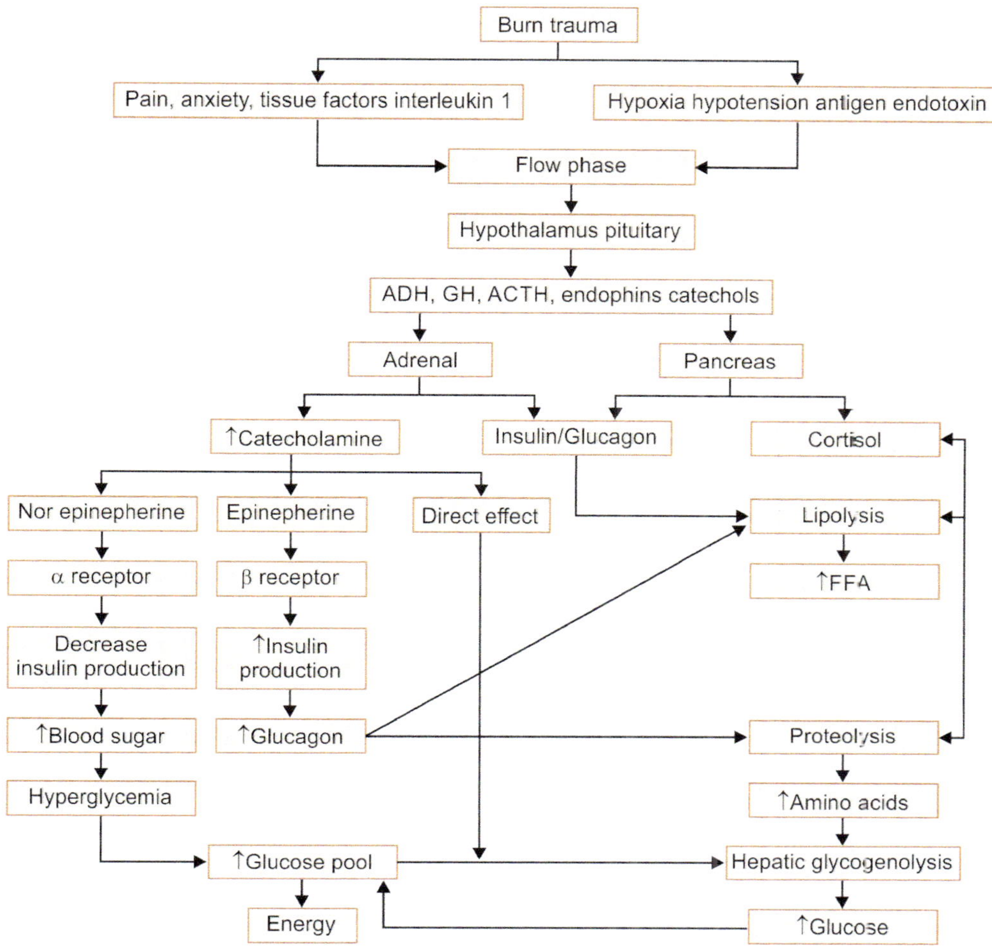

FLOWCHART 1: Hormonal changes following burns.

(ACTH: adrenocorticotrophic hormone; ADH: antidiuretic hormone; FFA: free fatty acid; GH: growth hormone)

Sources:

1. Adapted and modified from Herndon D (Ed). Total Burn Care. Philadelphia: WB Saunders; 1996.
2. Adapted and modified from Ramakrishnan M, Hanumadas M (Eds). Handbook of Burns Management. New Delhi: Jaypee Brothers Medical Publishers (P) Ltd.; 1991.

this period helps in preparing the patient physically for undergoing successful skin grafting. Rate of utilization of nitrogen does not differ in flow or anabolic phase, but the obligatory nitrogen loss and the requirements for nitrogen equilibrium decrease as the postburn course progresses through convalescence.

PARAMETERS TO ASSESS THE NUTRITIONAL STATUS OF BURN PATIENT

The acute phase of burn injury is driven by various inflammatory mediators such as catecholamines and counterregulatory hormones. In burn patients, the nutritional status usually deteriorates regardless of the initial baseline. Though the body weight which is a reasonable marker of fat and lean tissue is the most useful assessment tool for nutritional status, it has limitations as postburn weight is usually increased due to resuscitative fluid administration, dressings, edema, etc.

Upper arm anthropometry (upper arm circumference, triceps skin fold thickness) is not a valuable assessment tool in massive burns with edema. This is especially so if burn wound eschar and underlying wound edema involve the areas to be assessed.

Circulating proteins or visceral proteins are good indicators of nutrition.[3,4] Serum albumin <3.5 g/dL and prealbumin < 1.2 g/dL indicates malnutrition. However, they are also affected by various other factors such as rate of protein synthesis and breakdown, exudative wound losses, and blood transfusion(s).

TABLE 1: Predictive formulas to calculate ideal body weight.

	Men	Women
Devine	50 kg + (2.3 kg/inch over 5′ height)	45.5 kg + (2.3 kg/inch over 5′ height)
Hamwi	106 lb + (6 lb/inch over 5′ height)	100 lb + (5 lb/inch over 5′ height)
Hammond	48 kg + (1.1 kg/cm over 150 cm height)	45 kg + (0.9 kg/cm over 150 cm height)

The investigations which can be done to assess the nutritional status are:

- Nitrogen balance (NB) studies
- Urinary creatinine excretion
- Estimation of total body potassium and nitrogen
- Serum transferrin estimation
- Indirect calorimetry

They have their own limitations. Preinjury height and weight of patient or daily body weight and clinical appearance is the most effective index of nutritional balance. Estimation of hemoglobin, serum proteins, albumin-globulin (A/G) ratio, immunological markers–total lymphocyte count, and delayed hypersensitivity are other investigations used to evaluate the nutritional status.

There are multiple formulas to calculate the ideal body weight (IBW) in adults **Table 1**.[5]

Body mass index (BMI) is also used, which is calculated by dividing an adult's weight in kilograms (kg) by their height in meters (m) square [W (kg)/H (m^2)]. While it can overestimate the status of nutrition in a patient with edema, it is still considered a good tool for nutritional status assessment.[6]

Serial evaluation of resting energy expenditure, as measured by indirect calorimetry, is the best method available to assess the nutritional status as energy requirements vary not only from one patient to other.[7]

NUTRIENT REQUIREMENT AND DIETARY MANAGEMENT

After resuscitation and assessment of nutritional status, the patient is examined for the presence of diabetes, hyperlipidemia, any bowel or liver disease, alcohol abuse, lactose intolerance, etc.

Early feeding, i.e., within 24–48 hours after an acute event is preferred, but we usually rely on intravenous (IV) fluids or clear oral liquids for first 2 days as the narcotics used for pain relief during resuscitation may cause nausea, vomiting, and anorexia. Fluid and electrolyte requirements are calculated considering the daily maintenance, burn wound losses, losses due to fever, and through gastrointestinal tract (GIT) losses.

TABLE 2: Nutrition in intensive care unit (ICU) patients after the patient is out of shock.

Main food groups	Weight/Measures	Calories
Clear liquids:		
Water + glucose (1 tsf)	100 mL	20 kcal
Orange juice	200 mL	100 kcal
Tomato soup	200 mL	60 kcal
Soft drink	200 mL	120 kcal
Switch on to other liquids if patient tolerates clear liquids, i.e., 2,500 mL/day		
Other liquids:		
Milk + 2 tsf sugar + 2 tsf protein rich powders (commercially available)	100 mL/h	1800/24 h
Lentil soup	200 mL	137 kcal
Vegetable soup	200 mL	100 kcal
Semisolids:		
Khichdi (rice with lentil)	150 g	190 kcal
Porridge (*daliya*)	2 bowls	410 kcal

Early parenteral nutrition (PN) has no role in intensive care units (ICUs) and in patients who do not have pre-existing malnutrition. Early enteral nutrition is proven to be beneficial in patients with major burns. When the patient becomes hemodynamically stable and gut mobility returns, liquids and semisolids are started, setting a tolerable level of intake which supports adequate wound healing and weight gain.

Protein and Energy Requirements

By the time the flow phase ends, the hydration of the patient is usually adequate and the body weight becomes close to the preburn injury weight. The return of bowel movements indicates that the patient can be slowly introduced to the nutritional support in the form of oral or enteral feeds or PN **(Table 2)**.

IV fluids after 24 hours (maintenance fluid) = 50 mL/kg + evaporative water loss (evaporative water loss = 4 mL/kg × 20 × % burn/100)

Intravenous alimentation till patient is on full-diet dextrose 10% 1,000 mL = 400 kcal

IV fat preparation 10% 500 mL = 450 kcal

Amino acid preparation 3.5–5% (200 mL) = 1 g nitrogen, total volume = 1,900 mL

Nonprotein calories = 850 kcal

Calorie-protein ratio = 150/200: 1 g nitrogen, 6.25 g protein = 1 g nitrogen

A burn patient can be provided nutrition via oral, enteral, or parenteral form. A combination of any two of these aforementioned routes is used on a daily basis depending upon the clinical parameters of the patient and severity of burns. The objectives of dietary management are:

- Prevention of weight loss by providing sufficient calories
- Prevention of fluid and electrolyte imbalance
- Minimizing stress response to pain and anxiety
- Maintenance of positive NB
- Replenishment of vitamins and minerals lost
- Prevention of complications such as Curling's ulcers and ileus.

Energy

Burn injury causes a severe disturbance of metabolism.[8] The energy needs of the burn patient are variable and depend upon the depth and size of the burn.

The requirement of energy in a patient with burns is quite high. But it is important to provide nutrition judiciously and not to overload the patient with excessive calories. The excess calories are not assimilated in the body but are accumulated as a fat layer beneath the skin. If the amount of energy provided is in excess, it leads to greater complications and increased mortality in burn patients.[9]

Energy requirement varies during the course of burn and is highest in third-degree burn. Several formulae have been developed to determine the energy needs of burn patients. Fixed formulae lead to underfeeding initially, while leading to overfeeding later in the course of treatment.[10]

Various formulae have been devised for calculating the energy requirements in burns as described in **Table 3**.

Calculating Nutrient Requirement

For calculating the nutrient requirements in adults, Toronto formula is used commonly: −4343 + 10.5 [total body surface area (TBSA)] + 0.23 (calorie intake in last

TABLE 3: Formulae for calculating energy requirements in burns.[11-13]

Formula	Kcal/day	
Harris–Benedict formula	• *Men*: 66.5 + 13.8 (weight in kg) + 5 (height in cm) – 6.76 (age in years) • *Women*: 655 + 9.6 (weight in kg) + 1.85 (height in cm) – 4.68 (age in years)	• Basal energy expenditure is calculated • Multiplied by 1.5 for burn stress adjustment • Long's modification of Harris–Benedict formula can be used for calculation of energy needs. But the results obtained are not definite as the TBSA burns, depth, location, and presence/absence of infection are not included in the formula
Toronto formula	–4343 + 10.5 (%TBSA) + 0.23 (calorie intake in last 24 hours) + 0.84 × REE(Harris–Benedict estimation without adjustment) + 114 (temperature degree celcius) – 4.5 (number of postburn days)	Accurately predicts the resting energy expenditure in clinically stable and mechanically ventilated burn patients
Davies and Liljedahl	20 (weight in kg) + 70 (TBSA)	It overestimates caloric needs, especially for large injuries
Curreri	• *Age 16–59 years*: 25 (weight in kg) + 40 (TBSA) • *Age > 60 years*: 20 (weight in kg) + 65 (TBSA)	It overestimates energy needs
Modified Schofield	Estimated energy requirements: BMR × injury factor *Men*: • 10–18 years = (0.074 × weight) + 2.754 • 18–30 years = (0.063 × weight) + 2.896 • 30–60 years = (0.048 × weight) + 3.653 • 60 years = (0.049 × weight) + 2.459 *Women*: • 10–18 years = (0.056 × weight) + 2.898 • 18–30 years = (0.062 × weight) + 2.036 • 30–60 years = (0.034 × weight) + 3.538 • >60 years = (0.038 × weight) + 2.755	Calories are adjusted according to the stress level

Continued

Continued

Formula	Kcal/day	
	Injury factors: • <10% TBSA = 1.2 • 11–20% TBSA = 1.3 • 21–30% TBSA = 1.5 • 31–50% TBSA = 1.8 • >50% TBSA = 2.0	
ASPEN	For all patients, 25–35 kcal/kg/day	Frequently leads to underfeeding
Ireton–Jones formula	For spontaneously breathing patients, • *Estimated energy requirements*: 629 – (11 × age in years) + (25 × weight in Kgs) – (609 × O) • *Ventilator dependent*: 1784 – (11 × age in years) + (25 × weight in Kgs) + (244 × S) + (239 × T) + (804 × B)	
Pediatric formulae		
Galveston	• *0–1 year*: 2,100 (body surface area) + 1,000 (body surface area × TBSA) • *1–11 years*: 1,800 (body surface area) + 1,300 (body surface area × TBSA) • *12–18 years*: 1,500 (body surface area) + 1,500 (body surface area × TBSA)	Focuses on maintaining body weight
Curreri junior	• *<1 year*: Recommended dietary allowance + 15 (TBSA) • *1–3 years*: Recommended dietary allowance + 25 (TBSA) • *4–15 years*: Recommended dietary allowance + 40 (TBSA)	Commonly overestimates caloric needs
Mayes	For children, estimated energy requirements: • *Male and female < 3 years*: 108 + (68 × weight in kg) + (3.9 × %TBSA) • *Male and female 3–10 years*: 818 + (37.4 × weight in kg) + (9.3 × %TBSA)	
WHO	For children: • Male < 3 years (60.9 × weight in kg) – 54 • Male 3–10 years (22.7 × weight in kg) + 495 • Female < 3 years (61 × weight in kg) – 51 • Female 3–10 years (22.5 × weight in kg) + 499	

(ASPEN: American Society of Enteral and Parenteral Nutrition; BMR: basal metabolic rate; TBSA: total body surface area; WHO: World Health Organization)

O= Obesity (present =1, absent = 0), S = Sex (male = 1, female = 0), Temperature degree celcius, (one point for every degree > 37) , B = Burn (present = 1, absent = 0)

24 hours) + 0.84 (Harris-Benedict estimation without adjustment) + 114 (temperature) – 4.5 (number of postburn days).

This formula is useful in acute stage of burns and should be adjusted with changes in clinical parameters.

While for pediatric patients, Schofield equation is used:

Schofield equation = Baseline calorie requirement ± other adjustments = [25 + 30 kcal/g/day + other adjustments according to stress level **(Tables 4 and 5)**].

TABLE 4: Protein and energy requirement according to stress level.

Stress level	Proteins in g/kg/day	Energy in kcal/kg/day
Unstressed	0.8	25
Mild	1.2	25–30
Moderate	1.3–1.75	30–35
Severe	2	35–40
Burns	2.0–2.5	25 kcal/kg/day + 20 kcal/% body surface area (BSA)

TABLE 5: Other calorie adjustments (NPC).

Undernourished	+10%
Age 18–30 years	+10%
Fever	+10%/°C rise
Mobile in bed	+5%
Mobile	+10%
Obesity	–10%
Age > 70 years	–10%

Note: For optimal utilization of proteins, adequate calorie supplementation is essential.

Contribution of Various Macronutrients Toward the Total Energy

Carbohydrates

To fulfill calorie requirements, the first priority is given to carbohydrates which should provide 60–65% of total energy. Adequate carbohydrates in the diet reduce protein requirement for gluconeogenesis and protein is spared for wound healing and to enhance the immune status. Rate of administration of glucose should not be above 7 mg/kg/min. Glucose administration above this rate is not used to provide energy but is converted to fat. Blood glucose levels should be closely monitored to prevent hyperglycemia and its associated complications.

After entering the anabolic phase, when the patient starts oral intake and has normal bowel movement, a combination of simple and complex carbohydrates is given. Providing adequate nutrition rich in mono and disaccharides and starches is necessary. Nutrient-dense meals, small in volume, and easily digestible are given. Thus, rice, refined wheat flour, semolina, sago, arrow root rice, rice-based meals, pasta, dextrose, glucose, honey, and potato are incorporated liberally in the diet.

Carbohydrates provide 4.1 kcal/g. The number of nonprotein calories given should bear a definite relationship to the nitrogen intake (NI). The mix should provide approximately 150 kcal/g of nitrogen or a calorie to protein ratio of 20:1.

Fats

Fats are excellent source of calories (9 cal/g) with polyunsaturated fats, providing 4% of the total calories and avoiding a FA deficiency. There is an ample evidence to show that the total number of calories is not the critical issue, but the composition of the mixture is important. For instance, both carbohydrates or amino acid administration have the desirable protein-sparing effect. Lipid administration is done carefully in all critically ill patients. Attempting to give all calories by peripheral IV fat preparations does not spare protein. Not more than 20% of nonprotein calories in the catabolic phase should be fat. Increasing fat and decreasing carbohydrate percentage in the diet is particularly helpful in trying to wean a patient from the ventilator as carbon dioxide (CO_2) production is decreased. When lipid is administered, monitoring of immune function, tolerance to feed, and measurement of serum triglyceride levels are required. Lipid administration can lead to thrombogenesis and immunosuppression. Burn patients benefit from the use of structured lipids and medium-chain triglycerides and hence are preferred. As GIT function among many burn patients is impaired, emphasis is placed on foods rich in emulsified fat and medium-chain triglycerides. Nutritional support with lipids helps in wound healing, maintenance of cellular integrity, and absorption of the fat-soluble vitamins.

Proteins

Proteins are one of the most important macronutrients which determines the ultimate outcome of burns. Amino acids are required in the diet so as to prevent their efflux from the skeletal muscle and to maximize protein synthesis required for optimal wound healing and immune function.

There may be considerable amount of fluid loss from a burn wound. The fluid contains up to 4–6 g protein/100 mL, constituting about 25–50% of total nitrogen loss, while fecal nitrogen loss is approximated to be around 1–3 g N/day. Hence, 20–25% of total calories should be provided as protein in adult patients. To achieve a net balance between synthesis and breakdown, the protein intake should be approximately 1.5 g/kg/day.

Protein food sources with high biological value (BV) include meat, poultry, legumes, pulses, milk, cheese, yogurt, and seafood. These should be included liberally in diet but should be given in an easy-to-digest form.

Contribution of Vitamins and Minerals

Micronutrients

Major burns frequently lead to micronutrient deficiencies.[14] Burn patients suffer from depletion of trace elements such as copper, selenium, and zinc because of exudative losses. These trace elements are required in wound healing and in maintaining immune defenses.

These patients benefit from the use of antioxidant nutrients such as vitamins A, C, and E and trace elements. The benefits include decrease in infection rates, rapid wound healing, and reduced length of stay in hospitals.[15]

The supplementation of micronutrients is provided to correct a state of deficiency. Whenever oral intake is possible, it is advisable to give plenty of fresh fruits and vegetables.

Wound healing includes four stages: Hemostasis, inflammation, proliferation, and maturation. This process includes hemostasis followed by infiltration of neutrophils and macrophages with proliferation and migration of fibroblasts, leading to the remodeling/maturation of collagen. These molecular events are mediated by various chemokines and cytokines such as platelet-derived growth factor (PDGF), transforming growth factor-beta (TGF-β), vascular endothelial growth factor (VEGF), interleukins (ILs), and tumor necrosis factor-alpha (TNF-α).[16] Vitamins help by acting as cofactors in various stages of wound healing.

Vitamin C

Whenever a person suffers from burn injuries, there is an increase in the levels of reactive oxygen species and reactive nitrogen species in the body. When this exceeds the host's innate antioxidant defenses, it leads to oxidative stress. Vitamin C has antioxidant properties which protects against oxidative stress.[17] It functions as a cofactor for many enzymatic reactions, suppresses proinflammatory processes, and promotes anti-inflammatory activity in macrophages. It prevents the autoinactivation of lysyl and prolyl hydroxylase which are two main enzymes in collagen biosynthesis. It also leads to a dose-dependent increase in collagen type I deposits by normal human fibroblasts. Humans are dependent on dietary supply of vitamin C because they lack functional L-gulono-γ-lactone oxidase which is the final enzyme for vitamin C biosynthesis.[18]

Multiple studies have demonstrated a link between higher dosage of vitamin C and reduced mortality in burns. The definition of high dose varies among the studies. Vitamin C when used in doses of 66 mg/kg/h I/V was shown to decrease fluid requirements and improvement in outcomes.[19-21] A dose 10–24 g/day decreases mortality in patients with severe burns.[22]

Vitamin E

Vitamin E includes α-, β-, γ-, and δ-tocopherol and α-, β-, γ-, and δ-tocotrienols. Due to burn injury, triphenyl phosphonium cations accumulate within the negatively charged mitochondrial inner membrane and lead to oxidative stress.

Vitamin E and its various conjugated forms protect mitochondria from this oxidative stress. Vitamin E acts as an antioxidant and reacts directly with free radicals and transforms them into more stable, nonradical products.

At a dosage of 400 mg/day, it reduces the incidence of infection, leads to rapid wound healing time, and decreased mortality rate.[17]

Vitamin D

Vitamin D exerts most of its physiological effects via 1,25-dihydroxyvitamin D [$1,25(OH)_2D$]. The actions of vitamin D include modulation of the innate immune system (monocytes, macrophages, and dendritic cells) with regulation of antimicrobial peptides such as cathelicidin and β-defensin. It also facilitates the autophagy of intracellular microbes and regulation of antigen presentation in dendritic cells, monocytes, and macrophages.[23]

Vitamin D deficiency is seen in approximately 85–90% of burn patients. It may lead to delay in healing of wounds and increase in the duration of hospital stay.[24] Supplementation is provided based on vitamin D levels, in blood. At levels <25 ng/mL, 50,000 IU once a week for 8 weeks is given, with a follow-up measurement after completion of course. Once the levels reach >25 ng/mL, 2,000 IU daily is given.[12]

Vitamin A

Vitamin A plays an important role in all stages of wound healing. It stimulates the growth of epithelium and fibroblasts, promotes angiogenesis and formation of granulation tissue, while enhancing collagen synthesis. It acts via nuclear retinoic acid receptors, retinoid X receptors, and peroxisome proliferator-activated receptors (PPARs) and enhances the synthesis of extracellular matrix,[25] thus playing an important role in wound healing and growth of epithelium. Vitamin A should be given in dosage of 5,000 IU daily for ages < 3 years and 10,000 IU daily for ages > 3 years.[26]

The recommended dosage for other nutrients are:

- *Zinc sulfate*: 75 mg/day[17]
- *Vitamin K*: 10 mg/week
- *Iron*: 10–15 mg/week

Electrolytes

- Na^+: 1–2 mmol/kg/day
- K^+: 0.5–1 mmol/kg/day
- Mg^{++}: 0.35–0.45 mEq/kg/day
- Ca^{++}: 0.2–0.3 mEq/kg/day
- PO_4^{3-}: 20–30 mmol/day

Fluid requirement in adults may be taken as 30–35 mL/kg/24 h (25 mL/kg/24 h for those who are above 65 years).

Additions must be made for fever approximately 300–500 mL/kg/24 h/°C above normal and other losses. Fluid restriction may be indicated in certain disease states such as cardiac, liver, and renal malfunction.

TIME TO START NUTRITION

Early enteral nutrition can be defined as oral nutrition being started within 24 hours of admission of the patient.[27]

The effectiveness of early enteral nutrition versus late enteral nutrition following burn injury in adults remains unclear in terms of clinical outcomes such as duration of hospital stay and mortality.[28]

Early enteral nutrition leads to the blunting of hypermetabolism and early positive NB.[29]

It also has other benefits including the maintenance of gastrin hormone secretion and gut motility, reduction in the permeability of intestinal wall, and maintenance of mucosal integrity, with a decrease in infections.[30,31]

Oral route is preferred, supplemented with enteral or parenteral supplementation. Feeding via the parenteral route can be used in patients with prolonged ileus or as an adjunct to enteral feeds so as to meet the increased requirements of energy.

Our aim is to prepare the wound for cover and patient for surgical stress. Vigorous nutritional support is started as early as possible to achieve positive energy and NB.

Early versus Late Enteral Nutrition

The time of initiation of nutrition plays a decisive role in the ultimate prognosis of burn patients. Proponents of early nutritional support say that oral feeding started within 24 hours of burns is safe and effective. It also rapidly mitigates several of the important metabolic and hormonal consequences of burns.[27]

Depending on the gut status, nutritional supplementation should begin as early as possible, preferably with appearance of bowel movements and should be increased in a gradual way to achieve an adequate caloric intake.[32]

During the treatment of severe and deep burns, the problems of wound coverage due to inadequate donor areas arise. Early enteral nutrition counters these problems by reversing the major metabolic and hormonal effects of burns.

First studies on early nutrition in burns were done in 1994. Gianotti showed that early enteral nutrition decreased the intestinal translocation of bacteria.[33] While the study published by Wang (1997) showed decreased catabolism after burn with early enteral feeds. The study evaluated the requirement of energy in burn patients along with the levels of glucagon, serum insulin, urine cortisol, and catecholamines. Decrease in the levels of these indices is statistically significant in the early enteral nutrition group when compared to the late enteral nutrition group.[34]

Studies in children with burns have also shown that early enteral nutrition decreases duration of hospitalization and mortality.[35] In a study by Venter et al., improved outcome and betterment of the hormonal stress response were seen in children. This study evaluated the concentrations of insulin, insulin-like growth factor 1 (IGF-1), glucagon, cortisone, and growth hormone in pediatric burns.[36]

The enteral feeds are started with low volume and provided in a continuous manner. They are increased slowly to reach the desired volume so as to ensure patient tolerance.[11]

The recommendations are to start enteral nutrition with a hypocaloric mixture (0.5 kcal/mL) at the rate 25 mL/h. If this is tolerated well by the patient, the rate is increased to 25 mL 8 hourly initially to 100–120 mL/h later on.

MODES OF PROVIDING NUTRITIONAL SUPPORT

Oral Dietary Support

Oral feeding should always be encouraged and attempted. If tolerated by the patient, this is the most convenient and natural way of feeding. Other modes of feeding should be used only if this route is ineffective or cannot be used. Diets should be designed to give the calculated calorie value and protein.

Acceptable protein intake can be obtained with selective high-protein, high-calorie diet, and with additional supplements between meals. Oral liquids concentrated with protein hydrosulfates or amino acids should be provided so as to provide adequate calorie intake (See **Appendices 2.1 to 2.3**).

Depression is frequently present in the burn patients and they may need regular encouragement by family members and the medical team to ensure adequate food consumption. Food should be palatable and tasty and individual's likes and dislikes must be respected. It should fulfill all the nutritional requirements of the patient.

Meals should be served at regular intervals. Small meals 5–6 times a day should be given. The importance of adequate nutrition should be explained and stressed to the patient and his/her relatives.

We should start with liquid diet and gradually switch to semisolids and then solid foods in 4–5 days. Cleanliness in the preparation and serving is of paramount importance to avoid GIT infections. Moribund patients and patients with burned upper extremities require assistance. Excessive lactose in diet may precipitate post-traumatic lactose intolerance, leading to bloating of the abdomen, flatulence, cramps, and diarrhea. Burns of oral cavity may preclude feeding by oral route and may require alternate route of nutrition. Moreover, oral feeding solely cannot meet the elevated calorie requirement.

Enteral Nutrition by Tube Feeding

Administration of feeds with nasogastric tube is recommended as it is more physiological. Nasogastric tubes have the advantages of having a bigger diameter, which decreases clogging and providing bolus feeds becomes easier. But the stomach becomes more prone to develop ileus with nasogastric feeds.

Small postpyloric tubes can be used as a more comfortable option, but they are more prone to blockage and malposition. Patients undergoing surgical procedures can continue postpyloric feedings without an increased risk of aspiration.[37]

If large amounts of enteral mixtures need to be administered, nasoduodenal or nasojejunal tubes can be used. Percutaneous gastrostomy may be planned for providing long-term enteral nutrition.

In patients with more than 20% BSA burns and good bowel function, enteral nutrition has to be used judicially to meet the extra calorie and protein requirement. It is also indicated in patients who are unable to eat due to sepsis, endotracheal intubations, and following anesthesia.

Maximum calories that can be provided through this method are limited to 3,000 kcal/day, combining the calories from protein and nonprotein sources. Optimum-bore tube, which is well tolerated and allows for oral feed, is preferably used in our center. Small amount (0.5–1 mL/kg/h) of low bulk iso-osmolar formula is started initially and gradually, the amount is increased. Most of the tube-feeding formulae contain a high-protein diet, homogenized in a blender with milk and supplemented with some type of commercial protein preparation. Eggs, honey, butter may be added to it. Small feeds should be prepared and given at frequent intervals till calculated volume for 24 hours is achieved.

Feeds exposed to room temperature for >8 hours should be discarded. Gastric contents should be aspirated every time the feed is given. Gastric residue after 4 hours should not exceed 150 mL or else the feeding should be postponed.

Enteral nutrition can be administered as bolus feeds or by a constant delivery pump. Ideally, enteral nutrition can be started at a rate of 15 mL/h of full strength formula and increased stepwise by 15 mL/h every 12 hours to reach up to 100 mL/h. An antiemetic may be added to decrease gastric residual volume.

Instructions to be followed during enteral nutrition are:

- Feeding tube is to be placed by expert.
- Check position of feeding tube by X-ray.
- Head is to be elevated to 30° during feeds.
- Aspirate the tube before every feed or 4 hourly if on continuous drip.
- If aspirate <150 mL, return aspirate and start feeding.
- If >150 mL, reduce feeding amount or increase the time interval.
- Irrigate tube with water after every feed or 4 hourly.
- Intake/output charts are to be maintained.
- Serum electrolytes, proteins, kidney and liver function tests are to be done twice a week.
- Weigh the patient on alternate days.
- Once the iso-osmolar formula is tolerated, hyperosmolar formula may be tried to attain 1 kcal/mL. Continuous drip using a mechanical pump may be used for feeding. The feedings are changed to oral dietary support as soon as the patient can take adequate oral diet.

Adverse effects of tube feeding include vomiting, diarrhea, abdominal distention, dehydration, gastric dilatation, and aspiration. Monitoring of fluid balance, osmolality, and electrolyte status is required to avert the adverse effects. Rectal examination should be done to exclude fecal impaction which may lead to overflow diarrhea. Adequate nursing care to administer tube feeding without complications is absolutely essential.

Bowel function is monitored daily. Immobility or opioid pain medications can cause constipation for which prokinetic drugs such as metoclopramide may be used.

Intolerance to enteral feeding should be monitored carefully. It manifests itself in the form of physical symptoms such as distention of abdomen, nausea, vomiting, bloating, diarrhea, and GIT bleeding or as metabolic derangements including electrolyte disturbances and hyperglycemia.[38]

Enteral feeding offers many advantages over parenteral feeding. Oral feeds help in maintaining integrity of mucosal cell mass which prevents endotoxins and bacterial translocation to the systemic circulation. It also maintains the secretion of digestive enzymes and trophic hormones, particularly gastrin which promotes insulin secretion and anabolism.

Parenteral Nutrition (Appendix 2.4)

Parenteral feeds are required in the following situations:

- In combination with oral/enteral feeds and extensive burns, >40% TBSA or deep burns > 20% BSA to meet high calorie needs

- GIT dysfunction or paralytic ileus
- Patients with septic complications or inhalation injury
- Patients on ventilatory support
- Patients at risk for decreased intestinal perfusion due to aggressive fluid resuscitation

Parenteral nutrition can be given by:
- Peripheral vein
- Central vein

Parenteral support via a peripheral vein is considered while increasing the oral/enteral support to the desired goal. For PN, a central vein is preferred over the peripheral veins because of nonavailability of peripheral veins in chronic burn patients and early development of thrombophlebitis in peripheral veins following administration of hyperosmolar solution.

The advantages of peripheral vein cannulation are:
- Convenient insertion and maintenance
- Lower incidence of mechanical and infectious complications
- Short-term PN of <7 days
- Partial (supplementary) PN
- Temporary in the absence of technical expertise
  Choose a large vein away from injury.

Advantage of parenteral feeding via central vein are:
- When calorie intake via other routes is insignificant or nil or when hyperosmolar liquids have to be given to meet the calorie requirement in extensive burn patients, it is easier to give via central vein as it does not cause thrombophlebitis.

The ideal vein for central venous access is subclavian vein; internal jugular vein is second best choice and femoral vein is best avoided though still is used frequently.

One cannula or one lumen of cannula should be dedicated for PN only. No other medication should be given through it; blood should not be drawn from this (except for the purpose of culture).

Disadvantages of central vein catheterization are:
- Insertion and maintenance needs expertise
- Higher incidence of infectious and mechanical complications

Central veins are therefore used in:
- Prolonged PN of >7 days
- Total PN (TPN)
- Peripheral vein not accessible

Investigations to be done before starting TPN are:
Hematological:
- Blood sugar
- Blood urea/serum creatinine
- Serum albumin
- Magnesium, calcium, phosphorus, and lipid profile
- Prothrombin time
- Liver function tests (bilirubin and enzymes)
- Urine analysis
- Serum electrolytes (Na^+, K^+, Cl^-, and HCO^-)
- Coagulation profile

Optimization of fluid and electrolyte status is mandatory before starting TPN. Daily monitoring of blood chemistry is required along with body weight and fluid balance.

Total parenteral nutrition can be given as separate components of commercially available preparations of proteins, fats, and carbohydrates or as premixed multicomponent solutions which are now available and have reduced the potential for error and metabolic aberration, see **Appendix 2.5 (Tables 2.5A and B)**.

Maximum rate of glucose administration should be 4–6 mg/kg/min to avoid the risk of hyperglycemia.

If carbohydrates are given as the only source of energy, they can lead to:
- Deficiency of essential FAs
- Deficiency of fat soluble vitamins
- Excess CO_2 load
- Hepatic steatosis
- Increased osmolarity of solution

Instruction charts should be maintained stating the following details of PN:
- Total energy calculated on body weight basis
- Substrate distribution (volume of carbohydrate, fat, and protein)
- Fluid volume
- Rate of delivery
- Hang time
- Total time frame
- Steps to be taken in case of accidental change in rate of delivery

There are various complications of parenteral feeding, such as overfeeding of IV nutrients which may lead to hepatic disorders, fluid retention, and metabolic derangements. The rate of substrate utilization determines the volume of PN required, as opposed to a predetermined energy goal, because the demand of energy may reach up to 50 kcal/kg/day. It is important to maintain a rational balance when providing nutrients and the patient should not be overloaded with excessive amounts of energy.

The maximum oxidation of glucose in liver occurs when given at a rate of 4–6 mg/kg/min. If given beyond this rate, it is not assimilated but deposited as fat beneath the skin.[9]

Proteins at 2.5–4 g/kg can be given, increasing gradually to the desired goal.

Fat preparations (20%) are not given during acute phase of shock. Starting with 0.5 g/kg/h, the maximum rate of 1.0–1.5 g/kg/day should not be exceeded when given during the recovery phase.

The daily volume for TPN requirement is calculated on the basis of:
- All ongoing losses, including insensible loss
- Input–output chart
- Alternatively, 30–40 mL/kg body weight
- Caution in patients with renal dysfunction and congestive heart failure

For infants and children weighing < 20 kg = 1.7 mL/kg/h

For children > 20 kg = 1.5 mL/kg/h

Parenteral nutrition is started at 60 mL/h and increased to 80–100 mL/h after 4–6 hours. PN should ideally be given during the daytime. Lipid emulsions when given alone should be completely infused within 12 hours of hanging. Lipids when administered as total nutrient admixture can be hung for 24 hours.

If PN is interrupted due to any reason, clear instructions should be stated to administer 10% dextrose solution at the same rate to prevent sudden hypoglycemia caused by high endogenous insulin. Complications of IV hyperalimentation are greater than with enteral route.

Complications of PN:
- *Mechanical*: Related to catheter placement or thrombosis
- *Infectious*: Bloodstream or catheter site infections
- *Metabolic*:
    - Hyperglycemia
    - Hypertriglyceridemia
    - Fluid, electrolytes, and acid–base disturbances
    - Asymptomatic rise of serum hepatic transaminases
    - Refeeding syndrome

Refeeding syndrome: It is a rare life-threatening syndrome, seen when carbohydrate-rich feeding is started in severely malnourished patients. It is characterized by massive influx of electrolytes inside the cells, resulting in hypokalemia, hypophosphatemia, and hypomagnesemia. The precautions to be taken in such patients are providing only half the calorie needs of 1 day, administration of thiamine (250 mg in 100 mL 5% dextrose IV over 30 min) before starting PN, and aggressive electrolyte monitoring.

Side effects and precautions for PN use: Patients on PN may develop severe egg allergy or allergy due to high levels of triglycerides (>400 mg/dL). Rapid infusion of lipid emulsions can cause fever, chills, tachypnea, wheezing, palpitations, and vomiting. Discontinuation of PN is required in such conditions of severe allergy.

Weaning of PN and precautions for use:
- Stop TPN when enteral feeding can restart.
- Wean slowly to avoid hypoglycemia.
- Monitor hypoglycemia during weaning.
- Give IV dextrose 10% solution at 100 mL/h rate for at least 4–6 hours.
- Alternatively, wean TPN while introducing enteral feeding and stop when enteral intake meets total energy requirement.
- In case PN is to be stopped for some other reason (e.g., a complication), the same protocol of dextrose infusion (10% dextrose at 100 mL/h × 4–5 h) is followed.

Biological value related to how much of the protein consumed is actually absorbed, retained, and used in the body. More specifically, BV is the measure used to rate protein quality through nitrogen retention in human. Higher the quality of protein, more is the nitrogen absorbed and retained by the body.

NB: Of the three energy nutrients, carbohydrates, fats, and proteins, only proteins contain nitrogen. Everyday nitrogen is excreted in our sweat, urine, feces, and from open wounds when present. The human body is in state of continuous nitrogen flux. The body can either be in positive, negative, or zero NB. The state of zero NB is a state of equilibrium where the nitrogen ingested from protein equals the nitrogen loss. Before going into zero NB, the body is in a positive NB. At this stage, the nitrogen absorbed and retained in the body exceeds nitrogen used and lost. It is only during this period that the body can repair and rebuild itself.

In a burn patient, there is an excess of loss of nitrogen from the burn wound and if this excessive demand is not met with, the patient goes into negative NB, i.e., catabolic state.

Free Amino Acids versus Intact Proteins

The ingested free forms of amino acids compete with each other for their uptake through the intestinal lining, thus limiting their rate of absorption by overwhelming the available transport mechanisms. This reduces the total amino acid absorption. There are various drawbacks of these free amino acids. These free amino acids lead to poor nitrogen retention, and hence are the least anabolic. As they lead to increased osmotic pressure in the intestine, there is disturbance in the absorption of all the nutrients which leads to diarrhea and intestinal distress.

Partially hydrolyzed proteins, forming peptides, act as the most anabolic form of dietary supplements and are absorbed significantly faster than either single amino acids or whole proteins. They lead to highest degree of nitrogen retention and do not cause intestinal problems.

ASSESSMENT OF NUTRITIONAL SUPPORT

Evaluation of efficiency of the provided nourishment is important as insufficient nutrition impedes wound healing. Clinical analysis is done to evaluate the nutritional status of the burned patient. Fatigue during physiotherapy and while doing everyday work is usually the first sign of insufficient nutritional intake. Patients are continuously observed for intolerance to enteral nutrition. When tube feeding is given to the patient, measurement of the volume of residual food in the stomach is measured and intestinal transit is observed.

- Intake records give idea of daily protein and calorie intake.
- Daily weight record is a simple method of assessing effectiveness of nutritional support. However, it may be inaccurate due to bulky dressings, fluid shifts, excision, and amputations. Sometimes, it is difficult to weigh a sick patient.
- Immunological markers may be unreliable for assessing nutritional status.
- Serum albumin levels or transferrin can be easily assessed.
- NB studies—consistently elevated blood urea nitrogen (BUN) may indicate deterioration in renal function or increased protein catabolism. Very high BUN is an indication to reduce protein in the diet. If there is no renal insufficiency, evaluation of NB in the body is a good means to evaluate the nutritional state and efficiency of nutrition.

Nitrogen balance is the difference between it's intake (NI) and loss. Practically, excreted nitrogen is measured only in urine. But when other physiological ways of excreting nitrogen, for example, from hair and through skin exudates are included, it becomes necessary to specify nitrogen loss.

Nitrogen loss = Nitrogen lost in urine + 8 mg/kg body wt. + 0.2 g nitrogen/% body surface area burned

Nitrogen in urine = (urea in urine × 0.08)/2.14 + 4 g

Here, 0.08 is a coefficient to convert urea from g/L into mmol/L, 2.14 is a coefficient used to calculate the level of nitrogen in urine from the levels of urea in urine.

NB = NI - nitrogen lost in U + F + S (urine, feces, and skin)

On the first day, blood sugar is measured every 6 hours for 24 hours. During the first week, serum electrolytes, blood urea, sugar, and triglycerides are measured daily. Unstable patients may require their blood sugar and serum electrolytes measurements as often as twice a day. Serum calcium, bilirubin, alkaline phosphatase, phosphorus, magnesium estimations and blood counts should be done at least twice a week.

Liver profile estimation, trace elements, and serum transferrin are done once a week.

NUTRITIONAL ASSESSMENT CHART

See **Appendix 2.6** for stepwise calculation of nutritional requirement.

Surgeons and residents involved in management of burns should learn to prescribe a nutritional regimen in a methodical and scientific manner as follows:

- Before starting nutritional support, patients with shock should be adequately resuscitated and gross fluid and electrolyte imbalance should be corrected. Mild degree of fluid and electrolyte imbalance can be corrected with ongoing nutritional support.
- Decide on the route of administration for nutrition, plan the oral/enteral/PN or partial PN.
- Calculate the energy requirements of burn patients according to Curreri formula depending on the TBSA burn and the patient's age.
- These formulae or equations for calorie estimation often overestimate the calorie requirements.
- To avoid this and simplify it, one can easily calculate the calorie protein needs according to appropriate stress level taking the severity of disease into consideration.
- Calories are derived from three major substrates—carbohydrates, fats, and proteins. By and large, 50% of calories are derived from carbohydrates, 30% from fats, and 20% from proteins. In critically ill patients, certain adjustments are required as mentioned earlier.
- After finalizing the total calorie and substrate requirements, the total permissible liquid intake has to be calculated. Normal recommendation is 30–40 mL/kg/day. However, liquid intake has to be adjusted in specific conditions such as renal and cardiac failure, where volume load needs to be restricted. Consequently, total calories will have to be given in restricted volume of fluid. In patients on TPN, this becomes a challenge and one will have to resort to using more lipid emulsions as they give higher calories on weight to weight basis.

NUTRITION IN SPECIAL CONDITIONS

Pulmonary Conditions

Increased administration of glucose in burn patients (>4–6 mg/kg/h) results in increased CO_2 production. Hence, a patient with ventilatory impairment receiving high-carbohydrate diet will have harmful effect on pH and respiration. Instead, such patients are benefitted by low-carbohydrate and high-fat diet.[39]

Fat should provide 30–50% of nonprotein calories.

Renal Conditions

Due to massive catabolism in burn patients, there is increase in uric acid, potassium, and phosphorus nitrogenous wastes. BUN may increase and complicate the metabolic and nutritional management. BUN should be kept below 100 mg/dL with protein-restricted diets and dialysis. Protein-restricted diets containing only essential amino acids may be tried. 0.6 to1 g/kg/day protein is given initially and gradually increased each day to achieve the goal. Monitoring the daily increase of BUN levels, is important and if BUN levels increase >30 mL/dL/day, amino acids/proteins supply must be reduced and one may consider modified amino acid compositions.

Due to oliguria and hyperkalemia, fluid and potassium restriction is advised in renal failure. Citrus fruits and IV fluids with potassium, for example, Ringer's lactate is restricted. If IV fluids are required, 5% dextrose saline is preferred. Fluid requirement is calculated on the basis of loss due to burns plus previous day's output. Phosphorus and potassium binders may be used orally.

Because of fluid restriction, optimum nonprotein calories are provided with concentrated glucose and lipid solutions. There is reduced glucose tolerance and increased insulin resistance in presence of acute uremia and acidosis; hence, blood glucose levels should be monitored closely in patients with acute renal failure (ARF). Although there are benefits of using lipids as source of energy in patients with ARF, the intake should be limited to 25–30% of total energy.

Hepatic Conditions

In patients with chronic liver disease, aromatic amino acids may lead to hepatic encephalopathy. Supplementation with branched-chain amino acids (BCAAs) is beneficial in such patients. Milk (casein) and vegetable protein diet should be preferred to meat protein diet with rate of 0.6 g to 1 g/kg/day.

However, patients with alcoholic liver disease may benefit from early nutritional support by providing adequate calories, proteins, minerals, and vitamins. In the presence of hepatic encephalopathy, the total protein intake should be reduced to 0.5 g/kg/day or even less.

ADJUVANT THERAPIES TO MODULATE ENERGY REQUIREMENT AND PROMOTE WOUND HEALING

Environmental and clinical factors influence metabolism of the body and hence determine the energy requirements of a burn patient.

The severity of trauma determines the magnitude of inflammatory responses. The response is proportional to the severity of trauma and is not preventable. However, this metabolic rate can be modified by various clinical interventions which can affect or amplify it, influencing the energy requirements. Due to the added effects of inflammation and evaporation, the burn patients are among the most hypermetabolic. Occlusive dressings, early excision, and grafting help in minimizing this effect.

Various interventions can be undertaken to minimize the heat loss. Maintaining optimal temperature of the surroundings, vigorous pain management, sedation as and when required, and ventilator and nutritional support contribute to patient's overall energy expenditure. For instance, a patient with good pain control, proper sedation, and minimal efforts toward breathing while on ventilatory support may have lower requirements than a patient who is less critical, with spontaneous breathing, and with more participation in rehabilitation. Carbohydrate is more efficient in diminishing weight loss and protein degradation after injury.

Hormonal Therapy

Recombinant Human Growth Hormone

Burns involving >40% TBSA are associated with an increase in protein breakdown and a decrease in protein synthesis. This decreased protein metabolism leads to poor healing of the burn wounds and donor sites. Recombinant human growth hormone (rhGH) can be used in such patients to increase protein synthesis.[40]

Animal studies have shown that administration of rhGH during the acute burn phase influences the hepatic acute phase response favorably. Use of rhGH is associated with increase in hepatocyte mitosis and serum and total liver protein concentrations. It also decreases type I acute phase proteins and modulates IL-1-like cytokine expression along with increase in its secondary mediator IGF-1.[41] Muscular growth is maintained by rhGh along with beneficial effects such as improved muscle protein kinetics, early donor site healing, and improved resting energy expenditure.[42-45]

Anabolic effects of rhGH include increase in serum albumin and hemoglobin along with marked augmentation of nitrogen retention, decreased BUN, and increase in serum basal insulin. The beneficial effects of rhGH are mediated by IGF-1 and IGF-binding protein (IGFBP)-3.[46]

Basal insulin secretion is closely related to NB and increased insulin augmentation seems to be the control mechanism for the increased nitrogen retention.

Recombinant growth hormone supplementation is given in the doses of 0.5 IU/kg/day for 2 weeks to arrest severe catabolic state of burns and to avoid weight loss.[47]

Despite its beneficial effects, rhGH use is associated with an increased risk of hyperglycemia. Also, rhGH treatment is costly and long-term treatment could be an obstacle to its wide application.[40]

Oxandrolone

Oxandrolone is a synthetic testosterone analog used in burns to alleviate the hypermetabolic catabolic state. Use of oxandrolone leads to decreased loss of body mass and nitrogen in the burn patient and faster donor area healing.[48]

Oxandrolone given at a dose of 0.1 mg/kg every 12 hours shortens length of acute hospital stay, maintains LBM, improves body composition, and increases hepatic protein synthesis.[49]

When given to children for 1 year after severe burns, it improves LBM, bone mineral content, and muscle strength.[50]

As some studies differ and show no difference in metabolic rate and duration of hospital stay with oxandrolone treatment, further research is warranted.[48]

Oxandrolone can be used for patients with loss in body mass, increased nitrogen loss, or impaired burn wound healing. It can be used as an alternative to rhGH having similar effects but with less hyperglycemia.[51]

Propranolol

Catecholamines act as the primary mediators in the hypermetabolic response associated with burns.[52] Beta-blockers such as propranolol are known to reduce heart rate and blood pressure in addition to their effects on metabolism. Propranolol decreases gluconeogenesis, lipolysis, net catabolism, and the mesenteric blood flow.[53]

It reduces thermogenesis and resting energy expenditure in burn patients along with increased protein synthesis in wound, leading to improved wound healing and epithelization.[54] Propranolol is also shown to induce bactericidal effects in monocytes.[55]

Studies have shown that propranolol use in pediatric patients is associated with decreased heart rate and cardiac work. It reduces central body mass and trunk fat and improves LBM and bone mineral density.[56]

Williams et al. in 2011 in a study found that propranolol given at dosage of 1 mg/kg/day in pediatric and adolescent burn patients reduced heart rate by 15% as compared to basal heart rate.[54]

A combination of propranolol and oxandrolone known as "oxprop" has been used, which leads to a significant increase in muscle strength.[57]

Insulin in Burns

Insulin causes the uptake of blood glucose into skeletal muscles and adipose tissue. It enhances protein and FA synthesis and decreases proteolysis. ICU studies in sepsis and in critical patients show reduced mortality with insulin treatment.[58]

Insulin helps in wound healing and has promitogenic and antiapoptotic action on keratinocytes and fibroblasts.[59]

Maintaining normoglycemia in burn patients leads to better outcomes. Randomized control trials in pediatric patients also show beneficial effects of insulin treatment.[60,61]

Immunotherapy

Immune dysfunction in burn patients makes them susceptible to infections. In the postburn period, severe depression of immunoglobulin G (IgG) concentration occurs, which rises to normal within 1–2 months, while the levels of IgM and IgA remain relatively unaltered.[62]

Bacterial infections such as pseudomonas lead to a decrease in number and function of T cells mediated by an upregulation of programmed death-1 (PD-1) receptor on T cells and programmed cell death ligand-1 (PD-L1) on myeloid cells. This contributes to multiorgan injury and decreased survival. The blockade of PD-1/PD-L1 interactions serves as a potential mechanism to improve outcomes in burn patients.[63]

Studies have shown that prophylactic intravenous immunoglobulin (IVIG)-B in major thermal injury reduces the incidence of septic episodes and decreases hospital stay.[64]

Pentaglobin, i.e., IgM-enriched IV immunoglobulins, contains IgG and elevated concentrations of immunoglobulins A (IgA) and M (IgM). It has an antibacterial, antitoxic, antiinflammatory, and immune-modulating activity, having a broad spectrum of antibodies against various infectious agents and their toxins. It increases microvascular perfusion when used in patients with sepsis or septic shock.[65]

It is given at the rate of 3–5 mL (0.15–0.25 g)/kg body weight. It is repeated at weekly intervals, if required.[66]

The severity of trauma determines the magnitude of inflammatory responses. Adjuvant therapies such as giving immunoglobulins can help modulate inflammatory responses, hence affecting metabolic rate which further influences energy requirements. The rate of metabolism increases with onset of wound sepsis, leading to an increase in the consumption of protein and energy. Pentaglobin used concomitantly with antibiotics, especially against gram-positive and gram-negative bacteria and their toxins indirectly help in reducing rate of metabolism.

Role of Albumin in Burns

Albumin is a protein present naturally in plasma. It has been thought to be beneficial for patients and has also been defined as a "gold standard."[67]

Human albumin solutions available for commercial use must contain 95% of albumin.[68]

Purified protein fractions consist of 83% albumin. The molecular weight of albumin is 69,000 Daltons (approximately). 4% albumin is mildly hypo-oncotic and 5% albumin is iso-oncotic, whereas 20% and 25% solutions are markedly hyperoncotic. Whenever albumin is given, it expands the total plasma volume by shifting of fluid from the interstitial or the intercellular compartment to the intravascular compartment.[68]

The increase in intravascular volume after administration of albumin cannot be predicted as it depends on the volume of blood, level of proteins, and permeability of capillaries. The concentration of serum albumin depends on the rates of synthesis and degradation and also in its distribution between the intravascular and extravascular compartments. The body contains about 3.5–5.0 g/kg body weight of albumin, measuring up to 250–350 g for a healthy 70 kg adult. It is distributed in the plasma compartment (about 42%) and the rest being in extravascular compartment. Some part of it is bound to the tissues and becomes unavailable to the circulation.

The distribution of albumin between the two compartments (intravascular and extravascular) is altered by critical illnesses such as burns. When a patient suffers from burns, the rate of protein synthesis and degradation is also altered. The concentration of serum albumin decreases and it does not increase again until the recovery phase. The pharmacokinetics of IV albumin differ greatly between critically ill patients and the healthy subjects.

The altered distribution in critical illness is related to an increase in capillary leakage. This occurs in sepsis, burns, and after major surgical stress. It involves dysfunction of the endothelial barrier, resulting in capillary leakage and loss of protein, inflammatory cells, and large volumes of fluid into interstitial space.

In the critically ill patients, as an acute phase response to trauma, burns, inflammation, or sepsis, the gene transcription rate for the positive acute phase proteins such as C-reactive protein increases. There is a decrease in the rate of transcription of albumin messenger ribonucleic acid (mRNA) and the resultant synthesis of albumin. Inflammatory mediators such as IL-6 and TNF-α both lead to reduced gene transcription. A prolonged inflammatory response in severe illnesses can lead to continued inhibition of albumin synthesis. There may be alteration of albumin catabolism also.

Theoretically, use of exogenous albumin to raise the intravascular concentration of albumin during the course of a critical illness should be beneficial. But unfortunately, multiple studies over the years have failed to prove any benefit of administering exogenous albumin over other colloidal therapies in adult patients.[69]

Indications for Albumin Administration

- *Volume replacement therapy*: At present, there is no evidence from randomized controlled trials that resuscitation with albumin and plasma protein fraction (PPF) improves survival, compared with resuscitation with cheaper alternatives such as saline, in patients with hypovolemia, burns, and hypoalbuminemia, except in highly selected populations of critically ill patients.[70]
- *Support of colloid oncotic pressure*: It is believed that the oncotic force of concentrated human albumin may help reduce tissue edema. Recent literature states that albumin may exert a direct protective effect in the critically ill patient and its ability to sustain oncotic pressure may only be one of many possible mechanisms.
- *Maintenance of serum albumin levels*: The normal serum concentration of albumin is 35–50 g/L—albumin appears to be a nonspecific marker of the seriousness of an illness.
- As a transport molecule for various drugs and endogenous substances and also acts as an effective plasma buffer
- *To assist in coagulation*: Albumin is involved in the coagulation pathways and has an anticoagulant effect which is probably antithrombotic in nature.
- Free radical scavenging and maintenance of membrane integrity
- *Management of fluid shifts*:
  - As an osmotic agent
  - To redistribute fluid during dialysis
  - To improve oxygenation
- *Miscellaneous—to correct metabolic acidosis*:
  - Neonatology ICU
  - Liver disease, ascites, and malnutrition
  - Starvation
  - Nephrotic syndrome

- Severely burned ICU patients constitute a specific group in whom albumin can play a beneficial role. Though it is reported to be harmful in first 24 hours, its use may be justified after 24 hours in patients with severe hypoalbuminemia as it favors the resorption of edema.

The effectiveness of albumin in burns has been studied extensively. A Cochrane meta-analysis of randomized trials in 1998 attributed increased mortality to albumin among critically injured patients and burns. But the results of this study could not be reproduced.[68] While the 2011 update of the Cochrane meta-analysis continued to suggest an increase in the odds of death among patients receiving albumin, other studies showed no significant increase in mortality.[71]

A 2016 meta-analysis suggested improved outcomes with resuscitation of burn shock with albumin. Albumin infusion during the first 24 hours also leads to a decreased occurrence of compartment syndrome.[72]

After the criticism of albumin-only regimens, hybrid regimens combining crystalloids with albumin were used; such regimens mitigate fluid creep.[73]

Further, the use of human albumin supplementation is expensive, especially in a developing country such as India.

Side Effects of Albumin

The side effects of albumin supplementation are as follows:

- Rapid volume replacement with 20% albumin can lead to cardiac decompensation as it can lead to fourfold increase in volume.
- Albumin can cause or worsen pulmonary edema in the patients with capillary leak and can compromise tissue oxygenation and can finally lead to multiorgan dysfunction.
- It can lead to increase in blood loss in postsurgical or trauma patients due to its antihemostatic and platelet-lowering properties.
- It can lead to worsening of renal failure due to impairment of sodium and water excretion when used in the resuscitation of hypovolemic shock.
- Commercially available preparation of albumin contains aluminum and may lead to toxic concentration of ions. Despite a growing body of systematic reviews, evidence-based medicine analyses and consensus and conferences, the utility and safety profile of albumin is still under dispute.

Human Albumin Replacement Therapy in Burns

- In cases of extensive and severe burns with an increased hematocrit value, normalization of the circulatory conditions can be approached in a very efficient manner with human albumin 20% or 25% diluted with dextrose, levulose, or electrolyte solutions with recommended doses as follows:
    - Adults:
        - 200–400 mL human albumin 20% (40–80 g) diluted 1 in 4, corresponding to 800–1,600 mL of 5% albumin solution

          Or

          200–400 mL of human albumin 25% diluted to 1 in 5 with isotonic electrolyte or dextrose solutions (corresponding to 1–2 L of 5% of albumin solution)
    - Children: 4 mL human albumin 20% per kg body weight diluted 1 in 4 corresponding to 16 mL of 5% albumin solution

      The total dosage over 24 hours can be determined in accordance with the formula:

      $$2 \text{ mL} \times \text{body weight (kg)} \times \% \text{ of surface burn} + 1{,}500 \text{ mL}$$
- Once the acute stage is managed, considerable protein deficiency, especially of albumin may occur. This hypoalbuminemia can be managed by providing albumin as follows:
    - Adults: 50 mL human albumin 20% (10 g) twice a day
    - Children: 1 mL human albumin 20% (0.29 g) per kg body weight

Additional loss of protein and diminished albumin synthesis might lead to severe albumin deficiency. In debilitated patients, stabilization of the protein balance with human albumin 20% may considerably improve the general condition of the patient.

Role of Immunonutrition/ Immunomodulators in Burns and Critically Ill Patients

Malnutrition can lead to impaired immune function. The importance of certain nutrients known as immunomodulators in burns is proven and has got special attention in recent years. These substances have a positive effect on protein metabolism, immune state, and function of intestines. The "immunonutrients" include amino acids arginine and glutamine, omega-3 FAs, nucleotides and antioxidants, vitamins, and minerals.

The amino acid glutamine accounts for >60% of body free amino acid pool and can be synthesized by almost all the tissues. It is considered as a conditionally essential amino acid following injury and illness. During periods of starvation and stress, the glutamine pool reduces significantly.

Glutamine has many pharmacological effects. In catabolic conditions, glutamine is mobilized from muscle tissue to provide energy and substrate to the body. Its low levels correlate with increase in mortality and morbidity.[74]

Supplementation of glutamine enhances serum protein levels and improves the nutritional status of burn patients. It also has immunomodulatory effects, thus reducing burn wound infection and decreased burn wound culture positivity rates.[75]

The study of Zhou (1999) determined that supplementation of glutamine in early stage after burns in the dosage of 0.5–1 g/kg decreases the risk of complications and improves the healing of wound and reduced hospital stay.[76]

Ornithine ketoglutarate (OKG) is a salt which is the precursor to the amino acid glutamine made from the amino acid ornithine and alpha-ketoglutarate.

Its administration improves nutritional status in chronically malnourished (e.g., elderly) and acutely malnourished patients (especially, burn and trauma patients). It improves wound healing and increases liver and intestine protein synthesis.[77]

Ornithine ketoglutarate might change the way amino acids, the building blocks of protein, are used in the body. It also increases insulin. Enterally administered ornithine alpha-ketoglutarate supplementation is usually safe and well tolerated; it decreases protein hypercatabolism and significantly shortens wound-healing time in severe burn patients.[78]

As recommended by Cynober, alpha-ketoglutarate is administered twice a day, a total of 10 g (two bolus every 12 h); it leads to a decrease in the catabolism of muscles and myofibril proteins. This saves muscle glutamine, decreases its catabolism in intestine, and stimulates the synthesis of proteins in liver after burns.[79]

Omega-3 FAs have anti-inflammatory actions; they inhibit the interaction of the endothelium of blood vessels with leukocytes and inhibit synthesis of IL-1 and -6. Ratio of omega-6 FAs and general FA level is important because synthesis of prostaglandins or leukotrienes predominates depends on this ratio. But the effects on clinical outcome remain unclear.

Fish oil as a primary source of omega-3 FAs in nutritional support may be used in burn patients. However, various systematic reviews and meta-analyses do not support the advantage of omega-3 FA nutritional support over low-fat, adequate-protein diets.[80]

Branched-chain Amino Acids

There are nine essential amino acids among which leucine, isoleucine, and valine are considered as the BCAA. Reports (Bower 1986) suggest that administration of BCAA via the parenteral route improves nitrogen retention and leads to better hepatic protein synthesis when compared with standard amino acids.[81] However, the increase in visceral protein concentrations may not improve outcomes in terms of patient mortality and duration of stay.[82]

After burns, a stable mixture of immunomodulators consisting of glutamine, arginine, alpha-ketoglutarate, omega-3 FAs, selenium, and zinc can be used for enteral nutrition.[83,84]

When routine administration of immunonutrients is considered, it is seen that apart from glutamine no other intervention shows any effect on mortality or secondary outcomes. However, routine administration of glutamine is not recommended.[85]

Antioxidants

Antioxidants possibly reduce burn progression by neutralizing reactive oxygen species.[86]

Various compounds have been studied in burns care and need further research such as curcumin in a 2% concentration topically for healing of burn wounds,[87] lazaroids (21-aminosteroids acting as inhibitors of lipid peroxidation in membranes), N-acetylcysteine, metal chelator ethylenediaminetetraacetic acid (EDTA), and human recombinant copper–zinc superoxide dismutase (Hr-CuZnSOD).[88-91]

Role of Environmental and Clinical Factors

There are lots of environmental and clinical factors that influence metabolism and hence energy requirements. Skin acts as an interface and barrier between the patient and the surrounding environment. Hence, all efforts should be made to promote wound healing and re-establish the lost skin barrier.

Adequate nutritional support along with closure of wound is associated with a regain of lost body mass, weight gain, and the patient's return to an active life.

Burn patients are prone to hypothermia. Hypothermia in burns is related to prolonged hospital stay and poor clinical outcomes, which includes higher mortality rates.[92,93]

Role of Early Physiotherapy

Physical activity leads to deposition and assimilation of amino acids into skeletal proteins. With the help of a physiotherapist, early physiotherapy and a planned exercise program must be initiated as soon as possible in burn patients.

Early physiotherapy may reduce the effects of hypermetabolic response after major burns. The physiotherapy program should consist of early mobilization, ambulatory training, chest physiotherapy, and both active and passive normal joint movement exercises. Simple isometric exercises can be done to improve the strength of muscles and enhance the movement of nitrogen to skeletal muscle cells once the equilibrium of calories and nitrogen is achieved.

Early physiotherapy has been related with improvement in biochemical parameters of burn patients, which included reduced inflammatory response and early return to normal of acute phase reactants.[94]

SUMMARY

Apart from the medical and surgical needs of a burn patient, the nutritional aspect should also be given equal importance as nutritional care complements the medical and surgical treatment of any burn patient. Nutritional requirement is met not only by carbohydrates, fat and proteins but also by adjuvant hormonal therapy and immunotherapy. Protein catabolism and mobilization of body fat occurs due to hormonal signals that summons these substrates, apparently for wound healing and energy utilization following burn trauma. The signal for substrate utilization or storage is basically an interaction between insulin and catecholamines. Food intake by the patient stimulates insulin production which diminishes the catabolic effects of increased nervous activity and favors protein biosynthesis and glycogen storage. Judicious and early administration of enteral or parenteral feeds in a burn patient goes a long way in reducing the morbidity and mortality in major burns.

REFERENCES

1. Chang DW, DeSanti L, Demling RH. Anticatabolic and anabolic strategies in critical illness: a review of current treatment modalities. Shock. 1998;10(3):155-60.
2. Mathangi Ramakrishanan K. Handbook of Burns Management, 1st edition. Jaypee Brothers Medical Publishers (P) Ltd.; 1991. pp. 61-5.
3. Carlson DE, Cioffi WG, Mason AD, McManus WF, Pruitt BA. Evaluation of serum visceral protein levels as indicator of nitrogen balance in thermally injured patients. JOEN. 1991;15:440-4.
4. Rafuso CA, Dupertuis YM, Pichard C. The role of visceral proteins in the nutritional assessment of intensive care unit patients. Curr Opin Clin Nutr Metab Care. 2003;6:211-6.
5. Chichester S, Holmes TM, Hubbard J. Ideal body weight: A commentary. Clin Nutr ESPEN. 2021;46:246-50.
6. Nuttall FQ. Body Mass Index: Obesity, BMI, and Health: A Critical Review. Nutr Today. 2015;50(3):117-28.
7. Cunningham JJ, Hegarty MT, Meara PA, Burke JF. Measured and predicted calorie requirement of adult during recovery from severe burn trauma. Am J Clin Nutr. 1989;49:404-8.
8. Wolfe RR. Metabolic response to burn injury: nutritional implications. Keio J Med. 1993;42(1):1-8.
9. Hart DW, Wolf SE, Herndon DN, Chinkes DL, Lal SO, Obeng MK, et al. Energy expenditure and calorie balance after burn: increased feeding leads to fat rather than lean mass accretion. Ann Surg. 2002;235(1):152-61.
10. Natarajan M. Recent Concepts in Nutritional Therapy in Critically Ill Burn Patients. Int J Nutr Pharmacol Neurol Dis. 2019;9:4-36.
11. Clark A, Imran J, Madni T, Wolf SE. Nutrition and metabolism in burn patients. Burns Trauma. 2017;5:11.
12. Coffey R, Thomas S, Murphy CV, Bailey JK, Jones LM, Evans DC. Clinical Guide to Nutrition Therapy: One Center's Guide. Austin J Emergency Crit Care Med. 2015;2(6):1036.
13. Mendonça Machado N, Gragnani A, Masako Ferreira L. Burns, metabolism and nutritional requirements. Nutr Hosp. 2011;26(4):692-700.
14. Berger MM, Shenkin A. Trace elements in trauma and burns. Curr Opin Clin Nutr Metab Care. 1998;1:513-7.
15. Adjepong M, Agbenorku P, Brown P, Oduro I. The role of antioxidant micronutrients in the rate of recovery of burn patients: a systematic review. Burns Trauma. 2016;4:18.
16. Wilkinson HN, Hardman MJ. Wound healing: cellular mechanisms and pathological outcomes. Open Biol. 2020;10(9):200223.
17. Sahib AS, AlKaisy AA. Effect of anti-oxidants, on the incidence of wound infection in burn patients. Ann Burns Fire Disasters. 2010;23(4):199-205.
18. Mohammed BM, Fisher BJ, Kraskauskas D, Ward S, Wayne JS, Brophy DF, et al. Vitamin C promotes wound healing through novel pleiotropic mechanisms. Int Wound J. 2016;13(4):572-84.
19. Tanaka H, Matsuda T, Miyagantani Y, Yukioka T, Matsuda H, Shimazaki S. Reduction of resuscitation fluid volumes in severely burned patients using ascorbic acid administration: a randomized, prospective study. Arch Surg. 2000;135:326-31.
20. Kahn SA, Beers RJ, Lentz CW. Resuscitation after severe burn injury using high-dose ascorbic acid: a retrospective review. J Burn Care Res. 2011;32:110-7.
21. Tanwar B, Uppal D, Mittal RK, Kaushal S, Garg R, Shah S, et al. To evaluate the role of Vitamin C in reducing the resuscitation fluid volume requirement in burned patients. Indian J Burns. 2018;26:77-82.
22. Nakajima M, Kojiro M, Aso S, Matsui H, Fushimi K, Kaita Y, et al. Effect of high-dose vitamin C therapy on severe burn patients: a nationwide cohort study. Crit Care. 2019;23(1):407.
23. Al-Tarrah K, Hewison M, Moiemen N, Lord JM. Vitamin D status and its influence on outcomes following major burn injury and critical illness. Burns Trauma. 2018 6:11.
24. Cho YS, Seo CH, Joo SY, Ohn SH. The association between vitamin D levels and burn factors in different burn types. Burns Trauma. 2020;8:tkaa018.
25. Huang Z, Liu Y, Qi G, Brand D, Zheng SG. Role of Vitamin A in the Immune System. J Clin Med. 2018;7(9):258.

26. Rodruguez DJ. Nutrition in Patients With Severe Burns: State of the Art. J Burn Care Rehabil. 1996;17(1):62-70.
27. Mosier MJ, Pham TN, Klein MB, Gibran NS, Arnoldo BD, Gamelli RL, et al. Early enteral nutrition in burns: compliance with guidelines and associated outcomes in a multicenter study. J Burn Care Res. 2011;32(1):104-9.
28. Wasiak J, Cleland H, Jeffery R. Early versus delayed enteral nutrition support for burn injuries. Cochrane Database Syst Rev. 2006;(3):CD005489.
29. Chiarelli A, Enzi G, Casadei A, Baggio B, Valerio A, Mazzoleni F. Very early nutrition supplementation in burned patients. Am J Clin Nutr. 1990;51:1035-9.
30. Chen Z, Wang S, Yu B, Li A. A comparison study between early enteral nutrition and parenteral nutrition in severe burn patients. Burns. 2007;33:708-12.
31. Pu H, Doig GS, Heighes PT, Allingstrup MJ. Early enteral nutrition reduces mortality and improves other key outcomes in patients with major burn injury: a meta-analysis of randomized controlled trials. Crit Care Med. 2018;46:2036-42.
32. Gupta JL. Ten commandments of burn management. Indian J Burns. 2012;20:7-10.
33. Gianotti L, Nelson JL, Alexander JW, Chalk CL, Pyles T. Post injury hypermetabolic response and magnitude of translocation: Prevention by early enteral nutrition. Nutrition. 1994;10:225-31.
34. Wang S, Wang S, You Z. Clinical study of the effect of early enteral feeding on reducing hypermetabolism after severe burns. Zhonghua Wai Ke Za Zhi. 1997;35(1):44-7.
35. Khorasani EN, Mansouri F. Effect of early enteral nutrition on morbidity and mortality in children with burns. Burns. 2010;36(7):1067-71.
36. Venter M, Rode H, Sive A, Visser M. Enteral resuscitation and early enteral feeding in children with major burns—effect on McFarlane response to stress. Burns. 2007;33(4):464-71.
37. Jenkins ME, Gottschlich MM, Warden GD. Enteral feeding during operative procedures in thermal injuries. J Burn Care Rehabil. 1994;15(2):199-205.
38. Bernard AC, Magnuson B, Tsuei BJ, Swintosky M, Barnes S, Kearney PA. Defining and assessing tolerance in enteral nutrition. Nutr Clin Pract. 2004;19(5):481-6.
39. Cai B, Zhu Y, Ma Yi, Xu Z, Zao Yi, Wang J, et al. Effect of supplementing a high-fat, low-carbohydrate enteral formula in COPD patients. Nutrition. 2003;19:229-32.
40. Breederveld RS, Tuinebreijer WE. Recombinant human growth hormone for treating burns and donor sites. Cochrane Database Syst Rev. 2014;2014(9):CD008990.
41. Jeschke MG, Herndon DN, Wolf SE, DebRoy MA, Rai J, Lichtenbelt BJ, et al. Recombinant human growth hormone alters acute phase reactant proteins, cytokine expression, and liver morphology in burned rats. J Surg Res. 1999;83(2):122-9.
42. Aili Low JF, Barrow RE, Mittendorfer B, Jeschke MG, Chinkes DL, Herndon DN. The effect of short-term growth hormone treatment on growth and energy expenditure in burned children. Burns. 2001;27(5):447-52.
43. Hart DW, Herndon DN, Klein G, Lee SB, Celis M, Mohan S, et al. Attenuation of posttraumatic muscle catabolism and osteopenia by long-term growth hormone therapy. Ann Surg. 2001;233(6):827-34.
44. Herndon DN, Barrow RE, Kunkel KR, Broemeling L, Rutan RL. Effects of recombinant human growth hormone on donor-site healing in severely burned children. Ann Surg. 1990;212(4):424-9; discussion 430-1.
45. Klein GL, Wolf SE, Langman CB, Rosen CJ, Mohan S, Keenan BS, et al. Effects of therapy with recombinant human growth hormone on insulin-like growth factor system components and serum levels of biochemical markers of bone formation in children after severe burn injury. J Clin Endocrinol Metab. 1998;83(1):21-4.
46. Branski LK, Herndon DN, Barrow RE, Kulp GA, Klein GL, Suman OE, et al. Randomized Controlled Trial to Determine the Efficacy of Long-Term Growth Hormone Treatment in Severely Burned Children. Ann Surg. 2009;250(4):514-23.
47. Singh KP, Prasad R, Chari PS, Dash RJ. Effect of growth hormone therapy in burn patients on conservative treatment. Burns. 1998;24(8):733-8.
48. Real DS, Reis RP, Piccolo MS, Okamoto RH, Gragnani A, Ferreira LM. Oxandrolone use in adult burn patients. Systematic review and meta-analysis. Acta Cir Bras. 2014;29 Suppl 3:68-76.
49. Jeschke MG, Finnerty CC, Suman OE, Kulp G, Mlcak RP, Herndon DN. The effect of oxandrolone on the endocrinologic, inflammatory, and hypermetabolic responses during the acute phase postburn. Ann Surg. 2007;246(3):351-62.
50. Przkora R, Jeschke MG, Barrow RE, Suman OE, Meyer WJ, Finnerty CC, et al. Metabolic and hormonal changes of severely burned children receiving long-term oxandrolone treatment. Ann Surg. 2005;242(3):384-9; discussion 390-1.
51. Demling RH. Comparison of the anabolic effects and complications of human growth hormone and the testosterone analog, oxandrolone, after severe burn injury. Burns. 1999;25(3):215-21.
52. Wilmore DW, Long JM, Mason AD Jr, Skreen RW, Pruitt BA Jr. Catecholamines: mediator of the hypermetabolic response to thermal injury. Ann Surg. 1974;180(4):653-69.
53. Núñez-Villaveirán T, Sánchez M, Millán P, García-de-Lorenzo A. Systematic review of the effect of propranolol on hypermetabolism in burn injuries. Med Intensiva. 2015;39(2):101-13. [English, Spanish].
54. Williams FN, Herndon DN, Kulp GA, Jeschke MG. Propranolol decreases cardiac work in a dose-dependent manner in severely burned children. Surgery. 2011;149:231-9.
55. Kobayashi M, Jeschke MG, Asai A, Kogiso M, Yoshida S, Herndon DN, et al. Propranolol as a modulator of M2b monocytes in severely burned patients. J Leukoc Biol. 2011;89:797-803.
56. Herndon DN, Rodriguez NA, Diaz EC, Hegde S, Jennings K, Mlcak RP, et al. Long-term propranolol use in severely burned pediatric patients: a randomized controlled study. Ann Surg. 2012;256:402-11.
57. Chao T, Porter C, Herndon DN, Siopi A, Ideker H, Mlcak RP, et al. Propranolol and oxandrolone therapy accelerated muscle recovery in burned children. Med Sci Sports Exerc. 2018;50(3):427-35.
58. Finney SJ, Zekveld C, Elia A, Evans TW. Glucose control and mortality in critically ill patients. JAMA. 2003;290:20417.
59. Pierre E, Barrow RE, Sakurai Y, Wolfe RR, Herndon DN. Structural effects of insulin on wound healing. Plastic Surg. 1996;36:743-45.
60. Jeschke MG, Kulp GA, Kraft R, Finnerty CC, Mlcak R, Lee JO, et al. Intensive insulin therapy in severely burned pediatric patients: a prospective randomized trial. Am J Respir Crit Care Med. 2010;182:351-9.
61. Gauglitz GG, Toliver-Kinsky TE, Williams FN, Song J, Cui W, Herndon DN, et al. Insulin increases resistance to burn wound infection-associated sepsis. Crit Care Med. 2010;38:202-8.

62. Munster AM, Hoagland HC, Pruitt BA Jr. The effect of thermal injury on serum immunoglobulins. Ann Surg. 1970;172:965-9.
63. Patil NK, Luan L, Bohannon JK, Hernandez A, Guo Y, Sherwood ER. Frontline Science: Anti-PD-L1 protects against infection with common bacterial pathogens after burn injury. J Leukoc Biol. 2018;103(1):23-33.
64. Lyons JM, Davis C, Rieman MT, Kopcha R, Phan H, Greenhalgh D, et al. Prophylactic intravenous immune globulin and polymixin B decrease the incidence of septic episodes and hospital length of stay in severely burned children. J Burn Care Res. 2006;27(6):813-8.
65. Domizi R, Adrario E, Damiani E, Scorcella C, Carsetti A, Giaccaglia P, et al. IgM-enriched immunoglobulins (Pentaglobin) may improve the microcirculation in sepsis: a pilot randomized trial. Ann Intensive Care. 2019;9(1):135.
66. MIMS. Pentaglobin: Human normal immunoglobulin. [online] Available from https://www.mims.com/hongkong/drug/info/pentaglobin?type=full [Last accessed May, 2024].
67. Cochrane injuries Group Albumin Reviewers. Human Albumin administration in critically ill patients: Systematic review of randomized controlled trials. BMJ. 1998;317:235-40.
68. 5 Human Albumin. Transfus Med Hemother. 2009;36(6):399-407.
69. Liumbruno GM, Bennardello F, Lattanzio A, Piccoli P, Rossettias G; Italian Society of Transfusion Medicine and Immunohaematology (SIMTI). Recommendations for the use of albumin and immunoglobulins. Blood Transfus. 2009;7(3):216-34.
70. Eljaiek R, Heylbroeck C, Dubois MJ. Albumin administration for fluid resuscitation in burn patients: A systematic review and meta-analysis. Burns. 2017;43(1):17-24.
71. Roberts I, Blackhall K, Alderson P, Bunn F, Schierhout G. Human albumin solution for resuscitation and volume expansion in critically ill patients. Cochrane Database Syst Rev. 2011;11:CD001208.
72. Navickis RJ, Greenhalgh DG, Wilkes MM. Albumin in Burn Shock Resuscitation: A Meta-Analysis of Controlled Clinical Studies. J Burn Care Res. 2016;37(3):e268-78.
73. Hunter JE, Drew PJ, Potokar TS, Dickson W, Hemington-Gorse SJ. Albumin resuscitation in burns: a hybrid regime to mitigate fluid creep. Scars Burn Heal. 2016;2:2059513116642083.
74. Boelens PG, Nijveldt RJ, Houdijk AP, Meijer S, van Leeuwen PA. Glutamine Alimentation in Catabolic State. J Nutr. 2001;131(9 Suppl):2569S-77S; discussion 2590S.
75. Arora S, Shankar C. Effects of early enteral glutamine supplementation on the outcome of severe burns: A randomized control study. Indian J Burns. 2020;28:57-62.
76. Zhou Y, Jiang Z, Sun Y. Glutamine dipeptide enriched enteral nutrition improving gut permeability in severe burns. Zhonghua Yi Xue Za Zhi. 1999;79(11):825-7. [Chinese].
77. Cynober L. Ornithine α-Ketoglutarate as a Potent Precursor of Arginine and Nitric Oxide: A New Job for an Old Friend. J Nutr. 2004;134(10 Suppl):2858S-62S; discussion 2895S.
78. Coudray-Lucas C, Le Bever H, Cynober L, De Bandt JP, Carsin H. Ornithine alpha-ketoglutarate improves wound healing in severe burn patients: a prospective randomized double-blind trial versus isonitrogenous controls. Crit Care Med. 2000;28(6):1772-6.
79. Cynober L. Ornithine alpha-ketoglutarate in nutritional support. Nutrition. 1991;7(5):313-22.
80. Siritientong T, Thet D, Buangbon M, Nokehoon P, Leelakanok N, Methaneethorn J, et al. Nutritional Support with Omega-3 Fatty Acids in Burn Patients: A Systematic Review with Meta-Analysis of Randomized Controlled Trials. Nutrients. 2022;14:2874.
81. Bower RH, Muggia-Sullam M, Vallgren S, Hurst JM, Kern KA, LaFrance R, et al. Branched chain amino acid-enriched solutions in the septic patient. A randomized, prospective trial. Ann Surg. 1986;203(1):13-20.
82. Brown RO, Buonpane EA, Vehe KL, Hickerson WL, Luther RW. Comparison of modified amino acids and standard amino acids in parenteral nutrition support of thermally injured patients. Crit Care Med. 1990;18(10):1096-101.
83. Saffle JR, Webke G, Jennings K, Morris SE, Barton RG. Randomized trial of immune enhancing enteral nutrition in burn patients. J Trauma. 1997;42:793-802.
84. Gottschlich MM, Jenkins M, Warden GD, Boumer T, Havens P, Snook JT. Differential effects of 3 enteral dietary regimes on selected outcome variables in burn patients. JPEN. 1990;14:225-36.
85. Tan HB, Danilla S, Murray A, Serra R, El Dib R, Henderson TO, et al. Immunonutrition as an adjuvant therapy for burns. Cochrane Database Syst Rev. 2014;2014(12):CD007174.
86. Shupp JW, Nasabzadeh TJ, Rosenthal DS, Jordan MH, Fidler P, Jeng JC. A review of the local pathophysiologic bases of burn wound progression. J Burn Care Res. 2010;31:849-73.
87. Mehrabani D, Farjam M, Geramizadeh B, Tanideh N, Amini M, Panjehshahin MR. The healing effect of curcumin on burn wounds in rat. World J Plast Surg. 2015;4(1):29-35.
88. Clark WM, Hazel JS, Coull BM. Lazaroids. CNS pharmacology and current research. Drugs. 1995;50:971-83.
89. Deniz M, Borman H, Seyhan T, Haberal M. An effective antioxidant drug on prevention of the necrosis of zone of stasis: N-acetylcysteine. Burns. 2013;39:320-5.
90. Wang CZ, Ayadi AE, Goswamy J, Finnerty CC, Mifflin R, Sousse L, et al. Topically applied metal chelator reduces thermal injury progression in a rat model of brass comb burn. Burns. 2015;41:1775-87.
91. Vorauer-Uhl K, Furnschlief E, Wagner A, Ferko B, Katinger H. Reepithelialization of experimental scalds effected by topically applied superoxide dismutase: controlled animal studies. Wound Repair Regen. 2002;10:366-71.
92. Ziegler B, Kenngott T, Fischer S, Hundeshagen G, Hartmann B, Horter J, et al. Early hypothermia as risk factor in severely burned patients: a retrospective outcome study. Burns. 2019;45:1895-900.
93. Hostler D, Weaver MD, Ziembicki JA, Kowger HL, McEntire SJ, Rittenberger JC, et al. Admission temperature and survival in patients admitted to burn centers. J Burn Care Res. 2013;34:498-506.
94. Çınar MA, Bayramlar K, Erkılıç A, Güneş A, Yakut Y. The effects of early physiotherapy on biochemical parameters in major burn patients: A burn center's experience. Ulus Travma Acil Cerrahi Derg. 2019;25:461-6.

CHAPTER 33

Physiotherapy in Burns

R Raja Shanmugakrishnan

INTRODUCTION

Physiotherapy is a crucial component of burn management. As a vital member of the burn team, the physiotherapist ought to participate in multidisciplinary meetings and have conversations with the burn surgeons and other paramedics. They must be included from the beginning of the treatment regimen to promote proper wound healing, joint function and expedite the patient's recovery.

EVALUATION OF THE BURN PATIENT

Soon after the patient arrives, the physiotherapist should assess the patient based on the following parameters:

- History of how the accident occurred and whether there was inhalation injury.
- Interview the patient's caregivers to decide upon the patient's preinjury functional status and activity level.
- Note the burn injury's etiology, and total body surface area (TBSA) burned.
- Assess the edema, range of motion of the joints, strength, and sensation if appropriate.
- Look for positioning of the affected areas, including splinting.
- Note down the short-term and long-term treatment goals.

Finally, the physiotherapist should document the treatment plan clearly based on the above.

PHYSIOTHERAPY IN ACUTE BURNS

The Rationale Behind the Importance of Physiotherapy in Acute Burns

In major burns, a supranormal release of proinflammatory mediators, glucocorticoids, and catecholamines results in hypermetabolism, muscle wasting, and insulin resistance. Prolonged immobilization can also lead to disuse atrophy and severe muscle wasting. The skeletal muscle is responsible for 70–80% uptake of glucose. When the majority of the muscle is lost, this leads to glucose not being taken up and causing insulin resistance. Within days after injury, there is a noticeable loss of lean body mass due to increased protein breakdown and muscle atrophy. Lean body mass refers to the body's mass that is not fat. A 10% reduction of lean body mass results in impaired immunity. Additionally, a 20% loss of lean body mass leads to impaired wound healing with associated 30% mortality. Furthermore, a 30% loss of lean body mass leads to pneumonia and pressure sores with 50% mortality. Lastly, a 40% loss of lean body mass results in death in almost all 100% of cases. The injury can also result in various problems such as joint contractures, restricted range of motion, weakness, fatigue, poor wound healing, sepsis, and even death. Hence, exercise and physiotherapy are crucial for preserving and increasing muscle mass, maintaining muscle bulk, preventing contractures, preserving the full range of motion of joints, promoting good wound healing, and preventing insulin resistance.

THERAPEUTIC EXERCISE

Therapeutic exercise is the scientific supervision of bodily movement with or without apparatus to restore normal function to diseased or injured tissues. The goals of therapeutic exercise during burn rehabilitation include the following:

- Maintaining joint motion and muscle strength.
- Reduce the effect of edema and immobilization.
- Stretch the scar tissue.
- Return the patient to an optimal level of function as soon as possible.

Exercise prescription is a continuous process that is modified based on the patient's medical condition and individual requirements. The conservative treatment of burn management includes starting vigorous physiotherapy as soon as possible to maintain good function. Escharotomies, fasciotomies, allografts, and synthetic dressings do not contraindicate exercise, and the patient should be mobilized as soon as possible. Early mobilization is crucial for reducing edema. After surgery, exercises involving autografted skin over joints are typically paused for 4–5 days. During deep burn healing, shortening of immature connective tissue leads to scar contractures and limited joint mobility. Physiotherapy prevents joint deformities and preserves range of motion.

Exercise can be very painful for patients. So, physiotherapists must spend time with them, understand them, and communicate effectively with a positive attitude. This is essential for patients to succeed in physiotherapy, gain confidence, and improve compliance. The initial repetition of an exercise is typically the most challenging and painful. This is because the discomfort is primarily caused by stretching dry and tight skin that has lost its natural lubrication. However, as the skin stretches and the muscles pump, each subsequent repetition becomes easier and helps to reduce swelling and pain. Patients tend to do well when they have an achievable goal in mind. The physiotherapist should constantly motivate the patient to improve their outcomes and do more every time they do an activity. When provided with the desired incentives such as an age-appropriate game or activity, small children tend to do well. The patients may need frequent periods of rest due to their decreased endurance levels or pain. The physiotherapist needs to be considerate regarding this and probably needs to do it multiple times with short sessions. The goal is to make the patient move regularly, frequently, and progressively.

Exercise during the Active Rehabilitation Phase

The acute rehabilitation phase is defined as the time from burn admission until the patient's wounds are 50% closed, or skin grafting for wound closure has begun. The main goals of this period are to reduce edema, promote early ambulation, maintain joint mobility, and prevent lung complications. These objectives can often be achieved without interfering with other life-saving measures done during this period.

Mobilization

Prolonged immobilization can also result in decreased cardiovascular fitness, decreased endurance, increased risk of thromboembolism, pressure sores, pulmonary complications, osteoporosis, and disuse muscle atrophy. Hence, all efforts should be taken to mobilize the patient as frequently and early as possible. Impaired cognitive status, decreased motor control, weakness, pain, and risk of graft shearing can make ambulation difficult. It is a standard practice to immobilize a patient for an extended period after graft application. However, recent studies have shown that patients can be ambulated earlier.

All wounds should have a proper dressing done before ambulating. Wrapped bandages help to facilitate capillary drainage. The "figure of eight" pattern gives better pressure support than the spiral wrap, probably due to increased vascular support **(Fig. 1)**. Stiff hips, knees, and ankles may make ambulation difficult. Therefore, they need to be stretched and mobilized before ambulation is started.

Hence, many units apply Unna boot to prevent graft shearing early on. Unna boot is based on a bandage impregnated with zinc oxide and calamine lotion. When applied over the grafted lower limb, it hardens to a semi-rigid dressing resembling a total contact cast, providing uniform support to the fresh skin graft and enabling early ambulation. The Unna boot can be worn for 7 days. If an earlier inspection of the skin graft is desired, it can be removed and replaced with a new "Unna" boot.

Total contact cast can also be applied. In this, the assistant supports the patient with the ankle bent to a 90° angle. The leg is covered with a stockinette. Several layers of padding should be applied taking appropriate care of the bony prominences. Wrinkles and irregularities in the padding should be avoided. Above this, a shell cast composed of 6-inch plaster of Paris rolls is applied. The plaster of Paris rolls is applied from distal to proximal. Typically, 3–4 plaster of Paris rolls is applied. The casting material should be smoothened out to fill plaster voids, strengthen layer connections, and fit the extremity shape. The leg is held in the desired position until the

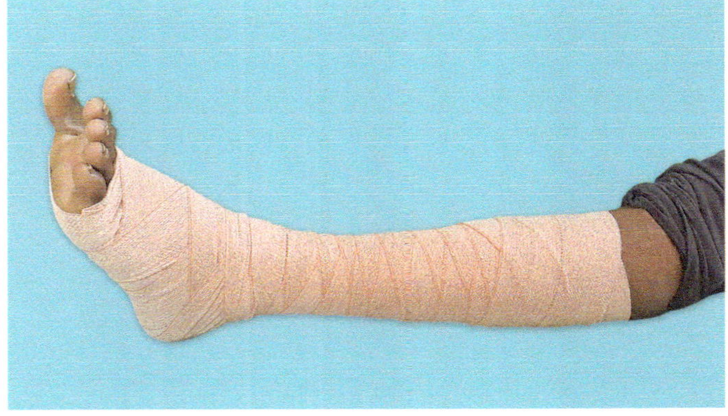

FIG. 1: Figure of "eight bandaging".

cast material hardens sufficiently. A fiber cast is added on top of the plaster of Paris cast to strengthen the cast sufficiently. The fiber cast has sharp edges and the edge of the cast should be a few centimeters within the shell cast margins and should not extend beyond it to avoid injuries during usage. We should allow sufficient time for the cast to be set before using it. The use of cast shoes is a must during weight bearing. Check for distal neurovascular status at the end **(Figs. 2A to E)**.

Range of Motion Exercises

Active exercises are exercises in which a person exerts a force to complete the action. For cooperative and understanding patients, active range of motion exercises should be initiated within 24 hours after a burn injury. These exercises are beneficial in reducing edema in the extremities, increasing muscle strength and bulk, stretching healed or healing skin, preventing joint contractures and stiffness, and providing overall strength-related benefits. However, active range of motion exercises may not be feasible for patients who are intubated or experiencing fear, anxiety, and pain. In such cases, active assisted range of motion exercises can be performed, where the patient exerts some force to complete a movement, and the physiotherapist passively assists in achieving the full range of motion. This exercise also helps to prevent joint

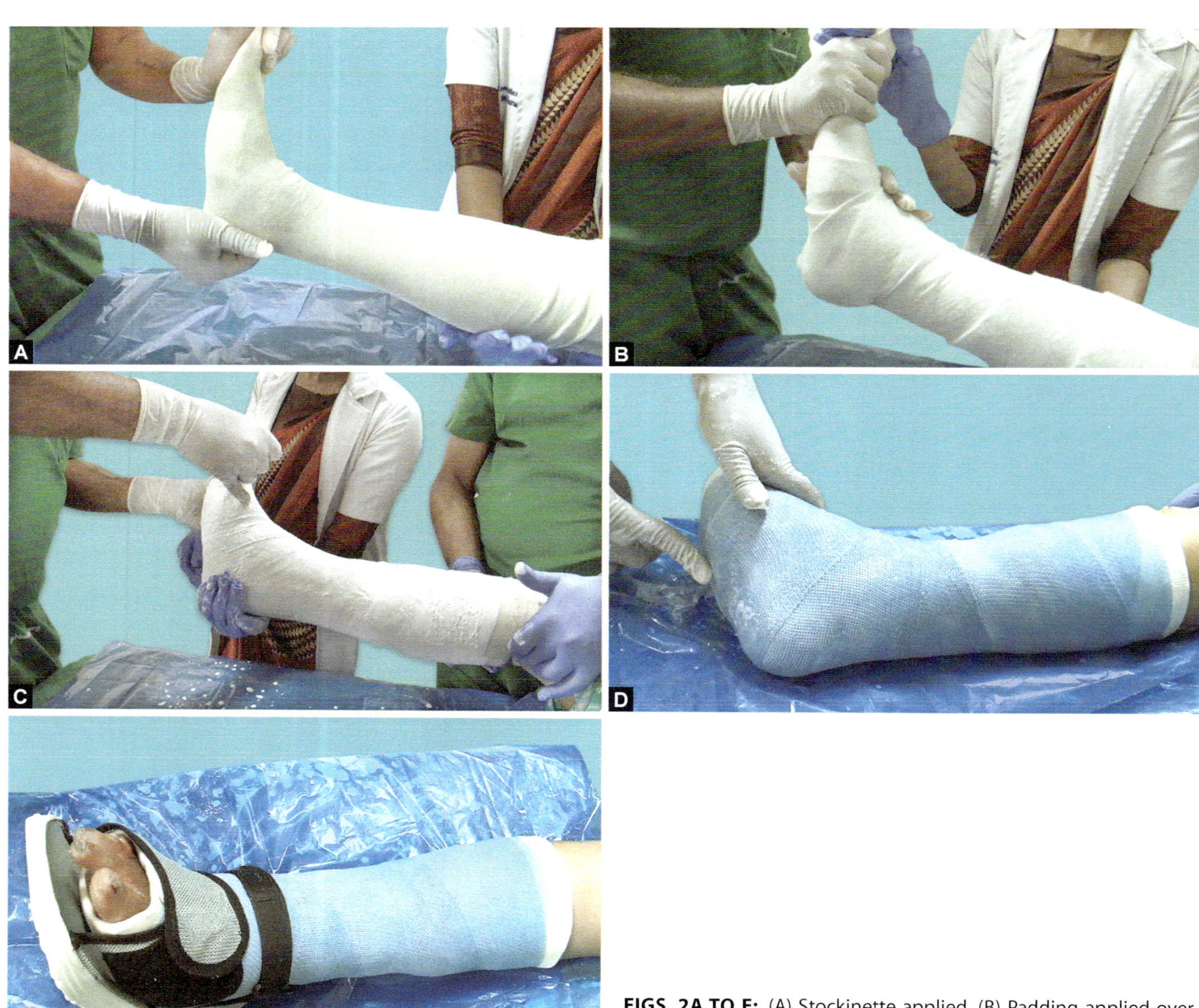

FIGS. 2A TO E: (A) Stockinette applied. (B) Padding applied over stockinette. (C) Plaster of Paris rolls applied over the stockinette. (D) Fiber cast applied. (E) Cast shoes applied at the end.

contractures and aids in attaining the complete range of motion. Critically ill, heavily medicated, septic, and intubated patients are unable to perform active or active assisted exercises. So, passive range of motion exercises is recommended. During passive range of motion exercises, the therapist moves each joint individually without active effort from the patient to maintain the full range of motion, prevent skin thickening, elongate tissues, and achieve optimal range of motion. Although the passive range of motion exercises requires less energy expenditure, they are inferior to active exercises as they do not strengthen the muscles. Modern continuous passive motion devices are also effective in improving joint range of motion and facilitating exercise.

Resistance Exercises

Resistance exercises increase muscle strength and bulk by making the muscles work against a weight or a force. As the patient's condition improves, it is essential to begin incorporating resistance exercises. The therapist can apply resistance while instructing the patient to flex their muscles against it. This technique effectively increases muscle strength and can be applied to both the upper and lower limbs.

The therapist gives resistance while the patient tries to actively flex the elbow to strengthen and build the flexors of the arm **(Fig. 3)**. Similarly, as the patient attempts to actively extend the elbow, the therapist gives resistance to increase the muscle strength and bulk of the triceps muscles **(Fig. 4)**. Similarly, a weight is tied to the leg, and the patient tries to actively extend the knee from the flexed position while sitting. This strengthens the quadriceps muscle. The ankle is dorsiflexed and plantarflexed against resistance to strengthen the muscles of the anterior and posterior compartments of the leg **(Figs. 5A and B)**.

Isometric Exercises

Isometric exercises are exercises in which a muscle or a group of muscles are tightened without reducing the length of the muscle or moving the joint. They help to maintain the strength of the muscle. Isometric exercises

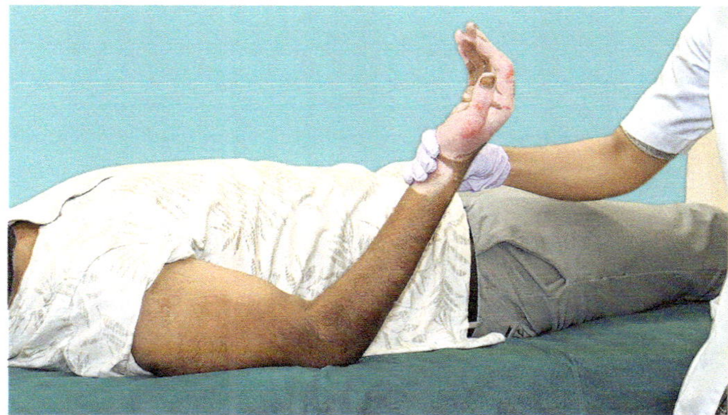

FIG. 3: The patient actively flexes the elbow against resistance while the physiotherapist offers resistance.

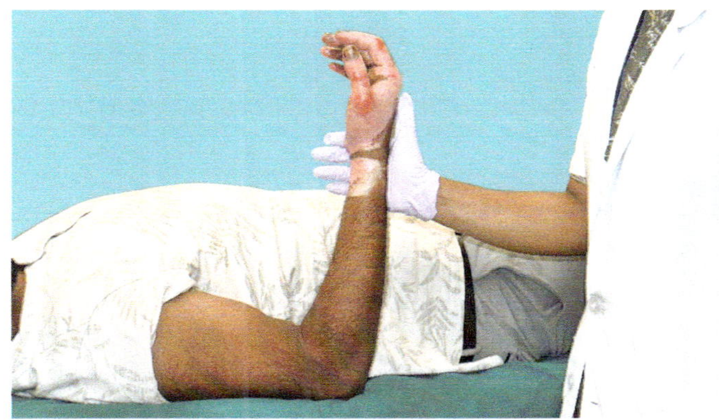

FIG. 4: The patient actively extends the elbow while the physiotherapist offers resistance.

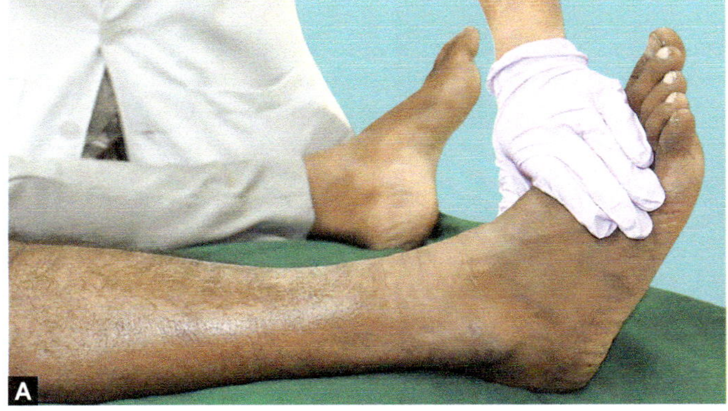

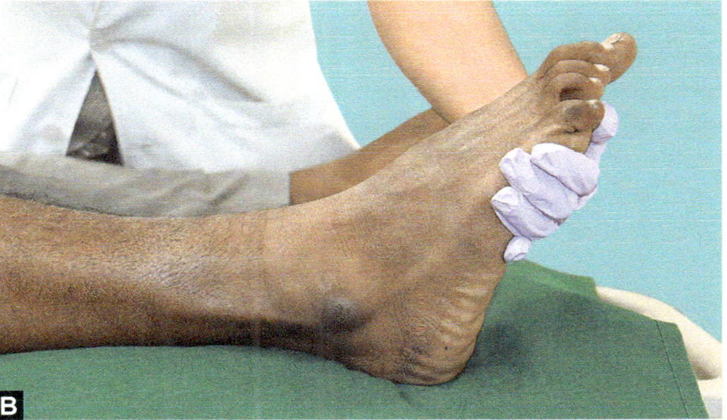

FIGS. 5A AND B: (A) The patient actively dorsiflexes the ankle against resistance. (B) The patient actively plantarflexes the ankle against resistance.

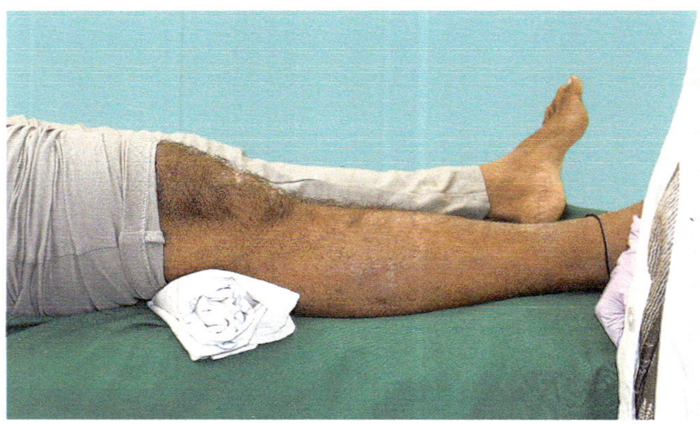

FIG. 6: Isometric exercises: The patient is advised to press a towel or hand placed beneath the extended knee to contract the quadriceps muscle.

can also increase muscle strength, but not as effectively as isotonic exercises. An example of isometric exercise is when the quadriceps muscles contract when we encourage the patient to contract the quadriceps muscles with the knee extended. A towel can be placed below the extended knee and the patient is advised to press the towel below **(Fig. 6)**.

Isometric exercises offer several benefits:

- They enhance muscle strength even when the patient is at rest and is comfortable.
- They require minimal energy expenditure.
- They prevent muscle contraction loss, which often occurs during prolonged immobilization.
- Patients do not "forget" how to contract the muscle, which is a common phenomenon that occurs with prolonged periods of immobilization.

Exercises during the Intermediate Rehabilitation Phase

The intermediate phase is the time between the start of the wound's closure and the final closure. The primary focus of this phase is to prevent the ill effects of skin contraction, such as contractures, which can limit the patient's functional status. The goals of exercise during this period are:

- Maintaining the full joint range of motion
- Increasing motor skills and coordination
- Promoting functional independence
- Increasing the endurance and strength to prevent muscle atrophy

During this period, as the patient's medical status improves, the sedation decreases, the operation becomes less frequent, and the patient becomes alert. The patient understands what is being done, and at this point of time, many patients go in for depression. We must spend a lot of time with the patient and understand the patient's problems, encourage them with a smile, show them how the previous patients have improved and keep encouraging them to do well. This is very important for them to do all the exercises and activities that we recommend. If the patient is not fully convinced of what we will do, the patient's compliance becomes poor, and appropriate rehabilitation may not be possible. Hence, talking to the patients is very important.

As the wounds heal, scars form and start contracting. Slow and sustained stretch is considered one of the best methods to combat scar contraction and contracture formation. Gentle, slow, and sustained stretch is more effective than multiple repetitive movements to gain the length of burnt tissues. Connective tissues tend to elongate under constant tension. Hence, sustained stretches are performed across joints to prevent joint contractures. However, this can be painful and discomforting to the patient. We must look into the blanching of the scar tissue and the patient's response. If the tissue blanches and if the patient is very uncomfortable, it is stopped. The exercise is paused for a short time and then restarted. It is imperative to impart the appropriate force to produce plastic elongation of the tissues without causing trauma to the tissues or the patient.

We should gradually strengthen the muscles further by increasing weights and applying resistance **(Fig. 7)**. We should concentrate on areas we find very weak during strength assessments and the muscles that oppose the scar tissue contractures.

The patient is encouraged to ambulate further **(Fig. 8)**. We need to set daily goals for the patient and encourage the patient to walk further while providing the least amount of support. While doing so, we must look for any gait disturbances. If there are any gait disturbances, they need to be corrected before they become lasting habits. As the patient ambulates more and more, the patients become more confident and have a sense of functional independence.

Long-term Rehabilitation Phase

The long-term phase is the time between the wound closure or discharge from the acute hospital setting until the patient has received maximum benefit from rehabilitation services.

We must encourage the patient to moisturize the skin well and continue exercising at home. Patient compliance is critical, and we need to monitor the compliance to get good results. We need to encourage the patient to keep walking for longer distances. We need to encourage them to do all the day-to-day activities. The ultimate rehabilitation is getting them back to work. We must

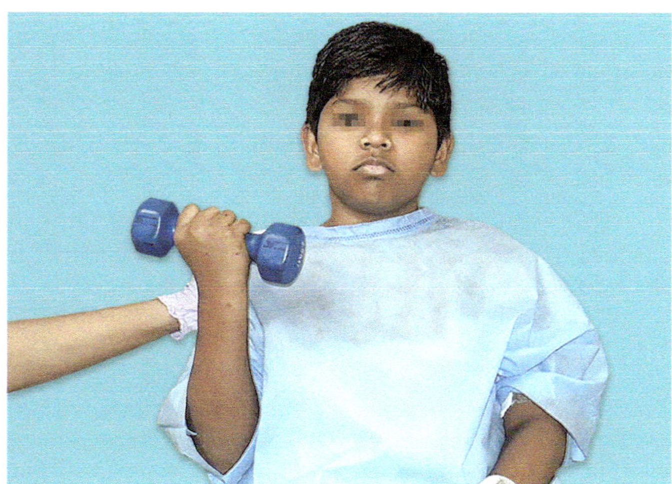

FIG. 7: Weight training muscles strengthened by increasing weights and applying resistance.

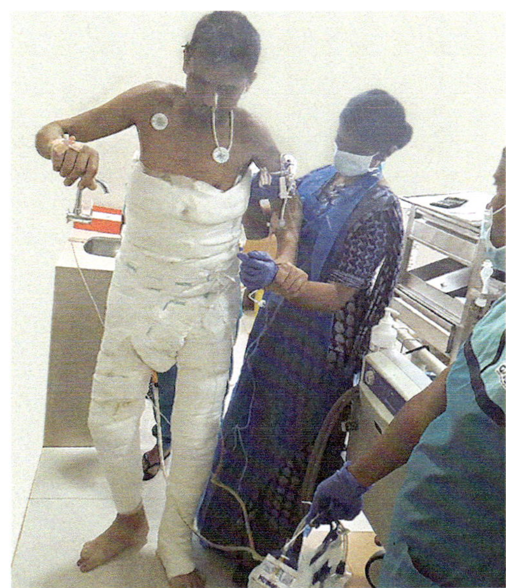

FIG. 8: Early mobilization of a patient.

encourage them to return to work as soon as possible. When the patient goes back to work, the patient feels better. We also need to encourage the patient to strengthen the muscles as hypermetabolism is present for almost 3 years after major burns. If the range of motion is limited due to various scar contractures, the patient needs contracture release surgery by the burn surgeon.

Positioning of the Patient

Proper positioning of the burn patient is crucial to bring about the best functional outcomes in burn rehabilitation. Proper positioning should begin immediately after admission and continue throughout the rehabilitative process. The reasons why we need to position the patient well are:

- To reduce edema.
- To enable good wound care and physiotherapy.
- Minimize the risk of peripheral neuropathy.
- Facilitate joint alignment.
- Maintain soft-tissue elongation to facilitate functional recovery and prevent bed sores.

The positioning of the patient should depend upon the patient's medical condition and consultation of the surgeon, nurses, and the entire burn team. It is often quoted that the "position of comfort is the position of deformity". This is very true in burns. The basic rule for positioning burnt areas is to place and maintain the body part in the opposite plane and direction to which it will potentially contract. Deformities can be prevented by various methods such as mechanical traction, splinting, cut-out foams and mattresses, pillows, strapping techniques, serial casting, and surgical application of pins.

Burn patients are kept in the intensive care unit for an extended period in the supine position. Hence, they must be placed on air beds and turned once every 2 hours to prevent pressure sores. In addition to lying down supine, two other positions are often required: the side-lying and the prone positions.

Side-lying Position

Patients at risk of developing a pressure sore need to be rotated frequently. The side-lying position can be done. The full side-lying position at 90° should not be done as it places a lot of pressure on the greater trochanter. Hence, a 30–40° tilt from the supine position, which distributes pressure more evenly between the head of the femur and the lateral portion of the sacrum, should be done. This can be done easily by placing a foam or a wooden block on one side below the mattress. By doing so, we need not disturb the patient at all. This can also be done by placing a pillow underneath one side of the patient.

Prone Position

Burn patients may need to be placed in the prone position to protect delicate skin grafts over the posterior aspect of the body, offload pressure sores in the sacral or scapular region, in some instances of acute respiratory distress syndrome (ARDS) and to aid in wound healing. The airway is a paramount issue that needs to be considered while designing a prone position mattress. The supporting surface is cut from a solid foam mattress that is placed on a wire mesh bed frame. Nasal and tracheal intubation are not contraindications for the prone position. A space should be provided through the open cell foam mattress to provide direct access for regular airway care and for comfortably using an ambu (artificial manual breathing unit) bag. If there is any problem regarding the airway, the prone position should be abandoned immediately until the patient can breathe properly. The facial opening should be so that it helps to distribute the weight of the face without allowing the head to enter the opening. Excess weight over the zygomatic arches, brow ridge and the anterior mandible should be avoided. Corneal abrasions can occur if one is not diligent, as the foam can contact the unprotected eye. The feet are placed in a neutral position, and one must be careful that the great toe is not in contact with the supporting frame to prevent pressure sores. The elbows are kept flexed to accommodate hand elevation. Frequent elbow positioning is recommended to avoid damage to the ulnar nerve.

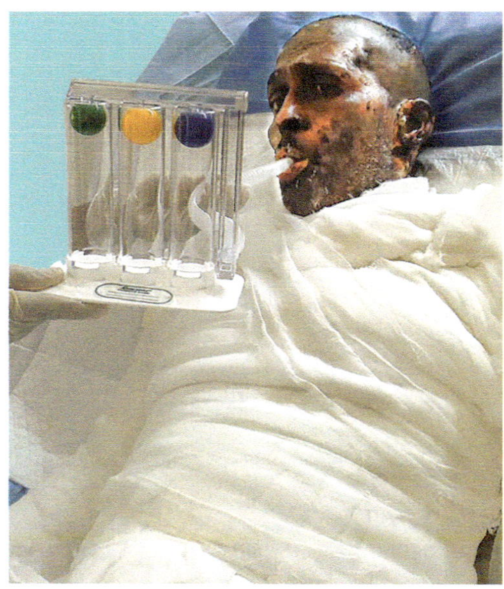

FIG. 9: Incentive spirometry.

Chest Physiotherapy

The lungs are commonly affected by inhalation injury, ARDS, and pneumonia. This, in turn, affects the oxygenation of tissues and wound healing. Hence, chest physiotherapy and respiratory care are extremely important for the patient to do well. The physiotherapist should start the chest physiotherapy from the first day onward. Chest physiotherapy mainly aims to clear the airway of secretions. This is done through therapeutic coughing, bronchial drainage or positioning, percussion, vibration, early ambulation, and airway suctioning.

Deep Breathing Exercises

Patients may take shallow breaths due to pain and anxiety. Shallow breaths reduce the dead space and increase the chances of atelectasis. Patients are advised to take deep breaths and slowly exhale. Incentive spirometry can be used to encourage the patients to take deep breaths **(Fig. 9)**. Patients can be encouraged to blow balloons. This would reduce atelectasis and increase the vital capacity of the patient.

Therapeutic Coughing

Coughing helps to clear the excess mucus and fibrin in the respiratory tract. Poor coughing may result in retained secretions, atelectasis, bronchial obstruction, and pneumonia. Hence, therapeutic coughing is essential, and we must encourage the patient to cough every 2 hours to remove the retained secretions. Some patients have a lot of pain while coughing due to surgery, chest injury, or other reasons. For these patients, a series of three coughs can be done. The patient is asked to take a small breath and a small cough, followed by a bigger breath, a hard cough, and finally a deep breath and a harder cough. This helps those who are in a lot of pain. For patients recovering from anesthesia and obtunded, the therapist gently places the index or the middle finger over the sternal notch and massages it in a circular fashion over the trachea. This makes the patient cough. Cough can be stimulated in the patient with an endotracheal tube or tracheostomy by inflating the cuff, manually giving a large and rapid inspiration, holding the breath for 1–2 seconds, and rapidly allowing the bag to release and ensure exhalation. When two therapists are present, this cough stimulation can be more effective when the other therapist performs vibration and chest compressions between the inspiratory hold and exhalation.

Bronchial Drainage or Positioning

Bronchial drainage or positioning is a therapeutic means by which the patient is positioned to help to move the secretions using gravity. Hence, it is common practice in intensive care units to turn the patient side by side every 2 hours to help to mobilize the secretions. Arterial oxygenation may fall during this procedure in certain positions, so it must be monitored.

Percussion

The physiotherapist rhythmically and alternately strikes the chest wall to remove the excess secretions from the respiratory tract. The physiotherapist cups the hand to allow air to enter between the therapist's hand and the patient. A popping sound is heard when the patient is percussed. Percussion is done over the surface landmarks of the bronchial segments being drained to mobilize the secretions. A towel can be placed between the patient and the therapist's hand to prevent skin irritation **(Fig. 10)**. One should be careful of skin grafts and bony prominences, which are to be avoided during percussion.

Vibration

Vibration involves rapid shaking of the chest during exhalation. The therapist places both hands over the surface landmarks of the bronchial segments and then forcefully vibrates the patient **(Fig. 11)**. This helps to loosen the secretions so they can be coughed up or removed by suctioning. Recently, mechanical vibrators have been used to do this function.

Early Ambulation

Early ambulation is one of the best ways to improve the condition of the lungs. Every effort should be made to make the patient sit as early as possible. For the patient to ambulate, the patient should not be highly sedated. Early tracheostomy can reduce sedation levels and facilitate earlier extubation for intubated patients. Once extubated, the patients are made to sit, stand, and mobilize early.

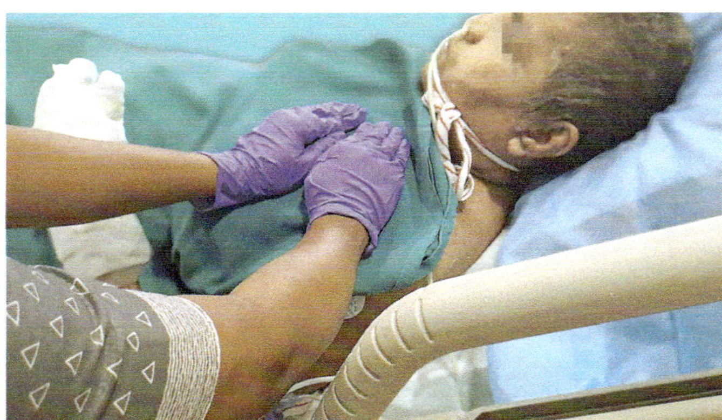

FIG. 10: Percussion.

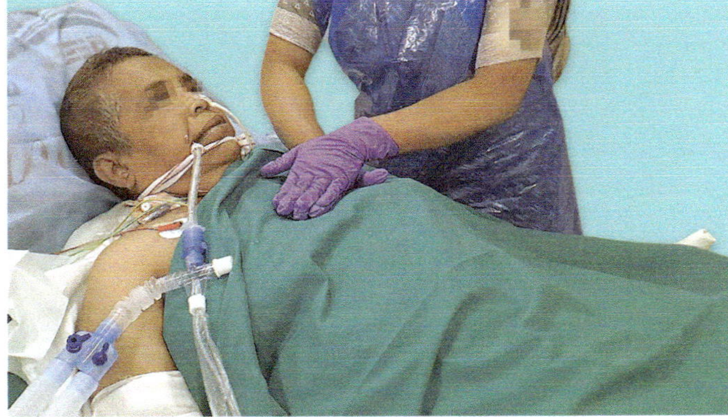

FIG. 11: Vibration.

Airway Suctioning

Suctioning helps to remove the accumulated secretions in the respiratory tract that cannot be removed by the patient's cough or other less invasive means. Before one suctions the respiratory tract, we should hyperoxygenate the patient with 100% oxygen. The patient should not be suctioned for >15 seconds without being reoxygenated. However, there can be potential problems with suctioning, namely respiratory tract irritation, bleeding, vagal stimulation, abrupt drop in saturation, and bradycardia. The fall in saturation can be decreased or eliminated by preoxygenating the patient and limiting the suction time. Suctioned sputum can be sent for microbiological analysis.

Secretions that cannot be removed by other means can be removed by passing a fiber-optic therapeutic bronchoscope. The bronchial tree can also be washed to remove the soot during inhalation injury and to reduce inflammation.

Splints

Splints are a rigid or flexible material used to protect, immobilize, or restrict motion in a part of the body. Splints are of three types, namely static, dynamic, and semi-dynamic splints. A static splint does not allow motion of that body part and keeps it in a particular position. Dynamic splint supports and permits movement of that part. Semi-dynamic splints support the part and allow little movement. Splints are designed to reduce edema, immobilize, protect and support joints, maintain and or increase range of motion, promote wound healing, relieve pressure points, protect grafts and flaps, and stabilize one or more joints so that other joints can function correctly. Splints should primarily be designed to support the joint and prevent the joints from going to a deformity, not cause pain, be cosmetically appealing, easy to remove and apply, be lightweight, allow ventilation to prevent wound or skin macerations, and should be made out of readily available and appropriate materials.

PHYSIOTHERAPY OF PARTICULAR REGIONS

Head

Head elevation above the level of the heart should be done to reduce edema in a patient with facial burns. To do this, the head end of the bed can be inclined at an angle of 30–45°, if the patient's hips are not involved with burns. If the patient's hips are involved in burns, then inclining the bed at 30–45° elevation may result in a hip flexion deformity. In this situation, the bed as a whole should be lifted at the head end **(Fig. 12)**. This can be done using wooden blocks with recessed slots for the bed (reverse Trendelenburg proposition). This allows the head to be kept elevated without the hips being flexed. The head should be moved frequently every hour to prevent pressure sores on the occiput. Pressure relief gel cushions can be placed underneath the occiput as a precautionary measure. Nasal obturators may be required to maintain the nostrils open **(Fig. 13)**. These obturators can be serially adjusted to gradually increase the nostrils' size. When the mouth is affected by burns, it can go in for severe microstomia. Hence, various mouth splints can be made to increase the horizontal, vertical, and circumferential mouth opening to prevent microstomia.

Neck

The neck is positioned in the neutral position or with a mild extension of 15°. This can be done by placing a rolled towel or a foam cushion behind the upper back. One should avoid using a pillow behind the occiput as this can result in flexion contractures of the neck. A conforming custom thermoplastic collar can be fabricated for anterior neck burns while the patient is in bed.

In cases of contracture release of the neck, after grafts have been applied, it is necessary to extend the neck as much as possible for at least 6 weeks. The grafted skin can easily contract, resulting in recurrent contractures. One or two pillows must be placed behind the upper back to keep the neck in full extension **(Fig. 14)**. The patient should lie like this as much as possible for 6 weeks after grafting. Gentle sideways movement can be done to relax the muscles. The patient should be taught to move the shoulders, elbows, and hands, and encouraged to mobilize. While getting up from the bed, the patient should be careful about how to get out of bed. One must first sit up in the bed, then put the legs down and stand up. During this movement, the neck should be kept extended. The patient may feel giddy and nauseous for a few days. This would soon normalize with neck exercises. Hard cervical collars can be worn **(Fig. 15)**. We use a thermoplastic splint placed behind the head, neck, and upper chest. This splint is stabilized using velcro straps, which are fastened over the head and the chest. Dressings

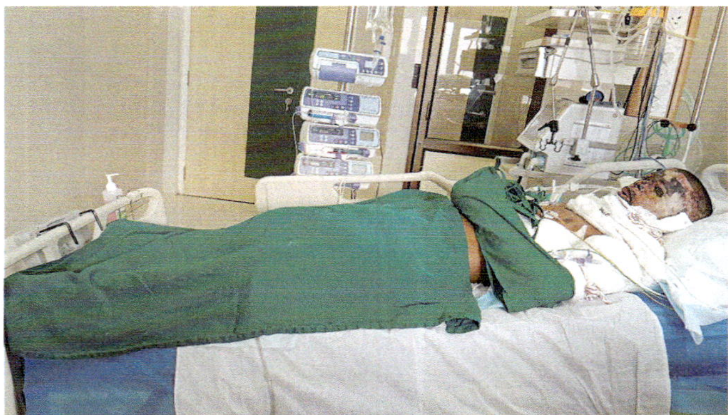

FIG. 12: Reverse Trendelenburg position to prevent hip contractures.

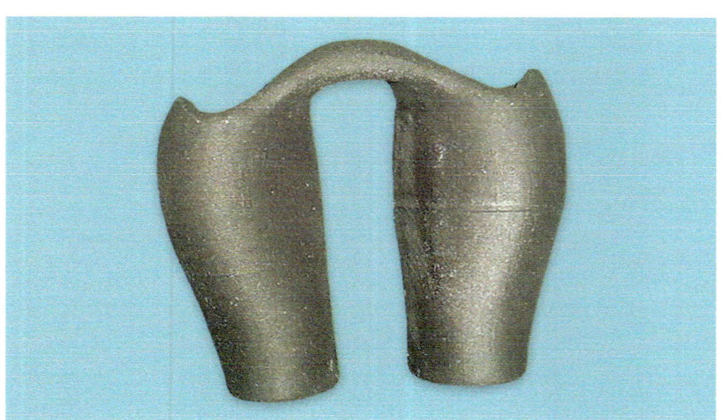

FIG. 13: Nasal obturators.

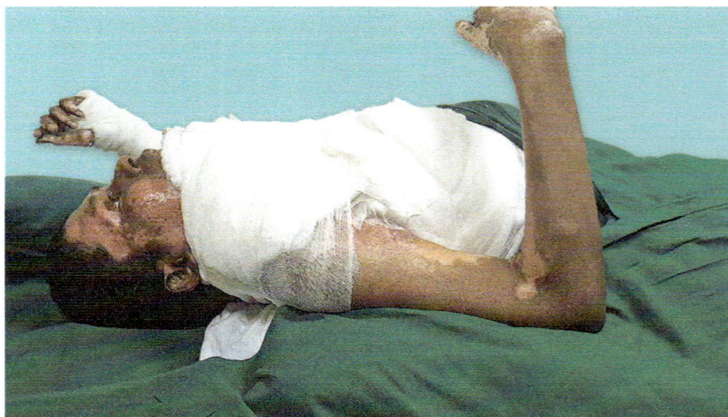

FIG. 14: Neck extended with two pillows beneath the shoulder after a neck contracture release.

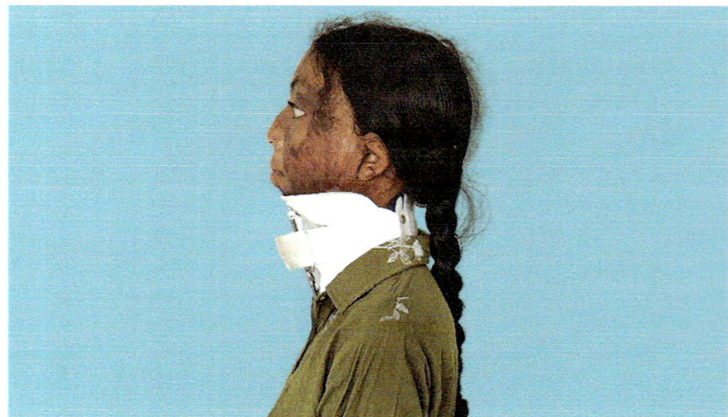

FIG. 15: Hard cervical collar.

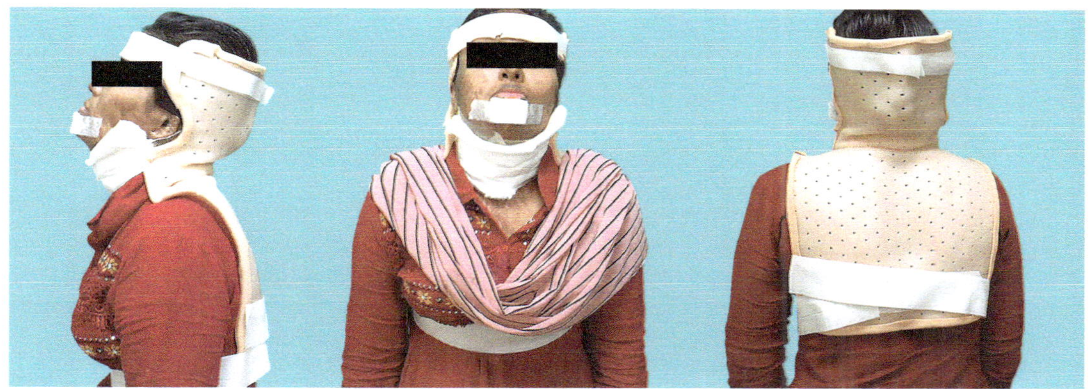

FIG. 16: Neck splint applied from the back.

and wound inspection can be done from the front while the neck is still extended **(Fig. 16)**.

Spine

Contracture from unilateral or asymmetrical burns of the axilla, trunk, neck and groin, and pelvic obliquity accompanying asymmetric hip or knee flexion can result in lateral curvature of the spine and scoliosis. As long as a patient is lying down, the lateral contracture can be prevented by straight alignment of the trunk and neck. The curvature may not be initially noticed but can be easily seen while walking. The other subtle signs of spinal curvature are asymmetry of the shoulder levels, asymmetry of the pelvic rim levels, scapular asymmetry, and asymmetry of the upper extremity. Once there is an established asymmetric contracture, it is difficult to stretch it out by physical therapy; hence, early surgery is better for even minor scoliosis.

Axilla

The recommended position for the burned shoulder and axilla is 90° abduction, 15–20° horizontal adduction and maximum external rotation. If the position of abduction alone is maintained for an extended period, there is a high chance of anterior subluxation of the glenohumeral joint. Horizontal adduction anatomically reduces the chances of brachial plexus or peripheral nerve compression. The shoulder joint is externally rotated to combat internal rotation deformities. The shoulder can be positioned through splints and thermoplastic slings suspended from above. After a release of axillary contractures, aeroplane splints can be given **(Fig. 17)**. The shoulder is abducted at 90° with 15–20° of horizontal adduction in these splints.

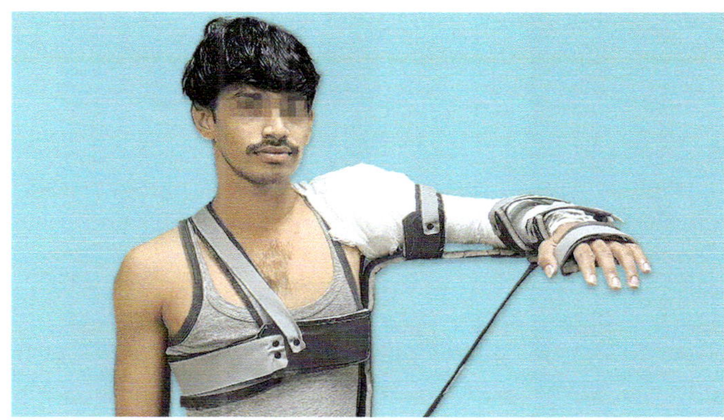

FIG. 17: Splint for axillary contractures.

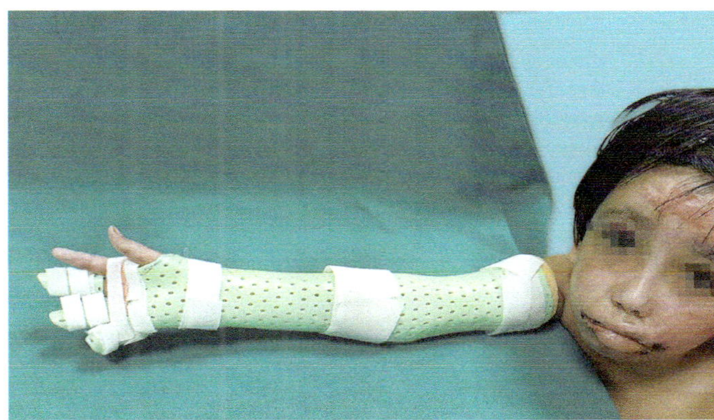

FIG. 18: Splint for elbow contractures.

Elbow

Burns involving the elbow can result in flexion contracture of the elbow and posterior exposure of the elbow joint. Hence, the elbow should be kept elevated and fully extended. An anterior elbow conformer can be used to keep the elbow in extension. Patients should be encouraged to actively flex the elbow often as the elbows can become very stiff if immobilized for an extended period. Elbows are prone to heterotrophic ossification and severe stiffness; hence, they should be actively flexed and extended. In the resting position, the elbows should be kept extended **(Fig. 18)**.

There can be problems in pronation and supination, especially in electric burns, as the pronators and supinators may be necrosed and have been removed during surgery. The forearm should be placed in the neutral or slightly supine position for these patients. During hand elevation, the palm should look toward the face. If the forearm is not correctly placed, the patient may keep it in the pronated position, making it challenging to supinate it later.

Wrist and Hands

After burns, the hand is initially swollen, painful, and the sensation at the fingertips can be blunted. The initial goal of hand physiotherapy is to reduce edema and facilitate mobilization to reduce the stiffness of the fingers. The edema can be prevented, reduced, and treated by elevating the hand above the level of the heart at all times. If there are circumferential eschar and deep burns over the hand and forearm, it may need an escharotomy. If the sensation at the fingertips is blunted, one might need to do a carpal tunnel release. The hand and wrist can get deformed if the hand and forearm edema are left unchecked. The dorsal skin is thinner than the volar skin. In addition, there are multiple septae from the palmar skin to the underlying structures compared to the dorsal skin. Hence, edema is more severe over the dorsum of the hand when compared to that of the palmar aspect of the hand. This differential edema over the dorsum of the hands pushes the metacarpal heads volarly, flattens the palmar arches, and hyperextends the metacarpophalangeal (MCP) joints. Due to hyperextension of the MCP joints, the tension imposed by edema forces the proximal interphalangeal (PIP) joints into flexion. The ring and little finger are affected 65% of the time **(Fig. 19)**. With time, the joints become stiff. The extensor tendons undergo adaptive shortening and the patient may go into a claw-like deformity with the wrist in flexion, MCP joints in hyperextension and the interphalangeal (IP) joints in flexion. Due to edema, the thumb lies in the plane of the palm and can reduce the first webspace. If the first webspace shortens, the thumb cannot oppose the fingers, and the hand function is impaired.

This claw-like deformity can be prevented by splinting the hand in the correct position. A dorsal slab can be applied over the hand, wrist, and forearm with the wrist in 30° extension, MCP joints in 70–80° flexion, IP joints in extension, and the thumb in palmar and radially abduction with the MCP and IP joints in slight flexion **(Fig. 20)**. This can be supplemented by a volar cock-up splint across the wrist joint up to the distal palmar crease. When applying this volar splint, one must be very careful not to cross the distal palmar crease **(Fig. 21)**. One should remember that the distal palmar crease is not straight and tends to be lower when one goes ulnarly toward the little finger.

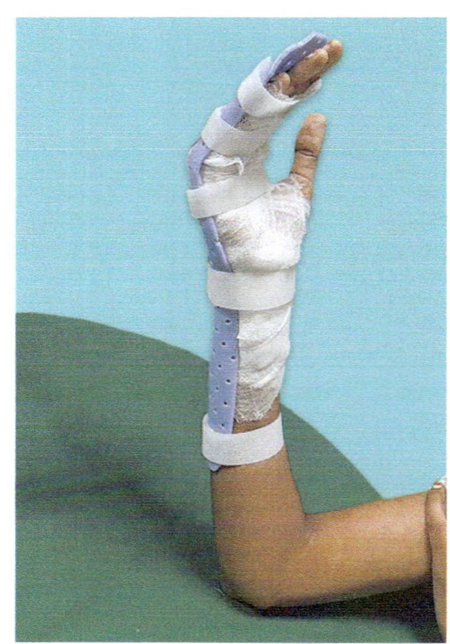

FIG. 20: Dorsal splint.

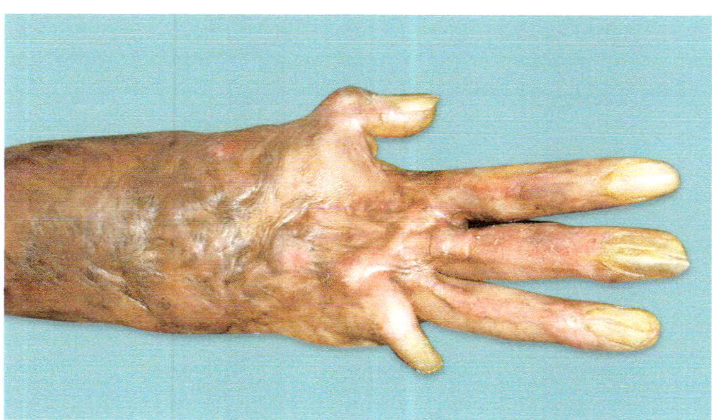

FIG. 19: Postburn contracture of the hand when left untreated.

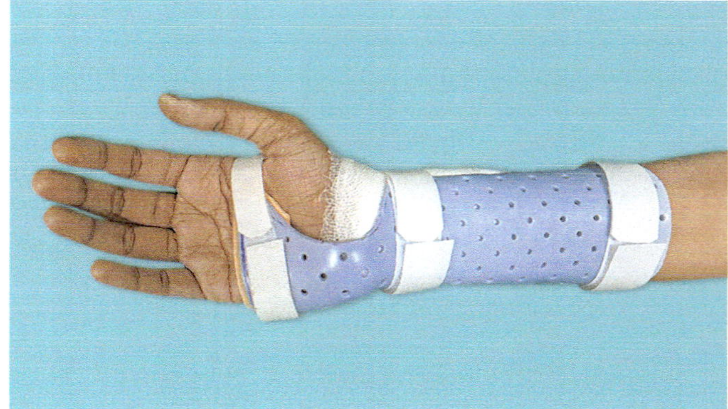

FIG. 21: Volar cockup splint.

If the splint crosses distal to the distal palmar crease, this splint itself will prevent the MCP joints from flexing. Early and regular mobilization of the fingers is very important to prevent hand stiffness. The importance of mobilization of the fingers has to be emphasized to the patient and the patient's caregivers so that they would mobilize well.

In superficial burns, the burns heal well conservatively with regular dressings. In superficial burns, the fingers need to be mobilized well. Mobilization can be painful, and appropriate analgesics should be given. In deeper burns, in addition to mobilization and elevation, the burns should be excised early and covered by autografts. If the deep burns are not excised early and covered by autografts, there would be increased inflammation, which would contribute to edema and decrease the mobilization. Hence, early surgery helps to reduce edema and enables mobilization. However, early surgery may not be possible in many circumstances due to extensive burns and poor general condition. In this situation, K-wires should be passed across the IP joints to prevent contractures. If there are residual raw areas after surgery or burns, it is better to heal those raw areas with grafts or flaps than conservatively healing them. This would reduce inflammation and edema. If the tendons and joints are exposed, a flap cover is required. The gains made by surgery must be maintained by appropriately splinting the joints **(Fig. 22)**. Grafts heal within 3 weeks, and the maximum graft contraction happens within 6 weeks. So, K wires have to be retained till then. Meanwhile, the grafts should be moisturized well, and the scars should be massaged. This moisturizing and scar massage should be continued for at least 6 months. After the wounds have healed well, Cobban bandages **(Fig. 23)** can be applied to the fingers and compression garments **(Fig. 24)** for the hands to reduce the edema and facilitate early mobilization. If a contracture or a deformity develops, an early surgical intervention is very important so that the deformities can be corrected early. If the deformity is not corrected early, it can increase the severity and the treatment for it becomes more difficult and with poorer resuts.

Mallet deformity of the fingers is characterized by flexion of the finger at the distal interphalangeal (DIP) joint. This can occur due to the rupture of the extensor tendon at the DIP joint. This can result in a swan neck deformity. A swan neck deformity is characterized by flexion at the DIP joint and hyperextension of the PIP joint. The swan neck deformity can also occur due to skin contractures across the dorsum of the PIP joint and tightening of the intrinsics due to ischemic fibrosis of the muscles in compartment syndrome. Mallet finger and swan neck deformities have to be corrected as they affect function. Mallet finger can be prevented when seen early by applying a mallet finger splint which is a volar splint across the DIP joint which would prevent the DIP joint from going into flexion **(Fig. 25)**. However, with time if the deformity gets fixed it would best be treated by arthrodesis of the PIP joint in the functional position from the index 25–30° to little finger 40–50°. If there is a mallet finger, a K-wire can be passed across the DIP joint in full extension and maintained for at least 6–8 weeks so that it can be corrected.

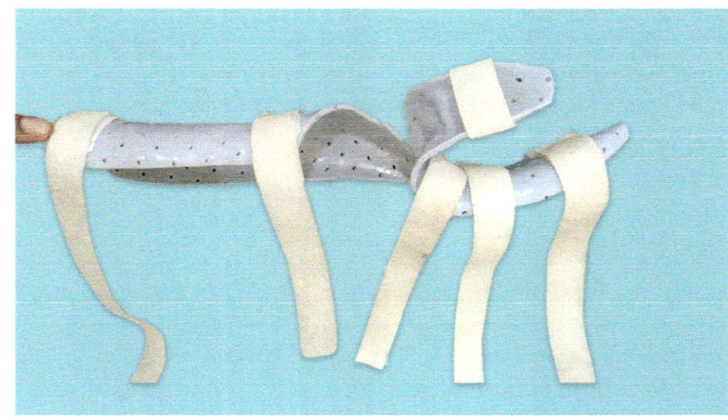

FIG. 22: The hand is splinted with the wrist slightly extended, metacarpophalangeal (MCP) joints in 70–80° flexion, interphalangeal (IP) joints extended and the thumb kept abducted.

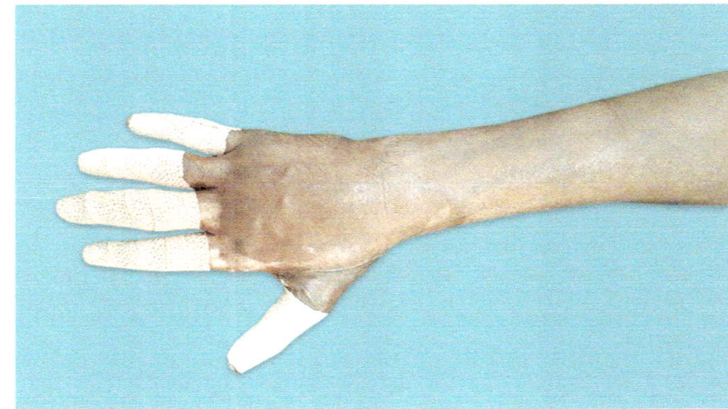

FIG. 23: Cobban application for the fingers.

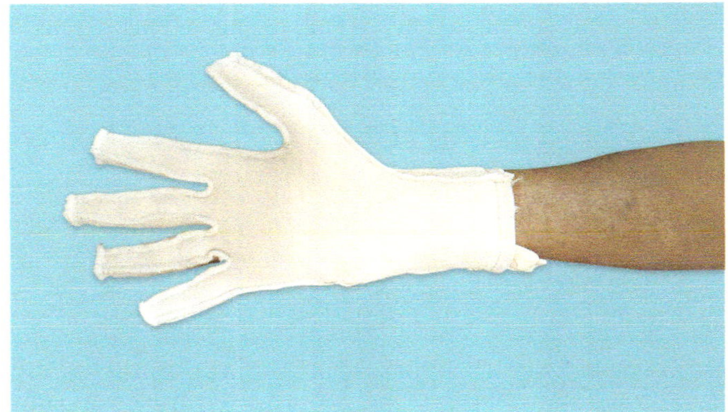

FIG. 24: Compression garment for the fingers.

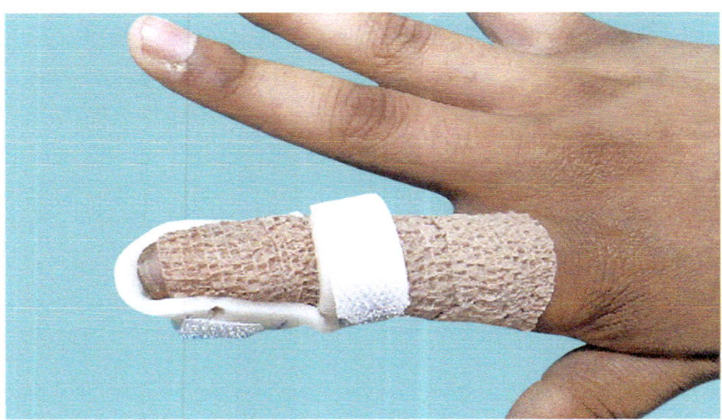

FIG. 25: Mallet splint keeping the distal interphalangeal joint extended.

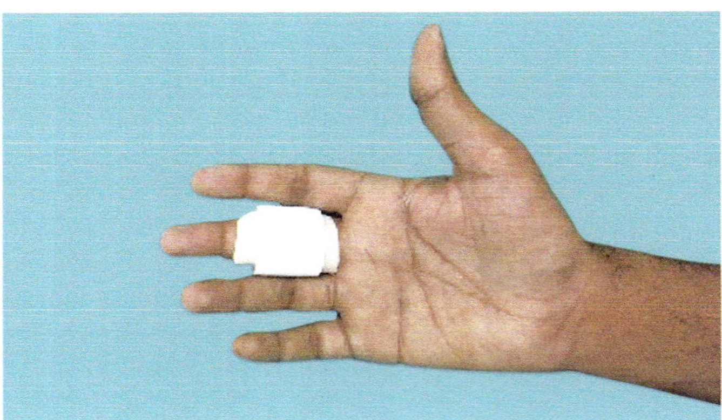

FIG. 26: Splint across the proximal interphalangeal joint (PIP) joint for "Boutonnière deformity".

Boutonnière deformity is characterized by flexion of the PIP joint and hyperextension at the DIP joint. This happens mostly due to the rupture of the central slip. This can be prevented by splinting the PIP joint in extension **(Fig. 26)** either by K-wires or splint across the PIP joint. If the joint becomes fixed, then if the thumb meets the fingers, then the deformity might be accepted. However, it is best that the deformity is prevented.

Burn, syndactyly, and web contractures occur when the fingers are not separated by dressings during healing. Dressings should be applied appropriately to separate the fingers. Attention should be given especially at the web as the dressings in between the fingers can slip. Hence, a gauze or tape can be placed across from the volar to the dorsum of the hand to prevent web contractures **(Fig. 27)**.

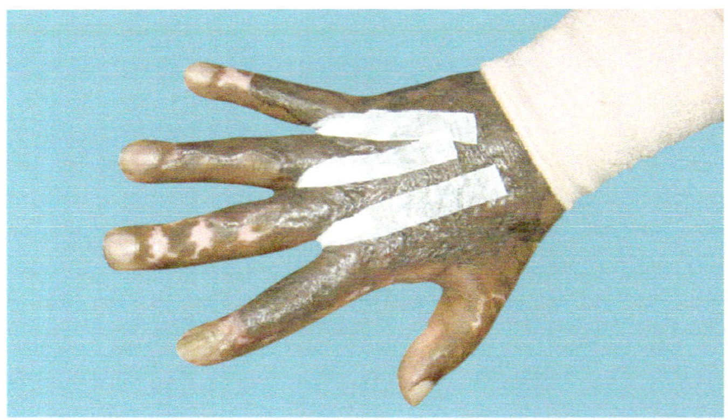

FIG. 27: Webspace strapping to prevent "burn syndactyly" between the fingers.

The first webspace is important as it allows the thumb to meet the fingers. The thumb should be placed in palmar abduction. A first webspace spreader helps to keep the first webspace in good palmar abduction **(Fig. 28)**.

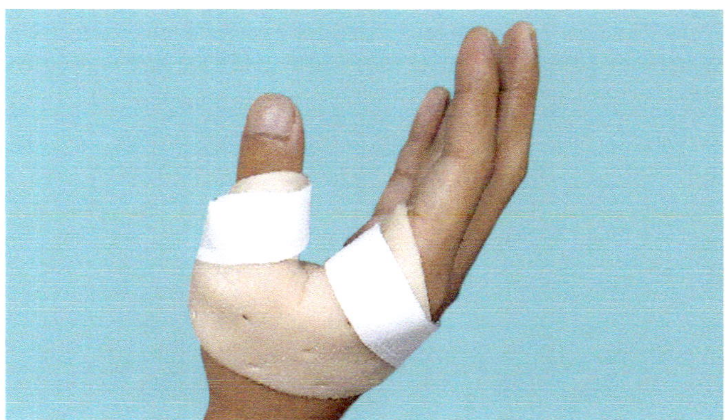

FIG. 28: First webspace spreader.

However, good surgery for burn contracture is done, unless physio is done preoperatively and post-operatively from day 1, one may not achieve a good result. Physiotherapy has to be done diligently multiple times per day and the joints will have to be splinted in between. Elevation, mobilization, appropriate surgery at appropriate time, splinting, mobilization, and patience from the patient, family, and caregivers can give a good hand function and make all the efforts worthwhile.

Hip

When burns extend anteriorly from the abdomen to the thighs, it can result in anterior flexion contractures of the hip. These flexion contractures of the hip are often accompanied by flexion contractures of the knee and lumbar lordosis when present bilaterally. When present unilaterally, it can result in pelvic obliquity and scoliosis. In addition to this, when deep burns extend across both hips, this can result in adduction contractures of the hips. In adults and older children, and in young infants who are non-ambulatory, the hips are often placed in abduction; hence, they can result in abduction contractures. Flat mattresses should be used as this can prevent hip flexion contractures. If a head-end elevation is also required, the whole mattress should be elevated with blocks of wood underneath the head end of the bed so that the head end is elevated and the hips are kept straight. Slight hip flexion contractures can be compensated by mild lordosis. However, these contractures should be treated aggressively to prevent back and hip pain. Extensions can be placed across the abdomen to the thighs to extend the hip fully.

Knee

Deep burns to the anterior or posterior surface of the knee can result in disabling contractures. Deep burns over the anterior aspect of the knee can expose the knee joint, the patella, and the patella tendon. Deep burns to the posterior part of the knee can result in functionally debilitating flexion contractures of the knee. Flexion contractures of the hip often accompany this. When this does happen, the patient is unable to stand or walk and is almost bedridden. And hence, this has to be corrected. The knee should be kept in full extension. A splint or skeletal traction can maintain this **(Fig. 29)**. When the patient is in a full extension splint, they are advised to keep contracting their quadriceps muscle and strengthen the quadriceps muscle. This can be done by asking the patient to imagine an object underneath the knee and telling them to keep pressing the knee down. When this happens, the quadriceps muscles contract. As in the hip, small contractures may result in pelvic obliquity and scoliosis. Hence, even a small contracture should be corrected as soon as possible to rehabilitate the patient quickly. While looking for a knee contracture, one must not miss the flexion contracture of the hips as well as the ankle equinus, which can frequently occur due to the shortening of the tendoachilles muscles.

Foot and Ankle

Ankle equinus is the most common deformity that occurs in the ankle after burns. This is often accompanied by hindfoot inversion and forefoot varus. The equinus deformity is most commonly due to the failure to support the foot in the neutral position, as the scars are tight over the posterior aspect of the leg. It can occur due to loss of deep and superior superficial peroneal nerve function, which will make the foot go into inversion and equinus because of the loss of dorsiflexion and eversion. The ankle equinus deformity can soon become a resistant deformity and be fixed in that position within a few days if it is not supported well. The scars, muscle and capsule contractures combine to make this deformity. Hence, the ankle should be placed and supported in 90° dorsiflexion **(Fig. 30)**.

The foot deformities can be prevented by supporting the foot and ankle well with a good splint with the foot kept in neutral alignment or slight dorsiflexion. If the patient is nursed prone, the patient's foot should be allowed to fall free from the mattress to keep it in proper alignment. The entire foot, ankle, and distal leg should be supported well while fabricating a splint in all parts because the foot's natural tendency is to plantar flex. If the patient's foot and the splint are not congruous and unstable, it can result in undue pressure over the heel, malleoli, and toes where the splint touches the skin and can result in ulcers. The equinus can be corrected or maintained by placing calcaneal pins and giving traction for extensive burns and those with long-standing burns. Transmetatarsal pins can also be used to connect with the calcaneal pins to correct the equinus.

For minor equinus defects, gradual heel lifts can correct the deformity. Serial corrective casts or splints can be used to correct minor contractures. Scar release

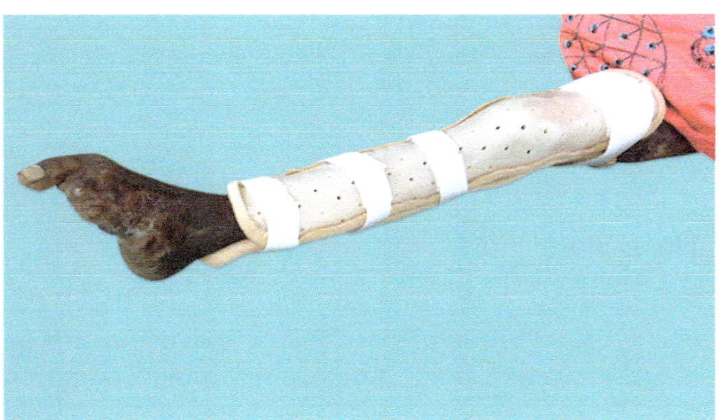

FIG. 29: Knee extension splint.

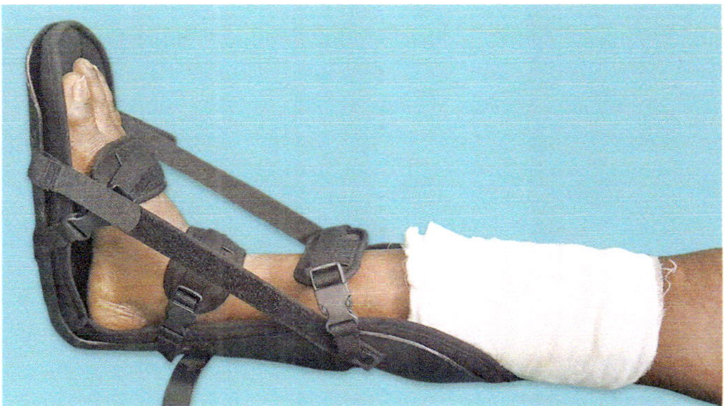

FIG. 30: Foot and ankle splint.

combined with tendoachilles lengthening or posterior capsulotomy can give good results for fixed, unyielding, and resistant contractures. In some instances, the Ilizarov technique has also been used to correct this deformity. If there are no ankle dorsiflexors available, as in cases of some electrical burns, ankle fusion may provide the best functional result.

Dorsiflexion of the toes is a common deformity seen in burns over the dorsum of the foot. This is often accompanied by MTP joint subluxation involving one or many toes. The metatarsal heads become prominent over the plantar aspect, and walking may become very painful. Splinting the toes is very difficult; hence, these deformities should be corrected early by surgery with contracture release and grafting. In severe cases, intrinsic or extrinsic pinning of the digits can be done to prevent this.

Scar contracture over the dorsum of the leg and foot can also pull the foot into marked inversion. This can result in undue pressure over the lateral aspect of the foot, callous formation, and painful gait. Scar contraction along the first and the fifth toes can pull the toes into abduction. This deformity prevents patient from putting their feet into regular shoes. These deformities should be corrected early by surgery.

ORTHOTIC TREATMENT OF THE LOWER EXTREMITY

Orthotics are specially designed shoe inserts that help to support the feet and improve foot posture. The ideal shoe should distribute all forces to the foot, reduce pressure on sensitive or deformed structures, and encourage total weight bearing over the foot. Shoe modifications such as arch pads, molded foot thermoplastics, metatarsal bars, and tongue pads can be used. Orthotic devices can position the foot appropriately, prevent plantar or dorsal contractures, and correct inversion and eversion of the foot. Limb length discrepancies can be managed with a shoe lift.

Serial Casting

Serial casting is a treatment option for mild burn contractures when the patient is noncompliant, does not tolerate splints, there is a persistent limitation of range of motion, or a skin graft requires immobilization or protection. Casting is based on the principle of stress relaxation in which a low-intensity force with a prolonged duration of stretching to connective tissues can help to elongate the tissues for correction of contractures. The casting technique involves cleaning and moisturizing the skin, dressing the wounds, applying orthotics or silicone inserts if necessary, and padding bony prominences and applying a good dressing. One therapist maintains the position while the other therapist helps to fabricate the cast. This may be painful in some patients and may need premedication with analgesics. Aggressive tightening can lead to compression neuropathies or vascular compromises. The casts are fabricated mostly with plaster of Paris or fiberglass casting materials. Plaster casts made of plaster of Paris are inexpensive and easy to fabricate. However, they can easily break when exposed to water and are not very strong. Fiberglass materials are lighter, more durable, and stronger. However, they are more costly than plaster. After cast fabrication, the clinician should check the firmness of the cast, sharpness of cast edges, neurovascular status of the extremity, and any signs of the cast rubbing adjacent structures. The cast can be changed approximately 1 week to 10 days apart. Serial casting is terminated when the desired range of motion has been restored, and no further gains are expected.

Therapy for Hypertrophic Scars

Hypertrophic scars are common in deep dermal burn wounds where they have been treated conservatively or healed with infection. Hypertrophic scars are mainly treated by pressure garments, scar massage, silicone sheets, lasers, and injections with intralesional steroids. (Refer to chapter on "Post burn sequelae and their management")

WHEN TO REFER FOR SURGERY?

Mild contractures of joints can be prevented and treated by scar massage, splints, orthotics, and exercises. However, as time progresses, the contractures can further worsen, which can be functionally very debilitating. Early release of contractures, and soft-tissue cover are very important. It is generally thought that one has to wait till the scar matures before contracture release surgery. However, when it is functionally debilitating and involves important structures such as the hands, face, and eyelids, then it is important that surgical intervention is done early.

SUMMARY

Physiotherapists are critical members of the burn multidisciplinary team. They should evaluate the patient well before therapy. Physiotherapy is essential to reduce the effects of hypermetabolism in burns, preserve and increase muscle mass, maintain muscle bulk, prevent contractures, preserve the full range of motion of joints, promote good healing, and prevent insulin resistance. The patients should be mobilized as early as possible. Active and passive exercises should be combined with isometric and resistance exercises to preserve the full range of motion and improve muscle mass. The patients should be positioned appropriately, and the joints should be splinted correctly. Physiotherapists should actively give chest physiotherapy to reduce the secretions, clear the secretions in the airway, and treat inhalation injury, ARDS, and pneumonia. The hypertrophic scars should be treated with scar massage, pressure garments, lasers, intralesional steroids, and silicone sheets. If the contractures worsen, the patients should be referred early for surgery.

BIBLIOGRAPHY

1. Al-Mousawi AM, Williams FN, Mlcak RP, Jeschke MG, Herndon DN, Suman OE. Effects of exercise training on resting energy expenditure and lean mass during pediatric burn rehabilitation. J Burn Care Res. 2010;31(3):400-8.
2. Esselman PC, Thombs BD, Magyar-Russell G, Fauerbach JA. Burn rehabilitation: state of the science. Am J Phys Med Rehabil. 2006;85:383-413.
3. Holavanahalli RK, Helm PA, Kowalske KJ. Long-term outcomes in patients surviving large burns: the musculoskeletal system. J Burn Care Res. 2015.
4. Jeschke MG. Postburn Hypermetabolism: Past, Present, and Future. J Burn Care Res. 2016;37(2):86-96.
5. Paratz JD, Stockton K, Plaza A, Muller M, Boots RJ. Intensive exercise after thermal injury improves physical, functional, and psychological outcomes. J Trauma Acute Care Surg. 2012;73(1):186-94.
6. Richard RL, Barzya MJ, Carr JA, Dewey WS, Dougherty ME, Forbes-Duchart L, et al. Burn rehabilitation and research: proceedings of a consensus summit. J Burn Care Res. 2009;30:543-73.
7. Sabapathy SR, Bajantri B, Bharathi RR. Management of post burn hand deformities. Indian J Plast Surg. 2010;43(Suppl):S72-9.
8. Sabapathy SR, Shanmugakrishnan RR, Vamseedharan M. Extremity Burns. In: Neligan P, Chan D, Hong JP. Eds. Plastic Surgery, Fourth Edition, Elsevier.
9. Serghiou MA, Ott S, Cowan A, et al. Burn Rehabilitation along the continuum of Care. In: Herndon DN. Total Burn Care, Fifth Edition, Elsevier.

CHAPTER 34

Postburn Sequelae and their Management

Arun Goel, Aakanksha Goel

INTRODUCTION

A severe burn injury is the most devastating injury a person can sustain and yet hope to survive! These injuries constitute the second common cause of all trauma-related deaths in the developing as well as the developed countries. Over the last 75 years, great advances have been made in the field of burns at basic as well as applied level. The pathophysiology of burn injury has been understood at cellular as well as molecular level in great detail. Treatment methods have been devised to counter and reverse these changes. Burns are now being treated scientifically in a well-standardized manner. The mortality rates and the morbidity from burns have diminished greatly so much so that a mere survival of an extensively burnt patient [say, 65% total body surface area (TBSA)] is no longer considered a great outcome. As is true for any other life-threatening injury, survival is the immediate concern for the burn patient, his/her relatives, and the treating clinician. Actually, it is the degree of restoration to preburn level, quality of life, and finally "return to society" as active functional citizen which are more important. Burn survival statistics can indeed be misleading! Unfortunately, the tremendous advancements in the field of burns have not benefitted a very large majority of burn victims in India and other developing/underdeveloped countries. It is not only life-threatening burns which are important. Even smaller burns may also be important. Thus, a deep dermal burn on dorsum of one hand or both cheeks may be the cause of more concern than say, a 5% TBSA burn of thigh because of severe functional loss in hand and aesthetic reasons on face. Postburn sequelae resulting in deformities with crippling contractures/amputations and disfigurement with grotesque appearance continue to be a great challenge to the modern burn surgeons in their attempt to restore the burnt patient to preinjury status **(Figs. 1A to D)**.

The immediate goal of burn treatment is restoration of the intact cutaneous barrier protecting the patient from his or her environment. Unfortunately, such a healed patient may be left with one or more of the various postburn sequelae in different permutations and combinations. These postburn sequelae have varying degrees of functional and aesthetic components. The actual prevalence of these disabling conditions in general population can never be assessed accurately, especially in a vast country like ours. However, it must be inversely proportional to the standards of initial treatment with patients receiving best of care having minimum number and severity of these sequelae. Conversely, it is also true that more the number of patients with massive burns salvaged, more will be the number of persons in society having some of these sequelae. In addition, there is a massive burden of burn patients who have minor burns but with a huge impact on one's quality of life.

For descriptive purposes, the various postburn sequelae have been considered under the following headings. An individual burn patient may have any number of them in varying severity. Surgical reconstruction of these sequelae requires the knowledge and expertise of the full spectrum of a plastic surgeon's armamentarium from local excision, serial excisions, tissue expansion, skin grafts, local flaps, regional flaps, and free flaps to prefabricated/prelaminated flaps.

- Postburn scars
- Postburn contractures
- Postburn losses
- Chronic unhealed areas and non-healing scar ulcers
- Bone and joint deformities

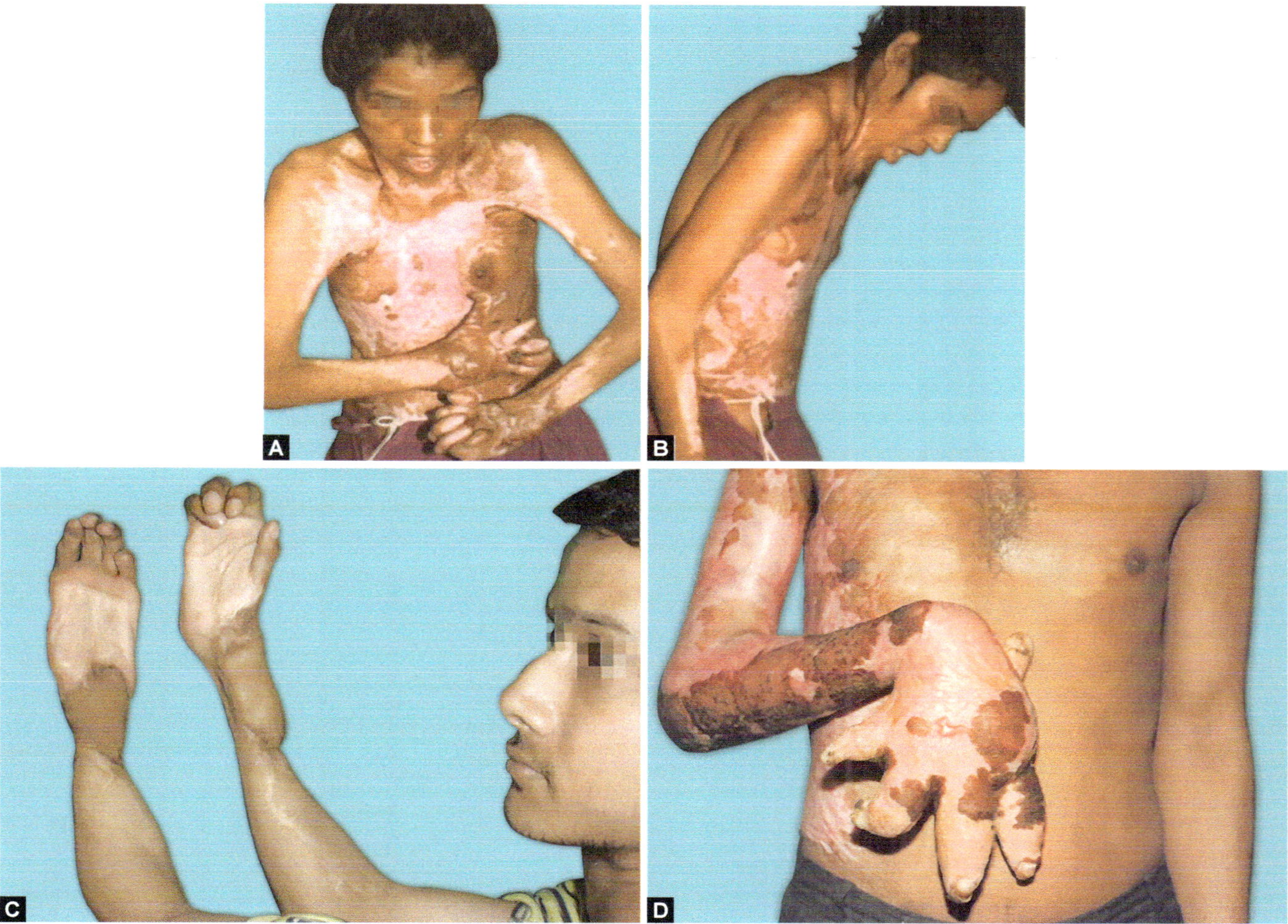

FIGS. 1A TO D: (A and B) Front and lateral view of a 28-year-old female with extensive post-thermal burn scars, severe, and multiple contractures of neck, axillae, wrists, and hands. Also note the kyphotic posture and loss of right nipple-areola complex. (C) A 16-year-old male with postelectric contact burns bilateral hand deformity with loss of digits and flexor tendons. Distant flap covers done to perform reconstructive surgery. (D) Grotesque deformity and loss of function of right hand in a 30-year-old male.

- Development of malignancy
- Miscellaneous
- Psychological disorders

POSTBURN SCARS

Postburn scars are inevitable even with the best of treatment. This is because they depend primarily upon the depth of burn injury. They not only cause psychological trauma but may also lead to severe functional impairment requiring prolonged and costly treatment to be borne by the individual or government exchequer. The role of a burn surgeon is to get the best outcome with all the reconstructive options at one's disposal.

It must be remembered that the term "scar" has a different meaning for a pathologist, a plastic surgeon, and the patient. For a pathologist, the normal response to a wound healing after birth is by the formation of scar. The appearance of even the best results of skin grafted/flap covered areas and the perfectly healed donor sites of these grafts/flaps is still a "scar" by the patient's definition of a scar.

An understanding of the burn wound healing is fundamental not only for the management of an acute burn wound, but also for the prevention, minimization and treatment of postburn scars and scar contractures.

Mechanism of Cutaneous Burn Wound Healing and Development of Scar and Scar Contracture[1-4]

Healing of the burnt skin is nature's attempt to restore the epithelial continuity by deposition of collagen and re-epithelialization. With the exception of healing in a growing fetus, all wounds heal by scar formation. Smaller amounts of transforming growth factor-β1 (TGF-β1, a scar promoting enzyme) and higher amounts of metalloproteinases in fetal skin are said to be the reasons for scarless healing. In superficial dermal burns which heal in < 14 days, healing may be so perfect as to resemble the normal skin and become indistinguishable from the surrounding unburnt skin. All other deeper burn injuries lead to healed "areas" which are clearly different from the surrounding unburnt skin with respect to their color, texture, dullness/shininess, stretchability, hair pattern, thickness, etc., even when the healing had proceeded "normally" **(Figs. 2A and B)**. In these as well as all other cases where healing has not proceeded normally due to one or more of the various factors affecting wound healing adversely, the final appearance of the healed burnt areas is definitely different from the surrounding unburnt skin.

Burn wound healing is a complex, dynamic, and interactive process involving various cellular elements and soluble mediators. There is cellular migration, proliferation, and synthesis of extracellular matrix with growth factors and cytokines to coordinate the healing. It occurs in three phases, namely, (1) the inflammatory phase, (2) the proliferative phase, and (3) the remodeling phase which overlap in time. Prolongation of the inflammatory phase is the most important factor in scar formation. The healing of a burn wound is accomplished in two ways, namely, (1) complete regeneration (restitution) and (2) substitution. Restitution is possible when the skin is burnt as deep as the stratum papillare and all the specialized cells of the organ are preserved. Re-epithelialization begins within 24 hours after burn and the epithelial cells, in these cases, are derived from the epidermal appendages such as pilosebaceous units and sweat glands in the central portion and wound edges at the periphery. These appendages extend into the deeper dermis and may even penetrate into the subcutaneous fat (as in beard area in males) and survive in partial thickness injuries. The sequence of cellular events that comprise epithelialization include cellular detachment, migration, proliferation, and differentiation. The epidermis and dermis no longer remain attached to each other because of dissolution of hemidesmosomes between the former and the basement membrane. This allows epidermal cells (or "buds") to move laterally and spread over the wound. They have a pink color due to loss of pigment and increased vascularity. Over a period of next 1 month or so, repopulation by melanocytes occurs in the basal layers. The hemidesmosomes take time to develop after healing. The superficial surface attaches to the basal keratinocytes through anchoring filaments while the deeper aspect attaches to the underlying dermis. Thus, blister/ulcer formation is commonly seen after minor sheering trauma in healed burns. The clinical significance is that the newly regenerated epithelium is delicate and must be protected for some time from even minor trauma, e.g., prefabricated pressure garments are to be either worn very carefully or else crepe bandages, etc., be used initially.

If the skin is affected deeper in the zone of stratum reticulare, the defect is covered by substitutive unspecialized connective tissue. Although the patient and the surgeon always desire that the result should be structurally and functionally identical to normal unburnt skin but actually it is not so. There is a lesser or more extensive formation of cicatrix. Dermal reconstitution begins 3–4 days after injury, characterized clinically by formation of granulation tissue. Remodeling consists of the deposition of the matrix and its subsequent changes over time. TGF-β is the most important cytokine involved in wound healing with its role in fibroblast proliferation,

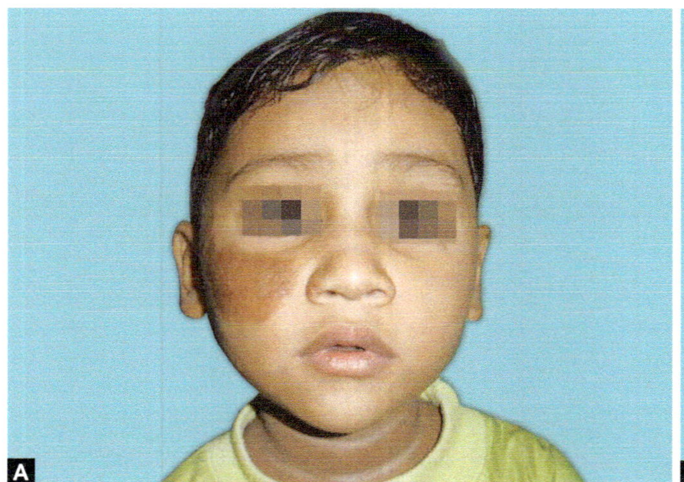

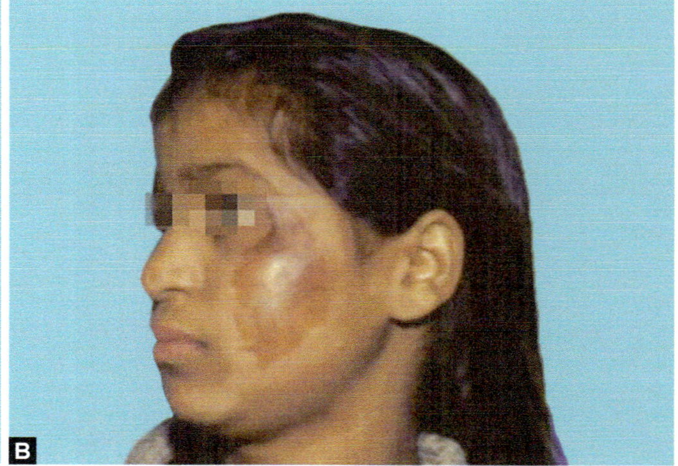

FIGS. 2A AND B: Well healed postburn scars on face. Note the difference in color, texture, and shininess. No deformity or functional deficit. Only aesthetic considerations.

collagen synthesis, and storage and reshaping of new extracellular matrix by stimulating inflammation and angiogenesis. Wound healing can be excessive leading to pathological scar formation (hypertrophic scar/keloid) or it may become dynamic or not heal and become a chronic wound. The hypertrophic scar, unlike a keloid, remains within its limits and regresses over a period of time. The fibroblasts derived from hypertrophic scars are different from fibroblasts which are from areas healed without excessive scarring or undamaged dermis. Excessive healing with hypertrophic scar (actually contraction) continues resulting in a functional (e.g., contractures across the joints) and/or aesthetic deficit. A scar contracture, thus, is the end result of the process of contraction occurring in a healed scar. The normal healthy skin in these patients is replaced by excessive scar tissue which lacks extensibility, resulting in decreased range of motion, and/or poor aesthetics.

With full thickness burn of skin, wound contraction and epithelialization from the margins occurs leading to contractures. However, migration from the wound edges is very limited (5 mm) which explains why there is more of contraction and scar formation than re-epithelialization. Wound contraction is an active biological process by which an area of skin loss in an open wound is decreased by concentric reduction in the size of the wound. It is a vital part of spontaneous healing of open wounds and perhaps nature's attempt to close them. A wound contraction, thus, also leads to a contracture. The reduction in size of wound causes lesser degree of connective tissue deposition. The amount of epithelialization needed has also decreased. The rate of wound contraction depends on degree of laxity of tissues (e.g., loose skin like that of neck, axilla, breast, and gluteal region contracts faster) and presence/absence of bone underneath (e.g., presence of calvarium, tibia, etc., hamper contraction). Presence of free margin (as in lips and eyelids) or a joint (e.g., cubital/popliteal fossa) allows the contraction to proceed faster. The square shape of a wound favors faster contraction as compared to circular wounds. When the contracture is opposite a joint, it leads to a functional deficit in its full range of motion. Thus, while contractures of the lower extremity interfere in upright ambulation and wearing of ordinary shoes, those of the upper extremity interfere in all the day to-day activities of the individual. The nonjoint contractures like ectropion of eyelids endangers vision and that of lips in normal eating and lip seal apart from poor aesthetic appearance. Similarly, contractures of the breast may pull it in one direction or the other leading to disfigurement. Wound contraction is a satisfactory mechanism when the tissue loss is small, in a noncritical area and surrounded by loose skin. A small full-thickness burn over upper medial thigh, gluteal region or lower abdomen may heal satisfactorily by contraction aided by epithelialization from the margins. In a fingertip injury or small scalp loss, contraction may be desirable so as to have specialized sensitive and hairy skin respectively to cover the wound. A full-thickness burn of axilla, anterior neck, or in the cubital/popliteal fossa region can be devastating because of diminished extension possible. Contraction is independent of epithelial migration and relies on the myofibroblasts with contractile elements present in the granulation tissue in the wound.

It is at this stage that most of these patients move on to the metropolitan cities in search of a plastic surgeon who can treat them. Patients of postburn scars, contractures, defects, and disfigurements constitute almost half of the workload of many general plastic surgeons, especially the ones in government institutions.

Types of Postburn Scars and their Management

Scarring is an imperfect evolutionary mechanism which compromises between restoration of tissue integrity and preventing infection at the expense of appearance. The only way to erase the postburn scars completely is to prevent the burn injury itself. "An ounce of prevention is better than a pound of cure" is no better exemplified than by a burn injury. Once burn injury has occurred, the scars can only be minimized and not prevented or removed completely. This can be done by appropriate patient and wound management in the acute phase (including first aid) and various physical therapy measures instituted and meticulously followed after the burn wound has healed completely till the complete maturation of the scar. These include:

- Prevention of increase in burn wound depth by taking measures to avoid hypotension, hypovolemia, infection, and trauma to regenerating delicate epithelium. Bringing down the temperature of the skin to normal body temperature in thermal burns as soon as possible by pouring water minimizes the depth of burn injury. Similarly, depth in chemical burns can also be minimized by diluting the chemical thoroughly at the earliest (by water, in general). Radiation burn injury to skin in cancer patients has been minimized by improved technology. Immediate correction of hypovolemic shock and hypoxia, not only benefits the patient as a whole but also allows for adequate perfusion of burnt tissues, especially in the zone of stasis. The desiccation of the burn wound, increased viscosity of the blood and hypoxia of the patient all lead to death of compromised tissues which could have survived if appropriate therapeutic measures were instituted promptly. Along with infection, they can convert a burn wound into a deeper injury leading to more scarring. In addition, trauma to regenerating neoepithelium must be prevented by delicate handling of tissues and use of nonstick paraffin gauge and antimicrobial ointments and moist dressings. It must be noted that for a given depth of burn, the scars formed are not only different in different parts of the body but also different individuals show different outcomes for a given site and depth.

- Taking appropriate care of factors which retard the rate of healing. Poor nutritional status is one of them. Apart from carbohydrates, proteins and fats, higher doses of minerals and vitamins are given to patients to take care of hypermetabolic state. Uncontrolled diabetes, smoking, alcohol intake, local wound infection with pathogens and local edema, etc., are some other treatable factors.
- Increasing the rate of healing using specialized dressing materials and topical growth factors.

Again, for purely descriptive purposes, the completely healed burn patients may be divided into two categories depending on the time of their presentation to a specialist burn surgeon:

1. The patient is being treated by the burn surgeon right from the acute stage and/or the scars are immature. The newly healed burn wound is immature, hypervascular and hence red in color. It changes in appearance, pigmentation, and gains strength to preinjury level over a period of time, generally 1–2 years or more and is amenable to various modalities used to change it toward desired outcomes.
2. The scars have already matured at the time of presentation to the burn specialist. A mature scar has become stabilized in its appearance and gained full strength. Its vascularity has now decreased to normal for the area. It is soft and supple (pliable), flat, and its color does not change any more. Other than surgical intervention(s) to change, it remains same throughout the life of an individual.

When the scars are immature **(Figs. 3 to 5)**, their maturation can be altered favorably by using a number of physical therapeutic and other measures.

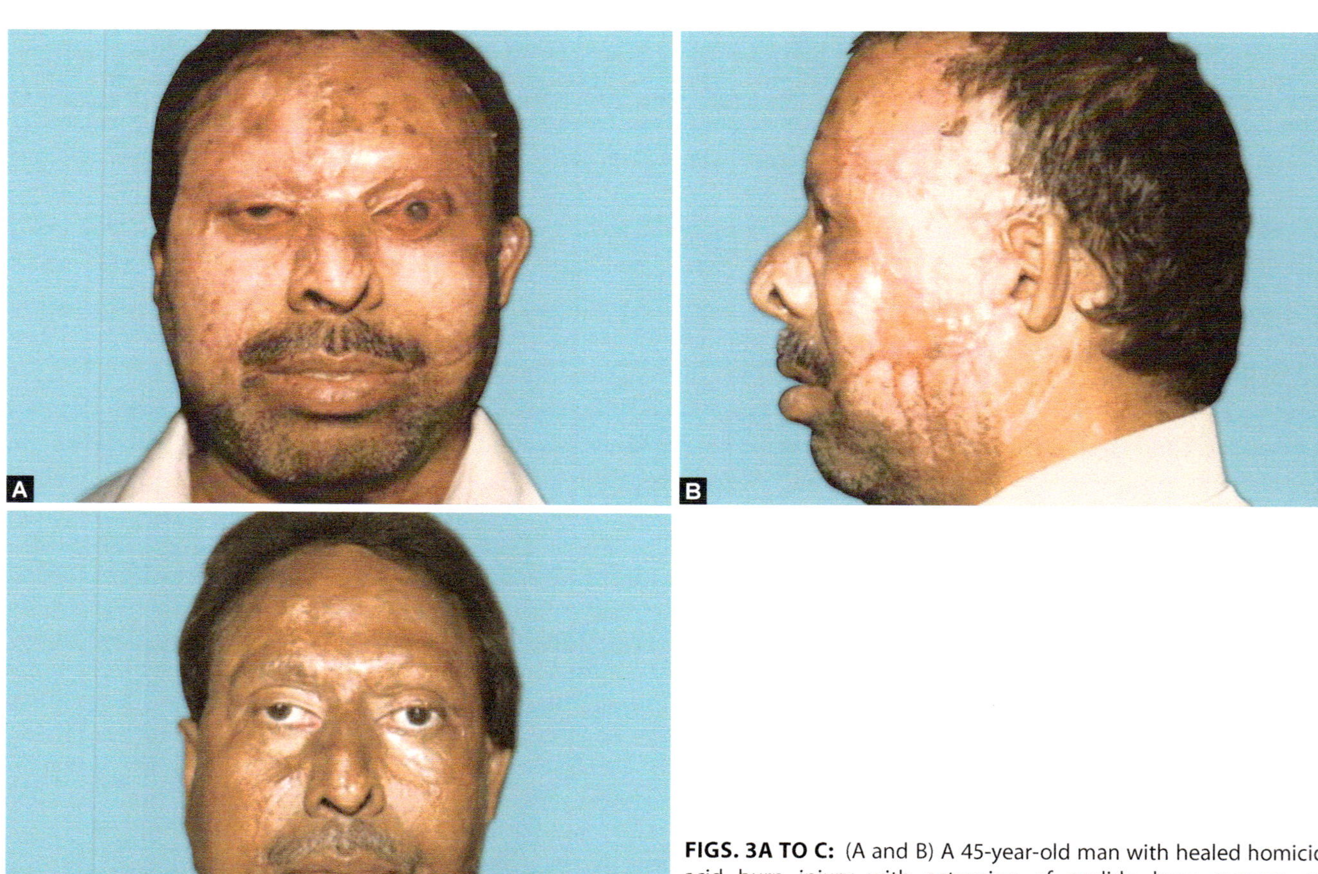

FIGS. 3A TO C: (A and B) A 45-year-old man with healed homicidal acid burn injury with ectropion of eyelids, hazy corneas, and immature facial scars. (C) Appearance after spontaneous maturation of scars by physical therapy. The only operative intervention done is release and grafting of eyelids ectropion. Also note the spontaneous clearing of corneas after restoration of eyelid function.

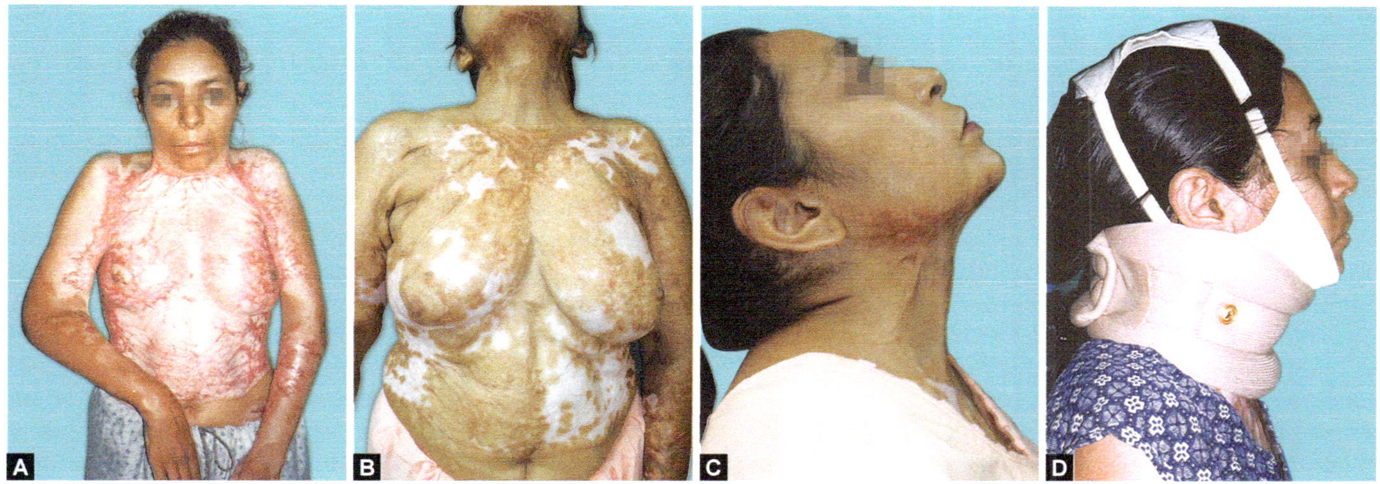

FIGS. 4A TO D: (A) A 27-year-old female with multiple contractures and immature, hyperemic scars. (B) Result 18 months later, the contractures have been treated and the scars matured with greatly diminished vascularity. Please note the improved breast contours due to diminished upward pull and softening of mature scars. No surgical intervention can be worthwhile for extensive hypopigmented areas. (C) Postoperative lateral view of neck. (D) Chin-neck pressure garment and cervical collar is worn for 6–9 months to provide splintage for favorable maturation of graft.

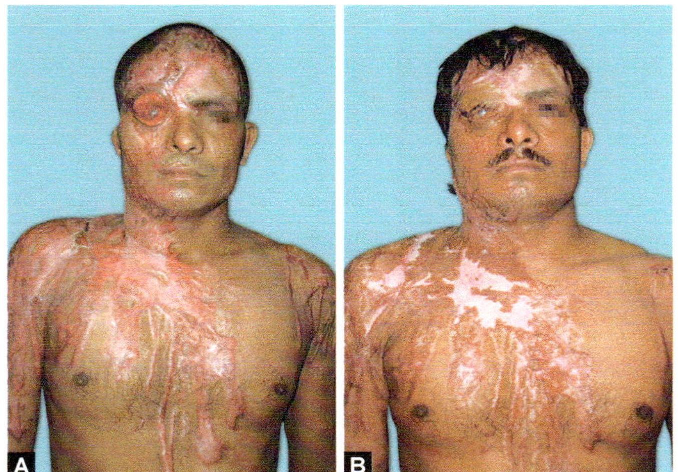

FIGS. 5A AND B: (A) Young adult with very severe ectropion of right upper and lower eyelids, loss of vision, with facial disfigurement. (B) Simultaneous release and split skin graft of both eyelids done without waiting for scar maturation. Result after 4 months. Please note the maturation of other scars with massage and passage of time.

Hyperpigmentation[5,6]

The just healed scars must not be exposed to sunlight till their color returns to normal or they have matured. Exposure to sunlight leads to hyperpigmentation of postburn scars, donor sites of split skin grafts, and recently applied grafts. This hyperpigmentation is extremely difficult to treat. Exposure can be prevented by covering with thick and dark clothes, avoidance of outdoor activities, use of wide brim hats, umbrellas, pressure garments, and sunscreen lotions with sun protection factor (SPF) of at least 30. This is because an SPF of 32 absorbs 96.9% of UV light. Since the burn patients have to avoid sun for several months to years, their vitamin D levels must be monitored and oral supplements prescribed, if required. The patients must also be forewarned on the use of various proprietary creams containing steroids for itching which is a common complaint in healing and recently healed burns. This is because steroids are photosensitizers and lead to hyperpigmentation, if exposed to sun.

Skin grafts have increased melanocyte numbers and increased melanocytic activity. A number of skin lightening agents have been developed. While several compounds target tyrosinase, the rate limiting enzyme of melanogenesis, there has been an increased interest in alternate hypopigmenting mechanisms. Hydroquinone containing creams are commonly used to inhibit tyrosinase activity. To have a synergistic effect, these also contain a steroid (e.g., mometasone to reduce inflammation) and tretinoin. The latter reduces atrophy associated with steroid, promotes penetration of hydroquinone, and decreases pigmentation by increasing keratinocyte turnover. Laser therapy is also being increasingly used to reduce pigmentation in burn patients.

Hypopigmentation[6-10]

Significant hypopigmentary changes can occur after a burn injury because the main pigment, melanin resides in the epidermis which is always affected in a burn. Similarly, whatever may be the thickness, a split skin graft always includes removal of whole of epidermis. Specialized cells called melanocytes, derived from melanoblasts, synthesize melanin which is stored in special cell organelles called melanosomes. Melanocytes are present in the basal layer of epidermis from where they spread dendrites which distribute melanosomes to keratinocytes present in the deepest two layers of epidermis. Each melanocyte links to about forty keratinocytes and forms an "epidermal melanin unit". Although all people have similar number of melanocytes, their pigmentation varies in number and size of melanosomes transferred to keratinocytes. Highly pigmented people have larger melanosomes filled with more melanin and greater density than those with lighter pigmentation. Melanin production is also increased in response to sun exposure. In fact, pigmentation has been considered to be a compromise between the need for sun exposure which is essential for vitamin D synthesis and the need to protect the skin from harmful effects of ultraviolet light. Thus, populations which are more exposed to sun (at equator) are pigmented more to protect from harmful effects of ultraviolet light as compared to those who have lesser sun exposure (more northern or southern latitudes). It is, thus, clear that in every burn injury, pigmentary changes whether temporary or permanent are bound to occur.

A number of patients have the chief complaint of hypo- or depigmented scars. These vitiligo patches are very unsightly and are a taboo in our society. It may not be possible to treat all of them if they are extensive. However, in areas such as face, neck, hands, and feet, which cannot be covered by clothes treatment has to be done. Similarly, if limited areas are present over the breasts or anterior abdomen in females, treatment has to be offered **(Figs. 6 and 7)**. The surgical treatment should begin after the maturation of scar and only after the patches have

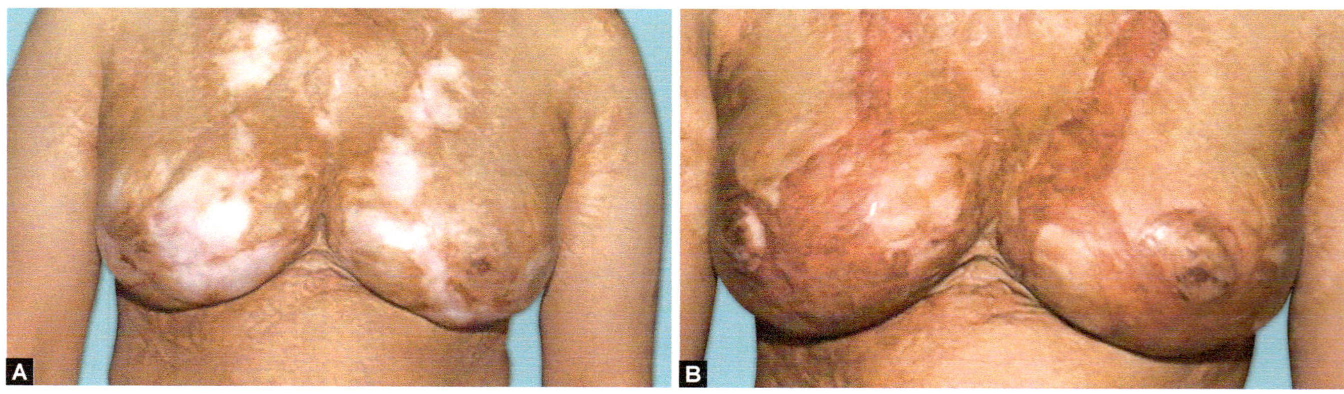

FIGS. 6A AND B: (A) A 22-year-old female with hypopigmented postburn scars over both breasts. (B) Early result after excision and overgrafting with thin split skin grafts.

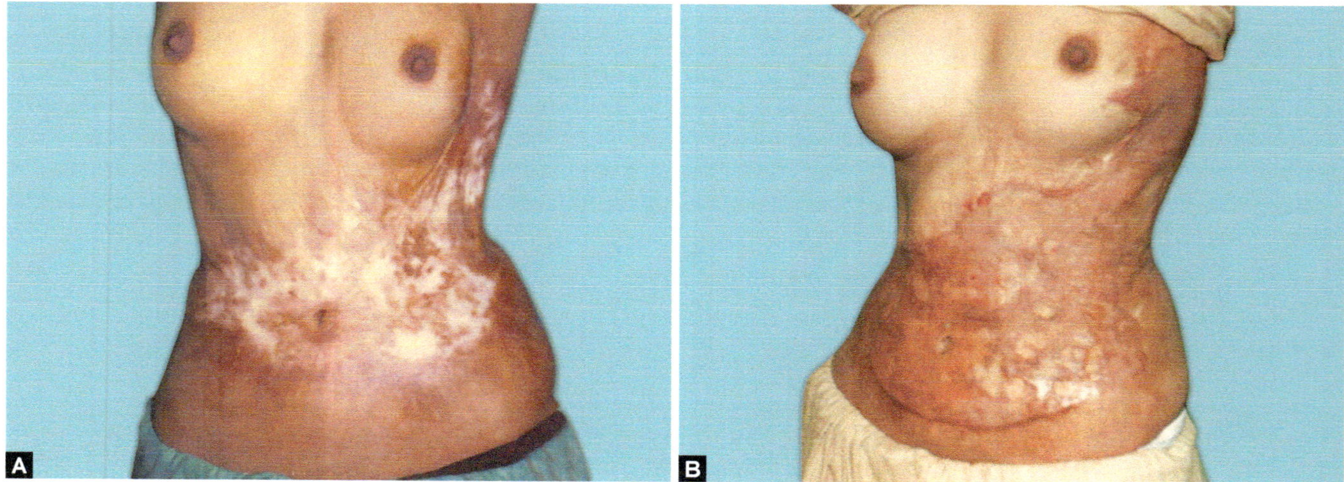

FIGS. 7A AND B: (A) A 25-year-old female with hypopigmented postburn scars over abdomen, an area usually exposed while in traditional Indian dress "*Saree*". (B) Result at 6 weeks after excision and overgrafting with thin split skin grafts.

stabilized. Excision/dermabrasion and over grafting with thin split skin grafts are commonly done. This excision can be done using Watson skin grafting knife or electric dermatome apart from scalpel blade. Another option is transplantation of melanocytes-keratinocytes by harvesting skin graft from a normal area, converting it into a cell suspension after digestion with trypsin and applying over the affected area after dermabrasion. Although color may not be exactly like the surrounding skin but the results are always very satisfying when compared to initial problem. Very small areas may be treated by excision and primary closure or by tattooing of appropriate pigment in the vitiligo area.

When the scars are mature, soft, and supple, physical therapy measures cannot alter their appearance **(Figs. 8A to D)**. These patients need surgical intervention purely to improve their aesthetic appearance and regain self-confidence. They are to be dealt with last after all the deformities have been taken care of and missing structures reconstructed. Thus, a full spectrum of a plastic surgeons' reconstructive armamentarium is required. Last but not the least, they need psychotherapy to boost their morale and return "back to society". Most commonly the exposed areas such as head and neck, upper limbs, and feet are treated. It must be remembered that improvement should be seen in totality and not in isolation. It is of no use making the neck look like normal while the lower lip or forehead is "ugly".

Apart from hypo-/hyperpigmented scars the postburn scars may be atrophic, hypertrophic, and stable or unstable. The atrophic scars need intervention because they may breakdown with minimal trauma (scar ulcers) especially when present over areas of stress, e.g., joints, subcutaneous bones, etc., and become unstable. They may be unaesthetic as well. The atrophic/unstable scars also need surgical intervention to prevent risk of malignant transformation. Generally, excision and cover with split skin grafts/flaps are required.

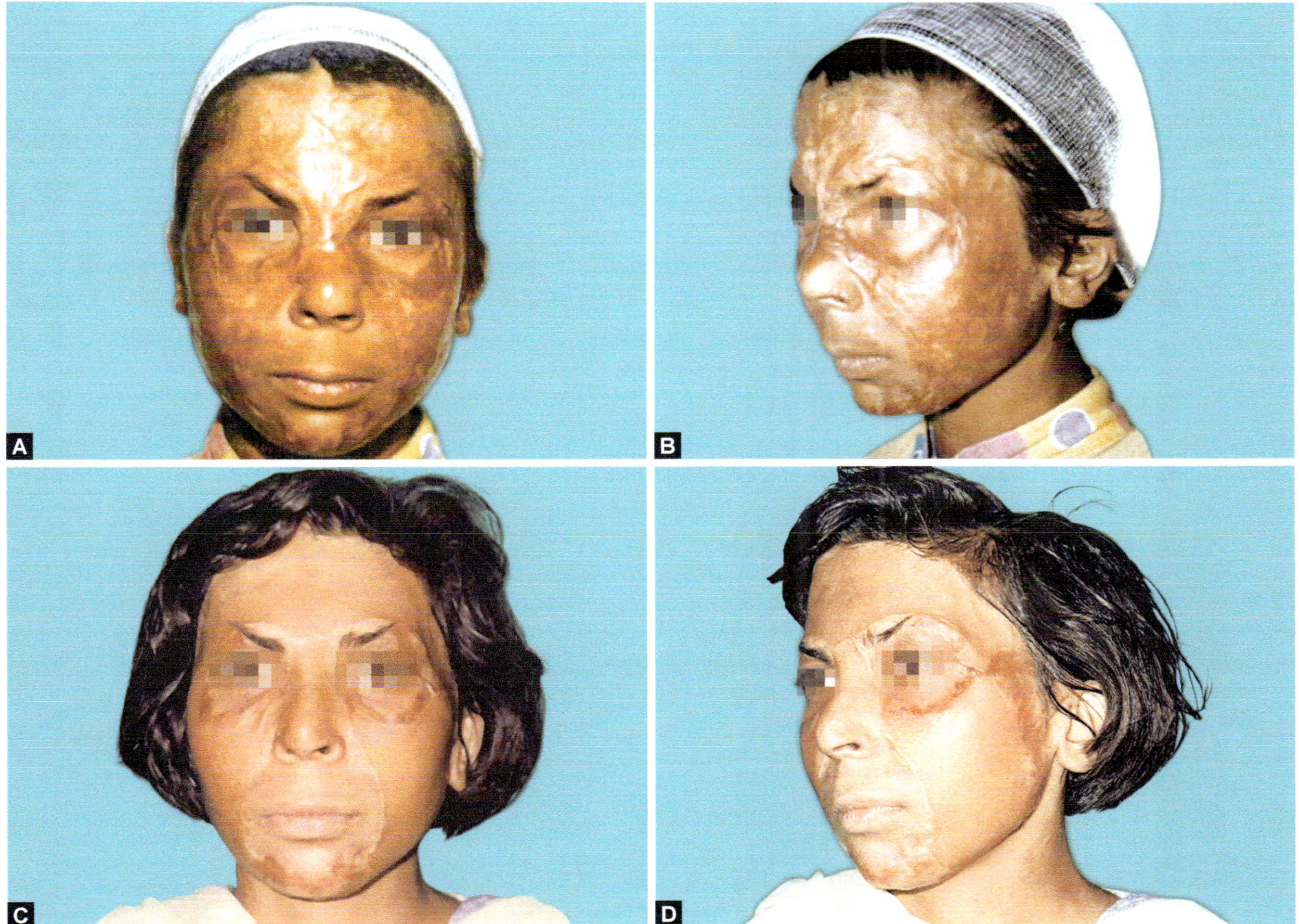

FIGS. 8A TO D: (A and B) Young girl with extensive postburn scars on whole of face. (C and D) Surgical correction by excision and cover with intermediate thickness split skin grafts from thigh on to cheeks, forehead and nose. Note good color and texture match on the face and excellent contour of the resurfaced nose. Patient opted for use of eyebrow pencil over surgical reconstruction of partial loss of eyebrows.

Hypertrophic Scars[11-13]

The deep dermal burn injuries and the donor sites of thick split skin grafts, both of which involve the reticular layer of dermis, usually heal by hypertrophic scar formation. Hypertrophic scarring is a fibroproliferative disorder of dermal tissue occurring after cutaneous injury and appears as hyperemic scar, red to deep purple in color, raised, firm to hard in consistency, and gradually increasing in thickness. These lesions are itchy and some patients may even complain of pain or both. There is an over-abundant synthesis and deposition of collagen coupled with its limited lysis during the remodeling phase of wound healing. They do not extend beyond the limits of original burn/skin graft donor site/operative injury and usually start developing within a month of complete healing. The natural history of these scars is of spontaneous resolution with diminishing redness, thickness and itching over a period of 1–2 years or more (rarely longer) and become mature. A number of factors influence the severity and time period of maturation. Age of patient, anatomical site and depth of burn/thickness of graft harvested, presence of continued infection especially sinuses due to retained hair follicles, and associated repeated tension due to joint movements are some of the important factors apart from individual genetic predisposition. The prevention and treatment of hypertrophic scars are discussed later along with postburn contractures.

Over the last more than three decades, it has become almost mandatory to have standardized measurements of outcome of any medical treatment. These measurements are first applied to existing treatment outcomes and then new treatment outcomes are compared with them. A number of scales have been devised to assess the burn scars, subjectively as well as objectively.[14-17] These scales can reveal the course of improvement over a period of next 1–2 years or more during maturation phase. "Vancouver Scar Scale"(VSS)[14] and "Patient and Observer Scar Assessment Scale" (POSAS)[15] are the two most commonly used out of more than a dozen proposed since Sullivan et al. first published VSS in their paper "Rating the burn scar" in 1990.[14] In VSS, the scar is assessed with respect to four parameters, viz., (1) vascularity, (2) pigmentation, (3) pliability, and (4) height as shown in the **Box 1** and marks are awarded. Lowest score of 0 means the best while highest score of 13 means the worst scar. The major shortcomings of this scale are that (1) it does not include pruritus and pain which are very important from the postburn patient's point of view, (2) it lacks the patient's own opinion, and (3) all the parameters are not given equal weightage.

BOX 1 Vancouver Scar Scale.[14]

- *Vascularity*:
  - 0: Normal
  - 1: Pink
  - 2: Red
  - 3: Purple
- *Pigmentation*:
  - 0: Normal
  - 1: Hypopigmentation
  - 2: Hyperpigmentation
- *Pliability*:
  - 0: Normal
  - 1: Supple
  - 2: Yielding
  - 3: Firm
  - 4: Banding
  - 5: Contracture
- *Height*:
  - 0: Normal/Flat
  - 1: >2 mm
  - 2: 5 mm
  - 3: >5 mm

In 2004, Draaijers et al. published POSAS scale which takes opinion of the patient also to assess the outcome.[15] In addition, pain and pruritus were also included. Here, the clinician assesses the scar with respect to vascularization, pigmentation, thickness, relief, and pliability and gives marks from 1 to 10 for each parameter. Score of 1 is considered as normal while 10 is the worst. The patient also assesses the scar with respect to 6 parameters as shown in **Table 1** and again scores are given to each parameter. Thus, a score of 11 reflects the best scar and 110 as the worst scar.

In both these scales, the site of scar has not been given any importance despite the fact that it is well known that some sites are of greater concern to a given patient or more prone to hypertrophy. VSS is more of a qualitative scale as compared to POSAS which is more quantitative.

Patients may also present late with mature scars along with one or more of other postburn sequelae. They need detailed assessment of the functional and aesthetic needs and planning of priorities and order of surgical interventions.

POSTBURN CONTRACTURES

A patient, who receives the best of the modern burn treatment, is expected to heal without any contracture.

TABLE 1: Patient and Observer Scar Assessment Scale (POSAS).

Observer Scar Assessment Scale (OSAS)												
	Normal skin	1	2	3	4	5	6	7	8	9	10	Worst scar imaginable
Vascularization		O	O	O	O	O	O	O	O	O	O	
Pigmentation		O	O	O	O	O	O	O	O	O	O	
Thickness		O	O	O	O	O	O	O	O	O	O	
Relief		O	O	O	O	O	O	O	O	O	O	
Pliability		O	O	O	O	O	O	O	O	O	O	
Observer scar rating												
OSAS summary score: ______________(minimum 5; maximum, 50)												
Patient Scar Assessment Scale (PSAS)												
	No, no complaints	1	2	3	4	5	6	7	8	9	10	Yes, worst imaginable
Is the scar painful?		O	O	O	O	O	O	O	O	O	O	
Is the scar itching?		O	O	O	O	O	O	O	O	O	O	
Is the color of the scar different?	No, as normal skin	O	O	O	O	O	O	O	O	O	O	No, very different
Is the scar more stiff?		O	O	O	O	O	O	O	O	O	O	
Is the thickness of the scar different?		O	O	O	O	O	O	O	O	O	O	
Is the scar irregular?		O	O	O	O	O	O	O	O	O	O	
Overall patient scar satisfaction												
PSAS total score: ___________ (minimum, 6; maximum, 60)												

However, contractures, an inability to perform full range of motion of a joint, like bed sores, do form even in the best of facilities. This is because contraction is a strong natural force and difficult to counter. Moreover, life-threatening complications in acute stage may compromise on problems which can be tackled later. Unfortunately, the incidence of postburn contractures is extremely high in our country. Quite often, they are not only multiple in a given patient but also very severe and diffuse. This is because the majority of the millions of burn victims in our country have no access to a trained burn specialist. The incidence and severity are likely to be less if postburn raw areas are split skin grafted in time. The number of trained burn and plastic surgeons is too small in our country. It is around 2,500 for >1.4 billion population. The burn patients are treated not only by a general surgeon but also by general practitioners of all systems of medicine, quacks **(Fig. 9)** and even patients and their relatives themselves. In this scenario, the aim and endpoint of a burn injury management is unfortunately a healed wound only.

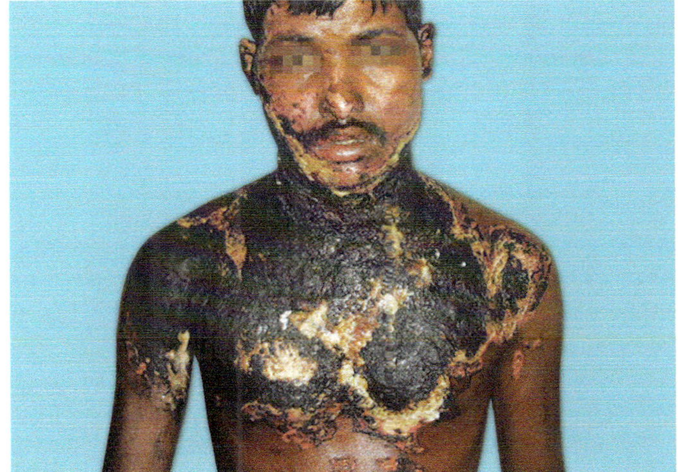

FIG. 9: Patient being treated by quacks with application of indigenous mixture of "Ratnajyouti" (an edible coloring agent) and camphor in coconut oil.

Associated Local Conditions in Patients with Contractures

A postburn contracture may be associated with additional problems on the skin and/or in the deeper tissues.

On the Skin

There may be:

- A hypertrophic scar which may have sinuses and be infected in addition
- An atrophic scar
- An unstable scar over flexor aspects of joints/chronic nonhealing scar ulcer(s) over nonjoint areas which

may or may not heal over prolonged periods of time and may recur. There may be chronic postburn massive raw areas which are not expected to heal of their own.

- Depigmented/Hyperpigmented scar
- A Marjolin ulcer

Presence of one or more of above along with a contracture may alter the physical therapy and/or surgical treatment of a contracture. For example, an unstable scar or chronic nonhealing scar ulcer(s) needs their surgical excision, release of contracture, and provision of skin cover. Physical therapy in the form of exercises, massage, and pressure garments prior to surgery is not possible in these cases. Bigger raw areas need wound closure with skin grafting before contracture can be subjected to physical therapy. Wide excision of Marjolin ulcer needs to be combined with release of contracting bands. A postburn contracture associated with a hypertrophic (especially, if infected) or an atrophic scar or a depigmented scar needs excision-release of all to achieve best results not only functionally, but also aesthetically.

In the Deeper Tissues

The deeper tissues may be affected either due to their involvement in the initial burn injury (e.g., electrical burns) or secondary to the presence of a skin contracture over a prolonged period of many years which leads to shortening of musculotendinous units and neurovascular structures. Contractures of fingers following electrical burns are invariably associated with loss of underlying flexor tendons and need flap cover, even if a split skin graftable bed is present, because of the need for tendon grafting later. In addition, there is greater risk of digital circulation becoming compromised on straightening the finger as compared to patients with thermal burns. The joints may be subluxated or dislocated with joint capsule and ligaments becoming tight in the direction of the contracture especially when adult patients present for treatment of burns sustained in early childhood. The bones may be deformed specially in growing children, e.g., mandible may be deformed due to chronic pull in cases of severe postburn contractures of the neck (mentosternal contractures) **(Figs. 10 A and B)**.

The shortening of deeper structures has great clinical significance. It may not be possible to release the contracture fully at the time of operation because the neurovascular structures and musculotendinous units may stand out as bowstrings limiting any further release. Moreover, the vessels may also go into spasm with compromise of distal limb or digit circulation if subjected to excessive stretch. There may be prolonged neurapraxia due to nerve stretch. The musculotendinous units may resist any lengthening by forceful pull even under general anesthesia. Such contractures need maximal release possible and dressing of the wound followed by sustained traction using various methods for complete correction. This can generally be achieved within 2 weeks. Skin cover is provided only after complete or maximum possible correction is achieved. In occasional circumstances, when the patient presents with severe postburn contractures of elbow, wrist, knee, etc., several years or even decade(s) after sustaining the burns in childhood, it may not be possible to achieve complete release and correction at all **(Figs. 11A to D)**. When bones and joints are also affected, orthopedic consultation may be needed. When mandible is deformed along with loss of normal dental occlusion in severe and untreated postburn contractures of neck in children, orthodontic/orthognathic measures are needed after the contracture is fully treated.

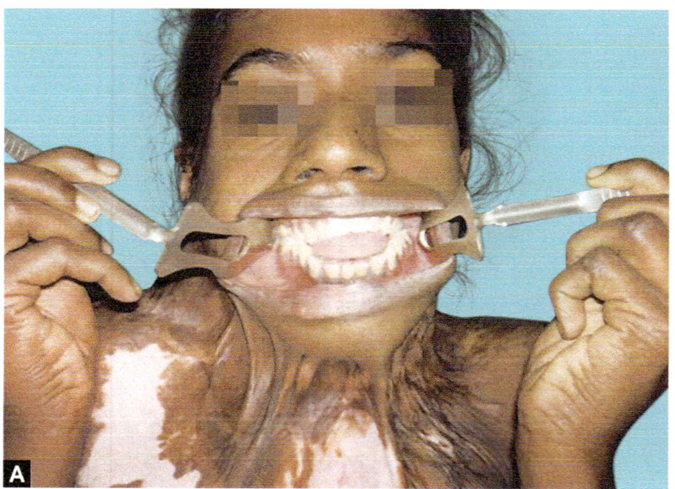

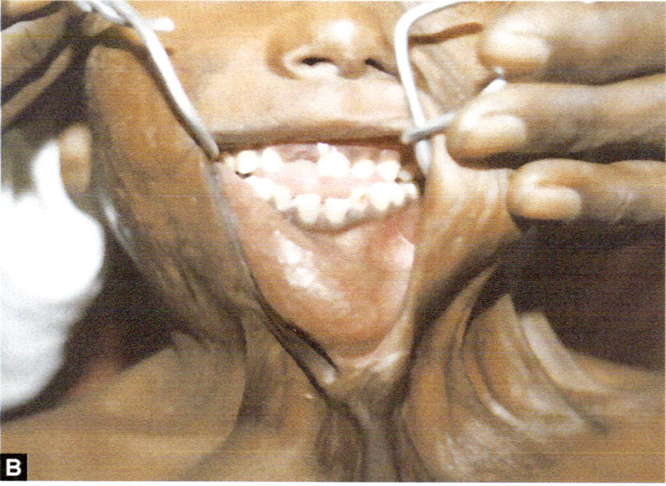

FIGS. 10A AND B: Deformed mandible with severe malocclusion due to untreated mentosternal contracture following burns sustained in very early childhood.

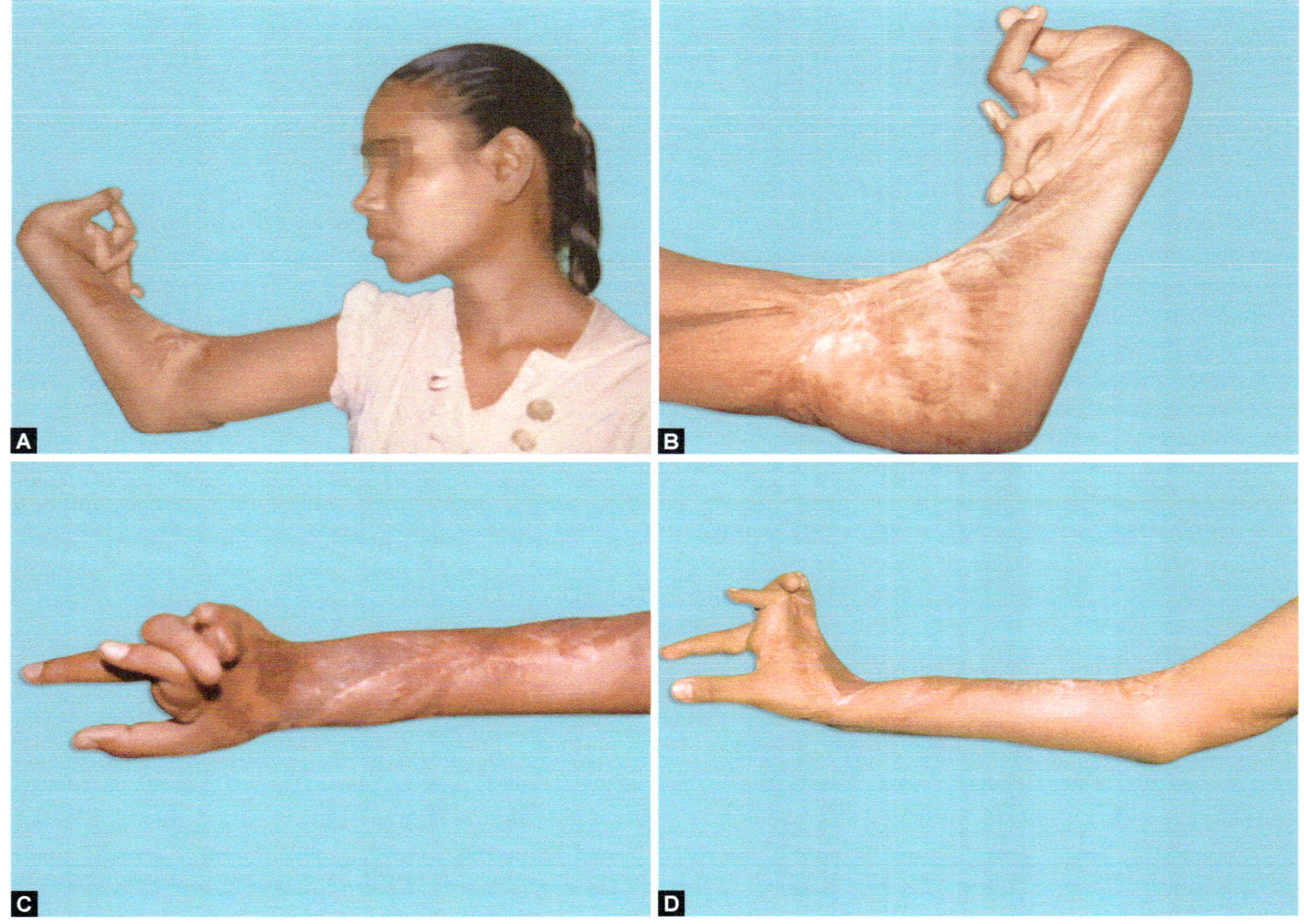

FIGS. 11A TO D: (A and B) Severe contracture of elbow and wrist secondary to burns sustained at the age of 1 year; (C and D) Suboptimal result after release and skin grafting is attributed to bony deformity and contracted ligaments, joint capsule and musculotendinous units.

Timing of Surgery in Postburn Contractures

As a rule, surgical intervention for postburn contractures should not be undertaken during the active phase of healing and scarring, i.e., as long as the scar is immature and highly vascular. This usually takes 1 year or so. One must allow the scar to become mature, soft and supple, and "avascular" before undertaking surgery for contractures. This is because a highly vascular scar bleeds more during operation with difficulties in achieving perfect hemostasis resulting in poorer skin graft "take" leading to healing by further contraction or hematoma under a flap leading to its loss. Secondly, operation on an active, highly vascular scar with wound bed still in active phase of contraction, adds insult to already traumatized tissues with vigorous local response in the form of further contraction. All these lead to a less than perfect result. Lastly, an immature scar is amenable to physical therapy measures resulting in significant improvement even nonsurgically. With the passage of time, some mild contractures may improve with a better final result than if they had been surgically managed. Hence, one must get benefit from this therapy before any operative intervention. Time is a great healer, not only of the emotional trauma but also of the wounds and scars of the skin! The patients also develop more realistic expectations during this waiting period, due to their interaction with other patients who are in their last stage of reconstructions. Lastly, it must be remembered that physical therapy is the mainstay of achieving best results even after surgical intervention. A patient who is noncompliant prior to operation is likely to get a poor or an average result postoperatively with all the blame being put on the surgeon especially in this era of Consumer Protection Act.

A burn surgeon must never be guided or influenced by the patient, his or her relatives, and higher authorities to do "something operative" at the earliest. However, there are many exceptions to this "general rule" of scar maturation. In these cases, the results may be compromised and they may need another surgery at a later date.

- Ectropion of the eyelids, especially the upper eyelid with constant danger of keratoconjunctivitis, corneal ulceration, scarring, or perforation with loss of vision
- Incapacitating contracture of the neck with inability to look forward
- Severe microstomia interfering with adequate nutrition and maintenance of orodental hygiene
- Crippling contractures of hand, especially dorsal contracture with metacarpophalangeal joints going in hyperextension leading to permanent damage to extensor mechanism with various deformities
- Contractures of both the knees, which force the patient to be on "all the fours" and endangers the very dignity of being an upright human being
- Postburn contractures with associated adjoining chronic raw areas needing skin cover
- Contractures with infected hypertrophic scars and abscesses, which need excision/drainage for their recovery
- Any severe, incapacitating contracture unlikely to improve at all with physical therapy measures

Priority of Release in Cases of Multiple Contractures

A large percentage of patients coming to a burn surgeon have multiple contractures in different parts of the body. It is obvious that all of them cannot be released in one stage. In addition, there may be other reconstructive needs, e.g., reconstruction of scalp, nose and pinna, etc. Quite often, there may be limitations due to paucity of healthy donor sites for skin grafts and flaps. Release of contractures and reconstruction in such patients may take many years. Therefore, a definitive strategy is essential in planning to reduce the number of anesthetic and surgical procedures and yet provide the best functional and cosmetic result safely. The patient and all his/her operative needs must be considered as a whole. The traditional reconstructive ladder advises the simplest to achieve the reconstructive goal. While it remains the guiding principle, a number of its modifications have come up because of great advances in the field of reconstructive surgery since it was first described.[18] In the present-day scenario, one is free to choose the best and straightaway reach even the top of ladder depending on the age and sex of patient, extent and depth of initial burn injury and consequently reconstructive needs, availability of best donor sites, wishes of the patient, facilities available and expertise of the surgeon, etc. Thus, a microsurgical free flap can be done in a selected case where this would be ideal and possible in the given scenario. Another principle of replacing "like tissues with like" (in color, texture, and pliability and use of adjacent areas) is sometimes not possible and has to be compromised especially in patients who had extensive burns in extent and depth with scarcity of ideal donor sites because of scarring.

With each stage, the patient must be able to appreciate the result and improvement. This adds to the patient's compliance and morale. It is ideal that this plan of action is put in black and white before the treatment is started and kept in patient's records along with a copy to patient. It must be remembered that the association of a burn patient with one's surgeon is a very protracted journey, sometimes extending to several decades especially for burnt children. The patients require not only surgeon's professional competence but also their time and compassion. A photographic record of the patient is to be kept for comparison with later improvements and failures, if any. This is also of use for the surgeon to perform audit of one's own results, changing practices over a period of decades, medicolegal issues, and last but not the least, teaching trainee residents, presenting in conferences and discussing with peers.

An ectropion of the eyelids, especially the upper eyelid, with its attendant risks needs to be dealt with first to prevent irreparable damage. One must remember that loss of vision due to burns per se is rare except for chemical burns. It may even be managed under local anesthesia in case of an adult. Similarly, a severe contracture of the neck or microstomia leading to difficulties in intubation should be corrected before planning any other contracture release or reconstructive procedure requiring general anesthesia. This takes care of repeated intubation difficulty with its all the attendant risks. Additionally, the complete release of a neck contracture removes the extrinsic pull from the facial structures (lips, chin, and even lower eyelids) and contractures of the axilla and the breast. For full release, the neck contractures need division of platysma and fascia until the strap muscles are seen.

Contractures of the hand need to be addressed after the neck is treated. They are not only crippling and interfere in the day-to-day life, studies, and earning, but may also cause permanent damage to the delicate balance of tendon movement. This is especially true of contractures on the dorsum of hand. A dorsal contracture of the hand with metacarpophalangeal joints in extension not only stops the function, but also wrecks the machinery (extensor apparatus) **(Figs. 12A to D)**. Here, it must be noted that both hands should rarely be operated together (except in small children) to allow the patient his/her daily needs of feeding and toilet care

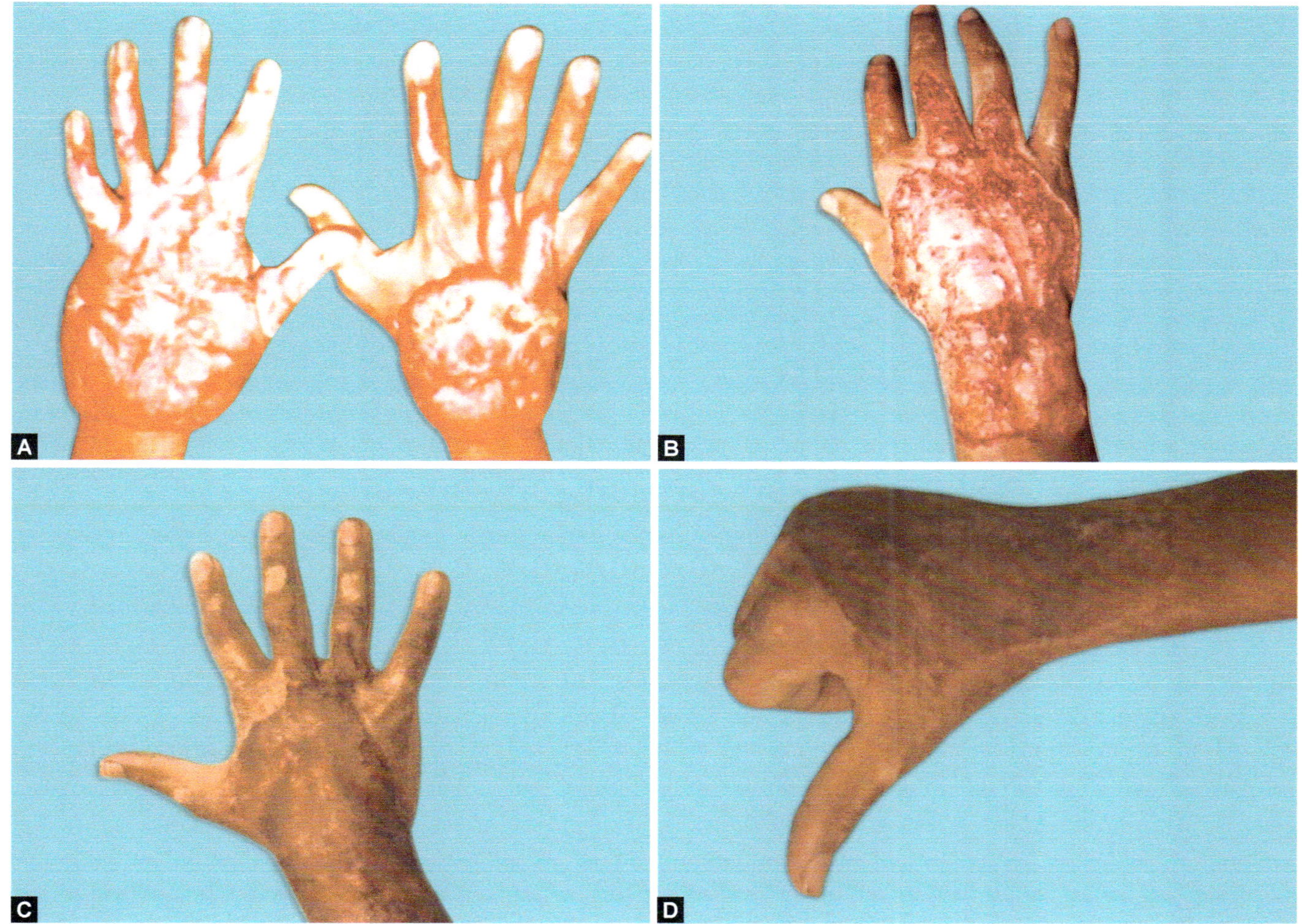

FIGS. 12A TO D: (A) Postburn contracture and severe hypertrophic scar on dorsum of both hands and wrist. (B) Intraoperative: Complete excision of hypertrophic scar and release of contracture (right hand); (C and D) Result at 1 year with full range of movement at metacarpophalangeal (MP) joint with pleasing aesthetics.

(Figs. 13A to D). Also, the hand with greater likelihood of becoming more functional should be treated first rather than the right hand (in a right-handed person), which may be almost irreparably damaged. Conversely, the hand which may be retrievable today and significant damage is expected with any further delay, should be operated first. When ipsilateral axilla, elbow, and hand are all affected, it may not be possible to operate on the hand (inability of application of tourniquet and positioning the hand on a hand table) till the axilla and elbow are released. Contractures of the popliteal fossa also need early intervention as they are also highly incapacitating **(Figs. 14 and 15)**.

The order of management of other contractures depends upon the surgeon's evaluation of the remaining reconstructive needs, feasibility of combining multiple procedures in the same surgical sitting, availability of donor sites, scope of improvement, and the patients' desires.

Prevention and Management of Hypertrophic Scars and Contractures

In a healed burn patient, the healing may have been achieved by one or more of the following:

- Spontaneous healing with epithelialization and contraction
- Split-skin grafting over granulating raw areas after spontaneous eschar separation
- Early excision and split-skin grafting

In all these patients, various physical therapy measures are immediately instituted for the healed burnt areas and split-skin graft donor sites to minimize scars and scar contractures. It should be noted that physical therapy in a burn patient actually begins on the day of admission. This may take the form of limb elevation, crepe bandages to reduce edema, active and passive joint movement, splintage and positioning of the body parts in anti-deformity posture, functional position, etc.

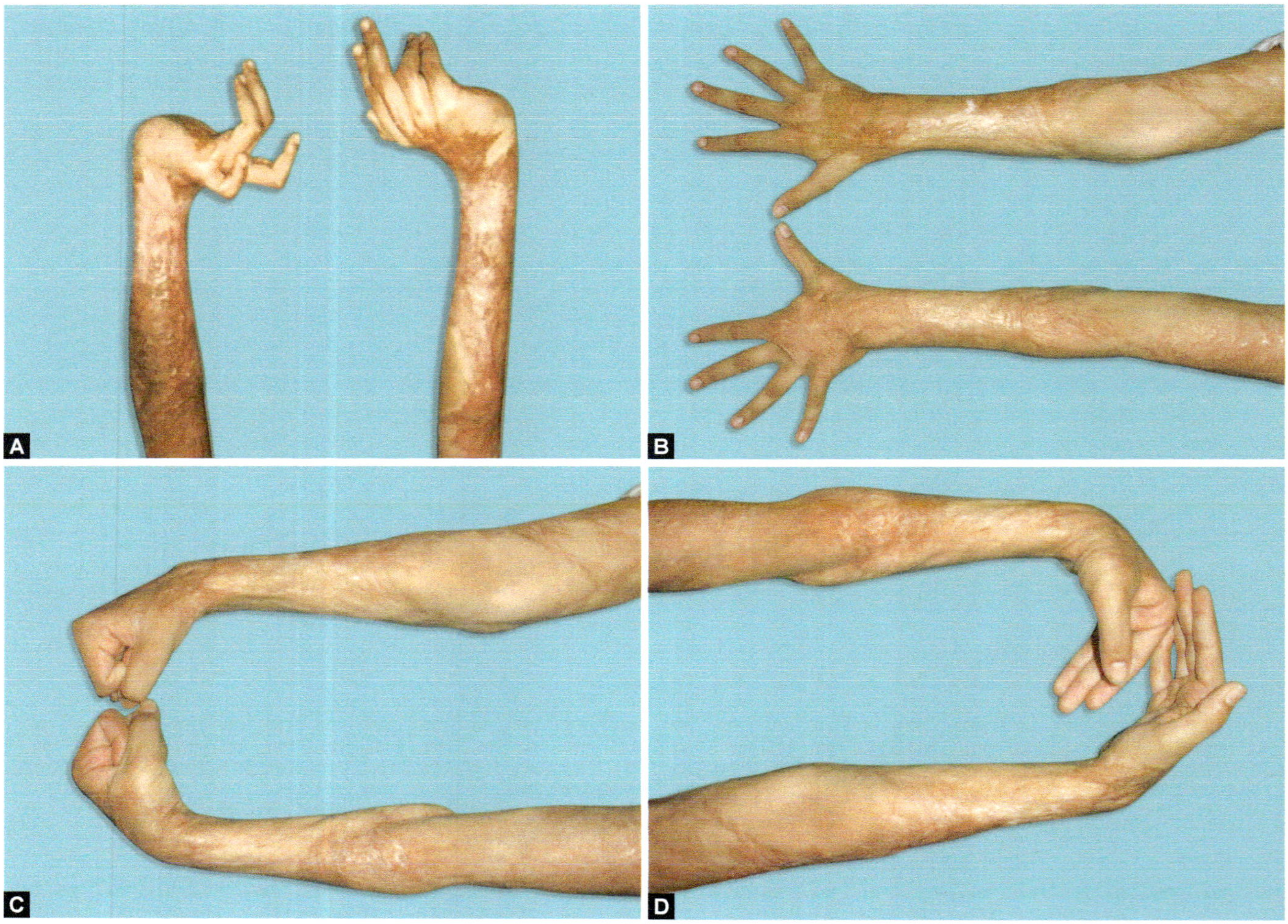

FIGS. 13A TO D: (A) A postburn contracture on dorsum of both hands and wrist in an 8-year-old-child. (B to D) Release and split skin grafting with complete restoration of hand and wrist function. Result after 5 years.

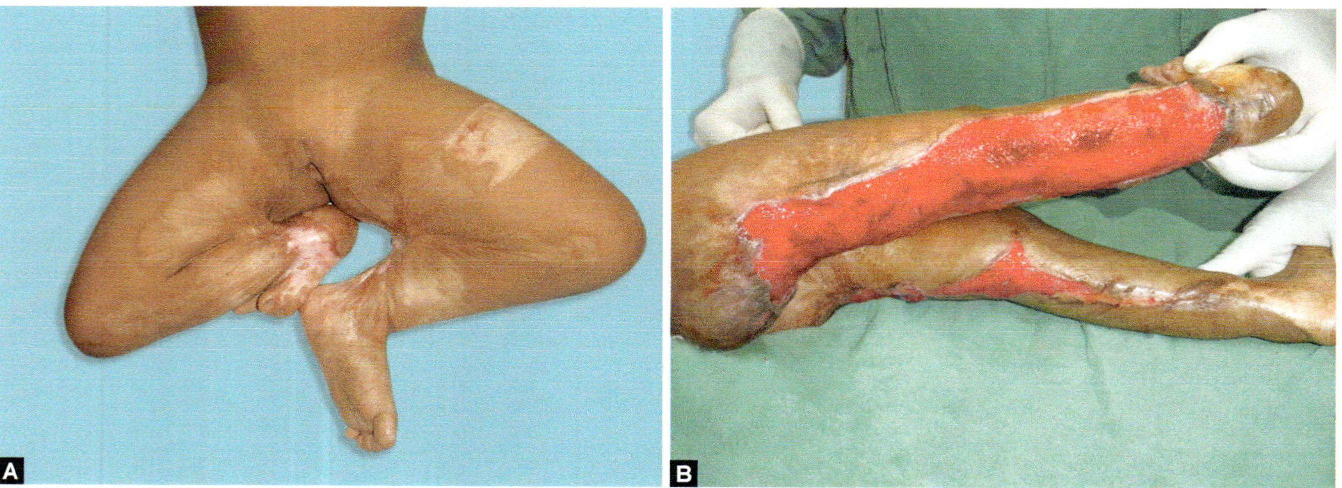

FIGS. 14A TO D: *Continued*

Continued

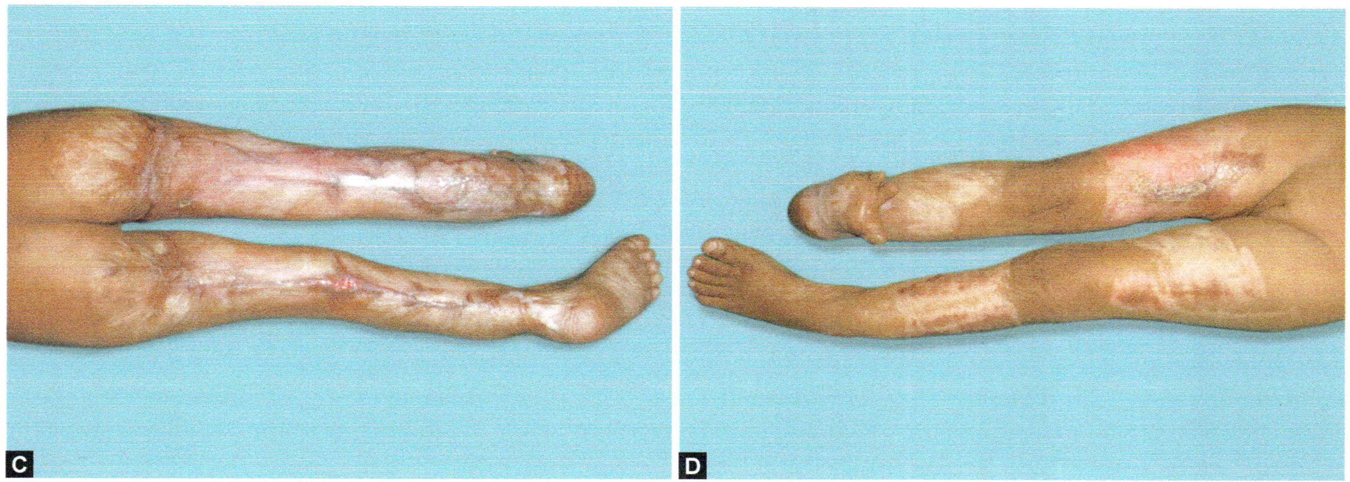

FIGS. 14A TO D: (A) Severe contracture of both knees and right ankle in a 3-year-old girl precluding ambulation. (B) Complete release was not possible in one go; serial splintage done over 2 weeks. Please note the straight limbs and healthy granulations. (C and D) Grafted and all wounds healed.

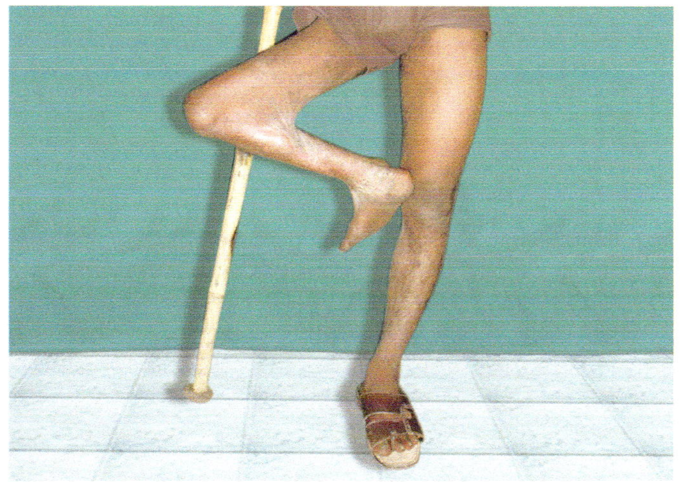

FIG. 15: An untreated popliteal and ankle contracture due to burns sustained in infancy leading to limb shortening with subluxated knee joint.

Due to prolonged contractile nature of the burn wound, a patient who heals initially with full range of motion may develop severe deformities as the healed skin/scars mature and hypertrophic scarring occurs. Dermatological problems, e.g., blister formation, its repeated breakdown, excessive dryness, and cracking of skin can occur or a gradual build-up of hypertrophic scar tissue can lead to a rapid decrease in motion and functional ability. Thus, the physical therapy measures have to be continued till the scars have matured and no further change is expected. During continuation of this therapy, various surgical interventions may also be needed and undertaken. It is only when all the scars have matured, the correctable deformities looked after, reconstructive surgeries performed and no further reasonable improvement is expected that the treatment of a burn patient is called off (except probably continued psychological support and aid for "return to society").

The healed burn wounds and both the recipient as well as donor sites of split-skin grafts need care till they are mature. The scar maturation is a natural process and will occur any way without any intervention over a period of 1–2 years or more in general. The focus of just healed burn patient now changes from "how to heal fastest" to "how to get rid of all scars at the earliest". It is quite reasonable for them to expect that their clinician does and/or advise something to expedite the process with the best possible outcome. The deep dermal burns, especially the ones which take 4–6 weeks to heal and donor sites of intermediate to thick and thick split skin grafts are at a great risk of hypertrophy.

The modulation and control of burn wound/scar contraction and scar contracture are done by the following surgical and nonsurgical techniques.

Skin Grafting

The single most important and effective method of controlling the wound contraction is to close the wound at the earliest. This is done using split-skin grafts in selected deep dermal and all full-thickness burns. Contraction can be inhibited by applying grafts to fresh burn wounds (as in early excision) or over healthy granulating areas (after spontaneous eschar separation). Full-thickness skin graft (FTSG) inhibits contraction almost completely.[19] Unfortunately, in a clinical setting, the raw areas of burns have to be covered with split-skin grafts so that the donor sites can heal on their own and may even be reharvested.

The split skin grafts may have to be expanded with meshing. Although this leads to complete healing of the wound, the latter is largely covered with epithelium in the interstices of the meshed graft.

It is widely believed that thicker the graft, greater will be the inhibition of contraction. This holds good only if the grafts are harvested from a given site. The fact is that when split-skin grafts are harvested from different sites, it is the total percentage of dermal thickness grafted which determines how much contraction will be inhibited. Delayed application of skin graft does not inhibit contraction as effectively as immediate grafting.

In the presence of even mild contractures on or near a joint or even nonjoint areas and surrounding immature scars, the progression of hypertrophy does not stop unless the tension is relieved by release of scar and closure by readjustment of local skin as in Z-plasty, etc., or with skin graft/flap. Tension free wound closure and removal of infective foci which are a source of continued inflammation are the two most important considerations to be taken care of by a burn surgeon for early scar maturation and better results.

Massage[20-22]

Massage of an area consists of manipulation of skin and subcutaneous tissues with varying degrees of hand pressure. Being a noninvasive and nonsurgical intervention, burn surgeons and therapists all over the world advise massage therapy to their patients once their wounds have healed. Despite so much of research, there is still no foolproof clinical data regarding their beneficial effects and how these are obtained. A great number of variables can be blamed as to why a clear answer in not available. Amongst them are whether the massage is done by a trained therapist (with or without a gadget) or by patient and/or attendant, severity of scar when the therapy is commenced, time it took for the burn to heal, genetic predisposition of the patient to develop hypertrophy, age of patient, any associated tightness/contracture, how the outcomes are measured, etc. Moreover, in today's scenario, all patients are treated by multimodalities and it is practically not possible to withhold any treatment method. However, it is clear that there are definite psychological benefits as it helps to relax the patient and creates an overall feeling of well-being. It also buys time for the surgeon before the time is appropriate for surgical intervention by involving the patients in their own treatment.

The effects of massage can be due to stimulation of afferent peripheral nerves to central nervous system producing relaxation of muscles. The massage causes an increased flow in the veins and the lymphatics thereby increasing the absorption of metabolic wastes. There is an increase in capillary circulation and mobility of subcutaneous soft tissues. Massage has also been shown to decrease itching, anxiety, depression, and pain. Massage is said to cause mechanical disruption of fibrotic tissues thereby increasing the softness in the scar. The expression of extracellular matrix proteins and proteases may be altered by mechanical forces. Lower levels of urinary cortisol while higher levels of serotonin and dopamine after massage support its role in decreasing anxiety and improving mood. Pain alleviation may be due to release of endogenous opioid peptides and neurotransmitters.

The scars are massaged manually twice a day with lubricants such as coconut oil or one of the various proprietary moisturizers and oils which should be nonirritating and free of any sensitizers. These are applied lightly and rubbed in gently on a clean skin after a thorough bath. Massage should initially be done with care to avoid damage to superficial layers of skin (neoepidermis/scar epithelium) by friction leading to formation of blisters/ulcerations. This is due to the absence of desmosomes between neoepithelium and underlying tissues. Gradually as the scar epithelium "toughens", enough pressure should by applied so that blanching occurs. Obviously, massage cannot be done in the presence of infection and ulceration or allergy to any component of the lubricant. Heavy lubrication is avoided as their build-up on the skin blocks the pores and causes development of furuncles. The massage is continued till the maturation of scar. This prolonged time period also means that the role of reconstructive burn surgeon/therapist is only to guide as to what and how it is to be done and review from time to time with respect to improvement or any complication, while the massage itself is done by patient and/or attendants at home.

Once all the areas which were being massaged have matured, lubrication of some larger areas may still be needed at least once daily with some oil or cream for whole life. This is because all the grafted areas and most of the healed deep dermal areas are without any sweat and sebaceous glands and hair follicles and tend to become dry, pruritic, and crack with risk of infection.

Pressure Garments[23-26]

Deep dermal burns and donor sites of intermediate and thick split-skin grafts frequently develop hypertrophic scars due to uncontrolled synthesis and deposition of collagen. They remain confined to the affected area and do not encroach upon normal skin. Although the exact cause is still being elucidated, overproduction of TGF-β has been blamed to cause excessive deposition of scar tissue and fibrosis. Levels of cytokines such as interleukin 6 (IL-6), IL-13, and IL-15 may be abnormal and play a role. The hypertrophic scars definitely need prevention/treatment. Pressure garments, made from elasticized fabric, are very commonly used to reduce the mass of immature hypertrophic scars **(Figs. 16 to 18)**. The effectiveness of these garments decreases after the development of mature hypertrophic scars. Pressure garments are also prescribed after treatment of contractures with skin grafts to support the graft till its venous drainage is well established. Otherwise, hemorrhages may occur underneath with resultant loss of graft especially in lower limbs. They also prevent hypertrophy at junctions of two graft pieces and between graft and surrounding skin.

Ambroise Paré, a 16th century French barber surgeon, described pressure therapy for scarring. Almost six decades back, Larson, from Shriners Hospitals was the first to introduce the custom-made modern elasticated pressure garment, as we know it today. Since then, it has been popularized all over the world and its mechanisms of action studied. A reduction in fibroblast content, total chondroitin-4-sulfate and cohesiveness of collagen fibers have been noted. A reduction in intralesional mast cells and their histamine production and release has also been demonstrated. Pressure therapy diminishes the number of myofibroblasts, erythema, thickness, and firmness of hypertrophic scar and accelerates its maturation.

The exact mechanism(s) whereby the pressure therapy works, is still not known. In present scenario, it is very difficult to conduct any controlled trial on them because the patients themselves have an expectation of being prescribed a pressure garment which may be a barrier to join the trial. However, the various explanations

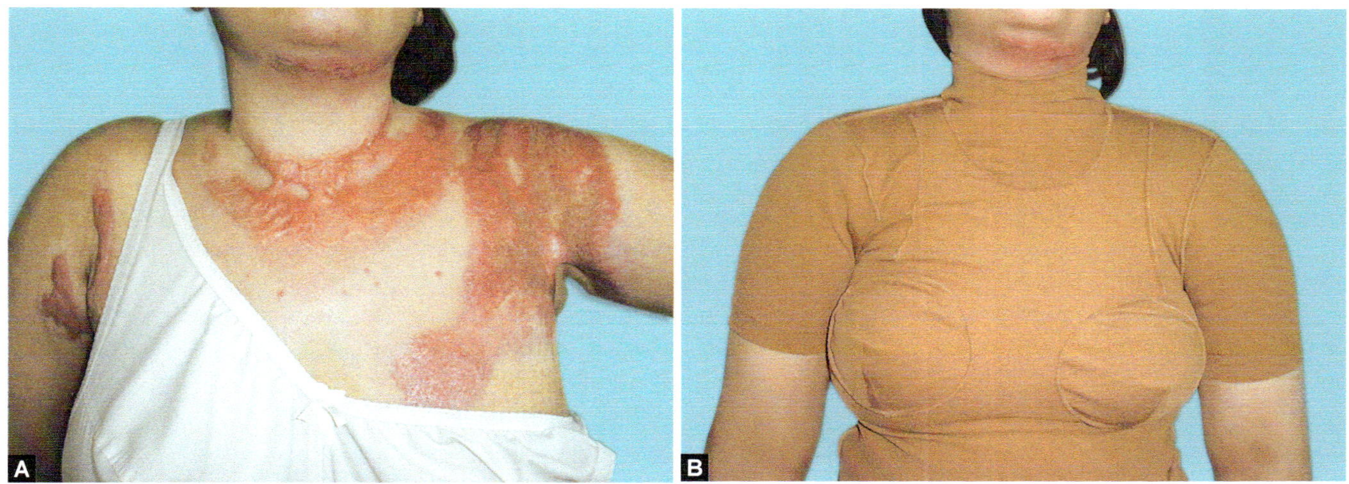

FIGS. 16A AND B: (A) Postburn hypertrophic scar in healed deep dermal burns. (B) Pressure garment.

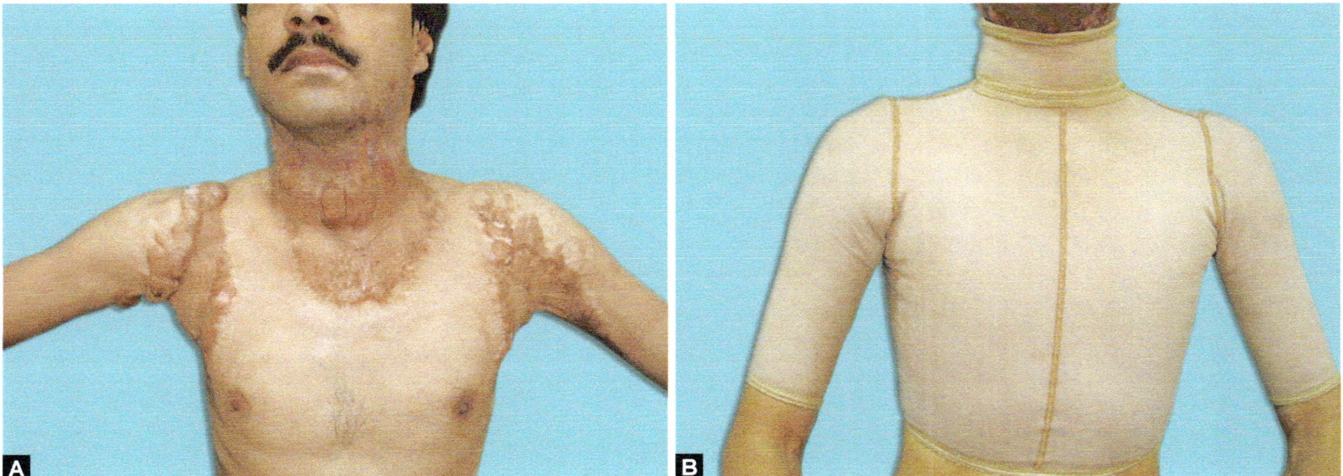

FIGS. 17A AND B: (A) Postburn hypertrophic scar in healed burns. (B) Pressure garment.

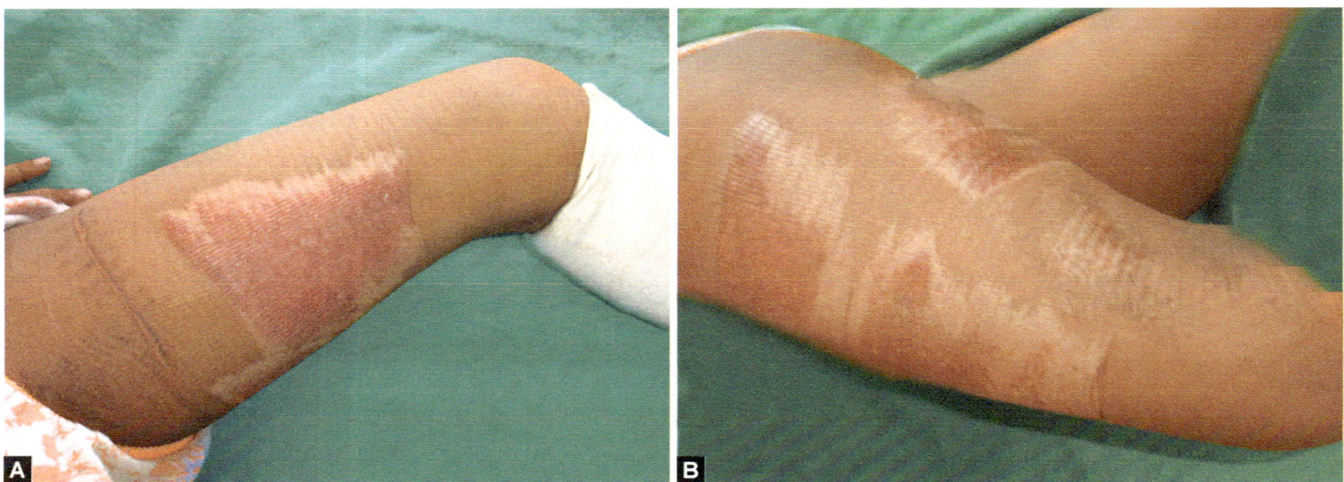

FIGS. 18A AND B: Hypertrophic split skin graft donor site being treated with pressure garment. Note the markings of the garment cloth on the skin on turning down the pressure garment.

put forward for these changes are (1) hypoxia of the scar tissue by occlusion of the microvasculature, (2) increased collagenase mediated collagen breakdown due to pressure induced decrease in capillary blood flow, (3) reduction in tissue edema with less ground substance due to compression, (4) neutralization of local venous hypertension by preventing leakage of plasma proteins and improving tissue oxygenation (5) elevation in skin temperature by 1–3° by blockage of heat loss from the cutaneous surface, etc. With pressure therapy, collagen nodules present in the hypertrophic scar tissue disappear and the collagen bundles become aligned parallel to the skin. The ideal pressure required is not clear but it must be from 24 to 30 mm Hg for capillary pressure to be countered. While significantly lower pressures may not work, a pressure above 40 mm Hg may not be tolerated with appearance of paresthesia and maceration.

Before prescribing commercial pressure garments, the newly healed skin must be preconditioned to accept the stress and pressure exerted by the garments as otherwise scar breakdown may occur. For this, initially gentle pressure is applied with crepe bandages. As the skin "toughens", the commercial pressure garments "tailor made" to the individual patient measurements may be prescribed. They have to be worn for almost 24 hours a day (except during bath, massage, and exercises) for a period of at least 9–12 months to be of benefit. Two sets of pressure garments are made available to the patient for washing of one set when the other is being worn by the patient. In addition, it must be remembered that they tend to lose their elasticity over a period of 2.5–3 months or more and hence, a new set must be ready before they become ineffective and need to be disposed of.

In the hot and humid conditions of our country, it is difficult to wear them continuously. Some patients simply find them unattractive when going to school/office or other social gatherings. Many patients simply cannot bear the high cost of good quality garments. Hence, compliance is a great problem not only in children but also in adults. These garments have also been said to delay growth of face and other skeleton in children. In some areas of the body, e.g., presternal region, axilla, clavicle or over the spine, etc., a pressure garment may not be able to deliver desired pressure and flexible conformers have to be used under them to get the effect. In order to get the benefits of both, silicone-lined pressure garments are also available.

Splintage and Exercises

Ebers papyrus, an Egyptian textbook on medicine (1500 BC), mentions the use of splints made of copper to treat burn patients. Today, they are an integral part of burn patient management from the day of burn till the day when no further improvement is anticipated and burn surgeons' treatment stops. They have been used prophylactically to prevent deformities, therapeutically to treat/improve mild/moderate deformities and as part of split skin graft immobilization and prevention of secondary graft contraction **(Figs. 4 and 19)**. They are also used to prevent damage to critical structures from injury, e.g., neurovascular bundles and exposed vessels. The scar collagen and elastin are relatively uncross-linked and malleable during their initial deposition. Gentle, passive, and sustained stretching using various dynamic and static splints exploits this malleability and is an effective technique for the lengthening of bands of scar tissue and

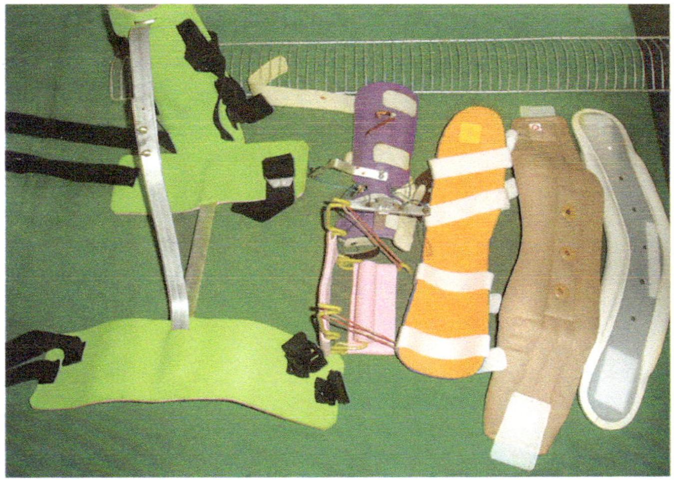

FIG. 19: Various splints used for postburn patients.

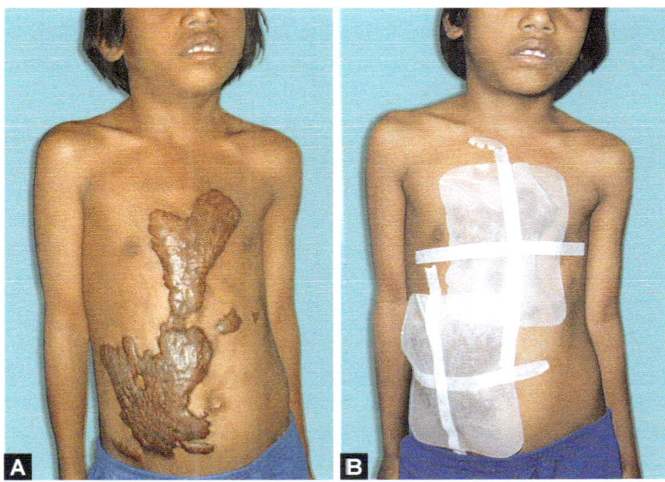

FIGS. 20A AND B: (A) Postburn hypertrophic scars over anterior trunk; (B) Application of silicone gel sheet.

increasing the range of motion. Combination of paraffin wax bath (as a form of heat therapy) application with positions of sustained stretch using serial splintage is highly effective. It increases blood flow, relaxes muscles, and decreases joint stiffness. When several joints are involved, the contractile nature of the scar must be remembered and body positions devised that provide stretch along the length and breadth of the area involved. Thus, in patients with scars involving both of the upper limbs, axillae, anterior chest, and neck, a pillow is placed under the shoulder and upper limbs are kept in maximum abduction. The paraffin is applied to the patient in this position and left in place for 20–30 minutes of sustained stretch. It is to be noted that, in general, patients who heal in <3 weeks do not require any splintage as they are unlikely to develop contractures.

Silicones

Silicones have been used in various forms for prevention and treatment of hypertrophic scars and have been available for four decades **(Figs. 20A and B)**. These are synthetic polymers based on dimethylsiloxane monomer with polydimethylsiloxane (PDMS) being the most common in use.[27,28] Silicone gels having lightly cross-linked chains of PDMS are available as sheets with nylon mesh backing, the latter to take care of its fragility, increase durability and life and ease of handling. They have to be kept in contact with scarred area for almost 24 hours a day for 6 months or more. Particular care must be taken of local hygiene of the area as well as the cleaning of the silicone sheet to avoid the development of contact dermatitis and folliculitis due to accumulation of sweat and dead exfoliating cells. This also means that there should not be any wound under the silicone sheet. The biggest drawback of silicone gel sheets is the practical difficulty in keeping the sheet in contact with the scar all the day and night, especially in areas with high range of movements (e.g., joints). Their application on exposed areas of the body such as face and hands is unsightly/impractical. To overcome this problem, silicone-lined pressure garments were made available to get the benefit of both forms of therapy. It was also found that the benefit of these garments is more than either therapy alone. The silicone reduces the erythema and makes the scar soft and supple while pressure garment decreases the thickness of hypertrophic scar. Another alternative was found in the silicone being developed and made available as gels, creams, and ointments containing short, straight, and unbound chains of PDMS. These are being increasingly promoted as they are simple to use, do not need any tapes to hold them, and are not unsightly and maintaining hygiene is easy. A very thin film is applied over the hypertrophic scar and allowed to dry over 4–5 minutes. On drying, it forms a thin, impervious and almost invisible film. A number of pharmaceutical companies have made both, sheets as well as gel, available in the Indian market. A real practical difficulty in their use in burn patients is when the scarred areas are extensive say, following a 40% TBSA injury. The cost is highly prohibitive by any standards apart from difficulty in keeping sheets in contact. Hence, they are generally prescribed for smaller scars.

Although the silicone therapy has not been considered as "gold standard", it is definitely noninvasive, preventive as well as therapeutic and evidence-based. Its exact mechanism of action is not known. Instead, what is more known is that it does not exert its actions by exerting pressure, lowered oxygen tension, and diffusion of silicone into the scar (as biopsies do not show any foreign body reaction).

Silicone is said to exert its effects by increasing the temperature of the scar, thereby enhancing the activity of collagenase, which is known to increase several folds over 1–1.5°C increase of body temperature. Hydration of the stratum corneum has been shown to increase because of formation of an impervious layer occluding the evaporation of water. This has been considered to be the primary mechanism of its action because even nonsilicone containing products, with appropriate extent of water impermeable properties, have given equally good results.

Intralesional Steroids[25,26,29]

Intralesional injections of triamcinolone acetonide have been in use for over 60 years and found to be effective for control of hypertrophic scars and keloids. Triamcinolone, a synthetic glucocorticoid, is a very powerful steroid that exerts strong anti-inflammatory activity. The regression in size occurs due to a decrease in collagen and glycosaminoglycan synthesis, reduction in inflammation in scar, decreasing fibroblast proliferation, and increasing hypoxia. Reduction in plasma protease inhibitors allows collagenase to degrade collagen. Triamcinolone has also been shown to inhibit expression of TGF-β1 and induce apoptosis in fibroblasts.

It can be used in early stages of hypertrophic scar formation when the scar is comparatively soft and easy to inject. It can also be used in mature scars but because of their hardness, it may be very difficult to inject especially in first couple of sittings. On being injected into a hypertrophic scar, it activates the endogenous collagenase to degrade the mature collagen to more soluble forms. Unfortunately, the total dose and volume injected at any one time are limited and adequate for a very small lesion only. Not >80–120 mg is injected in adults in one sitting in a concentration of 10–40 mg/mL every 4–6 weeks. The available vial of 40 mg/mL. can be diluted with 3 mL of 2% lignocaine to decrease the pain of injection. It is preferable to use a Luer-Lock syringe as otherwise the needle tends to get detached from syringe, spilling all the drug. The therapy is generally continued for 6–8 months or less when the desired result has been obtained. With continuation of therapy, there is softening, flattening, decreased redness, and improved appearance of the scar apart from the relief from pruritus.

While the effectiveness of intralesional steroids for hypertrophic scars cannot be questioned, they are of very limited use in burn patients because the extent of scars is too much. The main complication of atrophy, sometimes leading to necrosis and ulceration, is due to overdosage and spillage into normal skin or subcutaneous tissues. Telangiectasia and hypo- or hyperpigmentation can also occur. Although the systemic absorption is minimal, hirsutism can be an annoying problem in young females and hence this therapy is better avoided or used minimally and cautiously. Very rarely Cushingoid features may be seen. They are better avoided in growing children, diabetics, and tuberculosis patients. Because of multiple injections, it is scary to many patients.

Although intralesional steroids are highly effective of their own, they have been combined with pressure garments and silicones as all of them have different mechanisms of action. They have also been combined with other intralesional drugs [e.g., 5-fluorouracil (5-FU) and bleomycin] which have been found to have beneficial effects on these scars in last few decades. They are also used to prevent recurrence after surgical excision of lesion by injecting into a recently healed wound in patients who are at high risk.

Laser Therapy[30-32]

Castro et al. first described the use of neodymium-doped yttrium-aluminum-garnet (Nd:YAG) laser in 1983 for scar treatment and since then a number of other laser systems have been shown to be effective in the management of hypertrophic scars. The pulsed dye laser (PDL) has shown good results over the last more than two decades. It is a safe and efficacious modality in the prevention and treatment of postburn hypertrophic scars. They can be used even before burn surgery. PDL therapy (wavelength 585–595 nm) reduces erythema/inflammation based on the concept of selective photothermolysis. Thus, it is selectively absorbed by oxyhemoglobin and gets converted into thermal energy causing coagulative necrosis and microvascular damage with thrombosis of vessels. There is flattening of the hypertrophic scar and an increase in its pliability. Pliability refers to elastic texture of the scar surface on touch by the clinician. A reduction in pruritus is also seen which may be due to diminished mast cell count, decreased substance P and calcitonin gene-related peptide which is said to mediate the vascular response of the skin. The vascular patterns of the normal skin and hypertrophic scars are different in that the latter have larger number of dilated vessels in both layers of dermis, papillary as well as reticular. An interval of 5–6 weeks between two sessions gives better results. However, it is more prone to cause complications in dark-skinned individuals. Also, as its effects are not dose-related, higher doses are likely to cause irritation rather than remission. Common side effects of this therapy are blisters, hypo- or hyperpigmentation and purpura (usually lasting for 7–10 days), especially in darker patients. As the depth of penetration of PDL is limited (<2 mm), it is often combined with other modalities to get optimum results. Thus, better results can be obtained with initiation of therapy early when the hypertrophic scars are thin. Most patients show improvement by 50% or more after two sessions of laser therapy. Up to six sessions may be required to get desired and sustained results. PDL reduces the expression of TGF-β, proliferation of fibroblasts, an increase in collagenase-3 (MMP-13) activity, and decreased deposition of type III collagen. The collagen metabolism may also be affected by release of histamine and interleukins from mast cells. The disulfide bonds break due to heating of collagen fibers and their realignment and remodeling takes place.

Ablative lasers such as Nd:YAG (wavelength 1,064 nm) cause deepest photothermal effect (5–6 mm), leading to a decrease in collagen production, erythema, and the scar. However, its absorption by hemoglobin and ultimately its efficacy, is lesser as compared to PDL. They also have a very high recurrence rate.

A number of different lasers have been developed, e.g., fractional ablative CO_2 laser and are at the disposal of a clinician dealing in laser treatment of various problems. A burn surgeon may have to refer these patients to a laser expert for opinion and treatment for the best outcome. Also, extensive areas of postburn scarring may not be treatable by this method. Unrealistic expectations of patients from a "fancy" name must be addressed beforehand. No form of treatment can guarantee "complete scar eradication".

Antipruritic Therapy[33,34]

Itching is an extremely common complaint of patients with healing and healed burn wounds and donor sites of split skin grafts especially at night. Weisshaar et al. (2003) wrote, "The definition of pruritus as an unpleasant sensation that provokes the desire to scratch was introduced in 1660 by the German physician Samuel Hafenreffer".[35] This definition has remained unchanged for the last >350 years. The biological purpose of pruritus (Latin for "itch") must have been to remove a pruritogen, a response likely to have originated when most pruritogens were parasites. Patient's scratching the area to get relief causes breakdown of recently formed neoepithelium with consequent ulceration, the healing of which again causes itching, thus forming a vicious cycle. The ulceration(s) may become infected which prevent application of many of the measures for minimizing scar contraction and optimizing its maturation. Although the prevalence of pruritus decreases with maturation of scars, some patients may still complain of this problem after many years. Pruritus is a highly disturbing sensation and a "quality of life issue" affecting the daily life and emotional well-being reminding the traumatic event again and again. In some patients, this is perceived as pain although the mechanism for both is same.

The treatment of postburn pruritus is difficult and frustrating to the patient and the surgeon alike. A number of pharmacological and other measures have been advocated. It is an observation of many burn surgeons that wool and synthetic (e.g., nylon) clothes lead to more itching and hence their direct contact is forbidden. Cotton clothes are best. The dry skin is especially prone to itching and the spontaneously healed/grafted areas may be deficient in production of sweat and sebum due permanent loss or temporary functional failure of sweat and sebaceous glands and hair follicles in these areas. Keeping the skin well lubricated with moisturizers and oils (such as coconut oil) at least once a day is beneficial. This is because this softens and restores the barrier function of stratum corneum and the itch is relieved. A number of other modalities for scar maturation which are being used simultaneously, e.g., massage, pressure garments, intralesional steroids, silicone sheets, laser therapy, etc., are also effective in varying degrees in decreasing the patient's desire to scratch. Any single modality is unlikely to be sufficient in eradicating the itch and probably a judicial, multimodal approach may be able to provide the necessary relief in majority of patients. However, a simple single therapy should be started and then built up reasonably fast to prevent chronicity, till satisfactory relief is obtained.

Cooling of the itchy areas by bathing/showering has been shown to relieve itching. However, excessive bathing may lead to drying of skin. Similarly, application of topical medicaments such as menthol, which induces a feeling of cold can provide relief by reducing the sensation of itching.[36] Both cooling and menthol have been shown to activate A-delta afferents which in turn activate an ion channel, namely, transient receptor potential cation channel, inhibiting unmyelinated C-fibers carrying itch signals. Creams and lotions containing menthol, urea, and camphor are available for local application three to four times daily.

A number of other topical drugs have been used to relieve the symptom over a period of last several decades with varying success and side effects. Topical application of steroid containing creams, if at all used for local massaging, must be avoided over areas exposed to sunlight for fear of hyperpigmentation. Only very small areas should be treated lest its absorption leads to systemic side effects. Doxepin, a tricyclic antidepressant and potent histamine receptor blocking agent, has been used on postburn scars <20% TBSA with good effects.

Transcutaneous electrical nerve stimulation (TENS) had been introduced as a modality for pain treatment and pruritus is now considered as a form of pain only. It is noninvasive, nonpharmacological, and nonaddictive. It applies controlled low voltage, high intensity electrical impulses to the nervous system with transcutaneous electrodes placed on the itchy skin. This blocks the A-delta fibers carrying pruritus signals. Short duration (150 seconds) of TENS at a high frequency (180 Hz) yields nonpainful tingling sensations with no muscle contraction.[37]

The mainstay of systemic antipruritic therapy is still antihistamines over last several decades. They have been divided into two types, namely, (1) H-1 receptor antagonists or H-1 blockers and (2) H-2 receptor antagonists or H-2 blockers. While the former is used to treat pruritus, the latter is used to treat gastrointestinal diseases. The H-1 blocker can be first-generation and second-generation antihistamines. The first-generation antihistamines work on histamine receptor in the brain by crossing the blood–brain barrier and act centrally by their sedative actions. Drugs such as pheniramine, chlorpheniramine, hydroxyzine, diphenhydramine, and promethazine are commonly prescribed. Psychomotor impairment can persist throughout the next day following administration. The second-generation antihistamines do not cross the blood–brain barrier to the extent that first generation do and therefore do not cause drowsiness. Being nonsedating, they are more suitable for daytime relief. Examples are loratadine, fexofenadine, cetirizine, and levocetirizine, etc.

Gabapentin and its analog pregabalin have also been used to relieve the postburn itch in adult patients.[38] Last but not the least, psychological support by the treating burn surgeon and psychologists helps a lot in the amelioration of pruritus.

Miscellaneous Products

As is usual for any medical problem with less than desired outcomes to any form of therapy, everything under the sun gets proposed for its relief. Scars in general and hypertrophic scars in particular are no exception. As triamcinolone has undesirable side effects of a steroid, intralesional injection of 5-FU, bleomycin, verapamil, enalapril and interferon (INF), etc., have been introduced.[29] Even when effective, most of these drugs are not of much use in moderately and extensively burnt and scarred patients because of dose constraints and consequently the extent of area which can be injected.

Bleomycin and 5-FU are both antineoplastic agents in common use for several malignancies for a very long time. They have been used alone or in combination with triamcinolone in the hope of getting results better than if they had been used alone. They inhibit rapidly proliferating fibroblasts by blocking DNA synthesis and transcription. Use of bleomycin for intralesional injection does not cause systemic side effects and is quite safe. 5-FU is known to inhibit TGF-β signaling in collagen production. Each vial of bleomycin containing 15 mg (15U) of lyophilized powder is diluted with 10 mL of sterile 0.9% saline. A maximum of 4 mL is injected intralesionally, 0.2–0.4 mL/cm^2 at 4-week intervals. 5-FU is used in a concentration of 50 mg/mL and not >2 mL is injected every 2–4 weeks. Both 5-FU and bleomycin have also been used in combination with triamcinolone.

Intralesional injection of verapamil (2.5 mg/mL, not >1.5 mL every week for 4 weeks), a calcium channel antagonist, has been reported to be effective as the activity of fibroblasts is calcium related. It suppresses the intracellular calcium ion concentration by blocking its entrance from extracellular matrix to intracellular cytoplasm and thus decreases the hypertrophy. It reduces extracellular matrix production/secretion, induces fibroblast procollagenase synthesis, and inhibits IL-6, vascular endothelial growth factor (VEGF), TGF-β1, and cellular proliferation of fibroblasts.

Enalapril, an angiotensin-converting enzyme (ACE) inhibitor, is commonly used as antihypertensive and for treatment of congestive heart failure. It has been suggested that ACE-inhibitor is related to fibrous tissue formation and thus, may reduce scar mass.

Cryotherapy, or freezing of scar tissue, causes ischemic damage to microcirculation of scar tissue with consequent anoxia and cell destruction leading to its shrinkage.

Interferons, naturally occurring antifibrotic cytokines, cause a decrease in synthesis of collagen type I and III by fibroblasts and an increase in collagenase activity.[29] Classified as an antiviral, treatment with INF-alpha 2b (INF-α2b) slows induction of myofibroblast apoptosis, a decreased number and activity of fibrocytes and reduction in serum TGF-β concentration. Human recombinant IFN-α2b (1 × 10^6 units) injected subcutaneously daily for 7 days and then 2 × 10^6 units three times a week for 6 months has been shown to be useful. Although INF therapy is effective, it is highly expensive and not suitable for large postburn scars. Adverse effects include fever, chills, headache, arthralgias, fatigue, and confusion.

Commercial products containing 10% onion extract (extractum cepae), 50 units/g of sodium heparin and 1% allantoin for topical mild massage as gel are available for several decades and promoted for prevention and treatment of hypertrophic scars. Onion extract has been reported to have anti-inflammatory, antimicrobial, antioxidant, antiproliferative, and regenerative properties.

The primary component of onion extract is flavonoids (quercetin and kaempferol) which inhibit fibroblast proliferation and collagen production.

Despite great advances in burn wound healing and burn scar research, at fundamental and clinical levels in the last half a century, the treatment of fresh scars following a healed moderate and extensive burns, is still done by massage with bland oils, pressure garments, and surgical intervention. Silicones, intralesional steroids and other drugs, laser therapy, and various topical compounds cannot be used either because of dose limitations (size of area which can be treated) and/or tremendous costs involved.

Medical Makeup

Medical makeup can camouflage the postburn scars in exposed areas of the body in normal dress of the patient. It is different from ordinary cosmetic makeup because in medical makeup, the burn patient tries to look normal and attempts to save oneself from the "intrusive" eyes of the public. On the other hand, in cosmetic makeup a normal individual wants to look still more beautiful as per trends prevalent in a given society and wishes to be seen/noticed more. This medical make up can have a highly positive impact on the mental well-being of the burn patient and increase one's happiness tremendously. Despite using all the armamentarium of a plastic surgeon, a patient may ultimately be left with tell-tale evidences of burns. Burn scars are a permanent visible reminder of the unfortunate incident on a daily basis. The stigmata of burn scars are more than skin deep. The burn victim's mental anguish needs to be diminished by camouflage for successful "return to society". Over the years, burn surgeons have concentrated more on treatment of wounds, disfigurements, and deformities amenable to medical and surgical means only. Whole of face and neck and distal half of forearms and hands are the areas which cannot be concealed by any dress when the patient moves out in society for studies, a job or say, shopping, tourism etc. The camouflage therapy can be considered as a smooth step-down from burn surgeon's active intervention to the patient leading an independent life. It is inexpensive, reversible, and cheap. A change in hairstyle, use of an eyebrow pencil, lipstick, tinted glasses, use of simple cheap products like calamine lotion applied over whole of face/neck or henna over the dorsum of hand/forearm in various designs, etc., are some of the ways. Any product used should be hypoallergenic, noncomedogenic with high SPF apart from easy to apply and easy to wash. It should also preferably serve for the whole day after one application. A patient can find them useful as they do not require the services of a beautician and are possible on daily basis. Permanent tattoos made over scars by professionals also help a lot. Thus, makeup does not only conceal scars but actually may make a patient look more beautiful/presentable. Males can have their face clean shaven to disguise irregular hair pattern on beard/moustache areas, etc.

Surgical Management of Postburn Contractures

The surgical management of any postburn contracture involves the following steps given here.

Release of Contracture

At the outset, it must be remembered that as a rule rather than exception, contracture release opens up a larger area than expected by a novice burn surgeon. This is especially true if a small area surrounding the contracture needs to be excised as well. Hence, the raw area must be created first before committing to any particular reconstructive technique. Also, a contracture can be intrinsic or extrinsic, i.e., the skin of the area itself may be burnt and scarred leading to a tightness or the skin itself may be normal and there may be pull from the surrounding structures. These two considerations are to be kept in mind before marking/planning an incision and assessing the amount of skin cover required. Complete release of contracture should be done avoiding damage to any important underlying structure, e.g., arteries, nerves, tendons, etc. Although contraction occurs in all directions, the incision should begin across the point of maximum tension, i.e., where the contracture is maximally tight. This point is usually opposite the joint line. The incision is deepened all the way to the unscarred, healthy tissues. After the complete release of contracture, multiple darts are made at appropriate points along the periphery of the defect created to take into account the contracture along other directions. Fishtailing of the incision line at either end is inadequate and inferior to the multiple darts especially when the former is marked on the skin at the beginning of operation. Darts are "cut as you go" while the fishtails are predetermined. No attempt should ever be made at undermining the surrounding healthy/scarred skin and advancing it to decrease the defect. Incision line can be infiltrated with 1:200,000 adrenaline solution either alone or preferably mixed with lignocaine to get a concentration of 1% to have a relatively bloodless field. Maximum dose of adrenaline is 5 μg/kg body weight and that of lignocaine is 7 mg/kg body weight. The limb contractures, especially distal to arm/thigh, should be released under pneumatic tourniquet control, wherever possible. Bipolar cautery should be used to achieve accurate hemostasis during release incision. When a contracture is released under tourniquet, hemostasis is done once again after deflation of tourniquet. The raw area should now be covered with1:200,000 adrenaline solution soaks and skin graft/flap harvested.

Incision versus Excision

In general, a contracture should be released by incision rather than by excision. This is especially true for patients who have received adequate preoperative physical therapy and their scars have become soft and pliable. Incision alone decreases the requirement for skin cover. A marginal release incision is given all around to allow retraction of the scarred/heathy skin. This also increases the raw area and the required amount of skin graft or size of flap. When the scars are extensive, it is futile to excise a small amount, if whole of scar cannot be excised for fear of creating an extensive raw area. Excision may, however, be required in certain circumstances, e.g., (1) adjoining small depigmented or hypertrophic areas, excision of which will add to the final aesthetic result, (2) atrophic/unstable scars/chronic nonhealing ulcer(s) should be excised along with release of contracture to obtain healthy bed for split-skin graft "take", (3) scars may also be excised so as to apply the graft/flap in accordance with principles of aesthetic units. Partial excision of hypertrophic scars may sometimes be done, e.g., in a case of postburn contracture of neck, the scars may extend from chin, neck on to the chest, and even abdomen. Here, only neck scars are excised. When excision release is planned, the size of the defect created must be estimated beforehand, and availability of required donor site for skin graft/flap assessed.

Immediate versus Gradual Release

In general, a contracture should be released completely in one go. However, in severe long-standing contractures, there is considerable shortening of musculotendinous units and neurovascular structures. Hence, it may not be possible to achieve complete release. Their exposure may limit any further release and vessels may go into spasm or even rupture if forceful extension is attempted, especially in contractures of limbs. The tendons and neurovascular bundles may also get separated from the bed as bowstrings with exposure/rupture of subcutaneous fat globules. In all these cases, contracture is released as much as possible and the raw area created is dressed. Full correction is achieved gradually over a period of up to a couple of weeks using serial splintage with Crammer wires, skin/skeletal traction, or any other modern device. Once full/maximum correction is achieved, skin cover is provided **(Figs. 14A to D)**. If split skin graft is applied immediately, the size of the graft applied limits the further extension and/or else a halo of raw area appears around the graft on attempted serial splintage. The graft "take" on uneven raw area may also be less than satisfactory as compared to that on 10–14 days old granulating wound. In addition, any future attempt at release may not be possible because these structures will be lying just under the graft.

Provision of Skin Cover

After the complete release of a postburn contracture, the recreated defect is covered using skin grafts or a skin flap. Commonly, the raw areas resulting after release of postburn contractures are covered with split skin grafts. Skin grafts are the workhorse for postburn reconstruction, especially for very large defects. Flap covers are required/used in special situations only.

Skin Graft

When using split skin grafts, sheet grafts are to be preferred and no attempts should be made to expand the graft by meshing. However, making a few cuts in the form of "piecrusting" to permit drainage is allowed. As far as possible, one must try to feed in graft more than the size of the defect to take care of the postoperative, inevitable secondary contraction. The junction line of the sheets of skin grafts should preferably lie parallel to the axis of joint motion. Ordinarily, the skin grafts are applied immediately after complete release. Sometimes, delayed application after 5 days, once the granulations form, is done. The delayed approach is required when release of contracture results in exposure of fat which is a poor bed for graft "take". When the raw areas are oozing a lot or when the contracture is associated with infected area, delayed application gives a better result. When skin grafts have been used, rigid immobilization is done by one or more of the various techniques namely, "tie-over" dressings, plaster of Paris splints, crepe bandages, elastoplasts, etc., depending upon the site. Fibrin glue, an expensive product, has also been used and advocated for its advantages of reduced hemorrhage and consequently lesser incidence of hematoma/seroma and improved graft adherence. Skin staplers or cyanoacrylate adhesive can be used to fix the graft to bed. Negative pressure wound therapy has been used successfully for graft immobilization, especially on irregular surfaces.

Donor sites of split skin grafts have been managed in different ways by different workers. Any dressing over the site should prevent trauma to the regenerating neoepithelium and wound infection. Additionally, it should provide pain relief as these wounds are quite painful for a week or so after the harvest. The simplest, commonly used and cheap technique consists of immediate application of nonstick paraffin gauze followed by layers of gauze wrung out in adrenaline 1:200,000 solution and bandage. After the graft is stitched to the recipient wound and immobilized, the adrenaline-soaked gauze is replaced by multiple layers of absorbent gauze, Gamgee pads, and bandage. This dressing is not disturbed for a period of 10–14 days depending on the thickness of the graft harvested. The nonstick gauze is allowed to come off of its own lest there is a damage to recently formed neoepithelium. Thereafter, the dressing is repeated every 2–3 days till the donor site has healed. The biggest disadvantage of this technique is that it does not lessen pain. A number of newer dressing materials, e.g., hydrocolloids, alginates have been devised which not only relieve pain but are also said to enhance the rate of epithelialization. Any unexplained increase in local pain, fever, and foul smell/discharge emanating from the dressing calls for an early inspection of the wound and appropriate steps are taken with administration of topical antimicrobials and systemic antibiotics based on wound swab culture-sensitivity.

The biggest advantage of donor sites of skin grafts as compared to that of flaps is minimal morbidity especially if the latter itself requires closure by skin grafts.

- *Split skin graft versus FTSG*: In general, all contractures are treated with split-skin grafts of intermediate or thick variety. This allows the donor site to heal spontaneously. Moreover, extensively burnt patients with multiple contractures have paucity of donor sites because of split skin grafts having been used during management of acute burns as well. Full-thickness grafts, although better than the split skin grafts in most of the properties, have poorer chances of "take" and their donor sites, in turn, need split skin grafts. Their use is limited to very small defects resulting after release of contracture in aesthetically important areas, e.g., ectropion of the upper lip, lower eyelid, etc. Larger FTSG may be harvested after tissue expansion of a suitable unburnt area. Very rarely, a burn patient may be in need of aesthetic procedures like abdominoplasty where the excised tissue becomes the donor site for FTSG. This confers the dual benefit of a purely aesthetic procedure being combined with burn reconstruction.

  Dermal replacements, in the form of products such as Integra (a bioengineered dermal regeneration template), have been used to provide a thick layer of regenerated dermis which in turn is covered with thin split skin grafts after it gets vascularized in approximately 4 weeks. Apart from the need for two-stage procedure, unpredictability with respect to its vascularization, nonpigmentation of its surface and the highly prohibitive cost prevents its routine use.
- *Donor sites.* The split skin grafts are usually harvested from thighs. However, in a severely burnt patient, with extensive scarring, the burn surgeon may have limited or no choice and the grafts may have to be harvested from legs, upper limbs and abdomen, back, or even scalp. If possible, the donor area should match the recipient area with respect to color and texture and should be from an inconspicuous site as well. While grafts from the limbs can be harvested using Watson's skin grafting knife, electrical dermatome is needed for abdomen, back, and scalp. It should be noted that in every patient who presents with multiple postburn problems which need to be addressed surgically, one must look for the donor sites available. In a case with multiple, massive contractures, the donor sites should be checked and a plan charted out for "which donor site for which contracture". This is important as large sheets are usually required for neck, axilla and facial resurfacing, etc., while comparatively smaller pieces of grafts are adequate for contractures of fingers, eyelids, etc. Moreover, in burn patients, the donor sites are limited.

One must remember that both the defects as well as the donor site must be given equal importance with respect to final outcome, functional as well as aesthetic. Careful selection of the tissues and their donor site(s) must be done lest one problem is exchanged with another. If Peter must be robbed to pay Paul, Peter must have it. A burn patient is already having unacceptable scars and must not be given more by the surgeon, if possible.

Skin Flaps

There are a few situations where a skin flap is a must. If the contracture release is likely to open up the joint, especially of the dorsum of hands and feet, or tendon/nerve surgery is planned in the same stage or at a later date, e.g., old healed electrical burns, a flap cover must be provided after release of contracture. Irradiated areas also need flap cover. If release of contracture results in a moderate defect in a cosmetic area, which if covered with a flap will give a better aesthetic appearance, a flap cover may be provided. For example, an ectropion of the upper lip in an adult male can be released and covered with a flap from the scalp or upper neck to restore moustaches. In a female, the same ectropion requires a graft cover. A groin contracture, after release, may be treated using a tensor fascia lata flap transposed into the defect with graft on the flap donor site **(Figs. 21A and B)**. This decreases the need for postoperative splintage to prevent secondary graft contraction.

If a local flap in the form of Z-plasty, V-Y plasty or, V-M plasty, etc. (for linear/webbed contractures), will be sufficient in itself to treat the contracture, there is no reason why they should not be used alone **(Figs. 22A and B)**. However, these flaps are always in danger of necrosis when raised in scar tissues. Moreover, they are possible only in cases which fulfil the requirements for these local tissue adjustments. They are also useful when massive diffuse contractures are treated with split skin graft and later on, after graft maturation, contracting bands form at the junction of graft with surrounding skin. The flaps used for provision of cover may be local, regional or distant. They may be free or pedicled.

Local perforator-based flaps can be designed if sufficient normal skin is available. One big advantage of using a flap for treating a postburn contracture is that prolonged postoperative splintage is not required. However, in a practical clinical scenario with patients of extensive burns with multiple sequelae, the appropriate flap may not be available. Moreover, the healthy unscarred skin of the flap may stand out prominently in the midst of surrounding spontaneously healed, scarred, or skin grafted areas. Their donor sites may also need split skin grafts for closure. The grafts blend far better in such surroundings. In patients with smaller burns and limited needs for reconstructive surgery, an appropriate local, regional, or distant flap may be used to provide cover after release of contracture. It must be remembered that most of the contractures result because the postburn raw areas were not split skin grafted in acute stage. At that stage, nobody would have thought of putting skin flaps!

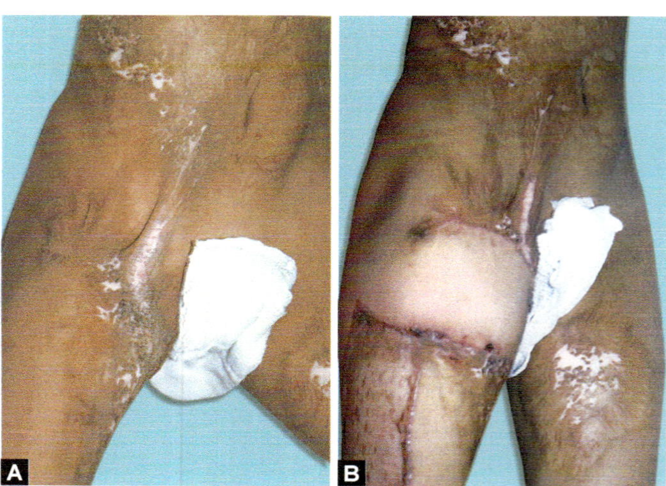

FIGS. 21A AND B: (A) Young adult female with contracture of right groin region with umbilicus pulled downward and laterally. (B) Release and cover with transposition of tensor fascia lata flap whose donor site was split skin grafted. Postoperatively the patient does not require any splintage.

Use of Prefabricated Flaps in Burn Reconstruction[39-41]

The term, prefabricated flaps was first used by Shen in early 1980s to describe a flap wherein a vascular pedicle is ligated at its distal end, isolated, mobilized, and buried under a preselected donor tissue for a period of 8 weeks. At the end of this period, this tissue starts receiving the blood supply from this new source and can be raised and transferred on it as a pedicled or free axial pattern island flap. These prefabricated flaps are especially useful in postburn reconstructions, especially head and neck region, where the desired flaps, available in nonburnt individuals, may not be available because of damage due to burns. Before selecting out of the probable sites available, color, texture, and other features similar the recipient site are compared so as to replace "like with like". The vascular pedicle can be either trans-

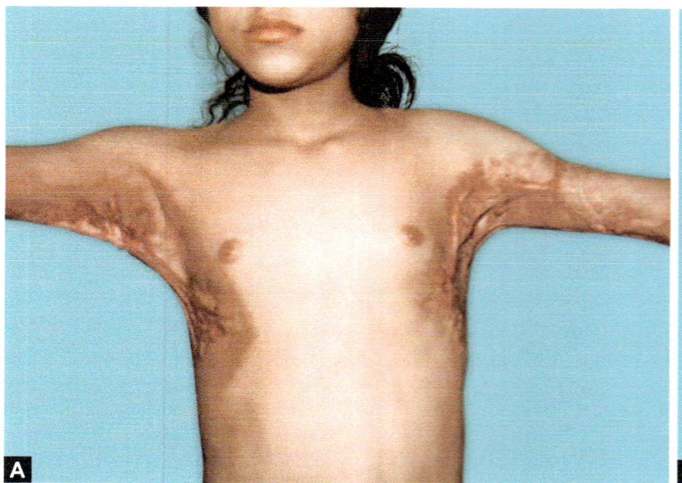

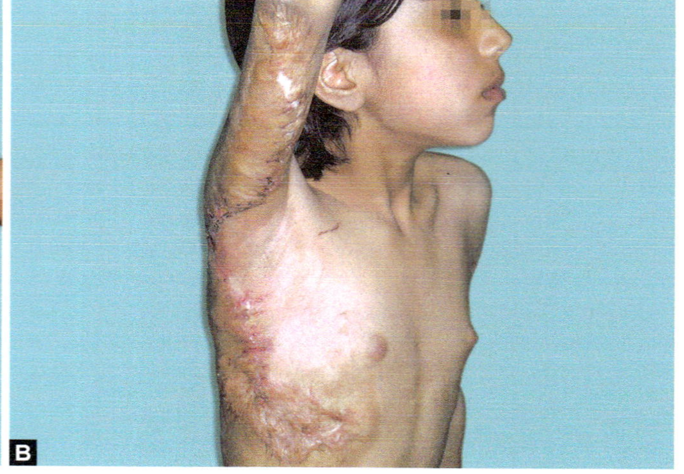

FIGS. 22A AND B: (A) Contracture of both axillae; (B) Right axilla treated by release—excision of scar contracture and multiple Z-plasty.

posed locally or by microvascular transfer as a free flap. A tissue expander can also be inserted deep to the mobilized vascular pedicle and benefit of larger tissues can be obtained. Sometimes, to avoid risk of congestion, a delay procedure is done before the flap is raised and used for reconstruction.

Use of Prelaminated Flaps in Burn Reconstruction

Flap prelamination was first described by Pribaz et al. 1994.[42] It consists of a reconstructive process in which a three-dimensional tissue mass is built at a remote site by laminating different layers of desired components as composite grafts into a reliable existing axial vascular bed. Once all the tissues start getting the blood supply based on a pedicle, the whole of reconstructed body part is transferred to the defect based on this pedicle. It is very useful in postburn nose and pinna reconstructions when all the contouring is done on the forearm after the skin, cartilage, etc., are layered and then transferred to head and neck region as a free radial artery forearm flap.

Microsurgical Reconstruction of Burn Patients

Free tissue transfer in the management of burns is not new. In the present-day scenario, the armamentarium of a burn surgeon has included microsurgical free tissue transfer for management of acute burns as well as reconstruction of postburn sequelae to achieve the best of outcomes.[43-45] In acute burns, they may be required for closure of wounds such as exposed neurovascular structures, exposed bone, joints, and tendons. In the reconstruction of postburn sequelae, they are usually required for complex tissue defects and aesthetic restorations. Nasal reconstruction which cannot be done from forehead flaps because of bad scarring were earlier treated by arm tubes in stages. This has now been replaced by free radial artery forearm flap. Similarly, it is almost impossible to reconstruct pinna if there is no healthy skin and subcutaneous tissue present for cartilage framework insertion. A prelaminated radial artery forearm free flap can again rescue the burn reconstructive surgeon. Out of all the contractures, postburn neck contracture is the one which has been most commonly resurfaced with free tissue transfer for aesthetic considerations even when split skin grafting was possible. It is also sometimes required if wide excision of Marjolin ulcer bares the neurovascular bundles especially in cubital or popliteal fossa and no locoregional flaps are available. In reconstruction of thumb and other digits in a badly destroyed hand, microsurgical transfer is required. Microsurgery is obviously required when composite allogeneic homotransplantation is considered, e.g., full face or hand transplantation. Flaps have also been preexpanded and then transferred as free flaps.

Tissue Expansion

The technique of tissue expansion is now available for almost half a century. In burns the tissues are completely lost while in tissue expansion there is generation of healthy tissues. Hence, the appeal of this concept. There is no donor defect and it can produce some specialized tissues such as hair bearing scalp. Additionally, the expanded skin has increased vascularity and thus a safer mobilization of flaps. It has been used to expand adjacent tissues or else distant tissues may be expanded and then transferred as free flaps. However, it is a two-staged surgical procedure with expansion being carried out for around 3 months when the patient has to visit the clinician at least twice a week. It is not without complications and has its own set of morbidity which may extend to complete failure.

Postoperative Care

Maintenance of released/corrected position is mandatory until the graft has become stable (usually 3 weeks) or till the flap margins have healed.

Postoperative use of static or dynamic splints, interspersed with a routine of daily physical therapeutic exercises is required to keep the joints in full range of motion (especially if static splintage is used). This therapy is continued till the grafts have matured (usually a period of 1–2 years or rarely more) and complete range of motion is achieved.

The grafted skin needs to be taken care of till its maturation which is aided by using massage with lubricants, use of pressure garments and silicone gel sheets, etc. Lubrication of the split skin grafts applied over large areas should be advised indefinitely because of absence of sebaceous and sweat glands and hair follicles in the grafted skin.

Examination of several physical characteristics of the graft is required to know its status of maturation. A mature skin graft is soft and supple, mobile over the bed, pinchable, and wrinkle free with a stable color. When a skin graft is applied to a raw area, it sticks to bed for its nourishment. With maturation, it becomes mobile over the bed. This can be checked clinically by pulling and pushing the graft tangentially in all directions over its bed. Pliability is mechanical property of firmness and extensibility of the graft and can be judged by pinching it between index finger and thumb and pulling it away from its bed. As decreased pliability can affect the range of motion of a joint, a nonpliable graft in front of a joint can diminish it. The junctional hypertrophy at surrounding skin and graft junction or between two pieces of grafts also becomes flat. Lastly, with diminution of hypervascularity and hyperpigmentation, the color of the graft stabilizes and becomes best since grafting procedure was carried out.

Planning of a Contracture Release and Provision of Skin Cover in a Clinical Case Scenario

From time-to-time, a number of classifications have been proposed by various workers with respect to contractures of some major and common areas, e.g., neck, axilla, and hand.[46-49] Some classifications have been given here for the sake of completion **(Boxes 2 to 4)**. However, they have a number of shortcomings and not really useful in patient's management or comparison of outcome of different studies or even in communicating/sharing a patient's problem with another colleague. The present senior author has not found them useful at all in treating his patients.

Most commonly, in day-to-day clinical practice, a contracture is labeled as mild, moderate, or severe. While it is obviously an oversimplification of the problem and subjective assessment only, it simply means what is the extent of functional loss and trouble to the patient in daily life. It also sometimes means how much difficult it is for the surgeon to correct the deformity and whether full recovery will be possible or not (prognosis). For contracture of the neck/microstomia, it may also mean how much intubation difficulty will be faced by the anesthesiologist. A mild contracture (ectropion) of lower eyelid causes epiphora while that of upper eyelid may endanger cornea (and vision). A mild tightness in popliteal fossa leads to an unstable scar-ulcer and even risk development of malignancy. On the other hand, a moderate flexion contracture of fingers or axilla may allow normal daily functions to be carried out and not even visible/noticeable to others. Moreover, it is difficult to quantify what constitutes mild, moderate, or severe for different areas and for different individuals.

No classification takes into account whether the patient can be managed by local adjustment of skin (as in Z-plasty, V-Y plasty, etc.), or a graft is required or requirement of a flap (locoregional/distant and pedicled/free) or a combination of reconstructive paraphernalia is absolute. A mild contracture may need skin graft while a moderate/severe contracture may be treatable by say, Z-plasty. If the surrounding area is scarred and/or transverse laxity is unavailable, raising any flaps may not be possible/desirable or else it may lead to their necrosis. A Z-plasty in axillary region can move the axillary dome/hair from its normal position or in case of angle of mouth, the oral mucosa may come out and facial skin may become intraoral. Similarly, even classifying on the basis whether the contracture is linear or diffuse does not always mean that the former can be treated by a local arrangement of skin, e.g., Z-plasty or similar other technique. While a mild contracture of neck/elbow may wait, any delay in dorsal contracture of hand may lead to severe permanent deformity. There may be associated

BOX 2 **Classification of burn scar contractures of neck.[46]**

- *Grade I*: Symptomatic; no limitations in range of motion; and no facial distortion
- *Grade II*: Symptomatic; may have mild limitations in neck extension and/or rotation; distortion of lower one-third of face may be noted on extension
- *Grade III*: Symptomatic; cannot extend head past neutral position; limited extension; and distortion of lower one-third of face
- *Grade IV*: Symptomatic; loss of cervicomental angle; severe facial distortion; and possible fusion of chin to anterior chest wall

BOX 3 **Classification of burn scar contractures of axilla.[48]**

- *Type 1A*: Injuries of the anterior axillary fold
- *Type 1B*: Injuries of posterior axillary fold
- *Type 2*: Injuries involving both anterior and posterior axillary folds (sparing the axillary dome)
- *Type 3*: Injuries involving both anterior and posterior axillary folds along with the axillary dome

BOX 4 **Classification of burn scar contractures of hand.[49]**

- *Grade I*: Symptomatic tightness but no limitation in range of motion, normal architecture
- *Grade II*: Mild decrease in range of motion without significant impact on activities of daily living, no distortion of normal architecture
- *Grade III*: Functional deficit noted, with early changes in normal architecture of hand
- *Grade IV*: Loss of hand function with significant distortion of normal architecture of the hand

Subset classification for grade III and grade IV contracture:

- *A*: Flexion contractures
- *B*: Extension contractures
- *C*: Combination of flexion and extension contractures

surrounding chronic nonhealing ulcers, hypopigmented areas, etc., which may also need to be taken care of during surgery for contracture. Some scarred areas may need excision to get better final appearance by bringing the junctional lines in accordance with aesthetic zones. How much time it will take to recover and what are the chances of recurrence are some other considerations?

The classifications also do not take into account whether the scars are mature or not. The status of the surrounding skin, healthy unburnt, or spontaneously healed deep dermal burn, is also not considered. They also do not take into consideration whether this is the only postburn sequela or part of a large number of problems. Whether usual/adequate donor sites for grafts or the best flap for that contracture (local/regional/distant) are available or not. Whether the release is likely to expose the neurovascular and/or musculotendinous units or even open up a joint or not. An arthrotomy always needs a flap cover for wound closure. Whether there is requirement of more than one operation.

Hence, the present authors look at the classifications with a pinch of salt. The above discussion actually enumerates the factors which a burn surgeon should take into account when planning operative treatment for contracture(s) in a given patient.

The detailed account of surgical technique for the correction of each and every individual postburn contracture/deformity and various local, regional, and distant flaps described in literature for providing cover is beyond the scope of this chapter. However, management of some of the commonly seen contractures, namely, ectropion of the upper and lower eyelids, microstomia, neck, axilla, elbow, wrist, breast, trunk, groin, perineum, knees, ankle, and toes are given below. Management of postburn scars and principles of contracture release given above, along with the specific discussion of a few contractures which follows, read together can be a guide to help manage any contracture in the body.

Ectropion of the Eyelids

It is the most important contracture which should not wait for scar maturation for its correction. In ectropion, the free margin of the eyelid is everted outside with palpebral conjunctiva becoming visible. There is damage to the skin and may be a minimum of involvement of orbicularis oculi during acute burn. Apart from an unaesthetic look, it leads to a number of functional problems like irritation of the conjunctiva, burning sensation, redness, dryness (due to exposure to air) of the eye, and epiphora (due to eyelid margin being away from globe), resulting in inadequate lubrication of the cornea leading to its desiccation, ulceration, and finally threatening the vision (exposure keratitis). As for any sequela of burn, prevention/minimization of the complications is very important. Unfortunately, in the case of ectropion of eyelids, of the several measures in acute stage, e.g., tarsorrhaphy which invariably leads to irreversible damage to lid margin due to stitches cutting through the inflamed tissues apart from not being effective, early grafting of raw area with poorer "take" of graft or operating on immature scar with greater risk of skin graft contraction, etc., none have been found to be effective. It is useful to take care of cornea using antibiotic eye drops and ointment, ocular lubrication with artificial tears (carboxymethyl cellulose 1%) four times daily, pad and bandages, etc. Since loss of vision due to thermal burns is extremely rare because of protective blink reflex, it will really be tragic, if vision is lost because of a potentially preventable cause. A good Bell's eye phenomenon is a patient's and surgeon's friend.

Both upper as well as lower eyelid ectropion can be intrinsic or extrinsic, meaning thereby that while the former can be due to upward pull by the forehead skin tightness, the latter may be getting pulled down by the contracture of the cheek/neck skin. The ectropion may be totally extrinsic or intrinsic or a combination of the two. In patients with completely extrinsic ectropion, the skin of eyelid itself is normal. Since it is the upper eyelid which covers and protects the cornea, it is obvious that it should be taken care of first.

For ectropion correction in immature contracture, it does not even need the patient being fit for general anesthesia. It can be very easily done under infiltration with a local anesthetic agent in adult patients. It should be remembered that eyelid burns are not isolated but part of larger facial burn injury. The local infiltration with adrenaline is required even if the operation is being done under general anesthesia as the tissues are very vascular. The amount of split skin graft required is very small and can be harvested under local anesthetic infiltration or even simple application of EMLA cream (a eutectic mixture of 2.5% lignocaine and 2.5% prilocaine applied as a thick layer over the donor area for 2 hours before harvesting). A point should be marked at the site of maximal deformity and a paramarginal skin incision is made 2–3 mm away from the eyelashes toward medial and lateral canthi. In severe, almost symmetrical contractures, the incision generally extends beyond the canthi (up to 5 mm.) and fish-tailing may open up a larger area for grafting. However, in milder cases, eccentrically placed toward one side or the other, a lesser incision may be sufficient. With the help of gentle traction on the stay sutures applied at the lid margin, the contracting bands are gently incised with a slight touch of No. 15 blade and the ectropion released and overcorrected. Once the area opens up, a gentle marginal release is done all around. An intermediate-thickness split skin graft is harvested and grafted with "tie-over" sutures. Overcorrection is very important as the postoperative graft and scar contraction cannot be prevented due to free margin of the eyelids. If both the eyelids have ectropion, both are released with overcorrection and then grafted **(Figs. 3 and 5)**. The conjunctival sac is washed with saline, an antibiotic ointment instilled into it and dressing done. When this operation is carried out in acute stage as is generally the case, re-ectropion although less severe is almost inevitable and has to be accepted. However, the cornea gets protected and the second definitive operation can be delayed.

In cases where the scar is mature at the time of operation, thick split skin graft can be applied after upper eyelid release and full-thickness graft can be used for lower eyelid to provide mobility/flexibility to upper and stability/rigidity to the latter. The FTSG is usually harvested from postauricular/medial arm region. One eye should be operated at a time as operating on both the eyes together leads to temporary blindness due to dressings for a period of a week or so. This is highly distressing and frightening to any person with otherwise normal vision. However, if there is vision in only one eye, both eyes can be treated together. It is traditionally believed that the ipsilateral upper and lower eyelids should not be treated in a single stage because of inability to achieve the required overcorrection in these cases. The senior author's experience of four decades is contrary to that. It is also possible to perform release and grafting on both upper eyelids simultaneously as even after tie over dressing, the patient can still see from the narrowed palpebral fissure. After 3 days of operation, any bandage applied over the tie-over sutures should be removed, medial canthus cleaned of all secretions with squeezed saline cotton swabs and fresh antibiotic ointment applied without any further bandage. Tie-over dressing can be removed completely after 6–7 days and graft dressed again.

A V-Y plasty can be done only for lower eyelids when the eyelid skin is soft and supple and correction required is only 5–6 mm.

A number of patients lose eyelashes also due to burn injury. Follicular unit hair transplantation offers a delicate and aesthetically pleasing outcome for them. The eyebrows can be used as the donor site.

Mentosternal or Flexion Contractures of the Neck

These are very common because the skin of the anterior neck is very loose and patients tend to use pillows under their head either unknowingly or even otherwise. These may become combined with ectropion of the lower lip and may be severe enough as to bring the vermilion border of lower lip and chin to the level of manubrium sterni. Very commonly they are diffuse and may extend to mid-lateral line on either side. They may involve skin of one half of the neck so that the neck is flexed to one side or else there may be linear band(s) as may occur after chemical burns. All severities of postburn neck contractures are seen from very mild cases with almost no disability to the severest ones who have microstomia, deformed mandible and poor occlusion, and kyphoscoliotic cervicothoracic spine in addition to being unable to see in front. Some mild and linear contractures of the neck can be managed by Z-plasty. Most cases are diffuse and need release (with or without excision) and skin cover. These patients pose the problem of endotracheal intubation to the anesthesiologist. In earlier times, blind nasal intubation was tried under ether and the success depended on the competence of the anesthetist and the luck of the patient. If it failed, the surgeon used to help his colleague by releasing the contracture under local anesthetic infiltration. The release was also sometimes attempted under ketamine especially in children and intubation attempted. Once the intubation was done, complete release was done and skin cover provided. With the availability of laryngeal mask airway (LMA), intubating laryngoscopes and fiberoptic intubating bronchoscopes and the technical knowhow, anesthetizing a severe postburn contracture has got comparatively easier and safe. The patient is positioned by placing a large positioner under the shoulder and a stack of two to three positioner rings under the head. The neck contracture is released at the point of maximum tension and the extra rings gradually removed from under the head so that finally the patient's neck becomes hyperextended at the time of skin cover. The severe mentosternal contractures may need release from one mid-lateral line to other. The strap muscles may also need division to gain better release and contours. Any unsightly scars or infected skin pockets are excised and complete hemostasis achieved. The severest mentosternal contractures may open up an extensive area.

For the last several decades, a controversy repeatedly comes up with the publications in literature and presentations in burn conferences as to the superiority of skin flaps and split skin grafts over one another for postburn neck contracture management. As has been said above, there is no absolute indication for skin flap application as the bed is excellently graftable. The reasons given for use of flap cover are—(1) it does not require postoperative splintage as it does not contract, (2) it is one stage, (3) it has better color/texture and hence better aesthetic result, (4) long-term follow-up is not required.

After going through the published literature and the photographs therein [without doubt the best results of the author(s) of those articles], the following facts become obvious to the present authors (the authors have intentionally omitted the references). (1) The main aim of the operation was excision of the postburn scar in the neck (which had a mild element of contracture) rather than a severe mentosternal contracture; (2) even when the contracture was very severe, no importance was given to the scars on the surrounding areas of lower face, chin, shoulders, and upper chest; (3) the healthy normal skin of the flap stood out conspicuously from the surrounding scarred skin like an island in the ocean. This appearance of the patient can be compared to that of a poor beggar wearing a highly expensive neck-tie! Consequently, the patient as a whole does not have a pleasing appearance; (4) the donor site morbidity of the flap itself was never taken into consideration; (5) any flap, even a relatively thin one, tends to conceal the details of the neck contours and gives the neck a "milk can" appearance. When free flaps are used, the circular suture line contracts and gives the flap a "biscuit" or "cookie" appearance obscuring the underlying contours further. When local pedicle flaps are used, they may become very thick even after many years when the patient gains weight spoiling the initial good result; (6) the flaps may be hairy depending on the donor site as well as the "hairiness" of the individual patient. While presence of hair is obviously undesirable in females, it is no good either even in males because of totally different appearance from the normal male in shaven as well as nonshaven state; (7) all flap operations, including free microvascular flaps, were only theoretically single-staged. Actually, they required two to four thinning procedures in addition, to get the desired contours, over a period of time requiring frequent patient visits. Some flaps were raised after tissue expansion. (8) Most of the articles are reports of a few patients; (9) secondary graft contraction in split skin grafts and the need for splintage, pressure garments, massage, etc., have been presented as something highly unmanageable. This is not true; (10) in the unfortunate event of a pedicled flap failing partially, use of a split skin graft to close the resultant wound leads to a very poor aesthetic result. Failure of a free flap will necessitate the use of large sheets of skin grafts which may not be now available.

The present senior author has exclusively and extensively used skin grafts for management of postburn mentosternal contractures over the last four decades in a center with an extensive workload of postburn sequelae and special interest in treating them and has achieved excellent results. Following are the reasons for using split-thickness skin grafts for diffuse neck contractures **(Figs. 4 and 23 to 28)**. (1) As a rule, it is a single-staged procedure, very rarely requiring a second stage to improve the result; (2) the graft fits better into the surrounding postburn scars and grafted raw areas without any sudden changes in color and texture, etc.; (3) there is minimal donor site morbidity; (4) far less operating time is required; (5) excellent contours with finer details can be achieved; (6) it is suitable for mild as well as the most severe cases; (7) microsurgical skills and operating microscope are not required; (8) in the unfortunate event of a partial graft loss, minor graft losses heal by conservative management whereas bigger areas, even if grafted again, do not spoil the aesthetics of the final result; (9) most patients have multiple contractures, scars, losses and other reconstructive needs out of which neck is the first major one to be addressed (next only to upper eyelid). Improvement after neck release tremendously improves the appearance of the patient and his/her confidence in the treating surgeon. Hence, there is no question of poor compliance or lengthy follow-up; (10) the contractures formed as a result of deeper forms of second degree deep dermal or full-thickness burns which were not treated by split skin grafting in acute initial stage. After release of contracture neck, a split skin graft only is required; and (11) last but not the least, a split skin graft only can take care of the 1.4 billion populations. Thus, while more and more articles with newly discovered/modified old flaps will continue to appear in journals, the massive load of burn victims will continue to be benefitted only by the skin graft. It must be made amply clear to the reader that the author is not "antiflap" and has no objection to treat the patient shown in **Figures 29A and B** using an appropriate flap as the scar contracture was limited, surrounding region normal, and overall other reconstructive needs nil.

The sheets of skin grafts are applied with their junction lines horizontally placed and immobilized using tie-over sutures. Postoperatively, after the graft is taken up, the patient is given simple neck collars and chin-neck pressure garments and other care as detailed above for grafts. Patient's compliance in postoperative care of the graft is surgeon dependent. Better the surgeon in his doctor-patient relationship, better is the result!

Postburn Microstomia

Microstomia, abnormal narrowing of oral aperture, due to perioral cicatricial contracture, causes severe morbidity to the burn victim with regard to feeding, orodental hygiene, drooling, speech, and cosmesis.[50] Removable dentures can also not be used. It may involve one or both angles of mouth or may be circumoral. The sphincteric action of orbicularis oris muscle and the free lip margins along with inability to prevent scar hypertrophy and

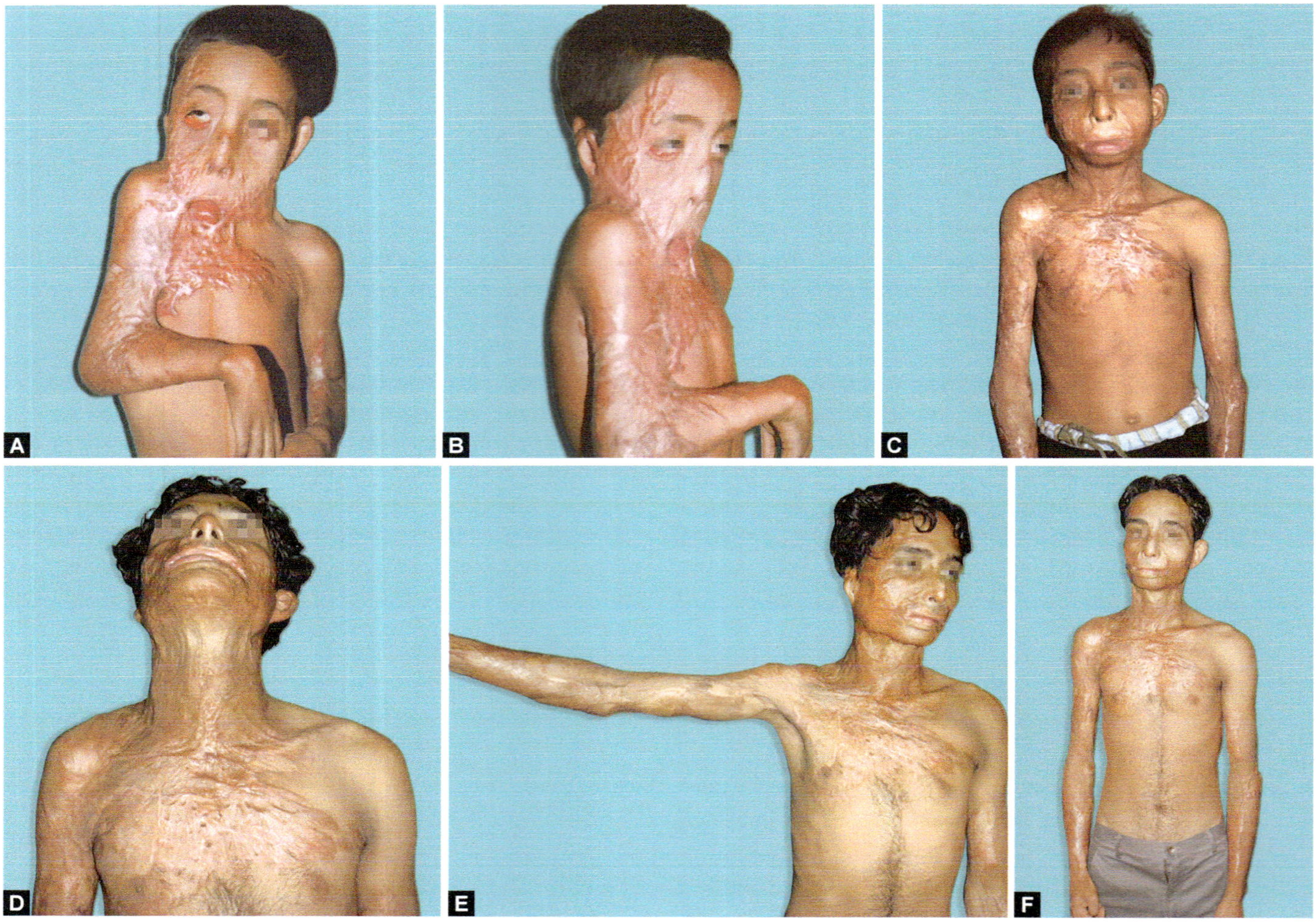

FIGS. 23A TO F: (A and B) A 7-year-old boy with severe contracture of neck, right axilla, and both elbows along with ectropion of lower lip with microstomia and extrinsic ectropion of lower eyelids. (C) A timely sequential release of all contractures. (D to F) Follow-up at 18 years of age.

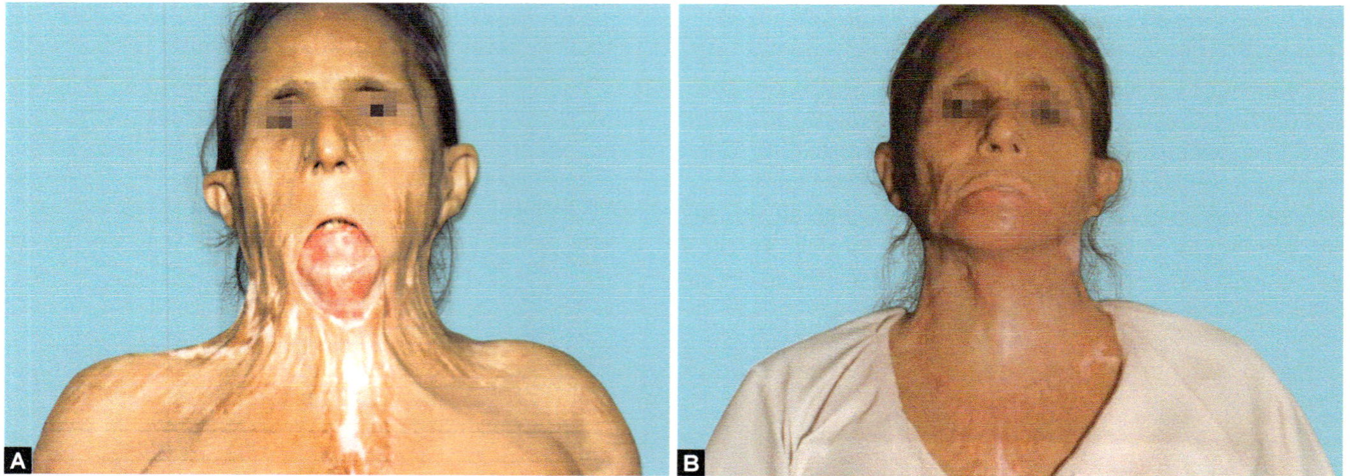

FIGS. 24A AND B: (A) A 50-year-old female with severe mentosternal contracture with completely everted lower lip. (B) Result after 1 year with adequate lip seal (pre- and postoperative view).

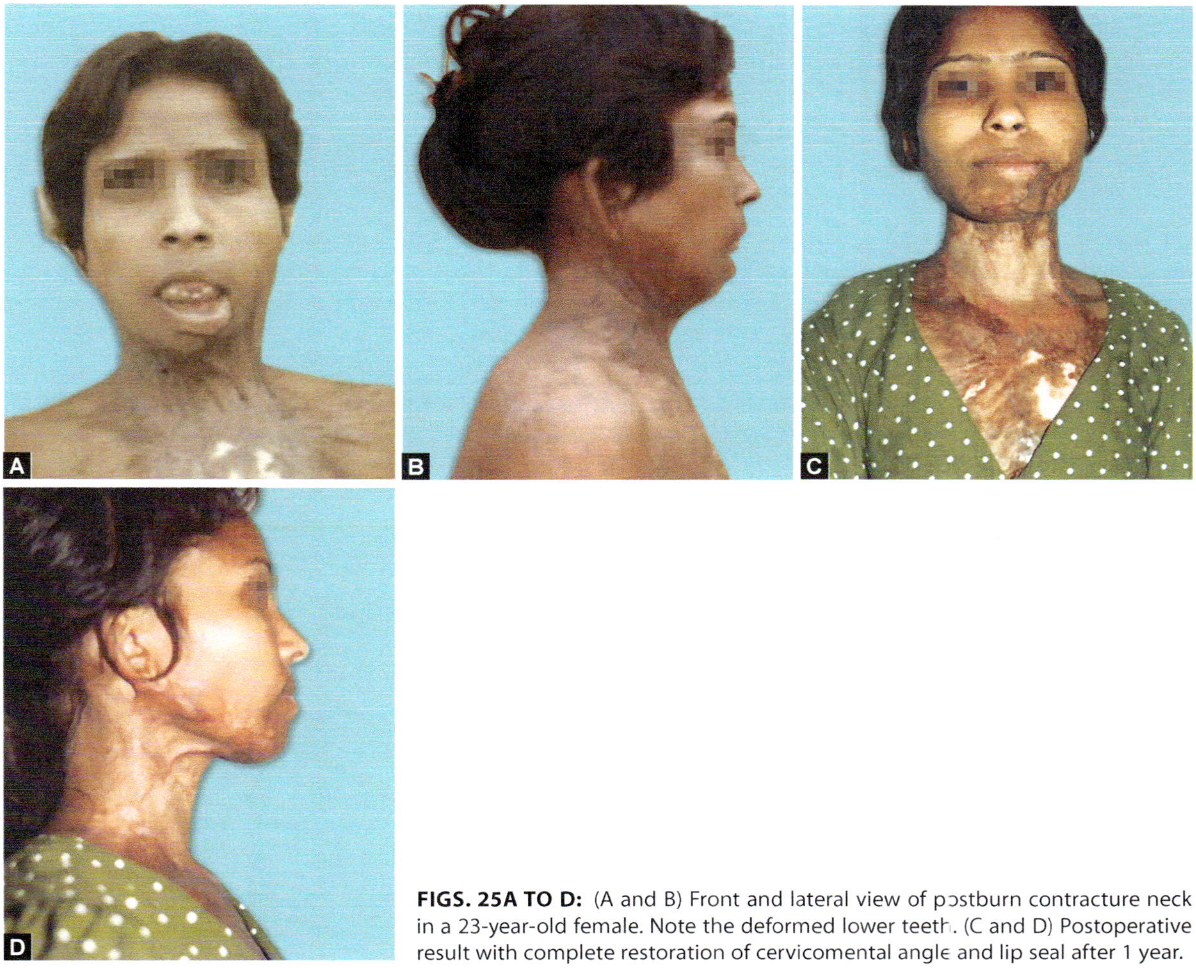

FIGS. 25A TO D: (A and B) Front and lateral view of postburn contracture neck in a 23-year-old female. Note the deformed lower teeth. (C and D) Postoperative result with complete restoration of cervicomental angle and lip seal after 1 year.

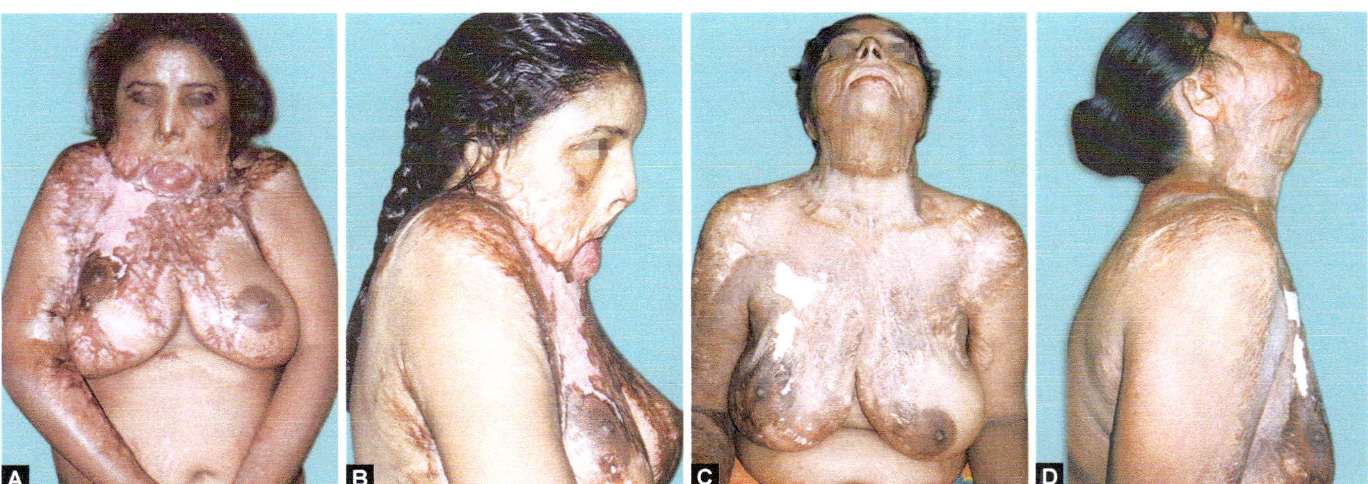

FIGS. 26A TO D: (A and B) A 25-year-old female with severe contracture of neck, right axilla, right elbow, and breasts. (C and D) 2 years after release and split skin grafting. Note the improvement in breast contours without any surgical intervention on breast.

contracting forces successfully are the reasons for many of the very severe cases seen following facial burns. The mean maximal mouth opening (inter-incisor distance) for Indian males and females was found to be 51.3 ± 8.3 and 44.3 ± 6.7 mm respectively.[51]

Postburn microstomia involves the upper lip superiorly, lower lip inferiorly, and angles of mouth and cheek skin laterally in various permutations and combinations. It may even involve the external naris and become a nightmare for the treating surgeon and the anesthesiologist because of intubation difficulty. It may continue to be an extubation difficulty at the end of operation as well because of bulky tie-over dressings which may still not allow easy access to oral and nasal passages with risk of inhalation of vomitus/blood and consequent choking, etc. In general, thermal burns involve only the skin with sparing of orbicularis oris and cheek mucosa. However, in electrical burns, especially in small children due the chewing of end of a "live" wire, it may involve full thickness of lips. In burns due to swallowing of a chemical, mucosal scarring may be more as compared to that of skin. The aim of microstomia correction is the ability to feed normally and provision of symmetry and aesthetics in mouth closed as well as mouth fully open. Additionally, the intervention makes the patient safe for any future requirement of general anesthesia or need for intubation for any other reason in whole of one's life. Anesthetists with experience

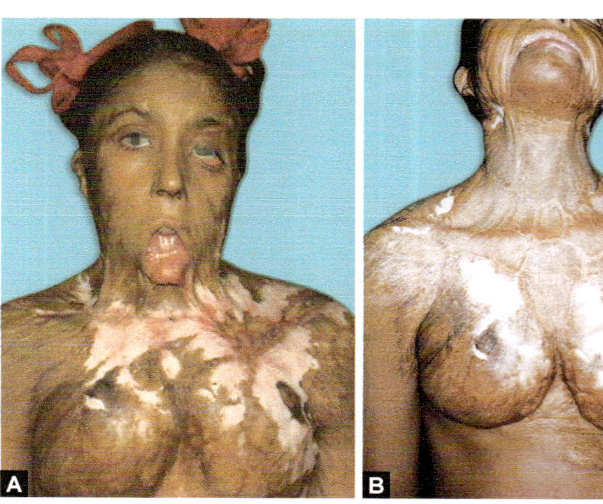

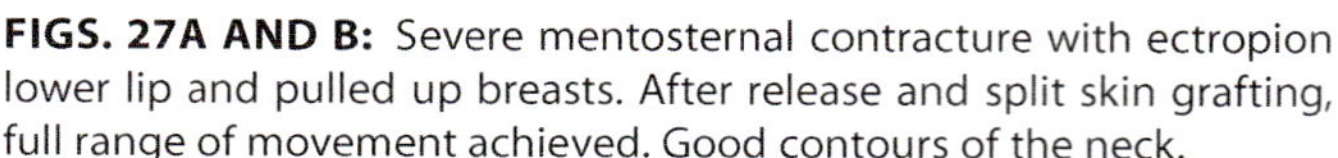

FIGS. 27A AND B: Severe mentosternal contracture with ectropion lower lip and pulled up breasts. After release and split skin grafting, full range of movement achieved. Good contours of the neck.

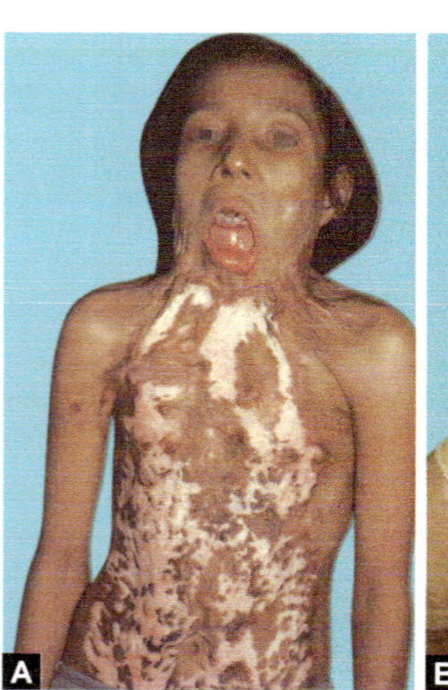

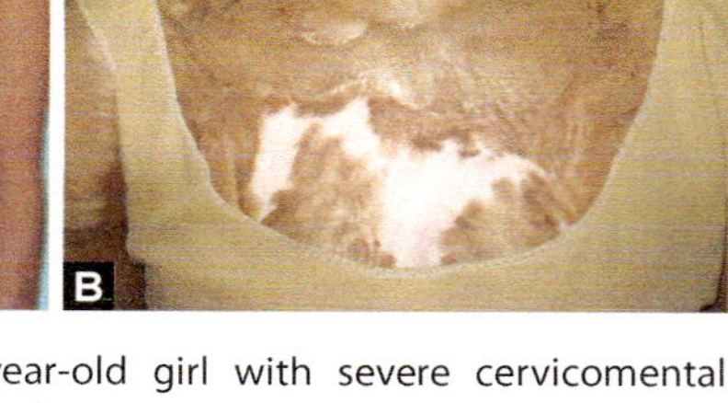

FIGS. 28A AND B: A 9-year-old girl with severe cervicomental contracture and depigmented scars on anterior trunk. Postoperative result after 8 years. Release of contracture and split skin grafting done.

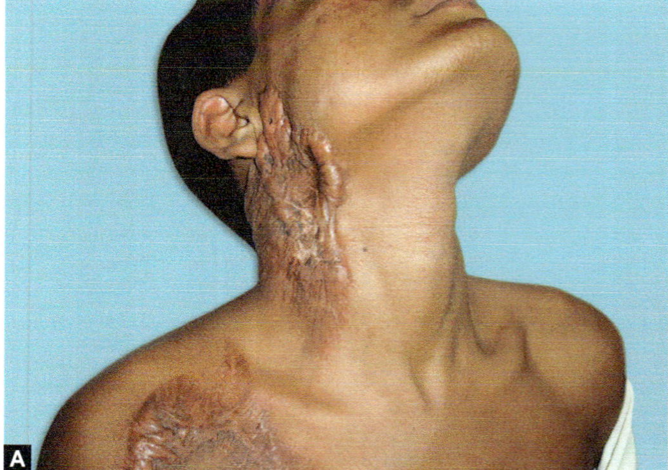

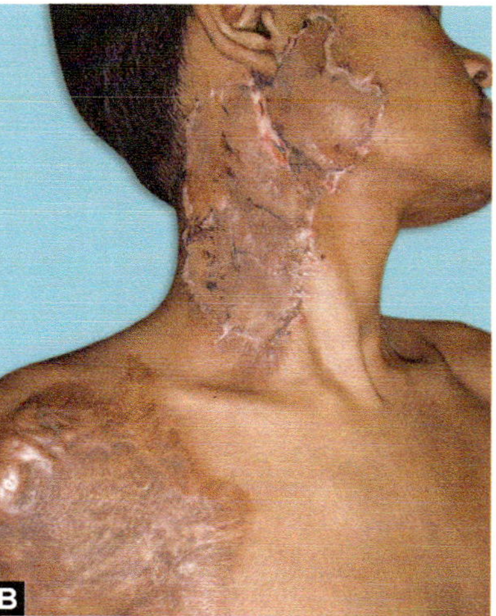

FIGS. 29A AND B: Hypertrophic scar lateral neck with mild contracture. Pre- and early postoperative result (see text).

of intubating such cases, (with intubating bronchoscope and other gadgets/facilities available with them), can only intubate these patients and are hard to be found.

In early milder cases with immature scars, splinting, exercises, and massage are started. In moderate and severe cases, surgical intervention is needed without waiting for scar maturation. The basic principles of contracture release demand that a transverse incision be made on one or both sides of angles of mouth till the normal stretchable, soft-supple mucosa is reached and complete mouth opening is achieved aided by a Denhardt mouth gag. A number of surgical methods are used either alone or in various combinations depending on the involvement of lip/cheek skin, orbicularis oris muscle and intraoral mucosa, or a full-thickness loss of all the three. In patients with minor restrictions in opening the mouth, a Z-plasty, V-Y plasty, etc., are designed in such a manner that neither the mucosa comes out abnormally nor the facial skin goes intraorally. Ectropion of the lips is also released one at a time and preferably lower lip in first stage if chin and neck are also involved. Scars are excised, if required. The skin release should take into account that the lateral limit of angle of mouth is up to a vertical line dropped from the pupil on either side. Iatrogenic macrostomia should be avoided. In burns of thermal origin, the release exposes healthy muscle fascia. At the end of release, the oral aperture all around should be soft and stretchable like in a normal individual. The whole of raw area is grafted with thick split skin graft preferably from medial arm, if unburnt.

Electrical burns of the oral commissure which have full-thickness loss of tissues, sometimes require local or distant flaps to reconstruct the loss.

Contractures of the Axilla

Contractures of the axilla (shoulder adduction contracture) commonly follow the burns of the upper trunk, shoulder and arm region. Similar to neck, the axillary skin is thin and loose and the patient tends to keep the arm adducted. Also, it is quite difficult to really keep the patient in aeroplane splints, especially if bilateral. This is not only because they tend to slip or even break but also because the patient becomes totally dependent on the attendants for even the most minor daily needs. This is not liked by the victim especially if the forearms and hands are at least partially functional.

A contracture of the axilla may involve only the anterior or posterior axillary folds or there may be a diffuse contracture involving both folds and the axillary apex, leading to a complete adhesion of the lateral chest wall with the medial arm skin **(Figs. 22, 23, and 26)**. Sometimes, the anterior and posterior folds are extensively involved but a part or whole of the normal hairy skin in the apex of the axilla is unburnt and healthy. In the latter case, there may be a very narrow access to apex so that even a finger cannot be introduced and the secretions from the sweat glands and hair follicles accumulate. In the absence of hygiene, there may be foul smell, infection, and discharge. Such patients may be advised to cleanse the area by flushing using the nozzle of a 10 mL syringe with soap solution, clear water and finally, may be povidone iodine solution. It should be done several times daily starting 3–4 days before surgery to avoid graft loss due to infection. A swab culture/sensitivity may be done and appropriate action taken. Additionally, while releasing the contracture in such cases, the incision has to be made in such a way that neither the normal skin of the apex of the axilla is divided nor its anatomical position altered. One has to be very careful in prepubertal children with no axillary hair to guide. During contracture release, assistant constantly abducts the arm synchronous with the surgeon. Once the contracture is released and the arm can be raised above the head fully (almost up to 170°), thick split skin graft is applied with "tie-over" sutures but the arm is splinted using an aeroplane splint abducted at an angle of 100–110° only lest brachial plexus may be stretched and damaged. This splint is continued till the graft is mature and there is no risk of graft contraction.

As a rule, most of the cases, especially severe type 3 with extensive healed surrounding burn scars/grafted areas, do require, and have to be managed with split skin grafts after release. The skin grafts are also required if some surrounding areas need excision because of atrophic/limited hypopigmented skin to achieve better final aesthetic outcome. The donor sites of local flaps which cannot be closed primarily because either they are too wide or scarred to be undermined and advanced, need skin grafts for their closure.

Other than the use of skin grafts, axillary contractures have been treated by any one or more of the vast armamentaria of a plastic surgeon.[52] In selected cases, scapular or para scapular flap and other fasciocutaneous flaps if available and sufficient, can be planned preoperatively to provide cover and may obviate the need for prolonged postoperative cumbersome splintage. Sometimes, patients present with linear axillary contractures with healthy skin on either side and a single or multiple Z-plasty or other multiple interdigitating flaps (e.g., V-M plasty and W-plasty) may be designed and contracture treated. Propeller flaps based on a subcutaneous pedicle in the center can be designed in patients with normal axillary apex and moved by 90°. Partial flap necrosis is the most common complication if the flap has been raised from healed burnt areas. Use of latissimus dorsi flap, tissue expanders (pre-expanded perforator flaps), and free flaps is certainly an overkill.

Flexion Contractures of the Elbow (Cubital Fossa), Wrist and Knee (Popliteal Fossa)

Flexion contractures of the elbow (cubital fossa), wrist and knee (popliteal fossa) are similar in many respects. In all these areas, a large number of major nerves, vessels, and musculotendinous units are concentrated under a soft thin skin without much subcutaneous fat and at high risk of injury. This risk is not as much by incision of knife but by stretch on any attempt at undue/careless force in an eagerness to achieve complete range of motion in one go. The vessels may go into spasm or even rupture. In addition, none of these structures can be sacrificed. As a rule, application of pneumatic tourniquet is possible in almost all these patients and local infiltration of adrenaline, as detailed above, is done. A severe contracture developed in any of these sites in early childhood and presenting for corrective surgery after many years in adulthood is very difficult to correct completely because the shortened musculotendinous units and neurovascular structures stand out as bow-strings and any further attempt to straighten them forcefully may injure and damage them or simply not possible **(Figs. 11 and 12)**. Moreover, the joint may be subluxated or deformed so as not to allow the limb to straighten fully despite complete release. A release incision is given opposite the point of maximum tension, usually opposite the joint line and maximal possible release is done just short of musculotendinous units/neurovascular structures getting separated from the bed. Hemostasis is achieved and the raw area is covered with nonstick tulle gauze followed by multiple layers of absorbent gauze, gamgee pads and bandage, and finally a crammer wire splint (two to three layers thick covered by cotton) or any sophisticated progressively adjustable device (made of thermoplast, etc.). The patients also need to be given narcotic analgesics (e.g., pentazocine) postoperatively for 2–3 days to take care of pain of stretching. It also helps in relaxation of skeletal muscles. Thereafter, it is replaced with one of nonsteroidal anti-inflammatory drugs (e.g., aceclofenac) plus paracetamol along with skeletal muscle relaxants (e.g., methocarbamol) in appropriate doses till required, usually a period of 7–10 days or less. The dressing is changed every 2–3 days and splint is gradually straightened over a period of 10–14 days. This helps in gradual lengthening of structures. By this time, the operative raw area gets covered with a layer of healthy granulation tissue which is split skin grafted. Since rigid postoperative splintage (to counter secondary graft contraction) is easier in a straight limb, an intermediate-thickness skin graft can suffice for excellent results **(Figs. 14A to D)**. By this two-staged technique, any damage to critical structures is avoided in addition to any need for lengthening procedures. The later will force the surgeon to use a flap for cover which may not be easily available in burn patients with multiple scars and other reconstructive needs.

In bilateral elbow/wrist contractures, both sides should not be operated together (except may be small children and completely incapacitated adults) to allow the patient some self-reliance in day-to-do activities. However, bilateral knee contractures should be operated simultaneously to make the patient ambulatory as soon as possible. Sometimes, a preoperative trial of straightening with Crammer wire or traction and counter-traction by hanging weights in lower limb may help in decreasing the deformity with better outcome at the time of contracture release operation.

For all other patients with contractures of these regions, a large number of options from the vast armamentarium of a plastic surgeon are available. Since all the contractures have a shortage of skin, split skin graft fulfils the need for provision of skin cover after release in most patients. Again, as for neck region, the grafts are ideally placed in such a way that the junction of two unexpanded sheet grafts are at right angles to the long axis of the limb to avoid contracting bands later. Some contractures may allow their correction using local arrangement by Z-plasty. Some workers, in an attempt to avoid need for postoperative splintage, make two parallel release incisions proximal and distal to the axis of elbow/knee joint leaving a strip of nonundermined mature scar/skin over the joint itself and apply split skin grafts proximal and distal to it in the arm/thigh and forearm/leg. Although it may diminish the need for splintage but the final appearance is unaesthetic and limb looks somewhat like Zebra stripes. In some cases, flaps from the lateral forearm/leg are transposed to lie across the joint axis and the donor defect split skin grafted. If an island of healthy skin is available, it might be possible to raise it as a propeller flap and the joint area covered with this tissue. A disadvantage of flap cover is that they stand out as a bulge surrounded by flattened healed scarred skin/split skin grafts.

Contractures of the Hand

Management of postburn hand deformities has been devoted a full chapter (No. 27) in this book and hence, not discussed here.

Contractures of Groin/External Genitalia and Perineum

Contractures of groin, when unilateral, may cause difficulty in normal standing/walking. When they are bilateral, the contracting band usually goes from one thigh across groin and pubis to the other groin and thigh (perineal contractures) leading to difficulty in abduction of hips with consequent problems in defecation, normal walking, and sexual activities **(Figs. 30A to C)**. They are more common in patients burnt in childhood. There may be disfigurement and pulling of external genitalia to one or the other direction, sometimes leading to their apparent concealment. Quite obviously, they have greater psychological effects as compared to contractures/scars, etc., in other body regions. The release incisions are to be planned in such a way that the umbilicus moves back to its normal position, the genitals are centralized, the pubic hair position is restored and full abduction of hip joints is possible. Some bilateral cases have webs running transversely in front and/or back of anal verge. In these patients, it may be difficult to clean the perineal region after defecation leading to infections, ulcerations, and increased hypertrophy. These scars may also extend onto thigh(s) and unstable scar-ulcers may also be present. These patients also come under the category where earlier intervention may be required before the scars have matured. Many of bilateral cases open up with extensive raw areas, in the shape of a butterfly, especially if umbilicus was also pulled down. If there are associated limited areas of hypopigmented scars and sufficient grafts are available, they should also be excised to have better final aesthetic result. In extensive cases, the areas need to be covered with split skin grafts These patients need a Foley catheter insertion and liquid diet for a week or so to prevent graft loss by contamination from urine and feces. In many such cases, a preoperative routine of 3–4 days of bowel cleaning and local hygiene prior to surgery may be of help. Some cases may be amenable to release in the form of a Z-plasty/W-plasty/V-Y plasty, etc. In patients

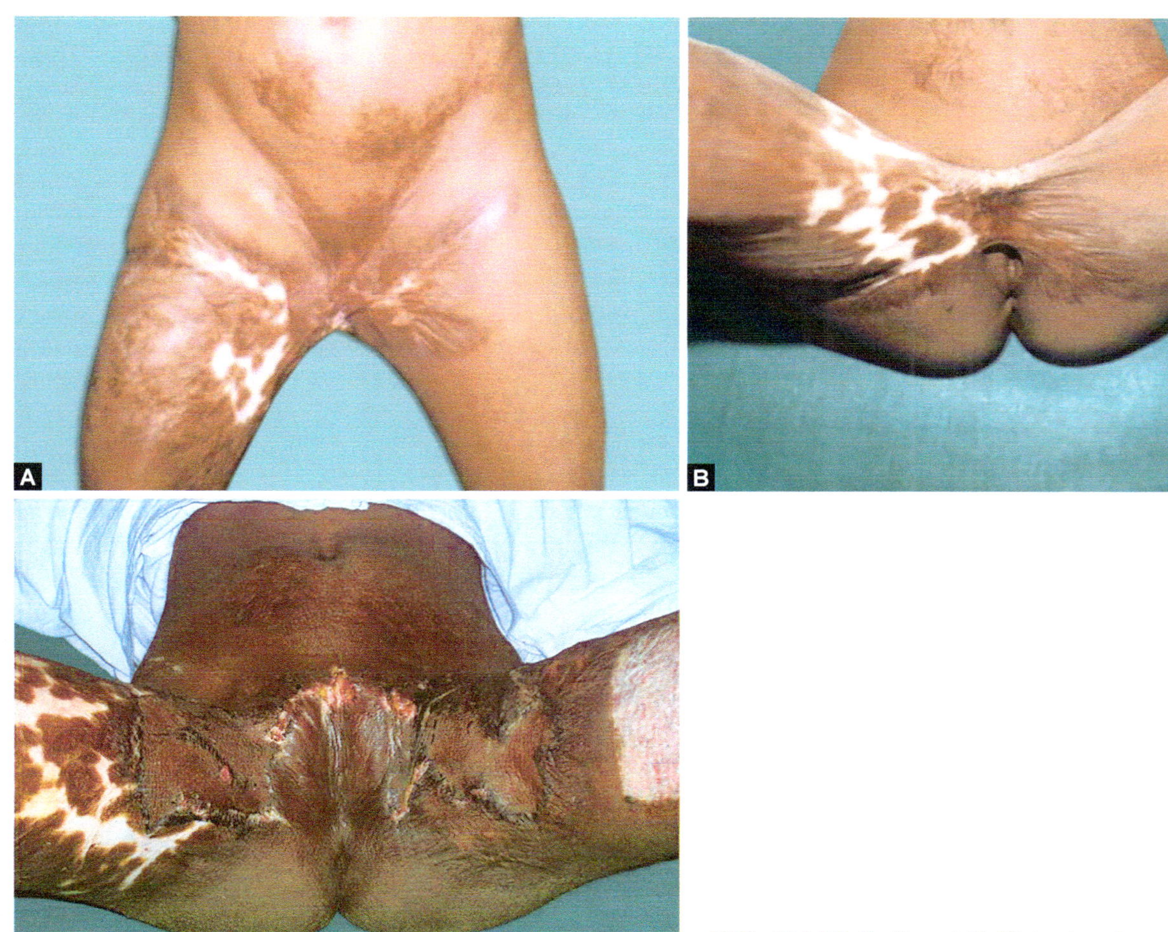

FIGS. 30A TO C: (A and B) Bilateral groin contracture. (C) After release and split skin grafting.

with involvement of groin only, release with tensor fascia lata flap cover and skin graft on its donor site may be possible.

Contractures of the Anterior Abdominal Wall

Tightness of skin of the anterior abdominal wall may or may not cause any problem to a male patient or a female who has completed her family but may be of serious concern during pregnancy when the enlarging uterus is not getting space to bulge out.[53-55] The tight scars may involve the anterior central region or lumbar region on one or both sides, uniformly or eccentrically and may be patchy as well. The parents of a female child must be advised that the tightness of the scars in abdomen must be reassessed before marriage so that if any surgical intervention is needed, it can be done before pregnancy. There is an inability for the abdominal wall to stretch/expand in response to enlarging uterus, especially during the later period of pregnancy with displacement of uterus to one side or the other depending upon the scar position. The patient may also complain of tightness.

How much a scar will cause trouble during pregnancy in future depends on its extent, location (infra- or supra-umbilical region, flanks, etc.), diffuse or a circumferential "constriction band", etc. As a rule, these scars are mature because the burns were sustained during childhood several years ago. Any release of anterior abdominal wall scars during later months of pregnancy subjects the patient and the fetus to risks of anesthesia/surgery, various drugs and premature termination of pregnancy may occur. Conversely, if the scars were such that they allowed successful full-term pregnancy and delivery, immediate postpartum period (within 2–3 days) may be utilized to release the scar contracture and the cover is provided with expanded skin of pregnancy in the form of local flaps/Z-plasty, etc. It is preferable to perform incision-release because it opens up a large area to be grafted. If possible normal healthy skin should be interdigitated with scars/grafts because even the FTSGs are not as extensible as normal abdominal skin. If a cesarean section is done through this scar, it may be equivalent to contracture release and the wound closure may have to be done by a burn surgeon with skin grafts immediately. Despite complete release of contracture and well-settled grafts/flaps in the nonpregnant stage, the skin may still fall short during pregnancy.

Male as well as female patients also present with complaints of malpositioned umbilicus which needs release to bring it back to its normal anatomical position. Several patients also demand removal of hypopigmented vitiligo patches, especially because these scars are visible in their ordinary dress. Excision and application of Thiersch skin grafts can provide the necessary color.

Contractures of the Foot and Ankle

Burns of the ankle and foot (unilateral or bilateral) are quite common and lead to various deformities which hamper the normal gait of the patient and make wearing the footwear difficult apart from poor cosmesis. There may be a diffuse contracture of ankle leading to its dorsiflexion or plantarflexion. It may also take the form of band(s) from distal leg to dorsum of foot. The contracting scars on the medial or lateral ankle going toward the foot may lead to varus or valgus deformity of foot which may be difficult to correct (due to changes in bony contour) if the patient presents several years later after getting burnt in early childhood. The scars may deform the growing bone while joints may subluxate/dislocate. They may have to be operated earlier than the complete scar maturation for this reason. Some very severe deformities may need external fixators or distractors for their management. The contracting scars on the dorsum of distal forefoot cause dorsiflexion at metatarsophalangeal (MTP) joints level (which may even be subluxated) with plantar protrusion of the head of metatarsals and flexion at interphalangeal joints (due to powerful long flexor tendons) forming a Z-deformity (clawing). There may be associated syndactyly or overriding/deviation of toes with narrowing of transverse foot dimensions. Overriding of toes may lead to difficulties in maintaining hygiene in web spaces with consequent bacterial and fungal infections. While contractures at ankle level can usually be treated by release (with/or without excision of scar) and skin grafting or Z-plasty, the dorsal contractures at MTP level, if very severe and long standing, have shortened musculotendinous units which do not allow complete release. In such cases, unlike contractures of dorsum of hands, wrist and popliteal fossa, the extensor tendons can be sacrificed without any functional loss. Their lengthening is not easy and will be an overkill. A sharp cut is made in tendons of all those toes, which are not amenable to sustained stretching on the table, at the MTP joint level. This leads to retraction of tendons in their sheath and allows the toes to straighten up. Kirshner wires of appropriate sizes are inserted from the tips of toes toward the metatarsals to maintain their position for 4 weeks. All unaesthetic hypopigmented, atrophic or hypertrophic scars are excised, syndactyly released and the whole area split skin grafted. A good deep first web is a must for the patient to be able to wear "'*Chappal*", commonly used by our population. Sometimes, a badly damaged toe may need removal (patient consent to be obtained beforehand) and its skin can be used as fillet flap. Very rarely, a patient may need a flap cover not only because the area is unfit for a good graft "take" but also because the orthopedic surgeon wants to carry out some bony correction in the same or later stage.[56] Hence, one must keep a plan ready for this situation in selected cases.

POSTBURN LOSSES

Burn victims may be left with losses of one or more specialized structures or body parts which may be either extremely difficult to reconstruct or else may not be possible to restore. Thus, there may be loss of scalp, eyebrows, moustaches, nose, pinna, nipple-areola complex, penis and testis, etc. Loss of testis(es) need prosthetic restoration. Amputations of limbs at various levels, especially after electrical burns, are beyond the realm of reconstruction (except probably by allotransplantation in bilateral cases). Loss of thumb and digits may be reconstructed with one of the many available techniques including toe transfers by microsurgical techniques. Loss of vision is very common after chemical burn injuries to eye.

These losses are also dependent on the depth of burn. However, they may sometimes be prevented, e.g., by timely escharotomy in full-thickness circumferential burns of limbs or fasciotomy in electrical burns or by prevention of chondritis (with eventual loss of pinna) by appropriate management of burns of pinna in the acute stage.

Scalp, Eyebrows, Moustaches, and Beard

Scalp

Deep dermal thermal burns of the scalp often heal with alopecia patches due to damage to hair follicles and scarring. On the other hand, electrical burns of the scalp often involve full thickness of scalp and even the calvarium. These wounds do not heal without appropriate surgical intervention. The initial intervention may leave the patient with patch of split skin graft over the calvarium. Later on, these patients present for restoration of hair bearing scalp. A number of patients reach a plastic surgeon after long periods of 6 months to 2 years or more following electrical burns of scalp. They have a chronically exposed calvarium. Typically, these patients had no access to specialized treatment of burns and were treated by dressings alone. Their wounds heal by formation of multiple contractures. However, since contraction is limited on rigid skull, they are ultimately left with an area of exposed calvarium with dried up outer table of skull or sequestrum formation **(Figs. 31A to F)**. These patients with chronically exposed calvarium should be treated by removing (chiseling out) the sequestrum of the outer table of skull and wound closure by application of a split skin graft over the diploe. Only very small wounds can be closed primarily using local rotation flaps in the same stage. Transposition flaps are not advisable in these situations as they leave the alopecic areas in the form of split skin graft over donor site and greatly jeopardize the adjacent areas which may be needed later for tissue expansion for ideal scalp restoration.

The restoration of hair bearing scalp has been revolutionized over the last four decades with the introduction and availability of tissue expansion and expanders, respectively **(Figs. 32 and 33)**. They truly allow the surgeon to reconstruct "like with like" tissues. Restoration of the anterior hair line only using repeatedly delayed strips of available hairy scalp is no longer done. Presently, the surgeon tries to excise all of nonhair bearing areas. Except for very small alopecic areas which can be excised and primarily closed either by simple under-mining and advancement or by local rotation flaps, all other larger areas are treated by tissue expansion.

It is the author's practice to get scalp completely shaved at the time of insertion as well as the removal of expander. The former has shown many unexpected scars in the scalp which have changed the plan of tissue expander placement. This also allows proper part preparation which is so very essential when one is inserting a foreign body. It is also possible that the ideal size and shape of the expander is not available (very common in a developing country). In such circumstances, use of a less than ideal expander may give excellent results if the entire scalp is shaved and the expander has been inflated a little more than the calculated amount. At the time of removal, one may have to change the plan of movement of the expanded tissue because the expansion did not proceed in the desired direction. It proves handy if the whole scalp is shaved and prepared. The tissue expander is inserted in subgaleal plane. The incision should be in the healthy skin, 1.5–2 cm away from the scar/graft with healthy skin junction, to avoid break down of the incision at the time of expansion. The port should be as far away as possible to avoid overlapping with the expanding implant and getting punctured unintentionally. The incision is closed in two layers with deeper layer of polyglactin 910 and skin with prolene. A small amount of sterile normal saline is injected in the expander at the time of insertion to flatten out the folds.

After a period of 2 weeks, once the wound has healed, gradual inflations are started. The inflations are done biweekly till the required scalp has been generated, usually

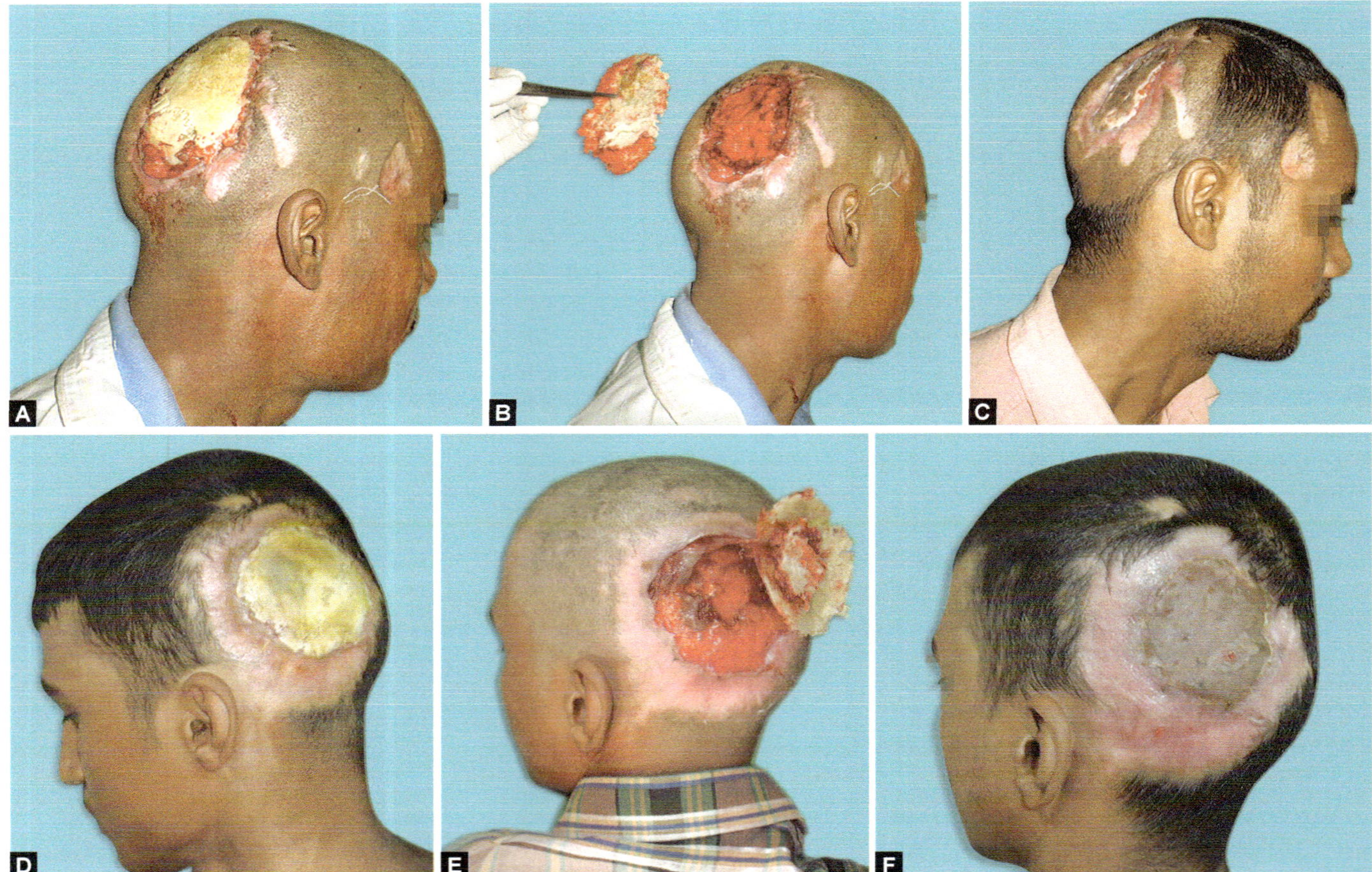

FIGS. 31A TO F: (A) Chronically exposed calvarium (15 months postburn). (B) Sequestrum removed exposing underlying granulation tissue. (C) 4-weeks later, healed with split skin graft. (D) Chronically exposed calvarium (12 months postburn). (E) Sequestrum removed exposing underlying granulation tissue. (F) 3 weeks later, healed with split skin graft.

a period of 3 months. The amount injected in any one sitting should neither blanch the overlying skin nor should cause undue discomfort to the patient. A record must be made of the dates and the amount injected. One must also observe for any thinning of the suture line or the skin being expanded. The expansion may be stopped for a while till recovery occurs and then, proceed slowly and cautiously. Strict asepsis and antiseptic precautions must be taken at all times to avoid any infective complication. After complete expansion has been achieved, the expander is removed through the old incision and expanded skin moved over the alopecic area.

Eyebrows

Facial burns are very common and so are the burns of eyebrows leading to loss of hair bearing supraorbital region. The loss of eyebrows may be unilateral or bilateral. Also, it may be complete, i.e., no hair is left or it may be incomplete and a significant number of hairs may still be present. Eyebrows are very important landmark on face without which the latter looks bland. However, the eyebrow reconstruction is usually the last operative intervention on the patient. This is because their restoration is purely aesthetic in nature and they are to be restored only after the scars and contractures of the surrounding facial region have settled well so that the reconstructed eyebrows do not change their position. Thus, one can rightly term the eyebrows restoration as providing a "finishing touch" to face. In the intervening period, the patient is advised to use an eyebrow pencil. Many patients, especially females, may opt for continued use of pencil rather than go ahead with reconstructive surgery. In this nonoperative option, the patient has to take the trouble of constructing the eyebrow daily. In the surgically reconstructed eyebrow as well, the patient has to take the trouble of regularly trimming the hair as they grow. This gives a waxing and waning of the eyebrow density and bushiness as compared to the uniformity of eyebrow pencil use. The male patients, however, should preferably be offered surgical reconstruction.

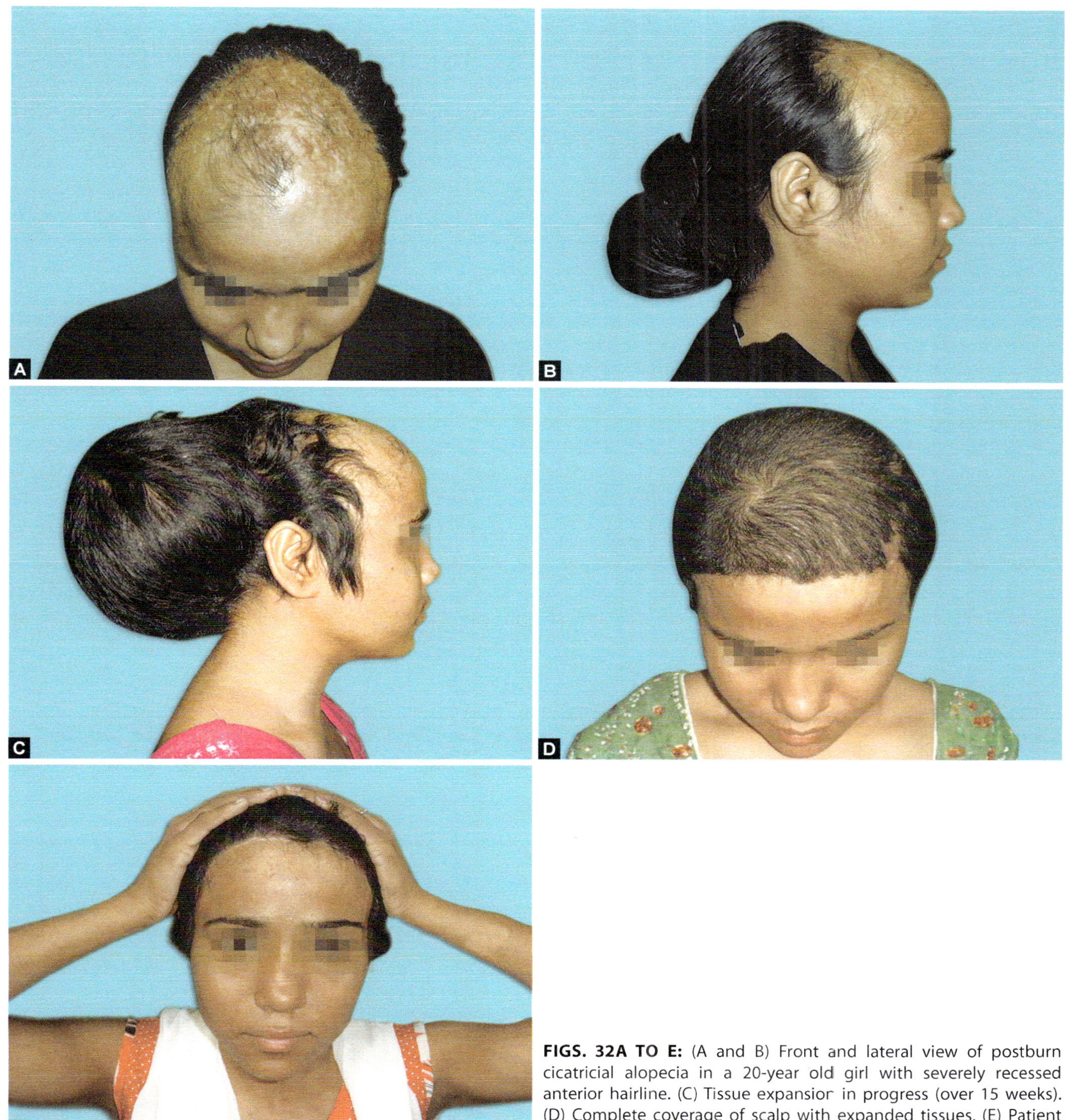

FIGS. 32A TO E: (A and B) Front and lateral view of postburn cicatricial alopecia in a 20-year old girl with severely recessed anterior hairline. (C) Tissue expansion in progress (over 15 weeks). (D) Complete coverage of scalp with expanded tissues. (E) Patient trying to show complete restoration of normal anterior hairline.

A number of operative techniques are available to restore the eyebrow when a normal healthy skin is available in the region. In postburn cases, however, the brow region is generally scarred or split skin grafted and a pedicled flap from the scalp is ideal. It must be added here that excisional surgery is absolutely forbidden in this region in acute stage, even if the burn appears full thickness as the eyebrow hairs have very deep-seated roots and may survive the burn injury giving a reasonable result.

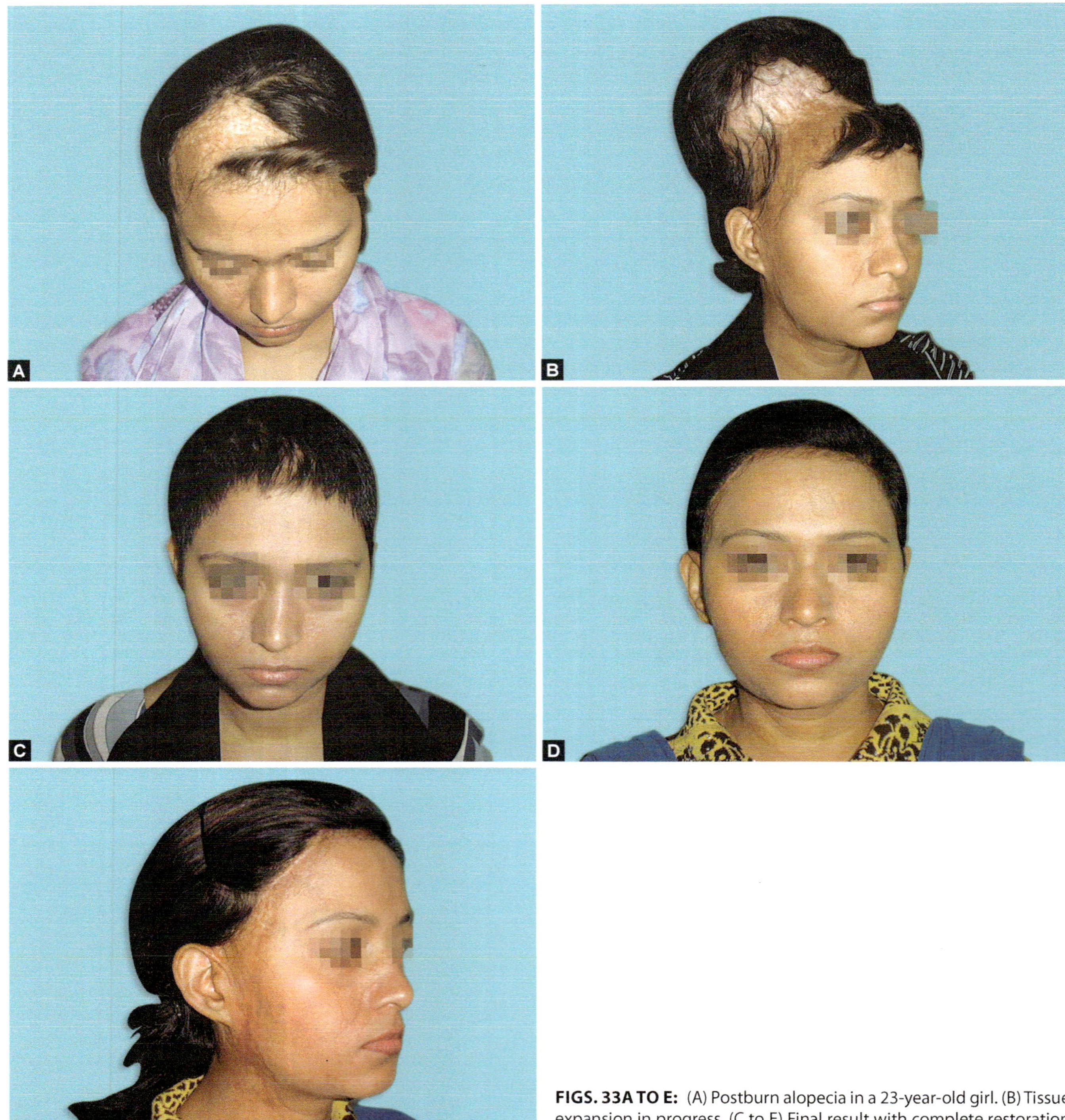

FIGS. 33A TO E: (A) Postburn alopecia in a 23-year-old girl. (B) Tissue expansion in progress. (C to E) Final result with complete restoration of scalp hair.

An island pedicle flap from the scalp based on the ipsilateral superficial temporal artery (temporal branch) is marked. The position of artery is found by light palpation and confirmed by Doppler, if available. Planning in reverse is done to mark the skin island on the scalp. The flap can be raised in two ways. The skin island is raised on an almost skeletonized superficial temporal artery and vein, and then transferred to the supraorbital region with the pedicle being tunneled through the intervening skin from the preauricular region to the recipient site. This method always has a danger of partial or complete loss due to island being not supplied or drained adequately or compression of the pedicle in the tunnel. A safer, although two-staged, technique followed by the author is to take a broad pedicle artery and vein and intervening fascia with the skin island being 1.5 times the width of desired eyebrow and transferred over intact skin with interpolation. This is an excellent and safe technique for the novice or the surgeon who performs this operation only occasionally. Since the initial inset is 100%, the pedicle is divided without any delay at the end of 3 weeks. Once the tissues have settled completely after a period of several months, the desired eyebrow width and shape are marked at appropriate place on the hairy island and excess excised. The newly created eyebrows require frequent trimming for aesthetic appearance apart from a brush looking appearance and an inappropriate hair direction **(Figs. 34 and 35)**.

Moustaches and Beard[57]

When a patient presents with a severe ectropion of the upper lip, a release and thick split-thickness skin graft application may restore the normal appearance in a child or an adult female. However, in adult males where facial hair are a sign of masculinity, absence of the moustaches may be resented and one may request for its restoration to have a more natural and masculine appearance and his self-esteem. Similarly, a patient may have patches of spontaneously healed burnt areas in beard area with alopecia due to damage to hair follicles or there may be split skin grafted areas following grafting for postburn raw areas or following contracture release, etc. Hair-bearing skin to upper lip can be transferred from the scalp or from the neck. A bipedicled flap from either of these sites can be transferred as a "visor" flap ("bucket handle"). Pre-expanded scalp has also been used as visor flap to restore beard.[58] The neck flap needs appropriate delays as they are not axial pattern and do not contain any named vessel in their pedicles. However, a scalp flap may be raised on both superficial temporal vascular pedicles and needs no delay. An L-shaped pedicled flap based on a single superficial temporal artery incorporating the parietal and occipital scalp with primary closure of the donor site has been described to restore whole of the moustache.[59] A free flap

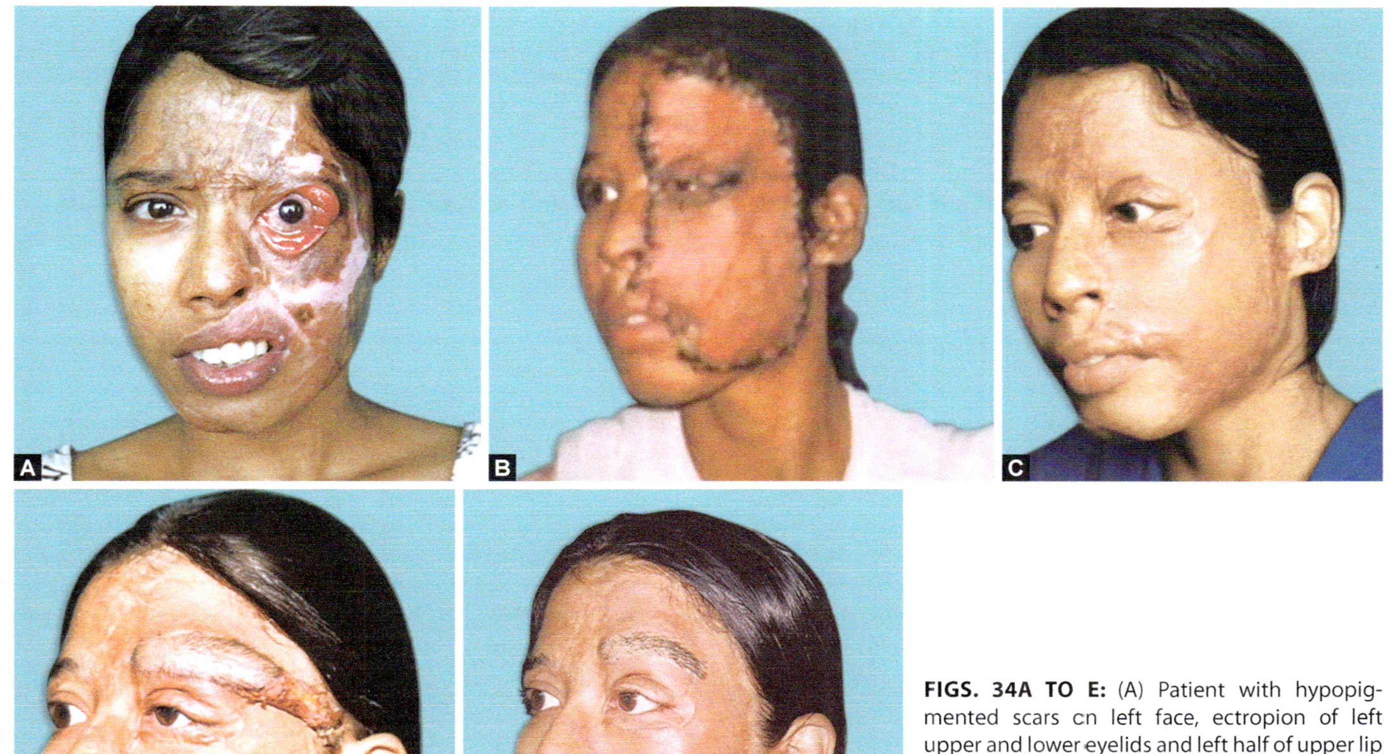

FIGS. 34A TO E: (A) Patient with hypopigmented scars on left face, ectropion of left upper and lower eyelids and left half of upper lip with loss of ipsilateral eyebrow. (B) Appearance after release of ectropion of both lids and lip and excision of scar and cover with a single sheet of graft from thigh in one stage. At 8 days. (C) At 6 months. (D) Eyebrow reconstruction being done by pedicled superficial temporal artery flap. (E) Final result—2 years follow-up. Well settled graft and symmetrical eyebrows.

based on one superficial temporal artery or an occipital artery has also been described to restore the moustache with anastomosis being done with facial vessels.

Hair Grafting for Scalp, Eyebrows Moustaches, and Beard[59-63]

Scalp, eyebrows, moustaches, and beard all have one thing in common, i.e., they need restoration of hair. There may be complete loss of hair or partial loss where intervening nonhairy areas can be seen. Over a period of last more than a decade, with increasing number of patients getting treated by hair transplant surgery for male pattern baldness, more and more attempts are being made by surgeons to treat postburn scalp, eyebrows, moustache, and beard with the same technique and have reported good success. Follicular unit extraction (FUE) and follicular unit transplant (FUT), both the techniques have been used. In these patients, the cause of concern is stiff recipient bed of healed postburn scar/healthy skin graft, poor blood circulation, and thinning of skin. Hence, hair transplantation is more challenging because of a fear of poor survival of hair grafts. However, >75–80% survival has been seen. It must be noted that all burn patients are not suitable for hair restoration surgery either because the donor sites are not available or the recipient sites are not suitable. The hair must be grafted in matured soft supple scars/skin grafts to obtain best results. Immature areas may ooze and the hair may be lost. The natural "grab" of the normal skin to hold the transplanted hair is missing/decreased in these areas. There is an overall satisfaction for the patient and surgeon alike because there is no risk of flap loss and the operation is done under local anesthesia. Usually, 2–3 sittings are required. The newer techniques of microfollicular or single hair grafting produce a more natural-looking result especially for eyebrow and moustaches because of desired hair direction and density. In addition, they can add on to hairs where more hair is required.

Nose

The nose occupies the most prominent position on the face making it vulnerable to almost every burn injury involving the upper part of the body and there may be associated inhalational injury as well. A partial thickness burn injury can lead to scarring of the skin of the nose with essentially preserved shape. It may lead to narrowing or eversion of external naris (nasal stenosis or ectropion respectively). A full thickness burns of skin or a still deeper injury may lead to a subtotal loss of nose, requiring lining, support, and cover for its reconstruction. Total loss of nose, i.e., loss of bony framework is extremely uncommon. The restoration of nasal structure, function, and cosmesis is vital to restore the self-esteem of the burn victim. Here again, whole of the plastic surgeon's armamentarium for reconstructive rhinoplasty in various permutations and combinations along with his ingenuity is needed to achieve the goal of "return to society". In most of the patients who come for reconstructive rhinoplasty to a plastic surgeon, the cause is either a human bite or other trauma or else they have a postexcisional (malignant tumors) defect. The reconstructive options of using forehead flap or nasolabial flaps which give excellent results in these patients are generally not available in burn patients. Commonly, the "less than ideal" options of restoring the nose from medial arm or other distant regions have to be chosen.

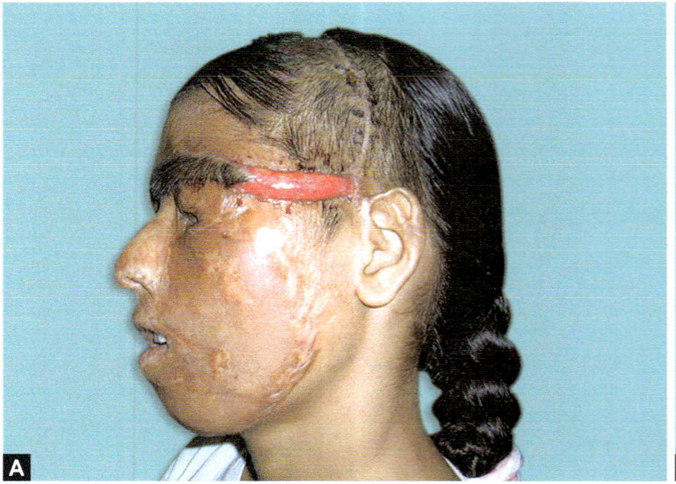

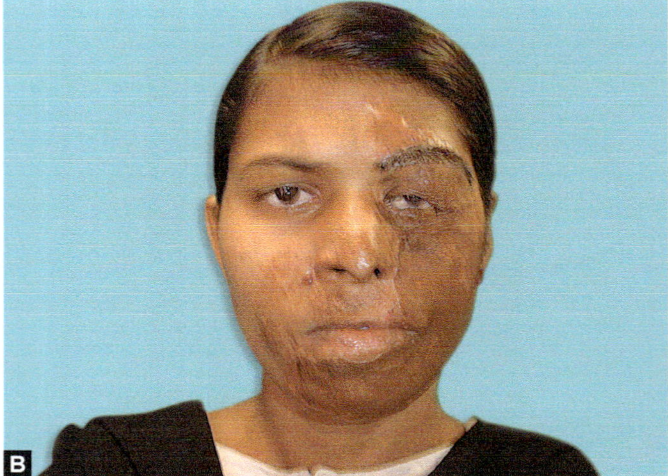

FIGS. 35A AND B: (A) Eyebrow being reconstructed by pedicled flap from scalp. Note the width of flap. (B) Result after trimming of flap and hair.

In patients with scarred nasal skin cover only, the latter can be replaced as a whole with a sheet graft or expanded thin skin from the forehead, if available. The aim should be a result that mixes well with the surrounding face which has healed spontaneously or after application of skin grafts or flaps, etc. Before this excision of scar is done, it is preferable that the surrounding scars/grafts/flaps have settled well and will not cause any extrinsic pull on the nose. Thus, ectropion of the eyelids and upper lip, microstomia, tight skin of the cheeks, bands passing from nose to cheeks, etc., should have been corrected. The scar should be excised thinly, preserving whatever subcutaneous tissues are available to prevent a "skeletonized" look to the nose. When cover is being provided with a graft, the incision at nasofacial junction must be slightly on to cheek as well as with a slight bulge toward the face to take care of secondary graft contraction. One must try to feed excess of graft as well. These measures prevent the junction line between nose and face to come over the nose and spoil the outcome. The graft can be harvested from the medial arm or groin **(Figs. 8 and 36)**.

The management of nostril stenosis is difficult and every effort should be made in the acute stage for its prevention or minimization by using molded splints till scar maturation. Once the scars have matured, the stenosis should be corrected by excision-release of scar and use of interdigitating or local flaps and thick skin grafts. The ectropion of the external naris, again, needs release and cover either with thick skin graft or local flaps, may be from the nasolabial region, if available. Whenever grafts are used at free margin of the nose, postoperative molds must be worn by the patient till graft maturation (Refer to Chapter 26 on 'Facial Burns').

The patients with subtotal loss of nose require recreation of the defect and assessment of the available donor site(s) for provision of lining, cover and support. For smaller defects, local flaps from nose or nasolabial region, if available, can be used. For larger defects forehead skin, if healthy and sufficient, can be used for cover with lining being provided by turn down flaps. They do not need a support as the forehead tissues are sufficiently tough to maintain their shape. Forehead flap rhinoplasty using one of its various modifications like midline or oblique forehead flap or after tissue expansion is commonly done procedure performed by every plastic surgeon for nonburn indications. Detailed of techniques are available in modern plastic surgical literature.[64,65]

Very commonly, however, a patient with postburn loss of nose does not have the forehead tissues fit for use and it is in these patients that the medial arm tube has to be constructed and transferred in stages for reconstructive rhinoplasty. To avoid multistaged operations and their attendant morbidity, microvascular free tissue transfer has been done by various workers using flaps based on radial or dorsalis pedis artery, etc. As stated above, nasal reconstruction with a prelaminated free radial artery forearm flap can also be done.[66]

The detailed technique of arm tube rhinoplasty is not covered in modern plastic surgical books as it is considered old-fashioned and outdated **(Figs. 37 and 38)**. Also, it does not give as good results as forehead flap. The author has, however, found this donor site to be an excellent source in those burnt patients where forehead

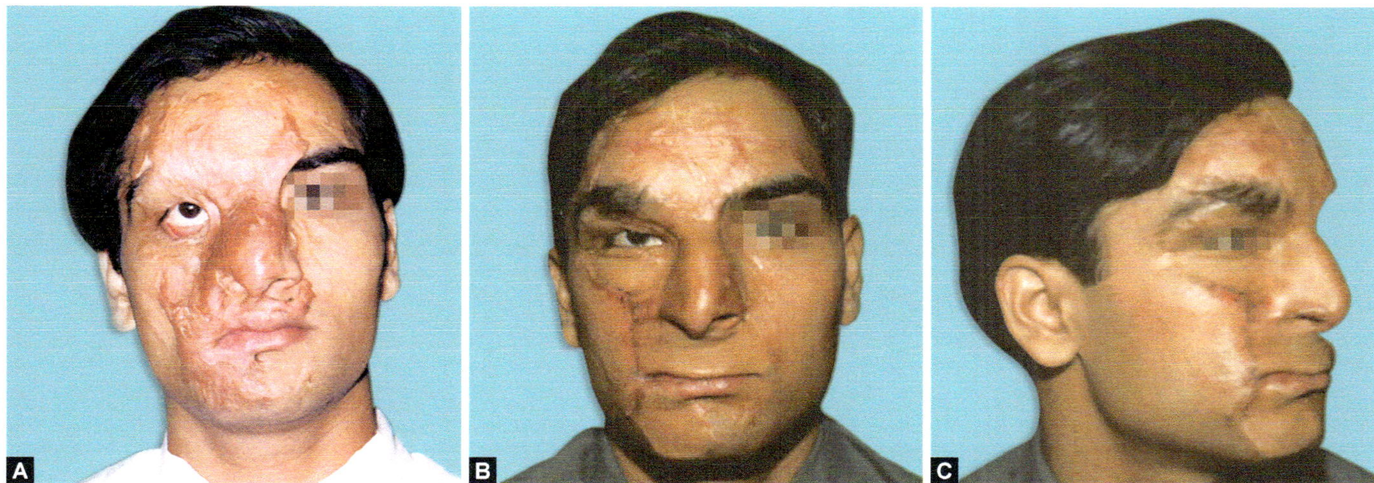

FIGS. 36A TO C: (A) A 23-year-old male with postacid burns hypertrophic scars on face and nose, ectropion of upper lip, and loss of right eyebrow. (B and C) Release and split skin graft to cover the upper lip. Nose has been resurfaced with a skin graft as an aesthetic unit. Eyebrow has been reconstructed from scalp flap (front and right lateral views).

is scarred or grafted. Although multistaged in itself, one must remember that construction of tube may not add any stage as it is usually combined along with some other reconstructive need of the burnt patient. The only real morbidity is for a period of 3 weeks when the first inset is done on the nose and the arm has to be fixed to head. The delay and division of the tube flap from the arm, inset on the nose, and return of pedicle to arm can all be done under local anesthesia. The skin of the medial side of the arm is chosen as it is fair colored, nonhairy, easily covered by elbow level sleeves and is mostly in contact with chest wall and hence not visible.

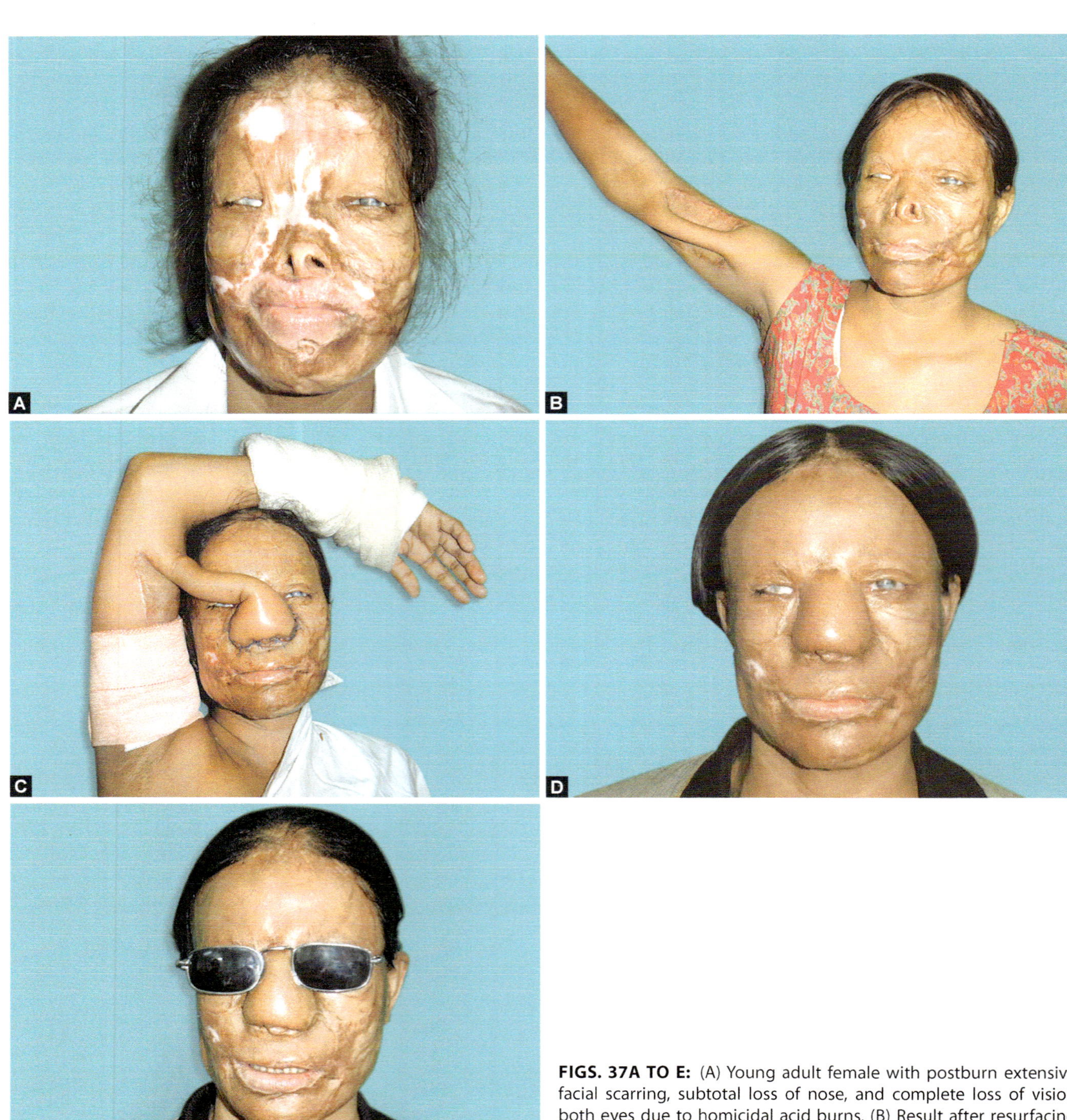

FIGS. 37A TO E: (A) Young adult female with postburn extensive facial scarring, subtotal loss of nose, and complete loss of vision both eyes due to homicidal acid burns. (B) Result after resurfacing of forehead, release of upper lip ectropion, and arm tube construction. (C) Arm tube inset on to nose. (D) Final result after nasal reconstruction. (E) Successful return to society.

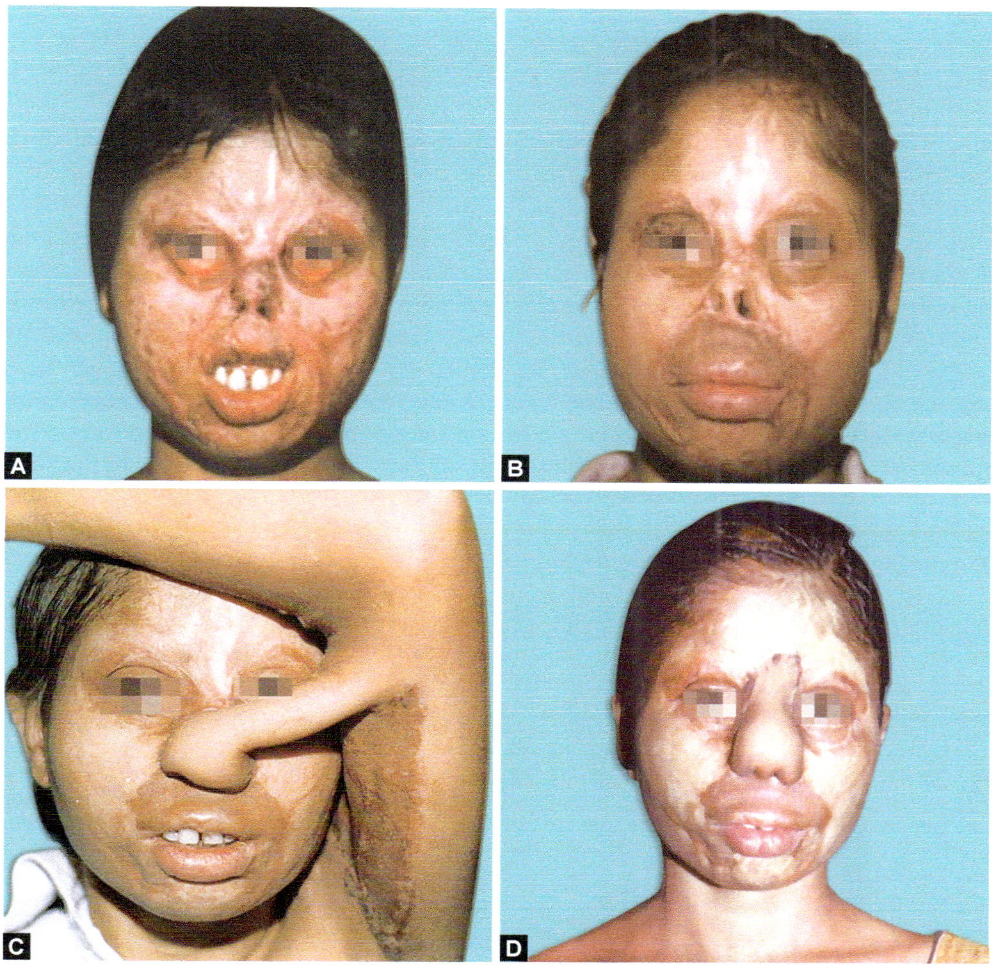

FIGS. 38A TO D: (A) 20-year-old female with bilateral ectropion of eyelids and upper lip, subtotal loss of nose and complete loss of both eyebrows. (B) After release of upper lip and eyelids. (C) Arm tube inset on nose. Note the small and scarred forehead. (D) Nasal reconstruction completed.

Two parallel incisions, about 8 cm apart and 16 cm long, are made in the long axis of the arm and deepened till the whole of subcutaneous tissues. Undermining is done in this plane and a bipedicled, random pattern skin flap (2:1 ratio) is raised. The longitudinal cut margins of the flap are stitched to each other forming a sort of suit-case handle. It is not possible to stitch the ends of the tube. The triangular raw areas on the under surface of the ends of skin tube and the donor bed are split skin grafted with a single sheet graft using tie-over sutures. Once the wounds have healed and the graft taken up, the tube is allowed to "mature" and become soft and supple over a period of 10–12 weeks. The proximal end of this tube is, then, delayed by a transverse incision and the first inset on to nose is done in 7–10 days. The lining is provided by turn over flaps from the defect margin and/or from the nasolabial flaps. The tube is opened at the seam for the required length and the first inset is done to form the ala, the columella, and the lower part of the nose as much as possible. The width of the adult male nose is around 7.5 cm at the broadest part; hence the width of tube was kept at 8 cm to allow for tissue loss in scarred seam. At the end of 3 weeks, the tube is divided at appropriate level keeping the tissues required on the nose. Final inset is done on the nose and pedicle is returned back after excising the skin graft on the donor site equal to the length of pedicle available for return.

Pinna

Reconstruction of pinna or auricle in patients of microtia is a challenging task for a plastic surgeon with a select few doing the job and producing reasonably good results. One can imagine the challenge when healthy skin cover of microtia is replaced by scarred skin or skin graft in a burn patient.[67-70] The results are bound to be far from satisfying the patient and the surgeon alike. The pinna is burnt as a part of extensive burn injuries involving face and upper parts of the body. The skin of the pinna is very thin with almost no subcutaneous tissue especially on its anterolateral aspect. The underlying cartilage is directly dependent on overlying skin for its nutrition. The pinna may be lost directly due to a very deep burn injury or else following chondritis of auricular cartilage leading to its resorption and deformation of the three-dimensional architecture.

The postburn deformities of the pinna may range from minor helical margin irregularities, loss of ear lobule, and auriculocephalic adhesions to complete loss of pinna **(Figs. 39A to D)**. In patients with loss of helical rim, skin tubes can be constructed in pre- or postauricular region or even in the neck and transferred in stages. Loss of ear lobule can be dealt with one of the various techniques like Zenteno Alanis, etc. Adhesions between pinna and scalp need simple release and application of thick split skin graft.

The reconstruction of total loss of pinna involves framework fabrication from autogenous costal cartilage or use of one of the various commercially available implants (Silastic, Medpore®, etc) and provision of skin cover. It is the poor quality with respect to texture and elasticity and shortage of skin that makes the draping of costal cartilage framework or auricular implants extremely risky with ever present danger of their exposure and a catastrophe. Undermining of the scarred skin is dangerous in itself. The temporoparietal fascial flap has solved the problem of coverage to some extent.[71] In case the skin is reasonably healthy and can withstand tissue expansion, the procedure can be done to regenerate sufficient skin in case of its shortage. Ear reconstruction is necessitated not only for aesthetic reasons but also to support the spectacles. In India, wearing ornaments in the pinna is almost a rule in females of all age groups.

When pinna is reconstructed using an autogenous costal cartilage, the synchondrotic portion of the sixth, seventh, and eighth ribs is harvested using extra-perichondrial dissection to obtain a complete graft. Cartilage framework fabrication is done with the help of a template and helical and conchal margins are

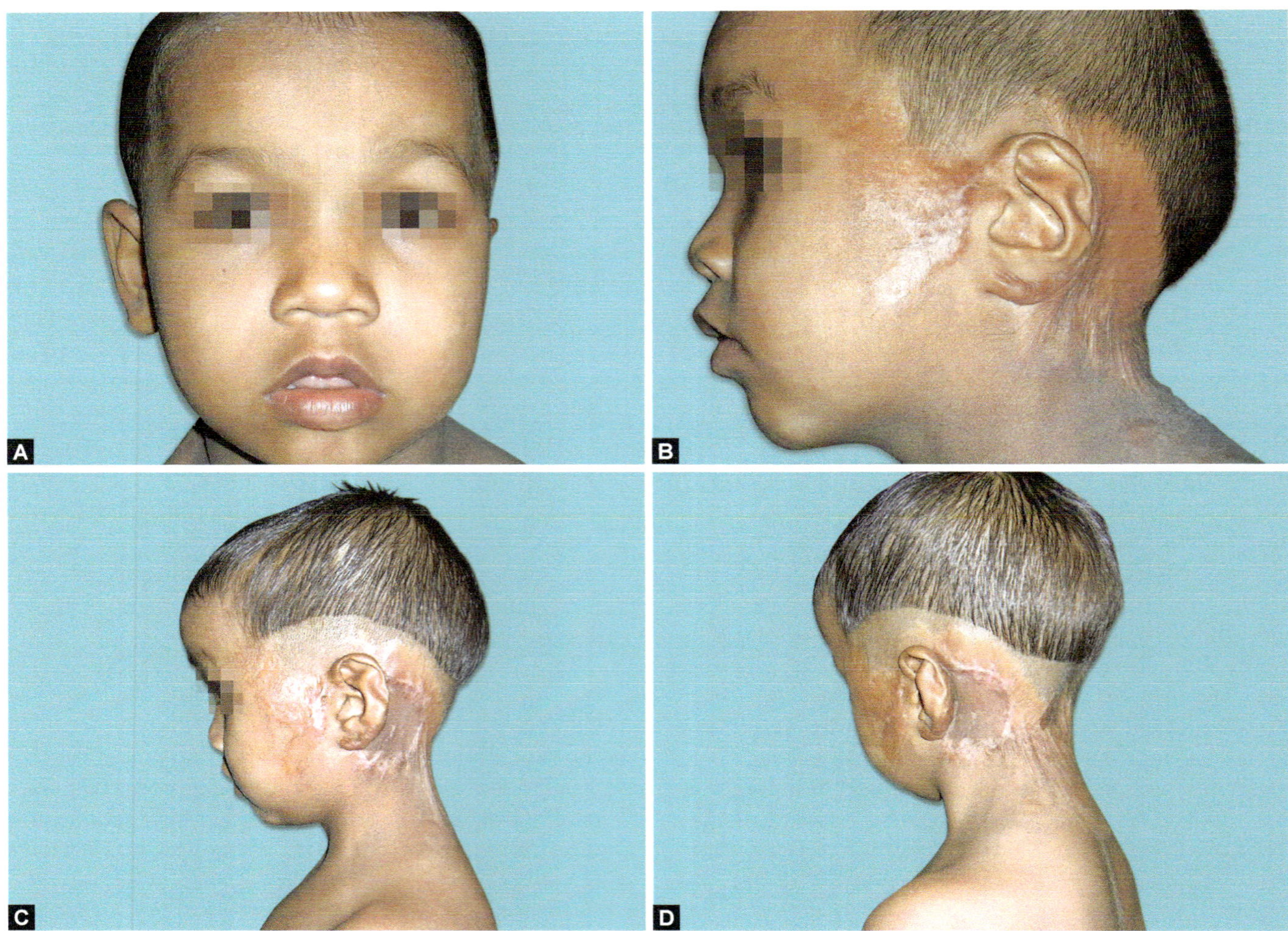

FIGS. 39A TO D: Preoperative and postoperative views of child with postburn auriculocephalic adhesions. Release and thick split-thickness skin graft (SSG) done.

augmented.[67] If local cover is available, a thin pocket is created or else after an incision at the appropriate place, the framework or an implant is covered with temporoparietal fascial flap which, in turn, is split skin grafted.[71] As stated above, pinna reconstruction can also be done by prelaminated free radial artery forearm flap. Prosthetic ear reconstruction with spectacle supported prosthesis or osseointegrated implant-retained prosthesis are the last resort for patients who do not want surgical options.[72]

Breast

Burns of the anterior chest region are very common in female children as well as adults. They are generally part of the extensive burns of the surrounding areas, i.e., head and neck, abdomen, arms, and axillae. In a prepubertal female child, the mammary gland which is 4–8 mm in size is located deep in the subcutaneous tissues. The bud is connected to the nipple by the mammary ducts which are lined by epithelium. Even in burns involving full thickness of skin, the breast bud gets spared and the proliferating epithelium of the milk ducts regenerates a nipple-like structure over the developing mound. There may be lack of areola in such cases and the nipple may be hypoplastic and of the same color as of the surrounding skin. It is to be noted that complete lack of development of breast, i.e., mound as well as nipple and areola complex (NAC) occurs only when the NAC region has been removed energetically but unfortunately during excisional surgery or else burnt deep up to the muscles in a prepubertal child as is possible in contact electrical burns **(Fig. 40)**.

Sloughing of NAC in a conservatively managed prepubertal female child does not mean that the mound

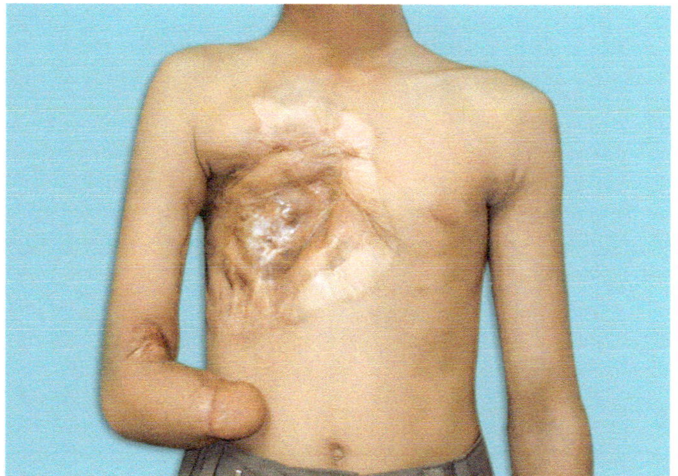

FIG. 40: Contact electrical burns of right anterior chest wall up to rib cage in a10-year-old girl with gangrene of right upper limb necessitating below elbow amputation. She needs breast reconstruction at appropriate time using myocutaneous flaps with silicone implant.

will not develop at the time of puberty. Hence, any form of surgical excision or debridement is absolutely contraindicated in this region. These areas must be managed conservatively with repeated dressings till eschar separation and the raw areas should be split skin grafted after the granulation tissue forms over the region. After complete healing of the wounds, the grafted and spontaneously healed areas are taken care of as usual with massage, pressure garments, etc. Surgical intervention of any sort is to be started only after the onset of puberty when the breast development begins (thelarche).

Reconstruction of the Burned Breast

Reconstruction of the burnt female breast is challenging because it affects the emotional well-being of a growing adolescent girl. Burns of the anterior chest wall in females can result in a variety of deformities which are dependent not only on the depth and extent of the burn but also on the age at the time of burn. In patients who got burnt after the full development of the breasts, there can be deformed breast(s) with or without partial or complete loss of NAC. In prepubertal children, on the other hand, the problem may not even be identifiable fully and/or treatable till the child shows some signs of breast development at the time of thelarche. The breasts may be pulled upward toward the neck, laterally toward the axilla, inferiorly toward the upper abdomen, or medially toward the opposite breast. Due to tight skin scars over the entire anterior chest, the two breasts may move medially toward each other with breast tissue directly over the sternum (symmastia). There may be bands across the sternum. In adult females, the presence of loose breast skin heals many raw areas with contraction without any need of skin grafting leading to "mastopexy" and sometimes better contours. This situation, if unilateral, may call for improving the unburnt side by appropriate operation to achieve symmetry of contours in consultation with the patient rather than "surgically deteriorating" the burnt side by releasing and inserting more graft. Also, in teenagers, more stages are required as compared to adults due to continued growth of the breast mound resulting in graft falling short in amount again and again.

Reconstruction of the Mound

The reconstruction of the breast mound in postburn cases differs greatly from that in postmastectomy cases. Whereas in the latter case, the breast has been totally removed, in postburn cases the apparent projection of the mound has been suppressed by the tight scarred skin over the breast tissue. Thus, the bulk of breast mound is only apparently absent. It is actually present beneath the tight scar **(Figs. 41 to 44)**. It is only in an extremely rare case that the breast was burnt right up to the costal muscles or when it was unfortunately excised completely by the surgeon during acute management that reconstruction of the mound is required. In these cases, the techniques used for postmastectomy reconstruction such as use of myocutaneous flaps, pedicled or free, tissue expanders, and silicone breast implants may be used. In patients who have postburn contractures of the neck or axilla in addition, the breast reconstruction should begin only after the former are released and their grafts/flaps well settled. This is especially true in patients who have their contracting bands of breast, neck, and axilla in continuity. The breast mound and its position improve considerably after the neck and axilla return to normal and the scars over the mound itself become soft and supple in the intervening period.

Release alone versus excision-release: Except for hypopigmented scars, which need de-epithelialization and cover with thin grafts, scars need not be excised. One should try to release and feed more and more of skin graft. As the breast grows, the graft always falls short in amount and another stage is needed. The hypertrophic scars improve with time and ultimately blend with the grafted areas and other scars due to spontaneously healed burns over the breast. Most of these patients have contiguous scars and/or contractures of the neck, axilla, and abdomen, etc., or have these areas split skin grafted during the management of acute burns. Hence, the removal of scars on the breast alone may not be of any

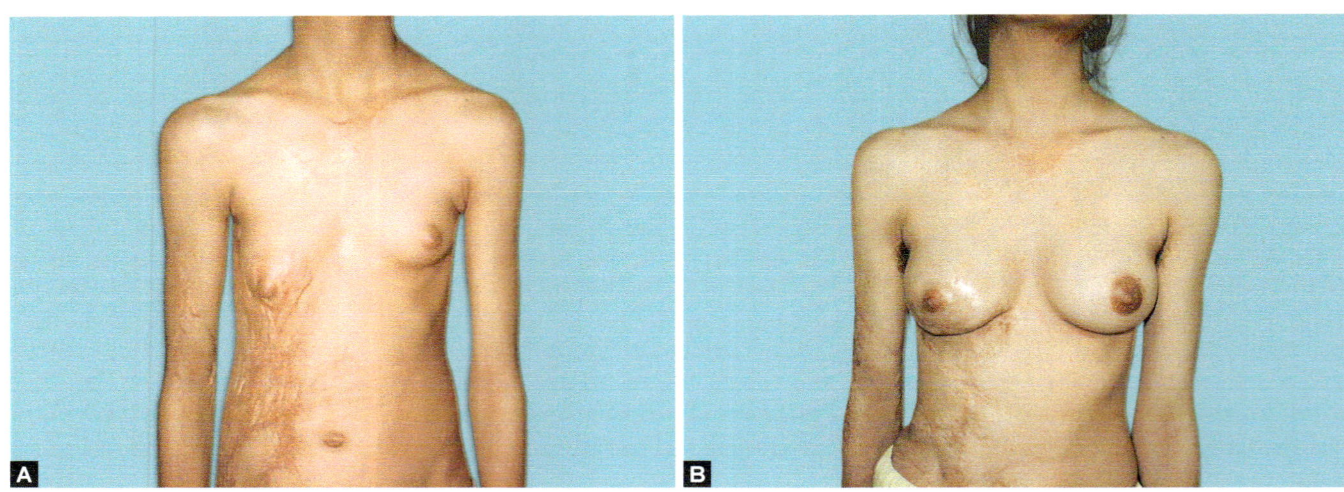

FIGS. 41A AND B: (A) A 15-year-old girl with postburn contracture of right breast. (B) Release and split skin graft done achieving normal contours and size of breast (result after 6 years).

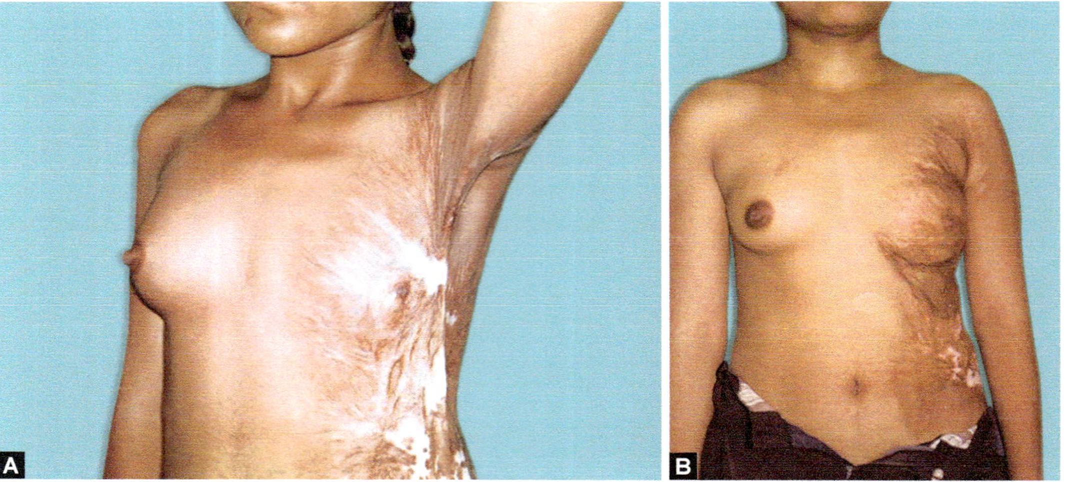

FIGS. 42A AND B: (A) A 15-year-old girl with postburn contracture of left axilla with apparently absent/undeveloped breast mound. (B) Postoperative result after release of axilla and skin envelop over the breast covered with split skin grafts. No augmentation was required. Please note the symmetry with respect to size and contours of both the breasts.

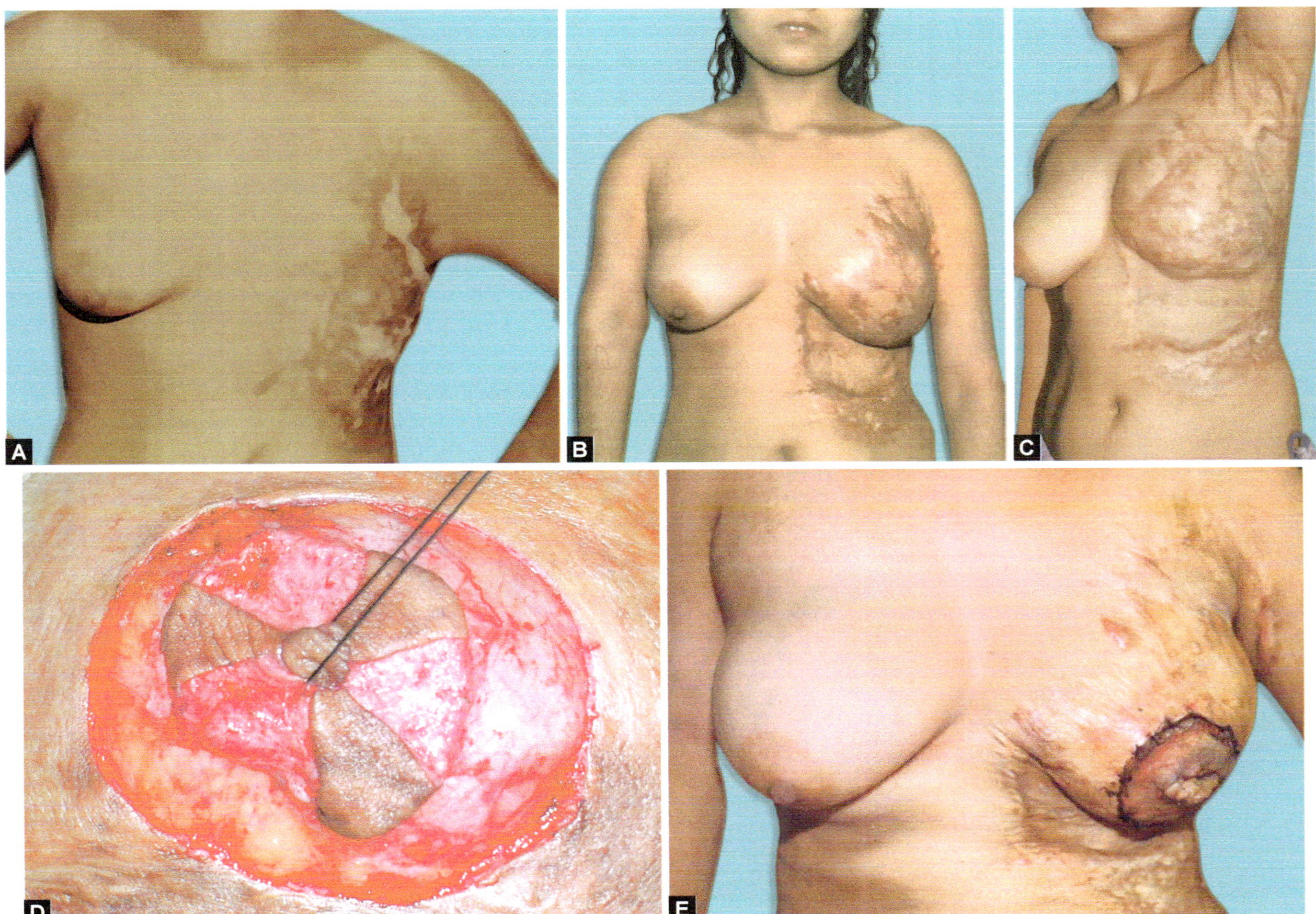

FIGS. 43A TO E: (A) A 14-year-old girl with contracture of left axilla and apparently absent left breast mound and nipple-areola complex. (B and C) Release and skin grafting were done for axilla and breast envelope. The breast envelope required release twice to accommodate the enlarging breast mound. No augmentation was done. The operated breast appears slightly larger than the normal breast. Front view and lateral view with arm abducted. Postoperative result after 4 years. (D) Nipple being reconstructed with modified Little's quadrapod technique. (E) Result after 1 week.

significance. In general, it is futile to excise scars and apply grafts as the patient is given good aesthetics in contours only under the clothes. Even excellently taken up and well-settled sheet grafts are bad enough for the patient so as not to allow her to wear revealing clothes. Vitiligo skin is a taboo in our Indian society. Moreover, they may be visible through the clothes specially when wet. Hence, they need treatment especially in younger age group. When the vitiligo scars are very limited, plenty of donor sites are available and the surgeon is sure that their replacement with a skin graft will improve the overall cosmesis, one can excise the scars in continuity with release incisions and graft one larger area with sheet grafts. In patients with extensive vitiligo scars on the anterior trunk, it may serve no purpose by treating those on the breasts only. Once again, the author would like to emphasize that the postburn patient should be treated as a whole and not in bits and pieces.

Where to Place the Release Incision?

The patient is examined with both arms by the side, then abducted at right angles and finally full abduction with arms parallel to each other and by the side of the head. The position of nipple and areola when present, its position with respect to opposite NAC whether above or below, movement of the mound with arm movements, etc., all determine the site of release incision. If the NAC is at proper position, it is better to encircle the areola and give long multiple darts in radial directions to release the mound fully. When release incisions are given, it is of utmost importance that the surgeon does not cut into the mammary gland. This is especially important in

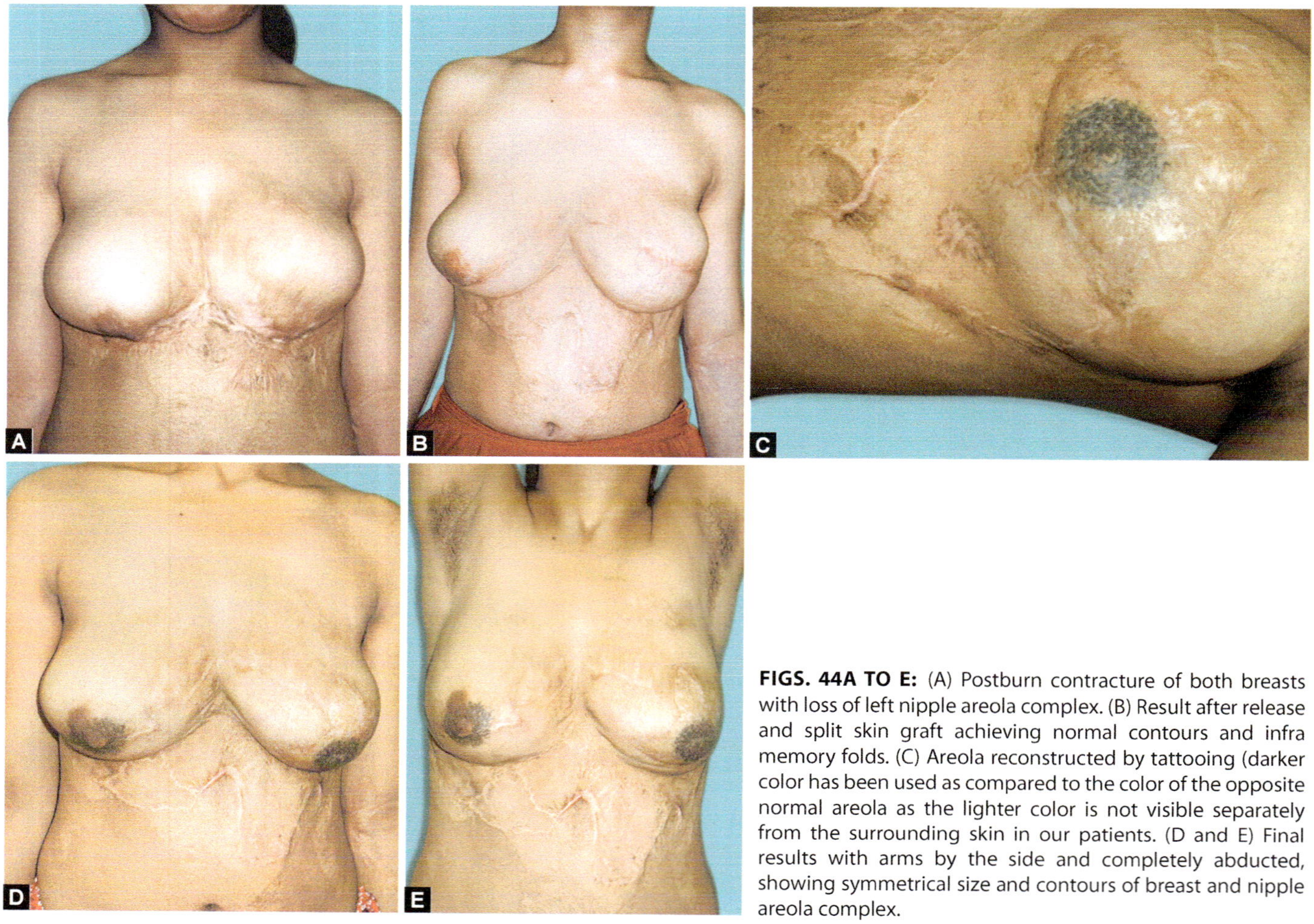

FIGS. 44A TO E: (A) Postburn contracture of both breasts with loss of left nipple areola complex. (B) Result after release and split skin graft achieving normal contours and infra memory folds. (C) Areola reconstructed by tattooing (darker color has been used as compared to the color of the opposite normal areola as the lighter color is not visible separately from the surrounding skin in our patients. (D and E) Final results with arms by the side and completely abducted, showing symmetrical size and contours of breast and nipple areola complex.

incisions made below the areola where the breast fat and the inframammary subcutaneous fat should be identified and the incision deepened between the two. In patients of symmastia, a midline incision is made over the sternum, the breast mounds pushed laterally on either side, and graft applied over the sternum. In patients with absent inframammary folds, this midline incision is curved laterally on both sides for their restoration. Fortunately, the breast tissue (fat) and the subcutaneous tissue over the ribs have different color, texture, and appearance. Breast fat is lighter in color **(Fig. 45)**.

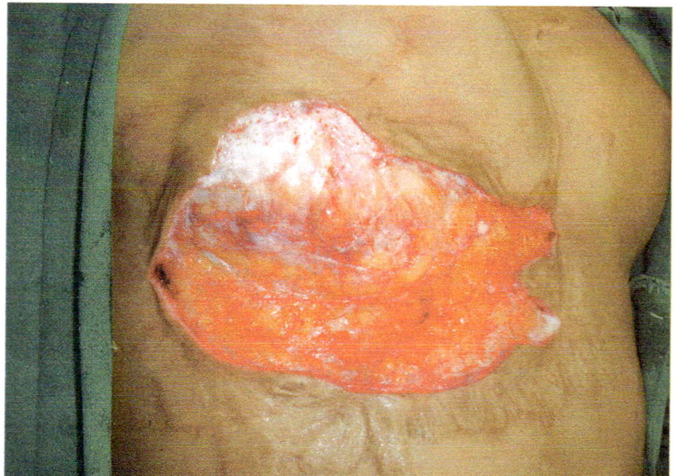

FIG. 45: Please note the lighter color and different texture of breast fat in the upper part of the photograph.

Nipple and Areola Complex Reconstruction

Nipple and areola complex reconstruction is the final surgical step of breast reconstruction. A large number of techniques have been described and more are being reported. This proves that no technique is totally satisfactory on a long-term basis. Some may not be possible in every case. The biggest problem with all the techniques is deterioration in nipple projection or reduction in the height of the nipple. Reconstruction of NAC in postburn cases differs from that in post mastectomy cases in many respects. Reconstruction of NAC is an integral part of postburn reconstruction. This is because most of the postburn cases are children and young adults in premarriage age group with a long life ahead of them. This is in sharp contrast to postmastectomy patients, most of whom are middle aged or even elderly and are more concerned about survival and cure from a dreaded disease rather than undergoing another surgery for breast reconstruction. Also in postburn reconstruction, an excellent mound is restored with rather simple and short operations. It is but natural to complete the reconstruction. It is also to be noted that many of the techniques that give excellent results in postmastectomy cases either give poor results or are not at all possible/desirable in postburn reconstruction.

In unilateral cases, the goal of NAC reconstruction is to match the opposite NAC with respect to site, size (projection), shape, color, and texture. In bilateral cases, the aim is to restore NAC's which looks similar to each other and to that of a normal female of that age and must be situated at appropriate site. In cases, where the nipple is apparently absent, an effort is made to find it out by pinching the skin at various places over the probable site and finding out whether the skin is tethered to underlying mound by ducts at any place. If the site of nipple is found, the reconstruction of NAC is done at this site. However, if the site is not found, the NAC is reconstructed at a site corresponding to the opposite normal breast in unilateral cases or at appropriate symmetrical site in bilateral cases.

Timing of NAC Reconstruction

The NAC should be reconstructed only in a stable mound. If a mound is still increasing in size or changing shape because of normal pubertal changes or because of surgical interventions, the reconstruction of NAC should be deferred till the breast size appears normal for the physique of the patient. An earlier reconstruction can be attempted when the site of NAC on burnt breast is clearly shown by the remnants of the NAC so that the surgeon does not have to select the appropriate site. In cases where the NAC is completely absent and the surgeon needs his own judgment and measurements to find the site, the stability of the mound assumes greater significance. One stage reconstruction of the mound and the NAC is simply not possible in postburn reconstructions. In postburn reconstructions, if one breast is unburnt, it is the author's firm belief that this breast must not be interfered with for various functional, aesthetic and sexual reasons. Moreover, these patients being teenagers and young adults, the normal NAC is never too big to donate.

Reconstruction of Areola

A number of techniques have been described in literature to reconstruct the areola in postmastectomy cases and have been extrapolated to postburn reconstruction. Grafts have been taken from upper medial thigh and labia minora for their darker color as compared to normal skin. These hyperpigmented areas become further pigmented on grafting and may give appropriate color match in postmastectomy cases. However, when the whole breast skin is burnt and there are areas on the breast that have spontaneously healed mixed with grafted areas, the color match of the existing grafts and scars is not much different from these donor areas and they do not stand out. Moreover, in unmarried and adolescent girls even the upper inner thigh skin is of same color as the rest of the thigh from where grafts have earlier been harvested to resurface the postburn raw areas or later to release the contracture of the breast mound. In addition, the darkening of grafted skin, after its "take", depends on its exposure to sun (ultraviolet light) in early postoperative period. This exposure is not there in these patients for obvious reasons. The best technique that is applicable for these patients is tattooing using appropriate colors inserted deep intradermally **(Figs. 44 and 46)**. More than one stage is required and any fading at a later date may need retattooing to augment the color. No donor site is required and opposite breast is not interfered with.

Reconstruction of Nipple

This is the most difficult and frustrating part of postburn breast reconstruction. It differs greatly from nipple reconstruction in postmastectomy cases. Almost all the techniques of nipple reconstruction have been described primarily for postmastectomy cases and extrapolated directly or with slight modifications to postburn cases. Again, in almost all the described techniques, the reconstructed nipple tends to lose height or projection over a period of time. The availability of a very large number of techniques is a testimony to the fact that none is universally successful. A number of techniques described for postmastectomy cases are not possible/desirable in postburn cases. For example, nipple sharing technique should not be used as most of these patients are young and their nipple is not large enough to donate. Moreover, one would not like to spoil the only normal nipple in this age group. Composite grafts from the ear lobule or toe pulp are bound to have an unacceptably high failure rate because of the poor vascularity they get from the skin grafted areas. The techniques where the nipple protrusion is obtained by burying a piece of autologous conchal cartilage or silastic implant, etc., are not desirable because of the risk of jeopardizing the vascularity of overlying split skin graft. Many of the techniques described using local skin flaps to reconstruct nipple projection rely on the dermal and subdermal base which are highly deficient in skin grafted areas. The only techniques which

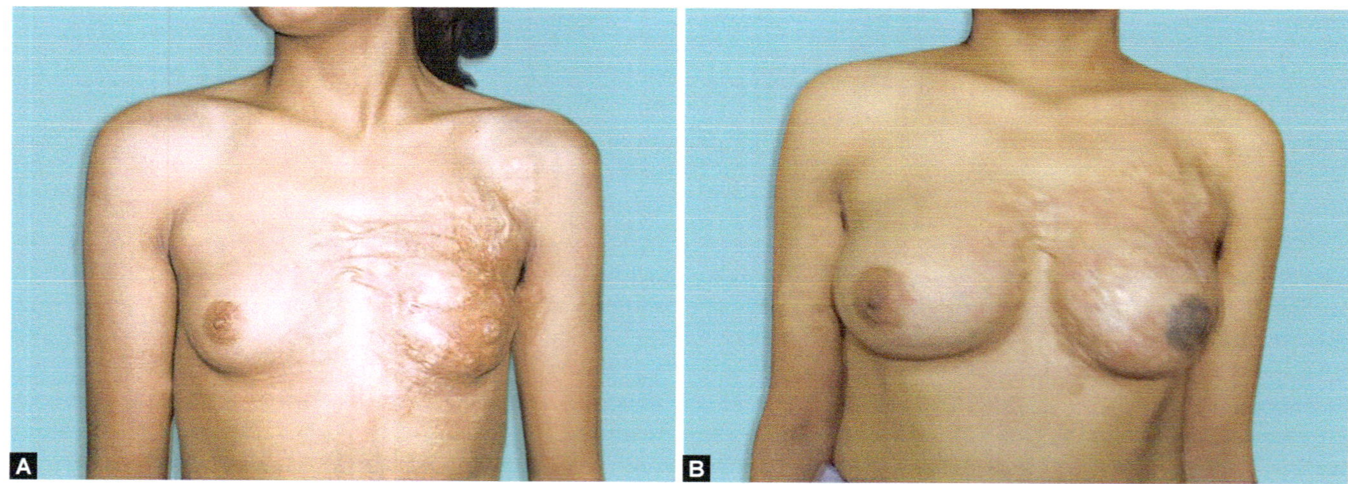

FIGS. 46A AND B: (A) Postburn loss of left nipple areola complex. Note the reconstructed nipple. (B) Tattooing done to reconstruct areola.

are possible are the ones which do not raise the local skin (actually skin graft) from its bed so that the vascularity of the skin does not suffer. The author reconstructs the nipple by the following techniques.

Two concentric circles of 1 cm and 4 cm diameter are marked with their center at the site where nipple is to be made. Three V-shaped areas are marked in the area between two circles as shown for de-epithelialization. A cut is made in the outer circle and deepened till and slightly into the breast tissue. The de-epithelialized areas are closed by stitching together the adjacent non de-epithelialized skin areas. With a stay suture in the center of the smaller circle, the newly formed nipple is pulled out and the raw area is grafted with thick split skin graft using tie over sutures. Theoretically, this will give a projection of around 1.5 cm. This over correction takes care of partial flattening over a period of time. After the wounds have healed and the graft settled, size of the areola required is marked with nipple as the center and tattooing done to complete the NAC reconstruction. This technique does not undermine any area and is modified from Little's quadrapod technique **(Figs. 43A to E)**.

Another technique involves construction of two adjacent "dog-ears" which together give a semblance of a papilla. 3 squares of 1 × 1 cm size (A, B, B′) are drawn as shown in **(Figs. 47A to H)** with square "A" over the site of nipple. Two triangular areas are also marked in the vertical axis as shown. Along with outer two squares B and B′, the triangles are thinly de-epithelialized. Two thick dermal flaps are raised with their base toward the nipple, i.e., square "A" and allowed to contract toward the latter. When stitching of the raw areas is started from either apex, a dog ear forms toward the square "A". The dog ears along with dermal flaps help in forming a nipple at site "A".

Male External Genitalia (Penis and Testes)[73,74]

Although penoscrotal region is very commonly burnt as part of extensive burns, it is highly unlikely for a thermal burn injury to result in loss of penis and/or testis. Contact electrical burn injuries, on the other hand, are known to result in a complete loss of penis and one or both the testes. Their reconstruction is a must not only for restoration of form and function but also for the psychosexual health of the victim. However, one has to wait for the scars in the region to become mature, soft, and supple. The reconstructive techniques for phalloplasty have seen great advances since the time of Bogoras who reported the first such operation in 1936. The penis being a tube within a tube and the tube flap having been described by Gillies during World War I, the penile restoration has seen the transformation from multistaged, random pattern tube flaps to axial pattern musculocutaneous and fasciocutaneous, and then free flaps which even included nerves and bone to provide sensation and stiffening. However, as yet there is no suitable replacement for erectile tissues. At present, state of the art neurosensory fasciocutaneous free flaps are used to reconstruct a phallus in a single stage which is acceptable not only functionally and cosmetically but also psychosexually.

For the last four decades, the free radial artery forearm flap has remained the flap of choice for phalloplasty. The basic design consists of construction of a tube within a tube and various modifications have been done to improve the appearance and sensation and to decrease the complications. The most important drawback of unsightly grafted donor site in the forearm may not be of much concern to a burn patient (compared to patients of gender reassignment surgery) as he already has plenty of such areas and scars due to initial burn injury itself. However, as the flap is hairy, free ulnar artery forearm flap has been described in its place. The use of fibular osteocutaneous flap for phallic construction has been advocated to achieve rigidity. Anterolateral thigh flap and latissimus dorsi myocutaneous flap have also been used to reconstruct phallus.

The photographs **(Figs. 48A to I)** show the staged reconstruction of phallus of a burn victim using a

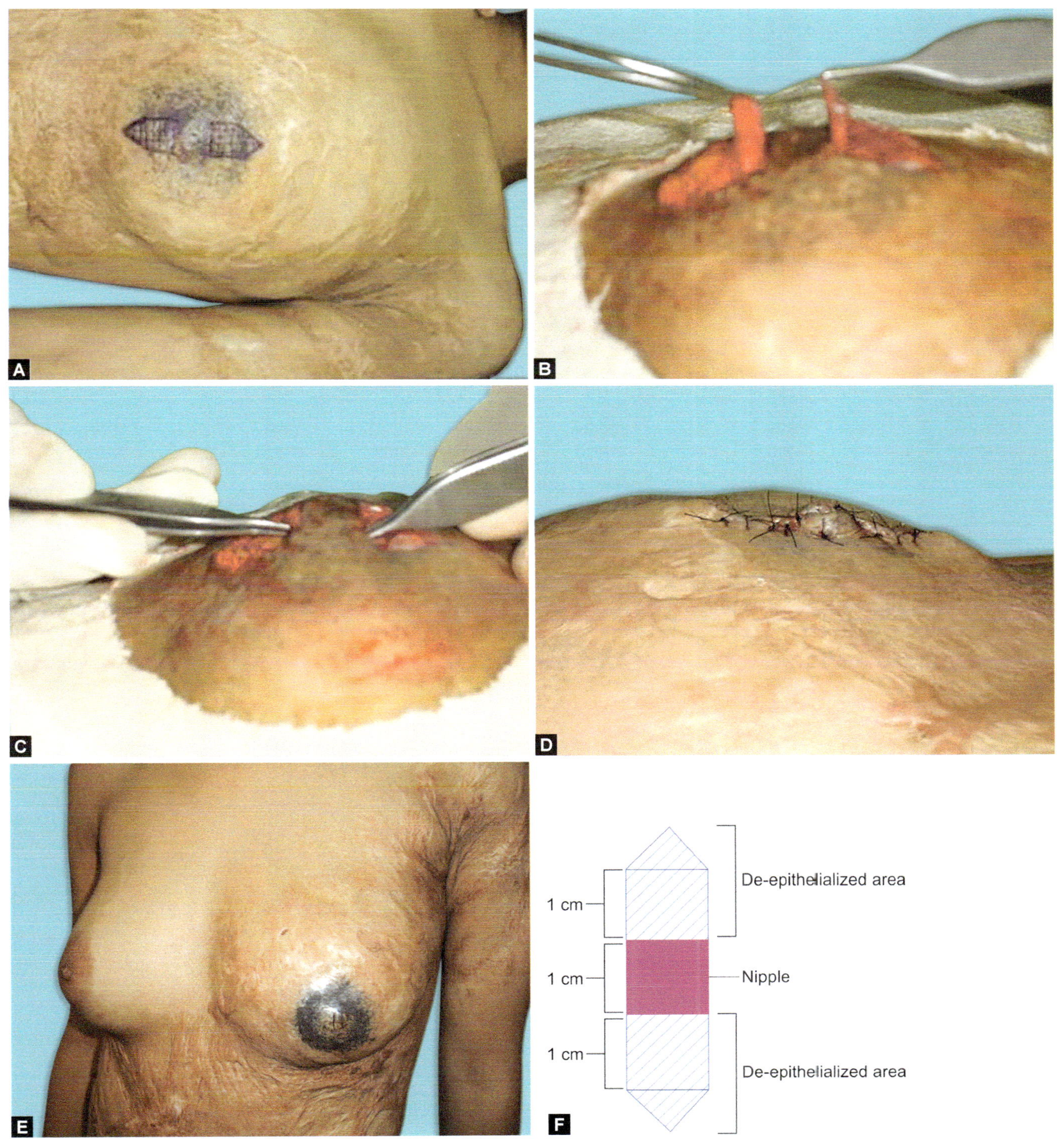

FIGS. 47A TO H: *Continued*

Continued

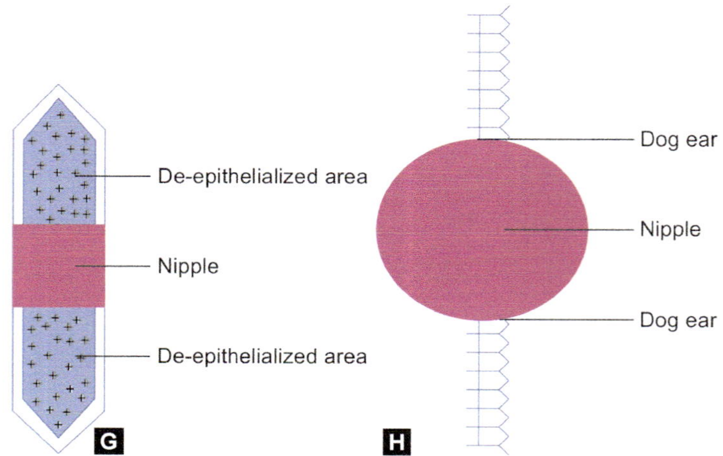

FIGS. 47A TO H: (A to E) Nipple reconstruction. Areolar tattooing done (F to H).

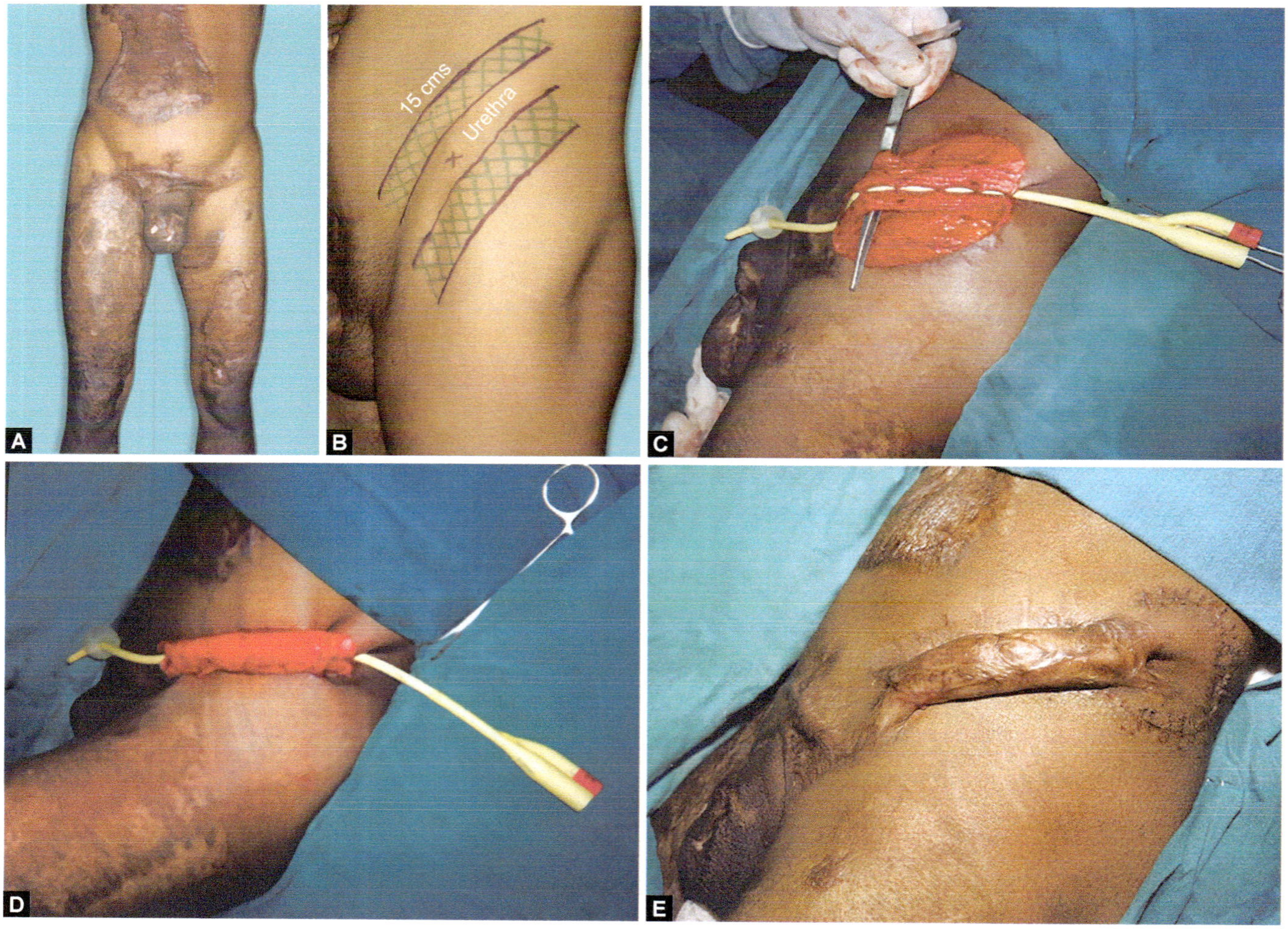

FIGS. 48A TO I: *Continued*

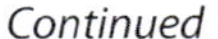

Continued

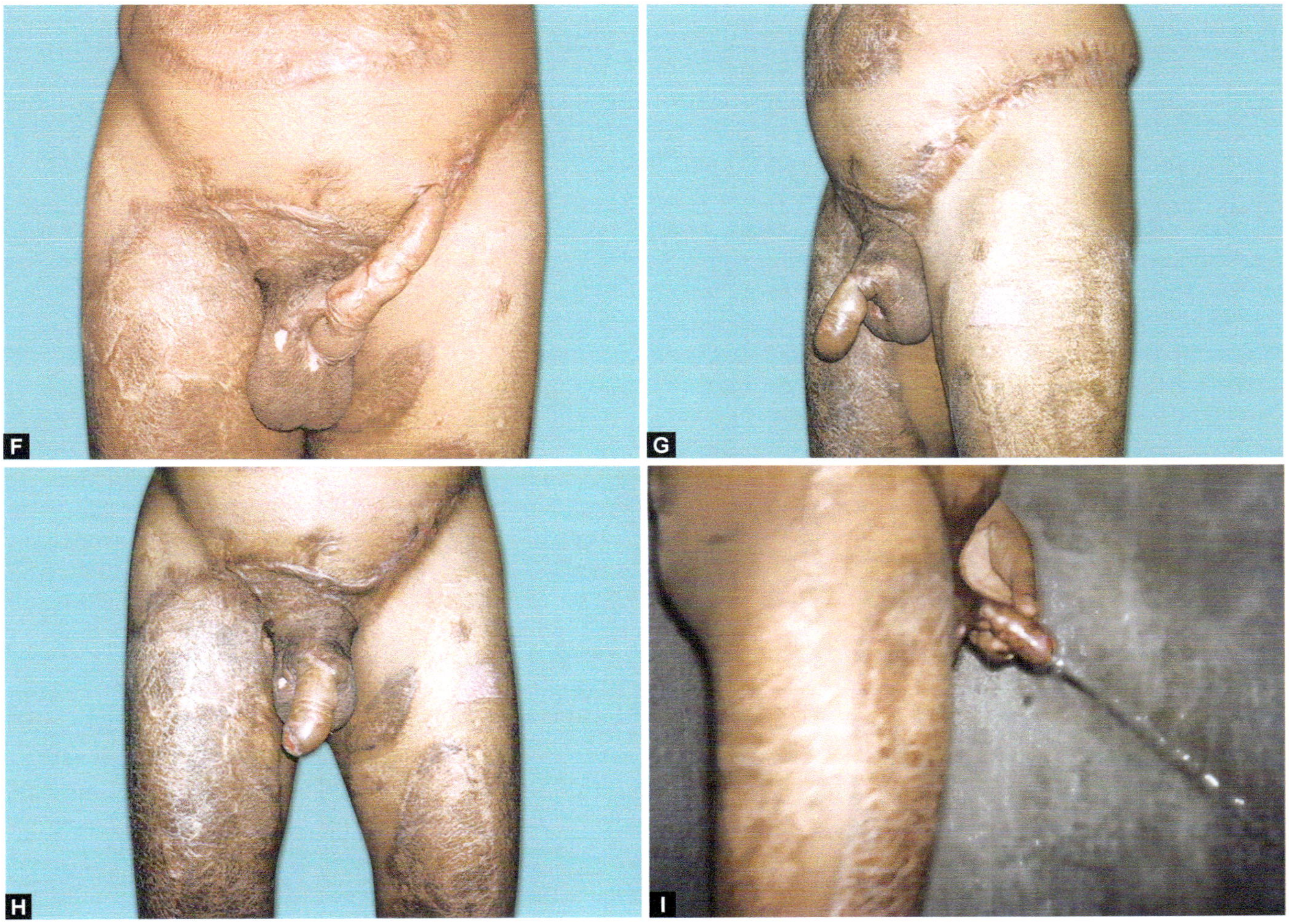

FIGS. 48A TO I: Postburn loss of penis in a 30-year-old male. Reconstruction done in stages by constructing tube in tube from groin region. Patient passing urine normally (Markings on a model).

bipedicled, tubed extended groin flap. The urethra has been made from the in-turning of nonhairy skin in the long axis of the center of the flap while the remainder of the flap skin is de-epithelialized. The dimensions of the flap are based on the length of penis desired (15 cm approximately) and width is based on the maximum donor site which can be closed primarily by undermining and advancement with hip flexed. The outer tube is made by stitching the flap margins together over the urethra in such a way that the under surface of the groin flap forms surface of the outer tube. This necessitates the covering of the raw area with a split skin graft. When the graft and the tube have matured over a period of 3–4 months, division and inset over the region of native penis is started. The use of graft to make the skin of the neophallus lends it some rigidity by virtue of secondary graft contraction. The silicone testicular implant(s) may be inserted into scrotal skin, if available, or the scrotum is reconstructed from locally available flaps from the upper inner thigh.

Amputations

Electrical contact burn injuries are known to kill the victim instantaneously. The "fortunate" survivors very commonly end up in multiple and major amputations at various levels leading to a lifelong disability to the victim and a liability on the family and the society. Contact with high tension wires often leads to gangrene of one or more limbs. They may need multiple fasciotomies for relieving compartment syndromes. Circumferential full-thickness burns of the extremities with tight eschar, if not treated timely by appropriate escharotomy incisions, may also end up in distal gangrene necessitating amputation(s). Most of these patients with amputations at higher levels in upper and lower limbs are offered prosthesis to improve function as well as overall appearance. These patients may have stump instability, poor soft tissue coverage over the bone end, joint contracture, atrophic scars, painful neuromas or improper stump length, etc., which may pose difficulties in fitting the prosthesis. These problems must be addressed to achieve successful rehabilitation. In upper limb if thumb alone is lost, "pollicization" of index finger may be done. Microvascular transfer of great or second toe to reconstruct the thumb can give excellent function and cosmesis. Web spaces may be deepened and "phalangization" done.

CHRONIC UNHEALED AREAS AND NONHEALING SCAR ULCERS

In India and several other developing nations, the only treatment received by a large number of burn patients is in the form of simple dressings with some of the commonly available antibacterial creams or even indigenous substances. These patients heal by contracture formation. However, some chronic raw (unhealed) areas may remain over nonjoint regions after all the natural limits of the force of contraction have been exhausted **(Figs. 49 and 50)**. Typically, these areas are over the sternum, rib cage, long bones and calvarium, etc. Depending on the time that has elapsed between the date of burn and reaching a burn surgeon, the wound bed has more and more of fibrous tissue and consequently poor vascularity. These areas have pale granulation tissue and do not accept split skin grafts well. They may need excision of all the fibrous tissue down to soft and supple healthy bed (apart from release of contracting elements) for a complete graft "take". In the scalp region and over the subcutaneous bones, the bed may be formed of the dried-up bone which needs chiseling till bleeding bone or diploe in the case of calvarium before wound closure with skin graft or flap.

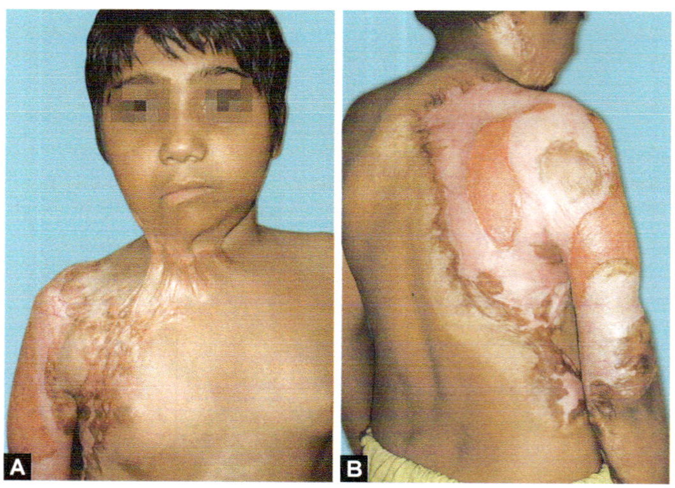

FIGS. 49A AND B: Chronic raw areas over lateral arm, shoulder, and scapular region along with contracture neck.

BONE AND JOINT DEFORMITIES

A burn injury may lead to a number of musculoskeletal deformities even if the burn injury was no more than skin deep. Many of these deformities are due to the strong contractile forces which tend to heal a full-thickness burn injury in the absence of skin grafting **(Figs. 10A and B)**. When the burns are sustained in early childhood and not treated appropriately, the deformities get accentuated with growth of the child. Thus, the joints may be subluxated or dislocated. The bones and joints may bend in an abnormal direction. When such patients come to a plastic surgeon after many years in late teenage or adulthood, it may not be possible to release the joint contracture not only because of shortened musculoskeletal units but also because the growing age has molded the bone and joint in an abnormal shape/position. Postburn contractures on the dorsum of hand may spoil the extensor apparatus giving rise to deformities such as boutonnière and swan-neck. When untreated for a long time, there may be irreversible damage to the joints of hand and permanent lifelong deformities result. Severe mentosternal contractures in children may lead to deformities of mandible, alveolus, and teeth with disturbed occlusion.

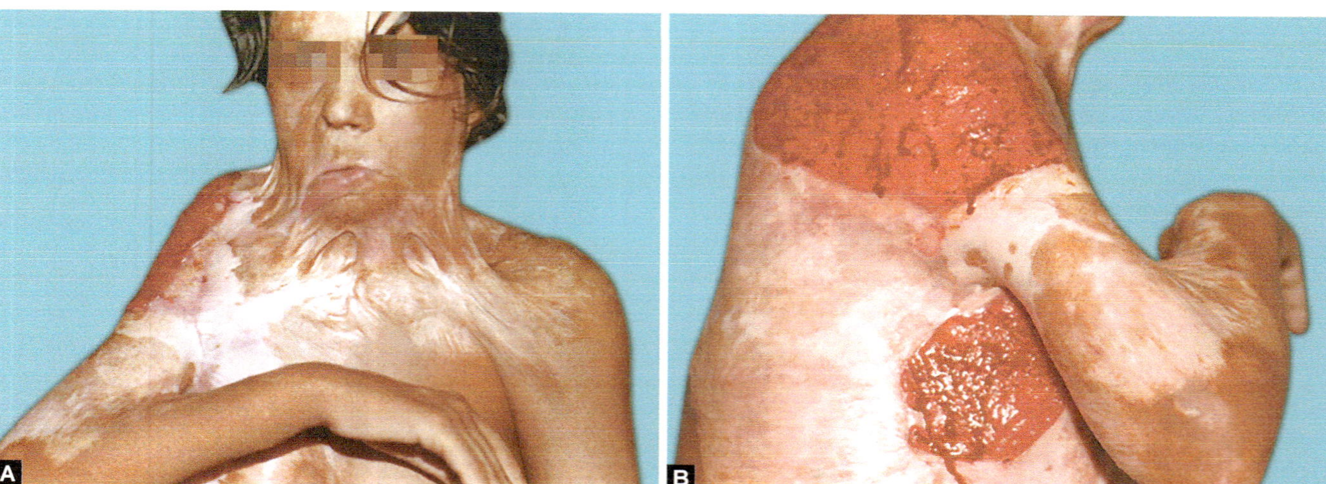

FIGS. 50A AND B: Chronic raw areas over shoulder, scapula, and lateral rib cage where healing by contracture formation is not possible along with postburn contracture of neck, axilla, and elbow.

DEVELOPMENT OF MALIGNANCY (MARJOLIN ULCER)

Once the reconstructive surgery of a burn patient is over, all the scars have well settled and matured and the patient has returned back to society, he/she is still at risk of development of malignancy even after several years **(Figs. 51 to 54)**. The fact that thermal burn scars can degenerate and develop into malignancy was known to Celsus in AD 100. However, Jean Nicholas Marjolin has been widely acknowledged as to provide with the first description of skin cancers in postburn scars in 1828.[75,76]

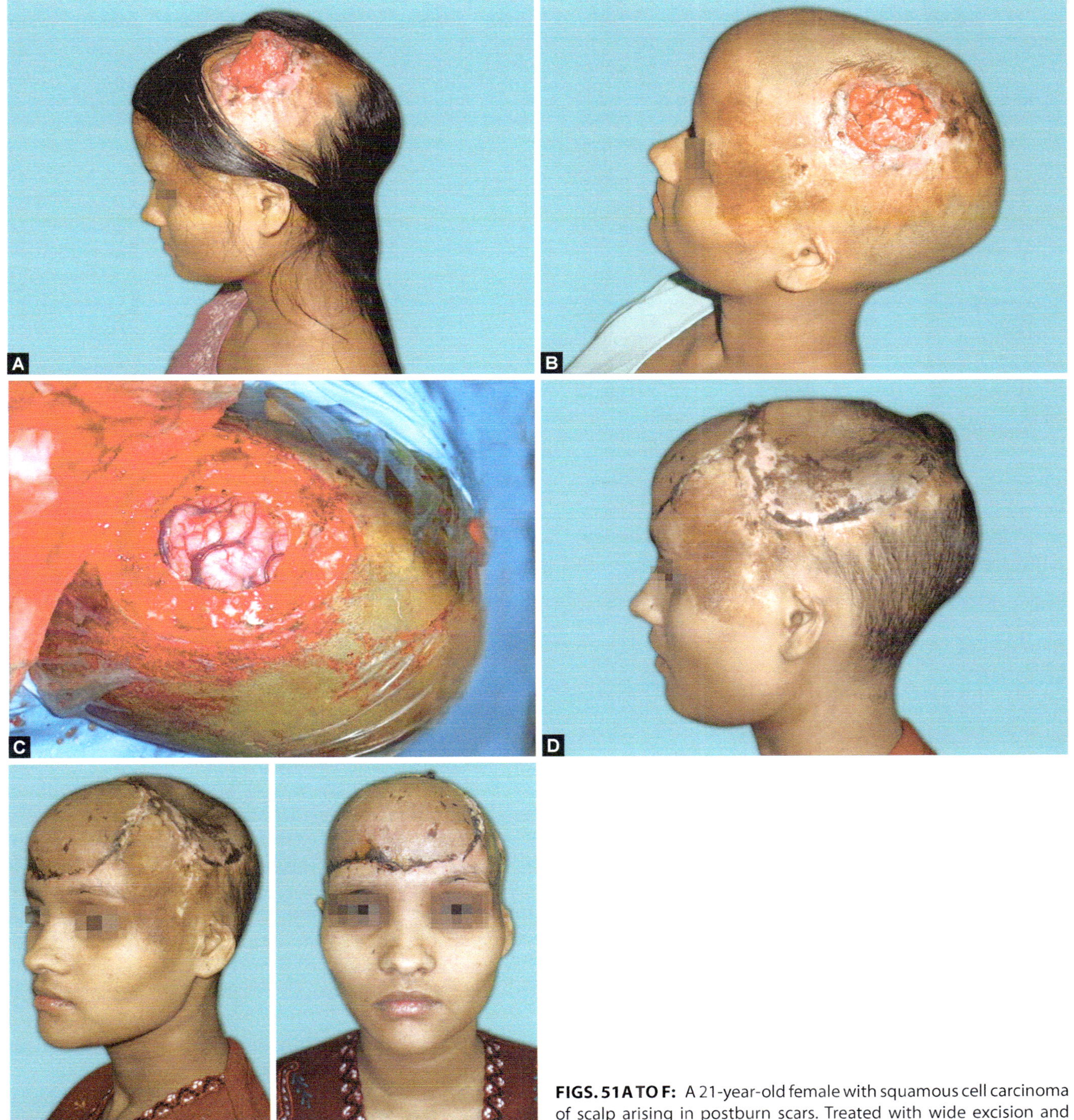

FIGS. 51A TO F: A 21-year-old female with squamous cell carcinoma of scalp arising in postburn scars. Treated with wide excision and local transposition of remaining scalp and split skin graft.

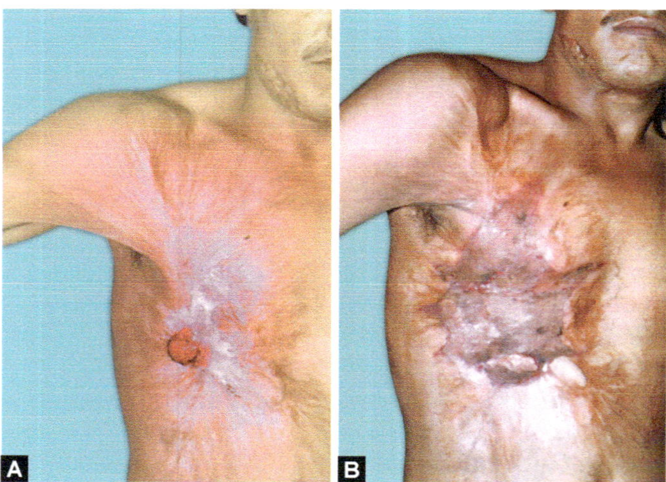

FIGS. 52A AND B: A 38-year-old male with squamous cell carcinoma over anterior ribs arising in postburn scars treated with wide excision and split skin graft.

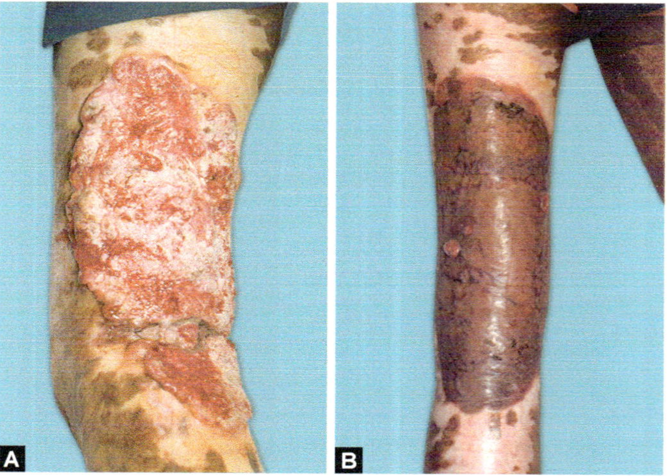

FIGS. 53A AND B: (A) Squamous cell carcinoma arising out of post burn scar in popliteal fossa region. (B) Wide excision and split skin grafting done. Result after 2 months.

De Costa in 1903 coined the term "Marjolin ulcer" and applied it to tumors arising in simple leg ulcers. The term Marjolin ulcer is used for malignant degeneration of burn scars as well as other cutaneous scars, chronic venous ulcers, sinuses of chronic osteomyelitis, pressure sores, scar tissue around colostomies, frost bite, etc.

The exact mechanism whereby a malignant change occurs in a postburn scar is still not known. It has been observed that a cutaneous scar subjected to continuous irritation has increased potential for malignant change. Slow initial healing and scar instability are very important in the development of cicatricial cutaneous malignancies. Repeated trauma, when applied to any tight scar situated over the joints, is an important factor in neoplastic change. The relationship between skin cancer and repeated/prolonged thermal injury is best exemplified by the unique examples of "Kangri" cancer in India, "Kairo" cancer in Japan and "Kang" ulcers in China. The "Kangri" is an earthenware bowl heated by charcoal and worn against the skin of the abdomen and thighs for warmth by Kashmiris in India. In the "Kairo" burn cancer of Japan, the person keeps a light tin box (with hot coal inside) that fits snugly against abdomen for at least 3 hours at a stretch to keep warm. Malignant ulcers on the buttocks known as "Kang" ulcers have been seen in North-Western China from the practice of warming the bed with external heat.[75] Owing to the continued application of heat, the skin in these areas becomes dry and horny and shows chronic dermatitis leading to malignant neoplastic changes.

To begin with, postburn skin cancers are very slow to grow and metastasize as has been observed and reported by a number of workers. Most patients are free of regional or distant metastasis at the time of presentation. However, once the tumor breaks into the surrounding normal skin or is excised, it becomes aggressive and there is a high incidence of local recurrence and regional/distant metastasis. This led some workers to suggest the theory (although unproven) of Marjolin ulcers developing in an "immunologically privileged site".[77] The presence of relatively avascular dense scar tissue and almost absent/obliterated lymphatics allows the primary tumor to grow unrestricted by host immunological mechanisms. This significant delay may be the reason for the aggressive behavior of the tumor once the malignant cells reach the lymph nodes as this is their first encounter with the immune system.

There is currently no clear explanation as to the exact cause(s) of Marjolin ulcers. It has been considered to arise primarily from longterm chronic inflammatory stimulation that leads to mutations in focal cells.[78-80] There may be release of mutagens from the breakdown of scar tissue directly influencing the *p53* and *Fas* genes, which subsequently disrupt apoptosis, homeostasis, and deregulate controls on proliferation. Several studies have also identified nuclear factor-κB as a key modulator of inflammation-induced tumors. A nonhealing wound represents a chronic inflammatory microenvironment that may facilitate angiogenesis and promote the uncontrolled growth leading to malignant change. Prolonged irritation and persistent attempts to heal the wound causes proliferative stress leading to continual secretion of cytokines, chemokines, and growth factors. They in turn, stimulate cellular proliferation and increase the probability of acquired mutations. Nthumba et al. and Bazaliński et al. have discussed various theories/hypothesis proposed to explain malignant degeneration.[81,82]

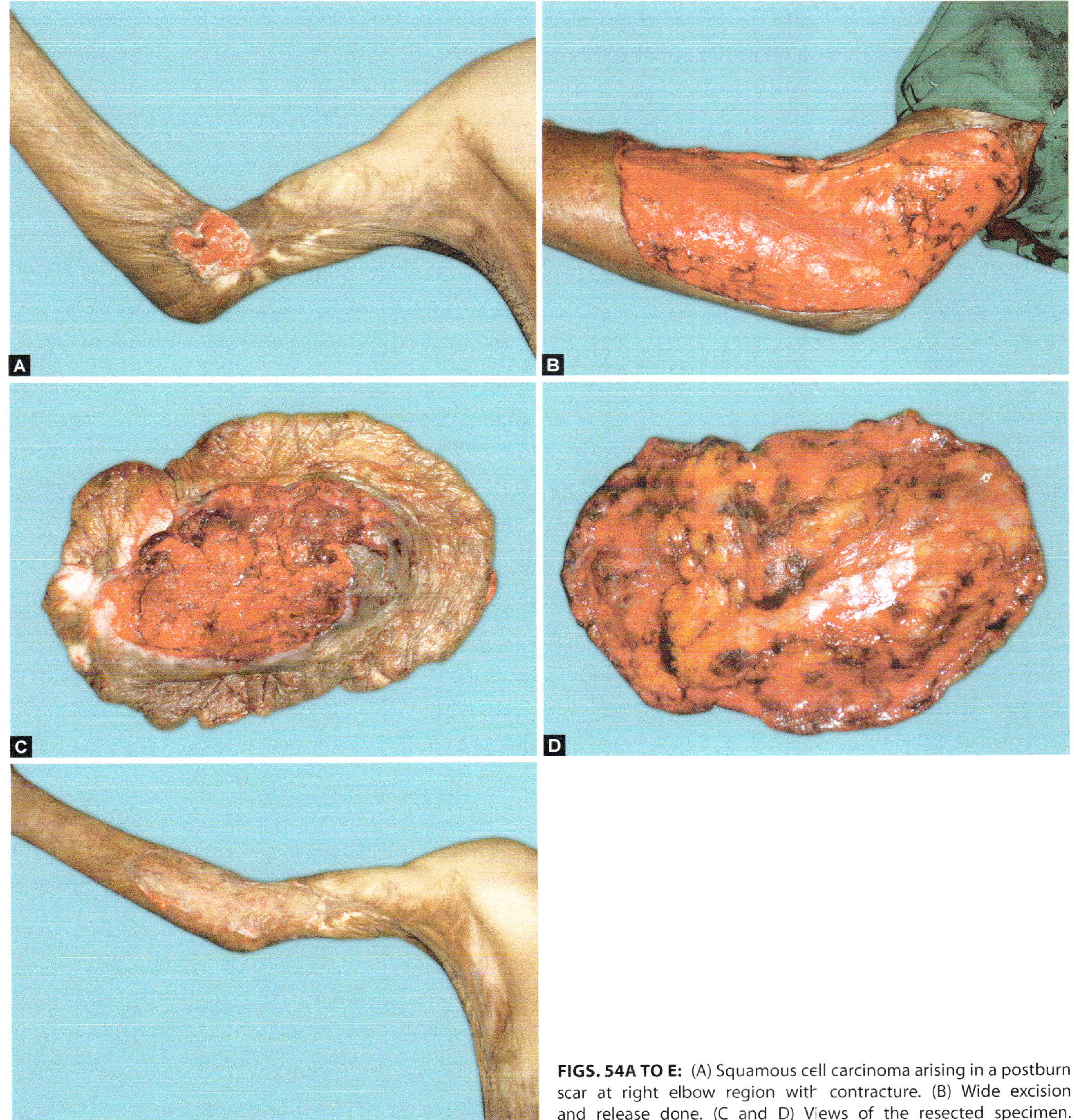

FIGS. 54A TO E: (A) Squamous cell carcinoma arising in a postburn scar at right elbow region with contracture. (B) Wide excision and release done. (C and D) Views of the resected specimen. (E) Postoperative result.

The most common malignant neoplasm to develop in postburn scars is the squamous cell carcinoma (SCC) with basal cell carcinoma (BCC) being the next. Case reports of various other cancers including sarcomas (e.g., melanoma, adenocarcinoma, liposarcoma, leiomyosarcoma, fibrosarcoma, malignant fibrous histiocytoma, even extraskeletal osteogenic carcinoma, malignant schwannoma, etc.), developing in postburn scars have also been reported. The relatively deep position of mesenchymal cells of the dermis and subcutaneous tissues making them less vulnerable to trauma and their lesser tissue regeneration than the superficial epidermis has been put forward as the explanation for rarer occurrence of sarcoma as compared to carcinoma in burn scars. Marjolin ulcer is three times more common in men as compared to women. Roughly, it involves lower limbs, head and neck, upper limbs, and trunk in a ratio of 4:3:2:1. All postburn cicatricial malignancies develop with a prolonged latent period, i.e., the time interval between the acute burn injury and the onset of malignancy. This period has been reported to vary from 8 to 63 years with a mean of 32.5 years. Rarely, early arising Marjolin ulcer cases have been reported with a latent period of 1 year or less. In addition, the latent period has been found to be inversely proportional to the patient's age at the time of burn, i.e., the younger the victim at the time of burn, longer is the interval for malignant change. Older the patient, shorter is the latent period.

The postburn scar malignancies are to a great extent preventable by instituting early treatment of unstable and tight scars and ulcers especially over the joints where repeated trauma occurs. The grafted as well as spontaneously healed burnt areas must be kept soft and supple by application of bland oils and creams. Once all the reconstructive treatment is over, all patients must be advised about the possibility of developing a malignancy in burn scar and report any ulceration at the earliest to the burn surgeon. Any patient presenting with a nonhealing ulcer in an earlier healed burn area, especially if there is history of recurring breakdown, must be looked upon with suspicion. Clinical findings include exophytic growth, everted edges, and irregular ulcer base in a postburn scar apart from contracting bands. If possible, an excisional biopsy with wide margin is done. If not, an incisional biopsy from appropriate representative area(s) should be taken.

Treatment of biopsy proved malignancy depends on the histopathological type and the status of lymph nodes draining the area.[76,83,84] For squamous cell and BCCs, a wide local excision with a 3–4 cm margin of normal skin including the muscle fascia and release of contracture should be done. Although some workers have done prophylactic lymph node dissection, most recommend this surgery only when they are palpable. It is to be noted that the enlarged lymph nodes palpable at the time of initial presentation may be due to chronic infection. Fine needle aspiration cytology (FNAC) examination may be done after a course of broad-spectrum oral antibiotics. The nodes tend to settle after the local wound heals in 2–4 weeks' time. A regular life-long follow-up is essential because metastatic recurrences are common within a 3-year period. SCCs arising in burn scars have always been considered as more aggressive than arising otherwise. Poor prognostic features are lymph nodal involvement and local extension of disease at the time of presentation. Involvement of the regional lymph nodes is followed by metastasis to brain, liver, kidney, and lungs. Lower extremity lesions have higher rates of nodal metastasis. A patient who has been metastasis free for 3 years has an excellent prognosis. Malignant lesions which involve deeper structures like bone and joint are treated by amputations at appropriate levels. Amputations are also required if wide excision involves major neurovascular structures whose loss will leave a nonfunctional distal limb. The management of the rare sarcomas in burn scars is no different from those which arise without any such history of burn or other scar.

Supplementary radiotherapy has been tried for further locoregional control while chemotherapy has been given to patients with unfavorable prognosis or distant metastases. Cisplatin, 5-FU, methotrexate, bleomycin, and paclitaxel have been used for inoperable cases or in the presence of distant metastases. However, they often produce unsuccessful results.

MISCELLANEOUS

It is said that a major burn is a systemic disease and affects the physiology of each and every system in the body. It is not surprising, therefore, that the list of postburn sequelae is almost unending and cannot be classified adequately. Each and every sequela described in the vast burn literature cannot be covered even in a book devoted to same. A number of problems must, therefore, have been left out in this chapter.

For example, electrical burns are known to lead to cerebral, spinal, and peripheral nerve injuries with a long latent interval between the injury and the neurological dysfunction or deficit. They may cause hemiplegia, quadriplegia, paraplegia, and neuropathies. These patients need the consultation of a specialist neurologist or neurosurgeon. Electrical burns are also a major reason for amputations of extremities at various levels. Many of such patients can be rehabilitated with use of appropriate artificial limb prosthesis. Cataract can also occur requiring an ophthalmologist's intervention. Heterotopic ossification or myositis ossificans is a rarely encountered complication of burns. Although elbow is the most common region involved shoulder, hip, and knee may also be affected and requires surgical treatment by an orthopedic surgeon. Respiratory and inhalational burn injuries may lead to long-term lower respiratory tract instability and need management by a respiratory physician.

PSYCHOLOGICAL DISORDERS

Beyond physical sequelae, a burn injury can also result in severe psychological and emotional distress due to the traumatic event itself and due to the scarring and deformities left even after the exhaustion of a plastic surgeon's armamentarium. It is said, "Time is a great healer". A burn surgeon realizes the truth of this statement not only in the healing of even extensive wounds but also in the recovery from emotional trauma. However, scars whether physical or psychological do remain to a greater or lesser extent. In contrast to other injuries and adult victims, the burn injuries in children do cause psychological problems in parents as well. This is because of their concern for the child's future, especially with respect to matrimony, when they grow up. Not only for victims who have postburn sequelae on the face is it difficult to find a match but also for patients who have scars in usually covered areas especially on the breasts as this fact cannot be disclosed to all prospective life partners. Parents of girls in marriageable age group do move from one plastic surgeon to another in the hope that some "cosmetic surgery operation" may solve their problem or at least there must be some cream or lotion the application of which will fade away the scars. The large number of proprietary creams available in the market for the purpose and their high turnover in amount of cream and money is a testimony to the fact that the patient and their parents are ready to do anything to achieve scar less skin. Expression of inability to do any further by the plastic surgeon leads to depression.

SUMMARY

The burn is a devastating injury with a lot of immediate morbidity and mortality to the victim, great financial implications to the patient, his/her family, and to the government and an unending list of postburn sequelae and the ever-changing improvements in techniques to manage them. This chapter attempts to present the most common problems and principles of their management over which the reader can build up from his own experience and study of further literature.

REFERENCES

1. Robson MC, Barnett RA, Leitch IOW, Hayward PG. Prevention and treatment of postburn scars and contracture. World J Surg. 1992;16:87-96.
2. Li J, Chen J, Kirsner R. Pathophysiology of acute wound healing. Clin Dermatol. 2007;25(1):9-18.
3. Wilkinson HN, Hardman MJ. Wound healing: Cellular mechanisms and pathological outcomes. Open Biol. 2020;10: 200223.
4. Gushiken LFS, Beserra FP, Bastos JK, Jackson CJ, Pellizzon CH. Cutaneous Wound Healing: An Update from Physiopathology to Current Therapies. Life (Basel). 2021;11:6659(p.1-15).
5. Ebanks JP, Wickett RR, Boissy RE. Mechanisms regulating skin pigmentation: the rise and fall of complexion coloration. Int J Mol Sci. 2009;10(9):4066-87.
6. Greenhalgh DG. A primer on pigmentation. J Burn Care Res. 2015;36(2):247-57.
7. Tyack ZF, Pegg S, Ziviani J. Postburn dyspigmentation: its assessment, management, and relationship to scarring–a review of the literature. J Burn Care Rehabil. 1997;18(5):435-40.
8. Chadwick S, Heath R, Shah M. Abnormal pigmentation within cutaneous scars: A complication of wound healing. Indian J Plast Surg 2012;45:403-11.
9. Maranda EL, Wang MX, Shareef S, Tompkins BA, Emerson C, Badiavas EV. Surgical management of leukoderma after burn: A review. Burns. 2018;44(2):256-62.
10. Grover R, Morgan BDG. Management of hypopigmentation following burn injury Burns. 1996;22:627-30.
11. Tredget EE. Pathophysiology and treatment of fibroproliferative disorders following thermal injury. Ann N Y Acad Sci. 1999;888:165-82.
12. Berman B, Maderal A, Raphael B. Keloids and Hypertrophic Scars: Pathophysiology, Classification, and Treatment. Dermatol Surg. 2017;43 Suppl 1:S3-S18.
13. Kwan PO, Tredget EE. Biological principles of scar and contracture. Hand Clin. 2017;33(2):277-92.
14. Sullivan T, Smith J, Kermode J, McIver E, Courtemanche DJ. Rating the burn scar. J Burn Care Rehabil. 1990;11(3):256-60.
15. Draaijers LJ, Tempelman FR, Botman YA, Tuinebreijer WE, Middelkoop E, Kreis RW, et al. The patient and observer scar assessment scale: A reliable and feasible tool for scar evaluation. Plast Reconstr Surg. 2004;113(7):1960-5;1966-7.
16. Nguyen TA, Feldstein SI, Shumaker PR, Krakowski AC. A review of scar assessment scales Semin Cutan Med Surg. 2015;34: 28-36.
17. Lipman K, Wang M, Berthiaume E, Holloway J, Da Lio A, Ting K, et al. Evaluating current scar assessment methods. Ann Plast Surg. 2020;84(2):222-31.
18. Janis JE, Kwon RK, Attinger CE. The new reconstructive ladder: modifications to the traditional model. Plast Reconstr Surg. 2011;127 Suppl 1:205S-212S.
19. Harrison CA, MacNeil S. The mechanism of skin graft contraction: an update on current research and potential future therapies. Burns. 2008;34(2):153-63.
20. Cho YS, Jeon JH, Hong A, Yang HT, Yim H, Cho YS, et al. The effect of burn rehabilitation massage therapy on hypertrophic scar after burn: a randomized controlled trial. Burns. 2014;40(8): 1513-20.
21. Ault P, Plaza A, Paratz J. Scar massage for hypertrophic burns scarring-A systematic review. Burns. 2018;44(1):24-38.
22. Nedelec B, Couture MA, Calva V, Poulin C, Chouinard A, Shashoua D, et al. Randomized controlled trial of the immediate and long-term effect of massage on adult postburn scar. Burns. 2019;45(1):128-39.
23. Atiyeh BS, El Khatib AM, Dibo SA. Pressure garment therapy (PGT) of burn scars: evidence-based efficacy. Ann Burns Fire Disasters. 2013;26(4):205-12.

24. Macintyre L, Baird M. Pressure garments for use in the treatment of hypertrophic scars-a review of the problems associated with their use. Burns. 2006;32(1):10-5.
25. Arno AI, Gauglitz GG, Barret J, Jeschke MG. Up-to-date approach to manage keloids and hypertrophic scars: A useful guide. Burns. 2014;40(7):1255-66.
26. Finnerty CC, Jeschke MG, Branski LK, Barret JP, Dziewulski P, Herndon DN. Hypertrophic scarring: the greatest unmet challenge after burn injury. Lancet. 2016;388(10052):1427-36.
27. Momeni M, Hafezi F, Rahbar H, Karimi H. Effects of silicone gel on burn scars. Burns. 2009;35(1):70-4.
28. Meaume S, Le Pillouer-Prost A, Richert B, Roseeuw D, Vadoud J. Management of scars: updated practical guidelines and use of silicones. Eur J Dermatol. 2014;24(4):435-43.
29. Loordhuswamy AM, Elango S. (2021). Interferon therapy for hypertrophic scars and keloids. [online] Available from https://www.intechopen.com/chapters/75901 [Last accessed May, 2024].
30. Parrett BM, Donelan MB. Pulsed dye laser in burn scars: Current concepts and future directions. Burns. 2010;36(4):443-9.
31. Brewin MP, Lister TS. Prevention or treatment of hypertrophic burn scarring: A review of when and how to treat with the Pulsed Dye Laser. Burns. 2014;40(5):797-804.
32. Kuehlmann B, Stern-Buchbinder Z, Wan DC, Friedstat JS, Gurtner GC. Beneath the Surface: A Review of Laser Remodeling of Hypertrophic Scars and Burns. Adv Wound Care (New Rochelle). 2019;8(4):168-76.
33. Goutos I, Clarke M, Upson C, Richardson PM, Ghosh SJ. Review of therapeutic agents for burns pruritus and protocols for management in adult and paediatric patients using the GRADE classification. Indian J Plast Surg. 2010;43(Suppl):S51-62.
34. Goutos I. Burns pruritus--a study of current practices in the UK. Burns. 2010;36(1):42-8.
35. Weisshaar E, Kucenic MJ, Fleischer AB Jr. Pruritus: A review. Acta Derm Venereol Suppl (Stockh). 2003;(213):5-32.
36. Bromm B, Scharein E, Darsow U, Ring J. Effects of menthol and cold on histamine-induced itch and skin reactions in man. Neurosci Lett. 1995;187(3):157-60.
37. Hettrick HH, O'Brien K, Laznick H, Sanchez J, Gorga D, Nagler W, et al. Effect of transcutaneous electrical nerve stimulation for the management of burn pruritus: A pilot study. J Burn Care Rehabil. 2004;25(3):236-40.
38. Chung BY, Kim HB, Jung MJ, Kang SY, Kwak IS, Park CW, et al. Post-Burn Pruritus. Int J Mol Sci. 2020;21(11):3880.
39. Pribaz JJ, Fine N, Orgill DP. Flap prefabrication in the head and neck: a 10-year experience. Plast Reconstr Surg. 1999;103(3):808-20.
40. Guo L, Pribaz JJ. Clinical flap prefabrication. Plast Reconstr Surg. 2009;124(6 Suppl):e340-50.
41. Daugherty THF, Pribaz JJ, Neumeister MW. the use of prefabricated flaps in burn reconstruction. Clin Plast Surg. 2017;44(4):813-21.
42. Pribaz JJ, Fine NA. Prelamination: defining the prefabricated flap--a case report and review. Microsurgery. 1994;15(9):618-23.
43. Jabir S, Frew Q, El-Muttardi N, Dziewulski P. A systematic review of the applications of free tissue transfer in burns. Burns. 2014;40(6):1059-70.
44. Ibrahim AE, Skoracki R, Goverman JG, Sarhane KA, Parham CS, Abu-Sittah G, Best al. Microsurgery in the burn population - a review of the literature. Ann Burns Fire Disasters. 2015;28(1):39-45.
45. Seth AK, Friedstat JS, Orgill DP, Pribaj JJ, Halvorson EG. Microsurgical burn reconstruction. Clin Plast Surg. 2017;44:823-32.
46. McCauley RL. Correction of Cervical Burn Contractures. RL McCauley (Ed). Functional and Aesthetic Reconstruction of Burn Patients. Boca Raton: Taylor and Francis; 2005. pp. 347-57.
47. Onah II. A classification system for postburn mentosternal contractures. Arch Surg. 2005;140(7):671-5.
48. Kurtzman LC, Stern PJ. Upper extremity burn contractures. Hand Clin. 1990;6(2):261-79.
49. McCauley RL Reconstruction of the pediatric burned hand. Hand Clin. 2000;16(2):249-59.
50. Zweifel CJ, Guggenheim M, Jandali AR, Altintas MA, Künzi W, Giovanoli P. Management of microstomia in adult burn patients revisited. J Plast Reconstr Aesthet Surg. 2010;63(4):e351-7.
51. Khare N, Patil SB, Kale SM, Sumeet J, Sonali I, Sumeet B. Normal mouth opening in an adult Indian population. J Maxillofac Oral Surg. 2012;11(3):309-13.
52. Karki D, Mehta N, Narayan RP. Post-burn axillary contracture: A therapeutic challenge! Indian J Plast Surg. 2014;47(03):375-80.
53. Aykan A, Ozturk S, Dede M, Keskin U. Constricting wide abdominal burn scar and pregnancy. Euro J Plast Surg. 2012;36(7):463-6.
54. Mitsukawa N, Saiga A, Satoh K. Protocol of surgical indications for scar contracture release before childbirth: women with severe abdominal scars after burn injuries. J Plast Surg Hand Surg. 2015;49(1):32-5.
55. Van Gelder ZJ, Snoeks A, van Zuijlen PPM, de Vries R, Pijpe A. Complications during Pregnancy after Abdominal Burn Scars: A Review. Euro Burn J. 2023;4:35-54.
56. Lee SH, An SJ, Kim NR, Kim UJ, Kim JI. Reconstruction of Postburn Contracture of the Forefoot Using the Anterolateral Thigh Flap. Clin Orthop Surg. 2016;8(4):444-51.
57. Dua K, Verma V, Dua A. Beard and moustache reconstruction. Indian J Plast Surg. 2021;54(4):483-8.
58. Gabilondo Zubizarreta F, Meléndez Baltanás J. Expanded visor flaps for post-burn beard reconstruction. EJ Plastic Surg.1998;21:399-401.
59. Kumar P. L-shaped scalp flap for moustache reconstruction in a patient with an acid burn of the face. Burns. 1996;22:413-6.
60. Rajput R. Postburns hair restoration of eyebrow, eyelash, moustache, beard and scalp areas. Indian J Burns. 2015;23:26-31.
61. Epstein J. Facial Hair Restoration Hair Transplantation to Eyebrows, Beard, Sideburns, and Eyelashes. Facial Plast Surg Clin N Am. 2013;21:457-67.
62. Farjo B, Farjo N, Williams G. Hair transplantation in burn scar alopecia. Scars Burns Heal. 2015;1:2059513115607764.
63. Yoo H, Moh J, Park JU. Treatment of postsurgical scalp scar deformity using follicular unit hair transplantation. Biomed Res Int. 2019;2019:3423657.
64. Menick FJ. Nasal reconstruction. Plast Reconstr Surg. 2010;125(4):138e-150e.
65. Menick FJ. Nasal reconstruction with a forehead flap. Clin Plast Surg. 2009;36(3):443-59.
66. Sinha M, Scott JR, Watson SB. Prelaminated free radial forearm flap for a total nasal reconstruction. J Plast Reconstr Aesthet Surg. 2008;61(8):953-7.
67. Bhandari PS. Total ear reconstruction in postburn deformity. Burns. 1998;24(7):661-70.

68. Bos EJ, Doerga P, Breugem CC, van Zuijlen PP. The burned ear, possibilities and challenges in framework reconstruction and coverage. Burns. 2016;42(7):1387-95.
69. Ray E, Wu T, Nazarian Mobin SS, Reinisch J, Urata MM. Review of options for burned ear reconstruction. J Craniofac Surg. 2010;21(4):1165-9.
70. Yamada A, Imai K, Nomachi T, Fujimoto T, Morimoto K. Total reconstruction of the burned auricle. Burns. 2007;33(1):112-20.
71. Guo P, Jiang H, Yang Q, He L, Lin L, Pan B. Burned Ear Reconstruction Using a Superficial Temporal Fascia Flap. Ear Nose Throat J. 2021;100(10_suppl):1134S-8S.
72. Louis PJ, Aponte-Wesson RA, Fernandes RP, Clemow J. Autogenous and prosthetic reconstruction of the ear. Oral Maxillofac Surg Clin North Am. 2013;25(2):271-86.
73. Gottlieb LJ, Pielet RW, Levine LA. An update on phallic construction. Adv Plastic Reconstr Surg. 1994;10:267-83.
74. Kropp B, Cohn JE, Wang W, Sokoya M, Ducic Y. Free tissue transfer penile reconstruction. Semin Plast Surg. 2019;33(1):24-9.
75. Kowal-Vern A, Criswell BK. Burn scar neoplasms: A literature review and statistical analysis. Burns. 2005;31(4):403-13.
76. Khan K, Schafer C, Wood J. Marjolin Ulcer: A comprehensive review. Adv Skin Wound Care. 2020;33:629-34.
77. Futrell JW, Myers GH. The burn scar as an "immunologically privileged site". Surg Forum. 1972;23:129-31.
78. Korniluk A, Koper O, Kemcna H, Dymicka-Piekarska V. From inflammation to cancer. Ir J Med Sci. 2017;186(1):57-62.
79. Conlon C, Pupa L, Reece EM, Chu CK, Yu JZ, Vorstenbosch J, et al. When Benign Becomes Cancer: Malignant Degeneration of Chronic Inflammation. Semin Plast Surg. 2021;35(3):159-163.
80. Sinha S, Su S, Workentine M, Agabalyan N, Cheng M, Gabriel V, et al. Transcriptional Analysis Reveals Evidence of Chronically Impeded ECM Turnover and Epithelium-to-Mesenchyme Transition in Scar Tissue Giving Rise to Marjolin's Ulcer. J Burn Care Res. 2017;38(1):e14-e22.
81. Nthumba PM. Marjolin's ulcers: Theories, prognostic factors and their peculiarities in spina bifida patients. World J Surg Oncol. 2010;8:108.
82. Bazaliński D, Przybek-Mita J, Barańska B, Więch P. Marjolin's ulcer in chronic wounds - review of available literature. Contemp Oncol (Pozn). 2017;21(3):197-202.
83. Kanth AM, Heiman AJ, Na r L, Giammarin A., Carpenter C, Ricci JA, et al. Current Trends in Management of Marjolin's Ulcer: A Systematic Review. Journal of Burn Care & Research. 2020;42(2):144-151.
84. Bozkurt M, Kapi E, Kuvat SV, Ozekinci S. Current concepts in the management of Marjolin's ulcers: outcomes from a standardized treatment protocol in 16 cases. J Burn Care Res. 2010;31(5):776-80.

CHAPTER

35

Medicolegal Aspects of Burn Injuries

Chandrakant, Sujata Sarabahi, Manish Kumath, Reisha Rijal

INTRODUCTION

Fire has played a multipurpose role in the Indian history. It has been used not only for cooking food but also for religious purposes (like "*havans*"), for blessing couples during marriage ceremonies, and also for sterilizing instruments for surgery (*Sushruta*). Over the years, it has been very often misused for committing homicide or suicide or even for destruction of evidence of the crime committed. Even though "dowry deaths" due to modes other than burns were prevalent in the West in the Middle Ages, "bride burning" or "dowry deaths" has continued to plague the Indian society even in the twenty-first century. Thus, burns in any female within 7 years of marriage are considered significant and culpable before the law until proved otherwise.

The Webster's dictionary of English language has described "burns" as the injuries caused by application of dry heat, moist heat, abnormal cold, chemical substances, poison, electricity, or lightning and characterized by reddening, blistering, or charring. For medicolegal purposes, injuries caused by lightning, electricity, X-rays, radiation, friction of body tissues, and ultraviolet radiation are also included in burn injuries.

Scalds are a kind of burn injuries resulting due to the application of a liquid object, usually hot water and other liquids at or near their boiling point or from steam. There is no singeing of hair or charring of tissues. It resembles like a second-degree burn showing reddening with formation of blisters with different shapes and sizes, with a well-defined, demarcated line of differentiation. If punctured, there is a red base.

Chemical burns are caused by corrosive substances like acids or alkalis, characterized by redness of skin, formation of ulcers, acute inflammation, and discoloration and staining of skin.

In all burn cases, the extent and pattern of the burn injury should be assessed and documented, if possible, on line diagram of a body. The extent and pattern of the burn injury is of particular interest for treatment and prognosis. Those are equally helpful in understanding and determining the cause of death and in reconstructing the case (e.g., clue as to how the burn occurred). Pattern is assessed by examining the body that sustained the burn injury. The extent of the burn is assessed by measuring the percentage of burnt surface. To give a clear picture of the degree of severity, burn injuries are classified in various ways depending on the depth of burn or on percentage of the body surface area involved. Some of the important classifications are given in the following text.

CLASSIFICATION OF BURNS

Classification of burns is based on the depth of burn injury severity is defined on basis of percentage of body surface area involved. There are various classifications for assessing burn depth but usually the following types are used.

Dupuytren's Classification

Burn injuries were divided by Dupytren into six categories depending upon the loss of external and internal tissues of the body.

- *First-degree burns*: There is simple redness of skin, erythema, and no scar formation on healing.
- *Second-degree burns*: There is acute inflammation and formation of blisters. Burns are very painful. There is no scar formation on healing.
- *Third-degree burns*: There is destruction of cuticle and part of true skin. Subsequently, healing results in scar formation.

- *Fourth-degree burns*: There is loss of whole skin with loss of nerve endings so burns are not painful. There is scar formation on healing.
- *Fifth-degree burns*: There is loss of deep fascia and internal tissues, and there is scar formation on healing, associated with deformities.
- *Sixth-degree burns*: There is charring of external and internal tissues with injuries to whole limbs including bones and other organs of the body.

This classification is no longer used because it is difficult to differentiate the various degrees clinically and they do not relate well to the prognosis.

Wilson's Classification (Modern Classification)

Wilson's classification is also known as "modern classification" and is based on the *depth* of the injury. Here, Dupuytren's classification has been grouped into three types:

1. *Epidermal (first- and second-degree burns)*: The burned part is red and there is formation of blister which is covered by pale, avascular epidermis surrounded by a thin bright area of inflammation, but on healing no scar formation results.
2. *Dermoepidermal (third- and fourth-degree burns)*: There is loss of cuticle and part of true skin (whole thickness). On complete healing, there is formation of scars. These types of burns are very painful due to the irritation of nerve endings surrounding the affected tissues.
3. *Deep (fifth- and sixth-degree burns)*: There is charring of external and internal tissues including bones with destruction of nerve endings. Burns are relatively less painful. Healing results in formation of scars, contractures, and deformities.

Clinical Classification for Medicolegal Purposes

According to this classification, depending upon the destruction or damage to epidermis or dermis (*depth*), burns are grouped into two categories:

1. *Partial-thickness burns*: When there is loss of epidermis and part of dermis. These burns are very painful.
2. *Full-thickness burns*: When there is loss of whole of epidermis and dermis. These burns are painless.

Extent of Burn Area Estimation

The Rule of Nine is used to estimate the *total body surface area* (TBSA) involved in burn. It estimates the percentage of body surface burnt. The whole body is taken as 100% and specific part of the body is given 9% or multiple of 9% as follows:

Part of body	% of body surface
Head and neck	9%
Right upper limb	9%
Left upper limb	9%
Right lower limb	18%
Left lower limb	18%
Anterior trunk	18%
Posterior trunk	18%
Perineum	1%
Total	100%

Lund and Browder Chart

It is regarded by most authors as the most accurate one for burn TBSA assessment as it takes into consideration the age of the person, where the percentage of body surface area for head and neck decreases and that for lower limbs increases as the child ages. It is considered more useful in pediatric burns. Practically, Rule of Nine is as accurate in adults as Lund and Browder chart but in pediatric cases, the latter holds more accuracy.

Rule of Palms

Rule of Palms is used in case of scattered and isolated burns where the palmar surface of the victim (including digital surface area) is roughly equal to 1% of his/her own *body surface area*.

Crow–Glassman Scale

Severely burned bodies are best classified by the Crow–Glassman scale, as given in **Table 1**.

TABLE 1: Crow–Glassman scale.

Level	Features
1	Second-degree burns, sometimes with singeing of the hair; visual identification is possible
2	Burns of varying severity, sometimes with thermal destruction/amputation of ears, genitals, hands, or feet; visual identification may still be possible
3	Consumption by fire with partial amputation of arms and/or legs; cerebral cranium is intact
4	Bony lesions of the cerebral cranium; residual extremities still present
5	Fragmented skeletal remains without soft tissue

EFFECTS OF BURNS

Effect of heat transmission in burns leads to the following consequences:

- *Burns of the tissues*: External findings include burns of skin, singeing of hair, and tissue destruction by fire. Internal findings include burns and consumption of internal organs including bones, edema, mucosal bleeding, and destruction of the airway mucosa.
- *Changes in the content and distribution of tissue fluid*: Externally, blisters are present. Internally, there is vaporization of body fluids, rupture of abdominal wall with prolapse of intestinal loops, fluid leakage from mouth and nose, heat hematoma, and accumulation of fat in body cavities, vessels, or heart.
- *Fixation of the tissue*: External findings include leather-like, brownish fixation of the skin. Internally, there is induration of organs and muscles, and fragmentation of red blood cells (RBCs).
- *Shrinking processes*: Externally, there is tightening and splitting of skin, protrusion of tongue, petechial hemorrhages of neck and head, and development of pugilistic attitude. Internally, there is development of so-called puppet organs (shrinkage of organs).

The effects of burns mainly depend on the following factors:

- *Duration of exposure*: The greater the duration of exposure, the more severe the burns.
- *Age*: Young children, infants, and older individuals suffer from burns more severely than adults.
- *Temperature*: The higher the temperature, the greater the damage and severe the burns as the human skin is tolerant to a very narrow range of external temperatures, usually between 20 and 44°C. Lower temperatures which can be tolerated for short periods can cause burns if exposure is prolonged. Similarly, an object at 44°C can cause burns if applied for 5 hours or more. On the other hand, at 60°C, only 10 seconds of exposure is sufficient to cause a burn injury. "Kangri burns"are very commonly seen in Kashmiris due to the close contact of lower abdomen with cisterns called "kangris" for the purpose of warmth.
- *Extent and part of body*: Surface area and part of the body are more important than the degree of burns. Burns on the head, neck, trunk, and genitals are relatively more dangerous than on other parts of body.
- *Clothing*: Presence of clothing, layers, type, and fit of fabric can alter the outcome of a burn injury.

OBJECTS PRODUCING BURNS

Objects producing burns are: (1) Highly heated solid objects or molten metal; (2) flames causing singeing of hairs and blackening of skin; (3) kerosene oil, petrol, etc., produce sooty blackening; (4) explosives produce tattooing and blackening; (5) X-ray and radiation cause redness of the skin with shedding of hairs and pigmentation of the surrounding skin; (6) ultraviolet rays cause acute eczematous dermatitis; (7) corrosive substances cause ulcerated patches; (8) microwave burns, which do not ionize, so its primary effect is heating which heats the body tissues with more water content (like muscle) than those with lower water content (like fat). There may be erythema and blisters on the skin, and muscles show similarities with electrical burns. For a forensic expert, the causative agent of burn is required to be known after death. Based on the details of the appearance, the causative agent can be identified with certainty.

The most common burns all over the world are the ones sustained due to dry heat which cause damage due to conduction or radiation. If applied beyond a certain time, they cause charring or coagulative destruction in the body. Burns from flames usually leave shadow areas of unaffected skin like in the creases (axilla, groin), which are spared from direct exposure.

If exposure to flames is for very short duration, only the tips of the hair all over the body are singed (eyelashes, eyebrows, and pubic and scalp hair). The melting of the keratin at the distal end of the hair and its resolidification on cooling leaves a blob at the end of the hair shaft. If the duration of exposure is prolonged, there is complete burning of the hair.

Corrosive burns: These are rarely accidental. Usually, they are associated with a homicidal intent, as seen in the Indian scenario. Death due to corrosive burns is uncommon, and homicidal attacks are done with the intention to maim the victim and not to kill. The most common agent used is sulfuric acid which is also called "oil of vitriol" and the act is, therefore, called "vitriolage".

The burns due to acids and alkalis usually give a trickle-like pattern. The nature of injury produced in the skin is usually typical for different corrosive agents, and hence the appearance of the wounds is an indication of the nature of the causative agent. Sulfuric acid-destroyed areas show a gray or black appearance; nitric acid produces yellow-brown discoloration of the skin. Strong alkalis react with skin and tissue lipids to give the wounds a soft, slippery, and slimy look which is initially grayish and later on attain a brown tinge. Prolonged exposure to petrochemicals like kerosene and petrol results in blistering. The blisters are initially creamish and turn yellow after a short time.

Indian Penal Code sections 326A and 326B are used in cases of acid attacks. IPC section 326A deals with voluntarily causing grievous hurt by use of acid and 326B deals with cases where acid is thrown or an attempt is done to throw acid. Punishment under section 326A is

10 years (not less than 10 years) but may extend to life imprisonment with fine and under 326B, it is 5 years (may extend to 7 years and also be liable to fine).

Scalds: If burns are due to splashing of hot liquids, a trickle pattern is seen which indicates the posture of the patient at the time of contact. The worst scalds are seen in the area of initial contact, and it decreases in intensity as the cooling liquid flows away, whereas in case burns are due to immersion in hot liquids, the severity of damage is uniform till the sharply demarcated margin. Scalds do not cause singeing of hair as in case of burns due to dry heat. Scalds particularly become important in cases of children where there can be suspicion of neglect or torture apart from homicide. One such case is immersion burns where the child is immersed in hot water in a tub or any vessel in order to punish or torture him. When the child is forcibly placed in the water, and the child reflexively withdraws from the water toward his body, a characteristic pattern of burn is produced where knee, popliteal fossa, and a portion of abdomen are spared **(Fig. 1)**. Spill burns can occur when a child pulls a vessel of hot water spilling the liquid over its body. It is important to correlate the history with the pattern of burns.

BURN INDEX

This index system was developed by the Brook Army Medical Centre, Burn Unit of the US Army, for ascertaining the effectiveness of treatment and prognosis of burns. According to this system, 0.5 point is denoted for each percent area of second-degree burns and 1 point for each percent of third-degree burns. At about 45 points, the mortality rate is calculated to be approximately 50%. However, this system is not used anymore. Details of newer methods is given in Chapter 3.

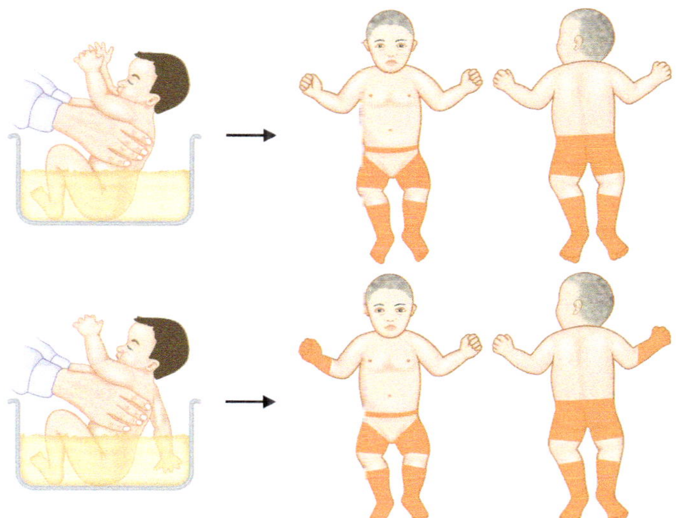

FIG. 1: Scald injury pattern in a case of immersion burn of a child.

ANTEMORTEM AND POSTMORTEM BURNS (FIGS. 2 TO 5)

Many times, burnt or charred bodies are discovered and the question arises whether the victim succumbed to burns or otherwise. Also, burning of the bodies can be done to conceal a homicide. Determining the actual cause of death becomes even more important in such cases. Victims may have died due to inhalation of toxic fumes or due to some other reason like strangulation or other violent acts and then burned later. It is, therefore, essential to differentiate the antemortem burns from postmortem burns by their characteristic features **(Table 2)**.

When burn injury is sustained before death, immediate and late reactions of inflammation and healing

TABLE 2: Differentiating features of antemortem and postmortem burns.

	Antemortem burns	Postmortem burns
Evidence of vital reaction, line of redness	Present	Absent
Vesicles	Fluids present containing albumins, chlorides	No fluid; only air present
Inflammation	Signs of inflammation, formation of granulation tissues, pus, and sloughs	Absent
Healing	Process of reparative changes present	Absent
Enzymes estimation	Increase in enzymes estimation	Nil
Carboxyhemoglobin in blood	Present	Absent
Carbon soots in upper respiratory tracts	Present	Absent
Pugilistic attitude/boxer attitude	Present	+/−
Carbon soot in stomach due to reflex swallowing	Present	Absent

set in which will be absent if a dead body is burnt. To check for the vitality of the injury, the burn wound should be inspected for gross and microscopic changes. Grossly, erythematous margins and blisters with proteinaceous fluid can be present. There can be other signs of inflammation and healing as pus and granulation tissues. Microscopic changes such as separation of dermoepidermal junction and epithelial breakage can be appreciated by histological examination in antemortem burn cases. However, inflammatory reactions may take a few hours to be evident.

Apart from the burn injury on the skin, there are other vital signs which are present in cases when a person has sustained burn injuries when alive. These are as follows:

- *Soot inhalation*: Presence of soot into the bifurcation of the bronchial tree is considered a definite vital reaction. Abundant mucous secretion can be present in the lung airways.
- *Soot swallow*: Soot may be swallowed by a living person during burn and particles may be found in the stomach or upper part of the small intestine.
- *Smoke inhalation*: If someone is burnt alive, positive carbon monoxide (CO) findings are expected. However, one should keep in mind the age of the victim, circumstances, and site of fire as well as normal CO levels (as it varies among smokers and nonsmokers).
- *Crow feet*: Presence of crow feet could be regarded as the sign of vitality. These are areas in forehead, around eyes, or nasolabial folds which are deprived of burns or soot deposits. It is mainly thought to occur due to wrinkling of skin because pain and smoke cannot penetrate into the base of wrinkles. However, another mechanism suggested is shrinkage of skin due to heat causing the wrinkle.
- *Heat shock protein (Hsp) expression*: Hsp27 and Hsp70 are expressed in pulmonary tissue, renal tubules and vessels, and cardiovascular tissue after heat exposure in fire-related fatalities. Both are present in short-term survivors, and Hsp70 are greatly expressed in long-term survivors.
- *Respiratory tract*: Coagulation necrosis or severe edema of mucosa, capillary, and venous hyperemia with microhemorrhages and pulmonary edema

In case a body is burned after death, the vital reactions mentioned above are not present in skin or internally in most cases. If the skin actually catches fire, black brittle masses of dead burnt skin are formed. Postmortem drying of weeping serum in a burnt area may lead to a parchment-like surface which can be mistaken for third-degree burn. Underlying muscles may show redness and cooked appearance in both antemortem and postmortem burns.

When a body is burnt, either dead or alive, muscle contractures occur from prolonged heat exposure. This is more commonly seen in the flexor muscles which produces a "boxer's" or pugilistic attitude. On the other hand, contracture of paraspinal muscles produces opisthotonus. Pugilistic attitude of a burnt body can occur in both antemortem and postmortem burnt bodies. However, if pugilistic attitude is not seen in a charred body, postmortem burns should be suspected because body could have been burnt after rigor mortis had set in. In cases where a body is burnt after the death of the victim, the area of body in contact with the ground (in lying-down position) will remain unburnt as opposed to an alive victim where they try to escape burn and are in upright position.

Besides these, there are certain *postmortem artifacts* seen in burn cases which may mimic antemortem injuries in a way that these artifacts may be mistaken as a cause of death and burn injury as concealment of homicide. These artifacts are as follows:

- *Postmortem external wounds or splitting of skin*: Skin, if heated after death, contracts markedly leading to splits in the body surface called "heat ruptures". These mimic antemortem wounds and are seen on the extensor and flexor surface of the joints. These may also be seen following forceful attempt to straighten a limb after death. They can, however, be differentiated from the antemortem wounds by absence of bleeding in the deeper tissues. It may, however, be difficult to differentiate between antemortem skin injury and postmortem skin splitting due to burn if the burns are very deep and involve the deeper tissues also.
- *Heat hematoma*: This is found following prolonged application of intense heat to the head which causes the brain to compress into a cooked mass; the dura may split and blood may boil out of the diploe or venous sinuses. At times, even the brain may ooze out as a frothy paste. The skin as well as underlying skull bones may be totally charred. These changes must be differentiated from antemortem skull fractures. Heat hematoma appears as a chocolate-brown spongy mass which is brittle and has a honeycomb appearance. In case of doubt as to whether the hematoma is antemortem or postmortem artifact in burn, one can preserve the hematoma for determination of carboxyhemoglobin. If the person was alive during burn (meaning the hematoma is due to burn), the person would have inhaled the smoke and carboxyhemoglobin level in blood would rise, which would in turn be increased in the hematoma. In case the person was burnt after sustaining the head injury (leading to hematoma), the blood level of carboxyhemoglobin would not be high, and

thus, hematoma CO level will not be high. The most common site for heat hematoma formation is the parietotemporal region.

- *Heat fractures*: On postmortem, some charred bodies often show skull fracture and intracranial hemorrhages. These arise either due to violence before death or due to action of heat on skull and brain or injury to head after death. Antemortem fractures can be differentiated from postmortem fractures by the presence of tissue reaction at the margin of the fractured bone on microscopy, which would occur only if the victim survived for at least an hour after injury. In case the victim dies in lesser time, these changes will not be seen; instead, there will only be external signs of trauma. Heat fractures of skull have been described as two types by Mortiz:
  1. Increased intracranial pressure forcing contents of skull outward leading to an explosive fracture. These fractures are seen along suture lines along with brain matter exploding out in a circular pattern.
  2. Drying and shrinkage of outer table leading to stellate fractures and fragmentation of outer table which cracks on handling, during postmortem, thus mimicking a depressed fracture. However, in antemortem depressed fractures, the outer table shows shelving along the edges of the fracture.

DEATH CAUSED BY HEAT AND FLAMES WITHOUT VITAL SIGNS

In the literature, the frequency of such kinds of death is mentioned to be around 3–10%. If natural death and homicides are excluded, the following causations can be taken into consideration:

- *Cyanide intoxication*: It can rapidly develop in the victim depending on the materials burnt in the surrounding. In such cases, even increased CO-Hb concentrations may not be present.
- *Flashfire*: In flashfire, death may occur due to apnea from laryngeal spasm, bronchial spasm, vagal reflex, or inhalational heat shock.
- *Oxygen deficiency*: Oxygen depletion by the fire source may cause death.
- *Heat shock*: Reallocation of circulating blood volume due to skin exposure to heat

CAUSES OF DEATH IN BURNS

The death in burn injuries may occur from:

- Primary shock/primary neurogenic shock due to pain, fear, or inhibition
- Secondary shock due to loss of fluids is the most common cause of death in the first 24 hours.
- Acute renal failure with associated biochemical disturbances
- Asphyxia or due to inhalation of smoke, carbon dioxide, or toxic gases like CO, cyanide, acrolein, nitrogen dioxide, etc. Inhalation of toxic gases should be suspected in any case where soot is readily visible in nares or mouth.
- Respiratory failure and development of acute respiratory distress syndrome (ARDS)
- Toxemia
- Septicemia—when the patient survives for some duration, it is the most common cause of death in the later period. It may be due to infection of widespread burn injury or secondarily due to pneumonia.
- Pulmonary embolus secondary to prolonged immobilization or thrombosis in vessels due to direct effect of thermal injury
- Gastrointestinal disturbances including Curling's ulcers
- Other complications, like tetanus, gangrene, amyloidosis, Marjolin's ulcer, etc.
- Nonburn injuries (e.g., in cases of fall from height while trying to escape fire)

Spontaneous combustion of the human body cannot occur as the human body is composed of 75% of its own weight of water.

Preternatural combustibility is rare. Inflammable gases like hydrogen sulfide, methane, or hydrogen are sometimes formed in the alimentary tract due to bacterial fermentation during the digestive process. These gases are belched out from the anal region and if a flame or flame-producing object is nearby the body, it may cause burns at the site. Similarly, during surgical procedures on large bowel or near that area, while using electric cautery a mild explosion may occur due to ignition of these gases. However, complete combustion of body is impossible.

MEDICOLEGAL ASSESSMENT OF A BURN VICTIM

A medical officer, forensic expert, forensic pathologist, or any other doctor, who is authorized by the concerned state government by issuing a Gazette Notification under subsection 3 of Section 174 of the Criminal Procedure Code, can conduct Medicolegal autopsies. Basically, the following facts are required to be determined in case of alleged deaths due to burn injuries: (1) Identification of the deceased—age, sex, height; (2) whether the burn injuries are antemortem or postmortem in nature; (3) what are the causes of death in the deceased; (4) whether the burns are accidental, suicidal, or homicidal; and (5) whether any contributing factors are present, such as alcohol/drug intoxication. A visit to the crime scene or at least a proper history and description of the setting of the crime scene is equally important.

Identification

In majority of the cases of burns, bodies are already identified prior to medicolegal autopsy. But in cases of unidentified bodies, detailed examination of bones, jaws, pelvic bones, status of teeth, and obtaining fingerprints from less damaged hands or feet need to be done. In cases of charred bodies, marks of external wounds may be destroyed and determination of age, sex, and height may be difficult. However, even at 2,000°F temperature, all body parts are not destroyed. Fragments of remaining muscles, long, short bones, pelvic bones, teeth, and jaw are carefully examined and X-rays are evaluated. Teeth hold a significant place in identification because they are relatively preserved, especially posterior teeth, even in a charred body.

Accidental Burns (Fig. 2)

Setting: Accidental deaths due to burns are generally reported at the place of work like kitchen, factories, burning houses or buildings or shops, cinema halls (like in case of Uphaar Tragedy, New Delhi), fire in an exhibition (Shastri Park, Meerut, Uttar Pradesh), hotels (Siddhartha Hotel, now known as Vasant Continental Hotel, New Delhi), and rarely in train compartments. A large number of deaths in accidental cinema hall burn injuries also occurs among aged persons, infants, children, intoxicated or drugged persons, or persons suffering from epilepsy or sudden syncope. Mainly the women and men working in the kitchen sustain burn injuries due to leakage of cooking gas, bursting of kerosene oil stoves **(Fig. 4C)**, which is very common in India, falling of kerosene oil lamps, burning candles during sleep, warming during winter seasons from electric heaters or wooden fire in remote areas of smaller cities and villages.

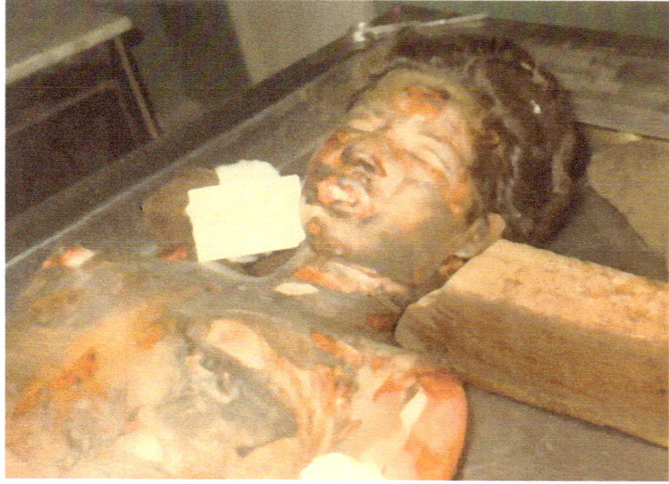

FIG. 2: Case of accidental 100% antemortem burns showing singeing of scalp hair and blackening of face, neck, and upper chest due to clothes catching fire following bursting of kerosene stove.

History: It is always important to find out the medical history of the victim such as epilepsy, muscular disorders, paralysis, peripheral neuropathies, cognitive disabilities, intoxication, etc., which can be the cause for predisposing a person to risk of burn injuries.

Appearance: Usually in cases of accidental burns, one area of body is burned more (than the other area where the body caught fire) and at varying depths. So, the burn is patchy and not uniform.

Suicidal Burns (Figs. 3 and 4)

Setting and history: Suicidal burns are relatively more common amongst Indian women than males due to increasing tension in day-to-day life with domestic problems, harassment by husband or his family members, financial crisis, chronic illness, loss of life of near and dear family member, depression, or suicidal tendencies. Self-immolation is also a way of public protest against some organization or government policies, in which the protestors, in public or other places which are in public view, pour kerosene oil on self and set themselves on fire. In suicidal burns, usually some inflammable material like kerosene oil or petrol is used.

Appearance: The material is poured on the head and other parts of body and then the body is set on fire producing characteristic features like burning/singeing of scalp hairs, eyebrows, and eyelashes, burning, or charring of scalp skin, ears, ear lobes, or temple region. Thus, the burn is mostly from top to bottom and there is usually sparing of soles of feet. It is usually difficult to differentiate between suicidal and accidental burns as in both the cases, victims may try to escape the burn. Careful evaluations of circumstances along with detailed postmortem examination findings are important to suggest suicidal burns.

Homicidal Burns (Figs. 5 to 7)

Cases of homicidal burns are common in India. Generally, kerosene oil, petrol, diesel, alcohol, hot metals, or corrosive substances have been used to inflict burn injuries. There is an increasing trend of homicidal burns in India with the sole intention of taking revenge or concealing

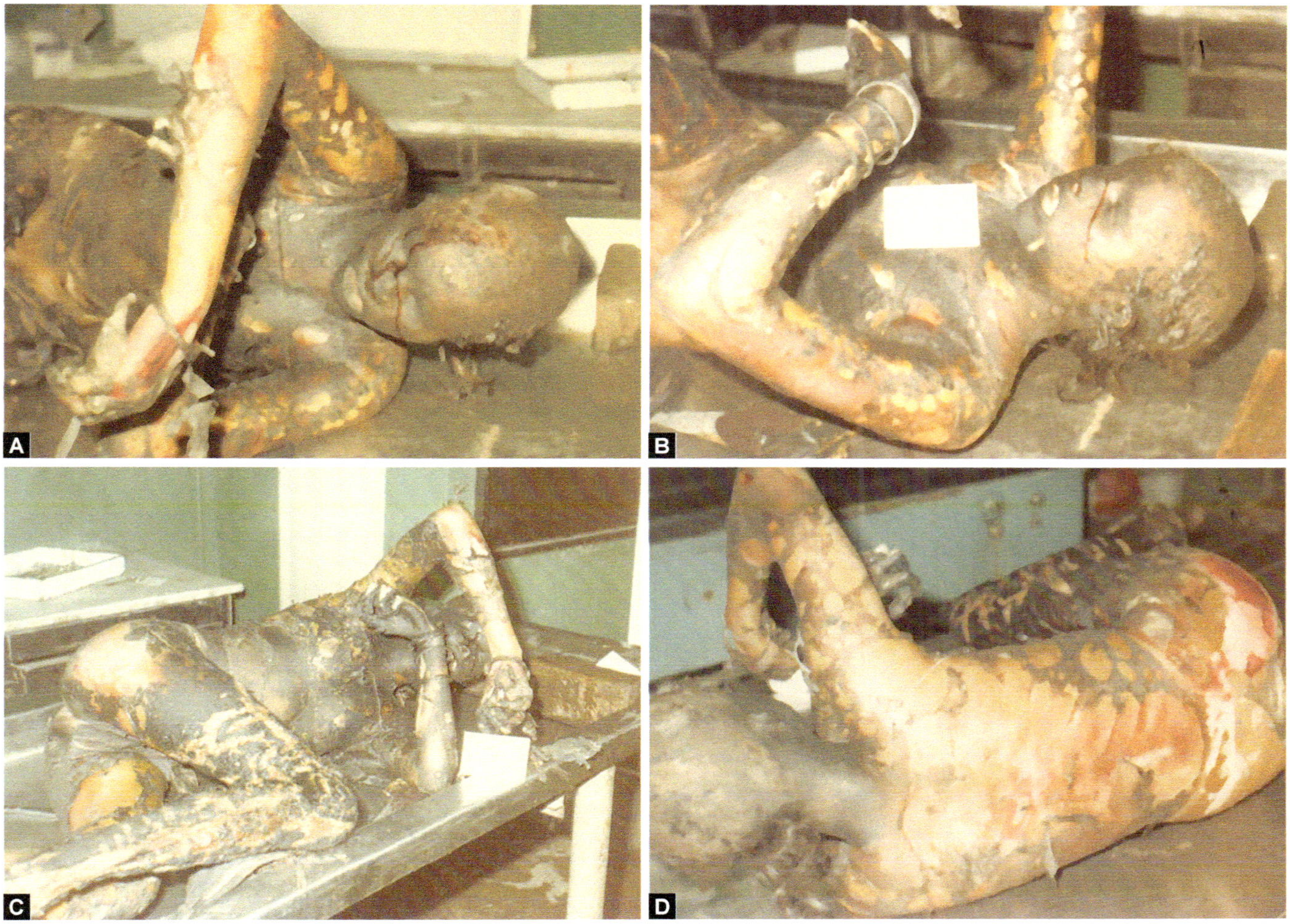

FIGS. 3A TO D: (A) 100% suicidal antemortem burns showing burned scalp hair and charring of both upper arms. (B) Same case in pugilistic attitude with heat rupture in the right inguinal region. Intact bangles indicate no signs of struggle. (C) Same case with pugilistic attitude, charring of skin of right forearm, chest, lower thigh, and knee with heat ruptures in the left lower leg. (D) Same case with charring of skin of scalp and tuft of scalp hair with area of redness over right hip.

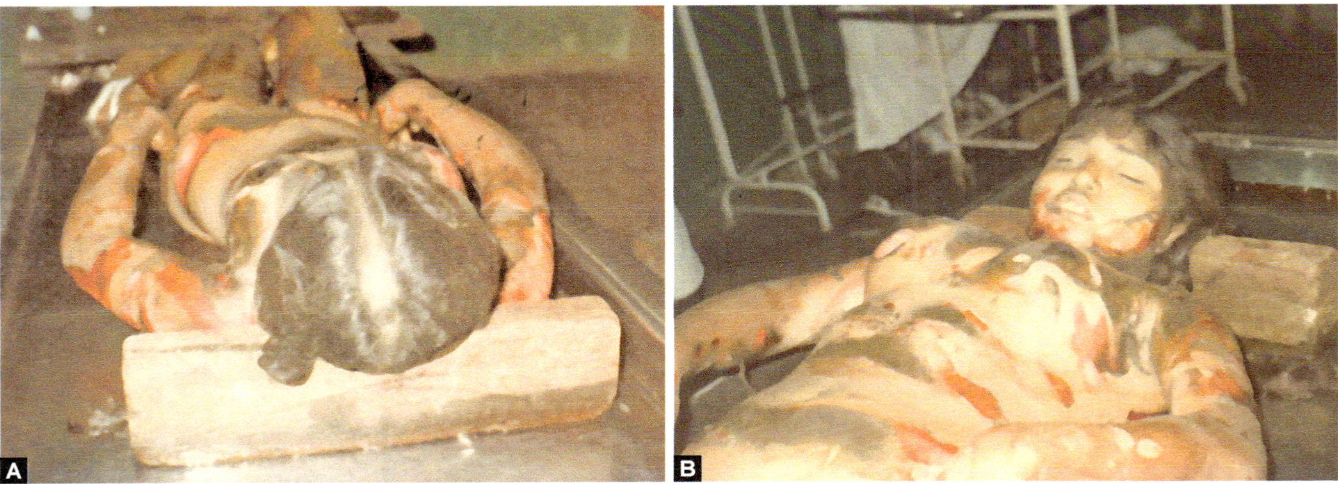

FIGS. 4A TO C: *Continued*

Continued

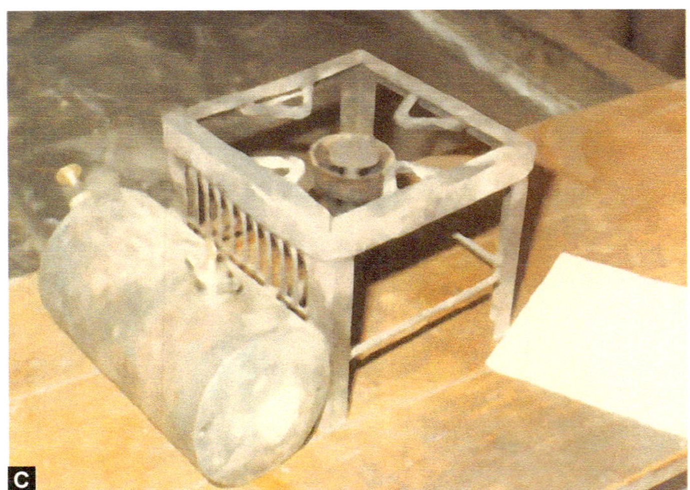

FIGS. 4A TO C: (A) Suicidal burns showing burning of scalp hair and scalp skin in the middle. (B) Same case with singeing of scalp hair anteriorly indicating suicide by pouring of kerosene oil on head also before igniting it. (C) In the same case nonfunctional kerosene oil stove allegedly blamed for accidental burns.

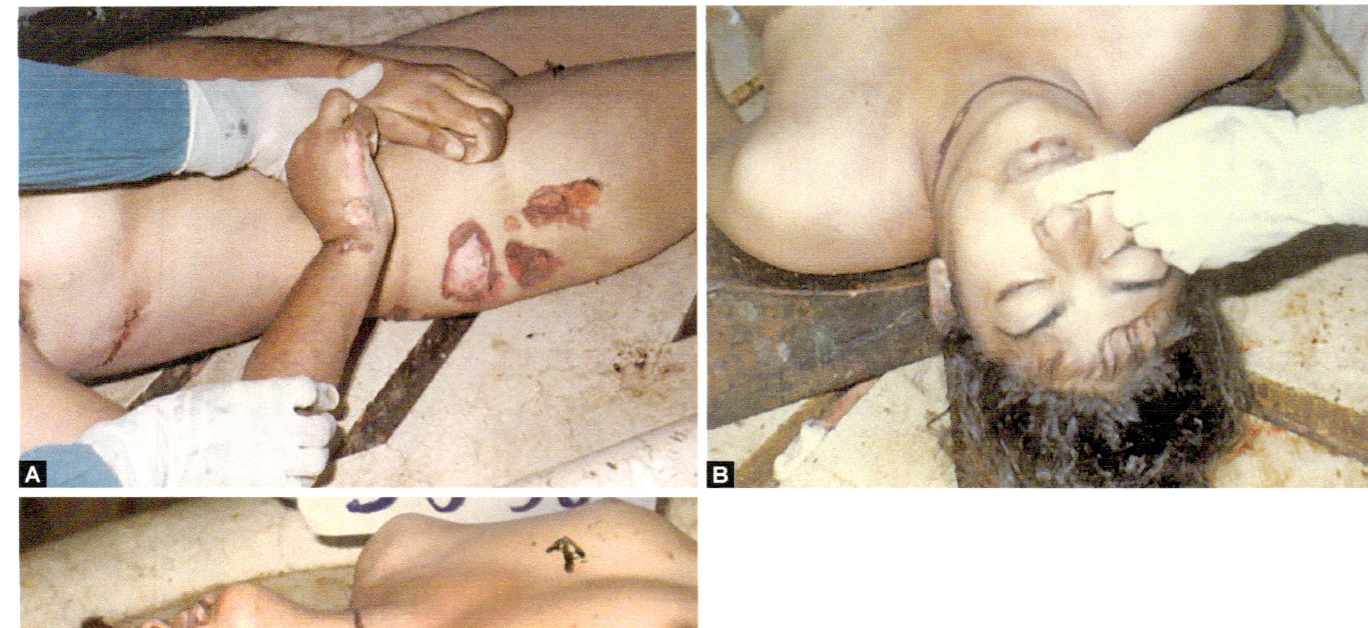

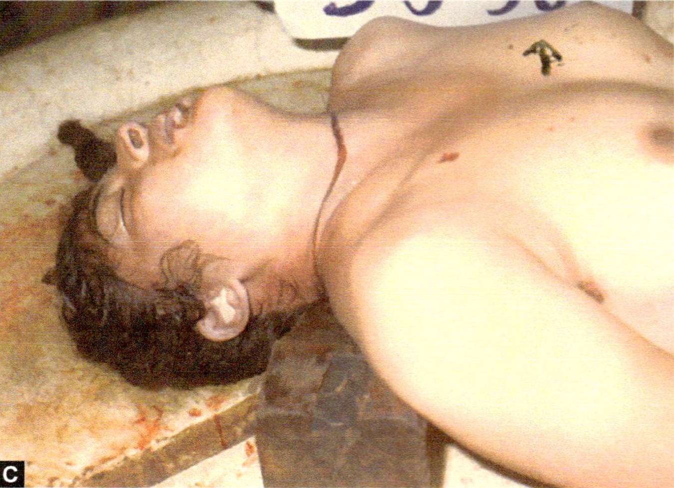

FIGS. 5A TO C: (A) Case of dowry burns with strangulation—deceased showing antemortem scalds on the left index finger and dorsum of right hand and hot metal antemortem burns on the right thigh indicating torture prior to strangulation. (B) Same case with antemortem cigarette burns on lower lip and right side of chest also indicating torture. (C) Same case with deceased showing sign of strangulation on neck.

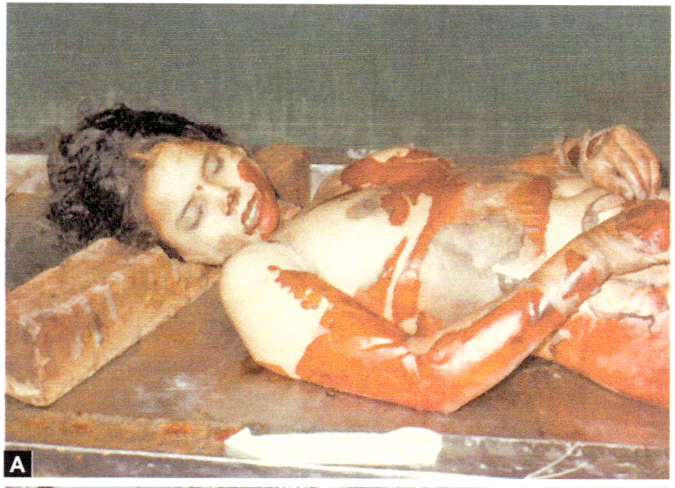

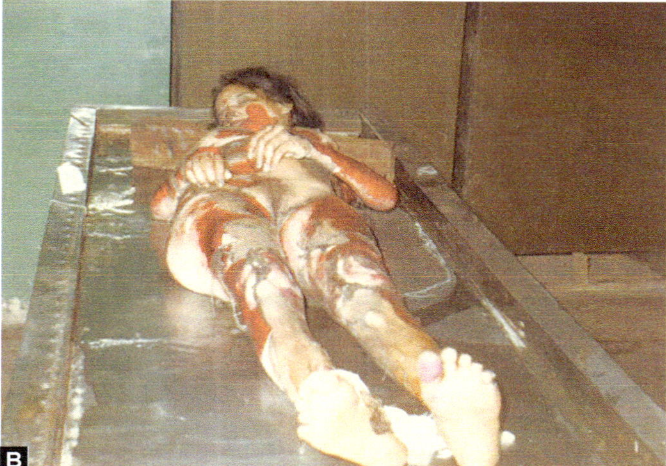

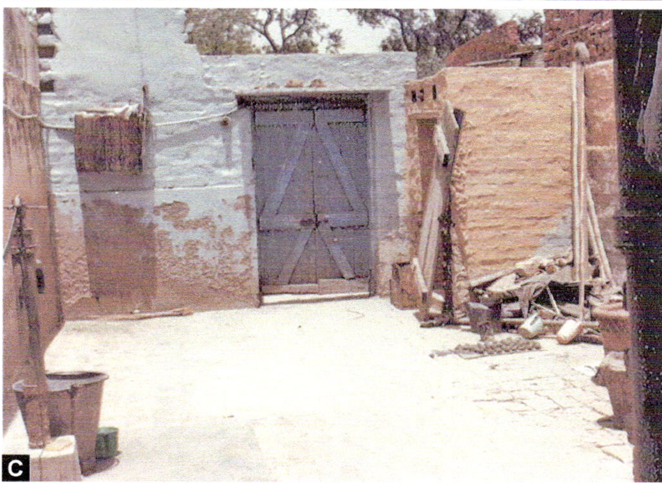

FIGS. 6A TO C: (A) Typical antemortem homicidal burns with normal hair and scalp. (B) Same case with ink impression on right big toe suggestive of recording of statement of the deceased prior to death. (C) In the same case, visit of the scene of crime by the autopsy surgeon who conducted the postmortem—showing door locked from inside.

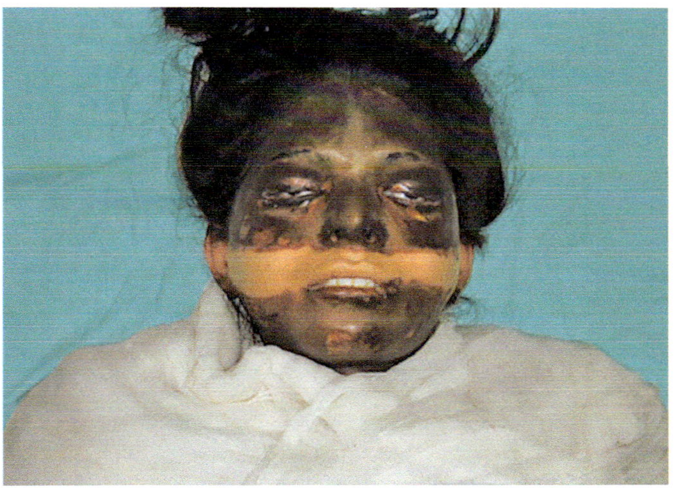

FIG. 7: Typical case of 100% homicidal burns showing intact skin as a white band on the face with surrounding burned skin indicating that the patient was gagged before setting her on fire.

the crime of murder and accordingly bodies are burnt to destroy these evidences. It can be in a closed room which is locked from outside or a secluded place. A detailed postmortem examination including evaluation of circumstances, even a visit to the scene of crime, will help in evaluating the nature of burn injuries and cause of death.

Appearance: If a victim is made unconscious by any other means before burning the body when still alive, one should seek out the signs of vital reactions and note the pattern of burn. In such cases, the body parts in touch with the ground (e.g., while lying) or other objects (e.g., while resting against a wall), remain unburnt or relatively less burnt than the rest of the body. One should also undoubtedly look for other causes of death. Although the skin may be charred, internal organs are relatively preserved even in seemingly charred bodies, which may show the evidences of stab injuries, bullet tracks, or poisons.

CHECKLIST FOR THE EXAMINATION OF BURNT BODIES

Apart from conventional external and internal autopsy findings in cases of burn, the followings should not be missed:

1. *History*: History of diseases which could prevent a person from escaping a fireplace as epilepsy, dementia, paralysis, etc.
2. *Presence of scene of crime on the body*: Certain traces or particles of materials from the crime scene could be found on the body and/or hand of the victim. These should be correlated with that in the crime scene. Traces of molten materials (metals, construction materials like ceiling liners, glass, plastics) can be present. Oddments of objects that may have fallen on the body such as construction material of collapsing building may be found.
3. Traces of oxidizing agents like fire starter or accelerants, inflammable liquids, and kerosene should be sought in clothes, body, and crime scene. When found on the body, clothes should be preserved for confirmation. Also, the bottles of such accelerants, matchsticks, lighters, etc., should be sought.
4. *Clothing*: Type of fabric, clothing layers, localization, extension, pattern, direction of thermal damage on the clothes should be done layer-wise. Correlate with the injuries present on the body.
5. Presence of injuries other than burn that can cause or contribute to death should be sought (e.g., injuries sustained while trying to escape a burning building).
6. *Additional examinations*:
    - Histological examination of the respiratory system for presence of signs of vitality, local heat damage, depth of damage, in an inhalation injury
    - Immunohistochemical investigation of Hsp
    - Examination of fractures by stereomicroscopy for differentiation between fractures caused mechanically from those caused thermally.
    - Toxicological examination of inhalation gas constituents (CO, CN, etc.), central nervous system (CNS) depressants and narcotics, blood alcohol levels

SUMMARY

Medicolegal aspects of burn injury is very important for burn surgeons as majority of the cases are medicolegal. Though it does not affect the management of the patient but accurate documentation at the time of admission of a burn patient is extremely important later for giving evidence in the court of law. Postmortem is a must in almost all these cases to investigate for any other associated cause of death.

BIBLIOGRAPHY

1. Aggrawal A. Textbook of Forensic Medicine and Toxicology, 1st edition. New Delhi: Avichal Publishing Company; 2014.
2. Brahmaji Master P, Chandra Sekhar V, Rangaiah YKC. Differentiating Perimortem and Postmortem Burning. J Evidence based Med Healthc. 2015;2(3):269-71.
3. DiMaio VJM, Dana SE. Handbook of Forensic Pathology, 2nd edition. Boca Raton: CRC Press; 2006.
4. Glassman DM, Crow RM. Standardization model for describing the extent of burn injury to human remains. J Forensic Sci. 1996;41(1):152-4.
5. Gordon I, Shapiro HA, Berson SD. (Eds). Death from burns, exposure to high and low environmental temperatures and electrical injuries. In: Forensic Medicine – A Guide to Principles, 3rd edition. London: Churchill Livingstone; 1988. p. 138.
6. Knight B. Forensic Pathology. London: Edward Arnold; 1994. p. 292 (Chapter 11).
7. Madea B. Handbook of Forensic Medicine, 2nd edition. Hoboken, NJ: Wiley; 2022.
8. Mortiz AR. Personal communication. In: Gordon I, Shapiro HA, Berson SD (Eds), Forensic Medicine – A Guide to Principles, 3rd edition. London: Churchill Livingstone; 1988. p. 149.
9. Polson CJ. Electrical injuries and lightening stroke. In: Polson CJ, Gee DJ, Knight B (Eds), Essentials of Forensic Medicine. Oxford: Pergamon Press; 1984. p. 282.
10. Tsokos M. Forensic Pathology Reviews. Totowa, NJ: Humana Press; 2004.

CHAPTER

36

Legal Requirements in Managing Burn Patients

Atul Kumar Shah

DISCLAIMER

Foregoing presentation is a personal view of the author, based on his personal experience. Any future legal amendments may change these views.

INTRODUCTION

Burn accidents usually take place due to failure to prevent. This trauma has an element of suspicion of a crime added to it in many cases. A treating physician has the responsibility of informing such incidences to legal authority.

Police is constantly engaged in keeping law and order in control. Society needs to support police in maintaining peace and in reporting crime. Police actually has to classify any mishap as crime and subsequently investigate the same. For collecting information, the police force will have to depend on various channels; one of them naturally is the body of citizens. Casualty doctors or treating physicians are duty bound to inform the police when they are managing trauma victims. Although this chapter deals with burn management and legal requirements in treating a burn victim, same procedures are equally applicable to other trauma, poisoning, drowning, suicidal, and homicidal victims.

INDIAN LEGAL SCENE

Indian Penal Code (IPC) enlists various body injuries. Code of Criminal Procedures in section 39 asks every citizen to inform police of any incidence which has harmed any human being. For a treating physician, informing police is, thus, an extension of his duty as a citizen. To the best of knowledge of the author, there is no requirement or compulsion specified in National Medical Commission Act, 2019, except in regulation 1.9 of Code of Medical Ethics 2002.

SOCIAL CIVIC AND MORAL DUTY

Except as required under section 39 (section 40 for village head, police patel or a villager) of the Criminal Procedure Code, the need for informing the police in case of a suspicious burn injury is social as well as moral rather than legal. However, the current sociolegal setup demands that police should be informed, whenever a trauma or burn case of nature, as enlisted here, is received by a treating doctor.

SITUATIONS

All major burns and other major trauma victims when received have to be notified to the police. Unexplained severity, not matching with the history or circumstances, needs reporting. Patients received after several days of burns and without proper treatment, patients likely to succumb to the injury, patients received dead, and mass casualties need to be notified to the police.

Usually, when a patient succumbs to injuries, a certificate of death is required to be issued. In this certificate, the cause of death has to be specified. When the treating doctor is not certain about the cause of death, demand for a medicolegal postmortem has to be made. Such a demand can only be made through a police officer. When the police officer is informed of such a request, his team has to visit the site where death has occurred. He carries out a report of the condition and situation of the body, known as "*panchnama*". He also fills an inquest for a medicolegal postmortem. Later, the body is handed over to this police officer, who takes it to nearby health establishment equipped with postmortem facilities. If the inquest has been filled in odd hours, the body is shifted to a morgue for postmortem later or else the body may be retained, at the request of the police officer, in the same room until shifted for postmortem next day morning. The police enter the scene and fill inquest without wasting time, only if they had been informed when the patient first came for treatment or got admitted.

Sometimes, the patients come from distant places and as per the police codes, the police officers of the area of incidence are required to carry out legal procedures. It is important to inform the nearby police immediately, so that at the time of the death of the patient, the nearby police do not waste time in procedural delays.

Similarly, in patients at extremes of age, extensive burns and evident homicide or suicide, it is better to inform police, as there is a likelihood of death and subsequent postmortem. All road traffic and industrial accidents are also to be reported to police and are governed by the Motor Vehicle Act and the Factories Act. It is the duty of the treating doctor, in his capacity as a citizen or as a person with the information of the mishap, to inform police.

HOW SOON TO INFORM?

The Supreme Court of India in a judgment has clarified that police activities can wait; the life of the victim is important and hence the treatment must be instituted immediately. Some judgments talk of "reasonable time". Therefore, one can conclude that as soon as the emergency care is over and the patient is stabilized, the process of informing the police may be started. Although it is not specified anywhere, we must make efforts not to make any delay in informing the police and this can be considered as within 4–6 hours or in case of very specific situations within 12 hours. Delays further than that may arouse suspicion in the mind of the investigating officers and their cooperation may get reduced.

WHOM TO INFORM?

This can be looked at from two different angles. In large cities, there are several police stations with area demarcations; it may so happen that the burn incident may have occurred in the jurisdiction of one police station and the treating hospital may be in jurisdiction of another police station. If the police station in which the area of accident falls is willing to take the information on phone or if it is not far away and written information can be sent without extra efforts, the same may be done. Doctor can decide to inform the nearest police station as an alternative.

The local police station may not be willing to take such information if the area of incidence is different and many times the approach of the local police station is variable depending on the current officers and their superiors. In case of such difficulties, in many places one can utilize services of police control number 100. Here, telephonic information can be given and it is one of the legal ways of registering information. From suburban areas also, one can call the district police control room and the connecting number is usually the same.

The burn victim comes from far-off places, which may fall in other districts and even other states. The treating doctor or hospital may not waste time in trying to find out contacts of the exact police station of the mishap area for passing on the information. The nearest police station, under whose jurisdiction the treating hospital falls, must, however, be informed without fail. If, for some reasons, the nearest police station shows inability to accept the information, informing police control at 100 is a legal alternative. At many places, police has announced e-mail addresses for accepting such information.

MODE OF INFORMATION

Calling the police station on phone and giving brief particulars of the victim as well as of the incidence is the accepted way of intimation now at most of the places. Each police station has one "on duty" PSO (police station officer) who usually attends the phone and writes down the details. This information is then passed on to the "on duty" IO (investigating officer). The doctor is required to obtain the name of the PSO and ask him as to what time of intimation he has entered in his records. Later, the police station converts this information into their procedural information and enters this into a special register which they call "station diary". On shifting the information to station diary, a diary number or FIR (first information report) number along with the date and year is generated and it may be of help for subsequent communication with the police.

Sometimes, the police insist on a written information, in which case if it is feasible, a letter stating name, age, gender, and address of the victim, address where mishap occurred, time when mishap occurred, time when patient arrived to current health establishment, and whether police has been informed by any other source(s) at any other health establishment(s) treating the patient previously must be sent in duplicate so that proof of receipt can be obtained. As an alternative, such a letter must be prepared in three copies and two copies are handed over to a willing relative of the patient, taking his signature on the third copy stating that he has received a letter for informing the police. The relative then goes to the police station and gets signature of the PSO on the duplicate, which must then be received back in the hospital. This exercise is necessary as it keeps a proof with the hospital that a process of informing the police has been initiated and it saves the hospital staff from running around. The larger and designated government hospitals have a satellite police post inside the hospital, and the information process is managed by specially appointed casualty doctors.

In case of paucity of time and manpower, unwilling relatives, unattended patients and when the nearby police station or the police station of the mishap area have not been reached by phone, call to police at control room number 100 would be sufficient. One must not forget to obtain the name of the person who attends your call at police control room and must register the time of such intimation in the case paper at appropriate place.

Police control room later identifies the responsible police station and transfers the information. Team from the concerned police station visits the hospital and takes note of the mishap as well as the health status of the victim.

BURN INJURIES IN MARRIED FEMALE

When a married woman is brought with extensive burn injuries, the police tend to treat this mishap as a dowry problem unless proved otherwise with circumstantial evidence. If the married life of the victim at the time of mishap is less than 7 years, the police investigation becomes stringent and under a senior officer of the rank not less than a deputy commissioner. Death in such cases would be governed by Section 304B, which became effective from November 19, 1986:

Dowry death

(1) Where the death of a woman is caused by any burns or bodily injury or occurs otherwise than under normal circumstances within seven years of her marriage and it is shown that soon before her death she was subjected to cruelty or harassment by her husband or any relative of her husband for, or in connection with, any demand for dowry, such death shall be called "dowry death", and such husband or relative shall be deemed to have caused her death.

(*Explanation*: For the purposes of this subsection, "dowry" shall have the same meaning as in section 2 of the Dowry Prohibition Act, 1961) (28 of 1961).

(2) Whoever commits dowry death shall be punished with imprisonment for a term which shall not be less than seven years but which may extend to imprisonment for life

CRIMINAL NEGLIGENCE

In a recent Supreme Court judgment, a guideline has been set up before applying section 304A against doctors. Rash or negligent act leading to death can attract imprisonment of up to 2 years and fine. However, the apex court has asked the investigating officers to first obtain sanction from senior government doctors to establish negligence in a particular case before arresting a doctor.

SUMMARY

Informing police is the duty of every citizen and so also of a doctor, when any mishap involving bodily injury is brought to their notice. With usage of electronic media, it has become less procedure oriented and less time consuming to inform police. Physicians treating burns must make sure that legal requirements have been properly met with.

BIBLIOGRAPHY

1. Indian Penal Code. New Code to be implemented from July 2024.
2. Code of Criminal Procedures. New Code to be implemented from July 2024.
3. Indian Medical Council (Professional conduct, Etiquette and Ethics) Regulations, 2002. New Code has been published in gazette but yet to be implemented.

CHAPTER

37

Burn Disfigurement and Physical Impairment Calculations

Atul Kumar Shah

INTRODUCTION

A burn victim is entitled to compensation for current and future medical expenses, lost wages, disfigurement, emotional sufferings, mental impairment, and physical disability. The concept of physical impairment has to evolve among the burn specialists so that the award of disability can become more meaningful. It must be realized that disability is not purely a medical condition. Burn disfigurement causes a lot of mental stress and undermines one's sense of self-worth and confidence. As their wounds heal, burn patients also endure agonizing pain. Burn victims endure excruciating pain during skin grafting operations and other surgical treatments to restore the harm caused by their injuries. Burn survivors may experience altered sensitivity to temperature, altered metabolism, and physical trauma. Emotional scars start to show as the physical wounds start to heal. As a wild guess based on the experience of the fellow burn specialist colleagues, approximately one million burn injuries could be occurring in our country per year. Approximately half of these injuries are treated by medical professionals; about one-tenth of them are hospitalized. Of those hospitalized, many have major burns involving at least 25% of their total body surface. Between 20,000 and 25,000 patients with burns die and approximately half a million sustain substantial or permanent disabilities resulting from their burn injury. There has to be a very extensive and collective efforts to bring out the burn incidence data in the country, and the use of census may also be taken to determine the prevalence of disfigured individuals.

Burn can result from negligence or inaction on the part of another person. Accidents are frequently the result of a combination of careless actions or inaction on the part of one or more people or organizations. There are numerous activities and causes that might cause burns. There are risks that one cannot always predict, whether at work or at home. According to law, everyone has an obligation to act in a way that would be expected of a reasonably prudent person in the same or comparable circumstances. A person or organization violating this obligation is accountable for any harm or damage resulting from their actions to the person or entity being harmed.

This obligation is established by statutes or earlier court rulings that have developed over time. As burn or trauma specialists, we need to be knowledgeable about the legal aspects of being granted a handicap by several agencies that are deemed qualified. To grasp the idea, we currently have to rely mostly on the Motor Vehicle Insurance Act and the Workmen's Compensation Act of 1923 in India. Any individual with a physical impairment may experience limits in their functional abilities, which are referred to as "disability to sustain" or "disability to earn livelihood." This may be evident from the World Health Organization (WHO) definitions. This chapter describes the difference between concepts of physical impairment and disability and guidelines to quantify permanent physical impairment (PPI).

IMPAIRMENT AND DISABILITY

A permanent or temporary loss of mental or physical abilities, as well as anomalies, constitute an impairment. Physical limitations include paralysis, amputation, diabetic retinopathy, and even burn disfigurement or contracture.

Functional limitation is the partial or complete incapacity to carry out tasks that are essential for motor, sensory, or mental functions within the range and style of a person's typical abilities, such as walking, lifting objects, speaking, reading, writing, counting, and showing interest in and interacting with the environment. Physical impairment is the source of functional limits, which can be temporary, permanent, or reversible. The idea is that these functional constraints should always be measurable. Thus, these restrictions can be classified as progressive or regressive.

A disability is an inability to do one or more tasks with ease. These are the "activities" that are widely acknowledged as fundamental and necessary elements of everyday life, such as self-care, social interactions, and economic activities, based on an individual's age, gender, and conventional social role. The underlying causes of this handicap are functional limits and physical impairment. The length of the functional limitation also plays a role in determining whether a handicap is permanent, long-term, or short-term. However, the majority of the time we can be dealing with permanent disability and PPI. The WHO has recently suggested revising the previous definitions and introduced new terms like "participation restriction" and "activity limitation." Activity is the degree to which a person operates on a personal level; it can vary in type, length, and quality. Participation refers to the kind and degree to which an individual engages in a given situation in life; limitations can be imposed on participation based on contextual considerations, health issues, or activity impairments. According to Webster's Dictionary, disability is defined as:

- *State of being disabled*: Absence of competent physical, intellectual, or moral power, fitness or the like; also, an instance of such lack
- Legal incapacity, incompetence, or disqualification

Disability also has an impact on one's physical, social, psychological, and professional life. Because disability is not just a medical condition, a trauma specialist is therefore ill-equipped and ill-qualified to determine an individual's level of disability. Thus, physicians must limit their practice to assessing and attesting to physical disability. The medical expert hopes that by doing this, the appropriate authorities will then take into account the social, psychological, and occupational factors when determining the individual's disability. Regretfully, at this time, the compensation authorities or the courts of law have limited understanding to demarcate between physical impairment and disability. Although facial burns would not be seen as a disability at all, imagine how someone with such a condition could ever work as a model, marketing executive, or TV news reader! A paraplegic, on the other hand, is regarded as severely disabled, but he makes a fortune performing vocally or giving talks on stress management, and he also gets the accommodations that are given to people with disabilities. Under the Workmen's Compensation Act, disability may be divided into three periods.

1. *Permanent disability:* When a person reaches the stage of maximal rehabilitation and their residual physical impairment remains constant, they are said to have a permanent handicap. This includes permanent damage or loss of use of a portion of their body. There is a temporal component to this, and it takes at least 6 months, if not more, to define persistent physical impairment. Partial or total temporary impairment is possible.
2. *Temporary total disability:* A person who is receiving therapy and is temporarily completely physically disabled is said to have a temporary total disability.
3. *Temporary partial disability:* The time after a person has fully recovered from a total physical impairment or when their physical impairment was initially only partial is referred to as a temporary partial disability. In most cases, irreversible physical impairment of a nonreversible nature resulting in permanent disability may be eligible for ultimate legal compensation. Therefore, a medical professional must assess any long-term physical impairment and might even be called as an expert witness in court. All medical graduates, who are recognized under Medical Council of India Act 1956's schedule I, are eligible to issue certifications of physical disability.

Contrary to what attorneys occasionally demand, a medical graduate does not necessarily need to be a specialist. But although the court relies on the medical professional's certified evaluation of physical disability, it always takes into account the specialization and experience of the certifying physician. The most widely used resource in the US for determining and classifying a person's permanent impairment is the American Medical Association's guides to the evaluation of permanent impairment. "Loss, loss of use, or derangement of any body part, organ system, or organ function" all come under the definition of impairment given in the 5th edition of the "Guides" (Chicago, IL: American Medical Association: 2000). At the organ system level, impairments are defined using objective measures like heart or lung function.

Based on medical expert's consensus, impairment ratings were created to represent a person's capacity to carry out fundamental everyday activities, such as grooming, speaking, standing, walking, sleeping, and engaging in social and leisure activities. The effects of accommodations are typically not taken into consideration in impairment evaluations (the usage of glasses for vision assessment is an exception).

Although there are frequently inadequate scientific data to back these ratings, the impairment ratings in the "Guides" try to link objective measures of organ function with the functional tasks of conducting activities of daily life. Even more challenging is estimating work ability from an impairment grade. Work is an intricate and personalized activity, even though many professional activities involve these aspects of daily living. Therefore, while the impairment ratings may be used to evaluate certain aspects of job ability, they do not represent an individual's capacity for work. A disability is a change in a person's ability to fulfill obligations in their personal, social, or professional life as a result of an impairment or functional limitation. The "Guides" discuss work competence rather than disabilities explicitly.

To the best of the author's knowledge, the only reliable Indian documents that currently available are (1) Workmen's Compensation Act, (2) "The Manual for Doctors to evaluate Permanent Physical Impairment" and (3) "Evaluation of Impairments, Disabilities in the case of Occupational and other Diseases and Accidents." In September 1981, a meeting of specialists was held on disability evaluation and the another in December 1981 National Seminar on Disability Evaluation and Dissemination were held in New Delhi and served as the foundation for the contents of the Manual for Physicians to Evaluate Permanent Physical Impairment. The Manual was released in March 1982 and had the support of the WHO, All India Institute of Medical Sciences (New Delhi), and Director General Health Services (Government of India).

- Simplified examination criteria helped in granting certifications of PPI. The assessment of PPI in burns of the head and neck **(Table 1)** and burns of the trunk and genitalia **(Table 2)** is outlined here. Guidelines for assessing physical disability in upper limb burns are:
- Objective assessment of functional impairment is a prerequisite for estimating permanent impairment; it is not a subjective judgment.

TABLE 1: Guidelines for the evaluation of physical impairment in burns of head and neck. Ten-point formula for evaluating postburn disfigurement of head and neck. Total 100 points and 8 equitable components.

Component	Equitable points	Split-up points
1. Scalp and vault (10)	10 (includes forehead)	
a. Scalp (disfigurement alone)	2.5	
b. Scalp and skull bone involvement	10	
2. Eye brows (10)	5 each, 10 for both	
a. Part of one	2.5	
b. Total loss of one	5	
3. Eyelids (20)	6 for upper, 4 for lower	
a. Upper—skin disfigurement alone	Per side	1.5
b. Upper—deformity or full-thickness loss	Per side	6
c. Lower—skin disfigurement alone	Per side	1
d. Lower deformity or full-thickness loss	Per side	4
4. Pinna (20)	10 per side	
a. Anterior or posterior—skin disfigurement alone	Per side	2.5
b. Deformity due to full-thickness involvement of skin and cartilage without obliteration of meatus	Per side	7.5
c. Deformity due to full-thickness involvement of skin and cartilage with obliteration of meatus		10
5. Nose (10)	10	
a. Skin cover disfigurement alone		2.5
b. Deformity due to full-thickness involvement with both nares patent		7.5
c. Full-thickness deformity with one nare obliterated (7.5 +1.25)		8.75
d. Full-thickness deformity with both nares obliterated		10
6. Cheek and lateral area of face (10)	5 each	
a. Skin cover disfigurement alone	Per side	1.25
b. Deformity or full-thickness loss	Per side	5
7. Lips—upper or lower (10)	5 each	
a. Lips—upper or lower skin cover disfigurement	Per side	1.25
b. Lips—upper or lower skin cover disfigurement crossing midline		2.5
c. Deformity or full-thickness loss of one lip alone		5
d. Deformity due to involvement of both lips leading to contracture of oral opening		10
8. Neck (10)	10	
a. Skin cover disfigurement alone	Per side	2.5
b. Deformity due to involvement of skin, muscles, or deeper tissues		10

TABLE 2: Guidelines for evaluation of physical impairment in burns of trunk and genitalia.

1. Front of trunk and abdomen excluding breasts	Female	10	Male	5
2. Breast each side	Female	20	Male	5
Total or as per detail below				
a. Only skin cover disfigurement each side	Female	5	Male	1.25
b. Involvement of skin, areola and nipple and/or deformity resulting in loss of function—per side	Female	15	Male	5
c. Involvement of skin, areola, Nipple and parenchyma and/or deformity resulting in loss of function per side	Female	20	Male	5
3. Total back	Female	5	Male	10
4. Groins—each side	Female	5	Male	5
5. Buttocks—each side	Female	2.5	Male	2.5
6. Genitalia total	Female	30	Male	60
a. Skin loss resulting in mild deformity	Female	7.5	Male	15
b. Severe contracture of orifices or sloughing of urethra or severe deformity of penis	Female	30	Male	60

- When the clinical condition reaches a point where the treatment is not going to improve, the estimation and measurement should be done. Usually, the medical professional assessing the case for the PPI Certificate will determine this time frame in accordance with the certificate's standard format.
- The arm component and the hand component separately make up the upper limb.
- Loss of motion, muscle strength, and coordinated movements are measured when determining the degree of function loss in the arm component.
- Determining prehension, sensation, and strength constitutes the measurement of hand component for loss of function. As indicated in the hand component portion of the assessment proforma for upper extremity, opposition, lateral pinch, cylindrical grasp, spherical grip, and hook grasp must be evaluated in order to assess prehension.
- The sum of the functional deficits in the two components determines the impairment of the entire extremity. The Ministry of Social Justice's released guidelines or The Manual for Doctors to Evaluate Permanent Physical Impairment can be used for extremities (http://disabled.socialjustice.nic.in). You can get a detailed format for evaluating extremities at http://socialjustice.nic.in/disabled/part2.htm.

The Workman Compensation Act bases the award on both the employee's earnings and the involved portions. **Table 3** provides a quick explanation of the current award of compensation. On January 4, 2018, the central government notified the public of the criteria for evaluating the degree of certain specified disabilities, including acid attack victims, under the Rights of Persons with Disabilities Act, 2016 (49 of 2016). The same has been published in Section 3 of Part II of Gazette of India No. 61. "Acid Attack Victims" are included in Section G on page 81 of this Gazette **(Table 4)**.

PLIGHT OF A BURN SURVIVOR

The entire family is affected when one of the wage earners has a serious burn. In contrast to other forms of trauma or illness, burn care is time-consuming, painful and expensive. The treatment depletes the family's financial resources. Victims of industrial burn accidents are no exception. Even after the wounds have healed, the burn survivor still has several ongoing issues:

- Physical and emotional trauma
- An injury that leaves one in pain
- Disfigurement
- Organ damage
- Metabolic and biochemical damage
- Sensitivity to temperature change

LEGAL RIGHTS OF BURN SURVIVORS TO COMPENSATION

Depending on the circumstances associated with burn injury, the burn victim may be eligible to receive any of the following compensation which heavily relies on the current level of legal and social assistance. Compensatory damages are meant to "compensate" the injured party for a variety of losses or damages. These can include disfigurement, any kind of physical or mental impairment or disability, current medical expenses, lost wages, anticipated future medical expenses, and anticipated future loss of wages.

- *Past and prospective medical expenses*:
  - In-patient hospital treatment
  - Surgical procedures

TABLE 3: Indicative compensation payable currently under the Workmen's Compensation Amendment Act (46 of 2000).

Instance	Minimum compensation
a. Where death result from injury	₹80,000
b. For permanent total disability	₹90,000
c. For permanent partial disablement	As per % of loss of earning capacity. It varies from 1 to 90%
d. Temporary disablement	An amount equal to 50% of monthly wages subject to maximum ₹1,000. For up to 3 days disablement, no compensation is payable. But if it is more than 3 days but less than 28 days, then 50% of the balance days wages are payable. If it is more than 28 days, then the 3 days wages are not deducted
After the 2,000 amendment, the maximum liability under the act for workman is limited to a monthly wage of ₹4,000. In such cases, the compensation based on actual last monthly wage is as follows:	
a. Where death result from injury	An amount equal to 50% of monthly wages of the deceased workman multiplied by the relevant age factor or ₹80,000—whichever is more
b. For permanent total disability	An amount equal to 60% of monthly wages of the deceased workman multiplied by the relevant age factor or ₹90,000—whichever is more

TABLE 4: Guideline for assessment in acid attack victims, Gazette of India no. 61 published on January 5, 2018.

Part of body affected	Deficit	% of permanent impairment
Scalp and vault including forehead	Disfigurement alone	5
	Deformity or full-thickness loss	10
Eyebrows (right and left)	Loss of part of one or both	3% each
	Total loss of one or both	5% each
Eyelids—Upper	Skin disfigurement alone	3% each, 5% each
Lower	Deformity or full-thickness loss skin disfigurement alone	2% each
	Deformity or full-thickness loss	3% each
Ear (pinna)	Skin disfigurement alone	2% each
	Deformity due to full-thickness involvement of skin and cartilage without obliteration of meatus	3% each
	Deformity due to full thickness involvement of skin and cartilage with obliteration of meatus	5% each, and 10%
Nose	Skin cover disfigurement alone	3%
	Deformity due to full-thickness involvement with both nares (nostrils)	5%
	Patent	10%
	Full-thickness deformity with one nares obliterated	20%
	Skin cover disfigurement one lip alone	3%, 5%, and 10%
	Deformity or full-thickness loss of one lip alone	
Cheek and lateral area of face	Skin disfigurement	5% each side
	Deformity or full-thickness loss	10% each side
Neck	Skin cover disfigurement	5%
	Deformity due to involvement of skin, muscle or deeper tissue	10%
Breast (female)	Only skin cover disfigurement	5% each
	Deformity resulting in loss of function due to involvement of:	
	• Skin, areola, and nipple	10% each
	• Skin, areola, nipple, parenchyma	15% each
Front of trunk and abdomen excluding breast	Only skin cover disfigurement	5%
	Deformity or full-thickness loss	10%

Continued

Continued

Part of body affected	Deficit	% of permanent impairment
Total back	Only skin cover disfigurement	5%
	Deformity or full-thickness loss	10%
Groins	Only skin cover disfigurement	2% each
	Deformity or full-thickness loss	5% each
Buttocks	Only skin cover disfigurement	3% each
	Deformity or full-thickness loss	5% each
Genitalia	Skin loss resulting in mild deformity	7%
	Severe contracture of orifices or sloughing of urethra or severe deformity of penis	20%
Thigh	Only skin cover disfigurement	3% each
	Deformity or full-thickness loss	5% each
Lower leg	Only skin cover disfigurement	3% each
	Deformity or full-thickness loss	5% each
Foot	Only skin cover disfigurement	3% each
	Deformity or full-thickness loss	5% each
Upper arm	Only skin cover disfigurement	3% each
	Deformity or full-thickness loss	5% each
Forearm	Only skin cover disfigurement	3% each
	Deformity or full-thickness loss	5% each
Hand	Only skin cover disfigurement	5% each
	Deformity or full-thickness loss	10% each

    - Medical managent
    - Psychological guidance
    - Cosmetic surgery for scar improvements
    - Rehabilitation through exercise
    - Rehabilitation through occupational therapy
- Payment for past and future income losses
- Job retraining through vocational rehabilitation
- *Pain and suffering compensation*: As a result of their injuries, burn survivors may be entitled to compensation for the pain and suffering they have already experienced and may experience in the future.
- *Loss of consortium*: This is a new idea for the Indian judiciary, and case legislation may include it shortly. In cases when an injury is so severe as to interfere with the wounded party's ability to maintain a marriage, the spouses of burn survivors may be eligible for compensation. A very real harm could come to the affected family member. In an appropriate instance, several courts acknowledge the spouse of the injured party's claim to compensation for loss of services, love, companionship, society, affections, sexual relations, and consolation through a loss of consortium action. A claim for loss of consortium is distinct from a claim made by an injured party. It is specific to the spouse of the injured person and is payable through a separate damage recovery.

INDIAN LEGAL ENFORCEMENTS

Survivors of burns who have irreversible contractures, keloids, grafted areas, deformity, and similar conditions may be eligible for assistance from the state. Experts in burn and trauma care must present a unified front in order to provide burn survivors with these advantages. One major accomplishment of the Indian disability movement is the passage of the "Persons with Disabilities (Equal Opportunity, Protection of Rights and Full Participation) Act, 1995" (also known as the "People with Disabilities Act"). The goals of this Act, which include full participation and equality for people with disabilities, are outlined in the Preamble. The Act seeks to uphold and advance the social and economic rights of those with disabilities.

"A person suffering from not less than forty percent of any disability as certified by a medical authority" is what is meant to be understood as a person with a disability under Section 2(t). Section 2 lists the following disabilities: Mental retardation, mental illness, low vision, hearing impairment, cerebral palsy, blindness, mental illness, and people who have recovered from leprosy. The "National Trust for Welfare of Persons with Autism, Cerebral Palsy, Mental Retardation and Multiple Disabilities Act, 1999" also provides coverage for autism and multiple disabilities.

The new "Rights of Persons with Disabilities Act, 2016 (49 of 2016)" came into force and included all the above specified disabilities.

Prevention of Disability

The current state of the law only serves to illustrate a limited interpretation of the right to health, placing a strong focus on measures to prevent, cure, improve, or eliminate disability. These are, after all, conditions that typically exist prior to the onset of disability and, as such, have no rational connection to the rights of the disabled. For instance, Section 25 of the Persons with Disabilities Act, 1995, says the following: "The appropriate governments and the local authorities, with a view to preventing the occurrence of disabilities, shall, within the limits of their economic capacity and development, (a) undertake or cause to be undertaken surveys, investigations, and research concerning the cause of occurrence of disabilities; (b) promote various methods of preventing disabilities"; (c) screen all children at least once a year to identify "at-risk" cases; (d) provide training facilities for primary health center staff; (e) sponsor or cause to be sponsored awareness campaigns and disseminate information about general hygiene, health, and sanitation; (f) take steps for prenatal, perinatal, and postnatal care of mother and child; (g) educate the public through preschool primary health centers, village-level workers, and "*anganwadi*" workers; and (h) raise public awareness about the causes of disabilities and the preventive measures that should be taken.

More susceptible than others, thus it was thought that a specific law would be needed to safeguard them, their belongings, and their well-being. The National Trust Act, also known as the National Trust for Welfare of Persons with Autism, Cerebral Palsy, Mental Retardation and Multiple Disabilities Act 1999, was enacted in response to a common request from families looking for a stable environment for their seriously disabled loved ones. The Act's specific goals are to:

- Empower and enable people with disabilities to live as independently and fully as possible in their community of choice
- Encourage policies that will provide care and protection for people with disabilities in the event that their parent or guardian passes away
- Offer assistance to registered organizations so that they can offer need-based services to families of disabled people covered by this act during times of distress. The establishment of a local-level committee (LLC) with the District Magistrate and other members required by the National Trust Act with one individual with a disability and one representative from a registered organization

Rehabilitation Council of India Act, 1992

In order to control and standardize training programs and policies in the area of rehabilitation for people with disabilities, the Government of India established the Rehabilitation Council of India in 1986. Since most people involved in education, vocational training, and counseling of people with disabilities lacked professional qualifications, there was an urgent need for minimal requirements. The prospects of disabled people thriving in the workforce are significantly impacted by subpar educational and training standards. Consequently, the council's status was raised to that of a statutory entity in 1992 by an Act of Parliament, which had the following objectives:

- Standardize training courses for professionals dealing with people with disabilities
- Prescribe minimum standards of education and training for various categories of professionals dealing with people with disabilities
- Regulate these standards in all training institutions uniformly throughout the country
- Promote research in rehabilitation and special education
- Maintain central rehabilitation, register for registration of professionals
- Training requirements for 16 different categories of rehabilitation workers are governed by the Rehabilitation Council of India (RCI). The Council is actively supporting research and training projects that make use of the expertise of both specialized and traditional academic institutions. In order to prevent the permanent incapacitation of government employees due to physical or mental disabilities, the Ministry of Social Justice and Empowerment amended Section 47 of the Persons with Disability (PWD) Act. This was done through order 6/17/2002-SCS/1925, which states that no employer may terminate or downgrade an employee who becomes disabled while they are employed. If the employee is deemed unfit for their position, they may be transferred to one with the same salary and benefits. If he cannot be placed in any job, he might be maintained on supernumerary duty until a position becomes available that suits him or he reaches the age of superannuation, whichever comes first. A person cannot be refused a promotion just because of their disability.

According to the Rights of Persons with Disabilities Act, 2016 (49 of 2016) rules, the Ministry of Social Justice and

Empowerment has issued several gazette notifications. Here, guidelines for evaluation of the following disability and process of certification are outlined:

I. Locomotor disability including cerebral palsy, leprosy cured, dwarfism, acid attack victims, and muscular dystrophy
II. Blindness and low vision
III. Deaf and hard of hearing and speech and language disability
IV. Intellectual disability and specific learning disabilities
V. Mental illness
VI. Chronic neurological conditions
VII. Hemophilia, thalassemia, and sickle-cell disease
VIII. Multiple disabilities

Only medical boards that have been officially established by state and federal governments are authorized to issue disability certificates. A medical board with a minimum of three members, at least one of whom must be an expert in the relevant field, may be established by the state government. in the event that there is any disagreement or dispute over how to interpret the definitions, classifications, evaluation tests, and the like, the Director General of Health Services at the Ministry of Health and Family Welfare, located in Nirman Bhawan in New Delhi, will be the ultimate authority.

SUMMARY

Advocates frequently challenge the quantification of PPI and the issuance of an authenticated certificate for the same by doctors within the medical and nonmedical communities, there is a lack of knowledge regarding the distinction between physical impairment and disability. The Medical Council of India (MCI) legislation gives medical professionals the authority to grant a certificate of PPI in accordance with the current national norms. Calculation of loss of the earning capacity of a person becomes the responsibility of the authorities appointed for the work. Guidelines for calculating physical impairment in burns of head and neck, face, trunk, and genitalia are based on the area and depth of involvement and calculation can be so based easily in arriving at the percentage of PPI of a particular anatomical component of the body. Efforts are going on at both the national and international levels to help and support disabled persons and burn survivors who would qualify for several of these services.

BIBLIOGRAPHY

1. American Medical Association's Guides to the Evaluation of Permanent Impairment. Chicago, IL: American Medical Association; 2000.
2. Ministry of Social Justice. Guidelines on Disability. online] Available from http://socialjustice.nic.in/disabled PWD Act, 1995.
3. Office of Chief Commissioner for Persons with Disabilities. The Persons With Disabilities (Equal Opportunities, Protection of Rights and Full Participation) Act, 1995. [online] Available from – http:// www.ccdisabilities.nic.in/Act%201.htm [Last accessed June, 2024].
4. Society for Participatory Research in Asia. (1996). Evaluation of impairments, disabilities in case of occupational and other diseases and accidents. Guidelines for the purpose of assessing the extent of specified disability in a person included under the Rights of Persons with Disabilities Act, 2016 (49 of 2016). Published in Gazette of India No. 61 on January 5, 2018, New Delhi.
5. The Employee's Compensation Act 8 of 1923. [online] Available from http://indiacode.nic.in/fullact1.asp? tfnm=192308
6. The Employee's Compensation (Amendment) Act, 2000 Act no. 46 of 2000. [online] Available from http://indiacode.nic.in/fullact1.asp?tfnm=200046
7. The Manual for Doctors to evaluate Permanent Physical Impairment. DGHS, New Delhi, March 1982.

SECTION

7

Organization of Burn Care

CHAPTER

38

Organization of a Burn Unit

Madhuri Gore, Shivangi Saha, Maneesh Singhal

INTRODUCTION

The optimal functioning of a burn unit demands commitment from the burn team and the hospital administration. A specialized burn unit can contribute significantly to the field of burn care as it offers the following advantages:

- Provides high-quality and holistic burn care
- Facilitates accrual of experience
- Permits implementation and evaluation of protocols
- Facilitates collection and analysis of data
- Provides stimulus for innovation and research
- Provides facility for training
- Opportunity to improve the quality of burn care leading to reduction in mortality and morbidity.

The main purpose of a burn unit is to minimize the incidence of infection in burnt patients and to provide comprehensive burn care. The design of a burn unit should be conducive for this purpose. A typical burn unit should have provision for 11–18 patients.[1] The actual number of beds depends on the available data about patient load.

MEMBERS OF BURN TEAM

The core of the burn team is formed by:

- Director of burn unit—He or she maybe a Plastic surgeon or General Surgeon with at least 2 years of experience in burn care.[2] Junior consultant surgeons and training surgeons complete the surgical contingent
- Nurse Manager—with at least 2 years of experience in acute burn care and 6 months of managerial experience.[2] Nursing staff and trainee nurses complete the nursing team
- Critical care intensivist
- Microbiologist
- Nutritionist
- Physical and occupational therapists and respiratory therapists
- Clinical psychologist
- Burn nurse coordinator or manager
- Social worker
- Dressing assistants
- Labor staff

The specialists from the following departments should be available for consultation:

Pediatrics, Ophthalmology, Obstetrics/Gynecology, Internal Medicine, Pulmonary Medicine, Anesthesiology, Radiology, Nephrology, Psychiatry, Neurology, Cardiology, Pathology, Microbiology, General Surgery, Orthopedics, Otorhinolaryngology, Neurosurgery, Hematology.

CASUALTY

The patient-receiving area may be a part of the burn unit or of the Accident and Emergency Department of the hospital. It should be easily accessible and should have an identified attending medical professional available 24 hours.

Facility size: A 12 ft × 12 ft area is comfortable for accommodating patient trolley, personnel, and equipment.

Equipment: Intensive care patient trolley, crash cart with lifesaving equipment, drugs, fluid warmer, shower trolley are essential components of the receiving area.

Weighing facility especially for trolleys should be available as most patients presenting to the emergency are brought on a stretcher or trolley.

Central suction and oxygen supply are desirable. A suction machine and oxygen cylinder with a regulator and humidifier may be an acceptable alternative **(Figs. 1A to D)**. The instrument sets for the following procedures should be available:

- Equipment to examine and secure airway—self-inflating bag, face mask, Guedel airways, supraglottic airways, endotracheal tubes, laryngoscope, and if possible a flexible fiberoptic laryngoscopy should be available

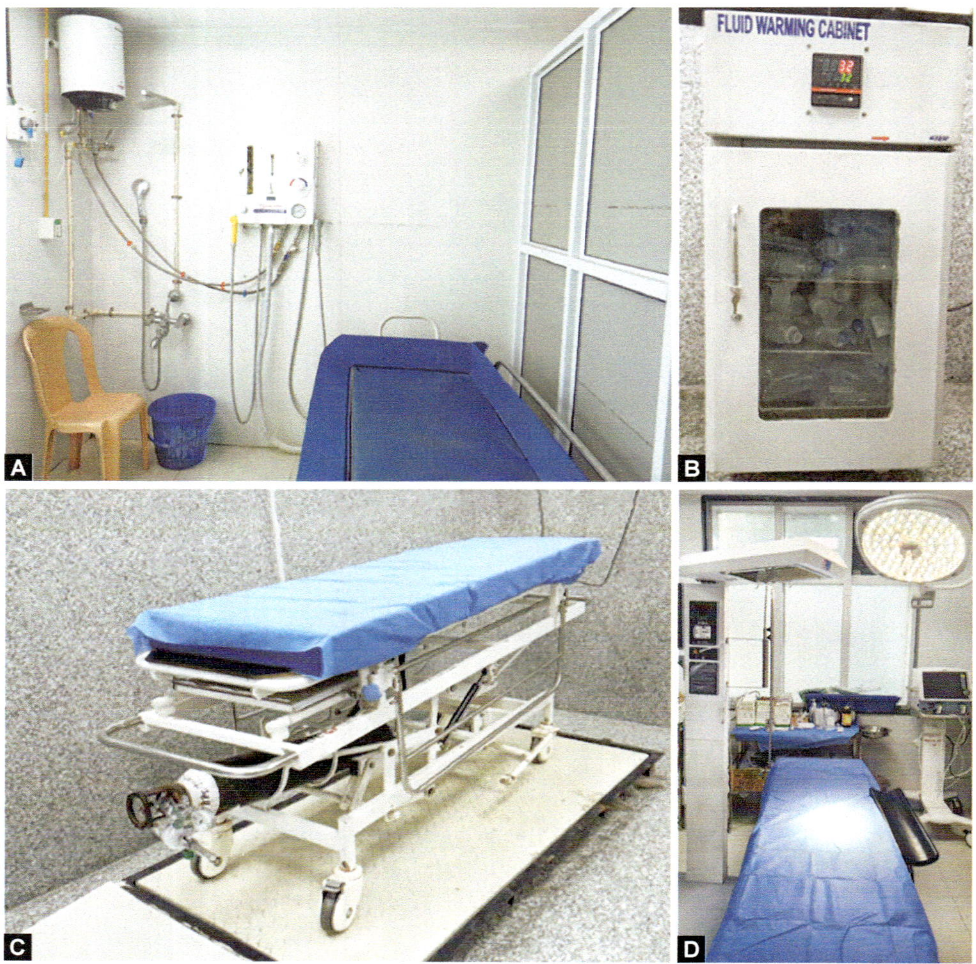

FIGS. 1A TO D: Essential equipment for the casualty area. (A) Burn wound washing area with shower trolley. (B) Fluid warming cabinet. (C) Weighing machine with patient-weighing trolley. (D) Overhead radiant warmer.

- Intravenous access including venesections and blood collection for investigations
- Tracheostomy
- Escharotomy/fasciotomy; an electrocautery will be useful
- Insertion of nasogastric tube
- Urethral catheterization

A dressing trolley with dressing materials in adequate quantity should be available if the receiving area is a part of the burn unit. If it is in Accident and Emergency Department, the patient can be wrapped in a sterile drape and transported to the burn unit for further wound management.

The following documents should be displayed or be readily available in the receiving area:

- Burn unit admission criteria
- Protocol for initial evaluation and management
- Chart for evaluation of the extent of burn and intravenous (I/V) fluid calculation
- I/V access protocol
- Contact telephone numbers
- Mass burn casualty action plan

An emergency facility designated for burn cases should have a well-defined standard operating procedure (SOP) in place to effectively handle mass burn disasters. Ideally, the facility should include a disaster-holding area equipped with trolleys, oxygen, medical air inlets, and suction facilities **(Fig. 2)**.

Furthermore, this emergency facility should be situated nearby or be a shared facility with a trauma emergency unit. This proximity enables swift treatment for burn victims with accompanying trauma. **Figure 3** illustrates a sample layout for such an emergency room.

DESIGN OF BURN UNIT

By definition, a burn unit is part of a multispecialty hospital and should occupy either a complete floor or a part of it. Control of infection should be the basic consideration while deciding the distribution of space in a burn unit. In order to minimize the transportation of micro-organisms, the necessity for the movement of healthcare workers, patients, and waste material within the unit should be reduced. This can be achieved by:

- Allocating zones within the unit for each category of patient condition (acute, infected, high dependency, nonacute/convalescent) and equipping each zone with all the patient-care requirements for daily routine (therapy, hygiene, staff areas, etc.). Depending on the available space, the convalescent care area may be located outside but in physical proximity of the acute and high-dependency care area of the burn unit.
- Keeping immunosuppressed, infected, and acute patients isolated in single rooms **(Fig. 4)**
- Employing appropriate measures for environmental control
- Organizing unidirectional traffic routes and corridors so that during routine procedures, there are no points of contact between the various zones

A concentric design has been proposed, featuring a central core dedicated to patient support and general services, an intermediate ring comprising patient care rooms, and an external visitors' corridor.[1]

Alternatively, a bottom-up approach can be adopted, organizing zones based on contamination levels.

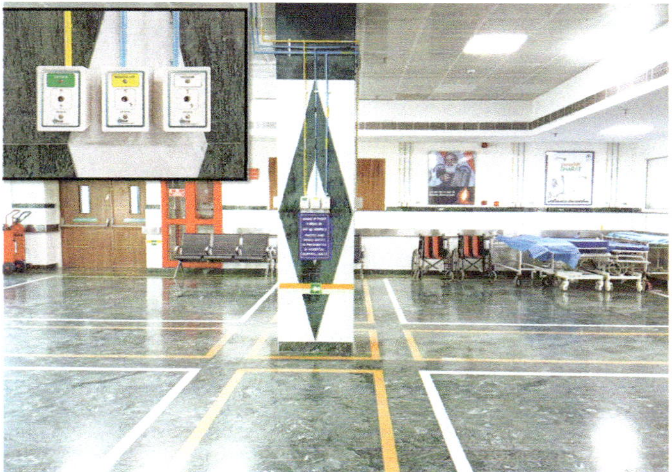

FIG. 2: Burn disaster holding area equipped with trolleys, oxygen and medical air inlets, and suction facilities (Inset).

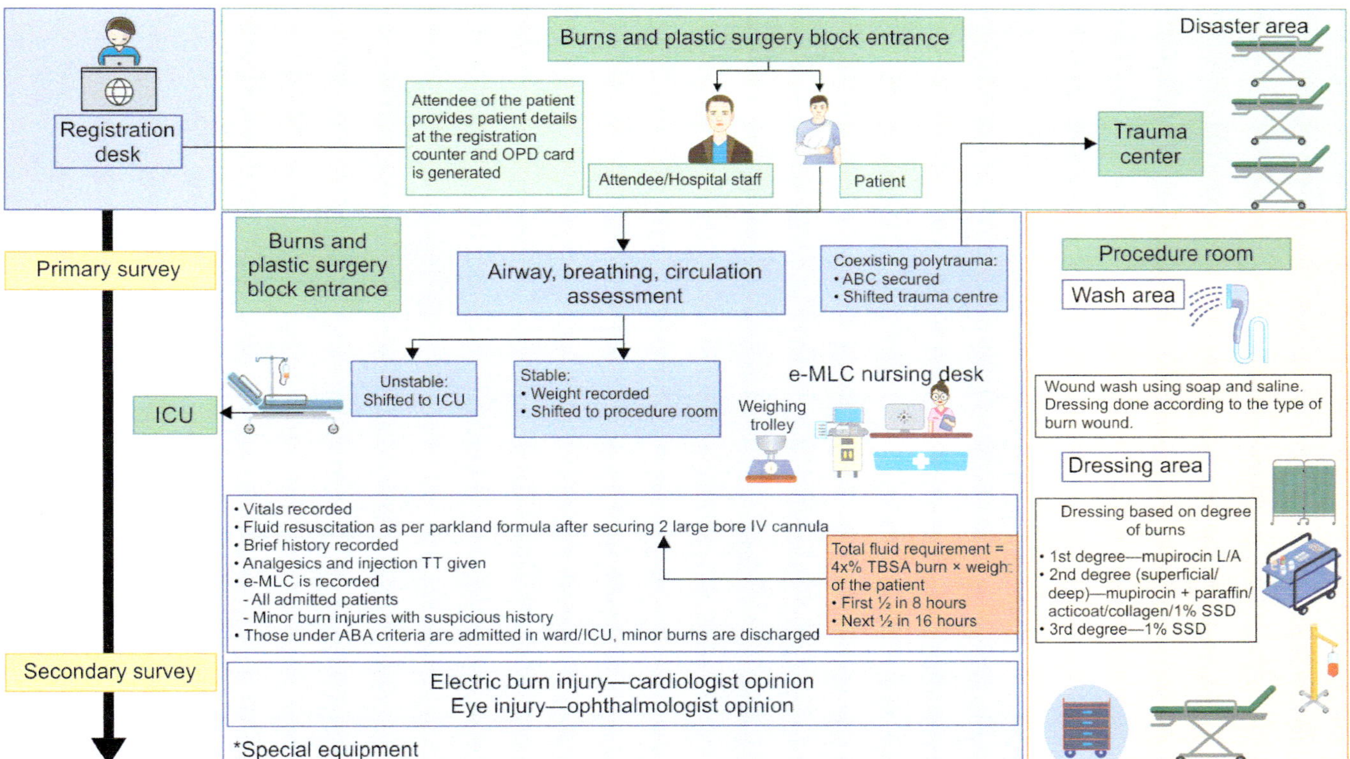

*Fluid-warming cabinets, burn bath area, infant radiant warmers; bedside warmers.

FIG. 3: Sample layout for burns emergency.

(ABA: American Burn Association; ICU: intensive care unit; MLC: medical legal case; TBSA: total burn surface area)

The layout begins with the bottommost level housing outpatient department (OPD) and emergency areas, followed by wards. Above that are the high-dependency unit (HDU) and intensive care unit (ICU), requiring higher sterility. The topmost level houses the OT, necessitating the highest level of sterility. This design is particularly well suited for standalone burn facilities.

The service areas should include:

- A nurses station
- A kitchenette/pantry
- An on-call restroom
- Staff changing room
- Stores
- An examination room for outpatients
- An operating suite, including a "clean" operating theater and a dressing room
- A procedure room/washing area
- A conference/meeting/classroom and a counseling room are desirable if the space permits.

The patient care rooms can be of different designs depending on the type of patient. The number of beds in each category will depend on the average number of admissions. (The numbers indicated here are considered appropriate for about 400 admissions per year).

- The patient at high immunological risk (acute and infected): 4 + 4 = 8 beds
- The patient without particular immunological problems, and in a nonacute but high-dependency state, that is, after complete resuscitation, between wound excision and closure procedures: 8 beds
- The patient in the convalescent phase with healing of more than 50% of the burnt area till the time of discharge: 8 beds.

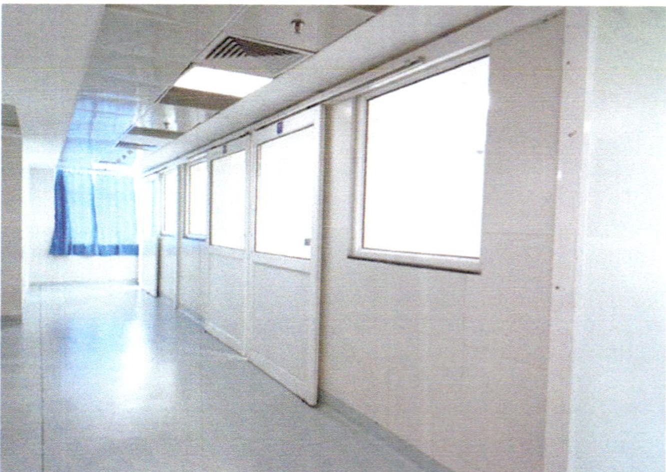

FIG. 4: Acute care area for keeping immunosuppressed, infected, and acute patients isolated in single rooms.

The Ministry of Health and Family Welfare (MOHFW) has provided guidelines for establishing burn units at medical colleges as part of the National Programme for Prevention and Management of Burn Injuries (NPPMBI). These guidelines serve as a reference for designing the sample layout and determining essential infrastructure, required manpower, and necessary equipment.[3]

Acute Care Area

For acute or septic patients, a single room is considered essential. Ideally, to limit still further the patient's transfer and the consequent dispersal of organisms, each room should have an adjoining **(Fig. 5)**:

- Water closet (WC) with sluice disposal (separate for each room)
- Hydrotherapy room (one between two single rooms, accessed through an air-lock from each side)
- Filter/anteroom (separate for each room, positioned between bedroom and access corridor and acting as air-lock to the tub room) would be ideal.

The minimum desirable dimensions of the acute care room are 10 ft × 10 ft × 10 ft. The room should have central oxygen supply and a central suction facility. The equipment needed for providing acute intensive care are as follows:

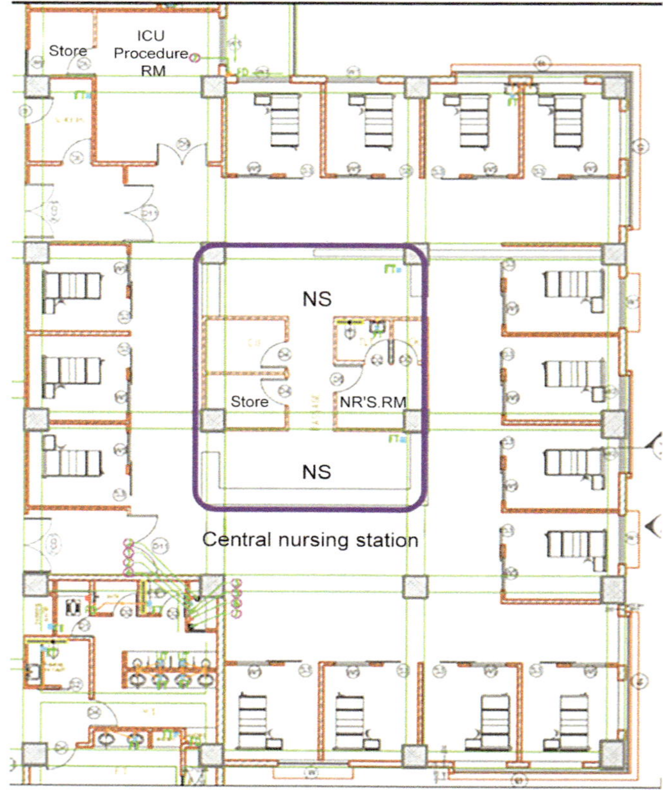

FIG. 5: Sample layout of an acute care area.
(NS: nursing station)

- Intensive care bed—1
- A set of resuscitation equipment including laryngoscope, endotracheal tubes, Ambu bag, connections, suction cannula, and emergency drugs
- Multipara monitor/capnometer/cardioscope with a pulse oximeter (depending on the availability of funds—1
- Syringe infusion pump—preferably 2, at least 1
- Nebulizer—1
- Deep vein thrombosis (DVT) pump
- Air mattress
- Chest physiotherapy/percussion device
- Splints to maintain position
- Dressing trolley with dressing drum
- Standby suction machine
- Patient care articles such as bedpan, kidney tray, etc.
- Hand disinfection facility should be provided in the anteroom or in the patient room in the absence of anteroom.

The acute care area should have:
- Sophisticated ventilators—ideally 8 (1 for each ICU bed) but at least 2, along with the required accessories
- Intensive care trolleys—2
- Crash cart—1
- ECG machine—1
- Portable X-ray machine—1
- A multipara monitor in each room connected to the central monitoring station at nurses' station and a closed-circuit television facility in each room for observing the patient from nurses' station would be an asset that can be procured at a significant cost.
- Vacuum cleaner—heavy duty—1
- A point-of-care laboratory with arterial blood gas (ABG) and carboxyhemoglobin measurement facility is preferred.
- A dialysis machine is a nonmandatory but good option to perform dialysis in patients with acute kidney injury (AKI) following burns as it is difficult to shift them to a dialysis facility since they are often in a very critical medical state.
- A portable ultrasonography machine can serve to perform point-of-care ultrasonography (POCUS) for airway, fluid status measurement, pulmonary edema, and I/V access.

Surgical residents: Two surgical residents should be assigned to this area.

Nurse:Patient ratio—1:1 is very desirable for all shifts.

A dressing assistant is necessary for the morning shift. Helper staff of a minimum of four ward attendants and four cleaners is necessary for every shift.

High-dependency Area

A room with two beds is desirable, with a WC and shower for each room. At least 5 feet should be available on either side of the patient bed for ease of procedures and infection control.

The equipment that should be available for each bed are:
- Intensive care bed
- Central suction and oxygen facility
- A set of patient care articles
- Dressing trolley with dressing drum
- Splints, extremity supports

Each room should have:
- Pulse oximeter—1
- Nebulizer—1
- Wheelchair—1
- Syringe infusion pump—1
- Volumetric infusion pump for continuous nasogastric tube feeds
- Simple physical therapy equipment
- Hand disinfection facility

In critical cases of pediatric burn patients, conscious sedation is often necessary to alleviate pain during dressing changes. To facilitate this, it is essential to ensure the presence of an intensivist or anesthetist during the procedure, along with the availability of necessary monitoring and airway equipment. The procedure room should be meticulously organized with suitable monitoring devices, airway management tools, and emergency medications. It is crucial to have equipment and supplies tailored to the child's specific age and weight, ensuring a safe and effective sedation process.

The high-dependency area should also have:
- Ventilators—2
- Intensive care trolleys—2
- Crash cart—1
- Vacuum cleaner-heavy duty—1
- Washing machine—1

Surgical residents: At least one surgical resident should be assigned to this area.

Nurse:Patient ratio: The ratio should be 1:2 for the morning shift and 1:3 for the other two shifts with patient allocation. A dressing assistant is necessary for the morning shift. Helper staff of a minimum of three ward attendants and two cleaners is necessary for every shift.

Convalescent Care Area

The convalescent care area **(Fig. 6)** should be in proximity to ICU and HDU. It should have at least eight beds. This

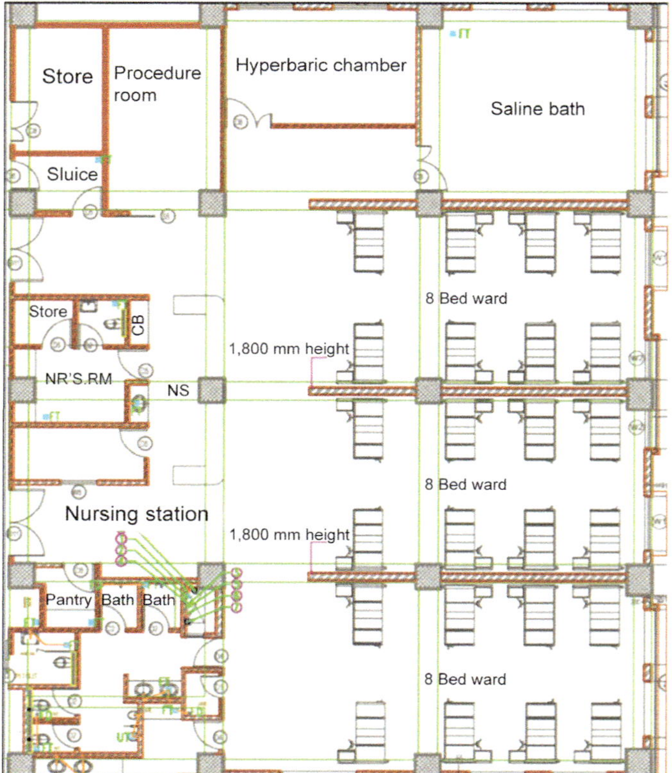

FIG. 6: Sample layout of a convalescent area.

can be a big hall with adequate space between the beds with a facility to isolate the patient with curtains. Each bed should be provided with a central suction and oxygen facility. Windows and exhaust fans can be used for providing good natural ventilation.

At least four showers and WCs should be provided in the toilet block of the ward. The WC should also be equipped with a grab bar. Indian WC is unsuitable for burnt patients as squatting can be extremely difficult.

Each bed should be furnished with a set of patient care essentials, including a chair, bucket, mug, and bedpan. It is highly recommended to have a dedicated dressing drum for each bed, and a separate dressing trolley is essential. If not by the bedside, there should be a trolley preparation area.

The significance of having a dedicated dressing trolley for each patient in a preparation area lies in the prevention of cross-contamination of wounds and the potential outbreak of wound infections. When each patient has their own designated dressing trolley, it ensures that the dressing materials and instruments used are specific to that individual, reducing the risk of bacterial colonization and subsequent infections. Maintaining sterile techniques in preparing these trolleys is crucial and having a designated dressing assistant responsible for this task further enhances infection-control measures. This approach not only prioritizes patient safety but also upholds stringent hygiene standards, ultimately contributing to the overall effectiveness and success of wound care and treatment.

Patient cabinets should be avoided, as they can attract pests and insects. Instead, a shelf should be provided for each bed to accommodate the patient's personal items. Additionally, a hand disinfection facility should be available for each bed.

The facility should encompass service areas like a nurses' station, changing room, pantry, store, dressing room, physiotherapy area, and recreation area within this section. The following equipment should be available in this area:

- Patient trolleys—2
- Wheelchairs—2
- Crash cart—1
- Nebulizer—1
- Suction apparatus—1
- Physical therapy equipment
- Vacuum cleaner—1
- Music system
- Television
- Pulse oximeter—1 (desirable
- Syringe infusion pump—1 (desirable)

Surgical residents: At least one surgical resident should be assigned to this area.

Nurse:Patient ratio: During the morning shift when maximum patient care activities are carried out, at least two qualified nurses should be available along with one dressing assistant. In the other two shifts, at least one qualified nurse should be posted. A dressing assistant is necessary for the morning shift.

Helper staff of a minimum of two ward attendants and two cleaners is necessary for every shift.

ENVIRONMENT CONTROL

The purpose of environmental control measures is to:

- Reduce the load of bacteria-carrying particles
- Impede the passage of air from areas with lower grades of asepsis (e.g., service areas) to those where the level of sterility is required to be high (e.g., patient room, dressing room) by maintaining pressure gradient
- Provide comfortable environmental temperature to help control the hypermetabolic state of the burn patients by reducing shivering
- Provide optimal humidity to control evaporative losses and to aid the wound-healing process
- Dilute the smells while keeping noise to a minimum

Air changes: An appropriately designed air treatment plant would serve this purpose by maintaining different levels of asepsis in the air according to the function of the space. The reduction of bacterial content in the air can be brought about by either filtration or sterilization. High-efficiency particulate air (HEPA) filters have the smallest pore size, but their use entails high recurring expenditure. Filters with 3–5 μm size pores are considered adequate for ICU. The sterilization is effected using ultraviolet lamps positioned either directly in the room or in the air conditioning ducts as a complement to the filters.[1]

Three systems of high-efficiency cleansing are:

1. Laminar flow
2. Directed vertical flow
3. Joubert system

Laminar flow systems exist with either horizontal or vertical orientation. In both cases, the airflow acts on the entire air volume and is characterized by its very high air-change rate (300–540 volumes/hour).

Directed vertical flow concentrates its action on the area in which the medical team is operating and in proximity to the patient. The system's capacity (20–25 changes/hour, which can drop to 15 when rooms are not in use), although notably lower than that of the laminar flow, is seen to reduce the content of colony-forming units (CFU) per cubic meter to a suitable level for delicate operations.

The Joubert system is a system based on directed vertical flow for operating rooms, introducing certain modifications: The air-change rate is around 50 volumes/hour; of these, 6 volumes/hour are fresh external air, while the other 44 are recycled from the room and filtered.[1] In the author's experience, directed vertical flow system with 20–24 fresh air changes/hour reduces the CFU/m^3 to < 10 which is considered adequate. Regular maintenance of the system needs to be carried out by cleaning/changing of filters, cleaning of ducts, and microbiological surveillance.

Temperature: Environmental temperature equal to normal body temperature, that is, 35°C, is optimal for controlling the metabolic rate and preventing shivering of burnt patients. This is most often perceived as uncomfortable by healthcare professionals as it causes sweating, fluid loss, and easy fatigue. In the author's experience, a temperature of about 30°C is an acceptable compromise for both patient and staff if maintaining different temperatures in the patient rooms and service areas is not possible due to resource crunch.

Humidity: Humidity of 55–60% is desirable.

Use of air curtains at identified entrances helps to maintain pressure gradient and thus aids control of the microclimatic conditions.

Odor control: Reducing odor in burns wards is important for maintaining a clean and comfortable environment for both patients and healthcare professionals. Here are several measures to help mitigate odors in burns wards:[5]

- Implement a strict and frequent cleaning schedule (at least twice a day) to ensure that all areas are thoroughly cleaned and disinfected.
- Ensure proper segregation, containment, and timely removal of waste, especially soiled dressings and bandages.
- Use sealed bins with lids to contain odors and prevent them from spreading. Have a dedicated sluice area which can be used for temporary waste disposal.
- Use deodorizers designed for healthcare settings to neutralize odors in the air.
- Ventilation and air circulation: Maintain frequent air changes throughout the burns ward to reduce stagnant air.
- Place odor-absorbing materials like activated charcoal or baking soda in key areas to help absorb odors.
- Emphasize personal hygiene practices among patients and visitors to minimize contributing factors to odor.
- Effective wound care reduces infection and minimizes odor associated with infected wounds.

CONSTRUCTIONAL CONSIDERATIONS

The material used for the floor and walls of the burn unit should be chosen with a thought about infection control, ease of cleaning, and durability. The cost of the material can be a major deciding factor in the presence of resource crunch.

Floor: The floor needs to withstand heavy load and traffic. It should be dust resistant, nonslippery, and easy to clean. Epoxy coating satisfies these criteria but is expensive. Among the natural stones, marble is unsuitable as its high porosity supports trapping of moisture and growth of organisms. Granite is slippery and expensive. Polished Kota or polished Shahabad stone is strong, durable, affordable, easy to clean, and with the least porosity. Use of large-sized slabs would reduce the number of joints.

Walls: The walls should be covered from floor to ceiling with suitable material which should be dust resistant, nonporous, and easy to clean. Large, marbogranite tiles are considered suitable as the porosity is less than that of the ceramic tiles and the surface is dust resistant.

Ceiling: If a false ceiling is planned, it should be of aluminum panels for ease of cleaning. If the ceiling needs painting, plastic emulsion or oil paint is recommended as both are moisture and dust resistant and easy to clean.

Cleaning: Use of a vacuum cleaner is strongly recommended for cleaning of floor, walls, and ceilings of all the areas in the burn unit. This sucks and removes the dust while sweeping displaces it.

Windows: If open ventilation is being used in the unit, the windows must have nets to prevent the entrance of flies, mosquitoes, and other insects. A strict protocol for cleaning of nets needs to be prepared and implemented.

OPERATION THEATER

The operation theater can be a part of the burn unit or may be an identified OT in the surgical OT block which would save space and personnel.

- *Size*: 20 ft × 20 ft
- Operation table with a facility to suspend extremities with the help of detachable rods or rails suspended from the ceiling
- All usual OT equipment, such as anesthesia machine, central gas supply and suction facility, and cautery machine
- Thermal blanket, patient warmer, on-line fluid warmer, and multipara monitor
- *Air changes*: 20–25 fresh air changes/hour, temperature: 35°C, humidity: 55–60%
- Surgical team should have two surgeons, two assistant surgeons, and two nurse assistants.
- Key instruments include the skin grafting knife or dermatome. It is essential to have a sufficient quantity of blades to facilitate the grafting process. Additionally, equipment like a skin graft mesher and dermacarriers are crucial for effective grafting procedures. An optional yet advantageous addition could be the MEEK micrografting device.

DRESSING ROOM

During a dressing procedure, the bacterial density in the dressing room increases significantly. About 8-10 air changes are needed to reduce the density to an acceptable level. This would need a time gap of 30 minutes between two dressing procedures. In a busy burn unit, it is impractical to follow this discipline. The author is convinced that doing dressings in the patient's own room is a convenient alternative. Selected dressings may be done in the dressing room with adequate time interval between the procedures. The dressing room should be of 12 × 12 feet for ease of manipulation of the patient trolley. The environment control specifications would be the same as for OT. It should have adequate supply of sterile dressing equipment and agents. A weighing machine can be conveniently placed in the dressing room for ease of implementing daily weight protocol.

HYDROTHERAPY FACILITY

A large number of burn units outside India use Hubbard tank for hydrotherapy. In the author's opinion, this is unsuitable for burn units in India for several reasons:

- The time taken for each patient is about an hour. Considering the number of patients in India, this would mean having multiple tanks which entails significant expenditure.
- In the absence of appropriate cleaning of the tank, the risk of endogenous as well as cross-infection is certainly increased. With a constant paucity of trained and committed personnel, this is a definite possibility.

The experience in India as well as abroad suggests that a shower bath (with a hand-held telephone shower) using an appropriately modified patient trolley is an effective alternative.[4] In contrast to the Hubbard tank, the shower trolley was observed to have the following associated advantages: (1) Quicker treatment sessions, (2) less pain to the patient, (3) elimination of patient exposure to contaminated water, (4) more comfort for the therapist, and (5) greater ease in patient handling, for example, rolling the patient onto a stretcher or bringing the patient into a sitting position. The use of the sterilized disposable plastic sheet was observed to be the most effective procedure to decrease the risk of contamination among patients during the shower.[5] The hydrotherapy facility should have adequate space and wide enough doors for manipulation of the trolley. A hot and cold water mixer with telephone shower attachment and appropriate drainage provision is necessary, inexpensive, and easy to use and maintain. In ICU and HDU, a trolley lined by a sterile plastic drape is appropriate while in the convalescent care area, the patients may walk or be taken on a wheelchair for hydrotherapy.

It is important to note that hydrotherapy may not be safe for patients with hypovolemia, sepsis, and hypothermia. For such patients, it is advisable to perform sponging of nonburnt body parts and wound cleaning and dressing on the patient bed.

Provision must be made for appropriate collection and disposal of waste generated in the hydrotherapy area without contaminating the patient care areas. Maintaining this unidirectional movement is crucial for infection control and needs to be incorporated in the unit design.

PHYSIOTHERAPY UNIT (FIGS. 7 AND 8)

A physical therapist should visit the unit twice a day for passive and active exercises for every patient. For patients in ICU, splints and extremity supports should be available for optimal positioning. The extremity supports can be prepared from thermoplastic material or aluminum sheet (cheaper). These have been observed to be effective and are easy to disinfect. Readily available aluminum splints for wrist and hand, elbow, ankle, and knee help in providing splinting and are easy to disinfect.

The physiotherapy equipment that should be available in HDU and convalescent care area are:

- Cycle pedals fixed on a stand
- Pulleys for upper extremity exercises
- Chronic passive motion (CPM) machines for different joint movements should be available, whenever needed.
- Parallel bars can be provided in the unit if the space permits. A walker should also be available.
- Simple games such as peg in the hole and building blocks provide valuable exercise for fingers and wrists.
- Toy cars and cycles provide excellent therapy to pediatric patients while they play.
- Group exercise therapy improves patient participation significantly. This can be effectively conducted in convalescent care area and for select patients in HDU.

It is necessary to ensure regular cleaning and disinfection of all the equipment. Besides the physical therapist, the nursing staff and surgical team should encourage the patients to perform activities of daily routine along with the exercises. The physical therapists also have to provide respiratory therapy not only to the patients with inhalation injury, but also to all the patients in the unit. The necessary equipment (nebulizer, incentive spirometer) should be available in the unit.

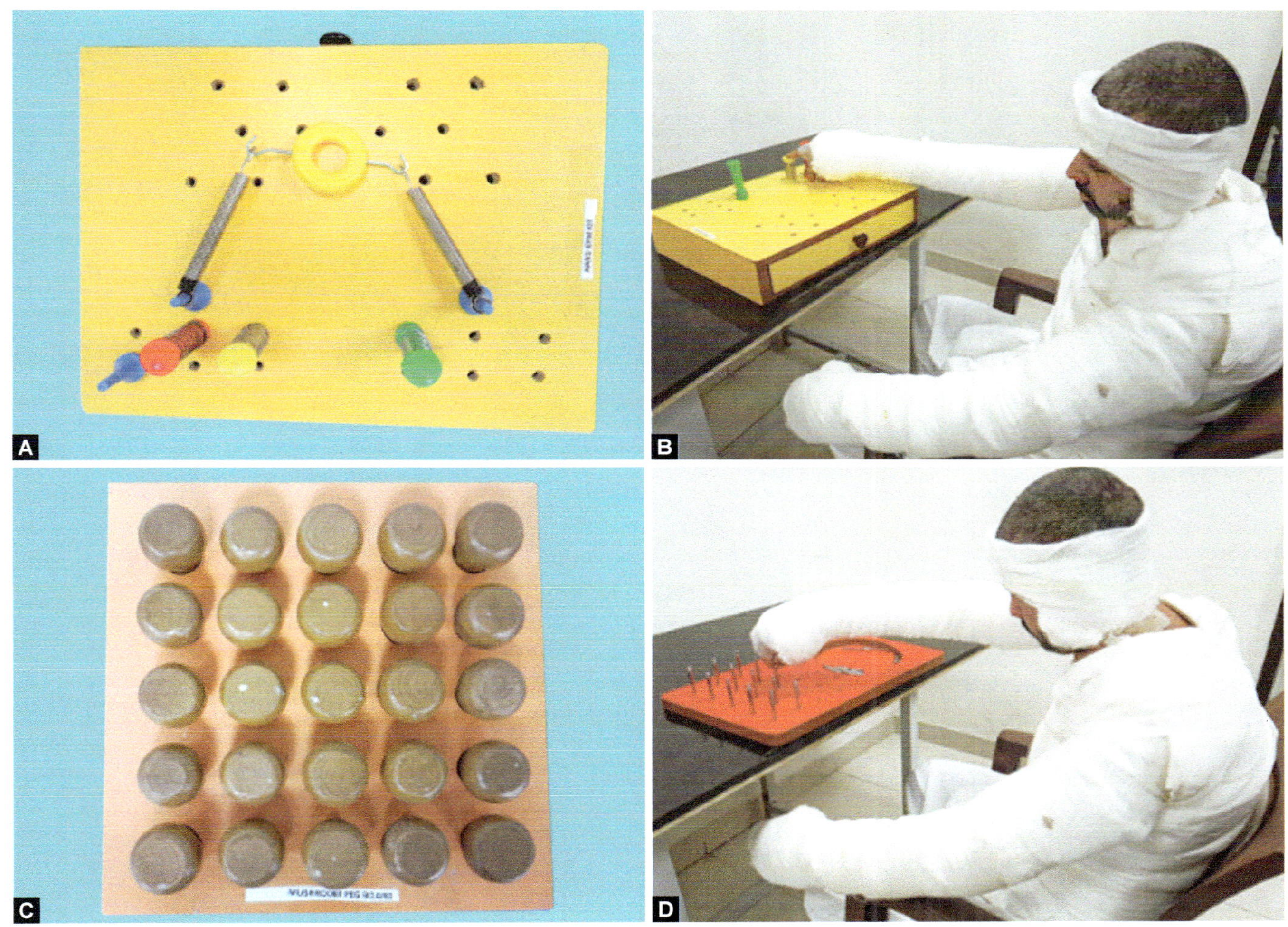

FIGS. 7A TO N: *Continued*

Continued

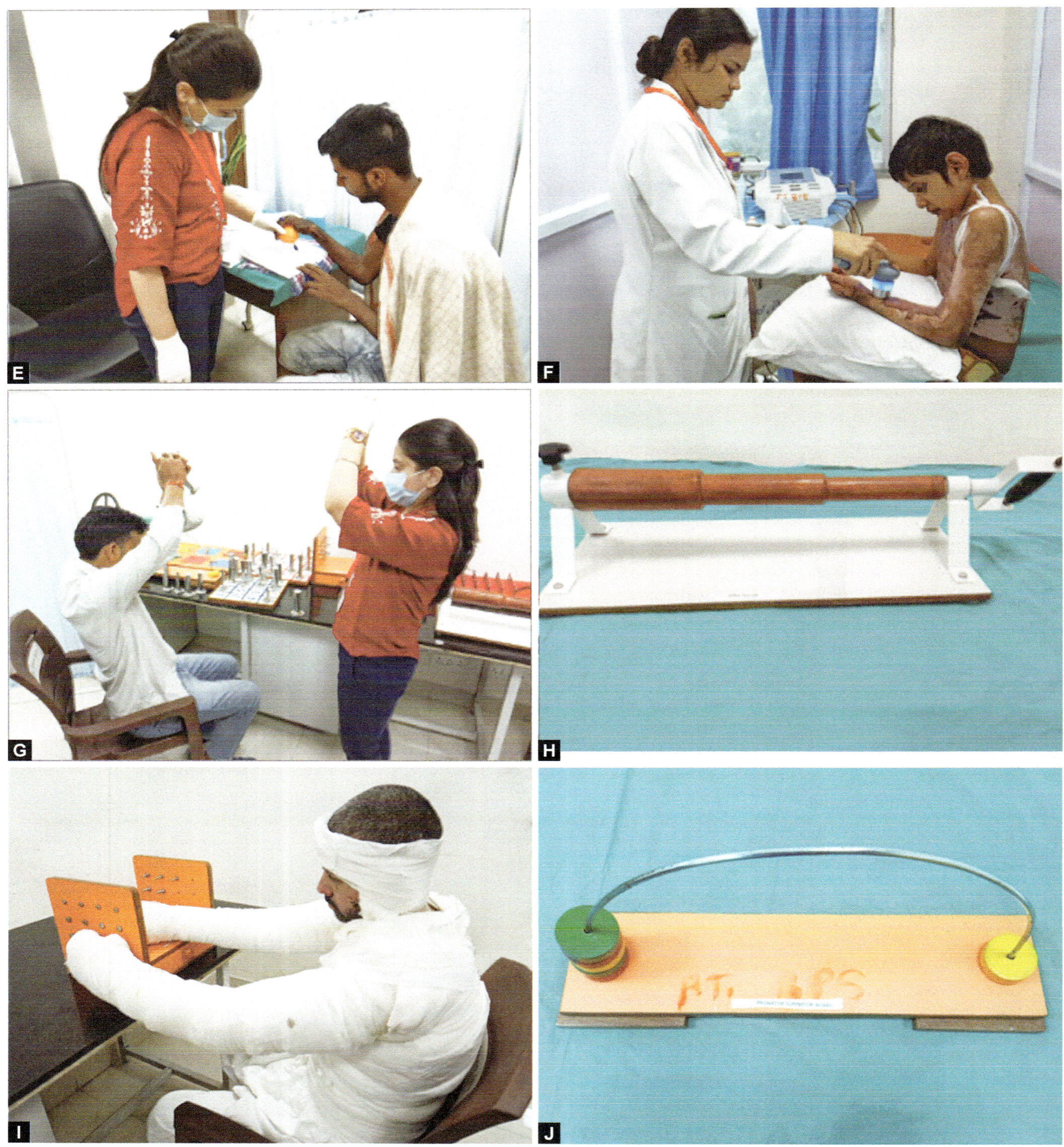

FIGS. 7A TO N: *Continued*

Continued

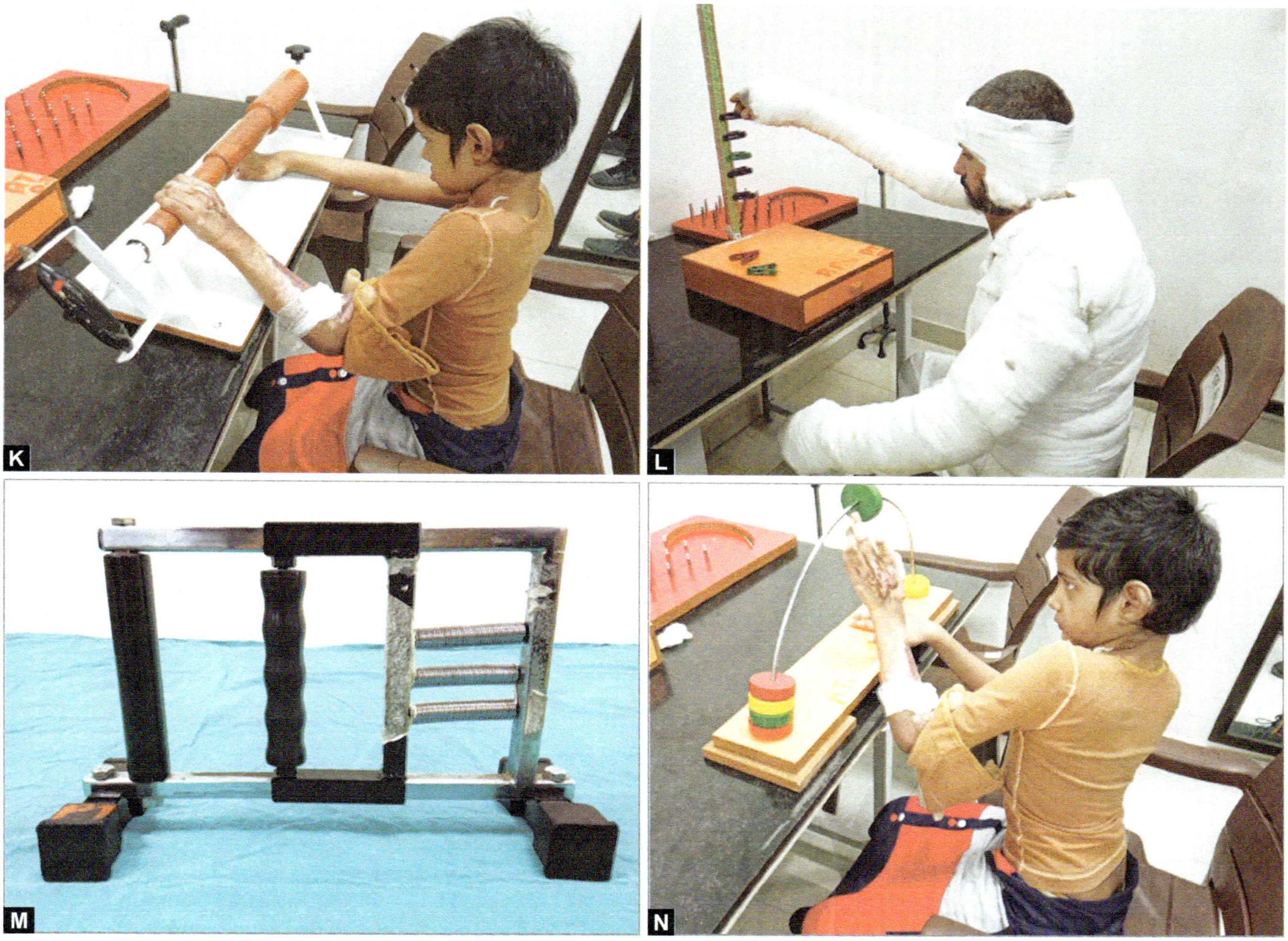

FIGS. 7A TO N: Essential occupational therapy equipment in rehabilitation of burn patients. (A) Hand gym kit; (B) Hand gym kit activity; (C) Mushroom peg board; (D) Metallic peg board. (E) Assistive device: Ball-shaped writing device; (F) Ultrasound therapy; (G) Bilateral integration activity of upper limb; (H) Wrist roller. (I) Nut and screw activity board; (J) Pronator supinator board; (K) Wrist roller activity. (L) Pinch tree activity; (M) Grip-strengthening activity; (N) Pronator supinator activity.

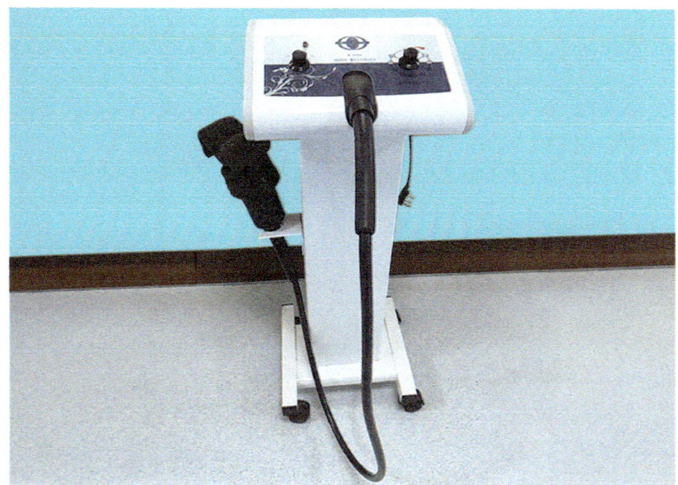

FIG. 8: Chest vibrator used in physiotherapy of critical burn patients.

UTILIZATION AND COST CONTAINMENT

The establishment of a burn unit is an expensive proposition. It should not be undertaken if optimum and appropriate utilization is not ensured. In our country, if a burn unit has to be closed for lack of patients, it would call for a celebration. But resource crunch is a major issue that plagues most of the burn units. To combat this problem, we must find our own solutions based on sound scientific principles. The burn team should discuss various shortfalls openly and the team leader must encourage suggestions from each and every member. Imaginative innovations and their critical evaluation would certainly lead to the development of methods that would take us ahead on the path of progress. The measures suggested here for environmental control are expensive, and available funds may not be sufficient. It should be realized that these are not solutions in isolation to the problem of hospital infections. These infections are the result of interacting causes, none of which should be undervalued or ignored and should be countered using interacting measures. For these reasons, surgical and nutritional treatment and, above all, the conscientious respect of hygiene discipline on the part of all members of staff are of fundamental importance and cannot be substituted by any of the expensive gadgets. Large, well-ventilated, multibed burn units can also generate impressive results with strict attention to cleaning protocols and barrier nursing. Excellent nutritional support can be provided using locally available inexpensive items of food instead of commercially available tube feeds or nutritional supplements. Paucity of funds should be considered as an opportunity to innovate. Burn care requires a high staff-to-patient ratio, and a hospital budget to support this is mandatory. The author strongly feels that the resource crunch should not compromise the number of healthcare professionals in the burn unit, especially the nursing staff. Such a step is extremely detrimental to the quality of care and may result in the loss of several valuable lives.

ACTIVITIES OF BURN UNIT

The burn unit should not be satisfied just with provision of burn care. The responsibility of the burn team and the unit extends much beyond to encompass the following.[2]

Performance Improvement Program

The burn unit should have a performance improvement program that is multidisciplinary. The burn unit multidisciplinary committee, which oversees the performance improvement program, should meet at least quarterly. Sufficient documentation should be maintained to verify problems, identify opportunities for improvement, take corrective actions, and resolve problems.

Morbidity and mortality conferences should be held at least monthly with physicians other than the immediate burn care team to ensure an objective review of the presentations. All significant burn complications and all deaths must be discussed. There must be open, candid discussion with high points documented and assessment of the death or complication classified as "caused by disease", "potentially preventable", or "possibly preventable" (or the equivalent thereof). Actions recommended must also be documented, and there must be documentation of loop closure. Records of this conference must be kept.

Patient care conferences shall be held at least weekly to review and evaluate the status of each patient admitted to the burn unit. Each clinical discipline should be represented in order to appropriately contribute to the treatment plan for each patient. Patient care conferences shall be documented in the minutes of the conference.

Audit

The burn service should conduct audits at least annually that should include, but should not be limited to, the severity of burn, mortality, incidence of complications, and length of hospitalization.

Educational Programs

The burn unit should have an educational program for the medical and nursing staff.

If residents rotate on the burn service, the burn specialist in the unit should be responsible for an orientation program for new residents.

Infection-control Program

It is imperative to have a dedicated hospital infection-control team within the burn unit to maintain a safe environment **(Fig. 9)**.

They are primarily responsible for conducting routine surface cultures to check the sterility of the surroundings and ensuring strict adherence to infection-control protocols during various medical procedures and dressing changes.

They also conduct regular inspections and audits to monitor and assess compliance with established infection-prevention protocols.

This team plays a critical role in the analysis of the nosocomial infection data, enabling them to devise antimicrobial sensitivity patterns and identify risk factors associated with outbreaks among burn patients.

Continuity of Care Program

The burn unit must provide the following services:

- Recreational therapy for children cared for in the unit
- Education in rehabilitation
- Support for family members or other significant persons
- Coordinated discharge planning
- Follow-up after hospital discharge
- Access to community resources
- Evaluation of the patient's physical, psychological, developmental, and vocational status
- Planning for future rehabilitative and reconstructive needs

Burn Prevention Program

The burn unit should participate regularly in public burn awareness programs.

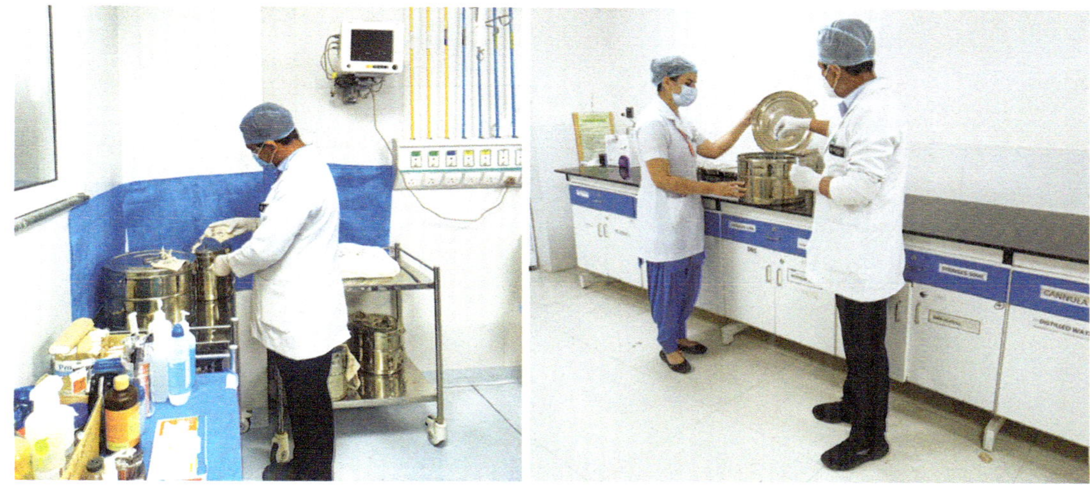

FIG. 9: Deployment of a dedicated hospital infection-control team within the burn unit to maintain a safe environment.

Research Program

The burn unit should participate in basic, clinical, community-based, and health sciences research.

Allograft Skin Bank Program

To initiate the registration and licensing process for a skin bank or any other tissue bank excluding eye banks, an application needs to be submitted through the head of the institution to the National Organ and Tissue Transplant Organization (NOTTO). This application should be meticulously prepared, providing comprehensive details about the tissue bank, its infrastructure, facilities, equipment, personnel, and adherence to regulatory guidelines outlined by the NOTTO.

The necessary infrastructure and equipment for a skin bank **(Fig. 10)** include the following:

- *Facility and space requirements*: Area of approximately 50 m^2
- Furniture and fixtures, such as tables, chairs, storage units, and workbenches
- *BSL 2 Biosafety Cabinet*: To maintain a sterile environment during the processing and handling of skin grafts
- Autoclave for the sterilization of instruments and equipment. It may be a shared facility with the OR.
- Walk-in refrigerator to store donated skin grafts at a temperature of 4°C to maintain their integrity and quality
- Mesher and dermatome for the harvest and processing of skin grafts
- An incubator to provide controlled temperature for incubation of tissue cultures
- Orbital Shaker for the gentle mixing of glycerol with the graft
- Computer, accessories, and AC

In terms of manpower, a skin bank requires two teams: A skin processing team, preferably consisting of microbiologists or biotechnologists, and a skin harvesting team, comprised of doctors, nurses, and paramedics. The skin processing team is responsible for:

- Processing donated skin
- Documenting the skin processing procedures
- Managing the quality of the processed skin
- Overseeing the overall management of the skin bank

On the other hand, the skin harvesting team consists of:

- A doctor as the team leader, overseeing the skin donation process and skin harvesting
- Nurses and paramedics as assisting staff, aiding in educating potential donors and their families, preparing donation kits, and providing logistic support for collecting donations

To ensure the continuous availability of trained manpower, it is essential for the skin bank to be integrated with the hospital setup, ensuring a 24/7 operational capacity in the campus at any time.

Funding

Burn care entails significant expenditure due to the need for intensive care, prolonged hospital stay, multiple procedures, expensive medications, long rehabilitation programs, and a high staff-to-patient ratio. Adequate budgetary provisions should be made by the administration to meet the exigencies.

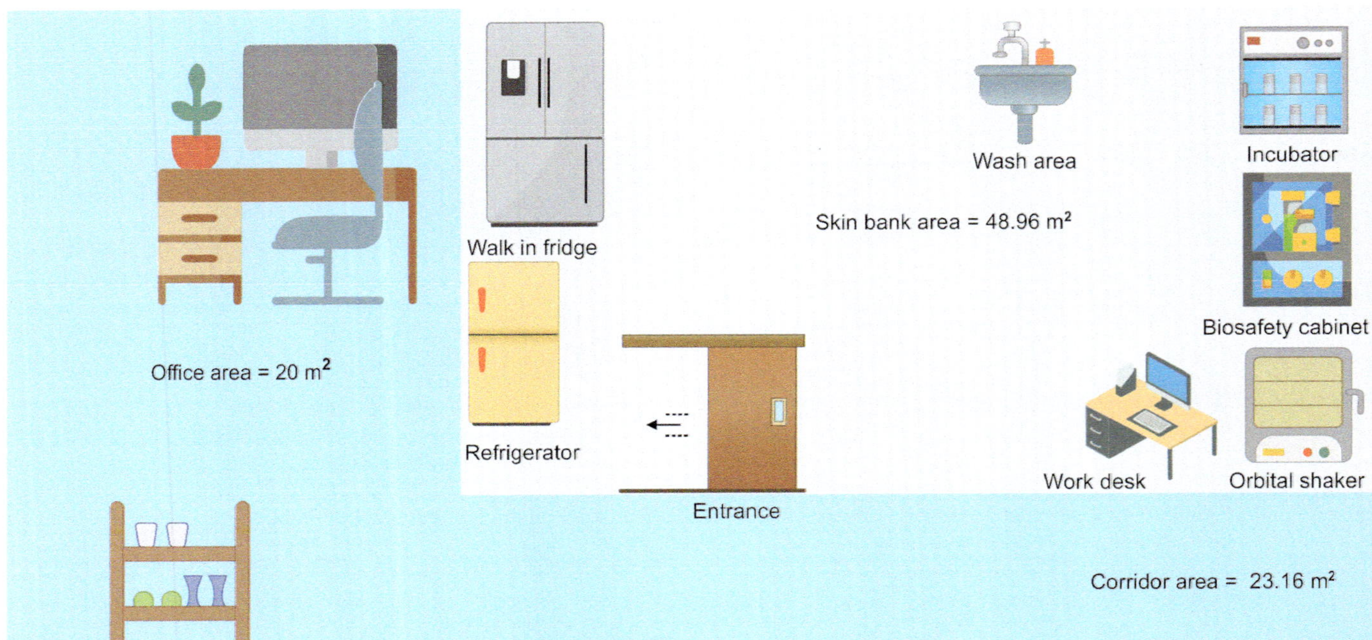

FIG. 10: Layout of skin bank.

As Curreri[6] said, the success or failure of the burn unit is based on managerial capability. Managers are responsible for accumulating resources, educating personnel, maintaining morale, and integrating the burn unit with the rest of the hospital. Moreover, it has become apparent that burn unit managers must become financial managers as well if we are to: (1) Maintain reasonable resources for the conduct of research, (2) participate in a variety of health delivery systems, (3) curtail health delivery costs, (4) maintain the current excellence of clinical care in an efficient manner, and (5) guarantee access of patients to the burn care delivery system at a cost that the country can afford.

It is the responsibility of the Director of the burn unit to garner funds needed for the smooth functioning of the burn unit and for conducting different activities. Procurement and maintenance of necessary equipment depends on the ability of the director to convince the management of the hospital and on the level of commitment of the management. In the author's experience, funding can be obtained from philanthropic individuals, organizations, and industry, for research and educational programs as well as for equipment. Besides the high quality of work; sincerity, commitment, and transparency in the utilization of funds are excellent advocates. The author truly believes that "If you have the purpose, means will follow."[9]

SUMMARY

A burn unit is only as good as its staff.[10] Trained experienced nurses, therapists, and surgeons accustomed to dealing with large open wounds are a major requisite for the care of burnt patients who have a multisystem disease. The field of burn care demands a high level of commitment, consistently excellent quality performance, and the ability to generate enthusiasm sometimes in the face of all adversities.

The burn unit's physical spaces and mechanical systems are designed to reduce infection, promote patient comfort, and improve staff efficiency and morale.[8] Patients and staff are the focal point of a burn unit and should continue to remain so for encouraging outcomes.

REFERENCES

1. Magliacani C, Teich Alasia S, Bormioli M, Stella M, Musci F, Holmes J. Structural aspects in a burn unit: Proposal of expanding models. Ann MBC; 1992;5(1).
2. Guidelines for the operation of burn units, resources for optimal care of the injured patient. Committee on Trauma, American College of Surgeons; 1999. (Chapter 14).
3. Gupta JL, Makhija LK, Bajaj SP. National programme for prevention of burn injuries. Indian J Plast Surg. 2010;43(Suppl):S6-S10.
4. Operational Guidelines for Establishment of Burns Units at Medical Colleges under National Programme for Prevention

& Management of Burn Injuries (NPPMBI). (n.d.). [online] Available from https://dghs.gov.in/WriteReadData/userfiles/file/Operational_Guidlines_Medical_College.pdf [Last accessed May, 2024].

5. Hayashida K, Yamakawa S. Topical odour management in burn patients. Burns Trauma. 2021;9:tkab025.
6. Neville C, Dimick AR. The trauma table as an alternative to the Hubbard tank in burn care. Burn Center, University of Alabama Hospital, Birmingham. J Burn Care Rehabil. 1987;8(6):574-5.
7. Akin S, Ozcan M. Using a plastic sheet to prevent the risk of contamination of the burn wound during the shower. Burns. 2003;29(3):280-3.
8. Curreri PW. 1984 American Burn Association presidential address: Burn unit success – a problem of management. J Trauma. 1985;25(1):1-10.
9. Snelling CF, Can J Surg. The comprehensive burn unit. Can J Surg. 1985;28(6):478-81.
10. Young SR, Thilliander BD. Patients, staff are focal point of new burn unit. Hospitals. 1980;54(4):93-9.

CHAPTER

39 Burn Injury Management in Disasters: Indian Perspective

Ravindra Tah

INTRODUCTION

Disasters: Definition and Impact

The Webster's dictionary defines a disaster as "a grave occurrence having ruinous results". The World Health Organization (WHO) defines disaster as "any occurrence that causes damage, economic destruction, loss of human life, and deterioration of health services on a scale sufficient to warrant an extraordinary response from outside the affected community or area".

The social and economic progress achieved over decades of initiatives by the people and advances in health can be significantly degraded by disasters.

Be it an act of God or an act of man, a mind boggling spectrum of disasters wreak havoc in the Indian subcontinent.

The disturbing fact is that even in a region like South Asia, where poverty, deprivation, and death due to disasters is a very common feature of life, India remains the worst-affected country. In fact, the frequency of all categories of disasters, varying from epidemics to road accidents, fires and perennial droughts and floods, increasing act of senseless terrorism has resulted in a multifold growth of injuries, disabilities, diseases and deaths, disrupting life-supporting systems and adding to the ill health, social and economic burden of already impoverished people.

According to the WHO publication fact, SHEET 2022 Burns are a global public health problem, accounting for an estimated 180,000 deaths annually. The majority of these occur in low- and middle-income countries and almost two-thirds occur in the WHO African and South-East Asia Regions.

In many high-income countries, burn death rates have been decreasing, and the rate of pediatric deaths from burns is currently over seven times higher in low- and middle-income countries than in high-income countries.

Nonfatal burns are a leading cause of morbidity, including prolonged hospitalization, disfigurement and disability, often with resulting stigma and rejection.

- Burns are among the leading causes of disability-adjusted life-years (DALYs) lost in low- and middle-income countries.
- The estimated annual burn incidence in India is approximately 6–7 million per year.
- Nearly 173,000 children in Bangladesh are moderately or severely burnt every year.
- In Bangladesh, Colombia, Egypt and Pakistan, 17% of children with burns have a temporary disability and 18% have a permanent disability.
- Burns are the second most common injury in rural Nepal, accounting for 5% of disabilities.
- In 2008, over 410,000 burn injuries occurred in the United States of America, with approximately 40,000 requiring hospitalization.

Experience and studies tell us that the actual figures greatly exceed the documented ones.

The cities are surrounded by industrial areas which have large stocks of inflammable materials like inflammable chemicals, gas storage fuel for furnaces and power generators, acrylic, woolens, textile yarn and fabrics, etc. The towns also have huge stocks of gadgets, and electrical instruments not maintained or scrutinized for safety. The extensive electrification is being done haphazardly which is prone to fire accidents due to short circuits.

The National Building Code of India lays down a set of minimum provisions according to which the buildings should be designed to protect the safety of the public. The regulations can be adopted immediately or enacted for use by various departments, municipal administrations, and public bodies. These guidelines become mandatory provisions once the state governments adopt the code through legislation. Many states like Tamil Nadu, Karnataka, etc., have passed fire service acts to ensure fire safety of buildings.

Through this act, the fire services are empowered to issue Fire License/No Objection Certificate to building owners which enables them to get clearance for occupation from Metropolitan Development Authority/City Municipal Corporation, etc. The fire safety license is issued based on the adherence to National Building Code provisions with respect to fire safety. In case of industrial buildings, the requirements of factories rules, Oil Industry Safety Directorate guidelines should also be complied with additionally, wherever applicable.

Despite the above mandatory requirements, implementation of fire safety in all buildings, residential as well as commercial, from the stage of planning is totally missing. Fires keep on happening frequently in less hazardous nonindustrial buildings in India.

Unregulated erection of temporary structures commonly known as "Shamianas" (make-shift tents) is done in India for all kind of functions from marriage to award giving ceremonies, including government functions. They extensively use inflammable material with loose, exposed, and temporary electrical wirings making them tinder boxes which go up in flames very easily.

A review of fire safety in India reveals that the available fire services are showing signs of "deficiencies in terms of manpower and infrastructure". Instead of growing and modernizing itself to ensure the safety of life and property, the usual fire services have depleted or become deficient for the growing population. We have, beyond doubt, made the world a dangerous place to live in.

Simply defined, a disaster occurs whenever the need exceeds resources. India does not have a very well-developed health infrastructure and has skewed distribution of available resources. There are a few fully equipped and staffed urban centers especially for burns injury. Therefore, any fire accident or act of terrorism resulting in large number of burn injury victims becomes a disaster. Worldwide, such a surge in burn injury causes significant morbidity and mortality. Developed and undeveloped health systems determine the response and humanitarian action. India remains a resource poor country where public health system has not paid any emphasis on special development of facilities. Burns cause significant morbidity and mortality and their prompt and swift management can reduce death and disability and, therefore, the need to have a plan for burn injury management in burn disaster. Lessons learnt from tackling various disasters have led to some improvement of public systems and realization of organized management for burn injuries. Preparation for burns disaster will help in improving and establishing burn care units. Therefore, every burns unit should prepare a burns disaster plan and it must be integrated with disaster planning of the emergency department and trauma care unit of the hospital. If possible, it should develop prehospital system or get linked with emergency prehospital system. It should be an integral part of the state and national disaster management plans.

The study and analysis of factors that cause a disaster, the characteristics that shape its evolution, the effects on the population and the natural environment, the instruments that can mitigate their effects and the various ways of re-establishing the optimal living conditions of the persons and communities involved have led to the creation of the new science of Disastrology. It studies disasters from all points of view and establishes guidelines for their management.

"Disaster medicine" considers the health aspects of disasters, in particular the study and collaborative application of the various health disciplines involved, i.e., from pediatrics, epidemiology, communicable disease, nutrition, public health, emergency surgery, social medicine, community care, humanitarian relief, and international health to the prevention, immediate response, and rehabilitation of the health problems arising from disaster, in cooperation with other disciplines involved in comprehensive disaster management. These approaches have led to the scientific elaboration of disaster planning and response. This has been gradually transformed from a combination of ad hoc and humane actions for the stricken persons into an efficient managerial system throughout all the phases and aspects of the disaster, from prediction and prevention to preparedness, immediate medical response, assistance, and rehabilitation.

Masellis described disaster as a serious and immediate threat to public health. He divided management and the rescue operations for (i) a fire disaster or thermal agent and (ii) a burn disaster.

Fire Disasters

It is a sudden vast ecological breakdown due to fire between man and his environment and needs extraordinary efforts to control this breakdown. This may not always result in a very large number of burn victims. Californian forest fires and Australian bush fires are the typical examples. Although a fire disaster need not necessarily reach catastrophic proportions, it will present some of the characteristic aspects of a disaster because of the highly destructive action of fire and the considerable number of victims. The surviving casualties will have mainly serious and extensive burns requiring immediate rescue procedures that cannot always be provided by local resources.

A fire of vast proportions can, moreover, cause damage to the surrounding environment by the massive production of heat and the emanation of burn gases and fumes. Smoke and gas, because of their suffocating action and their direct action on the airways, represent other specific danger elements. The danger of smoke and gas is generally underestimated by the population.

Stubble "parali" burning is a method of removing paddy crop residues from the field to sow wheat from the last week of September to November. It is a process of setting on fire the straw stubble, left after the harvesting of grains, like paddy, wheat, etc. It is usually required in areas using the combined harvesting method which leaves crop residue behind.

The process of burning farm residue is one of the major causes of air pollution in parts of North India, deteriorating the air quality causing epidemic respiratory ailments in cities like New Delhi and adjoining states.

With global climate change, the incidence of intense forest fires has risen ten-fold in India in the past two decades, according to a new study.

India ranked 7th among countries most impacted by climate change in 2019, according to the Global Climate Risk Index.

Wildfires were responsible for the death of some 310 people worldwide from January to September 2023, already putting 2023 as the year with the highest number of such deaths since 1990. In the past three decades, the global death toll due to wildfires surpassed 2,900.

Burn Disaster

It can be defined as the overall effect of the massive action of a known thermal agent on living beings. Burn disaster can be either part of a natural disaster like lightening, forest or bush fires, earthquake, volcanoes which are rare or manmade as airplane crash, building fires, explosions, fires in inflammable material industry, during transport of inflammable material or thermonuclear, and wars and terrorist acts. A burn disaster is characterized by a high number of fatalities and of seriously burned patients with a high potential for morbidity, mortality, and disability. Its extent may be aggravated if appropriate rescue operations are delayed. Some decisive factors involved here are the type of causal agent, the type of pathology caused, the overall characteristics of the harmful action of the thermal agent, the immediate evaluation of its gravity in relation to emergency care and the modalities of rescue operations.

In burn disaster, two concepts are, therefore, involved, viz., the pathological condition, i.e., extensive burns and the high number of persons injured. Its extent depends on the potentially large number of fatalities which is related to the considerably large number of persons involved, the seriousness of their condition and above all, the early initiation of emergency therapy. Advances in science and technology have increased the risk of accidents and transfer of energy to nearby population. We are confronted with possibility of use of harnessed powerful sources of energy and their accidental or malicious use to unleash the magnitude of destruction which can be appalling and shocking as in the case of World Trade Center terrorist attack. Such disaster terrorism and shift in war strategies have contributed to startling number of burn injuries or burn disasters. Therefore, a burn disaster is essentially a medical disaster for communities and the state and infrequently for the countries. It can be defined as any catastrophic event in which the number of burns victims exceeds capacity of local burn center(s) to provide optimal burn care. To tackle this disaster, one needs preparedness, planning, resource allocation, communication, and delegation of duties.

It can become a "humanitarian emergency" when the social, economic, and the medical infrastructure is disrupted or destroyed, and more and more victims of burn injury are generated which cannot be dealt with the already overburdened or poorly efficient and depleted medical systems. Such, ongoing humanitarian crisis exists today in several war affected countries because even small number of burn injuries constitutes a big disaster there.

What constitutes a burn disaster in terms of magnitude, number, and extent of burns is not defined. Few burn casualties may be a disaster in far flung places without medical facilities while a comparatively larger number of burn injuries may be dealt with satisfactorily in large cities because of large number of teaching institutes. In the USA, more than five victims of burn injury sustaining >20% total body surface area (TBSA) burn is a disaster and enough to trigger disaster response, while any fire incident causing >25 or more deaths is a major disaster (Masellis). As said earlier, if the local facility is overwhelmed by the number of burn injuries, then it is a disaster.

Most of the burn disaster are contained and local and rarely can be catastrophic as in case of war or large explosion nuclear leak. Study of epidemiology of burn disasters makes it unlikely. It is expected that the planning for general management of disasters will cope with such rare eventuality. But, even in countries which have such large-scale disaster plans, these plans remain untested.

From the burn physician's point of view, planning would essentially focus on medical treatment and intervention in case of large burn injury disaster. The most important aspect from public health planning would be to support medical infrastructure and develop burn care units to be operational in normal times.

EPIDEMIOLOGY OF BURNS DISASTERS IN INDIA

The greatest fire tragedy in India was the Bombay Docks explosion of April 14, 1944. A fire occurred in a ship called "Fort Strikine" in the Victoria Docks. The ship was carrying ammunition and explosives. A series of several explosions occurred, destroying about 14 ships. That day 336 people died and 1,040 were injured. The explosions were recorded over 1,000 miles away at Shimla. The total loss of property according to the then calculations was approximately rupees 100 crores. This was the worst explosion in the history of fire services in India which destroyed buildings in over 100 acres of Bombay Docks area. The death toll in the catastrophe was estimated at about 500, including 66 gallant officers and men of the Bombay Fire Brigade. Those gallant officers and men laid down their lives in the cause of safety, welfare, and prosperity of the community.

According to a conservative estimate of the Home Ministry, 4,000 human lives were lost along with the loss of property worth ₹ 588 crores due to fires in 1997. The actual figures may be much more, as the information collected was not exhaustive (Information Bureau, Government of India). Following are the details of major burn disaster in India since 1990.

April 16, 1990: 70 people were burnt to death as a shuttle train catches fire near Patna.

October 10, 1990: 40 persons were killed in a fire in a train near Cherpalli in Andhra Pradesh.

December 23, 1995: 442 people, majority of them children, were burnt to death at the Rajiv Marriage Palace in Dabwali town in Haryana. During the function of a local school there, the tent put up by the marriage palace, which had no permission to do so and flouted all fire safety norms, caught fire, and collapsed over 1,000 people.

June 13, 1997: 59 people died of asphyxia in Uphaar cinema hall fire, which broke out during screening of Hindi movie '*Border*'. Over 100 persons received injuries in the subsequent stampede.

February 27, 2002: 59 persons, including 25 women and 15 children charred to death in the S-6 coach of the train returning from Ayodhya at Godhra station.

May 15, 2003: A burst stove caused a devastating fire that swept through a speeding passenger train in Punjab, killing 40 people and injuring more than 50 persons.

January 23, 2004: 59 persons killed and injuring 60 people in a short circuit ignited fire in a marriage hall in Srirangam, a famous Hindu temple town 200 miles south of Chennai, Tamil Nadu.

July 2004: 94 children perished and 100 injured in a devastating school fire, Kumbakonam, Tamil Nadu.

April 10, 2006: Major fire killed at least 50 people, 115 people were injured in a blaze at a consumer fair in the industrial city of Meerut, Uttar Pradesh, 70 km from New Delhi.

December 10, 2008: An overloaded bus carrying 100 people broke down and caught fire. 63 people were killed due to fire and 40 severely burned.

October 29, 2009: A devastating fire/explosion accident occurred on 29th October 2009 at about 7.30 PM in the POL installation of M/s Indian Oil Corporation at Sitapura (Sanganer), Jaipur, Rajasthan, killing 11 persons and injuring 45 people.

March 23, 2010: Around 25 killed in an old mansion fire in Kolkata.

November 20, 2011: 15 persons died and more than 30 persons injured when a fire broke out at a community function of eunuchs in East Delhi.

December 9, 2011: At least 73 people died in fire at AMRI Hospital in Kolkata.

February 8, 2012: 11 workers were killed after fire broke out in an electronic factory in Haridwar.

July 30, 2012: 32 people killed in fire in Tamil Nadu Express bound for Chennai.

September 5, 2012: A catastrophic explosion happened in a firework factory at Mudalipatti near Sivakasi, a region known for its fireworks factories, that killed 54 workers and injuring 78 others.

December 28, 2013: At least 26 people, including two children, died after a fire broke out on a train. The blaze engulfed a carriage of the Nanded-Bangalore Express while it was traveling through southern Andhra Pradesh.

June 28, 2014: 15 people were killed and 20 persons injured in a blast in a GAIL **India** gas pipeline in Andhra Pradesh's East Godavari.

May 5, 2015: At least 21 people were burned to death after a bus fell into a ditch and caught fire in Central India.

April 11, 2016: Sunday's blaze at the 100-year-old Puttingal Devi temple complex in Paravur, Kerala, left 108 people dead and as many as 400 others injured.

December 28, 2017: Kamala Mills, Mumbai, in two rooftop pubs in Mumbai. The accident claimed 14 lives. The cause of the fire is claimed to be from a "hookah".

January 20, 2018: Around 6 PM, an illegal unit caught fire trapping laborers inside due to the exit being blocked by construction activity going around in the vicinity. The accident claimed the lives of 17 people.

June 19, 2018: A massive fire broke out at Viraat Hotel located in the Charbagh area of Lucknow. The accident claimed the lives of five people and injuring another five.

July 4, 2018: A fire cracker factory situated in Warangal, Telangana, was surrounded by fire on July 4, 2018. The fire caused the death of 10 workers who were trapped inside the factory.

December 17, 2018: Fire accident took place at ESIC Kamgar Hospital, Marol, Mumbai claiming the lives of 10 people on December 17, 2018.

February 12, 2019: 17 people, many of them sleeping guests, were killed in a *fire* at a *hotel* "Arpit Palace", in central *Delhi's* congested Karol Bagh area.

May 24, 2019: Fire had engulfed a tuition class running on illegally constructed 4th floor of *Takshashila* Arcade in Surat. A total of 22 students died and 19 others were injured in the incident.

December 8, 2019: A fire occurred at a factory building in Anaj Mandi area of Delhi, India. At least 43 people died and more than 56 people were injured.

August 9, 2020: A major fire broke out in at a coronavirus disease 2019 (COVID-19) facility located at the Hotel Swarna Palace in Vijayawada, Andhra Pradesh. The fire killed 11 people and wounded a further 22 people.

March 9, 2021: Nine people, including four firemen were killed in fire in Kolkata.

March 26, 2021: Ten patients died after a fire broke out at a hospital inside a mall in Mumbai where coronavirus patients were being treated.

June 7, 2021: In a major tragedy, at least 18 employees of a chemical factory located in Pune, Maharashtra, lost their lives while many missing as a massive fire broke out at the company's sanitizer manufacturing unit.

November 6, 2021: There were at least 11 COVID-19 patients died and several others sustained serious injuries after a fire broke out in the intensive care unit (ICU) of a civil hospital in Ahmednagar city, Maharashtra.

September 13, 2022: Eight people died and many were injured after a massive fire broke out at an electric scooter showroom in Hyderabad.

January 28, 2023: At least six persons, including a doctor couple, lost their lives due to suffocation after a massive fire broke out at Dhanbad in Jharkhand.

February 1, 2023: At least 14 people lost their lives, and many others were injured after a major fire broke out at a multistorey building at Dhanbad in Jharkhand.

March 17, 2023: Six people died when a massive fire broke out at the 10-storey commercial complex (Swapnalok Complex) in Telangana's Secunderabad.

July 29, 2023: Eight people were killed and several others sustained injuries after a massive explosion ripped through a firecracker factory in Krishnagiri, Tamil Nadu.

August 26, 2023: At least 10 people lost their lives, while over 20 people were injured after a massive fire broke out inside a stationary train compartment at the Madurai Railway Station in Tamil Nadu.

October 17, 2023: At least 11 people reportedly lost their lives in explosions at two separate firecracker units in Tamil Nadu's Virudhunagar.

Increasing incidents of terrorism involving explosions in recent times have resulted in multiple system trauma along with burn injuries.

The year 2008 claimed more than 210 lives and left more than 600 injured due to terrorist attacks in Jaipur (May 13th), Ahmedabad (July 26th), Delhi (September 13th), and Guwahati (October 30th). The worst terrorist attack on India occurred on 26th November 2008 and left 182 dead and more than 300 injured and torched several five-star hotels.

In India, during Diwali on 28th October 2008, more than 1,000 fires were reported from all over country and firecrackers, most of them unsafe, worth rupees 600 crores were burst. There were more than 5,000 injuries and at least 100 of them were very serious. The firecracker industry in India is 1,000 crores and as mentioned 600 crores worth crackers are spent around Diwali alone. The firecracker industry is becoming more and more unregulated and is experimenting with newer and dangerous combinations to compete with Chinese firecracker industry. We create and live this disaster every year.

We do not have records of burn injuries in India. It is estimated by extrapolation of population figures that there are 700,000 major burn injuries every year and about

120,000 die of burns. We do not have adequate facilities in terms of bed and personnel to provide them with optimal care. So, there is an ongoing burn disaster in India.

VULNERABILITY ASSESSMENT AND RISK ANALYSIS

Risk analysis and vulnerability assessment involves the creation of a scenario for each potential disaster in terms of exposure, loss of life, damage to property, and the geographic distribution of each hazard. Any monitoring facility, regulatory regimen, and counter measures available for each disaster are accounted for in this analysis.

Mass casualties from burns occur when fire and/or explosions interface with large numbers of people **(Figs. 1 to 3)**. In this context, the most likely hazards identified for India are fires, explosions, transport, train accidents, inflammable material trucks and tankers, mass gatherings especially in temporary structures, high-density urban dwellings, offshore oilrigs, and acts of civil disturbance and terrorism. The recent fire disasters show that in indoor fires where the victims are trapped, immediate morbidity and the very high rate of death were due to hypoxia (inhalation injuries). Intoxication due to carbon monoxide poisoning and other toxic fumes led to inability and incapacity to react and escape and, therefore, high indoor death rates as in Uphaar cinema fire tragedy.

Natural disasters such as rural fires and earthquakes fires are rare in India. In recent years, shift in terrorism to urban areas using unconventional ways to wrought destruction through explosion and fire as in the cases like 9/11 World Trade Center in New York (2001), Bali (2002), and Madrid (2004). All three events highlight the fact that many patients suffered significant burn injuries as well as other multiple system traumas. Indeed, in the Bali bombings, 62 patients were admitted across Australia, occupying all adult burn beds. This extra patient surge occurred on the background of normal operations where severe burn patients from other incidents also required care. As India is becoming the most common target of international terrorism with mass casualty burn disasters occurring with catastrophic consequences, it is important to have formal plans at both a State/Territory and national level.

Historical analysis of terrorist events, where improvised explosive devices (IEDs) have been used, consistently demonstrates that up to 10–15% of the total live casualties have severe burn injury and other multiple trauma injuries requiring critical care/tertiary level burn services.

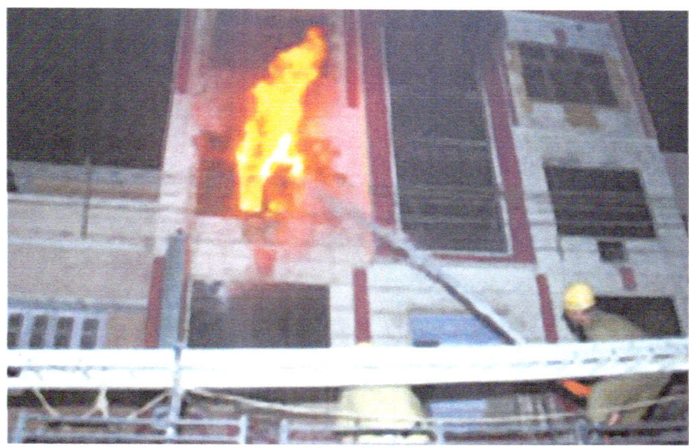

FIG. 2: Firemen in action during a fire in a high-rise building.

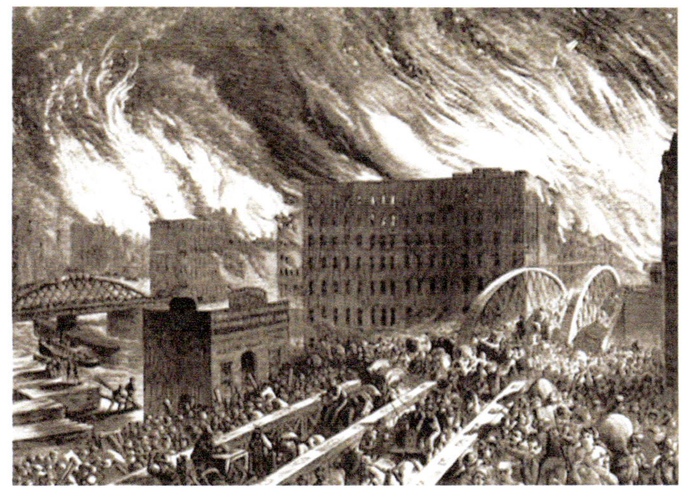

FIG. 1: Historical picture depicting a major fire.

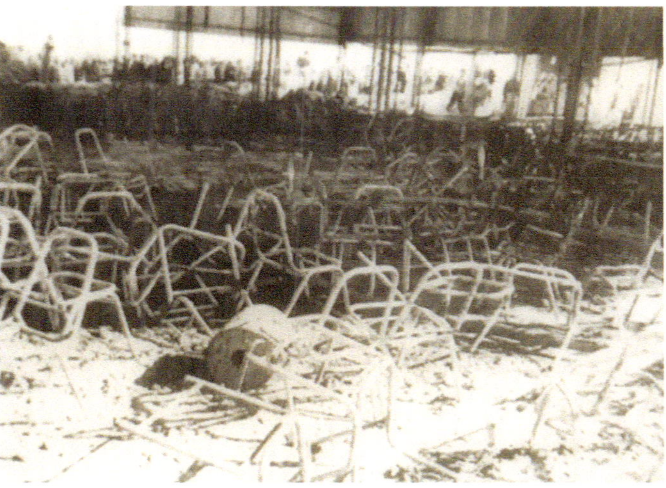

FIG. 3: Seen of the Dabwali fire disaster.

On the basis of scenario planning and historical precedent, in a worst-case scenario, with 2,000 live casualties, India will have to manage a surge of up to 300 severe burn injured patients in case of the worst explosive attack. This will significantly challenge existing systems.

Burns injuries in a disaster or burn injury disaster cannot be viewed only as a medical emergency and their management cannot be done in isolation. With the increasing awareness about scientific ways to manage a disaster, it becomes imperative that management of burn injury is an integral part of overall disaster management.

The limited scope of interpreting a burn injury disaster from hospital or healthcare point of view has to change to holistic disaster planning.

Therefore, all burns disaster plans have to be part of the comprehensive, multi-hazard disaster management plans, emphasizing disaster management response, disaster awareness, and education.

APPROACH TO DISASTER MANAGEMENT IN INDIA

The increasing frequency and fury of natural disasters have shaken the policy makers of India and a high-power committee has been established to address the multiple facets of natural and manmade disasters in India.

Till recently, the approach to disaster management has been reactive and relief centric. A paradigm shift has now taken place at the national level from the relief centric syndrome to holistic and integrated approach with emphasis on prevention, mitigation, and preparedness. These efforts are aimed to conserve developmental gains as also to minimize loss of lives, livelihood, and property.

A typical "Disaster Management" continuum as shown below, comprising six elements, i.e., (i) Prevention, (ii) Mitigation, and (iii) Preparedness in predisaster phase and (iv) Response, (v) Rehabilitation, and (vi) Reconstruction in postdisaster phase, defines the complete approach to "disaster management **(Flowchart 1)**".

Government of India (GOI), in recognition of the importance of disaster management as a national priority, set up a High-Powered Committee (HPC) in August 1999 and also a national committee after the Gujarat earthquake, for making recommendations on the preparation of disaster management plans and suggestions for effective mitigation mechanisms. The 10th Five-year Plan Document also had, for the first time, a detailed chapter on disaster management. Similarly, the 12th Finance Commission was also mandated to review the financial arrangements for disaster management.

On 23rd December 2005, the Government of India enacted the Disaster Management Act **(Flowchart 2)**, which envisaged the creation of the National Disaster

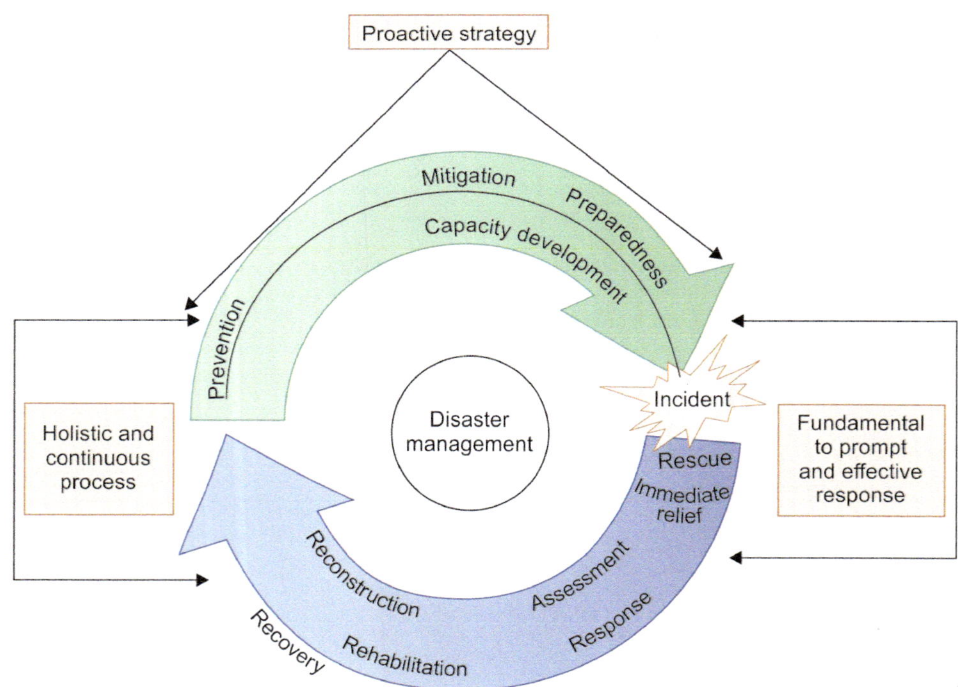

FLOWCHART 1: Disaster management continuum.

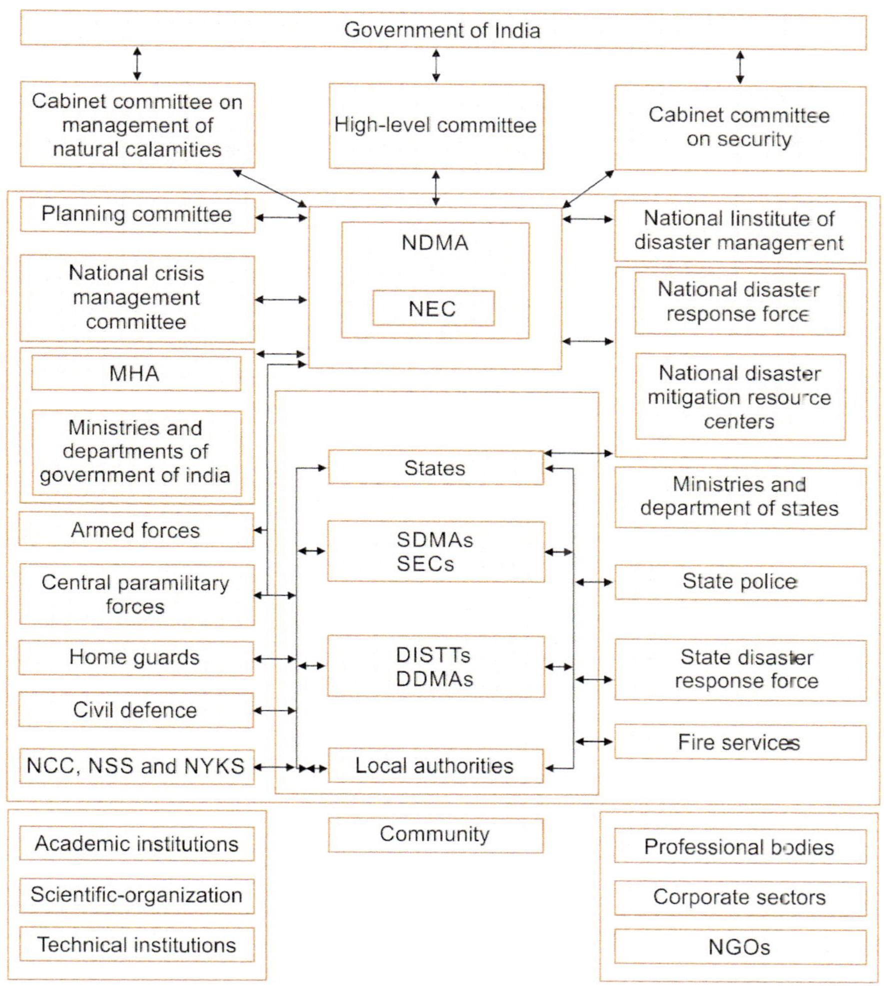

Notes:
- This diagram reflects interactive linkages for synergized management of disasters and not a hierarchical structure.
- Backward and forward linkages, especially at the functional level, are with a view to optimize efficiency.
- Participation of the community is a crucial factor.

FLOWCHART 2: National disaster management structure.

(DDMAs: District Disaster Management Authorities; MHA: Ministry of Home Affairs; NCC: National Cadet Corps; NDMA: National Disaster Management Authority; NEC: National Executive Committee; NGOs: nongovernmental organizations; NSS: National Service Scheme; NYKS: Nehru Yuva Kendra Sangathan; SDMA: State Disaster Management Authorities; SEC: State Executive Committee)

Management Authority (NDMA), headed by the Prime Minister and State Disaster Management Authorities (SDMAs) headed by respective Chief Ministers, to spearhead and implement a holistic and integrated approach to disaster management in the country.

National Institute of Disaster Management

Under the NDMA and through disaster management act, a National Institute of Disaster Management (NIDM) was created. It is a premier national organization working for human resource development at national level in the area of disaster mitigation and management. The NIDM came into existence on October 16, 2003 by the Government of India order upgrading the National Centre for Disaster Management (NCDM), which was located at Indian Institute of Public Administration, New Delhi. The NCDM was established by the Ministry of Agriculture, Department of Agriculture and Cooperation, Government of India, in March 1995. The NCDM had been functioning as a Nodal Center for the human resource development in the area of disaster management. NIDM will be gearing up the national, state, and district level administration to tackle natural calamities and will also be coordinating research projects, training programs, and will build a database on natural disasters with case studies.

India Disaster Resource Network

Under the national disaster plan, Ministry of Home Affairs, Government of India, established India Disaster Resource Network (IDRN). This is the network of networks. IDRN portal was launched in September 2003 in collaboration with United Nations Development Program (UNDP). Technical support was extended by UNDP to systematically formulate the resource inventory through an organized information system designed to collate and assimilate information from authorities in 563 district and 35 State/Union territories. The online inventory clearly lists out sequential details on specific equipment, types, their functions performed, human expertise in search and rescue operations and contact details of expertise and suppliers for prompt mobilization. IDRN was designed as a web-enabled information system to provide updated inventory of related items every quarter, entered at two levels, i.e., at district and state level. The portal has been hosted to the central server at the National Information Center (NIC), which is providing technical support to Ministry of Home Affairs. The portal has an online dual accessible interface system for users from state disaster management/relief and rehabilitation department officials (Relief Commissioners), district administrators (District Magistrate/Collectors), and other state and district nodal officers, corporate members, and public who can browse the portal. The user can obtain cataloged information as well as query-based data and list of resources available at district and state level. The online inventory user manual and details can be accessed at http://www.idrn.gov.in.

On the IDRN, nationwide availability of beds for burn injury can be listed along with trauma units and their surge capacity. National Academy of Burns-India (NABI) should provide authentic information after getting all the information from the public and private hospitals on IRDN to be used at the time of disasters. The list of burn care physicians should also be provided area-wise with their contact information for use during disaster.

Burn Disaster Response Team

At present no plan for burn disaster response team (BDRT) has been made in disaster planning in India a whole or in any other state. A burns disaster team can be raised in larger institutes, e.g., Safdarjung Hospital in New Delhi, as they are the repository of large number of trained burn care experts. At least one team should be readied with personnel, equipment, and resources to be dispatched at short notice from the Department of Burns and Plastic Surgery at Safdarjung Hospital, which is directly under Central Government. It will help dispatching such team promptly as sending an international and interstate humanitarian mission requires government permission.

Burn care is not optimal in all countries and even in India only very few centers provide desired optimal care. Therefore, there is a need to raise BDRTs. Government of India or National Academy of Burns India (NABI) and Burn Association of India (BAI) should prepare a plan to constitute such BDRTs and offer these teams for national needs in areas of deficient expertise or for international humanitarian missions.

Burn disaster response team can travel at short notice to the disaster site and carry out effective primary triage, first aid and execute safe transport. BDRT should have a designated leader and teammembers. The vehicles and resources should be planned and earmarked.

India Disaster Resource Network can also enlist information about individuals and agencies who can volunteer at the time of disaster and humanitarian crisis.

To build a safer and disaster resilient India by developing a holistic, proactive, multidisaster, and technology-driven strategy for disaster management, collective efforts of all governmental agencies, and nongovernmental organizations are required.

National Disaster Response Force

The concept: The Disaster Management Act has mandated the constitution of a Specialist Response Force to a threatening disaster situation or a disaster. This force will function under the NDMA which has been vested with its control direction, and general superintendence. This will be a multidisciplinary, multiskilled, high-technology force for all types of disasters capable of insertion by air, sea, and land. All the eight battalions are to be equipped and trained for all natural disasters including four battalions in combating nuclear, biological, and chemical disasters **(Fig. 4)**.

Present organization: Presently, this force is constituted of eight battalions, two each from the Border Security Force (BSF), Central Reserve Police Force (CRPF), Central Industrial Security Force (CISF), and Indo-Tibetan Border Police (ITBP). Each battalion will provide 18 self-contained specialist search and rescue teams of 45 personnel each including engineers, technicians, electricians, dog squads, and medics/paramedics. The total strength of each battalion will be approximately 1,158.

Deployment: These National Disaster Response Force (NDRF) battalions are located at 16 different locations in the country based on the vulnerability profile to cut

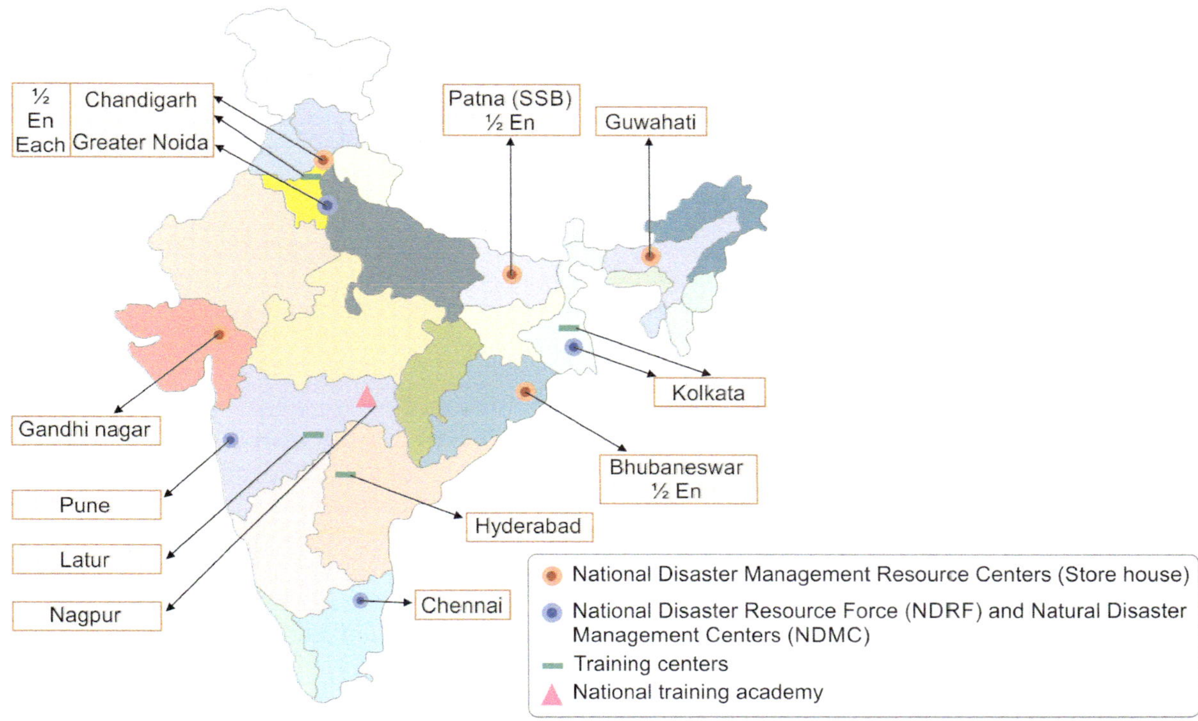

FIG. 4: National disaster response battalions and training centers.

down the response time for their deployment. During the preparedness period/in a threatening disaster situation, proactive deployment of these forces will be carried out by the NDMA in consultation with state authorities.

There is an urgent need to establish national burn injury response team which can be done as mentioned earlier at few large institutes in the country. One of the ideal centers to constitute such a team will be Safdarjung Hospital, New Delhi, as it is repository of largest number of burn specialists and paramedical and the trainees directly under Government of India.

National Disaster Mitigation Resource Centers

The National Disaster Mitigation Resource Centers (NDMRCs) will be co-located with the NDRF battalions. These will also serve as repositories for NDMR bricks of relief stores for 25,000 affected people, in each of the nine locations. These will cater to the emergent requirements especially for the first 72–96 hours. At Kolkata and Chandigarh, additional bricks of stores for 50,000 people each will be kept for high-altitude areas. These stores will supplement the reserves maintained by the respective States. In addition, these centers will assist in running mock drills and capacity development programs. During disasters, they will act as facilitators to the States/Union Territories in deployment of central resources and provide much needed additional link to the center.

NATIONAL DISASTER MANAGEMENT GUIDELINES-MEDICAL PREPAREDNESS AND MASS CASUALTIES MANAGEMENT

Medical Management of Mass Casualties is based upon "all hazard" concept where practically every Ministry/Department will be playing a role directly or indirectly with nodal ministry as Ministry of Health and Family Welfare, Government of India. As per the National Disaster Management Act, 2005, NDMA is required to prepare Guidelines, based on which, the Nodal Ministry will prepare a detailed action plan for the better and effective medical management of mass casualties. In view of evolving such guidelines, a National Workshop on Medical Preparedness and Mass Casualties Management was convened by NDMA in August, 2006 and various experts from the Center, State Governments and NGOs participated. In this workshop, the present status of the medical preparedness in the country was discussed and future course of action was set up. It was decided to articulate the MPMCM guidelines through a document called National Disaster Management Guidelines-Medical Preparedness and Mass Casualties Management (NDMG-MPMCM). A Core Group of the experts from the various fields related to medical management was constituted under a Chairman to assist NDMA in preparing National Guidelines for MPMCM. The core group has met for deliberations and has yet to finalize its recommendations. NDMA has observed some critical gaps in managing mass casualties and issued fresh guidelines for the disaster and need to adopt multidisciplinary and multisectoral approach for prevention/mitigation strategies so as to develop capacities to improve response. It envisages strengthening of about 200 hospitals from basic trauma care to advanced tertiary care, all networked with prehospital care ambulances to provide care during transit and hospitalize within the golden hour.

Essentially, apex bodies of central government are trying to associate other professionals. Surprisingly, no associates of medical fraternity, especially the burns care bodies like NABI or burns care experts have been nominated. There is an urgent need for NABI to take this issue with MP-MCM group. A model integrated plan applicable to all districts of India for management of burn injury mass casualty should be submitted. Making plans in isolation will not be effective as NDMA is planning disaster management to the level of districts through state government.

The Section 23 of the Disaster Management Act, 2005 provides that there shall be a disaster management plan for every state. It outlines the broad coverage of the plan as well as the requirements of consultation in the preparation of the state plans. It also provides for annual review and updating of the state plan, and enjoins upon the state governments to make provisions for financing the activities to be carried out under the state plans. It provides for the departments of the state governments to draw up their own plans in accordance with the state plan. The state plans shall be prepared by the State Executive Committee (SEC) in conformity with the guidelines to be issued on related matters by the SDMA having regard to the guidelines laid down in this regard by the NDMA and after such consultation with local and district authorities and the people's representatives as the SEC may deem fit.

With assistance of UNDP and United States Agency for International Development (USAID) under the State Disaster Management Plan document (SDMP), the states have been assisted to draw district and block level DMP through the Panchayati Raj Institution. The DMP has been prepared for 8,643 villages, 1,046 Gram Panchayats, 1,818 blocks, and 82 districts. More than 29,000 elected representatives have already been trained besides volunteers at village level who are being trained. Besides this, 18,000 government officials, 865 engineers, 425 architects, 600 master trainers, and 1,200 teachers have already been trained. 29 states have disaster management facilitates and plans finalized. Twenty eight of them have created training institutes. States such as Gujarat, Maharashtra, Assam, and Bihar have finalized their disaster plans and have published them **(Fig. 5)**.

In an effort to create awareness and plan for future management of disasters, disaster management has been introduced as subject in class eighth and ninth by Central Board of Secondary Education (CBSE), New Delhi.

In major cities (with a population exceeding 10 lakhs), municipal corporations have a large administrative system including departments like engineering, public health and revenue, and sometimes fire services. These should provide a good mechanism for coordinated response in case of any crisis/disaster. Therefore, management of major cities should be planned as a unit. In metropolitan cities, it is also advisable to make the urban metropolitan government directly responsible for DM.

Medical Preparedness and Mass Casualty Management

The following points must be reflected in the state plan:
- Listing of all hospitals and Primary Health Centers including private nursing homes and their capacities.
- Emergency casualty management plans at the local, district, and state level.
- For effective management of big cities like Delhi and Mumbai, nearby medical facilities must also be built into plans.
- Availability of mobile hospitals and/or plans for acquiring the same. The state plan may also adopt the Generic Categorization of Disasters with specific plans at the state level by various departments to handle different disasters.

COMPOSITION

National Disaster Response Force is a force of 16 battalions, organized on paramilitary lines, and manned by persons on deputation from the paramilitary forces of India: three BSF, three CRPF, two CISF, two ITBP, two Sashastra Seema Bal (SSB), and one of the Assam Rifles. The total strength of each battalion is approximately 1,149. Each battalion is capable of providing 18 self-contained specialist search and rescue teams of 45 personnel each including engineers, technicians, electricians, dog squads, and medical/paramedics.

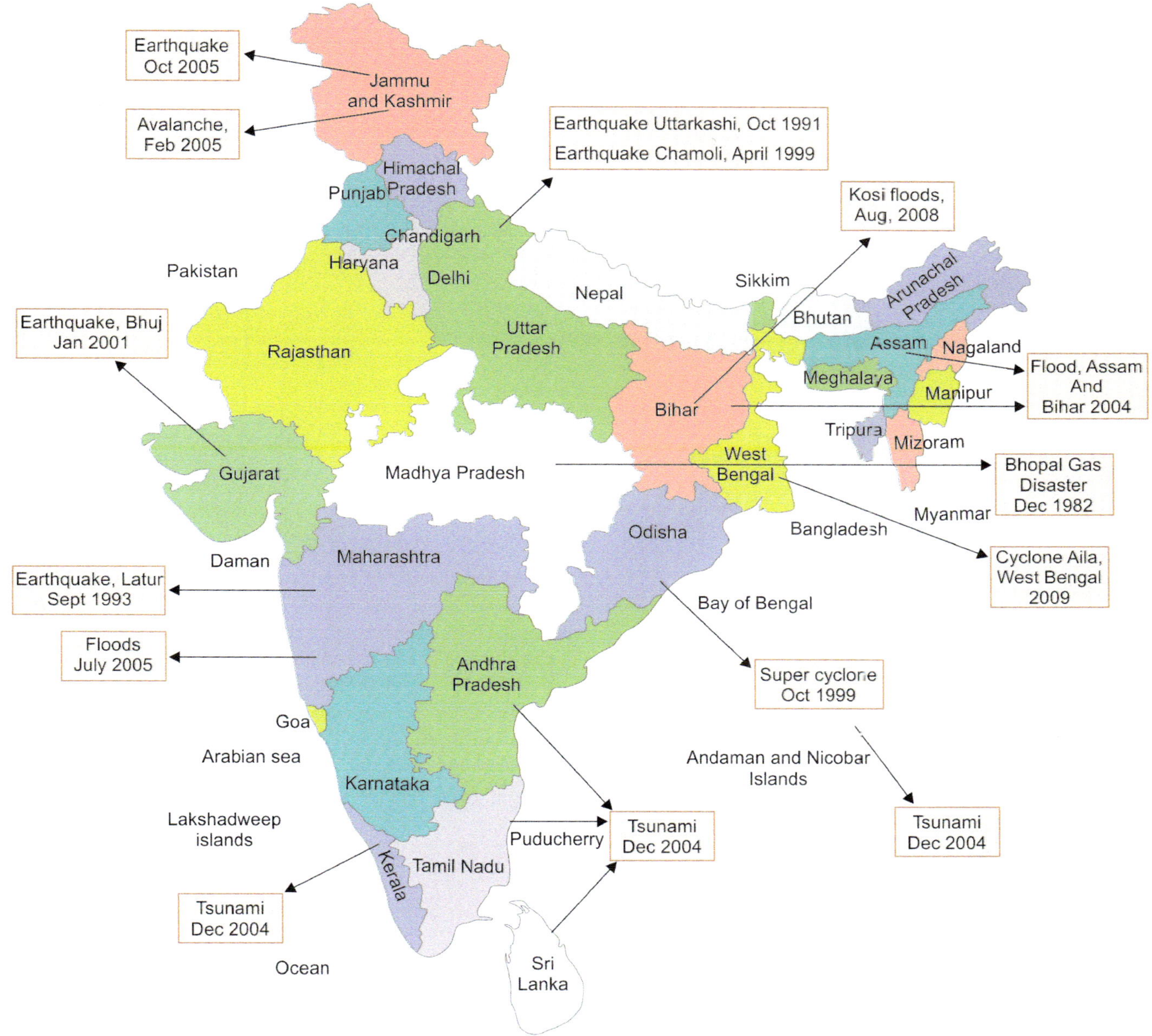

FIG. 5: Major disasters in India (1980–2009).

DEPLOYMENT

These NDRF battalions are located at 16 different locations in the country based on the vulnerability profile to cut down the response time for their deployment. During the preparedness period/in a threatening disaster situation, proactive deployment of these forces will be carried out by the NDMA in consultation with state authorities. The present location of NDRF battalions are as follows:

S. No.	NDRF unit	State	PMF
1	01 Bn NDRF, Guwahati	Assam	BSF
2	02 Bn NDRF, Nadia	West Bengal	BSF
3	03 Bn NDRF, Cuttack	Odisha	CISF
4	04 Bn NDRF, Vellore	Tamil Nadu	CISF
5	05 Bn NDRF, Pune	Maharashtra	CRPF
6	06 Bn NDRF, Vadodara	Gujarat	CRPF

Continued

Continued

S. No.	NDRF unit	State	PMF
7	07 Bn NDRF, Bhatinda	Punjab	ITBP
8	08 Bn NDRF, Ghaziabad	Uttar Pradesh	ITBP
9	09 Bn NDRF, Patna	Bihar	BSF
10	10 Bn NDRF, Vijayawada	Andhra Pradesh	CRPF
11	11 Bn NDRF, Varanasi	Uttar Pradesh	SSB
12	12 Bn NDRF, Itanagar	Arunachal Pradesh	SSB
13	13 Bn NDRF, Sambha	Jammu and Kashmir	Assam Rifles
14	14 Bn NDRF, Mandi	Himachal Pradesh	ITBP
15	15 Bn NDRF, Haldwani	Uttarakhand	ITBP
16	16 Bn NDRF, Najafgarh	New Delhi	BSF

(BSF: Border Security Force; CISF: Central Industrial Security Force; CRPF: Central Reserve Police Force; ITBP: Indo-Tibetan Border Police; NDRF: National Disaster Response Force; PMF: Para Military Force; SSB: Sashastra Seema Bal)

Levels of Disaster

The levels of disasters have been categorized and disseminated as L0, L1, L2, and L3, based on the ability of various authorities to deal with them. Various color codes relating to the level of alerts have also been designated.

- L0: denotes normal times which are expected to be utilized for close monitoring, documentation, prevention, mitigation, and preparatory activities. This is the planning stage where plans at all levels from community to the State shall be put in place. Training on search and rescue, rehearsals, evaluation, and inventory updating for response activities will be carried out during this time.
- *L1*: Specifies disasters that can be managed at the district level. However, the state and center will remain in readiness to provide assistance, if needed.
- *L2*: Specifies disaster situations that may require assistance and active participation of the state and the mobilization of resources at the state level.
- *L3*: Disaster situations arise from large-scale disasters where districts and the state may not have the capacity to respond adequately and require assistance from the central government for reinstating the state and district machinery.
- Even though there cannot be watertight compartmentalization of responsibilities between states and the center, especially in the case of man-made disasters, the participation by center will normally beat the L3 level. Most of the burn disasters would fall in L1 or L2 types. The burn care facility in the district has to coordinate with the district disaster plan (DDP). It has to become part of the community-based DDP. In case of absence of the burn care facility, the local government and private medical facility will have to be enlisted to provide initial care and plan evacuation to the nearby burn facility.

Role of the Emergency Operations Center

Timebound action plans must be indicated for creating facilities for environment scanning, intelligence gathering, operations, and logistics management under one roof for holistic and efficient management of disasters at the state and district level. Arrangements must be made and procedures must be laid down for manning the Emergency Operations Center (EOC) on 24 × 7 × 365 basis. The plan must also cover in detail the indigenized Incident Command System at the state, district, and local body levels.

The disaster specific plans for mining, oil spills, biological, chemical, and nuclear have been made by some states but no burn disaster specific plan has been made by any state or city administration. It is felt that bodies like NABI, with local burns care facilities, should develop burn disaster plans taking into consideration the local facilities, geographical conditions, etc. A model burn disaster plan for cities and rural area can be prepared and submitted to NDMA coordinating the activities of various health disciplines to prevent disasters, provide an immediate response to a disaster and help in rehabilitation of victims.

BURN INJURY SCENE IN INDIA

In India, specialized burns care is available for the last 60 years, but gloom prevails over this particular discipline, marked by alarming morbidity and mortality. On an average, burns center of a public hospital is able to save patients with burns below 40%. Those having burns close to 50% have 50% chances of survival and very few cases survive having burns beyond 60%. In West Bengal, the survival rate of a 50% burn is a dismal 25%. This is in stark contrast with the developed countries where patients with >70% burns also survive and the survival rate of patients with 50% burn is from 75–90%. There are approximately 70 burns units in India which are grossly inadequate. With around 700,000 major burn victims needing hospitalization and 120,000 succumbing to the injury, the meager 40 burns units in the country (of which only 19 are said to be up to the mark with a low mortality and morbidity rate) are not able to meet the demands and render quality care.

India with a population of >1.4 billion needs 10 times more number of burns units in the country. In the United States, there are about 120 burn care facilities for a population of <300 million.

Burns care in government hospitals is plagued by lack of infrastructure, whether it is sophisticated equipment, availability of medicines, spacing between beds or the manpower. With burns care needing the facilities of an ICU, some burns units are run without basic equipment like ventilator, pulse oximeter, infusion pump and patient weighing machine and skin graft mesher, etc.

The burns unit is not something that the private sector evinces interest with problems of high infection rates, medico-legal work (with every burns case to be reported to the police and requiring evidence in the court in case of complications) and a long hospital stay.

While the chances of survival of severe burns patient can be enhanced by skin grafting, burns surgeon rues that cadaver donation of skin cannot be practiced with the noninclusion of skin in "Transplantation of Human Organs (THO) Act, 1994". Though burns surgeon did lobby to allow cadaveric donation of skin, the government had turned down the proposal on the ground that skin is a tissue and not an organ and hence cannot be included in THO Act. Live skin donation is hampered by unavailability of donors, the risks associated with contacting acquired immunodeficiency syndrome (AIDS) and the pain and trauma that the donor has to undergo.

Since last few years movement to establish skin banks have gained momentum now, we have about 17 skin banks in India.

Although there are >2,600 plastic surgeons in India who constitute a useful resource of trained personnel in burns, most of them dedicate themselves to burns care only partially. Not >50 burns surgeons are exclusively dedicated to burns care. All the burns units in government hospitals are usually full. Therefore, there is hardly any surge capacity in specialized care units for burns injuries in India.

SURGE CAPACITY OF HEALTHCARE UNITS

Surge capacity has been defined as the "healthcare system's ability to manage a sudden or rapidly progressive influx of patients within the currently available resources at a given point in time. This term entered the disaster medicine lexicon after "9/11" 2001 in America, and has become a key feature of health disaster planning since the severe acute respiratory syndrome (SARS) outbreaks, the rising threat of pandemic influenza and the Madrid and London bombings in 2004 and 2005, respectively.

Mass trauma events in urban environments create surge problems for hospitals in the first 4 hours, with the majority of casualties likely to arrive at the hospital in the first 60–90 minutes. Health systems need to be able to meet this increased demand after acute mass casualty events, with an influx of patients who may require "specialized evaluation or intervention" specially burns, including surgery for penetrating trauma. As the epidemiology of traumatic events will differ depending on the cause, any preparations to manage a mass casualty event needs to be flexible enough to deal with a range of disaster types, including infectious disease emergencies and bioterrorism, with their more insidious and later-peaking surge.

Meeting the challenges of surge capacity enhancement calls for cooperative action at the complex interface between clinical practice, health systems management, logistics, facilities management, and personnel deployment.

The US Health Resources and Services Administration has set a minimum benchmark for surge capacity of 500 adults and pediatrics patients per million population for infectious disease events and at least 50 patients per million population sustaining trauma or burns in a mass casualty event. These figures have not been validated and based on other traumatic events, 100–300 patients per million may be more accurate for burns or trauma. The consensus from a series of articles on the "science of surge" in the November 2006 issue of Academic Emergency Medicine was that there is little or no quantifiable measurement for managing an acute "sudden impact" surge or the even less predictable surge resulting from infectious disease emergencies or obscure events.

Last COVID epidemic has seen dramatic increase in the surge capacity of all the medical facilities including ventilators, oxygenerators, oxygen plants which have seen at least three times increase. It leaves Indian medical facilities in urban and district hospitals manifold surge capacity to treat inhalation injuries due to smoke.

WORLD FIRST PORTABLE HOSPITAL

Another innovative and novel development of India and consisting of a set of "mini-cubes" which can be airlifted and deployed on any terrain, the "world's first portable disaster hospital" is now ready to be used shared with the world. This easy-to-use mobile medical facility can be swiftly deployed to save lives in the most challenging circumstances. It can provide critical medical care to 100 survivors for up to 48 hours, making it a lifeline on remote and tough terrains where immediate medical attention is needed. The cubes (which are self-sustained healthcare units) can handle bullet, burn, head, spinal and chest injuries, fractures, and major bleeding. India is now equipped and ready to supply this to any country in need.

The portable hospital was developed as part of Prime Minister Narendra Modi's ambitious "Project BHISHMA" (Bharat Health Initiative for Sahyog Hita and

Maitri) and consists of a fully equipped operation theater, mini-ICUs, ventilators, blood-testing equipment, an X-ray machine, and even a cooking station. It also includes a shelter facility and power generator, making it entirely self-sufficient during emergencies.

The lifesaving equipment are packed in a set of "mini-cubes" and a combination of these mini-cubes is used to set up a mobile hospital capable of performing life-saving surgery. The mini-cubes are carried in a "Aarogya Maitri Cube Cage", which has three frames, each accommodating 12 mini-cubes. An Aarogya Maitri Cube Cage can fit 36 mini-cubes overall.

Indian air force had deployed two Arogya Maitry Cubes hospitals with capacity to treat 400 patients of any disaster at Ayodhya.

Some of the measures which can be implemented in case of huge surge are:

- Creating temporary hospital facilities within public hospitals by having caches of medical supplies and equipment available.
- Using alternative health facilities, such as operating theaters, beds, and diagnostic resources in private hospitals and day procedure units for the "walking wounded" and "decanted" patients (patients already in hospital who can be transferred elsewhere to make way for disaster victims).
- Using general and private health practitioners to provide a range of care for the walking wounded and decanted patients; and
- Applying modified models of care, such as longer shifts and extended scope of practice for nurses, allied health practitioners and medical and other health students.

PREVENTION AND MITIGATION

Prevention is the most important public health tenet.

Pure disaster response alone is not sufficient and gives only tiding away and temporary results at a very high cost. Prevention and mitigation contribute to lasting improvement in safety and are essential to integrate in disaster planning.

To avoid a mass burn casualty disaster, planning from several key government areas is required in terms of legislation and strict implementation.

Industrial, high-density, urban fires—all buildings should have fire prevention strategies (sprinklers, smoke alarms, and fire egress). All residents of the buildings should be briefed on fire prevention and escape. This will be the responsibility of state-operated fire services.

It has been noted that although strict laws for buildings and other structures exist, it is the poor implementation and lack of will to maintain fire safety equipment which is the root cause of failure for prevention. Most of the Indian states have enacted their building codes and fire safety acts to meet the requirement of high-rise buildings.

Inspection of all buildings for their fire safety worthiness should be done on a regular basis. Fire escape plans must be displayed properly. Every room of a public building should have fire-escape plan displayed.

The fire departments under state governments are not well maintained and staffed. They need to have better allocation of funds to strengthen firefighting capacities.

Although there is national fire-safety institute in Nagpur but more needs to be done in the field of fire safety.

Forest fires—Although forest fires are rare in India, these fires have been reported sporadically from Himachal Pradesh in north India and Tamil Nadu and Karnataka in south India. Forest department, usually with district authorities, takes care of these fires.

Transport—All transport devices should meet the criteria for transport of hazardous materials. *Responsibility:* State Road and Transport authorities, Ports authorities, and Commercial Aircraft Safety Authority should implement the laws strictly.

Terrorism—To prevent a mass-burn disaster through an act of terrorism, intelligence from agencies such as newly created National Intelligence Authority, state intelligence, BSFs, and national body to fight terrorism is required. In the wake of terrorist attack from sea, strengthening of our coast by Coast guards and Navy is required.

Information should be freely available to all residents on what to do and where to go in the event of a major disaster.

Mitigation Strategy

The mitigation strategy and plan focus on the long-term planning for disaster reduction. It deals with the issues of continued commitment to hazard identification and risk assessment, applied research and technology transfer, investment incentives for mitigation and leadership and coordination for mitigation. The mitigation strategy makes an argument for better land use management, building codes, traffic standards, and health standards. These objectives are to be secured through disaster legislation, mitigation regulation, and incentives for mitigation.

At the state and district levels, the same structure is followed. The Disaster Management Plan calls for the creation of a variety of facilities and resources which provide support in the nature of infrastructure and organizational requirements.

FUNDAMENTALS OF BURN DISASTER PLANNING

- The burn injuries are common in mass disasters and terror attacks.
- The disaster plan is the best tool for preparedness.
- Burn center care is the most efficient and cost-effective care of burn injuries.

Burn centers are not same as trauma-care centers. Burn centers are unique national resources. NABI, has the capacity to be a key component in national disaster readiness for mass casualty.

Planning requires preexisting health and medical infrastructure and cooperation with local and state governmental agencies. Specialized burn care facility and the team are the key around which the plan must be developed. There has to be an active encouragement to layout plan for emergencies. All the stakeholders in burns mass casualty should be made partners. They are police, district civil authorities, fire department, emergency medical services, ambulance services, transport providers, health department, health centers, hospitals of burns care units, private physician, and NGOs.

The objective is to provide optimal treatment of disaster victim at the earliest. Though detailed plans through state disaster management to the level of district have been worked out, burn mass casualty management has not been included. The burn care organization and the specialized burn care units need to draw the attention of the state and national planners and get themselves included in the disaster plans. Scientific bodies like NABI should coordinate with state and national authorities.

Burn disasters are usually man-made, usually confined to local and limited geographical area. Consumption in terms of manpower and material are maximum for burn injury. Even three to four patients have the capacity to strain health facility. More than 20 patients will require intervention from multiple well-equipped facilities. In urban areas of India, it is possible to cope with 20–30 victims of burn injury. Magnitude of 100–200 victims will overwhelm the medical system, but we are not at all prepared for stronger surge. We need to plan for large-scale burn disasters, especially with increasing terrorism in recent times with trend of multiple bombing at multiple sites.

According to Masellis and Gunn, the following points should be considered when planning burn disaster plans.

- The time interval between the accident and initiation of care must be <2 hours.
- Triage of victims must be carried out by specialists, as specialist alone can evaluate the gravity of burn injury.
- Inhalation and combustion of gases, fumes, and hot air causing damage to airway alone can jeopardize survival.
- Hypovolemic shock is induced rapidly and tissue hypoxia induces irreversible changes in various organs. It should be addressed immediately.
- Burn may be associated with large wounds, fractures, electrical injuries, or blast injury lesions.
- The overall assessment should be made not only on the basis of dead but also on the number of injured and those likely to suffer disability.
- The place where disaster occurs may not be accessible and no disaster plan to respond exists.

Of the 14 burn disaster studied by Arturson, only in San Juanico tragedy of Maxico where LPG storage tanks caught fire, >600 people were dead with count of injured exceeding 7,000, the worst burn disaster on record in recent history, the disaster plan was in place.

Immediate care is provided by people present at the scene of the disaster, who may be survivors or passersby. These first responders are later guided by trained healthcare workers who arrive at the site. On-site management includes:

Immediate relief and first aid: Immediate assistance, provided in first 2–3 hours by the people preferably by trained nurses, physicians, and volunteers, is fundamental to prognosis of burn patients. More complex and organized relief may take 6–7 hours to reach. It may be too late for burn patient. When burn casualties exceed the local ability, a major disaster should be declared. DDP will take about 20 burn patients. In case of more casualties, the state plan should be activated. All the agencies should be utilized and educated about their roles and responsibility to avoid chaos at the scene.

UTILIZATION OF MEDICAL TRIAGE

- Ambulance staging with a basic aim of maximal use of resources, efficient and safe transport.
- Early notification and information to hospitals.
- Utilizing an existing point of entry to activate disaster plan.

TRIAGE

Sorting out and classifying casualty of war or any other mass casualty is known as triage. It is done to determine the priority and proper place for transfer. Triage is most aptly applied to burns as burn injury is to some extent quantifiable.

Triage is the cornerstone of effective burn disaster management and is done at the disaster site by staff with knowledge of burn treatment. Triage takes into consideration the total number of patients, bed availability, and transportation capacity. The guiding principle is to treat those who are most likely to survive or can benefit the most from treatment. Thus, triage standards assess who receives care and when care is provided or the urgency with which it is provided. Triage is performed most often by first responders. Triage begins in the field, if there is a fixed event site; however, it also occurs within care settings, such as hospitals and alternate care sites, where individual victims may present themselves for care independent of organized responses. Secondary triage also may be necessary within a facility, such as a hospital, as demands on the system grow. Several well-established standards for triage are currently in use. Triage systems include START; Jump START (a pediatric modification to START); and Sacco score system. Each system seeks to establish a small number of categories among victims that indicates the urgency with which they should be treated. Colors are often used to represent the categories—for example, red (immediate care); yellow (delayed); green or white (ambulatory and minor injuries); and black (dead and/or "expectant").

The adequacy of the triage system used depends on the nature of the event and the population affected. For example, systems such as START and Jump START are trauma-oriented and may be effective in an explosive event.

In case of burn disaster or a disaster with burn injuries, the most important aspect would be to segregate patient with only burn injury or burn injury associated with other injuries for examination and triage by burn specialist or physician trained in burn triage. If the incident is small with limited casualties, ambulance trained paramedical will carry out primary triage and transport.

Triage should be prognostic, and patients should be categorized on the basis of age, extent of burns and site of burns, and presence of inhalation injury. Although there are no specified triage criteria but recommendation for transferring patients to a burns unit for satisfactory management is the guiding principle, which are as follows:

- *Group I*—Minor burns (<10% of total surface area in children and <20% in adults) to noncritical areas.

  Assigned to—Outpatient care, dressing, and tetanus prophylaxis.
- *Group II*—Minor burns to critical sites (face, hands, and genitalia)

  Assigned to—Short hospital stay, special wound care or operation.
- *Group III*—Major burns (20–60%)

  Assigned to—Admission to burn unit, intravenous resuscitation.
- *Group IV*—Extensive burns (>60%)

  Assigned to—Lower priority for transfer.
- *Group V*—Minor burns with inhalation injury or associated injury.

  Assigned to—Oxygen, intubations, transfers to ICU.

The patients in groups III and V are evacuated first, followed by group IV. Group II cases are evacuated at the end. Group I cases are either discharged after first aid or asked to make their own way to the nearest primary care center. Once the surge capacity of nearest burn center is exhausted, transfer to another center. If the surge is too huge, then a trauma center serves as the next level to provide treatment.

Tele-triage can be done by getting in contact with any tertiary care unit where a burn specialist can guide in triage and initial management of the patients and the process of preferable transport can be initiated. There is a need to train primary physicians and all emergency medical officers in the early management of burns and the method of triage. An organization like NABI can play a very vital role in this education.

As mentioned earlier, ideally, the triage should be done at the site of accident itself or should be set up at a nearby dispensary or health unit. In India, there is no instance where the triage has been used or set up. Patients have been loaded and taken to nearby facility where some sort of triage-based transfer has been done.

COMMUNICATIONS

Communication during disaster is the most vital tool. It is desirable to have online voice communication to ambulance service to burns unit, hospital coordinator burns surgeon, and trauma center individually and collectively. In some developed countries, this aspect is already operational, e.g., INFOBRUL in France, NDMS in the United States, and Argo in Italy. Like USA, Germany has enhanced centralized system which communicates to fire ambulance service and hospitals and police at the same time. In India, none of the states or cities has tried to develop and use communication and command centers. The communication command centers should be developed and manned by police and civil administration. It should have central data bank about ambulances evacuation, transport availability, disaster teams locally, and hospital beds availability. It should be manned 24 hours by personnel trained in disaster management. The best way to keep this communication center developed is to use it on daily basis for routine distribution of patients of trauma and routine emergencies. In India, under disaster plan, district control room (DCR) and EOC are being developed. The state of Maharashtra has put communication network comprising wireless [very high frequency (VHF)] and satellite [very small aperture terminal (VSAT)] networks covering the entire state and computerized disaster management information system using geographic information system (GIS) applications.

District control rooms: District control rooms are to be established in each collectorate of the state. The control rooms serve as nodal facilities for directing operations in an emergency situation. The most important is to develop links to organizations capable of mobilizing carriers for transport of patients and send prior information to the hospitals for patients it is likely to receive. The first information usually received by these centers will trigger disaster management response.

Emergency operations center: The EOC is a well-equipped and modern facility located at the state government headquarters. The EOC is the hub of activity during a disaster. Its systems and procedures are designed in such a way that information can be promptly assessed and relayed to concerned parties. As the master coordination and control point for all counter-disaster efforts, the EOC is the center for decision-making under a unified command. It is to be linked with all district control rooms.

MANAGEMENT AT DISASTER SCENE

In an episode of disaster, the information should be passed on to police and district administration. In India, in all disasters the management is taken over by police and district civil authorities or in worst cases by the paramilitary and military forces.

Evacuation and transport: First task is to find, extricate and transport victims usually by first responders or by fire services who are professionally trained. The effort should be to recruit all those who can rescue because early rescue is the key to a greater number of lives saved. The response plan should take into consideration the activation plan for explosions and industrial accidents especially in districts having petrochemical and refinery industry. If the disaster occurs in a remote area or the district has hardly any capacity to deal with large number of burn victims, then establishing of field hospital should be considered. In India, as mentioned earlier, field hospital with the disaster management team is being readied. In normal circumstances, the response is to load and go to the nearest health facility. The "load and go" evacuation system must never be used, especially in burn disasters. It causes great hold-ups in transport, a chaotic use of specialized beds and considerable risks for patients who receive resuscitatory treatment only after long delays. If possible, the primary triage should be conducted near the scene of disaster and evacuation should be prioritized so that the scarce bed capacity at the hospital is not overburdened and low-priority patient may choke the system.

Modern disaster management plan should allow controlled and safe transportation of burn patient to meaningful destination. Early information and notification should be sent to potential burn facility to receive patient.

Emergency transport of burn patient is to be coordinated with rescue organization. It may be practical to transfer to the nearest medical facility for thorough assessment and life-saving treatment of respiratory and airway management. Burn injury tolerates transport best on the day of accident. Ideally, all victims should be transported within 60 minutes. Late transfer is best done on 3rd or 4th day before sepsis sets in. Mass burn casualty in urban areas must take into consideration traffic jams due to disaster. Therefore, corridors of fast transfer to hospital should be worked out beforehand and, if possible, civil authorities should keep access to hospitals clear. Traffic jams can also affect arrival of staff to the hospital for disaster management. In India, there is no provision of air or helicopter evacuation.

It is only rarely done for very important persons and in rare circumstances.

When military forces are involved, there is a need to establish regional helicopter evacuation services because it is rapid and is not hindered by chaos on the ground.

When the surge is large and in remote areas, establishing a field hospital should be considered. Field hospitals which can be flown rapidly and established are only available with army and paramilitary forces. As mentioned earlier, the national disaster plan is building and strengthening these field hospitals with special battalions.

Burn facility surge capacity and Hospital Emergency Incident Command System (HEICS): Burn patients are best treated in burn units and there would always be scarcity of specialized beds and expertise for the treatment of extensive burns. Traditionally, the role of burn units is to provide medical management to the patients who arrive or get admitted. With disaster planning, the extended role is to keep the team ready and send them to disaster scene to help evacuation, triage, and initial management, to coordinate and focus on leadership within medical component.

Burn units rarely have low occupancy. Therefore, there should be an emergency plan to shift and evacuate existing burn patients to accommodate mass burn casualties. The thumb rule should be to have at least 50% more capacity to accommodate. As the burn units are usually located in large hospitals, the hospital should develop and have Hospital Emergency Incident Command System (HEICS) in place and this should be tested for burns mass casualty. HEICS provides responsibility-oriented chain of command which is charted and available with every one following case of accident or emergency. It provides for prioritization of duties with the use of "job action sheets". The "job action sheets" are position job descriptions which have a prioritized list of emergency response tasks. The "job action sheets" also serve as reminders of the lines of reporting and promote the documentation of the incident.

- A dependable chain of command
- Improved communication through common language
- Flexibility
- Prioritization of tasks
- Organized documentation system
- Effective mutual aid planning
- All acute care hospitals should develop and begin using the HEICS structure.

Hospital Emergency Incident Command System commander should be in contact with EOC coordinating initial care and evacuation.

In India, except for corporate hospitals, the HEICS is not established. It should be mandatory for the hospitals to have HEICS system in place and its details available with EOC and the DDP.

All burn units should have plans to increase bed capacity by 50% in case of disaster and plan to evacuate more stable patients elsewhere in the hospital. If required, trauma facility can be utilized and all surgical beds can also be added to accommodate victims.

Personnel/Staffing

Staffing is the basic requirement for treatment of burns. Advance plan can include short summoning of resident staff. The plan should ensure that there are adequate numbers of trained personnel to give initial resuscitation to burn victim. Education regarding simple management of minor and moderate burns should be imparted to all doctors and nurses outside the burn units so that they become a great resource at the time of disaster. In the hospital, a mixed team of physicians is an asset as they can take care of initial care like establishing intravenous access, intubations, catheterization, initial dressings, etc. The senior surgeon should immediately calculate the requirement of staff in coming days, requirement of operation theaters and requirement of dressing change. Volunteers always come whenever there are disasters. "Goodness" in people is spontaneous. There should be planning to coordinate and supervise these volunteers. A team of hospital staff should be designated to do so, so that the requirements by the hospital can be communicated to the volunteers and NGOs. They can be a great asset and can serve as clean-up crew, help in transport, traffic control, stretcher bearers, managing relatives and friends, give information about victims, managing the dead, and help disposal of bodies.

Advanced Burn Life Support

Advanced burn life support (ABLS) developed by American Association of Burns is an excellent tool. It is desired that NABI develops such a course and through its own effort and the burns units all over the country imparts such training. Trained personnel are scarce in disaster; so, they should be used wisely. Having a single caregiver, usually a nurse or paramedic, taking initial care, intravenous fluids, pain control, tetanus toxoid, airway maintenance, ventilation and documentation is desirable. In case of remote places with nonavailability of burn expert, telemedicine facility can be used to give advice and consultation on daily basis. NABI, with Safdarjung Hospital, New Delhi and other burns centers which are adequately staffed, can establish burn telemedicine centers as national resource.

Arturson gave an analysis of San Juanico tragedy in which 7,000 people were injured, 2,000 people were hospitalized, 625 people had severe burns, 300 persons died immediately, 250 people died in hospitals, later. 6,000 people were evacuated and about 7,000 people were involved in rescue in the first 48 hours. Of these 200 were fire fighters, 1,000 were physicians, 1,300 were paramedics, 1,800 were nurses, 2,000 were military personnel, and 750 were drivers and helicopter pilots. The plan should have provision for such large mobilization response and coordination.

Handling of relatives and mass media should be relegated to noncaregiver personnel. Such resource persons should be identified and should be designated beforehand; they should be well-versed with press and multilingual. Handling of media and giving regular feedback to them about management is very important and it should be an integral part of the disaster management. It helps later in secondary mobilization of resources like blood donation and mobilization of volunteers.

Supplies, Equipment, and Stockpiles

It is recommended that the disaster plan should take into consideration the supplies and equipment available. In a resource rich country, supplies and equipment can be warehoused but in a country like India where health facilities are always under crunch, it is not possible to make such warehouse or stockpile. The burn disaster may increase the demand on supply and just on time supply system may not be able to keep pace with the demand. The concept of emergency kits for disaster should be an integral part of the plan and it must make provision for at least 50% surge and its maintenance for few days. It should include all necessary supplies for initial care of burn patient, and this involves investment of time and money to initiate and then maintain and rotate it.

Other concept is to maintain emergency kits at a regional or central stockpile depot. These can be used to air drop wherever the need of these kits arises including remote areas and where the rescue and emergency burn management team are dispatched, or field hospital has been set up. NABI and other burn experts should approve of such kits and get them stockpiled in regional response centers.

Exercising the Plan

Disaster plans usually fail because the dummy runs, or mock exercises are not conducted. The dummy runs help in identifying gaps and evolve methods to remedy them. These exercises are essential for role clarity of the stakeholders concerned at the district level and for synergizing coordination of various emergency support functions. A simulation of disaster should be carried out frequently to keep in preparedness. It should involve prehospital ambulance and evacuation services, hospital-based persons, application of HEICS and field teams which are supposed to reach disaster site. The entire system should be tested for seamless operation. The teams should meet frequently for desktop exercises. In India, now through disaster management planning at all levels the mass casualty training is being imparted although their coordination and actual application is yet to be tested.

Medical Response to Mass Burn Casualty

The most common burn mass casualty usually occurs in urban areas or nearby urban areas. It is only rare to have Ural train gas pipeline tragedy in Russia which occurred in remote inaccessible area. Sometimes, the tragedy can strike in a country or areas where there are no facilities to handle mass burn casualties as happened in Bali Night Club bomb explosions. In India, except for Dabwali fire tragedy, most of the fire accidents leading to burn casualties occurred in urban areas where rescue and transport was rapid but not organized. They all followed load and go policy to nearby medical facility without any triage. This leads to choking of emergency services which are not geared to mange such large numbers and the emphasis shifts to severe burn >60% TBSA. Lack of awareness about inhalation injury and being unprepared to handle large numbers of inhalation injuries led to high mortality in Uphaar cinema fire in Delhi.

Medical response depends on information reaching the hospital about the incident. It should happen through EOC. The other information is about the size of disaster and the type and number of casualties expected so that appropriate HEIC can be initiated.

The medical response through trained paramedics or trauma response team on the scene of incident is done in three phases:

1. Primary triage
2. Ambulance staging, and
3. Establishing first-aid post for severely burned

The rescue and extrication should be ideally handled by the fire department or other responders trained in entering buildings on fire and how to handle smoke and low visibility.

The guidelines as enumerated by Masellis for immediate care of burn patient are as follows.

Guidelines for Immediate Care of Burn Victim

- Self-control
- Self-protection
- Qualitative assessment of burn
- Quantitative assessment of burns
- IV fluid therapy
- Analgesic therapy
- Bladder catheterization
- Pressure relieving incision—escharotomy
- Reexamine the patient
- Hospital or burn center transfer
- Whosoever has been exposed to fire and have burns even minor to be examined for inhalation burns

After the primary triage, patients are shifted to nearby hospitals as there is no time to carry out expert secondary triage. The policy should be on first come first served basis because true priority cannot be actually assigned till the last patient has arrived there. Transfer to other centers, once the capacity of nearby center is full, should be organized through emergency control center.

TABLE 1: Triage criterion and care plan.

Triage criterion	Care plan
• Minor burns/noncritical site • <10% TBSA for children • <20% TBSA for adult	• Outpatient care, tetanus prophylaxis, dress the wound • Admit, early operation, special wound care, short hospital stay
• Minor burns at critical sites, hand face, perineum • 20–60% TBSA burned	• Admit burn unit, IV fluids, careful monitoring requires burn trained personnel
• Extensive burns >60% TBSA associated with inhalation injury trauma or medical illness	• High mortality, placed in expectant category, pain medication, psychological support
• Inhalation injury, minor burns, associated injuries	• Administer oxygen, intubate, ventilate, care of associated injuries needs to be in burn center

(TBSA: total body surface area)

Griffith has recommended the following triage and care plan. It can be of use in transferring and ambulance staging **(Table 1)**.

TRIAGE CRITERION AND CARE PLAN

Except for minor burns all patients, either in field or on reaching hospital, should receive prompt IV fluids. Prognosis depends on the initial fluid replacement. Effective fluid therapy during first 24 hours gives time for organization and secondary triage to determine further transfer.

The Baxter Shriners formula using Ringer lactate is the most straightforward and should be followed in all burns mass causalities. Avoid colloids in first 24 hours. The urine output should be maintained at 0.5–1 mL/kg/h. Adequate resuscitation is the key to better survival. Junior staff nurses and paramedics can set up IV infusion, catheterization, administer analgesics and document injury. In today's time, digital photography is an efficient way of rapid documentation.

Initially, burns can be covered with just a clean sheet. Care should be taken to prevent hypothermia, especially in children. Before any patient is dressed, he should be examined by a burn surgeon who makes assessment and documentation of burns. Only then, the patient should be dressed. Immediate coverage and dressing are a waste of time of nurses and other junior staff, if not examined in detail by a burn surgeon. This is the time when secondary triage is conducted and, if needed, the patient is transferred to another center.

The protocol for preparing patient for medical evacuation is as follows:

- Cannulation of several routes for IV fluids of which one should be central, followed by chest X-ray to rule out any complication.
- Monitoring of urine output
- Insertion of nasogastric tube
- Sedation, analgesia, and cleansing of wound
- Tracheal intubations, if required
- Prevent heat loss

The only surgical intervention is escharotomy. Early debridement is not done as the burn surgeon will be busy in life-saving measures for other victims. It should be carried out only within a burn unit and can be done till 5 days. Although many units do not start prophylactic antibiotics routinely, in case of mass casualty, antibiotics are started to protect the patients from hospital infection. It is also recommended to start prophylaxis against stress ulcers. Psychological support and counseling of the victim and relatives should be given.

DISASTER PLAN IN ACTION

The NDMA published final SDMP with details of guidelines in July 2007. The SDMP document included various disasters in its list but has not mentioned burn disaster. It is urgently required that NABI should bring this anomaly to the notice of NDMA. There should be planning for mass burn causalities at national level. The burn surgeon and burn units are important stakeholders in the disaster management. NDMG-MPMCM plan should recognize and include planning for burn mass casualty and recognize burn units in government and private hospital as national resource. Any plan for mass burn causality can basically be considered a generic plan for mass trauma casualties or any plan for mass casualty can have subplan catering to burn injury.

At district level in case of fire accident leading to burn injury disaster: What will be done? How it is to be done? Who will do it?

The logistics management details to be incorporated and documented in respective burn disaster plan.

The moot question is: How will the disaster plan be activated and who will trigger its implementation? This will depend on the first information from the site and as the police, fire department, and district authorities reach they will provide information to EOC. Under the guidance of a team of experts and leaders trained in disaster management, the disaster would be declared, and the plan shall be implemented with coordination and precision. In India, either it will be done by district collector or specially designated disaster management officer.

Establishing EOC is a must and should be done in every district as recommended in SDMP document.

The timebound action plan is must for creating facilities for environment scanning, intelligence gathering, operations, and logistics management under one roof for holistic and efficient management of disasters at the state and district level. Arrangements must be made and procedures must be laid down for manning the EOC on 24 × 7 × 365 basis. The plan must also cover in detail the indigenized Incident Command System at the state, district, and local body levels. Only states of Maharashtra and Assam have established such centers with satellite assisted communication. Without the EOC which is linked to live voice communication to the entire stakeholder in disaster management especially hospitals, ambulance, evacuation services, fire department, and police department, it is not possible to respond to any disaster in a coordinated manner.

At EOC, data should be available about hospitals, their capacity, and other health facilities. Some of the district medical officers or some medical personnel from the local hospital should be trained to act as field medical officers and act as link and liasoning for emergency management at the site and evacuation to various hospitals.

At hospital level, all hospitals should have emergency incident command system in place, i.e., HEICS and designated commander should be in constant contact of EOC. Once there is information about the incident:

- *Alert is declared*—liasoning done with various departments
- *Standby*—information confirmed, hospital concerned consultant put on standby
- *Emergency operations center* contacts hospital incident commander, ambulance, and evacuation agencies
- Disaster management team and BDRT readied.

Initial Response

Emergency teams sent to site, coordinate triage, transfer of patient to medical facility, create surge capacity at the hospital, HEICS activation, discharge patients, postpone routine surgeries, summon staff, nurses, paramedics, alert pharmacy, blood bank, and equipment for emergency care to be ready.

Ongoing Management

After initial resuscitation, carry out secondary triage; arrange "operation theater" for escharotomy and other emergency operation. Plan for long treatment of the patient requiring coverage. Schematic plan of burn disaster is given in **(Flowchart 3)**.

After action and review: After the burn mass casualty incident has been managed, a meeting will be arranged of all the participants and the plan should be reviewed. Otherwise also, all plans should be reviewed every 2 years. All the communication through EOC is transcripted and put on record. It can be evaluated for coordinating response. The benefit of such after action review is to bring practical changes in disaster plan. In the past, after action report of fire in Hilton Hotel, Las Vegas changed safety and fire prevention of high-rise buildings forever. This resulted in pressurized fire escapes systems, fire control centers in high-rise hotels, hospitals and other public buildings, fire sprinkle system, extensive alarm system, etc. Emphasizing disaster plan makes better disaster prevention.

In India, no analysis of fire disasters is available but from the judicial inquiries it is known that the worst accidents occurred in temporary structures erected without any safety precaution. We still have not been able to impose safety standards for the temporary structures erected.

National Burn Mass Casualty Management System

Training and Community Preparedness Programs: The government of India (GOI) has also taken up an extensive program of training for disaster preparedness and response. The training programs have been designed for the officials of the government at different levels, NGOs, and elected representatives of Local Bodies. The Disaster Management Centers are playing a pivotal role in developing the training literature and organization of training program. In the next 2–3 years, an intensive training schedule will be drawn up for orienting all the concerned agencies in different areas of disaster preparedness and response. The GOI also proposes to take up community disaster preparedness programs on a pilot basis in different areas of the state. This program will be implemented through the selected NGOs for identified disaster spots in the states and is aimed at building up the mitigation measures into community life.

Developing leadership is the most crucial and important aspect and the biggest asset a community can build for tackling mass casualty. This involves knowledge to initiate disaster plan and provides link between medical care system and incident response. A team of people should be trained to provide disaster-related leadership knowledge and skills and ability to match hospital and system specific resources, knowledge of surge plan, resources, and techniques in a particular part of the city or state.

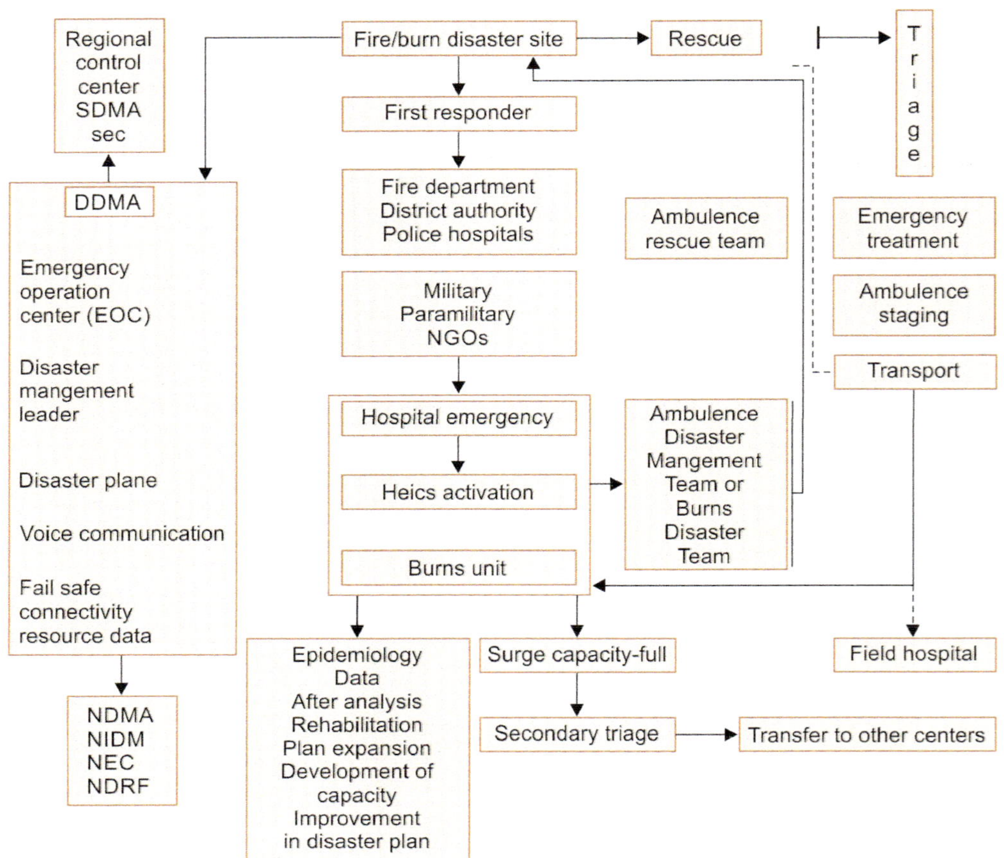

FLOWCHART 3: Burns disaster management plan (as suggested by the author).

(DDMA: District Disaster Management Authority; NDMA: National Disaster Management Authority; NDRF: National Disaster Response Force; NEC: National Executive Committee; NGOs: nongovernmental organizations; NIDM; National Institute of Disaster Management; SDMA: State Disaster Management Authority; SEC: State Executive Committee)

International Applications

In recent years, with rise of international terrorism which is transborders, it has been noticed that there has been more international cooperation in disaster management. Especially, in case of Bali bombings, large number of patients were shifted to Australia and treated there. In the past also, United States of America, United Kingdom, France, Israel, and Cuba have sent their teams for international medical relief. Sending such teams not only help in tiding away the disaster response need but also bring exchange of new ideas, learning, teaching, and sometimes upgrading the host countries medical systems. NABI along with Government of India should form such burn disaster international relief teams. These teams should be self-sufficient, should carry their own bulk supplies, and they should not be burden on host country. The required equipment should be stockpiled and kept ready to be retrieved and airlifted with the team on short notice. Such a team has to be in state of preparedness.

LEGAL FRAMEWORK

Although the disaster management has had paradigm shift with enactment of national *Disaster Management Act*, 2005 by Government of India which provides for the creation of a policy, legal, and institutional framework, backed by effective statutory and financial support, the details of the following relevant points remain to be worked out by states.

Authority to Declare Disaster

- Induction and triggering disaster management
- Legal responsibility to treat
- To admit and treat without questioning financial implications
- Liability of health department not to be held liable for any criminal and civil suits whosoever participates in disaster management.
- Power to quarantine or restrict movement

- Compelling provider to participate in disaster management
- Streamlined financial issues with provider and the victim

As the states develop their disaster management plans and enact it as law under Disaster Management Act 2005, most of these issues will be resolved.

Principles of disaster management: For preparing any burns disaster plan one should follow the principles. The disaster management and the principles are as follows:

- Prevention
- Preparedness
- Disaster profiles
- Disaster patterns
- Planning and preparation for effective multidisciplinary response
- Mobilization of multisectoral manpower resource
- Risk assessment
- Post-emergency phase
- Reconstructive phase
- Community and institutional involvement

SUMMARY

- India is developing its national disaster management.
- National Disaster Management Act, 2005 has been enacted.
- It is mandatory for the states to enact their state disaster management plans.
- NDMA and National Institute for Disaster Management (NIDM) are the key bodies for disaster management in India.
- There is a need to include burn disaster in the plans.
- Characteristics of the pathological conditions affecting burn victims, respiratory complications, and associated polytrauma in a burn disaster are different from other type of disasters.
- The burn disaster should be addressed systematically.
- Legislation of disaster management should include burn disaster.
- National Academy of Burns-India should become a stakeholder in disaster management plans. It has capacity to be the component in national disaster readiness for mass burn incidents.
- Emergency operation centers at district level are the basic building blocks of disaster management.
- All hospitals should develop their HEICS program and implement and rehearse it regularly.
- Recommendation for initial management, triage, and further treatment in burn units must be developed for our country.
- Physicians at all levels must be trained in triage and initial management of burns.
- Community at large and all stakeholders should be trained in disaster management.
- Awareness programs should be conducted regularly for community involvement; every citizen should have ability to deal with emergency.

This article is based on publications of Government of India, viz.,

- Disaster Management Act, 2005 document
- State Disaster Management Plan recommendations of NDMA published by Government of India, July 2007; and
- Disaster Management Plan, State of Maharashtra, and text and diagrams from the same have been used.

BIBLIOGRAPHY

1. Allister C, Hamilton G. Cardowan coalmine explosion: experience of a mass burns incident. Br Med J. 1983;287:403-5.
2. American College of Surgeons. Resources for the optimal care of the injured patient. Committee on Trauma Paper, 1999; Chapter 14.
3. Arnold JL, Tsai MC, Halpern P, Smithline H, Stok E, Ersoy G. Mass-casualty terrorist bombings: epidemiological outcomes, resource utilization and time course of emergency needs. Prehosp Disaster Med. 2003;18(3):220-34.
4. Arturson G. The Los Alfaques disaster: a boiling—liquid, expanding—vapour explosion. Burns. 1979;7(4):233-51.
5. Arturson G. The tragedy of San Juanico—the most severe LPG disaster in history. Burns. 1987;13:87-102.
6. Barclay TL. Planning for mass burns casualties. In: Wood C (Ed). Accident and Emergency Burns: Lesson from the Bradford Disaster, Proceedings of extended panel discussion held in Bradford 1985. London: Royal Society of Medicine Services; 1986. pp. 81-8.
7. Becker W, Waymack J, McManus A, Shaikhutdinov M, Pruitt B Jr. Bashkirian train-gas pipeline disaster: the American military response. Burns. 1990;16(5):325-8.
8. Benmeir P, Levine I, Shostak A, Oz V, Shemer J, Sokolova T. The Ural train—gas pipeline catastrophe: the report of the IDF medical corps assistance. Burns. 1991;17(4):320-2.
9. Bezuhly M, Gomez M, Fish J. Emergency management of minor burn injuries in Ontario, Canada. Burns. 2004;30148:160-4.
10. Cooper DM. Mass gatherings in a terrorist threat environment. Conference Presentation. Melbourne: World Congress of Emergency and Disaster Medicine; 2003.
11. Dove B, Del Guercio L, Stahl W, Star L, Abelson L. A Metropolitan Airport Disaster Plan—Coordination of a Multi-hospital response to provide on-site Resuscitation and Stabilisation before transfer. J Trauma. 1982;22(7):550-9.
12. Ehrlich P, Rockwell S, Kincaid S, Mucha Jr P. American College of Surgeons, Committee on Trauma Verification Review: Does it make a difference? J Trauma. 2002;53(5):811-6.

13. Eiseman B, Chandler G. Sheriff's Surgeon's Alert: A Trauma Surgeon's Responsibility. J Trauma. 2003;54.
14. Emergency Management Australia. Chapter 23: Australian Emergency Manual Disaster Medicine. Emergency Management Australia. (1996). Australia: Australian Emergency Manual, Disaster Recovery; 1999.
15. Emergency Management Australia. Australian Emergency Manual Emergency Risk Management. Applications Guide. 1999.
16. Emergency Management Australia. Bali Bombing: 2002 Bali bombings kill 88 Australians. National debrief 2002.
17. Frykberg ER. Medical Management of Disasters and Mass Casualties from Terrorist Bombings: How Can We Cope? J Trauma Lippincott Williams & Wilkins. 2002;53(2):201-12.
18. Griffiths R. Management of multiple casualties with burns. Br Med J. 1985;291:6500.
19. Hampson GV, Cook SP, Frederikson SR. Operation Bali Assist: The Australian Defence Force response to the Bali bombing, 12th October 2002. Med J Aust. 2002;177:620-3.
20. Harvey J. President Australian and New Zealand Burns Association. Personal correspondence 2004.
21. Hull D, Grindlinger G, Hirsch E, Petrone S, Burke J. The clinical consequences of an industrial aerosol plant explosion. J Trauma. 1985;25(4):303-8.
22. Jones K. Bulletin of the post-graduate committee in medicine. Australia: University of Sydney; 1979. pp. 180-7.
23. Keogh J. Management of mass burn casualties in a hospital with a burn unit. Med J Australia. 1991.
24. Leslie C, Cushman M, McDonald G, JoshiW, Maynard A. Management of multiple burn casualties in a high volume ED without a verified burn unit. Am J Emerg Med. 2001;19(6):469-73.
25. Mackie D, Koning H. Fate of mass burn casualties: implications for disaster planning. Burns. 1990;16:203-6.
26. Mackie D. Mass burn casualties: A rationale approach to planning. Burns. 2002;28(5):403-4.
27. Martinelli G. The ARGO satellite system: A network for severe burns and disasters. In: Masellis M, Gunn SWA (Eds). The Management of Mass Burn Casualties and Fire Disasters. Dordrecht/Boston/London: Kluwer Academic Publishers; 1992. pp. 7-12.
28. Masellis M, Ferrara MM, Gunn SWA. Immediate assistance and first aid on the spot in fire disaster—education of the public and self-sufficiency training. Arm Medit Burns Club. 1992;5:200-6.
29. Masellis M, Laia A, Sferrazza Papa G, Pirillo E, D'Arpa N, Cucchiara R, et al. Fire disaster in a motorway tunnel. Arm Burns Fire Disast. 1997;10:233-40.
30. Masellis M. Thermal agent disaster and fire disaster: Definition, damage, assessment and relief operations. Ann Medit Burns Club. 1991;4:215-8.
31. Mencka P, Hosek F. The importance of stored supplies of biological skin covers in territorial management of mass burn casualties. ACTA Chrurgiae Plasticae. 2002;44:3.
32. Morell G, Naif E, Domenech P, Sospedra C, Roda B. Burns caused by the terrorist bombing of the department store Hipercor in Barcelona. Part 1, 1990.
33. Nordberg M. Burn Free: Are you prepared for the fire of the future? Emerg Med Serv. 1995.
34. NSW Health. NSW Severe Burn Injury Service. Burn Transfer Guidelines. 39. NSW Health (2004) NSW Severe Burn Injury Service, Data Collection, Wingello Bushfire, Canberra Bushfire, 2004.
35. O'Hickey S, Pickering C, Jones P, Evans J. Manchester air disaster. Br Med J. 1987;294:1663-7.
36. Palmer D, Stephens D, Fisher D, Spain B, Read D, Notaras L. The Bali bombing: the Royal Darwin Hospital response. Med J Aust. 2003;179(7):358-61.
37. Pruitt B Jr, Goodwin C, Mason A Jr. Chapter 2: Epidemiological, demographic, and outcome characteristics of burn injury. In: Herndon D (Ed). Total Burn Care, 2nd edition. Kent, England: Saunders Publishing; 2001. pp. 16-29.
38. Pruitt B Jr. Editorial–Validation and verification. Burns. 1996; 22(3):36.
39. Southwick G, Pethick A, Thalayasingam P, Vijayasekaran V, Hogg J. Australian doctors in Bali: the initial medical response to the Bali bombing. Med J Aust. 2002;177(11-12):624-6.
40. Tran MD, Garner AA, Morrison I, Sharley P, Griggs WM, Xavier C. The Bali bombing: civilian evacuation. Med J Aust. 2003;179(6):353-6.
41. Wachtel L, Cowan M, Reardon J. Developing a regional and national burn disaster response. J Burn Care Rehabil. 1989;10(6):561-7.
42. Wedler V, Kunzi W, Meyer V. Care of burns victims in Europe. Burns. 1999;25(2):152-7.

Appendices

APPENDIX 1.1: COMPOSITION OF COMMON INTRAVENOUS (IV) FLUIDS

Crystalloids

Name	Na^+	K^+	Cl^-	HCO_3^-	Miscellaneous	CHO(g/L)	Pr (g/L)	MJ/L	Osmolarity	pH
Normal saline	154	0	154	0	0	0	0	0	308	5.0
Glucose 5%	0	0	0	0	0	50	0	0.84	280	4.0
Ringer's lactate	131	5	112	29	Mg: 1, Ca: 1 Lactate 28 mM	0	0	0.04	280	6.5
$NaHCO_3$	1,000	0	0	1,000	0	0	0	0	2,000	8.0
Glucose 4% Saline 0.18%	31	0	31	0	0	40	0	–	284	4
Glucose 5% Saline 0.45%	77	0	77	0	0	50	0	–	431	4

Note: Concentration of ions given as mmol/L.

Colloids

Name	Na^+	K^+	Cl^-	Miscellaneous	CHO (g/L)	Pr (g/L)	MJ/L	pH	Onc. Pres.	$t^{1/2}$
Human albumin										
4% solution	150	2	120	–	0	19	40	7.4	275	12 hours
Haemaccel (succinylated gelatin)	145	5.1	145	Ca 6.3 Gelatin 40 g	0	35	0	7.4	370	5 hours
Hydroxyethyl starch (HAES)	154	0	154	Starch 60 g	0	0	0	5.5	310	17 days

Notes:

- Concentration of ions given as mmol/L.
- $t^{1/2}$ half life in plasma

APPENDIX 1.2: BODY SURFACE AREA

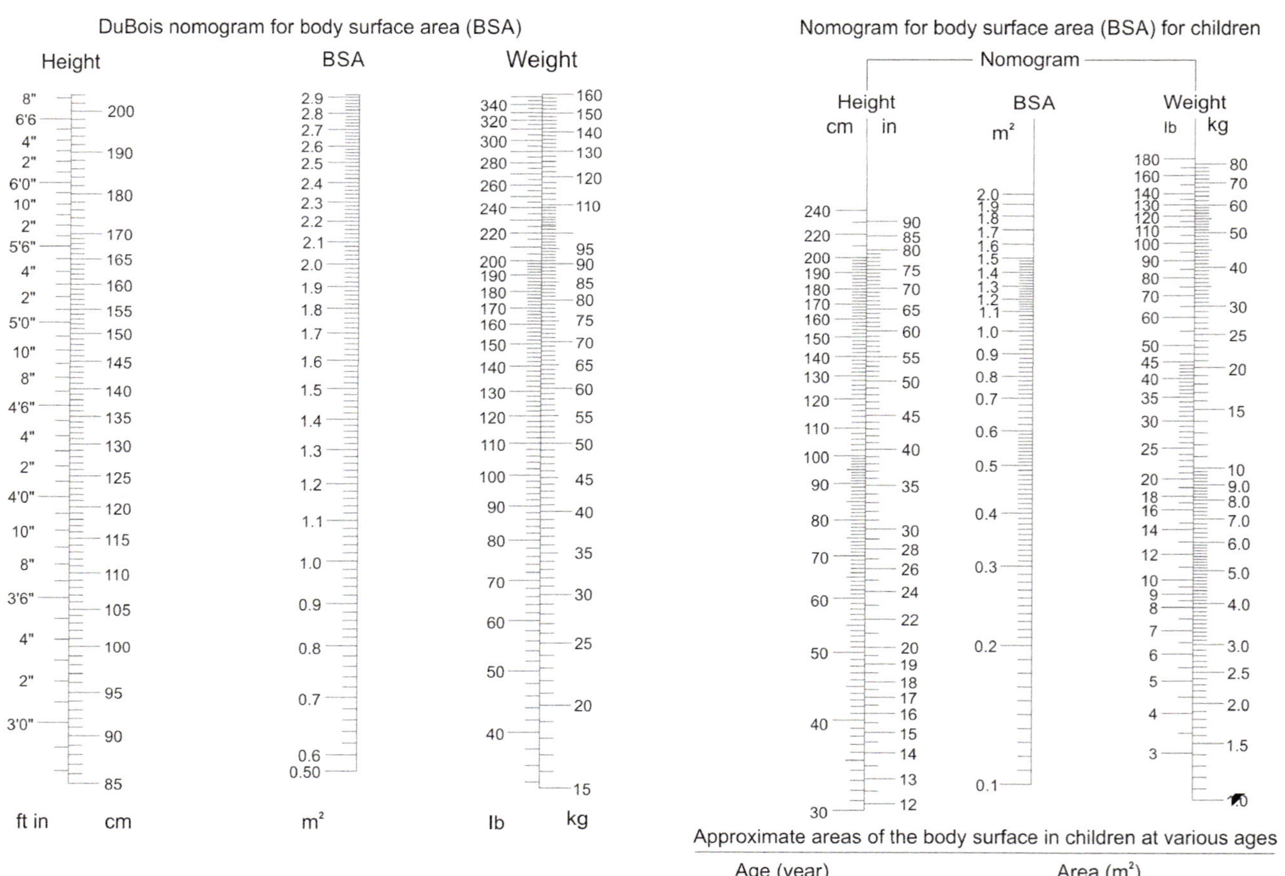

APPENDIX 1.3: NORMAL BIOCHEMICAL VALUES

Substance	Traditional units	SI units
Alanine aminotransferase (SGPT)	0–35 U/L	0–0.58 µKat/L
Albumin	4–6 g/dL	40–60 g/L
Alkaline phosphatase	F: 30–100 U/L	0.5–1.67 µKat/L
	M: 45–115 U/L	0.75–1.92 µKat/L
Amylase	0–130 U/L	0–2.17 µKat/L
Aspartate aminotransferase (SGOT)	0–35 U/L	0–0.58 µKat/L
Bicarbonate	22–26 mEq/L	22–26 mmol/L
Bilirubin		
Total	0.1–1.0 mg/dL	2–18 µmol/L
Conjugated	≤ 2 mg/dL	≤ 4 µmol/L
Blood urea nitrogen (BUN)	8–18 mg/dL	3–6.5 mmol/L

Continued

Continued

Substance	Traditional units	SI units
Calcium		
Total	8.5–10.5 mg/dL	2.2–2.6 mmol/L
Ionized	2.2–2.3 mEq/L	1.10–1.15 mmol/L
Chloride	95–105 mEq/L	95–105 mmol/L
Creatinine	0.6–1.5 mg/dL	0.05–0.13 mmol/L
Glucose—fasting	70–100 mg/dL	3.9–6.1 mmol/L
Magnesium	1.8–3.0 mg/dL	0.8–1.2 mmol/L
Osmolality	280–296 mOsm/kg	280–296 mmol/L
Phosphate	2.5–5 mg/dL	0.80–1.60 mmol/L
Potassium	3.5–5.0 mEq/L	3.5–5.0 mmol/L
Sodium	135–147 mEq/L	135–147 mmol/L
Total protein	6–8 g/dL	60–80 g/L

APPENDIX 1.4: BODY BUILD AND BLOOD VOLUME IN ADULTS

	Average blood volume (mL/kg)	
Body build	**Males**	**Females**
Thin	65	60
Normal	70	65
Muscular	75	70
Obese	60	55

APPENDIX 1.5: FLUID COMPOSITION OF BODY COMPARTMENTS

Estimates of blood volume	
Infant	90 mL/kg body weight
Child	80 mL/kg body weight
Adult male	70 mL/kg body weight
Adult female	60 mL/kg body weight
Total water content	
Adult male	60% body weight
Adult female	55% body weight
Extracellular fluid volume	35% total water content
Intracellular fluid volume	65% total water content

APPENDIX 1.6: COMPOSITION OF DIFFERENT BODY FLUIDS

Parameter	Males	Females
Total body water	600 mL/kg	500 mL/kg
Interstitial fluid	160 mL/kg	160 mL/kg
Blood volume	70 mL/kg	65 mL/kg
Erythrocyte volume	33 mL/kg	27 mL/kg
Plasma volume	37 mL/kg	38 mL/kg
Hematocrit	47% (mean)	42% (mean)
	40–54%	37–47%

APPENDIX 1.7: NORMAL VALUES FOR COAGULATION TESTS

Partial thromboplastin time	35–45 s
Prothrombin time	12–14 s
Bleeding time (platelet function)	2–9 min
Plasma fibrinogen	1.5–4.0 g/L
Fibrin degradation products (FDPs)	<10 mg/L

APPENDIX 2.1: AVAILABLE ENTERAL FORMULAE

Presently, a wide variety of ready-to-use commercially-prepared diets are available in the market to meet the requirements. However, ready-to-use feeds are expensive, and in our country, we still prefer to use blended home-made diets.

Example of Home-made Blended Feed

1,000 mL milk/buttermilk + 4 eggs + 4 bananas +10 tablespoons of sugar or honey

Final composition of the above is approximately 1,700 mL and it provides 1 Kcal/mL of energy, 60 g of protein and 350 g of carbohydrate.

Commercially-available Enteral Formulae (Tables 2.1A and B)

They include:

- Standard formulae (e.g., Fresubin) provide 1 Kcal/mL.
- Special formulae (Nutrilite) have high essential amino acids content.
- Fiber enriched formulae (Actibase)
- High lipid content formulae (Pulmocare)
- Glutamine enriched formulae

TABLE 2.1A: Commercially-available protein rich powder with nutritive values.

Food product	Dose	Nutritional value
Fresubin	50 g + 180 mL water	*Energy*: 220 Kcal
		Protein: 8.3 g
		Fat: 7.4 g
		1 Kcal/mL
Threptin diskettes	Approximately 5 g	*Protein*: 1.5 g
		Carbohydrate: –
		Fat: 0.7 g
		22 Calories/Diskette
Nutrilite	10 g 1 scoop	*Protein*: 8 g
		Carbohydrate: 0.5 g
		Fat: 0.3 g
		Calories: 36 Kcal
Actibase	2 scoops	*Protein*: 16.5 g
		Carbohydrate: 15 g
		Fat: 0.7 g
		Calories: 132 Kcal
GRD	100 g/2 teaspoon = 30 g	*Protein*: 18.5 g
		Carbohydrate: 63 g
		Calories: 425 Kcal/100 g

TABLE 2.1B: Commercially-available amino acids and lipids.

Trade name	Dosage	Protein	Nonprotein calories
Alamine-N	200 mL over 2–3 h	6 g	24 Kcal
Alamine-SE (in patients with oliguric renal failure)	20 mL	1.64 g	6.5 Kcal
Alamine-SN	20–500 mL	2 g	80 Kcal
Amino drip	200–500 mL	7.5 g/100 mL	30 Kcal/100 mL
Hermin	200–800 mL	100% essential amino acids	500 mL 10% = 450 Kcal
Lipofundin (5–10%)	100–500 mL 10–20 mL/kg/day start with 15–20 drops/min after 15 minutes increase to 45 drops/min		20% = 900 Kcal

APPENDIX 2.2: NUTRITIVE VALUE OF INDIAN FOOD

Average portion		Weight	Protein	Fat	Carbohydrate	Calories
Beverages						
Coffee: Cow's milk and sugar 2 teaspoons	1 cup	200	1.1	1.1	11.4	60
Lemonade: Fresh lime juice 2 tablespoons and sugar 3 teaspoon	1 glass	240	–	–	17.4	73
Tea: Cow's milk 2 tablespoons and sugar 2 teaspoons	1 cup	200	0.9	1.1	11.4	60
Cereals and cereal food						
Cornflakes	1 cup	25	2.1	0.1	2.1	95
Jowar (*Sorghum vulgare*, cholam)	1 small chapati	45	3.1	0.6	22.2	106
Maize 30 g flour	1 chapati	45	3.3	1.1	19.3	102
Ragi 30 g flour	1 chapati	45	2.1	0.4	21.5	98
Rice, milled, boiled (3 tablespoon dry)	1 cup	–	2.9	0.1	30.2	138
Wheat bread	1 slice	30	2.3	0.5	15	75
Wheat "chapati" (15 g flour)	1 thin	–	1.2	0.1	8	40
Wheat "*Parantha*" 60 g and fat 2 teaspoons	1	–	4.8	10.4	36	256
Milk and milk products						
Buttermilk, buffalo's (curd 1 cup making 3 cups of buttermilk)	1 cup	200	2.7	4.6	2.[illegible]	62
Cheese, cheddar	1 piece	28	7	9	0.6	111
Cheese cottage	1 round tablespoon	28	5.5	0.1	0.5	27
Cream light	1 tablespoon	30	0.8	5.4	1.2	56
Curd, buffalo milk	1cup	200	8	14	6.3	182
Ice cream	1 helping	100	4.1	11.3	19.8	196
Milk buffalo's	1 cup	200	8	14	6.3	182
Milk buffalo's skimmed	1 cup	200	8.4	0.2	10.8	78
Milk cow's	1 cup	200	7	9	9.6	160
Milk cow's skimmed	1 cup	200	7.2	0.2	10	70
Milk condensed sweetened	1 tablespoon	20	1.5	1.7	10.1	62
Milk goat's	Half cup	100	3.3	4.1	4.7	75
Milk whole powdered	1 tablespoon	7	1.9	1.9	2.7	35
Pulses, dried peas, and beans						
Bengal gram	1 cup cooked thin *daal*	200	7	2.3	14	105
Black gram	1 cup cooked thin *daal*	200	7	2.3	2.3	105
Green gram *(moong daal)*	1 cup cooked	200	7	2.3	2.3	105
Field bean *(val daal)*	Half cup	100	6	0.4	17.3	92
Lentil *(masur daal)*		100	22.9	11.4	58.1	340
Peas dried						
Red gram *(tur daal)*						
Beans baked						
Peas roasted						

APPENDIX 2.3: DIET CHART FOR BURN PATIENTS AND THEIR NUTRITIVE VALUE (TABLE 2.3A)

Calculations: 3,000 to 4,000 Kcal + 180 g of protein can be given by oral route.

According to Curreri formula:
For a 40% burns (50 kg weight)—calories required = 20 × body weight + 70 × % of burns
Calories = 20 × 50 + 70 × 40 = 3,800 Kcal protein = 1 g/kg + 3 g × % of burn
Protein = 50 + 3 × 40 = 170 g

TABLE 2.3A: Diet chart.

	Main food group	Weight and measures	Calories	Protein
Prebreakfast	Tea with sugar	125 mL	40	
	+			
	4 Marie biscuits	4	50	
Breakfast	Milk + 2 teaspoon sugar +2 teaspoon Protinex	200 mL + 30 g + 30 g	200 + 120	10 + 3 g
	Porridge/Cornflakes *Dalia*	2 *katori*	410	2 g
	Stuffed *parantha*	90 g + 40 g	210 + 100	20 g + 2 g
	Bread 2 slices + 2 egg	40 g	100	10 g
Prelunch	Sprout or roasted chana	1 *katori*	140	6 g
	Cheese	2 cubes	100	10 g
	Milk + 2 teaspoon	200 mL	320	13 g
	Protinex+ 2 teaspoon sugar			
Lunch	Cereal	Chapati 4 medium size 120 g +2 teaspoon ghee (30 g)	600	
	Leafy vegetables	2 cups	40	
	Daal or whole pulses/nonveg	3/4 *katori* cooked	100	6 g
	Curd/*Raita*/Buttermilk	1/2 cup	40	
	Fruit	Banana (big)	80	
Evening snacks	Milk + 2 teaspoon protinex + 2 teaspoon sugar	200 mL + 4–5 Marie biscuits	320	13 g
	Cereal	*Dhokla*/vegetarian sandwich/ sprouts/roasted chana	140	
Predinner	Chicken soup	1 cup 200 mL	185	10 g
	Corn soup (sweet)	1 cup	120	
	Daal soup	1 cup	169	6 g
Dinner	Cereal	Chapati (4 medium size)	600	
	Leafy vegetable	1 *katori* (30 mL)	50	
	Daal or pulses	1 *katori* (cooked)	100	6 g
	Curd	½ cup	40	

Continued

Continued

Main food group	Weight and measures	Calories	Protein
Desserts			
Rasgulla, or	1 (150 g)	140	
Gulab Jamun, or	25 g	200	
Laddoo, or	30 g	160	
Mango juice	200 mL (big glass)	150	
Use 4 teaspoon ghee/day			
Total calories = 4,000 Kcal; Total protein = 117 g			

APPENDIX 2.4: TOTAL PARENTERAL NUTRITION

Total parenteral nutrition (TPN) can be given as separate components like amino drip, *intralipid*, 10% dextrose or as premixed multicomponent solutions *like Clinomel*, which are now available and have reduced the potential for error and metabolic aberration.

Maximum rate of dextrose administration should be 4–6 mg/kg/min to avoid the risk of hyperglycemia.

If carbohydrate is given as the only source of energy, it can lead to:
- Deficiency of essential fatty acids
- Deficiency of fat-soluble vitamins
- Excess carbon dioxide load
- Hepatic steatosis
- Increases osmolarity of solution

Instruction charts should be maintained stating the following details of parenteral nutrition (PN):
- Total energy calculated on body weight basis.
- Substrate distribution (volume of carbohydrate, fat, and protein)
- Fluid volume
- Rate of delivery
- Hang time
- Total time frame
- Steps to be taken in case of accidental change in rate of delivery

It is said that to prevent the complications of parenteral feeding, like over feeding of IV nutrients, which may lead to hepatic disorders, fluid retention, and metabolic derangements, the required volume for the PN is determined by the rate of substrate utilization as opposed to a predetermined energy goal, as demand of energy may reach to 50 Kcal/kg/day. It is important to keep a rational balance and not overload the patient with huge amounts of energy.

The maximum oxidation of glucose in liver is when given at a rate of 4–6 mg/kg/min. If given beyond this rate, it is not assimilated but deposited as fat beneath the skin.

Proteins at 2.5–4 g/kg can be given, increasing gradually to the desired goal.

Fat at 20% intralipid is given but not during acute phase of shock. Starting with 0.5 g/kg/h, the maximum rate of 0.119 g/kg/h or 1.0–1.5 g/kg/day should not be exceeded.

Intralipid administration should not exceed >3.6 g/kg/day. Calculate *daily volume requirement* on the basis of:
- All ongoing losses, including insensible loss
- Input–output chart
- Alternatively, 30–40 mL/kg body weight
- Caution in patients with renal dysfunction and congestive heart failure
  For infants and children < 20 kg = 1.7 mL/kg/h
  For children > 20 kg = 1.5 mL/kg/h
  This is started at 60 mL/h and increased to 80–100 mL/h after 4–6 hours. PN should not be started out-of-hours (evenings and weekends). Lipid emulsions when given alone should be completely infused within 12 hours of hanging. Lipids when administered as total nutrient admixture can be hung for 24 hours.

If PN is interrupted due to any reason, clear instructions should be stated to administer 10% dextrose solution at the same rate to prevent sudden hypoglycemia caused by high endogenous insulin. Complications of IV hyperalimentation are greater than with enteral route.

APPENDIX 2.5: STANDARD PARENTERAL SOLUTION

Parenteral nutrition may be delivered through all-in-one system like *OliClinomel*, which is a preferred way of administering PN in author's unit, where all macronutrients and micronutrients required for 24 hours are infused from one bag or through multiple bottles. There are fewer chances of infection and metabolic aberrations in using a single-bag system.

Oliclinomel

Oliclinomel N4-550E emulsion for infusion:

- Qualitative and quantitative composition is given in **Tables 2.5A and B**.
- This medicinal product is presented in the form of a three compartment bag.
- It is available in four different presentations and volumes.

TABLE 2.5A: Qualitative and quantitative composition of oliclinomel.

Compartment	1,000 mL	1,500 mL	2,000 mL	2,500 mL
Lipid emulsion	200 mL	300 mL	400 mL	500 mL
Amino acid solution	400 mL	600 mL	800 mL	1,000 mL
Glucose solution	400 mL	600 mL	800 mL	1,000 mL

TABLE 2.5B: After the contents of the three compartments have been mixed, the final mixture composition for each of the bag.

Per bag	1 L	1.5 L	2 L	2.5 L
Nitrogen (g)	3.6	5.4	7.3	9.1
Amino acids (g)	22	33	44	55
Total calories (Kcal)	610	910	1,215	1,520
Nonprotein calories (Kcal)	520	780	1,040	1,300
Glucose calories (Kcal)	320	480	640	800
Lipid calories (Kcal)	200	300	400	500
Nonprotein calories/nitrogen				
Ratio (Kcal /g N)	144	144	144	144
Sodium (mmol)	21	32	42	53
Potassium (mmol)	16	24	32	40
Magnesium (mmol)	2.2	3.3	4.4	5.5
Calcium (mmol)	2	3	4	5
Phosphate (mmol)	8.5	13	17	21
Acetate (mmol)	30	46	61	76
Chloride (mmol)	33	50	66	83
pH	6	6	6	6
Osmolarity (mmol/L)	750	50	750	750

The final mixture allows PN for adults and children above 2 years of age when oral or enteral nutrition is not possible, insufficient, or contraindicated.

Dosage depends on metabolic requirements, energy expenditure, and the patient's clinical condition.

Maximum Daily Dose in Adults

The maximum daily dose is 40 mL/kg body weight (equivalent to 0.88 g of amino acids, 3.2 g of glucose, and 0.8 g of lipids per kg), i.e., 2,800 mL of the emulsion for a patient weighing 70 kg.

Maximum Daily Dose in Children Above 2 Years

The maximum daily dose is 100 mL/kg body weight (equivalent to 2.2 g of amino acids, 8 g of glucose, and 2 g of lipids per kg body weight).

As a general rule, do not exceed doses of 3 g/kg/day of amino acids and/or 17 g/kg/day of glucose and/or 3 g/kg/day of lipids, except in special cases. The dosage is based on fluid intake and daily nitrogen requirements.

Special Warnings

Water and electrolyte equilibration and metabolic disorders must be corrected before starting the infusion. This product does not contain vitamins or trace elements. They should be supplemented.

APPENDIX 2.6: NUTRITIONAL ASSESSMENT CHART (TABLE 2.6A)

Stepwise Calculation of Nutritional Requirement

Surgeons and residents involved in management of burns should learn to prescribe a nutritional regimen in a methodic and scientific manner as follows:

- Before starting nutritional support, patients with shock should be adequately resuscitated and gross fluid and electrolyte imbalances are corrected. Mild degree of fluid and electrolyte imbalance can be corrected with ongoing nutritional support.
- Decide on the route of administration for nutrition; plan the oral/enteral/or PN or partial PN.
- Calculate the energy requirements of burn patients according to Curreri formula, depending on the size of burn wound and age of the patient.
- This formula or equation for calorie estimation often overestimates the calorie requirements.
- To avoid this and simplify it, one can easily calculate the calorie protein needs according to appropriate stress level, taking the severity of disease into consideration.
- Calories are derived from three major substrates—carbohydrates, fats, and proteins. By and large 50% of calories are derived from carbohydrates, 30% from fats, and 20% from proteins. In critically ill patients, certain adjustments are required as mentioned earlier.

- After finalizing the total calorie and substrate requirements, the total permissible liquid intake has to be calculated. Normal recommendation is 30–40 mL/kg/day. However, liquid intake has to be adjusted in specific conditions such as renal and cardiac failure, where volume load needs to be restricted. Consequently, total calories will have to be given in restricted volume of fluid. In patients on total PN, this becomes a challenge and one will have to resort to using more lipid emulsions as they give higher calories on weight-to-weight basis.
- Let us now practically workout a stepwise prescription, taking an actual case scenario, a male patient aged 40 years, weighing 50 kg with 20% burns.

TABLE 2.6A: Nutritional assessment chart.

Name of patient:		Age/Sex:
Height and weight:	Ideal weight	
Date of burn:		
Date of arrival:		
Total body surface burnt:	% Full thickness	
Estimated energy requirement:	Kcal/day	
Estimated protein requirement:	g/day	
Kcal		
Oral		
Enteral		
Parenteral		
Protein		
Oral		
Enteral		
Parenteral		
Na^+/K^+		
Glucose		
Blood urea nitrogen (BUN)		

Step 1

Energy = (25 × weight in kg) + (20 × % burns)
E = (25 × 50) + (20 × 20)
E = 1,650 Kcal

Step 2

Protein requirement in 24 hours = 2 g/kg body weight
Protein = 2 × 50 = 100 g
Protein calories = 100 × 4 = 400 Kcal
So, nonprotein energy (NPE) = 1,650 - 400 = 1,250 Kcal

Energy values:
Protein = 4 Kcal/g
Carbohydrate = 4 Kcal/g
Fat = 9 Kcal/g

Step 3

For all age groups give 40–50% of nonprotein calories as fat, 50–60% as carbohydrate.
50% of 1,250 = 625 Kcal
Fat required = 625/9 = 70 g
Carbohydrate required = 625/4 = 156 g

Step 4

Daily requirement in 50 kg weight patient with 20% burn is:
Protein = 100 g
Carbohydrate = 156 g
Fat = 70 g
1 L of 5% dextrose = 50 g of monohydrate glucose = 200 Kcal
6.25 g of protein = 1 g of body nitrogen

Step 5

Calculate fluid intake in 24 hours.

Average requirement in an adult male is 40 mL/kg/day, i.e., 40 × 50 = 2,000 mL/day.

Step 6

Now, prepare standard nutrition (parenteral/oral/enteral) for 2,000 mL.

If >180 g of carbohydrate is given/day, frequent monitoring of blood glucose is required and insulin may be necessary.

100 g protein = 1,000 mL of 10% amino acids
150 g of carbohydrate = 750 mL of 20% dextrose
70 g of lipids = 350 mL of 20% lipofundin
Total volume = 2,100 mL giving 1,650 calories

The above composition can be conveniently delivered as an all-in-one solution, which is commercially available as *Clinomel* or as multiple bottles available as amino drip, lipofundin, and dextrose.

Step 7

If the above patient develops renal failure and his protein intake has to be decreased to 40 g of proteins and 1,000 mL of fluid intake/day:

40 g of protein = 400 mL of 10 % amino drip
150 g carbohydrate = 300 mL of 50 % dextrose
70 g lipids = 250 mL of 30% lipids
Final volume = 950 mL giving 1,470 calories

It can be given as 50% glucose solution, 30% lipid solution, and 10% amino acid solution.

Diabetics or patients with glucose intolerance require close monitoring of blood glucose levels and need correction. For them, reduce glucose as energy substrate and instead use lipid regimens.

Insulin may be given according to revised sliding scale by Dickerson **(Table 2.6B)**.

TABLE 2.6B: Sliding scale for insulin-dose management.

Finger stick glucose concentration (mg/dL)	Amount of regular human insulin (units)
<70	0
71–125	0
126–150	2
151–175	4
176–200	6
201–225	8
226–250	10
251–275	12
276–300	14
>300	16

NUTRITIONAL VALUES

NUTRITION READY RECKONER

These are average values for standard recipes found in most books.

Serving	Calories (Kcal)	Proteins (g)	Fats (g)	Carbo-hydrates (g)	Fiber (g)	Calcium (mg)	Iron (mg)	Carotene (µg)	Retinol (µg)	Vitamin B1 (mg)	Vitamin B2 (mg)	Niacin (mg)	Vitamin C (mg)	Portion
Beverages														
Hot tea	34	0.6	1.0	5.7	0.0	31.0	0.0	0.0	7.00	0.01	0.01	0.0	0	1 tea cup
Instant coffee	149	1.0	13.3	6.3	0.0	31.0	0.0	0.0	7.00	0.01	0.01	0.0	0	1 tea cup
Cold coffee (with cream)	279	3.9	17.0	27.7	0.0	144.0	0.3	487.0	183.00	0.06	0.23	0.1	2	1 tall glass
Banana milk shake	228	6.2	7.5	33.8	0.0	223.0	0.5	40.0	101.00	0.11	0.37	0.4	7	1 tall glass
Mango milk shake	237	6.2	7.7	35.6	0.8	227.0	1.3	2,067.0	608.00	0.15	0.41	9.0	16	1 tall glass
Lemonade	107	0.3	0.3	25.7	0.5	21.0	0.1	0.0	0.00	0.01	0.00	0.0	12	1 glass
Breakfast cereals														
Cracked wheat porridge	292	10.0	10.4	39.7	2.5	296.0	1.5	152.0	39.00	1.29	0.49	1.3	5	1 bowl
Semolina porridge	293	9.8	10.2	40.4	0.0	291.0	0.8	139.0	36.00	1.24	0.47	0.6	5	1 bowl
Vermicelli porridge	294	9.4	10.2	41.1	2.5	292.0	0.9	139.0	36.00	1.24	0.47	0.6	5	1 bowl
Oatmeal porridge	217	6.6	6.6	32.8	2.0	154.0	1.0	70.0	18.00	0.80	0.26	0.3	2	1 bowl
Cornflakes with milk	291	9.8	10.8	38.7	1.2	290.0	0.9	157.0	41.00	1.28	0.48	0.6	5	1 bowl
Semolina upma	147	2.3	7.7	17.1	9.9	11.0	0.5	1.0	0.00	0.04	0.01	0.4	2	1 bowl
Vermicelli upma	296	4.0	15.2	35.7	5.4	24.0	1.2	2.0	1.00	0.10	0.03	0.9	5	1 bowl
Vegetable upma	192	4.4	9.7	21.7	1.5	22.0	0.9	107.0	27.00	0.20	0.02	1.6	4	1 bowl
Poha	158	2.8	7.3	20.2	1.5	10.0	4.2	6.0	1.00	0.10	0.02	2.0	3	1 bowl
Vegetable with poha	202	4.9	9.3	24.7	2.1	21.0	4.6	111.0	28.00	0.18	0.03	3.1	5	1 bowl
Eggs														
Boiled egg	87	6.7	6.7	0.0	0.0	25.0	0.7	300.0	180.00	0.05	0.20	0.1	0	1 egg
Poached egg	87	6.7	6.7	0.0	0.0	25.0	0.7	300.0	180.00	0.05	0.20	0.1	0	1 egg
Fried egg	160	6.7	14.8	0.0	0.0	25.0	0.7	620.0	260.00	0.05	0.20	0.1	0	1 egg
Scrambled egg	172	6.7	15.8	0.8	0.0	57.0	0.7	620.0	267.00	0.06	0.22	0.1	0	1 egg
Baked egg	124	6.7	10.8	0.0	0.0	25.0	0.7	460.0	220.0	0.05	0.20	0.1	0	1 egg
Fluffy omelet	160	6.7	14.8	0.0	0.0	25.0	0.7	620.0	260.00	0.05	0.20	0.1	0	1 egg
Cheese and mushroom omelet	308	12.9	27.1	3.0	0.0	182.0	1.3	780.0	373.00	0.09	0.42	1.5	1	1 egg
Soups														
Minestrone soup	90	1.4	5.2	9.4	1.2	43.0	0.7	491.0	123.00	0.07	0.03	0.5	17	1 bowl
Chicken sweet corn soup	322	25.5	13.5	24.6	6.0	23.0	2.6	10.7.0	93.00	0.21	0.34	8.6	6	1 bowl
French onion soup	208	4.8	11.6	21.1	2.4	102.0	0.8	321.0	110.00	0.08	0.05	0.6	8	1 bowl

Continued

Continued

Serving	Calories (Kcal)	Proteins (g)	Fats (g)	Carbo-hydrates (g)	Fiber (g)	Calcium (mg)	Iron (mg)	Carotene (µg)	Retinol (µg)	Vitamin B1 (mg)	Vitamin B2 (mg)	Niacin (mg)	Vitamin C (mg)	Portion
Tomato soup	82	2.1	4.5	8.3	2.3	101.0	1.3	862.0	216.00	0.25	0.21	0.8	55	1 bowl
Green pea soup	186	9.0	6.4	23.1	2.2	70.0	1.9	375.0	109.00	0.28	0.08	1.1	11	1 bowl
Spinach soup	561	3.9	8.9	116.2	5.9	81.0	1.5	5,902.0	1,475.00	0.06	0.27	0.08	29	1 bowl
Mixed vegetable soup	146	3.3	9.2	12.5	1.4	124.0	0.9	779.0	225.0	0.11	0.16	0.6	23	1 bowl
Cream with tomato soup	245	5.4	16.6	18.5	2.3	180.0	1.5	984.0	287.00	0.32	0.25	1.0	45	1 bowl
Cream with spinach soup	307	8.5	23.2	16.0	5.1	200.0	2.2	6,214.0	1,644.0	0.20	0.52	0.9	32	1 bowl
Cream with carrot soup	250	4.6	16.2	21.5	2.0	172.0	1.4	1,935.0	531.00	0.17	0.17	0.9	6	1 bowl
Cream of pea soup	342	12.4	18.2	32.2	2.6	132.0	2.4	590.0	188.00	0.44	0.17	1.4	15	1 bowl
Cream with potato soup	282	5.4	13.1	35.7	3.1	118.0	1.1	415.0	144.00	0.24	0.17	1.6	21	1 bowl
Cream with mixed vegetable soup	263	7.5	13.4	28.0	3.2	179.0	2.0	1,160.0	331.00	0.33	0.24	1.5	45	1 bowl
Cream with mushroom soup	308	6.6	22.4	19.9	0.7	136.0	1.5	554.0	189.00	0.13	0.41	2.9	6	1 bowl
Hot and sour soup	181	11.2	9.3	13.2	1.6	65.0	2.8	86.0	22.00	0.22	0.25	23	6	1 bowl
Cereals														
Chapati	273	9.7	1.4	55.5	5.6	38.0	3.9	23.0	5.00	0.39	0.14	3.40	0	3 or 4
Plain Parantha	363	9.7	11.4	55.5	5.6	38.0	3.9	23.0	6.00	0.39	0.14	3.40	0	3 medium
Potato stuffed parantha	632	11.2	31.5	75.8	7.9	56.0	4.4	42.0	10.00	0.49	0.15	4.50	16	3 medium
Pea parantha	693	20.7	31.5	75.8	7.9	78.0	6.3	148.0	37.00	0.78	0.15	4.70	16	3 medium
Cauliflower parantha	577	12.0	31.7	60.9	7.1	74.0	5.0	47.0	12.00	0.44	0.22	4.30	47	3 medium
Radish parantha	574	10.8	31.5	61.8	8.2	90.0	4.5	27.0	7.00	0.48	0.16	4.10	20	3 medium
Daal parantha	665	16.2	33.1	75.6	9.0	65.0	5.6	62.0	15.00	0.55	0.19	4.20	3	3 medium
Sprouted daal parantha	727	22.1	32.0	87.6	10.2	85.0	6.0	48.0	12.00	0.64	0.24	4.70	2	3 medium
Paneer parantha	713	20.9	43.9	58.5	5.9	173.0	4.0	243.0	61.00	0.45	0.15	3.50	4	3 medium
Onion–green chilli parantha	594	10.9	31.5	66.6	7.1	85.0	4.5	23.0	6.00	0.57	0.15	3.80	11	3 medium
Keema parantha	712	24.8	42.1	58.4	5.9	169.0	6.2	25.0	13.00	0.55	0.25	9.00	3	3 medium
Methi parantha	652	14.2	32.4	75.8	8.1	293.0	7.2	1,230.0	303.00	0.52	0.32	4.50	0	3 medium
Pooris (10 g oil absorbed)	375	9.2	12.1	57.4	4.0	28.0	3.0	42.0	11.00	0.24	0.10	2.70	0	3 medium
Daal stuffed pooris	427	12.8	12.3	66.3	51.5	5.0	3.6	47.0	12.00	0.31	0.13	3.00	0	4 or 5
Palak pooris	388	10.2	12.4	58.8	64.9	6.0	3.6	2,832.0	708.00	0.26	0.23	2.9	14	4 or 5
Besan pooris	380	11.2	13.0	54.6	5.5	35.0	3.6	62.0	16.00	0.32	0.12	2.7	0	4 or 5

Continued

Continued

Serving	Calories (Kcal)	Proteins (g)	Fats (g)	Carbo-hydrates (g)	Fiber (g)	Calcium (mg)	Iron (mg)	Carotene (µg)	Retinol (µg)	Vitamin B1 (mg)	Vitamin B2 (mg)	Niacin (mg)	Vitamin C (mg)	Portion
Pea pooris	431	13.6	12.1	66.9	5.0	40.0	3.9	91.0	23.00	0.39	0.10	3.2	5	4 or 5
Pea *kachori* (10 g oil absorbed)	215	6.9	7.4	30.2	1.8	17.0	1.6	49.0	13.00	0.16	0.03	1.1	5	2
Khasta kachori (10 g oil absorbed)	441	11.4	18.9	56.3	3.2	45.0	2.4	163.0	41.00	0.16	0.8	1.8	0	2
Naan	200	6.7	2.1	38.5	1.5	60.0	1.4	31.0	9.00	0.19	0.10	1.2	1	1
Bhatura	176	5.6	3.8	29.9	1.2	28.0	1.2	51.0	27.00	0.06	0.07	0.1	0	2 or 3
Boiled rice	277	6.0	0.8	61.4	3.6	8.00	2.6	2.0	0.40	0.17	0.13	3.1	0	1 full plate
Curd rice	484	15.1	12.5	77.8	5.3	253.0	3.8	66.0	26.00	0.33	0.41	3.7	2	1 full plate
Zeera *pulao*	400	8.2	10.5	68.1	4.4	25.00	2.9	78.0	45.00	0.22	0.18	3.5	6	1 full plate
Mixed vegetable pulao	523	17.6	9.0	92.9	7.2	71.0	5.2	126.0	32.00	0.60	0.15	4.6	21	1 full plate
Pea pulao	510	12.1	9.1	94.8	8.1	108.0	4.6	1,033.0	258.00	0.44	0.17	4.8	28	1 full plate
Channa daal and vegetable pulao	529	15.1	10.1	94.3	8.5	102.0	5.3	1,014.0	254.00	0.47	0.19	4.6	14	1 full plate
Black channa pulao	464	10.9	10.2	82.1	7.5	82.00	4.0	49.0	11.00	0.28	0.17	4.1	6	1 full plate
Mushroom pulao	411	9.7	9.7	71.2	4.3	38.00	4.4	2.0	0.40	0.31	0.55	8.1	9	1 full plate
Paneer pulao	520	13.3	20.4	70.9	4.3	272.0	4.9	2.0	0.40	0.21	0.13	3.3	6	1 full plate
Mutton pulao	622	22.6	28.5	68.7	4.3	216.0	5.1	13.0	12.00	0.37	0.29	8.8	6	1 full plate
Chicken pulao	661	27.9	30.5	68.7	4.3	110.0	4.6	88.0	90.00	0.33	0.34	11.4	6	1 full plate
Idli	157	6.7	0.5	31.5	2.5	33.00	1.6	8.00	2.00	0.14	0.08	1.4	0	3 or 4
Plain dosa	261	7.1	4.6	47.8	3.2	28.00	1.6	166.0	41.00	0.17	0.08	2.2	0	2
Masala dosa	208	3.0	4.2	39.5	4.5	39.00	1.1	36.0	9.00	0.19	0.02	2.0	31	1
Mixed vegetable dosa	184	4.8	4.4	31.2	4.2	79.00	1.8	624.0	156.00	0.20	0.10	1.8	43	1
Paneer filling dosa	130	3.8	8.8	8.9	1.3	144.0	0.6	176.0	44.00	0.10	0.00	0.4	19	1
Uttapam	316	7.8	8.7	51.6	3.9	55.00	2.1	465.0	116.00	0.20	0.10	2.5	23	2
Beans and macaroni	352	12.1	16.8	38.0	3.7	243.0	2.2	673.0	242.00	0.20	0.20	1.5	40	1 Plate
Spaghetti Bolognese	346	14.6	14.9	38.3	33.0	174.0	3.2	867.0	236.00	0.28	0.21	4.8	30	1 shallow dish
Chicken Chowmein	542	31.4	24.2	49.6	3.9	104.0	5.6	9.8	333.00	0.39	0.36	8.1	59	1 shallow dish
Pulses														
Moong daal	104	7.3	0.4	17.9	2.6	23.0	1.2	15.0	4.00	0.14	0.06	0.7	0	1 curry bowl
Cumin seed baghar	47	0.0	5.0	0.5	0.0	0.0	0.0	100.0	25.00	0.00	0.00	0.0	0	1 curry bowl
Onion tomato *baghar*	59	0.4	5.1	2.8	0.5	17.0	0.2	153.0	38.00	0.03	0.01	0.1	6	1 curry bowl
Mustard seed baghar	45	0.0	5.0	0.0	0.0	0.0	0.0	100.0	25.00	0.00	0.00	0.0	0	1 curry bowl
Urad sp. dehusked dry	94	7.9	5.5	3.3	3.1	78.0	1.5	82.0	21.00	0.19	0.08	0.9	11	1 curry bowl

Continued

Continued

Serving	Calories (Kcal)	Proteins (g)	Fats (g)	Carbo-hydrates (g)	Fiber (g)	Calcium (mg)	Iron (mg)	Carotene (µg)	Retinol (µg)	Vitamin B1 (mg)	Vitamin B2 (mg)	Niacin (mg)	Vitamin C (mg)	Portion
Arhar daal with spinach	159	7.7	5.9	18.7	4.4	58.0	1.4	2,830.0	707.00	0.50	0.19	1.1	14	1 curry bowl
Channa daal with *ghia*	117	6.3	1.7	19.1	3.4	27.0	1.8	39.0	10.00	0.16	0.06	0.8	0	1 curry bowl
Sambar	119	5.6	2.5	18.4	3.2	45.0	1.7	88.0	22.00	0.13	0.08	0.9	19	1 curry bowl
Green gram whole	100	7.2	0.4	17.0	1.2	37.0	1.3	28.0	7.00	0.14	0.08	0.6	0	1 bowl
Dry *khatta* channa	232	6.0	11.7	25.6	4.8	83.0	1.9	369.0	91.00	0.16	0.07	1.3	14	1 bowl
Rajma curry	268	10.5	11.0	31.8	3.7	162.0	2.6	193.0	49.00	0.29	0.12	1.2	20	1 bowl
Lobia curry	259	10.9	10.9	29.3	2.8	89.0	4.1	182.0	46.00	0.31	0.12	0.9	19	1 bowl
Besan gatte curry	497	21.3	30.6	34.0	5.5	255.0	2.9	367.0	96.00	0.34	0.22	1.4	14	1 bowl
Besan kadhi with *pakoris*	408	9.9	30.2	24.1	3.7	140.0	2.2	73.0	23.00	0.21	0.19	1.0	1	1 bowl
Meats														
Keema matar	411	26.9	23.7	22.6	2.8	215.0	4.9	298.0	84.00	0.53	0.19	8.0	29	1 bowl
Roganjosh	404	25.0	30.6	7.2	0.8	276.0	4.0	114.0	45.00	0.31	0.27	8.0	12	1 bowl
Mutton *korma*	439	24.0	34.7	7.7	0.8	259.0	3.7	149.0	54	0.30	0.22	8.50	6.0	1 bowl
Palak meat	374	19.1	28.4	10.6	5.2	290.0	3.8	5,600.0	1,410	0.24	0.46	620	34.0	1 bowl
Shahi keema kofta curry	508	23.8	41.3	10.2	1.5	238.0	4.3	217.0	65	0.34	0.21	8.70	23.0	1 bowl
Boti kebab	365	23.6	27.8	5.0	0.5	232.0	3.6	8.0	19	0.24	0.22	8.30	9.0	1 bowl
Shammi kebab	435	25.0	25.8	25.8	3.6	180.0	3.4	890.0	58.00	0.29	0.21	7.4	3.7	1 bowl
Shepherd's pie	486	23.8	34.5	20.0	2.2	206.0	3.5	339.0	98.00	0.31	0.18	9.2	15	1 bowl
Roast chicken	297	25.3	21.8	0.0	0.0	18.0	2.0	334.0	166.0	0.13	0.20	10.0	0	1 bowl
Chilli chicken	464	27.3	35.5	8.8	1.9	46.0	3.1	222.0	135.0	0.35	0.31	10.9	50	1 bowl
Chicken sweet and sour	420	27.0	33.3	3.1	0.8	39.0	2.7	270.0	181.0	0.28	0.35	10.6	30	1 bowl
Chicken *korma*	493	28.1	36.4	13.2	2.1	188.0	3.2	94.0	127.0	0.23	0.32	10.2	11	1 bowl
Bengal fish curry	296	18.4	17.5	16.3	1.6	731.0	1.7	22.4	7.00	0.14	0.11	1.1	35	1 bowl
Tandoori fish	174	25.7	6.8	2.4	0.0	7.0	3.1	10.0	11.00	0.01	0.02	0.0	0	1 bowl
Fried fish with chips	443	26.3	26.2	25.4	2.3	307.0	3.3	165.0	94.00	0.09	0.11	0.9	9	1 bowl
Fish in coconut milk	371	27.0	17.1	27.2	3.2	150.0	3.2	4.0	1.00	0.06	0.03	0.5	7	1 bowl
Prawn curry	342	30.1	19.9	10.5	2.7	509.0	9.3	3.0	0.80	0.05	0.18	7.5	4	1 bowl
Crispy baked fish	390	32.3	15.1	31.2	4.1	461.0	4.1	496.0	153.00	0.13	0.13	1.3	16	1 bowl
Vegetables and paneer														
Nutri nugget sweet and sour	252	12.8	18.3	9.1	8.0	22.0	1.0	180.0	79.00	0.16	0.16	1.0	30	1 bowl
Nutri nugget korma	347	14.2	23.4	20.0	2.1	217.0	1.4	28.0	12.00	0.11	0.13	0.6	11	1 bowl
Mushrooom matar	239	10.3	10.8	25.2	2.8	68.5	3.3	298.0	75.00	0.41	0.30	4.1	31	1 bowl
Nutri nugget matar	283	18.4	10.5	28.6	2.8	68.5	2.4	298.0	75.00	0.35	0.05	1.0	29	1 bowl

Continued

Continued

Serving	Calories (Kcal)	Proteins (g)	Fats (g)	Carbo-hydrates (g)	Fiber (g)	Calcium (mg)	Iron (mg)	Carotene (µg)	Retinol (µg)	Vitamin B1 (mg)	Vitamin B2 (mg)	Niacin (mg)	Vitamin C (mg)	Portion
Palak mushroom	161	5.2	10.6	11.3	7.7	149.0	2.9	708.0	2,177.00	0.17	0.59	3.0	60	1 bowl
Vegetable *nargisi* kofta curry	394	17.1	33.1	6.8	6.7	188.0	2.0	146.0	103.0	0.30	0.06	2.6	43	1 bowl
Paneer makhani	659	9.5	61.3	17.4	3.0	305.0	2.9	2,046.0	580.0	0.36	0.19	1.3	64	1 bowl
Pea potato curry	267	8.9	10.3	34.6	4.1	62.8	2.2	165.0	41.00	0.37	0.03	1.7	30	1 bowl
Pea paneer curry	351	17.3	20.8	23.6	2.8	162.0	2.0	153.0	94.00	0.36	0.04	1.1	23	1 bowl
Pea curry	311	15.3	10.3	39.2	4.5	78.0	3.5	236.0	60.00	0.60	0.04	2.0	30	1 bowl
Pea/Cholia vadi curry	309	11.7	15.3	31.0	3.7	68.0	2.8	195.0	49.00	0.50	0.03	1.5	26	1 bowl
Potato curry	221	2.5	10.2	29.9	3.6	47.7	1.0	94.0	23.60	0.17	0.03	1.5	29	1 bowl
Egg curry	314	15.5	17.6	23.3	2.8	85.0	2.8	483.0	237.00	0.38	0.25	1.2	21	1 bowl
Dahi aloo	260	4.2	12.2	33.4	3.9	119.0	1.0	169.0	58.00	0.22	0.12	1.8	35	1 bowl
Dum aloo	291	2.1	21.1	23.2	2.5	41.5	0.5	29.0	8.00	0.11	0.03	1.2	17	1 bowl
Ghia *kofta* curry	273	3.6	20.9	17.5	2.9	70.0	1.9	122.0	31.00	0.17	0.05	0.9	15	1 bowl
Potato kofta curry	290	2.9	15.3	35.1	4.1	51.0	1.3	101.0	25.00	0.19	0.03	1.80	33	1 bowl
Cabbage kofta curry	297	5.9	21.0	21.0	4.0	85.0	2.1	210.0	52.00	0.20	0.14	1.1	136	1 bowl
Paneer kofta curry	383	11.2	30.7	15.5	1.5	149.0	0.9	74.0	74.00	0.13	0.04	0.6	15	1 bowl
Aloo methi	221	5.8	11.0	24.7	4.1	404.0	2.5	2,361.0	590.00	0.12	0.32	1.8	66	1 bowl
Gajar methi	180	5.2	11.0	15.0	3.5	460.0	2.8	3,854.0	963.0	0.08	0.33	1.3	55	1 bowl
Sarson ka saag	157	8.5	6.7	15.7	3.2	200.0	25.0	6,734.0	1,682.0	00.22	0.14	0.5	66	1 bowl
Palak paneer	240	11.2	17.5	9.4	7.7	228.0	2.1	8,545.0	2,180.00	0.16	0.43	1.1	59	1 bowl
Palak aloo	230	5.1	11.3	27.0	9.7	153.0	2.5	8,564.0	2,141.00	0.20	0.40	2.0	72	1 bowl
Mooli bhujia	144	4.6	10.6	7.6	2.3	294.0	0.8	5,300.0	2.00	0.23	0.49	1.2	91	1 bowl
Bathua bhujia	152	6.0	10.7	7.8	0.3	236.0	6.8	2,614.0	1.00	0.04	0.22	1.0	55	1 bowl
Peas and cabbage subzi	122	5.5	5.2	13.2	2.2	50.0	1.7	164.0	41.00	0.19	0.10	0.8	129	1 bowl
Dry arbi (fried)	254	3.6	15.2	25.6	1.6	62.0	0.9	79.0	14.00	0.14	0.04	0.6	8	1 bowl
Masala arbi	187	3.0	10.1	21.1	1.0	40.0	0.4	24.0	0.00	0.09	0.03	0.4	0	1 bowl
Bangan bhartha	192	2.8	15.5	10.4	4.5	55.0	0.9	216.0	54.00	0.12	0.19	1.6	29	1 small bowl
Stuffed tomatoes	233	6.0	15.6	17.1	2.8	138.0	1.5	829.0	228.00	0.27	0.08	1.1	41	2 tomatoes
Bhindi subzi	189	2.6	15.0	11.0	6.3	93.0	0.7	62.0	16.00	0.11	0.12	0.8	19	1 bowl
Stuffed bhindi	132	2.3	10.2	7.7	5.9	79.0	0.5	62.0	16.00	0.08	0.12	0.7	16	1 bowl
Stuffed karela (wet)	225	1.9	20.2	8.9	2.6	39.0	1.0	101.0	25.00	0.10	0.08	0.6	76	1 bowl
Stuffed karela (dry)	156	1.3	15.2	3.4	1.8	16.0	0.5	100.0	25.00	0.06	0.07	0.4	70	3 pieces
Kathal (dry)	300	2.2	20.3	27.0	7.1	89.5	1.3	201.0	51.00	0.15	0.02	1.1	12	1 bowl
Cauliflower, peas, and potato subzi	196	5.1	10.3	20.7	2.9	49.0	1.6	143.0	36.00	0.21	0.07	1.4	42	1 bowl

Continued

Continued

Serving	Calories (Kcal)	Proteins (g)	Fats (g)	Carbo-hydrates (g)	Fiber (g)	Calcium (mg)	Iron (mg)	Carotene (µg)	Retinol (µg)	Vitamin B1 (mg)	Vitamin B2 (mg)	Niacin (mg)	Vitamin C (mg)	Portion
Stuffed ghia	456	21.3	31.8	21.1	2.5	323.0	2.9	632.0	304.00	0.22	0.34	4.1	3	1/2 marrow
Roasted potatoes	191	2.4	5.0	34.0	3.8	15.0	0.8	228.0	57.00	0.15	0.01	1.8	26	1–2 potatoes
Stuffed baked potato	334	7.1	18.8	34.0	3.8	33.0	1.3	698.0	248.00	0.19	0.16	1.8	26	1–2 potatoes
Creamed spinach	429	21.4	29.8	18.8	9.3	458.0	3.5	11,812.0	3,195.00	0.25	1.00	1.4	58	1 small bowl
Creamed spinach and mushrooms	363	13.4	25.8	19.2	7.1	366.0	2.9	8,692.0	2,284.00	0.23	0.90	3.5	45	1 bowl
Salads														
Russian salad	959	19.7	85.6	27.5	3.3	100.0	3.8	879.0	333.00	0.38	0.33	5.4	39	1 small bowl
Beetroot and egg salad	366	8.9	30.8	13.4	3.6	62.0	2.1	300.0	180.00	0.12	0.29	0.6	15	1 small bowl
Tossed green salad	153	1.5	12.2	9.2	2.0	50.0	0.9	225.0	57.00	0.18	0.04	0.5	43	1 small bowl
Cucumber and yogurt salad	29	1.3	1.3	2.9	1.0	53.0	0.5	10.0	4.00	0.04	0.05	0.2	6	1 small bowl
French dressing	722	0.0	80.0	0.4	0.0	1.0	0.0	0.0	0.00	0.00	0.00	0.01	1	3/4 cup
Mayonnaise	1,220	7.1	131.8	1.3	0.0	56.0	1.4	380.0	229.00	0.08	0.26	0.0	4	1 cup
Mayonnaise without eggs	886	7.7	90.1	11.0	0.0	288.0	0.5	139.0	36.00	1.20	0.46	0.3	6	1 cup
Raitas														
Tomato onion raita	79	3.7	4.1	6.7	0.6	173.0	0.5	120.0	36.00	0.10	0.18	0.3	11	1 bowl
Cucumber raita	68	3.3	4.1	4.5	0.8	155.0	0.6	32.0	14.00	0.07	0.16	0.2	5	1 bowl
Carrot raita	85	3.6	4.1	8.3	0.9	189.0	0.7	977.0	250.00	0.07	0.17	0.4	3	1 bowl
Ghia raita	67	3.2	4.1	4.3	0.3	159.0	0.4	32.0	14.00	0.06	0.17	0.2	1	1 bowl
Potato raita	110	3.9	4.1	14.3	1.3	154.0	0.5	44.0	17.00	0.10	0.17	0.7	10	1 bowl
Spinach raita	143	7.7	8.7	8.5	4.9	231.0	1.6	5,616.0	1,410.0	00.17	0.43	2.6	29	1 bowl
Bathua raita	147	9.3	8.4	8.5	0.4	308.0	4.7	1,776.0	15.00	0.15	0.31	2.7	36	1 bowl
Sprouted green gram raita	105	5.8	4.1	11.2	1.2	166.0	0.7	37.0	15.00	0.11	0.18	0.4	3	1 bowl
Boondi raita	224	7.3	15.0	15.0	2.1	160.0	1.3	58.0	21.00	0.15	0.20	0.6	1	1 bowl
Pineapple raita	84	3.3	4.1	8.4	0.0	159.0	1.4	41.0	16.00	0.15	0.22	0.2	21	1 bowl
Banana raita	118	3.7	4.1	16.6	0.4	158.0	0.4	71.0	24.00	0.08	0.20	0.4	5	1 bowl
Mango raita	97	3.4	4.2	11.5	0.5	156.0	0.9	1,404.0	357.00	0.09	0.20	0.6	9	1 bowl
Grape raita	91	3.4	4.2	10.0	1.4	159.0	0.5	33.0	14.00	0.06	0.17	0.2	2	1 bowl
Desserts														
Rice kheer	257	7.2	8.3	38.3	0.4	241.0	0.7	12.0	104.00	0.12	0.40	0.6	4	1 bowl
Sevian kheer	271	7.9	9.2	39.2	1.2	273.0	0.6	12.0	111.00	0.12	0.40	0.4	4	1 bowl
Carrot kheer	218	6.9	8.3	29.0	0.9	280.0	0.9	957.0	340.00	0.12	0.38	0.5	6	1 bowl
Apple kheer	244	6.5	8.5	35.4	0.6	245.0	0.8	12.0	104.00	0.10	0.38	0.2	5	1 bowl
Phirni	258	7.1	8.3	38.8	0.4	241.0	0.5	12.0	104.00	0.11	0.39	0.4	4	1 bowl
Carrot halva	472	8.3	24.5	54.5	2.7	443.0	1.6	3,137.0	844.00	0.14	0.30	1.0	7	1 small bowl

Continued

Continued

Serving	Calories (Kcal)	Proteins (g)	Fats (g)	Carbo-hydrates (g)	Fiber (g)	Calcium (mg)	Iron (mg)	Carotene (μg)	Retinol (μg)	Vitamin B1 (mg)	Vitamin B2 (mg)	Niacin (mg)	Vitamin C (mg)	Portion
Suji halwa	380	3.6	23.2	39.1	0.8	16.0	0.7	400.0	100.00	0.04	0.04	0.6	0	1 small bowl
Moong daal halwa	545	13.8	28.2	59.0	2.7	310.0	1.2	415.0	149.00	0.22	0.27	0.9	2	1 small bowl
Vanilla ice cup cream	288	2.3	22.9	18.2	0.0	90.0	0.2	415.0	139.00	0.03	0.14	0.1	0	1 ice cream
Strawberry ice cup cream	288	2.3	22.9	18.2	0.0	90.0	0.2	415.0	139.00	0.03	0.14	0.1	0	1 ice cream
Chocolate ice cup cream	288	2.3	22.9	18.2	0.0	90.0	0.2	415.0	139.00	0.03	0.14	0.1	0	1 ice cream
Chocochip ice cup cream	288	2.3	22.0	18.2	0.0	90.0	0.2	415.0	139.00	0.03	0.14	0.1	0	1 ice cream
Coconut ice cream	460	5.5	30.5	40.8	0.0	106.0	1.0	411.0	414.00	0.10	0.18	0.4	2	1 sundae glass
Fruit ice cream	323	2.6	23.0	26.5	0.3	95.0	0.4	832.0	246.00	0.05	0.16	0.3	5	1 sundae glass
Cold lemon soufflé	534	6.9	41.9	32.3	0.4	41.0	0.8	1,000.0	355.00	0.05	0.20	0.1	8.8	1 soufflé dish
Cold orange soufflé	594	7.8	42.0	46.2	1.5	64.0	1.2	2,656.0	769.00	0.05	0.20	0.1	45	1 soufflé dish
Cold pineapple soufflé	525	6.7	42.0	30.00	0.0	25.0	0.7	1,000.0	355.00	0.00	0.20	0.1	0	1 soufflé dish
Cold vanilla soufflé	536	7.3	42.7	30.6	0.0	57.0	0.7	1,000.0	362.00	0.06	0.20	0.1	0.2	1 soufflé dish
Cold chocolate soufflé	536	7.3	42.7	30.6	0.0	57.0	0.7	1,000.0	362.00	0.06	0.20	0.1	0.2	1 soufflé dish
Bread and butter pudding	222	7.4	11.3	22.7	1.0	124.0	0.7	316.0	177.00	0.08	0.27	0.2	2	1 small plate
Snacks														
Gulab jamuns	329	6.7	12.9	46.6	0.2	279.0	0.2	145.0	36.00	0.23	0.17	0.3	2	2 pieces
Chena murki	275	9.3	10.6	35.6	0.0	110.0	0.0	186.0	47.00	0.06	0.02	0.0	2	10 pieces
Plain *barfi*	276	10.0	13.0	29.8	0.0	478.0	0.0	249.0	63.00	0.12	0.21	0.2	3	2 pieces
Coconut barfi	472	11.7	28.6	41.9	4.3	578.0	2.0	249.0	63.00	0.14	0.21	1.0	5	2 pieces
Besan barfi	266	5.3	13.9	30.0	2.7	14.0	1.3	282.0	71.00	0.12	0.05	0.6	1	2 pieces
Khoya *laddoo*	375	10.7	22.2	33.0	1.8	441.0	1.4	206.0	52.00	0.14	0.21	0.8	3	2 pieces
Besan laddoo	286	5.8	16.4	28.7	2.8	15.0	1.4	332.0	83.00	0.13	0.05	0.7	1	2 pieces
Suji laddoo with nuts	290	3.4	16.7	31.4	0.8	16.0	0.8	306.00	77.00	0.09	0.03	0.5	0	2 pieces
Suji laddoo with *khoya*	355	5.6	20.1	38.0	1.9	125.0	0.6	312.00	78.00	0.07	0.07	0.5	1	2 pieces
Til laddoo	158	3.2	7.2	20.0	0.0	256.0	2.0	10.0	3.00	0.18	0.07	0.8	0	6 pieces
Gujia	272	4.8	13.2	33.6	1.3	114.0	0.9	121.0	31.00	0.05	0.06	0.7	1	6 pieces
Peanut brittle *(chikki)*	229	5.2	8.1	33.7	0.9	44.0	1.3	7.00	2.00	0.20	0.06	4.1	0	5 pieces
Til and channa chikki	217	5.2	3.3	41.7	2.1	110.0	2.3	29.00	7.00	0.16	0.09	0.8	0	5 pieces
Murmura chikki	139	0.7	0.0	34.0	0.4	28.0	1.3	0.0	0.00	0.03	0.03	0.4	0	5 pieces
Vegetable *pakoras*	333	7.8	21.9	26.2	5.2	49.0	2.3	1,166.0	291.00	0.19	0.13	1.3	23	5 pieces

Continued

Continued

Serving	Calories (Kcal)	Proteins (g)	Fats (g)	Carbo-hydrates (g)	Fiber (g)	Calcium (mg)	Iron (mg)	Carotene (µg)	Retinol (µg)	Vitamin B1 (mg)	Vitamin B2 (mg)	Niacin (mg)	Vitamin C (mg)	Portion
Masala onion *pakoras*	343	7.5	21.8	29.1	4.7	64.0	2.2	39.0	10.00	0.20	0.06	1.1	11	5 pieces
Paneer pakoras	425	15.5	32.1	18.6	3.2	121.0	1.6	222.0	56.00	0.18	0.06	0.7	2	5 pieces
Bread pakoras	489	11.8	22.2	60.5	8.6	28.0	2.5	51.00	13.00	0.24	0.06	1.7	9	5 pieces
Egg pakoras	380	13.0	28.4	18.0	3.2	42.0	2.3	339.00	190.00	0.19	0.25	0.8	0	2 pieces
Chicken pakoras	451	22.6	31.8	18.7	3.2	29.0	3.0	1.1	78.00	0.23	0.18	7.2	1	2 pieces
Fish cutlets	373	19.7	22.8	22.2	3.2	538.0	2.6	41.00	10.00	0.19	0.11	1.3	18	2 pieces
Bondas	457	10.7	25.8	45.5	6.4	45.0	2.5	66.00	7.00	0.35	0.08	4.0	20	2 pieces
Vegetable cutlets	216	4.6	10.3	26.2	3.0	36.0	1.2	600.00	150.00	0.13	0.02	1.0	9	2 pieces
Paneer cutlets	330	14.5	24.7	12.3	1.2	148.0	0.3	257.00	65.00	0.07	0.02	0.2	2	2 pieces
Sago cutlets	293	1.7	10.2	48.7	2.5	13.0	0.9	24.00	6.00	0.10	0.01	1.2	17	2 pieces
Chirwa cutlets	325	6.8	10.7	50.4	2.6	41.0	9.1	593.00	148.00	0.19	0.03	2.2	4	2 pieces
Fish cutlets	470	19.1	31.6	27.2	2.3	658.0	1.6	13.00	3.00	0.12	0.08	1.5	31	2 pieces
Keema cutlets	307	1.8	23.6	21.9	1.1	155.0	3.0	1.00	9.00	0.21	0.14	7.2	0	2 pieces
Vegetable *samosas*	246	4.4	12.0	30.2	1.0	19.0	1.1	131.00	33.00	0.13	0.02	1.3	12	2 pieces
Paneer pea samosas	255	6.2	16.5	20.5	0.8	110.0	0.9	119.00	30.00	0.08	0.02	0.9	3	2 pieces
Keema samosas	262	10.0	17.0	17.3	2.8	80.0	1.7	164.00	45.00	0.13	0.08	3.3	6	2 pieces
Mathri	223	2.8	15.3	18.5	2.1	6.0	0.7	6.00	21.00	0.03	0.02	0.6	0	2 pieces
Masala vada	179	6.6	8.6	18.7	2.8	24.0	1.3	39.00	10.00	0.15	0.06	0.8	1	2 pieces
Plain urad daal vada	171	7.2	7.9	17.8	2.1	46.0	1.1	11.00	3.00	0.13	0.06	0.06	0	2 pieces
Masala urad daal vada	198	7.5	10.0	19.6	2.8	51.0	1.3	11.00	3.00	0.14	0.07	0.07	1	2 pieces
Mint and coriander chutney	17	0.6	0.1	3.4	0.3	28.0	1.7	43.00	108.00	0.01	0.02	0.1	8	1 teaspoon
Tomato ginger chutney	6	0.3	0.1	1.0	0.3	12.0	0.2	88.00	22.00	0.03	0.02	0.1	7	2 teaspoon
Sandwiches														
Tomato and cheese	268	7.2	11.8	33.3	4.6	88.0	0.9	460.0	145.00	0.09	0.06	0.6	11	2 pieces
Tomato and cucumber	231	5.2	8.6	33.1	4.9	28.0	1.0	460.0	115.00	0.10	0.02	0.6	12	2 pieces
Tomato grilled	313	9.6	15.0	34.8	5.0	160.0	1.2	530.0	192.00	0.12	0.12	0.6	16	4 pieces
French toast	443	14.6	27.6	34.0	4.6	144.0	1.7	1,088.0	407.00	0.15	0.20	0.6	11	2 pieces
Cheese open	340	11.7	18.6	31.5	7.4	196.0	1.1	328.0	168.00	0.14	0.11	1.5	0	2pieces
Danish luncheon	350	16.2	17.5	31.9	4.6	42.0	2.1	620.0	260.00	0.24	0.22	1.2	3	2 pieces
Chicken and corn open	340	15.6	15.0	35.6	5.5	18.0	1.8	362.0	124.0	0.12	0.11	4.6	3	2 pieces
Cakes														
Sponge cake	177	6.2	4.6	27.8	0.5	20.2	0.9	202.0	120.00	0.05	0.14	0.4	0	1 piece
Sponge chocolate cake	156	5.5	4.5	23.3	0.3	18.8	0.7	201.0	120.00	0.05	0.14	0.3	0	1 piece

Continued

Continued

Serving	Calories (Kcal)	Proteins (g)	Fats (g)	Carbo-hydrates (g)	Fiber (g)	Calcium (mg)	Iron (mg)	Carotene (µg)	Retinol (µg)	Vitamin B1 (mg)	Vitamin B2 (mg)	Niacin (mg)	Vitamin C (mg)	Portion
Pineapple pastry	279	7.1	13.2	32.9	0.6	23.1	1.0	390.0	176.00	0.06	0.16	0.5	0	1 pastry
Chocolate pastry	228	5.5	12.5	23.3	0.3	19.0	0.7	361.0	160.00	0.05	0.14	0.3	0	1 pastry
Chocolate cream cake	223	3.1	13.1	23.2	0.4	9.0	0.5	526.0	158.00	0.03	0.06	0.3	0	1 piece

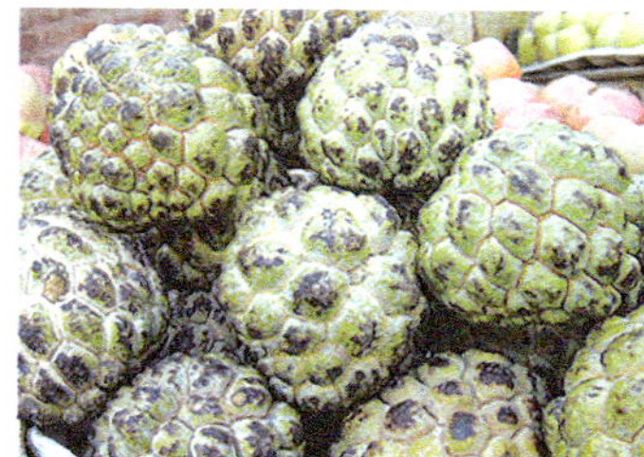
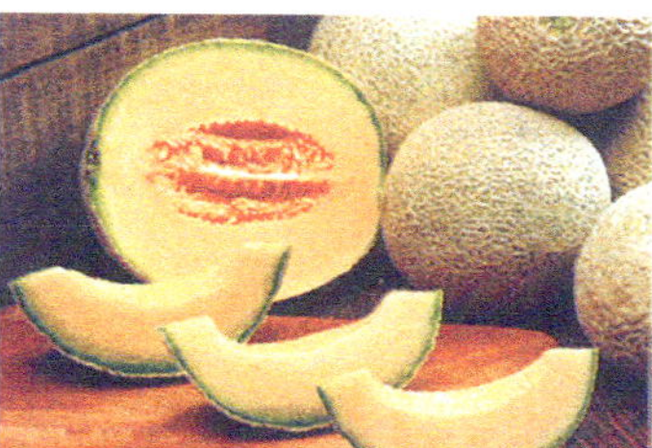
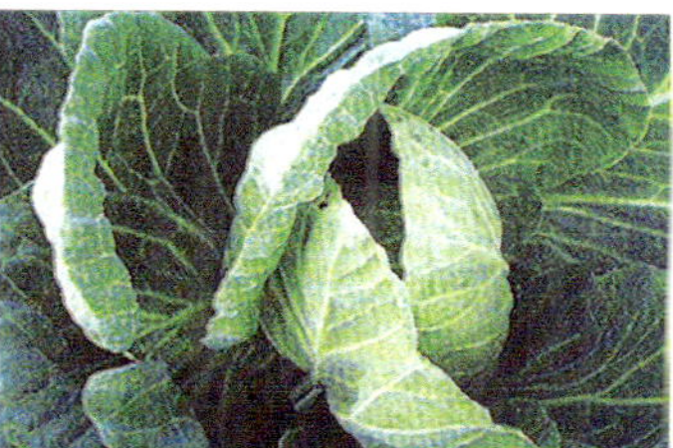
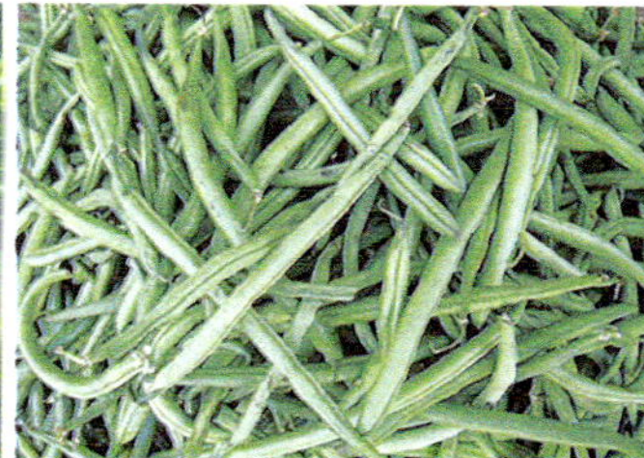

Index

Page numbers followed by *b* refer to box, *f* refer to figure, *fc* refer to flowchart, and *t* refer to table.

A

B

C

G

H

I

N

O

Q

R

S

T

U

V